图书在版编目（CIP）数据

1型神经纤维瘤病：从基础到临床 /（英）米娜·乌帕德亚雅（Meena Upadhyaya），（英）大卫·库珀（David N. Cooper）主编；王智超，李青峰主译. -- 上海：上海科学技术出版社，2025. 6. -- ISBN 978-7-5478-7129-4

Ⅰ. R730.264

中国国家版本馆CIP数据核字第2025FX9314号

First published in English under the title
Neurofibromatosis Type 1: Molecular and Cellular Biology, edition: 1
edited by Meena Upadhyaya and David Cooper
Copyright © Springer-Verlag Berlin Heidelberg, 2012
This edition has been translated and published under licence from Springer-Verlag GmbH, part of Springer Nature.

上海市版权局著作权合同登记号　图字：09 - 2024 - 0798 号

封面部分图片由译者提供。

1型神经纤维瘤病：从基础到临床

主　编　[英] Meena Upadhyaya
　　　　[英] David N. Cooper
主　译　王智超　李青峰
副主译　刘丕楠　倪　鑫　高兴华

上海世纪出版（集团）有限公司
上海科学技术出版社　出版、发行
（上海市闵行区号景路159弄A座9F-10F）
邮政编码 201101　www.sstp.cn
山东韵杰文化科技有限公司印刷
开本 889×1194　1/16　印张 28.75
字数 769 千字
2025年6月第1版　2025年6月第1次印刷
ISBN 978 - 7 - 5478 - 7129 - 4/R·3254
定价：350.00 元

本书如有缺页、错装或坏损等严重质量问题，请向印刷厂联系调换

1型神经纤维瘤病

从基础到临床

Neurofibromatosis Type 1
Molecular and Cellular Biology

主　编　［英］Meena Upadhyaya
　　　　［英］David N. Cooper

主　译　王智超　李青峰

副主译　刘丕楠　倪　鑫　高兴华

上海科学技术出版社

内容提要

本书由国际遗传学著名专家 Meena Upadhyaya 和 David N. Cooper 主持编写，共 44 章，系统探讨了 1 型神经纤维瘤病（neurofibromatosis type 1，NF1）从基础到临床的各个方面。本书从临床表现、并发症及鉴别诊断等角度切入，深入解析了 NF1 的分子基础，包括 *NF1* 基因的结构、突变机制、细胞起源、微环境等在 NF1 发病中的关键作用，并提出了最新的治疗策略。此外，书中总结了 NF1 相关动物模型的构建经验，深入分析了 NF1 给患者带来的心理和社会负担，强调了社会支持系统的重要性。

本书系统性强、图文并茂，是从事 NF1 治疗与管理的医务人员必不可少的实践指南，同时也适合相关研究人员参考使用。

献给 Lara Devi

译者名单

主　　译　王智超　李青峰

副 主 译　刘丕楠　倪　鑫　高兴华

主译助理　余　旋　郑婷婷

译　　者　（按姓氏汉语拼音排序）

陈敏亮　中国人民解放军总医院第四医学中心烧伤整形医学部
陈森敏　深圳市儿童医院血液肿瘤科
陈犹白　中国人民解放军总医院第一医学中心整形修复科
付瀚辉　北京协和医院神经科
高兴华　中国医科大学附属第一医院皮肤性病科
葛玲玲　上海交通大学医学院附属第九人民医院整复外科
顾　松　上海交通大学医学院附属上海儿童医学中心普外科
顾建英　复旦大学附属中山医院整形外科
顾熠辉　上海交通大学医学院附属第九人民医院整复外科
郭子桢　上海交通大学医学院附属第九人民医院整复外科
韩　岩　中国人民解放军总医院第一医学中心整形修复科
胡　杏　湖南省人民医院皮肤科；中南大学爱尔眼科研究院
黄　薇　中国科学院脑科学与智能技术卓越创新中心
黄景宣　上海交通大学医学院附属第九人民医院整复外科
黄雄梅　福建省立医院整形烧伤科
吉　毅　四川大学华西医院小儿外科
李海博　上海交通大学医学院附属第九人民医院整复外科
李青峰　上海交通大学医学院附属第九人民医院整复外科

李悦华	上海交通大学医学院附属第九人民医院整复外科
林志淼	南方医科大学皮肤病医院儿童皮肤科
刘　珺	上海交通大学医学院附属第九人民医院整复外科
刘昊天	天津医科大学肿瘤医院骨与软组织肿瘤科
刘丕楠	首都医科大学附属北京天坛医院神经外科
刘周亮	南方医科大学皮肤病医院儿童皮肤科
罗　蒙	浙江大学医学院附属第二医院整形外科
倪　鑫	首都医科大学附属北京儿童医院耳鼻咽喉头颈外科
彭　婕	上海交通大学医学院附属新华医院眼科
钱　闯	复旦大学附属儿科医院骨科
乔　军	南京大学医学院附属鼓楼医院脊柱外科
邱　勇	南京大学医学院附属鼓楼医院脊柱外科
孙　谛	华中科技大学同济医学院附属协和医院整形外科
孙家明	华中科技大学同济医学院附属协和医院整形外科
王　博	首都医科大学附属北京天坛医院神经外科
王　坚	复旦大学附属肿瘤医院病理科
王　薇	上海交通大学医学院附属第九人民医院整复外科
王　智	成都市妇女儿童中心医院神经外科
王达辉	复旦大学附属儿科医院骨科
王广宇	山东大学附属儿童医院神经外科
王生才	首都医科大学附属北京儿童医院耳鼻咽喉头颈外科
王旭东	上海交通大学医学院附属第九人民医院口腔颅颌面科
王智超	上海交通大学医学院附属第九人民医院整复外科
卫传元	复旦大学附属中山医院整形外科
魏澄江	上海交通大学医学院附属第九人民医院整复外科
吴　昊	上海交通大学医学院附属第九人民医院口腔颅颌面科
吴　浩	首都医科大学宣武医院神经外科
吴　南	北京协和医院骨科
吴祎炜	上海交通大学医学院附属第九人民医院神经外科
肖　杨	四川大学华西医院整形外科/烧伤科
谢婧怡	北京协和医院骨科
邢铭烟	中国科学院上海营养与健康研究所
徐　潇	中国人民解放军总医院第三医学中心眼科医学部眼眶病外科
徐学刚	中国医科大学附属第一医院皮肤性病科

许学文	四川大学华西医院整形外科/烧伤科
杨　军	上海交通大学医学院附属第九人民医院整复外科
杨吉龙	天津医科大学肿瘤医院骨与软组织肿瘤科
杨志国	河北省儿童医院神经外科
易成刚	浙江大学医学院附属第二医院整形外科
余　旋	上海交通大学医学院附属第九人民医院整复外科
袁晓军	上海交通大学医学院附属新华医院小儿血液肿瘤科
张　璠	陆军军医大学第一附属医院（西南医院）整形外科
张　雷	首都医科大学宣武医院神经外科
张　松	杭州市儿童医院神经外科
张　鑫	上海交通大学医学院附属新华医院小儿血液肿瘤科
张家平	陆军军医大学第一附属医院（西南医院）整形外科
张明路	北京协和医院神经科
张文川	上海交通大学医学院附属第九人民医院神经外科
张梓欣	四川大学华西医院小儿外科
章海兵	中国科学院上海营养与健康研究所
赵培泉	上海交通大学医学院附属新华医院眼科
郑胜武	福建省立医院整形烧伤科
郑婷婷	上海交通大学医学院附属第九人民医院整复外科
钟民衍	上海交通大学医学院附属第九人民医院整复外科
周宇红	复旦大学附属中山医院肿瘤内科
朱倍瑶	上海交通大学医学院附属第九人民医院整复外科
朱培培	复旦大学附属肿瘤医院病理科
朱以诚	北京协和医院神经科

中文版序一

医学，不仅仅是一门治病救人的科学，更是一项承载生命与希望的仁术。"医以活人为心，视人之病，犹己之病。"医者承载的不仅是健康的期望，更有"性命相托"的责任。这种精神，是每位医者的立身之本，也是推动医学进步的动力。在肿瘤学领域，尤以肝脏肿瘤为甚，我们在面临复杂的临床挑战的同时，也怀揣着这种信念不断追寻创新与突破。

我国是肝癌高发国家，随着经济社会的发展，目前大众对肝癌的认知度与关注度已显著提升，学界对肝癌的重视程度也达到较高水平。在健康中国建设的新时代背景下，结合国家对医疗行业的发展需求，学界也应将目光拓展到罕见病领域，这些尚未得到足够重视的疾病同样需要深入研究与关怀。

王智超医师是我指导的医学博士之一，他在读博期间接受了系统的肿瘤学培训，毕业后赴美国约翰斯·霍普金斯大学攻读并获得生物统计学方向的公共卫生硕士学位。学成回国后，我非常支持并鼓励他投身罕见病的临床与科研工作。1型神经纤维瘤病（NF1）是一种复杂的罕见病，它严重影响患者的生活质量，并对医生、学者提出了极大的挑战。长期以来，这种疾病缺乏有效的治疗手段。随着科技的持续进步，学界对NF1的认知也不断深化。在外科手术治疗的基础上，靶向治疗等综合治疗方案已逐步开发并应用于临床。随着精准医学的快速发展，在基因组学、单细胞测序等前沿技术的推动下，国内医疗界有望在NF1基础研究领域取得关键性突破，为临床诊疗提供新的理论依据。这正是译者引入 *Neurofibromatosis Type 1: Molecular and Cellular Biology* 一书的初衷。

该书由国际知名学者 Meena Upadhyaya 和 David N. Cooper 主编，系统阐述了NF1的分子机制及其在细胞层面的影响。通过引进这本书，我们希望国内的研究者能够从中汲取灵感，推动NF1在基础研究和临床治疗上的创新。同时，也期望更多的医生和科研人员加入到这一罕见病的研究中，共同为患者带来福音。

医学之道，终以济世为本。NF1综合诊疗之路道阻且长，基础研究与临床实践的紧密结合是推动医学前进的关键。我们不仅要继续提升技术，更要通过引进前沿的学术成果，激发新的思路与方法，不拘泥于现状，在与NF1搏击的擂台上使出最佳的组合拳，为更多患者带来治愈的希望。

最后，特别感谢王智超教授、李青峰教授及其团队为中国1型神经纤维瘤病诊治做出的卓越贡献，并感谢他们对本书翻译做出的组织工作。相信本书的出版将为更多医师、研究人员及患者提供宝贵的知识与参考，进一步推动国内NF1的研究与治疗发展。

樊嘉
中国科学院院士
2025年4月于上海

中文版序二

整复外科，不仅限于"锦上添花"，更是关乎重塑生命、恢复功能这类"雪中送炭"的学科。张涤生院士生前始终强调，整复外科的宗旨是"让伤者不残，残者不废，健者更美丽自信"。尤其是像1型神经纤维瘤病（NF1）这样复杂的罕见病，我们需要在形态和功能两个层面上进行双重改善。作为奋战在临床最前线的口腔颌面外科医师，我们同样能够深刻感受到每位患者背后蕴藏的生命重量与他们对康复的渴望。

NF1的诊疗涉及患者、医师及社会三方力量：患者去配合；社会去接纳；而作为医者，我们必须面对肿瘤患者的生理创伤，还要帮助他们恢复心理健康与生活尊严。NF1患者的治疗涉及多学科的协作，从外科手术到药物治疗，甚至是基因治疗的前沿探索，每一步都需经过严谨的研究与临床实践。

Neurofibromatosis Type 1: Molecular and Cellular Biology 正是填补国内NF1基础研究与临床治疗之间知识鸿沟的重要著作。在浏览本书之后，我总结出以下几点独特之处。

1. 书中详细回顾了NF1及其基因 *NF1* 的研究历程，涵盖了从早期的历史描述到现代的研究成果。此外，本书还提出了未来研究的方向和需要解决的问题，如对 *NF1* 基因的进一步研究和临床应用的扩展，特别是在成人NF1患者的研究和治疗上。最后，书中展示了如何将基础研究成果转化为临床应用，例如 $NF1^{+/-}$ 肥大细胞在神经纤维瘤发病机制中的作用以及智力损害的研究等，体现了临床与基础研究的紧密结合。

2. 书中突出了几种先进技术的应用，包括计算机磁共振神经成像技术和基因组学技术，这些技术在NF1研究中的应用提高了对丛状神经纤维瘤（PNF）、恶性外周神经鞘瘤（MPNST）等表征的理解和治疗的精准度。

3. 书中强调来自包括美国、欧洲各国、日本、加拿大、澳大利亚和巴西等地的研究人员和机构在NF1领域的重要贡献，把各自专长经验及创造性成果汇聚其中，对整复外科的进一步发展具有指导意义。

这些特点使得本书成为NF1领域的一个宝贵资源，不仅为医学专业人士和研究人员提供了深入的科学信息，也为患者和他们的家庭提供了关于疾病管理和支持的重要指导。

从书中传递的科学价值与人文关怀中，我们可以看到现代医学的核心追求——不仅是在治愈疾病，更是在帮助患者重拾生活的希望与尊严。这也呼应了医学的最终目标，不仅是战胜疾病，更是让每一个患者重新获得自信与幸福。我希望更多的医师、科研人员和相关领域的学者能够关注NF1这样的罕见病，为这些患者带来更多的希望与选择。我们将继续在这条充满挑战的道路上奋斗，为更多患者带来光明的未来。

中国工程院院士
2025年4月

中文版前言

1型神经纤维瘤病（NF1）是 *NF1* 基因突变导致的一种复杂多样的罕见病症，于2023年9月20日被纳入国家卫生健康委员会第二批罕见病目录。它不仅涉及皮肤、神经系统与骨骼等，更可能诱发一系列难以预见的并发症，尤以丛状神经纤维瘤、皮肤型神经纤维瘤等周围神经肿瘤为著。由于其遗传背景的错综复杂及表型的高度异质性，NF1的诊断、治疗与长期管理，对临床实践和科研探索提出严峻的挑战。

过去数年间，整复外科的神经纤维瘤病诊疗团队接诊了近万名NF1患者，他们所承受的身心痛苦不仅仅源于疾病本身，更源于社会对该病的普遍认知不足及缺乏有效的治疗手段。为此，我们与国内同行坚定不移地致力于推动国内NF1领域的研究与发展。通过不断努力，团队成功完成了国内首个神经纤维瘤孤儿药的临床试验，并促成其顺利上市。此外，我们与全国同道起草了中国首部《Ⅰ型神经纤维瘤病临床诊疗专家共识（2021版）》及《丛状神经纤维瘤的全病程管理专家共识（2025版）》，这些共识为NF1和丛状神经纤维瘤的规范化诊疗提供了有力依据，为全国临床医生提供了科学且系统的诊疗指导，有望显著提升我国对NF1的综合管理水平。在临床实践发展与科研前沿探索的过程中，多学科合作的重要性与迫切性日益凸显。基于此，国内整形外科、肿瘤外科、肿瘤内科、皮肤科和生殖医学科的权威专家联合创建了中国首个神经纤维瘤病多中心治疗协作组，旨在整合各学科的专业力量，以多维度、多层次的综合诊治方案为患者提供个性化的治疗选择。我们坚信，这种跨学科的协作模式将为NF1的精准医疗铺就更为坚实的基础。

这种多学科协作的探索不仅体现在临床实践中，更催生出学术研究领域的深度成果转化。*Neurofibromatosis Type 1: Molecular and Cellular Biology* 由国际NF1领域的领军人物 Meena Upadhyaya 教授与 David N. Cooper 教授主编。两位教授在NF1的分子与细胞生物学研究中积累了深厚的学术造诣，最终凝结成这部具有重要学术价值的著作。本书对NF1相关临床表现、分子机制、基础研究、病例总结等的内容介绍十分详尽，能为临床医师与研究人员深入理解NF1的致病机制、优化诊疗策略提供宝贵的理论依据。我们期望通过引进这部具有巨大学术价值的著作，助力国内NF1研究与诊治水平的提升。

除了期望本书为国内医学界带来全新的知识外，我们还期望这次翻译工作能促进全国各NF1医疗中心之间的密切合作，共同推动我国对这一疾病的认知与治疗水平迈上新台阶，使更多患者从病痛的阴影中解脱出来。在此，我向所有参与本书翻译工作的教授、同仁致以由衷的敬意，是他们的支持与帮助，才让这一成果得以呈现。

对于翻译中可能存在的疏漏与不足，我们恳请各位同道与读者不吝指正，以便我们不断精进。

2025年4月

英文版序

本书标志着我们对神经纤维瘤病的理解真正"成熟"。自首次准确描述这一疾病已经过去130年,但在过去的30年里才有了真正意义上的进展。正是在这30年间,我们才逐步深入理解这种常见且重要的疾病。1998年,Meena和David的第一本相关图书《1型神经纤维瘤病:从基因型到表型》(*Neurofibromatosis Type 1: From Genotype to Phenotype*,BIOS Scientific Publishers)面世,该书是一个里程碑,展示了分子遗传学的出现不仅帮助确定了相关基因,还指引我们理解该基因在疾病和正常状态下的功能。

这本新书(Meena和David的第二本书)向我们展示了这种全新观点的发展和延伸,揭示了这一复杂疾病的不同方面。从此,我们认识到基础分析和临床研究如何相互支持。本书还为我们展示了学者们在这一领域做出了各自不同但相互关联的贡献。

笔者不仅为主编在国际上的学术影响力感到自豪,更为主编成功地将这一领域的关键成员汇聚在一起并创作出这部代表作感到骄傲。本书将成为人类遗传性疾病的重要里程碑。所有在神经纤维瘤病领域的人,无论是患者,还是参与研究或提供服务的人,都将感激他们的成果。

Peter S Harper
Cardiff,UK
2012年7月

英文版前言

1型神经纤维瘤病(neurofibromatosis type 1，NF1)是一种常见的常染色体显性癌症易感综合征，由抑癌基因 *NF1* 的种系突变引起。本书的目的是以简明但尽可能全面的方式，呈现当前关于 NF1 分子遗传学和细胞生物学的知识。NF1 的分子和细胞生物学是一个快速发展的领域，相关文献庞大且分散，难以查阅。本书共包含 44 章，由国际公认的著名专家撰写，介绍了 NF1 分子和细胞生物学的最新进展。它不仅适合人类遗传学家、临床医师、全科医师、心理学家和遗传咨询师阅读，也适合医学与生物科学的本科生和研究生参考。我们希望本书在未来的多年里能成为有用的参考资料。

自我们在 1998 年首次出版关于这一主题的图书(Upadhyaya and Cooper 1998)以来，关于 NF1 不同特征发展背后的分子和细胞机制的认知大幅增长。在此期间，NF1 诊所的管理、分子诊断、体细胞嵌合现象的检测、基因型-表型关联以及 *NF1* 修饰位点的识别等方面取得了显著进展。过去 14 年的深入研究极大地扩展了我们对 *NF1* 基因及其蛋白质产物(神经纤维瘤蛋白)的功能作用、基因的种系和体细胞突变谱及其突变机制的理解。*NF1* 与错配修复基因之间的关系也得到了初步探索。

随着全身 MRI 和 PET 等灵敏的成像技术的出现，我们获得了大量关于体内肿瘤负荷及其管理的信息。我们对 NF1 患者骨骼和心血管异常的理解也得到了极大改善。认知功能障碍的临床、分子和细胞方面的研究已广泛开展，催生了治疗的可能性并推动了临床试验的进行。

关于 NF1 相关肿瘤[包括视路胶质瘤、嗜铬细胞瘤、皮肤和丛状神经纤维瘤、恶性周围神经鞘膜瘤(malignant peripheral nerve sheath tumours，MPNST)、血管球瘤和白血病]的发病机制，我们也学到了很多，使我们在管理这些肿瘤方面的能力得到了提升。NF1 相关肿瘤的起源细胞的鉴定对于设计新疗法至关重要。现有证据表明，皮肤型神经纤维瘤起源于皮肤衍生的前体细胞或其衍生物，而在施万细胞系中 *NF1* 的双等位基因失活导致丛状神经纤维瘤的形成。MPNST 的起源细胞尚不清楚。

我们对良性神经纤维瘤向恶性转化的机制仍然知之甚少，这可能涉及包括遗传和表观遗传改变在内的连续事件，且这些变化发生的顺序需要进一步阐明。肿瘤微环境在 NF1 肿瘤发生中起着关键作用，这也需要进一步探索。除了在 NF1 中发挥核心作用外，*NF1* 基因还作为一种重要的抑瘤基因在散发性癌症中崭露头角。

我们从果蝇、斑马鱼和小鼠等动物模型中学到了很多关于 NF1 的生物学的知识。这些模型有助于推进我们对疾病进展的理解，并有望促进生物标志物的鉴定、适宜疗法的开发以及临床试验中药物反应的预测。基于临床前工作的研究已经转化为针对各种 NF1 特征的治疗试验，包括丛状神经纤维瘤、胶质瘤、MPNST 和神经认知障碍。最近，一个新的发育综合征类别被命名为"RASopathies"，其由不同基因的胚系突变引起，这些基因参与调控 Ras/MAPK 信号通路。实际上，NF1 中存在位点异质性：其中一个 RASopathies——Legius 综合征，由 *SPRED1* 基因突变引起，并具有与 NF1 重叠的临床特征。

最新报道显示，不同癌症可能与不同的微小 RNA(microRNA，miRNA)表达模式相关，这可能可以为我们提供额外的预后和诊断标志物，并为MPNST的治疗干预开辟新途径。事实上，在人类原发性MPNST中已检测到表达CD133（肿瘤干细胞标志物）的细胞亚群。功能分析证实这些细胞是肿瘤干细胞（cancer stem cells，CSC），并已显示其在体外具有增强的耐药性（Borrego-Diaz et al. 2012）。

全球范围内的NF1公益基金会正在发展，成为NF1研究的重要推动力，为NF1社区提供了重要资源。书中还讨论了NF1患者面临的社会问题，最后探讨了NF1研究的潜在未来方向，强调了新的研究途径和治疗靶点。

David Cooper

Meena Upadhyaya

Institute of Medical Genetics

School of Medicine

Cardiff University

Cardiff，United Kingdom

参考文献

[1] Upadhyaya M，Cooper DN (1998) Neurofibromatosis type 1. From genotype to phenotype. BIOS Scientific, Oxford

[2] Borrego-Diaz E，Terai K，Lialyte K，Wise AL，Esfandyari T，Behbod F，Mautner VF，Spyra M，Taylor S，Parada LF，Upadhyaya M，Farassati F (2012) Overactivation of Ras signaling pathway in CD133+ MPNST cells. J Neurooncol 108：423-434

目 录

第 1 章　von Recklinghausen 病的 130 年 ············· 1
　　　　 von Recklinghausen Disease：130 Years

第 2 章　1 型神经纤维瘤病的临床诊断和非典型表现 ············· 11
　　　　 Clinical Diagnosis and Atypical Forms of NF1

第 3 章　"复杂 1 型神经纤维瘤病"的管理与治疗 ············· 19
　　　　 Management and Treatment of "Complex Neurofibromatosis 1"

第 4 章　1 型神经纤维瘤病死亡率 ············· 27
　　　　 Mortality in Neurofibromatosis 1

第 5 章　1 型神经纤维瘤病儿童的认知特征：治疗意义 ············· 33
　　　　 The Cognitive Profile of NF1 Children：Therapeutic Implications

第 6 章　单卵双胞胎中 1 型神经纤维瘤病的临床表现 ············· 42
　　　　 Clinical Expression of NF1 in Monozygotic Twins

第 7 章　全身 MRI 对 1 型神经纤维瘤病患者的价值 ············· 49
　　　　 Value of Whole Body MRI in Patients with NF1

第 8 章　1 型神经纤维瘤病患者的生命质量 ············· 54
　　　　 Quality of Life in NF1

第 9 章　NF1 基因：启动子、5′非翻译区和 3′非翻译区 ············· 61
　　　　 NF1 Gene：Promoter，5′ UTR，and 3′ UTR

第 10 章　1 型神经纤维瘤病的胚系突变谱及基因型–表型相关性 ············· 67
　　　　　The Germline Mutational Spectrum in Neurofibromatosis Type 1 and Genotype-Phenotype
　　　　　Correlations

第 11 章　*NF1* 基因的剪接机制和突变 ··· 80
Splicing Mechanisms and Mutations in the *NF1* Gene

第 12 章　*NF1* 基因型和体细胞嵌合现象 ··· 90
NF1 Germline and Somatic Mosaicism

第 13 章　*NF1* 的深部内含子突变以及潜在的治疗干预措施 ················· 107
Deep Intronic *NF1* Mutations and Possible Therapeutic Interventions

第 14 章　*NF1* 微缺失及其突变机制 ··· 117
NF1 Microdeletions and Their Underlying Mutational Mechanisms

第 15 章　*NF1* 基因的体细胞突变谱 ··· 131
The Somatic Mutational Spectrum of the *NF1* Gene

第 16 章　1 型神经纤维瘤病与构成性错配修复缺陷之间的关系 ············ 145
Relationship Between NF1 and Constitutive Mismatch Repair Deficiency

第 17 章　*NF1* 基因的进化论 ··· 156
Insights into *NF1* from Evolution

第 18 章　1 型神经纤维瘤病修饰基因 ··· 168
Modifier Genes in NF1

第 19 章　使用小鼠模型剖析影响 1 型神经纤维瘤病易感性的遗传和表观遗传的复杂相互作用 ······ 178
Dissection of Complex Genetic and Epigenetic Interactions Underlying NF1 Cancer Susceptibility Using Mouse Models

第 20 章　神经纤维瘤蛋白：蛋白质结构域及其功能特点 ······················· 189
Neurofibromin: Protein Domains and Functional Characteristics

第 21 章　1 型神经纤维瘤病骨骼异常的分子基础 ··································· 204
Molecular Basis of Bone Abnormalities in NF1

第 22 章　1 型神经纤维瘤病相关视神经胶质瘤 ······································· 213
NF1 - Associated Optic Glioma

第 23 章　1 型神经纤维瘤病患者心血管异常的分子基础 ······················· 221
Molecular Basis of Cardiovascular Abnormalities in NF1

第 24 章　血管球瘤的分子基础 ········· 231
Molecular Basis of Glomus Tumours

第 25 章　嗜铬细胞瘤和 1 型神经纤维瘤病 ········· 242
Pheochromocytoma and NF1

第 26 章　人皮肤型神经纤维瘤的分子和细胞基础及发生 ········· 250
Molecular and Cellular Basis of Human Cutaneous Neurofibromas and Their Development

第 27 章　体细胞拷贝数改变：1 型神经纤维瘤病相关的恶性周围神经鞘膜瘤中基因和蛋白质的表达 ········· 256
Somatic Copy Number Alterations: Gene and Protein Expression Correlates in NF1 - Associated Malignant Peripheral Nerve Sheath Tumors

第 28 章　1 型神经纤维瘤病相关周围神经鞘膜瘤的病理学和分子诊断特征 ········· 272
Pathologic and Molecular Diagnostic Features of Peripheral Nerve Sheath Tumors in NF1

第 29 章　恶性周围神经鞘膜瘤：预后和诊断标志物以及治疗靶点 ········· 280
Malignant Peripheral Nerve Sheath Tumors: Prognostic and Diagnostic Markers and Therapeutic Targets

第 30 章　血液恶性肿瘤中的 NF1 突变 ········· 295
NF1 Mutations in Hematologic Cancers

第 31 章　Legius 综合征：诊断与病理 ········· 306
Legius Syndrome: Diagnosis and Pathology

第 32 章　RAS 病：Ras/MAPK 通路失调的综合征 ········· 313
The RASopathies: Syndromes of Ras/MAPK Pathway Dysregulation

第 33 章　1 型神经纤维瘤病动物模型的进展和经验教训 ········· 323
Advances in NF1 Animal Models and Lessons Learned

第 34 章　果蝇：1 型神经纤维瘤病的无脊椎动物模型 ········· 329
Drosophila: An Invertebrate Model of NF1

第 35 章　1 型神经纤维瘤病的斑马鱼模型 ········· 337
Zebrafish Model for NF1

第 36 章　起源细胞及微环境因素在 1 型神经纤维瘤病肿瘤发生中的作用及治疗意义 ·············· 346
Cell of Origin and the Contribution of Microenvironment in NF1 Tumorigenesis and Therapeutic Implications

第 37 章　与 1 型神经纤维瘤病和其他 Ras 信号通路相关疾病相关认知障碍的分子学和细胞学研究方法 ················ 359
Molecular and Cellular Approaches to Cognitive Impairments Associated with NF1 and Other Rasopathies

第 38 章　恶性周围神经鞘膜瘤中 Ras 信号通路的生物学特点及相关疗法 ·············· 371
Ras Signaling Pathway in Biology and Therapy of Malignant Peripheral Nerve Sheath Tumors

第 39 章　miRNA 与 1 型神经纤维瘤病肿瘤发生 ·············· 385
MicroRNA and NF1 Tumorigenesis

第 40 章　儿童和成人 1 型神经纤维瘤病的转化/临床研究 ·············· 394
Translational/Clinical Studies in Children and Adults with Neurofibromatosis Type 1

第 41 章　1 型神经纤维瘤病民间基金会的作用：未来愿景 ·············· 415
The Role of NF1 Lay Foundations: Future Vision

第 42 章　1 型神经纤维瘤病中的社会污名化 ·············· 423
Social Stigma in Neurofibromatosis 1

第 43 章　1 型神经纤维瘤病的个性化诊疗 ·············· 429
Personalized Medicine in NF1

第 44 章　1 型神经纤维瘤病：未来的方向（我们该何去何从？）·············· 433
Neurofibromatosis Type 1: Future Directions (Where Do We Go from Here?)

第 1 章　von Recklinghausen 病的 130 年
von Recklinghausen Disease: 130 Years

Vincent M. Riccardi

1.1 引言

我是一名遗传学家，同时也是一名专注于研究 Recklinghausen 病的学者。在研究过程中，我力求运用我的遗传学知识，以深入理解并诠释这种被称为 von Recklinghausen 病的疾病，即 1 型神经纤维瘤病（neurofibromatosis type 1，NF1）。Recklinghausen 病的研究领域面临着一个问题：我们将全部注意力放在了 *NF1* 基因的突变或缺失而导致的疾病上，却忽视了更值得关注的部分——*NF1* 基因座上的正常野生型基因。本章中，我将首先简要回顾与 *NF1* 基因功能异常及其后果相关的研究历程，并介绍我个人参与的一些研究进展。另外，我希望能够深入探讨野生型 *NF1* 基因在人类进化和功能中的独特作用。整章内容（实际上包括整本书）都应明确一点："*NF1* 是抑癌基因"这一描述，更多的是针对发生基因突变的基因，而不是针对野生型基因本身。

我们对某种疾病了解得越多，就越能预防这种疾病，并提供有效的治疗方法。同样地，我们对引发特定孟德尔遗传病的基因了解得越透彻，也就越有可能开发出有效的治疗手段，无论是减轻突变基因的影响，还是直接替换或修改突变基因。因此，要理解并治疗遗传病，我们必须全面掌握在相关基因座上可能发生的所有突变。由此，我们引出两个问题：首先，我们应该专注于突变基因还是正常（野生型）基因？其次，基因到底是什么？在即将迎来 Friedrich von Recklinghausen 首次提出 NF1 概念 130 周年之际，我们认识到，虽然我们对 NF1 的自然史、发病机制和细胞生物学有了相对深入的了解，但对 *NF1* 突变的了解依然有限，对野生型 *NF1* 基因甚至几乎没有任何认识。部分原因在于，我们目前对"基因"的定义依然不够完善。

如前所述，在本书的引言部分，我们将分享截至 21 世纪初期我们对 NF1 疾病及 *NF1* 基因的现有知识和理解。我将从两个角度展开：一是回顾我们在这一领域取得的一些重要进展及其细节，二是探讨 NF1 以及 *NF1* 基因对我们理解基因和遗传病的启示。

1.2 历史

我们现在称之为"1 型神经纤维瘤病""NF1"的疾病，曾被称为"von Recklinghausen 病"，早在几个世纪前就已经为人所知了。相关资料多次提到，如 1988 年（第 1 章）(Mulvihill 1988) 和 1994 年（第 1 章）(Huson and Hughes 1994) 中的概述。Friedrich von Recklinghausen 在 1882 年发表的论文《多发性

V. M. Riccardi
The Neurofibromatosis Institute, 5415 Briggs Avenue, La Crescenta, CA, USA
e-mail: Riccardi@medconsumer.com

M. Upadhyaya and D. N. Cooper (eds.), *Neurofibromatosis Type 1*,
DOI 10.1007/978-3-642-32864-0_1, # Springer-Verlag Berlin Heidelberg 2012

皮肤纤维瘤及其与多发性神经瘤的关系》(Ueber die multiplen Fibrome der Haut and ihre Beziehung zu den multiplen Neuromen)是将这一疾病命名为 von Recklinghausen 病的基础。该论文的部分内容被译成英文,收录在 1981 年由 Riccardi 和 Mulvihill 编辑的 Advances in Neurology 第 29 卷(第 259 页)中。此外,该书还包括 Josef Warkany 撰写的 von Recklinghausen 的传记(第 251 页)。

因此,截至 2012 年,距离 1882 年 von Recklinghausen 首次将他的名字与我们现在称为 NF1 的疾病联系起来,已经过去了 130 年。然而,更准确地首次全面描述这一疾病应该在 1849 年,这意味着该疾病已有 160 多年的历史。1849 年,爱尔兰医师 R. W. Smith 发表了 A treatise on the pathology, diagnosis and treatment of neuroma 一文。该文在 1989 年重新出版(Smith 1989),其中指出,他关注的是神经周围的"结缔组织",而不是神经本身。2003 年的一篇出版物中也有类似的描述(Reynolds et al. 2003),而在 1992 年,另一篇文章的标题则提出了一个特别有力的问题:"神经纤维瘤病:为什么不叫 Smith 病?"(Neurofibromatosis: Why not Smith's disease?)(Lyons and Staunton 1992)。

从 19 世纪中叶到 20 世纪初期,关于 NF1 的综合性研究很少,直到 1951 年 Borberg 发表了一项大规模的丹麦人群研究(Borberg 1951;Mulvihill et al. 1983)。他的研究阐明了家庭成员之间的巨大异质性,并强调了 NF1 的成年人远多于儿童,且并非所有患者的临床问题都与肿瘤相关。换句话说,NF1 不仅仅是一种儿童肿瘤性疾病。1956 年,密歇根大学的 Crowe、Schull 和 Neel 的研究(Crowe et al. 1956)进一步强调了这些观点,尽管他们可能也因将现在称为 NF2 的疾病归为 NF1 的一个亚型而带来了某些混淆。1971 年和 1972 年,Brasfield 和 Das Gupta(Das Gupta and Brasfield 1971;Brasfield and Das Gupta 1972)提供了基于外科专家和机构的数据,强调了 NF1 的长期(即成人阶段)的发病率。

在此背景下,1972 年 2 月,我作为马萨诸塞总医院的一名遗传学研究员,被邀请在儿科大会上就我选择的主题发表演讲。我的导师 Lewis B. Holmes 建议我选择一个我愿意终身研究的课题。很明显,von Recklinghausen 病成为我的选择。在这一目标的引导下,当我在 1976 年被招募到贝勒医学院(Baylor College of Medicine)时,我明确表示,我搬到得克萨斯州休斯敦的条件是支持我建立一个以护理和研究为基础的神经纤维瘤病项目。因此,在 1977 年 2 月,贝勒神经纤维瘤病项目(Baylor NF Program,BNFP)成为现实,并在 1978 年 8 月迎来了第一位患者。同样在 1978 年,全国神经纤维瘤病基金会(National Neurofibromatosis Foundation, Inc., NNFF)由 Lynne Courtemanche 护士、Allan Rubenstein 医师和 Joel Hirschtritt 律师成立。1979 年 6 月,国家癌症研究所(National Cancer Institute,NCI)和 BNFP 主办了首届神经纤维瘤病国际会议,其会议记录如后所述被出版。

1980 年,得克萨斯神经纤维瘤病基金会成立。1981 年,Advances in Neurology 第 29 卷报道了 1979 年 NCI-BNFP 神经纤维瘤病国际会议的会议记录(Riccardi and Mulvihill 1981)。同年年底,New England Journal of Medicine 在其医学进展系列中发表了 BNFP 迄今为止对 NF 的概述(Riccardi 1981b)。1981 年,Winfrid Krone 等(1981)和 Juha Peltonen 等(1981)首次发表了关于 NF1 细胞生物学的初步研究。1983 年 11 月,BNFP 在首次国际推广活动中,于东京发表了关于超过一半 NF1 患者智力表现受损的重要数据(Riccardi 1984)。1985 年 3 月,BNFP 第二次重大国际推广活动在 3 周内访问了 5 个欧洲国家,最终在伦敦的"Let's Increase NF Knowledge"(LINK)会议上发表了关于 NF 的专题讲座。1986 年,NF1 的细胞生物学研究在 Nancy Ratner 的不懈努力下得到了进一步巩固(Ratner et al. 1986)。1987 年 7 月,NIH 共识会议采用了 BNFP 对 NF1 和 NF2 的命名法,并提出了两种疾病的具体诊断标准(1988)。同样在 1987 年,NF1 基因被定位于人类染色体 17 号长臂(17q)(Van Teinen et al. 1987;Barker et al. 1987;Skolnick et al. 1987;Pericak-Vance et al. 1987),而 NF2 基因被定位于人类染色体 22 号长臂(22q)(Rouleau et al. 1987)。1988 年,多个志同道合的

NF组织在州和地方组织成立了NF公司,以建立一个允许多个分组织保持地方独立,同时又在全国范围内进行合作的NF组织。1989年6月,部分日益壮大的国际NF组织在英国牛津会面,1989年11月,日本东京和意大利锡耶纳也举办了专门的NF会议,其中锡耶纳会议成为欧洲NF协会的模范会议。

1990年,研究者们鉴定出了NF1基因及其基因产物神经纤维瘤蛋白(Viskochil et al. 1990;Wallace et al. 1990;Daston et al. 1992;Hattori et al. 1992;DeClue et al. 1992;Daston and Ratner 1992)。1993年,又鉴定出了NF2基因及其基因产物默林(schwannomin)(MacCollin et al. 1993)。1994年,第一批关于NF1小鼠模型的研究成果开始显现(Jacks et al. 1994;Brannan et al. 1994),Parada和同事们则开始利用这些啮齿动物模型研究人类NF1基因突变(Smullen et al. 1994;Le et al. 2011;Li et al. 2012)。2005年,NNFF将其名称改为"儿童肿瘤基金会",这一举动令许多临床医师、受影响的家庭和患者感到困惑,因为他们认为NF1的负担远不止于儿童时期和肿瘤。

与此同时,NF领域的专家在日本、加拿大和欧洲也取得了显著进展。在日本,以Michihito Niimura为领导;在加拿大,由Jan Friedman引领;而在欧洲,则由欧洲NF协会和众多研究Recklinghausen病的学者领导的中心所推动,其中包括G. D. Evans、R. E. Ferner、A. Heiberg、S. M. Huson、D. Kaufmann、W. Krone、E. Legius、V.-F. Mautner、L. M. Messiaen、J. Peltonen、B. Samuelsson、R. Tenconi、M. Upadhyaya和P. Wolkenstein等。澳大利亚在K. North的领导下,巴西在L. O. Rodrigues的领导下,也在理解和治疗NF1的国际合作中做出了重大贡献。

在这些美国、欧洲和国际联盟的多项研究成果中,有七个方面尤为显著。当然,还有其他一些值得关注的领域。只要翻阅本书的目录就会发现,与理解NF1相关的所有重要领域都得到了充分的重视和探讨。可以说,从1882年到2012年,我们在这一领域取得了显著的进展。

第一值得注意的是计算机磁共振神经成像技术的应用,尤其是在神经纤维瘤体积测量和全身扫描方面,用于检测和追踪有症状及无症状的弥漫性和包囊性丛状神经纤维瘤(Dombi et al. 2007;Solomon et al. 2004;Mautner et al. 2008;Jaremko et al. 2012)。一方面,在阐明丛状神经纤维瘤的早期发育阶段及评估特定治疗对神经纤维瘤的抑制效果方面,这些策略取得了较大的成功。另一方面,神经纤维瘤的生长监测主要依赖于体积测量。然而,考虑到弥漫性丛状神经纤维瘤主要通过芽生的方式增大(Riccardi, 1992;Masson, 1970),如von Recklinghausen(1882)所述及Harkin和Reed(1969)图64所示,测量整个肿瘤的表面积可能对检测弥漫性神经纤维瘤的生长变化更加敏感,无论是与年龄有关,还是与治疗相关(Lebioda et al. 2008;Andea et al. 2004;Shahar et al. 2002;Videtic et al. 2001)。

第二个值得特别关注的领域是基因组学技术的应用,特别是在NF1基因全基因缺失的研究方面(Mautner et al. 2010;Zickler et al. 2011),以及对于全基因缺失(Pasmant et al. 2010;Vogt et al. 2011b)和基因内突变的基因型-表型相关性的研究(Upadhyaya et al. 2007)。德国汉堡的Mautner及其团队(Kluwe et al. 2004;Mautner et al. 2006, 2010)和亚拉巴马州伯明翰的Messiaen及其团队(Messiaen et al. 2000, 2010)在这一领域做出了巨大的贡献。如今,无论是在患者管理还是在胚胎移植前的选择上(Verlinsky et al. 2002;Spits et al. 2005),基因组诊断都已得到一致性和规范化的应用。

第三,除了在上文提到的基因型-表型相关性研究,临床异质性和自然史研究也得到了特别重视,尤其是体细胞嵌合现象(Ruggieri and Huson 2001;Maertens et al. 2007;Kaplan et al. 2010;Bottillo et al. 2010;Messiaen et al. 2010;Vogt et al. 2011a)和NF1与Legius综合征的重叠(Brems et al. 2007;Messiaen et al. 2009)。在2012年,我们已经有了为每位临床确诊为NF1的患者建立补充性的基因组诊断的依据。然而,尽管对自然史和纵向研究的重视有所增加,但成人NF1患者的诊所和治疗中心的数量却停滞不前。截至2012年初,针对成人NF1患者的项目建设投入仍然有限，而NF1细胞生物学和基因组学研究仍然集中于 NF1 基因产物神经纤维瘤蛋白的细胞生物学和生物化学，未能充分考虑其他遗传机制，如包括 miRNAs（如 miR-10b）在内的各种转录产物（Chai et al. 2010）。

第四，视路胶质瘤及其他脑部肿瘤的研究得出了明确的结论，这些肿瘤是 NF1 的关键组成部分，对疾病的慢性病程和早期病死率有显著影响（Lewis et al. 1984）。在此方面，Gutmann 及其团队的贡献特别值得一提（Bajenaru et al. 2002；Gutmann et al. 2000；Listernick et al. 2004；Rodriguez et al. 2008；Gutmann 2011；Banerjee et al. 2011）。他们对 NF1 基因产物神经纤维瘤蛋白各种异构体的研究也同样值得关注（Grand et al. 1993；Gutmann et al. 1993a，b，1995a，b）。

第五，虽然多名研究 Recklinghausen 病的学者已关注到 NF1 中普遍存在的骨骼影响（Riccardi，1992），但犹他州盐湖城的 Recklinghausen 病学小组在 D. A. Stevenson 领导下的研究还是值得关注（Stevenson et al. 2005，2006，2008；Kossler et al. 2011；Johnson et al. 2011）。理解骨骼组织细胞（软骨和骨）与施万细胞和黑色素细胞的共同特性，不仅对帮助 NF1 患者极有价值，也对理解正常骨生长和修复的动态具有重要意义。

第六，肥大细胞在理解神经纤维瘤的发病机制和治疗方法中的作用展示了临床研究与基础研究的高度融合。早在1981年，基于纯粹的临床观察以及病理学家对正常周围神经和神经纤维瘤（无论是否来自 NF1 患者）中肥大细胞的早期记录，V. M. Riccardi 便确认了肥大细胞在神经纤维瘤发展中的作用（Riccardi 1981a，1987，1990a；1993；Virchow 1857）。后续的病理学数据表明，两种基本类型的神经纤维瘤（包囊性与弥漫性，或束状与非束状）可以根据其中肥大细胞的数量和分布情况进行区分（Tucker et al. 2011）。与此同时，多个小鼠模型在细胞生物学水平上证实了肥大细胞在 NF1 神经纤维瘤起始和进展中的关键作用，这些肥大细胞在 NF1 基因位点上表现为单倍体剂量不足（Viskochil 2003；Badache et al. 1998；Staser et al. 2010，2011）。肥大细胞对靶向施万细胞微环境的修饰显然在神经纤维瘤的发育和生长中起着关键作用。早期使用酮替芬（一种口服肥大细胞稳定剂）治疗 NF1 神经纤维瘤的尝试有一些有限的疗效，但并未引起 Recklinghausen 病学组织的广泛关注（Riccardi 1990a，b，1993）。

第七，智力损害也是值得关注的领域，尽管名称和机制各异，但对患者、家庭以及神经纤维瘤症专家、遗传学家和脑科学研究者来说尤为重要。贝勒神经纤维瘤病项目（BNFP）特别重视 NF1 这一方面（Riccardi and Eichner 1986；Riccardi 1984，1992；Coleman 1987），尽管其他许多人也做出了重要贡献（Cutting et al. 2000b；Ozonoff 1999；Descheemaeker et al. 2005；Acosta et al. 2006；Barton and North 2007；Cutting et al. 2000a；Krab et al. 2008a；Said et al. 1996；Park et al. 2009；Pasmant et al. 2010），其中以 North 及其同事的工作尤为突出（North 1993；North et al. 1994，1997，2002；Hyman et al. 2003，2005；Payne et al. 2010；Sangster et al. 2011）。Silva 等集中研究了 $Nf1^{+/-}$ 小鼠模型，广泛使用 Morris 水迷宫测试，并在之后探索了他汀类药物治疗的潜在用途（Silva et al. 1997；Li et al. 2005；Shilyansky et al. 2010）。Krab 等验证了许多相关数据，并发起了一项直接测试辛伐他汀对 NF1 患者短期影响的研究，该研究目前尚无定论（Krab et al. 2008a，b，c；van Engelen et al. 2008）。其他研究者特别关注 NF1 患者的注意力及其相反现象——注意力缺失（Brown et al. 2010a，2011），Ribeiro 及其同事则专门研究了视觉注意力（Ribeiro et al. 2012）。在个人层面上，2007年4月，我在葡萄牙里斯本举行的欧洲 NF 协会会议上发表了一篇题为"*Prosody: The Real Learning Disability of NF1*"的论文。其目的是强调，在感知和运动技能方面，许多 NF1 患者往往缺乏注意力：他们无法充分利用周围环境中的所有可用信息。在同一场会议上，其他三位发言人（W. Li，P. Wolkenstein，L. C. Krab）也强调了注意力和专注力对 NF1 患者学习问题的重要性，无论是在小鼠还是人类中进行研究。同时，其他研究者也研究了嘌呤核苷酸，尤其是 cAMP、ATP 和 GTP，与 NF1 脑功能的相关性（Hannan et al. 2006；Tong et al.

2002，2007；Dasgupta et al. 2003；Guo et al. 2000；The et al. 1997；Ho et al. 2007；Hegedus et al. 2007；Xu et al. 2002；Kim et al. 1997；Brown et al. 2010b，2012；Park et al. 2009；Bland and Birnbaum 2011)。氧化应激、细胞生物学应激以及个体/患者应激之间的相互关系，作为 NF1 发病机制和野生型 *NF1* 基因功能的关键因素，是我在 BNFP 早期发展阶段的主要研究领域之一。具体来说，*NF1* 单倍体剂量不足的成纤维细胞对暴露于 3-硝基酪氨酸的代谢应激的适应能力，促使我们进一步沿着这条研究路径前进(Riccardi and Maragos 1980)。

在这个背景下，特别应该注意：在野生动物中没有发现带有 *Nf1* 突变的种群。尽管我们熟知有多发性神经纤维瘤的家畜(Doughty 1977；Canfield 1967；Canfield and Doughty 1980；Sartin et al. 1994；Omi et al. 1994)，但从未有任何记录过带有 *Nf1* 突变的野生动物能活到成年。可能除了一些表现出多个色素性神经纤维瘤的双色雀鲷种群，这些鱼表现出与 NF1 相似的病症(Schmale et al. 1983，1986；Schmale and Udey 1983；Lacson et al. 1988，1989；Fieber and Schmale 1994)。然而，这些鱼类中的 NF1 样疾病(目前称为 Stegastes partitus，以前被指定为 Pomacentrus partitus 或 Eupomacentrus partitus)似乎是由一种病毒或"类病毒"生物体感染所致(Schmale and Hensley 1988；Campbell et al. 2001；Schmale et al. 2002)。我反复提出，这种缺乏 NF1 野生动物的现象可能是因为随之而来的注意力损害严重影响了捕食者和猎物的生存能力；形象地说，猎物过早地"成为午餐"，而捕食者则"得不到午餐"，这种情况不断发生。要在野外生存，无论是作为捕食者还是猎物，都需要最高水平的注意力，而这种"最高水平"则需要一个完整的、野生型的 *NF1* 基因。

1.3 基因

我的研究起点在于 NF1 成纤维细胞对 3-硝基酪氨酸的抵抗力(Riccardi and Maragos 1980；Ma et al. 2007)，以及嘌呤核苷酸在 NF1 发病机制中所起的多种作用，尤其是 ATP 在生命起源和维持中的关键作用(表 1.1)(Saygin 1981；Galimov 2004，2009；Shelly et al. 2010；Bland and Birnbaum 2011)。随后，我推测人体中的野生型 *NF1* 基因是一个关键的感应基因，负责平衡机体(特别是中枢神经系统和周围神经)的营养/能量需求与可用的营养/能量供应之间的关系，类似于酿酒酵母中的对应基因[Ras 活性抑制因子(inhibitor of Ras activity，IRA)](Daston et al. 1992；Gutmann et al. 1993b；Russell et al. 1993；Dechant and Peter 2008；Hertz et al. 2007；Wallace and Fan 2010)。

表 1.1 ATP 是关键的嘌呤核苷酸

ATP 是嘌呤相互转化的枢纽(ATP、cAMP、GTP、cGMP)，也是核酸合成的重要参与者
ATP 在蛋白质激活中至关重要，是原型激酶辅因子(通过互补的磷酸酶调节来平衡)
ATP 是生物能量转移的关键成分，受 O_2 作用的影响
尽管大脑仅占体重的 2%~3%，却消耗了全身 20% 的氧气和 25% 的葡萄糖
周围神经系统有类似的需求，且一样脆弱
人体内的 ATP 不断分解为 ADP，随后又被转化回 ATP
尽管 ATP 和 ADP 的总量保持不变，但人体细胞的能量需求每天需要转换 50~75 kg 的 ATP，每个 ATP 分子每天循环利用 1 000~1 500 次

出于这种想法，我在 2009 年 11 月日本 Recklinghausen 病学会的首次会议上提出了以下观点(Riccardi 2010)："……我们必须认识到，*NF1* 不仅仅是 1 个'肿瘤抑制基因'，它实际上是一个嘌呤核苷酸平衡(Purine Nucleotide Balance，PNTB)基因。"换句话说，虽然 *NF1* 基因突变可能导致多种类型的肿瘤，但野生型 *NF1* 基因的主要功能是生成和维持嘌呤核苷酸的结合，以确保在极短的时间间隔(以秒计)内实现中枢神经系统和周围神经的最佳功能。这个基因确保大脑、脊髓和周围神经具备最佳的嘌呤核苷酸平衡，让生物体表现得最好，尤其是在注意力和运动反应方面。

简言之，作为遗传学家，我认为野生型 *NF1* 基因最应该从增强瞬时生存的脑和神经功能的角度来理解。是时候开始研究如何利用 NF1 野生型基因的这一(这些)特性了,我们是否可以增强它的功能?为了更深入地回答这个问题,我们需要了解哪些方面的知识?

(王智超,余旋 译)

参考文献

[1] (1988) NIH Consensus Development Conference Statement: Neurofibromatosis. Arch Neurol 45: 575 – 578

[2] Acosta MT, Gioia GA, Silva AJ (2006) Neurofibromatosis type 1: new insights into neurocognitive issues. Curr Neurol Neurosci Rep 6: 136 – 143

[3] Andea AA, Bouwman D, Wallis T, Visscher DW (2004) Correlation of tumor volume and surface area with lymph node status in patients with multifocal/multicentric breast carcinoma. Cancer 100: 20 – 27

[4] Badache A, Muja N, De Vries GH (1998) Expression of Kit in neurofibromin-deficient human Schwann cells: role in Schwann cell hyperplasia associated with type 1 neurofibromatosis. Oncogene 17: 795 – 800

[5] Bajenaru ML, Zhu Y, Hedrick NM, Donahoe J, Parada LF, Gutmann DH (2002) Astrocyte specific inactivation of the neurofibromatosis 1 gene (NF1) is insufficient for astrocytoma formation. Mol Cell Biol 22: 5100 – 5113

[6] Banerjee S, Crouse NR, Emnett RJ, Gianino SM, Gutmann DH (2011) Neurofibromatosis-1 regulates mTOR-mediated astrocyte growth and glioma formation in a TSC/Rheb-independent manner. Proc Natl Acad Sci USA 108: 15996 – 16001

[7] Barker D, Wright E, Nguyen K, Cannon L, Fain P, Goldgar D, Bishop DT, Carey JBB, Kivlin J, Willard H, Waye JS, Greig G, Leinwand L, Nakamura Y, O'Connell P, Leppert M, Lalouel JM, White R, Skolnick M (1987) Gene for von Recklinghausen neurofibromatosis is in the pericentromeric region of chromosome 17. Science 236: 1100 – 1102

[8] Barton B, North K (2007) The self-concept of children and adolescents with neurofibromatosis type 1. Child Care Health Dev 33: 401 – 408

[9] Bland ML, Birnbaum MJ (2011) Cell biology. ADaPting to energetic stress. Science 332: 1387 – 1388

[10] Borberg A (1951) Clinical and genetic investigations into tuberous sclerosis and Recklinghausen's neurofibromatosis. Acta Psychiatr Neurol Scand 71: 1 – 239

[11] Bottillo I, Torrente I, Lanari V, Pinna V, Giustini S, Divona L, De LA, Dallapiccola B (2010) Germline mosaicism in neurofibromatosis type 1 due to a paternally derived multi-exon deletion. Am J Med Genet A 152A: 1467 – 1473

[12] Brannan CI, Perkins AS, Vogel KS, Ratner N, Nordlund ML, Reid SW, Buchberg AM, Jenkins NA, Parada LF, Copeland NG (1994) Targeted disruption of the neurofibromatosis type-1 gene leads to developmental abnormalities in heart and various neural crest-derived tissues. Genes Dev 8: 1019 – 1029

[13] Brasfield RD, Das Gupta TK (1972) Von Recklinghausen's disease: a clinicopathological study. Ann Surg 175: 86 – 104

[14] Brems H, Chmara M, Sahbatou M, Denayer E, Taniguchi K, Kato R, Somers R, Messiaen L, De Schepper S, Fryns JP, Cools J, Marynen P, Thomas G, Yoshimura A, Legius E (2007) Germline loss-of-function mutations in SPRED1 cause a neurofibromatosis 1-like phenotype. Nat Genet 39: 1120 – 1126

[15] Brown JA, Emnett RJ, White CR, Yuede CM, Conyers SB, O'Malley KL, Wozniak DF, Gutmann DH (2010a) Reduced striatal dopamine underlies the attention system dysfunction in neurofibromatosis-1 mutant mice. Hum Mol Genet 19: 4515 – 4528

[16] Brown JA, Gianino SM, Gutmann DH (2010b) Defective cAMP generation underlies the sensitivity of CNS neurons to neurofibromatosis-1 heterozygosity. J Neurosci 30: 5579 – 5589

[17] Brown JA, Xu J, Diggs-Andrews KA, Wozniak DF, Mach RH, Gutmann DH (2011) PET imaging for attention deficit preclinical drug testing in neurofibromatosis-1 mice. Exp Neurol 232: 333 – 338

[18] Brown JA, Diggs-Andrews KA, Gianino SM, Gutmann DH (2012) Neurofibromatosis-1 heterozygosity impairs CNS neuronal morphology in a cAMP/PKA/ROCK-dependent manner. Mol Cell Neurosci 49: 13 – 22

[19] Campbell CE, Gibbs PD, Schmale MC (2001) Progression of infection and tumor development in damselfish. Mar Biotechnol 3 (Suppl 1): S107 – S104

[20] Canfield PJ (1967) A light microscopic study of bovine peripheral nerve sheath tumors. Vet Pathol 15: 283 – 291

[21] Canfield PJ, Doughty FR (1980) A study of virus-like particles present in bovine nerve sheath tumors. Aust Vet J 56: 257 – 261

[22] Chai G, Liu N, Ma J, Li H, Oblinger JL, Prahalad AK, Gong M, Chang LS, Wallace M, Muir D, Guha A, Phipps RJ, Hock JM, Yu X (2010) MicroRNA-10b regulates tumorigenesis in neurofibromatosis type 1. Cancer Sci 101: 1997 – 2004

[23] Coleman SL (1987) Neurofibromatosis and its relationship to school performance problems, learning disabilities, hyperactivity and intelligence. Master's degree thesis, Department of Psychology, University of Houston, Houston, TX

[24] Crowe FW, Schull WJ, Neel JV (1956) A clinical, pathological, and genetic study of multiple neurofibromatosis. Charles C. Thomas, Springfield, IL

[25] Cutting LE, Koth CW, Burnette CP, Abrams MT, Kaufmann WE, Denckla MB (2000a) Relationship of cognitive functioning, whole brain volumes, and T2-weighted hyperintensities in neurofibromatosis-1. J Child Neurol 15: 157 – 160

[26] Cutting LE, Koth CW, Denckla MB (2000b) How children with neurofibromatosis type 1 differ from "typical" learning disabled clinic attenders: nonverbal learning disabilities revisited. Dev Neuropsychol 17: 29 – 47

[27] Das Gupta TK, Brasfield RD (1971) Von Recklinghausen's disease. Cancer 21: 174 – 183

[28] Dasgupta B, Dugan LL, Gutmann DH (2003) The neurofibromatosis 1 gene product neurofibromin regulates pituitary adenylate cyclase-activating polypeptide-mediated signaling in astrocytes. J Neurosci 23: 8949 – 8954

[29] Daston MM, Ratner N (1992) Neurofibromin, a predominantly neuronal GTPase activating protein in the

adult, is ubiquitously expressed during development. Dev Dyn 195: 216-226

[30] Daston MM, Scrable H, Nordlund M, Sturbaum AK, Nissen LM, Ratner N (1992) The protein product of the neurofibromatosis type 1 gene is expressed at highest abundance in neurons, Schwann cells, and oligodendrocytes. Neuron 8: 415-428

[31] Dechant R, Peter M (2008) Nutrient signals driving cell growth. Curr Opin Cell Biol 20: 678-687

[32] DeClue JE, Papageorge AG, Fletcher JA, Diehl SR, Ratner N, Vass WC, Lowy DR (1992) Abnormal regulation of mammalian p21^{ras} contributes to malignant tumor growth in von Recklinghausen (type 1) neurofibromatosis. Cell 69: 265-273

[33] Descheemaeker MJ, Ghesquiere P, Symons H, Fryns JP, Legius E (2005) Behavioral, academic and neuropsychological profile of normally gifted Neurofibromatosis type 1 children. J Intell Disabil Res 49: 33-46

[34] Dombi E, Solomon J, Gillespie AJ, Fox E, Balis FM, Patronas N, Korf BR, Babovic-Vuksanovic D, Packer RJ, Belasco J, Goldman S, Jakacki R, Kieran M, Steinberg SM, Widemann BC (2007) NF1 plexiform neurofibroma growth rate by volumetric MRI: relationship to age and body weight. Neurology 68: 643-647

[35] Doughty FR (1977) Incidence of neurofibromas in cattle in abattoirs in New South Wales. Aust Vet J 53: 280-281

[36] Fieber LA, Schmale MC (1994) Differences in a K current in Schwann cells from normal and neurofibromatosis-infected damselfish. Glia 11: 64-72

[37] Galimov EM (2004) Phenomenon of life: between equilibrium and non-linearity. Orig Life Evol Biosph 34: 599-613

[38] Galimov EM (2009) Concept of sustained ordering and an ATP-related mechanism of life's origin. Int J Mol Sci 10: 2019-2030

[39] Grand RJA, Lecane PS, Roberts S, Grant ML, Lane DP, Young LS, Dawson CW, Gallimore PH (1993) Overexpression of wild-type p53 and c-Myc in human fetal cells transformed with adenovirus early region 1. Virology 193: 579-591

[40] Guo HF, Tong J, Hannan F, Luo L, Zhong Y (2000) A neurofibromatosis-1-regulated pathway is required for learning in Drosophila. Nature 403: 895-898

[41] Gutmann DH (2011) Molecular genetics of optic glioma—lessons learned from neurofibromatosis-1 genetically engineered mice. Expert Rev Ophthalmol 6: 363-369

[42] Gutmann DH, Andersen LB, Cole JL, Swaroop M, Collins FS (1993a) An alternatively-spliced mRNA in the carboxy terminus of the neurofibromatosis type 1 (NF1) gene is expressed in muscle. Hum Mol Genet 2: 989-992

[43] Gutmann DH, Tennekoon GI, Cole JL, Collins FS, Rutkowski JL (1993b) Modulation of the neurofibromatosis type 1 gene product, neurofibromin, during Schwann cell differentiation. J Neurosci Res 36: 216-223

[44] Gutmann DH, Cole JL, Collins FS (1995a) Expression of the neurofibromatosis type 1 (NF1) gene during mouse embryonic development. Prog Brain Res 150: 327-335

[45] Gutmann DH, Geist RT, Rose K, Wright DE (1995b) Expression of two new protein isoforms of the neurofibromatosis type 1 gene product, neurofibromin, in muscle tissues. Dev Dyn 202: 302-311

[46] Gutmann DH, Donahoe J, Brown T, James CD, Perry A (2000) Loss of neurofibromatosis 1 (NF1) gene expression in NF1-associated pilocytic astrocytomas. Neuropathol Appl Neurobiol 26: 361-367

[47] Hannan F, Ho I, Tong JJ, Zhu Y, Nurnberg P, Zhong Y (2006) Effect of neurofibromatosis type I mutations on a novel pathway for adenylyl cyclase activation requiring neurofibromin and Ras. Hum Mol Genet 15: 1087-1098

[48] Harkin JC, Reed RJ (1969) Tumors of the peripheral nervous system. In: Atlas of tumor pathology, Second series. Armed Forces Institute of Pathology, Washington, DC, pp 67-106

[49] Hattori S, Maekawa M, Nakamura S (1992) Identification of neurofibromatosis type I gene product as an insoluble GTPase-activating protein toward ras p21. Oncogene 7: 481-485

[50] Hegedus B, Dasgupta B, Shin JE, Emnett RJ, Hart-Mahon EK, Elghazi L, Bernal-Mizrachi E, Gutmann DH (2007) Neurofibromatosis-1 regulates neuronal and glial cell differentiation from neuroglial progenitors in vivo by both cAMP- and Ras-dependent mechanisms. Cell Stem Cell 1: 443-457

[51] Hertz L, Peng L, Dienel GA (2007) Energy metabolism in astrocytes: high rate of oxidative metabolism and spatiotemporal dependence on glycolysis/glycogenolysis. J Cereb Blood Flow Metab 27: 219-249

[52] Ho IS, Hannan F, Guo HF, Hakker I, Zhong Y (2007) Distinct functional domains of neurofibromatosis type 1 regulate immediate versus long-term memory formation. J Neurosci 27: 6852-6857

[53] Huson S, Hughes RAC (1994) The neurofibromatoses. Chapman & Hall, London

[54] Hyman SL, Gill DS, Shores EA, Steinberg A, Joy P, Gibikote SV, North KN (2003) Natural history of the cognitive deficits and their relationship to MRI T2-hyperintensities in NF1. Neurology 60: 1139-1145

[55] Hyman SL, Shores A, North KN (2005) The nature and frequency of cognitive deficits in children with neurofibromatosis type 1. Neurology 65: 1037-1044

[56] Jacks T, Shih TS, Schmitt EM, Bronson RT, Bernards A, Weinberg RA (1994) Tumour predisposition in mice heterozygous for a targeted mutation in Nf1. Nat Genet 7: 353-361

[57] Jaremko JL, Macmahon PJ, Torriani M, Merker VL, Mautner VF, Plotkin SR, Bredella MA (2012) Whole-body MRI in neurofibromatosis: incidental findings and prevalence of scoliosis. Skeletal Radiol 41: 917-923

[58] Johnson BA, Macwilliams B, Carey JC, Viskochil DH, D'Astous JL, Stevenson DA (2011) Lower extremity strength and hopping and jumping ground reaction forces in children with neurofi-bromatosis type 1. Hum Mov Sci 31: 247-254

[59] Kaplan L, Foster R, Shen Y, Parry DM, McMaster ML, O'Leary MC, Gusella JF (2010) Monozygotic twins discordant for neurofibromatosis 1. Am J Med Genet A 152A: 601-606

[60] Kim HA, DeClue JE, Ratner N (1997) cAMP-dependent protein kinase A is required for Schwann cell growth: interactions between the cAMP and neuregulin/tyrosine kinase pathways. J Neurosci Res 49: 236-247

[61] Kluwe L, Siebert R, Gesk S, Friedrich RE, Tinschert S, Kehrer-Sawatzki H, Mautner V-F (2004) Screening 500 unselected neurofibromatosis 1 patients for deletions of the Nf1 gene. Hum Mutat 23: 111-116

[62] Kossler N, Stricker S, Rodelsperger C, Robinson PN, Kim J, Dietrich C, Osswald M, Kuhnisch J, Stevenson DA, Braun T, Mundlos S, Kolanczyk M (2011) Neurofibromin (Nf1) is required for skeletal muscle development. Hum Mol Genet 20: 2697-27709

[63] Krab LC, Aarsen FK, de Goede-Bolder A, Catsman-

Berrevoets CE, Arts WF, Moll HA, Elgersma Y (2008a) Impact of neurofibromatosis type 1 on school performance. J Child Neurol 23: 1002 – 1010

[64] Krab LC, de Goede-Bolder A, Aarsen FK, Pluijm SM, Bouman MJ, van der Geest JN, Lequin M, Catsman CE, Arts WF, Kushner SA, Silva AJ, De Zeeuw CI, Moll HA, Elgersma Y (2008b) Effect of simvastatin on cognitive functioning in children with neurofibromatosis type 1: a randomized controlled trial. JAMA 300: 287 – 294

[65] Krab LC, Goorden SM, Elgersma Y (2008c) Oncogenes on my mind: ERK and MTOR signaling in cognitive diseases. Trends Genet 24: 498 – 510

[66] Krone W, Zorlein S, Mao P (1981) Cell culture studies on neurofibromatosis (von Recklinghausen). 1. Comparative growth experiments with fibroblasts at high and low concentrations of fetal calf serum. Hum Genet 58: 188 – 193

[67] Lacson JM, Riccardi VM, Morizot DC (1988) Possible genetic etiology of damselfish neurofibromatosis (DNF): generic differentiation of bicolor damselfish (*Pomacentrus partitus*) populations. Neurofibromatosis 1: 253 – 259

[68] Lacson JM, Riccardi VM, Calhoun SW, Morizot DC (1989) Hurricanes and genetic drift in populations of bicolor damselfish. Mar Biol 103: 445 – 451

[69] Le LQ, Liu C, Shipman T, Chen Z, Suter U, Parada LF (2011) Susceptible stages in Schwann cells for NF1-associated plexiform neurofibroma development. Cancer Res 71: 4686 – 4695

[70] Lebioda A, Zyromska A, Makarewicz R, Furtak J (2008) Tumour surface area as a prognostic factor in primary and recurrent glioblastoma irradiated with ^{192}Ir implantation. Rep Pract Oncol Radiother 13: 15 – 22

[71] Lewis RA, Riccardi VM, Gerson LP, Whitford R, Axelson KA (1984) Von Recklinghausen neurofibromatosis: II. Incidence of optic nerve gliomata. Ophthalmology 91: 929 – 935

[72] Li W, Cui Y, Kushner SA, Brown RA, Jentsch JD, Frankland PW, Cannon TD, Silva AJ (2005) The HMG-CoA reductase inhibitor lovastatin reverses the learning and attention deficits in a mouse model of neurofibromatosis type 1. Curr Biol 15: 1961 – 1967

[73] Li Y, Li Y, McKay RM, Riethmacher D, Parada LF (2012) Neurofibromin modulates adult hippocampal neurogenesis and behavioral effects of antidepressants. J Neurosci 32: 3529 – 3539

[74] Listernick R, Ferner RE, Piersall L, Sharif S, Gutmann DH, Charrow J (2004) Late-onset optic pathway tumors in children with neurofibromatosis 1. Neurology 63: 1944 – 1946

[75] Lyons JB, Staunton H (1992) Neurofibromatosis: why not Smith's disease? J Hist Neurosci 1: 65 – 73

[76] Ma TC, Mihm MJ, Bauer JA, Hoyt KR (2007) Bioenergetic and oxidative effects of free 3-nitrotyrosine in culture: selective vulnerability of dopaminergic neurons and increased sensitivity of non-dopaminergic neurons to dopamine oxidation. J Neurochem 103: 131 – 144

[77] MacCollin M, Mohney T, Trofatter J, Wertelecki W, Ramesh V, Gusella J (1993) DNA diagnosis of neurofibromatosis 2: altered coding sequence of the *merlin* tumor suppressor in an extended pedigree. JAMA 270: 2316 – 2320

[78] Maertens O, De Schepper S, Vandesompele J, Brems H, Heyns I, Janssens S, Speleman F, Legius E, Messiaen L (2007) Molecular dissection of isolated disease features in mosaic neurofibromatosis type 1. Am J Hum Genet 81: 243 – 251

[79] Masson P (1970) Human tumors: histology, diagnosis, technique. Wayne State University Press, Detroit

[80] Mautner VF, Hartmann M, Kluwe L, Friedrich RE, Funsterer C (2006) MRI growth patterns of plexiform neurofibromas in patients with neurofibromatosis type 1. Neuroradiology 48: 160 – 165

[81] Mautner VF, Asuagbor FA, Dombi E, Funsterer C, Kluwe L, Wenzel R, Widemann BC, Friedman JM (2008) Assessment of benign tumor burden by whole-body MRI in patients with neurofibromatosis 1. Neuro Oncol 10: 593 – 598

[82] Mautner VF, Kluwe L, Friedrich RE, Roehl AC, Bammert S, Hogel J, Spori H, Cooper DN, Kehrer-Sawatzki H (2010) Clinical characterisation of 29 neurofibromatosis type-1 patients with molecularly ascertained 1. 4 Mb type-1 NF1 deletions. J Med Genet 47: 623 – 630

[83] Messiaen LM, Collens T, Mortier G, Beysen D, Vandenbroucke I, Van Roy N, Speleman F, De Paepe A (2000) Exhaustive mutation analysis of the *Nf1* gene allows identification of 95% of mutations and reveals a high frequency of unusual splicing defects. Hum Mutat 15: 541 – 555

[84] Messiaen L et al (2009) Clinical and mutational spectrum of neurofibromatosis type 1-like syndrome. JAMA 302: 2111 – 2118

[85] Messiaen L, Vogt J, Bengesser K, Fu C, Mikhail F, Serra E, Garcia-Linares C, Cooper DN, Lazaro C, Kehrer-Sawatzki H (2010) Mosaic type-1 NF1 microdeletions as a cause of both generalized and segmental neurofibromatosis type-1 (NF1). Hum Mutat 32(2): 213 – 219

[86] Mulvihill JJ (1988) Neurofibromatosis: history, nomenclature, and natural history. Neurofibromatosis 1: 124 – 131

[87] Mulvihill JJ, Sorensen SA, Nielsen A (1983) Four decades of neurofibromatosis (NF) Recklinghausen disease in Denmark: incidence of cancers. Am J Hum Genet 35: 68A

[88] North K (1993) Neurofibromatosis type 1: review of the first 200 patients in an Australian clinic. J Child Neurol 8: 395 – 402

[89] North K, Joy P, Yuille D, Cocks N, Mobbs E, Hutchins P, McHugh K, De Silva M (1994) Specific learning disability in children with neurofibromatosis type 1: significance of MRI abnormalities. Neurology 44: 878 – 883

[90] North KN, Riccardi VM, Samango-Sprouse C, Ferner RE, Legius E, Ratner N, Moore BD III, Denckla MB (1997) Cognitive function and academic performance in neurofibromatosis 1: consensus statement from the NF1 Cognitive Disorders Task Force. Neurology 48: 1121 – 1127

[91] North K, Hyman S, Barton B (2002) Cognitive deficits in neurofibromatosis 1. J Child Neurol 17: 605 – 612

[92] Omi K, Kitano Y, Agawa H, Kadota K (1994) An immunohistochemical study of peripheral neuroblastoma, ganglioneuroblastoma, anaplastic ganglioglioma, schwannoma and neurofi-broma in cattle. J Comp Pathol 111: 1 – 14

[93] Ozonoff S (1999) Cognitive impairment in neurofibromatosis type 1. Am J Med Genet 89: 45 – 52

[94] Park CS, Zhong L, Tang SJ (2009) Aberrant expression of synaptic plasticity-related genes in the $NF1^{+/-}$ mouse hippocampus. J Neurosci Res 87: 3107 – 3119

[95] Pasmant E et al (2010) NF1 microdeletions in neurofibromatosis type 1: from genotype to phenotype. Hum Mutat 31: E1506 – E1518

[96] Payne JM, Moharir MD, Webster R, North KN (2010) Brain structure and function in neurofibromatosis type 1: current concepts and future directions. J Neurol Neurosurg Psychiatry

[97] Peltonen J, Marttala T, Vihersaari T, Renvall S, Penttinen R (1981) Collagen synthesis in cells cultured from v. Recklinghausen neurofibromatosis. Acta Neuropathol 55: 183-187

[98] Pericak-Vance MA, Yamaoka LH, Vance JM et al (1987) Genetic linkage studies on chromosome 17 RFLPs in von Recklinghausen neurofibromatosis (NF-1). Genomics 1: 349-352

[99] Ratner N, Bunge RP, Glaser L (1986) Schwann cell proliferation in vitro: an overview. Ann NY Acad Sci 486: 170-181

[100] Reynolds RM, Browning GG, Nawroz I, Campbell IW (2003) Von Recklinghausen's neurofibromatosis: neurofibromatosis type 1. Lancet 361: 1552-1554

[101] Ribeiro MJ, Violante IR, Bernardino I, Ramos F, Saraiva J, Reviriego P, Upadhyaya M, Silva ED, Castelo-Branco M (2012) Abnormal achromatic and chromatic contrast sensitivity in neurofibromatosis type 1. Invest Ophthalmol Vis Sci 53: 287-293

[102] Riccardi VM (1981a) Cutaneous manifestations of neurofibromatosis cellular interaction, pigmentation, and mast cells. Birth Defects 17: 129-145

[103] Riccardi VM (1981b) Von Recklinghausen neurofibromatosis. N Engl J Med 305: 1617-1627

[104] Riccardi VM (1984) Neurofibromatosis as a model for investigating hereditary vs. environmental factors in learning disabilities. In: Fukuyama Y (ed) The developing brain and its disorders. University of Tokyo Press, Tokyo, pp 171-181

[105] Riccardi VM (1987) Mast cell stabilization to decrease neurofibroma growth: preliminary experience with ketotifen. Arch Dermatol 123: 1011-1016

[106] Riccardi VM (1990a) Mast cell stabilization to minimize the symptoms of enlarging neurofibromas. Am J Hum Genet 47: A74

[107] Riccardi VM (1990b) The potential role of trauma and mast cells in the pathogenesis of neurofibromas. In: Ishibashi Y, Hori Y (eds) Tuberous sclerosis and neurofibromatosis: epidemiology, pathophysiology, biology and management. Elsevier, Amsterdam, pp 167-190

[108] Riccardi VM (1992) Neurofibromatosis: phenotype, natural history and pathogenesis. Johns Hopkins University Press, Baltimore

[109] Riccardi VM (1993) A controlled multiphase trial of ketotifen to minimize neurofibroma associated pain and itching. Arch Dermatol 129: 577-581

[110] Riccardi VM (2010) New approaches to von Recklinghausen disease: nonclonal origin of neurofibromas, S100 proteins and purine nucleotide balance. Jpn J Recklinghausen Dis 1: 8-10

[111] Riccardi VM, Eichner JE (1986) Neurofibromatosis: phenotype, natural history, and pathogenesis. Johns Hopkins University Press, Baltimore

[112] Riccardi VM, Maragos VA (1980) The pathophysiology of neurofibromatosis. I. Resistance in vitro to 3-nitrotyrosine as an expression of the mutation. In Vitro 16: 706-714

[113] Riccardi VM, Mulvihill JJ (1981) Advances in neurology, vol 29. Neurofibromatosis (von Recklinghausen disease): genetics, cell biology and biochemistry. Raven, New York

[114] Rodriguez FJ, Perry A, Gutmann DH, O'Neill BP, Leonard J, Bryant S, Giannini C (2008) Gliomas in neurofibromatosis type 1: a clinicopathologic study of 100 patients. J Neuropathol Exp Neurol 67: 240-249

[115] Rouleau GA, Wertelecki W, Haines JL, Hobbs WJ, Trofatter JA, Seizinger BR, Martuza RL, Superneau DW, Conneally PM, Gusella JF (1987) Genetic linkage of bilateral acoustic neurofibromatosis to a DNA marker on chromosome 22. Nature 329: 246-248

[116] Ruggieri M, Huson SM (2001) The clinical and diagnostic implications of mosaicism in the neurofibromatoses. Neurology 56: 1433-1443

[117] Russell M, Bradshaw-Rouse J, Markwardt D, Heideman W (1993) Changes in gene expression in the Ras/adenylate cyclase system of Saccharomyces cerevisiae: correlation with cAMP levels and growth arrest. Mol Biol Cell 4: 757-765

[118] Said SM, Yeh TL, Greenwood RS, Whitt JK, Tupler LA, Krishnan KR (1996) MRI morphometric analysis and neuropsychological function in patients with neurofibromatosis. Neuroreport 7: 1941-1944

[119] Sangster J, Shores EA, Watt S, North KN (2011) The cognitive profile of preschool-aged children with neurofibromatosis type 1. Child Neuropsychol 17: 1-16

[120] Sartin EA, Doran SE, Riddell MG, Herrera GA, Tennyson GS, D'Andrea G, Whitley RD, Collins FS (1994) Characterization of naturally occurring cutaneous neurofibromas in Holstein cattle: a disorder resembling neurofibromatosis type 1 in man. Am J Pathol 145: 1168-1174

[121] Saygin O (1981) Nonenzymatic photophosphorylation with visible light: a possible mode of prebiotic ATP formation. Naturwissenschaften 68: 617-619

[122] Schmale MC, Hensley GT (1988) Transmissability of a neurofibromatosis-like disease in bicolor damselfish. Cancer Res 48: 3828-3833

[123] Schmale MC, Udey LR (1983) Epizootiology of malignant tumors of the bicolor damselfish (Eupomacentrus partitus) from reefs within the Key Largo and Looe Key National Marine Sanctuaries. University of Miami, Miami

[124] Schmale MC, Hensley GT, Udey LR (1983) Multiple schwannomas in the bicolor damselfish, Pomacentrus partitus: a possible model of von Recklinghausen neurofibromatosis. Am J Pathol 112: 238-241

[125] Schmale MC, Udey LR, Hensley GT (1986) Neurofibromatosis in the bicolor damselfish (Pomacentrus partitus) as a model for von Recklinghausen neurofibromatosis. Ann NY Acad Sci 486: 386-402

[126] Schmale MC, Gibbs PD, Campbell CE (2002) A virus-like agent associated with neurofibromatosis in damselfish. Dis Aquat Organ 49: 107-115

[127] Shahar KH, Solaiyappan M, Bluemke DA (2002) Quantitative differentiation of breast lesions based on three-dimensional morphology from magnetic resonance imaging. J Comput Assist Tomogr 26: 1047-1053

[128] Shelly M, Lim BK, Cancedda L, Heilshorn SC, Gao H, Poo MM (2010) Local and long-range reciprocal regulation of cAMP and cGMP in axon/dendrite formation. Science 327: 547-552

[129] Shilyansky C, Lee YS, Silva AJ (2010) Molecular and cellular mechanisms of learning disabilities: a focus on NF1. Annu Rev Neurosci 33: 221-243

[130] Silva AJ, Frankland PW, Marowitz Z, Friedman E, Laszlo GS, Cioffi D, Jacks T, Bourtchuladze R, Lazlo G (1997) A mouse model for the learning and memory deficits associated with neurofibromatosis type 1. Nat Genet 15: 281-284

[131] Skolnick MH, Ponder BAJ, Seizinger B (1987) Linkage of NF-1 to 12 chromosome 17 markers: a summary of eight concurrent reports. Genomics 1: 382-383

[132] Smith RW (1989) A treatise on the pathology, diagnosis and treatment of neuroma. Clin Orthop 245: 3-9

[133] Smullen S, Willcox T, Wetmore R, Zackai E (1994) Otologic manifestations of neurofibromatosis. Laryngoscope 104: 663-665

[134] Solomon J, Warren K, Dombi E, Patronas N, Widemann B (2004) Automated detection and volume measurement of plexiform neurofibromas in neurofibromatosis 1 using magnetic resonance imaging. Comput Med Imaging Graph 28: 257-265

[135] Spits C, De Rycke M, Van Ranst N, Joris H, Verpoest W, Lissens W, Devroey P, Van Steirteghem A, Liebaers I, Sermon K (2005) Preimplantation genetic diagnosis for neurofibromatosis type 1. Mol Hum Reprod 11: 381-387

[136] Staser K, Yang FC, Clapp DW (2010) Mast cells and the neurofibroma microenvironment. Blood 116: 157-164

[137] Staser K, Yang FC, Clapp DW (2011) Pathogenesis of plexiform neurofibroma: tumor-stromal/hematopoietic interactions in tumor progression. Annu Rev Pathol 7: 469-495

[138] Stevenson DA, Moyer-Mileur LJ, Carey JC, Quick JL, Hoff CJ, Viskochil DH (2005) Case-control study of the muscular compartments and osseous strength in neurofibromatosis type 1 using peripheral quantitative computed tomography. J Musculoskelet Neuronal Interact 5: 145-149

[139] Stevenson DA, Zhou H, Ashrafi S, Messiaen LM, Carey JC, D'Astous JL, Santora SD, Viskochil DH (2006) Double inactivation of NF1 in tibial pseudoarthrosis. Am J Hum Genet 79: 143-148

[140] Stevenson DA, Schwarz EL, Viskochil DH, Moyer-Mileur LJ, Murray M, Firth SD, D'Astous JL, Carey JC, Pasquali M (2008) Evidence of increased bone resorption in neurofibromatosis type 1 using urinary pyridinium crosslink analysis. Pediatr Res 63: 697-701

[141] The I, Hannigan GE, Cowley GS, Reginald S, Zhong Y, Gusella JF, Hariharan IK, Bernards A (1997) Rescue of a Drosophila NF1 mutant phenotype by protein kinase A. Science 276: 791-794

[142] Tong J, Hannan F, Zhu Y, Bernards A, Zhong Y (2002) Neurofibromin regulates G protein stimulated adenylyl cyclase activity. Nat Neurosci 5: 95-96

[143] Tong JJ, Schriner SE, McCleary D, Day BJ, Wallace DC (2007) Life extension through neurofibromin mitochondrial regulation and antioxidant therapy for neurofibromatosis-1 in Drosophila melanogaster. Nat Genet 39: 476-485

[144] Tucker T, Riccardi VM, Sutcliffe M, Vielkind J, Wechsler J, Wolkenstein P, Friedman JM (2011) Mast cell densities and distributions distinguish two types of neurofibromas in patients with neurofibromatosis 1. J Histochem Cytochem 59: 584-590

[145] Upadhyaya M et al (2007) An absence of cutaneous neurofibromas associated with a 3-bp in-frame deletion in exon 17 of the Nf1 gene (c.2970-2972 delAAT): evidence of a clinically significant NF1 genotype-phenotype correlation. Am J Hum Genet 80: 140-151

[146] van Engelen SJ, Krab LC, Moll HA, de Goede-Bolder A, Pluijm SM, Catsman-Berrevoets CE, Elgersma Y, Lequin MH (2008) Quantitative differentiation between healthy and disordered brain matter in patients with neurofibromatosis type I using diffusion tensor imaging. Am J Neuroradiol 29: 816-822

[147] Van Teinen P, Rich DC, Summers KM, Ledbetter DH (1987) Regional mapping panel for chromosome 17: application to neurofibromatosis type 1. Genomics 1: 374-381

[148] Verlinsky Y, Rechitsky S, Verlinsky O, Chistokhina A, Sharapova T, Masciangelo C, Levy M, Kaplan B, Lederman J, Kuliev A (2002) Preimplantation diagnosis for neurofibromatosis. Reprod Biomed Online 4: 218-222

[149] Videtic GM, Gaspar LE, Zamorano L, Stitt LW, Fontanesi J, Levin KJ (2001) Implant volume as a prognostic variable in brachytherapy decision-making for malignant gliomas stratified by the RTOG recursive partitioning analysis. Int J Radiat Oncol Biol Phys 51: 963-968

[150] Virchow R (1857) Uber eniem Fall von vielfachen Neuromen (Faser-Kern-geschwultsen) mit ausgezeichneter localer Recidivfahikeit. Virchows Arch [A] 12: 144

[151] Viskochil D (2003) It takes two to tango: mast cell and Schwann cell interactions in neurofibromas. J Clin Invest 112: 1791-1793

[152] Viskochil D, Buchberg AM, Xu G, Cawthon RM, Stevens J, Wolff RK, Culver M, Carey JC, Copeland NG, Jenkins NA, White R, O'Connell P (1990) Deletions and a translocation interrupt a cloned gene at the neurofibromatosis type 1 locus. Cell 62: 187-192

[153] Vogt J, Kohlhase J, Morlot S, Kluwe L, Mautner VF, Cooper DN, Kehrer-Sawatzki H (2011a) Monozygotic twins discordant for neurofibromatosis type 1 due to a postzygotic NF1 gene mutation. Hum Mutat 32: E2134-E2147

[154] Vogt J, Nguyen R, Kluwe L, Roehl AC, Mussotter T, Cooper DN, Mautner VF, Kehrer-Sawatzki H, Schuhmann M (2011b) Delineation of the clinical phenotype associated with non-mosaic type-2 NF1 deletions: two case reports. J Med Case Rep 5: 577

[155] Von Recklinghausen F (1882) Über die multiplen Fibrome der Haut und ihre Beziehung zu multiplen Neuromen. August Hirschwald, Berlin

[156] Wallace DC, Fan W (2010) Energetics, epigenetics, mitochondrial genetics. Mitochondrion 10: 12-31

[157] Wallace MR, Marchuk DA, Andersen LB, Letcher R, Odeh HM, Saulino AM, Fountain JW, Bereton A, Nicholson J, Mitchell AL, Brownstein BH, Collins FS (1990) Type 1 neurofibromatosis gene: identification of a large transcript disrupted in three NF-1 patients. Science 249: 181-186

[158] Xu Y, Chiamvimonvat N, Vazquez AE, Akunuru S, Ratner N, Yamoah EN (2002) Gene-targeted deletion of neurofibromin enhances the expression of a transient outward K^+ current in Schwann cells: a protein kinase A-mediated mechanism. J Neurosci 22: 9194-9202

[159] Zickler AM, Hampp S, Messiaen L, Bengesser K, Mussotter T, Roehl AC, Wimmer K, Mautner VF, Kluwe L, Upadhyaya M, Pasmant E, Chuzhanova N, Kestler HA, Hogel J, Legius E, Claes K, Cooper DN, Kehrer-Sawatzki H (2011) Characterization of the nonallelic homologous recombination hotspot PRS3 associated with type-3 NF1 deletions. Hum Mutat 33(2): 372-383

第 2 章　1 型神经纤维瘤病的临床诊断和非典型表现
Clinical Diagnosis and Atypical Forms of NF1

Sirkku Peltonen and Minna Pöyhönen

2.1　1 型神经纤维瘤病的临床诊断

NF1(MIM 162200)的临床诊断基于 1987 年 NIH 共识发展会议中概述的诊断标准(表 2.1)(Stumpf et al. 1988)。几乎所有(95%)NF1 患者在 8 岁时都可以使用这些标准进行诊断(DeBella et al. 2000)。

NF1 的诊断根据不同年龄组中略有不同的表现决定。幼儿的诊断通常具有挑战性，因为大约半数散发性 NF1 病例在 1 岁时尚未达到 NIH 的诊断标准(DeBella et al. 2000)。在罕见的情况下，如镶嵌型 NF1(第 12 章)或 Legius 综合征(第 31 章)，仅根据 NIH 的诊断标准可能导致 NF1 误诊。因此，明确诊断需要结合分子诊断。针对怀疑有 NF1 但尚不符合临床诊断标准的情况时，对 *NF1* 基因的突变分析可能有助于明确诊断。

两项诊断标准：6 个或更多的咖啡牛奶斑和腋窝/腹股沟区雀斑，在皮肤上很容易观察到。然而，在常规临床检查中，皮肤褶皱处的检查往往容易被忽视。皮肤型神经纤维瘤可能与其他良性皮肤肿瘤

表 2.1　NF1 的 NIH 诊断标准。需要满足以下两项或更多项才能进行诊断

(1) 青春期前个体有 6 个或 6 个以上最大直径>5 mm 的咖啡牛奶斑，青春期后个体至少有直径>15 mm 的咖啡牛奶斑
(2) 2 个或 2 个以上任何类型的神经纤维瘤，或者 1 个丛状神经纤维瘤
(3) 腋窝或腹股沟区雀斑
(4) 视神经胶质瘤
(5) 2 个或 2 个以上虹膜 Lisch 结节
(6) 特征性骨病变，如蝶骨畸形或长骨皮质变薄，伴或不伴假性关节病
(7) 符合上述标准的诊断为 NF1 的一级亲属

(特别是当表面覆盖咖啡牛奶斑时)相混淆，如皮内痣。因此，诊断为皮肤型神经纤维瘤可能需要对其中 1 个或 2 个结节进行组织学检查。当出现面部、四肢或躯干的轮廓不对称时，通过临床检查可以发现丛状神经纤维瘤。尤其是面部肿物，在出生

后的几年里会越发明显。Lisch结节的识别需要使用特定显微镜检查(如裂隙灯),并建议将具有这一问题的患者转诊给眼科医师。根据胫骨向前外侧弯曲可以推测儿童是否具有假性关节的疾病。因此,大多数诊断表现都可以通过仔细的临床检查找到。由于NF1不同表现的发展遵循不同的时间表,在不同年龄组考虑不同的NF1诊断表现是切实可行的。

2.1.1　5～6岁以下儿童的NF1诊断

2.1.1.1　咖啡牛奶斑

咖啡牛奶斑(简称"咖啡斑")是NF1最常见的临床表现之一,95%的患者到1岁时都会出现(DeBella et al. 2000)。有的咖啡斑在出生时就可出现,但主要在出生后几个月开始出现,并在3岁时明显。早期出现咖啡斑这个临床特征对于鉴别诊断非常重要(表2.2)。咖啡斑略深于人的正常肤色,并且颜色均一。由于它们是色斑,意味着它们仅在颜色方面与周围皮肤有所不同,无法通过触摸感觉到不同。NF1中典型的咖啡斑直径超过5 mm,呈椭圆形,具有清晰、平滑的边界(图2.1)。咖啡斑的轮廓也可能不规则。然而,孤立的咖啡斑,即通常所说的"胎记",在一般人群中的发生率为10%～15%。

表2.2　咖啡牛奶斑的鉴别诊断

诊　断	临　床　特　征
色素痣	从浅褐色到深褐色不等。其他特征:可能有不同颜色的区域和多毛表现。先天性痣最初可能是平滑的,但几年后可能会突出于皮肤表面
老年斑	主要出现在阳光照射的部位,在儿童中很少见
贝克痣	浅褐色。位置通常在青春期出现在上胸部或肩部区域。常见多毛现象
斑痣	色素沉着的色斑,可能有清晰或不清晰的轮廓,在斑块内可能有黑色小痣
炎症后色素沉着	可能是由各种炎症性皮肤疾病(如特应性皮炎或水痘)引起的。边界不如咖啡牛奶斑明显
花斑糠疹(汗斑)	皮肤表面的真菌(马拉色菌)感染。浅褐色斑点局限于躯干,如果擦伤可能会出现轻微的脱屑
荨麻疹性色素斑	浅褐色斑点,边界有时非常清晰。除斑点外,还可见淡粉色丘疹和丘疹斑。组织学检查可以看到斑点内存在肥大细胞

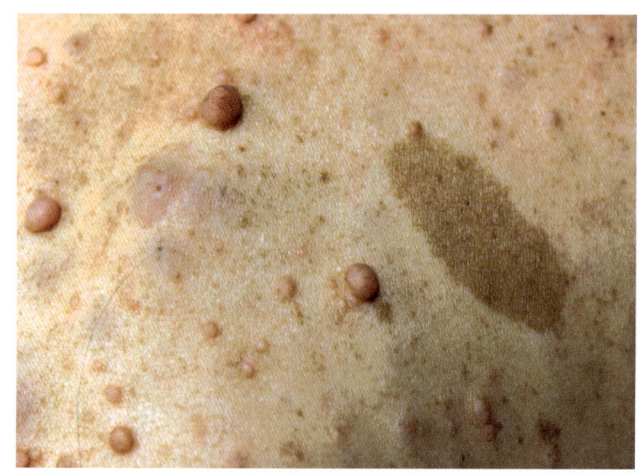

图2.1　咖啡牛奶斑和皮肤型神经纤维瘤。典型的咖啡斑色素均匀,轮廓清晰。皮肤型神经纤维瘤可隆起,也可呈紫红色斑点(photo, Eeva-Mari Jouhilahti)

咖啡斑是任何了解它们作为诊断意义的专业医疗人士都容易察觉的表现。由于约一半的NF1病例是散发性的,诊断可能会延迟。当儿童身上出现4～6个咖啡斑时应引起对NF1诊断的怀疑,但如果父母中没有人患有NF1,初级保健医生往往会忽视这些咖啡斑作为综合征的迹象。咖啡斑的鉴别诊断并不简单,因为其他病变也可能会存在这些斑点(Shah 2010)。如果怀疑为NF1,需要仔细检查父母是否有咖啡斑、腋窝或腹股沟雀斑,以及皮肤型神经纤维瘤等,因为即使在成年人身上,轻度的NF1表现可能也会被忽视。因此,仅仅通过父母有没有NF1,并不能排除其子女是否可能患有遗传性NF1。咖啡斑的鉴别诊断见表2.2。

2.1.1.2　神经纤维瘤

25%～30%的NF1患者具有可被发现或有症状的丛状神经纤维瘤,但全身MRI可显示更多的该类型肿瘤:在65名参与研究的儿童NF1患者中,超过 50% 的患者存在 1 个或多个丛状神经纤维瘤（Nguyen et al. 2011；第 7 章）。该肿瘤在下肢最常见，其次是胸部、脊旁和盆腔（Nguyen et al. 2011）。面部丛状神经纤维瘤通常在出生后的最初几年表现出症状（Ferner et al. 2007）。头颈部肿瘤可能在新生儿身上很容易看到，但也可能最初只导致面颊或唇部轻微不对称。在临床检查中，可以通过注意身体的不对称性来判断是否存在丛状神经纤维瘤，但不要忘记观察手掌和脚掌（图 2.2）。从脊神经根经过腹壁生长的丛状神经纤维瘤可能会表现为腰部线条的不对称，当存在肢体病变时，患侧则会出现更为饱满的外观。丛状神经纤维瘤上覆盖的皮肤有时看起来略呈紫红色，易误诊为血管畸形，覆盖的皮肤有时也可能存在多毛和（或）色素沉着现象，或在瘤体周围形成一圈色素减退的晕。丛状神经纤维瘤在儿童时期已经具有恶性转化的风险（Evans et al. 2002；第 28 和 29 章）。瘤体的大小和分布最好通过 MRI 检查去判断，但全身 MRI 并不是常规的诊断流程。

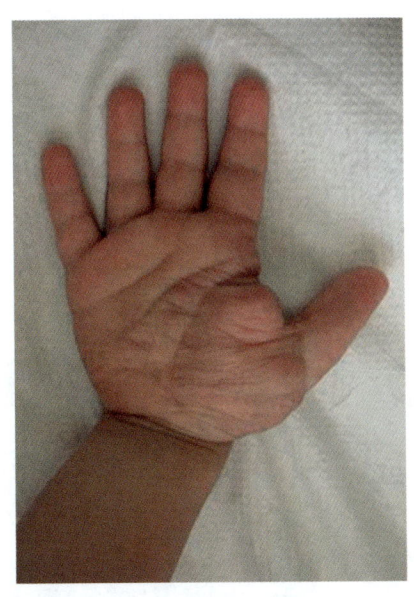

图 2.2 儿童手掌上的丛状神经纤维瘤

2.1.1.3 假性关节病

长骨发育不良在 NF1 患者中占 3%～5%（Friedman and Birch 1997，Stevenson et al. 1999；第 21 章）。而假性关节病在胫骨中最常见，在孩子学会站立和行走后症状变得明显。胫骨或胫腓骨可能向前外弯曲，进而可能导致骨折。假性关节病在罕见情况下可能发生在其他长骨，如尺骨或桡骨。骨折后的假关节进行手术治疗具有挑战性，目前尚无足够的大型研究来确定治疗方法（Elefteriou et al. 2009）。由于至少一半的儿科假关节患者有 NF1，因此应检查所有儿科假性关节病患者的皮肤是否同时存在咖啡牛奶斑。

2.1.1.4 视神经胶质瘤

对于视神经胶质瘤的儿童，超过一半患有 NF1（Nicolin et al. 2009）。在 NF1 患者中，视神经胶质瘤在组织学上表现为 I 级毛细胞星形胶质细胞瘤（Listernick et al. 2007），约占 NF1 患儿的 15%（Listernick et al. 1994）。大多数视神经胶质瘤在出生后的最初几年出现，但在青春期或成年期也可能出现。发生有症状的视神经胶质瘤的风险，在 7 岁以下的儿童中最大，平均诊断年龄为 5 岁（Nicolin et al. 2009）。视神经胶质瘤引起的最常见症状包括视力下降、眼球突出以及伴有头痛和呕吐，通常需要进行 MRI 检查。视神经胶质瘤还可能通过影响垂体分泌而引起性早熟。然而，与 NF1 相关的视神经胶质瘤大多数情况没有症状，其自然病史比非 NF1 患者更为缓慢。视神经胶质瘤儿童可以在麻醉后进行 MRI 检查。对于无症状的儿童，虽然不建议常规进行 MRI 检查，但也需要进行视力评估。然而，如果进行 MRI 检查，T2 加权成像通常会显示高信号病变，有时会误认为脑错构瘤。这一发现可以帮助 NF1 的诊断，但不建议仅为此进行麻醉下的 MRI 检查。

2.1.1.5 儿童 NF1 的其他特征

表 2.3 列出了儿童 NF1 可能出现的其他临床特征，需要进行仔细评估。

表 2.3 需要关注的儿童 NF1 的其他临床特征

症 状	临 床 表 现
身材矮小和巨颅[a]	13% 的患者身材矮小（身高低于人群平均值 2 个标准差以上），24% 的患儿存在巨颅（枕额径大于人群平均值 2 个标准差以上）
认知缺陷和学习困难[b]	NF1 儿童中最常见的并发症（超过 50%）。所有 NF1 患儿都应进行评估
营养不良型脊柱侧弯	约 5% 的儿童在数月内脊柱某一段出现角度急剧的侧凸。潜在的影响较大，需要进行手术干预

续　表

症　状	临床表现
运动和语言发育迟缓[c]	应该对所有 NF1 的儿童进行评估
性早熟	8 岁以下出现青春期迹象。可能是视神经胶质瘤所致的表现
皮肤颜色	全身轻度色素沉着
幼年型黄色肉芽肿	黄红色结节，好发于头部和颈部。通常在出生后的前 6 个月出现。据报道患幼年型粒-单核细胞白血病的风险增加[d]
先天性青光眼	单侧眼球巨大是新生儿时期的罕见并发症
癫痫	NF1 患者中癫痫发作和婴儿痉挛很少见
肾动脉狭窄	高血压
肺动脉狭窄和高血压	具有不明原因的心脏杂音和畸形特征的儿童应接受心脏评估

注：[a] Szudek et al.（2000）。[b] Hyman et al.（2006）。[c] Alivuotila et al.（2010）。[d] Raygada et al.（2010）。

2.1.1.6　突变分析

如果父母没有 NF1，并且咖啡牛奶斑是幼儿唯一的表现，那么在出现其他临床表现之前无法做出 NF1 诊断。这可能需要观察长达 5 年的时间，在此期间需要进行随访和眼科评估。这种不确定性也会给家庭带来压力。通过对患者的血样进行 NF1 基因的突变分析，可以更早明确诊断。当前的突变检测方案可以在 90% 以上的 NF1 患者中识别出致病突变（第 10 章）。突变阴性的患者几乎可以排除 NF1，并解除对专科随访的需求。考虑到后续医疗费用，NF1 突变分析被认为是具有成本效益的（Tsang et al. 2012）。此外，排除 NF1 对于提高生命质量也具有重要意义。

2.1.2　5～6 岁以上儿童的 NF1 诊断

2.1.2.1　腋窝和腹股沟的雀斑

典型的 NF1 特征，如腋窝/腹股沟区雀斑，大多在 3～5 岁时开始出现，到 7 岁时约 80% 的 NF1 患者可观察到。因此，雀斑在 5～6 岁以上的儿童中是一个有效的诊断标志。在多个皮肤区域如颈部和躯干出现更广泛的雀斑也是 NF1 患者常见的情况。

腋窝和腹股沟区域的雀斑与咖啡斑的颜色相同，但面积更小（图 2.3），在一般人群中不会出现。通常在一般医学检查中容易忽视这种皮肤褶皱处，但对于 NF1 的诊断，该部位需要仔细检查。

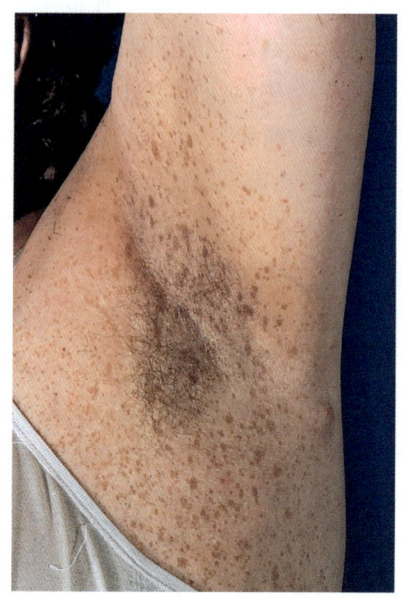

图 2.3　成年 NF1 患者的腋窝雀斑

2.1.2.2　Lisch 结节

Lisch 结节（图 2.4）是虹膜的无症状病变，通常在 5～6 岁时出现。超过 90% 的成年 NF1 患者有 Lisch 结节。如果没有透镜显微镜检查（裂隙灯），就无法有效地诊断它们，因此该临床表现通常由眼科医师来诊断。

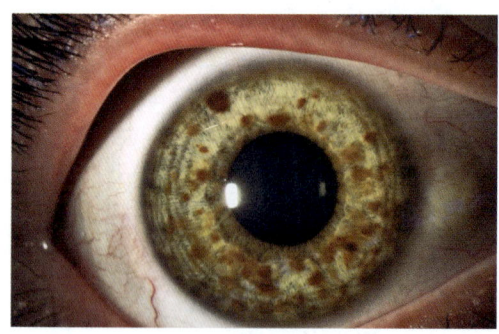

图 2.4　虹膜上 Lisch 结节的诊断需要眼科医师的检查（photo, Vesa Aaltonen）

2.1.3　青春期和成人的 NF1 诊断

2.1.3.1　神经纤维瘤

2 个或 2 个以上的神经纤维瘤是 NF1 的诊断标

志,但应该认识到单发的神经纤维瘤可以是健康成年人的常见表现。神经纤维瘤作为一种良性肿瘤,包含正常周围神经的组成结构(Peltonen et al. 1988;第26章)。皮肤型神经纤维瘤在青春期开始生长,一般首先在腹部和背部以稍微隆起的软结节形式出现。当它们进一步生长时,会变得更加明显并凸出于皮肤表面之上(图2.1)。它们也可呈紫红色斑块,会被误认为是淤血。这种表现下的神经纤维瘤往往不会隆起,当触摸时感觉比周围的皮肤更软(按钮样征)。如果对NF1的诊断不明确,可以对皮肤型神经纤维瘤进行组织学检查。除非这些肿瘤对患者造成困扰,否则通常不需要进行手术治疗,因为这些肿瘤不会发生恶性转化。成年NF1患者的皮肤型神经纤维瘤的数量从几个到数千个不等。当数目众多时,瘤体会导致美学问题和社交障碍,给成年患者带来重要的疾病负担。而NF1基因微缺失的患者往往有较重的肿瘤负担(见下文)。

皮下型神经纤维瘤也在青春期开始生长。它们表现为可在皮肤下移动的硬结,对触碰敏感。触摸时,瘤体也可能引起受牵连神经的疼痛或刺痛感。在对皮下神经纤维瘤进行手术切除之前,需要专家进行仔细的问诊和考虑,因为没有细致分析的手术可能会损伤穿过肿瘤的神经。

2.1.4　NF1的鉴别诊断

咖啡斑除了与NF1相关外,还与其他几种综合征有关。表2.4列出了以咖啡斑为特征的各种综合征。

表2.4　咖啡斑相关综合征

综合征	症状
Legius综合征(MIM 611431)	咖啡斑类似于NF1,有腋窝雀斑,但没有肿瘤[a]
NF2(MIM 101000)	40%的患者有与NF1相似的咖啡斑表现,但通常数量更少
McCune-Albright综合征(MIM 174800)	面积较大的咖啡斑,边界呈锯齿状。可能沿Blaschko发育线和沿中线分布。此外,还可伴有骨纤维发育不良、性早熟和其他内分泌功能紊乱等表现[b]

续表

综合征	症状
LEOPARD综合征(MIM 151100)	咖啡斑,雀斑,肺动脉狭窄,眼距增宽,听力损失[c]
错配修复癌症综合征(MIM 276300)	咖啡斑,儿童癌症,血液系统恶性肿瘤,脑肿瘤,早发性结肠癌[d]
神经皮肤黑变病(MIM 249400)	新生儿期出现,发生在躯干和颈部双侧、大面积多毛痣,伴有卫星痣[e]
Peutz-Jeghers综合征(MIM 175200)	发生在口周、结膜和生殖器黏膜的色斑。可出现消化道息肉,消化道、胰腺、乳房、卵巢和子宫的肿瘤
卡尼综合征(MIM 160980)	色斑、原发性色素性结节状肾上腺皮质疾病、心脏、乳房和皮肤黏液瘤、神经鞘瘤和睾丸肿瘤

注:[a] Brems et al. (2007)。[b] Dumitrescu and Collins (2008)。[c] Digilio et al. (2002)。[d] 第16章。[e] Lodish and Stratakis (2011)。

神经纤维瘤的最重要的鉴别诊断包括黑色素细胞痣、脂肪瘤和神经鞘瘤。在对只有少量皮肤肿物的患者进行NF1诊断时,有必要对至少1~2个神经纤维瘤瘤体进行组织学诊断。皮下神经纤维瘤在临床上的表现类似于脂肪瘤,而脂肪瘤在人群中比神经纤维瘤更常见。表2.5列出了可能与神经纤维瘤诊断相混淆的肿瘤相关综合征。

2.2　非典型的NF1

NF1的表型-基因型相关性是基于一代或两代以上家庭成员之间不寻常的表型或临床结果,去探究其相似性。然而,只有少数突变类型与典型的临床特征组合相关联(见第43章)。

2.2.1　微缺失

NF1基因微缺失是大片段缺失,涵盖整个NF1基因和多个相邻基因。已知存在3种不同类型的NF1微缺失(见第14章),总共约占NF1基因突变的10%。大多数微缺失源于母亲,该突变比其他类型的NF1突变更易引起严重的表型。NF1微缺失患者表现为颅颌面畸形,面部粗糙,手脚增大。有时,这些畸形特征被描述为类似于努南综合征(见第32章)。

表 2.5 多发性肿瘤综合征

肿瘤类型	综 合 征	临 床 表 现
神经瘤	NF2(MIM 101000)	施万细胞瘤：皮肤、真皮下、表皮下和双侧前庭神经。也可出现神经纤维瘤、脑室管膜瘤和脑膜瘤
	神经鞘瘤病(MIM 162091)	多发性皮肤、脊柱和周围神经中的多发性神经鞘瘤
脂肪瘤	多发性脂肪瘤(MIM 151900)	躯干和四肢中的多个包膜下脂肪瘤
	PTEN 错构瘤综合征（PTEN hamartoma tumor syndromes，PHTS）[a]［Cowden 综合征(MIM 158350)］	巨颅畸形、多发性脂肪瘤、面部毛囊外层瘤、末梢角化症、乳头状丘疹，并增加发生乳腺、甲状腺和子宫内膜恶变的风险
	Bannayan‐Riley‐Ruvalcaba 综合征(MIM 153480)	男性阴茎头脂肪瘤、血管瘤和色素斑，小头畸形，发育迟缓
脂肪瘤和(或)其他结节性皮肤或黏膜病变	MEN1(MIM 131100)	咖啡斑(1～3个)、面部血管纤维瘤、胶原瘤、脂肪瘤、各种内分泌肿瘤(甲状旁腺增生、胰腺和垂体腺瘤)[b]
	MEN2A(MIM 171400)	咖啡斑(1～3个)、皮肤苔藓淀粉样变性、甲状腺髓样癌(伴或不伴嗜铬细胞瘤)、甲状旁腺功能亢进
	MEN2B(MIM 162300)	黏膜和肠道神经瘤、马凡体征、侵袭性甲状腺髓样癌、嗜铬细胞瘤
	FAP+结肠外特征（Gardner 综合征）(MIM 175100)	皮肤囊肿结节[c]、脂肪瘤、纤维瘤、硬纤维瘤、骨瘤、FAP
过度生长综合征	Proteus 综合征(MIM 176920)	四肢不对称过度生长。线状疣状表皮痣，在足底通常有结缔组织痣，数枚小咖啡斑[d]
	Klippel‐Trénaunay‐Weber 综合征(MIM 149000)	皮肤毛细血管畸形(葡萄酒色斑)、静脉曲张或静脉畸形，以及四肢的骨或软组织增生
	先天性泛发性纤维瘤病(MIM 228550)	各种组织中的多发性纤维母细胞瘤

注：[a] Blumenthal and Dennis (2008)。[b] Almeida and Stratakis (2010)。[c] Juhn and Khachemoune (2010)。[d] Nowak (2007)。

NF1 微缺失患者身材较高，通常肿瘤负担较重，并且与其他 NF1 患者相比，罹患 MPNST 的风险增加。认知缺陷包括学习障碍及智力低下等在微缺失患者中更为常见，他们的平均智商略低于其他类型的 NF1 患者群体(Descheemaeker et al. 2004)。

2.2.2 脊柱神经纤维瘤

家族性脊柱神经纤维瘤或遗传性脊柱神经纤维瘤病(familial spinal neurofibromatosis, FSNF, MIM 162210)是 NF1 的一种罕见形式(Messiaen et al. 2003)。所有受影响的成年家庭成员都具有多发性对称分布的脊柱神经根神经纤维瘤和咖啡斑，但没有其他 NF1 的诊断征象。据报道，只有 12 个两代或三代家系中出现了脊柱神经纤维瘤并确定同时存在 NF1 突变。报道中的 NF1 突变为剪接或错义突变，但没有明确的基因型-表型相关性(见第 10 章)。然而值得注意的是，在 NF1 患者中，孤立的、无症状的脊柱肿瘤是常见的发现，但只有少数患者会出现症状(见第 7 章)。

2.2.3 外显子 17 中的 3 个碱基缺失

一些家族患有非常轻微的 NF1，只有咖啡斑、皮肤褶皱处雀斑和 Lisch 结节，在多代人中均并没有神经纤维瘤表现（Upadhyaya et al. 2007；第10章）。在这些家族中，已发现存在外显子17中的3个碱基AAT缺失。在该患者群体中，NF1症状非常轻微，以至于许多这样的家庭可能仍未被诊断出该疾病。另外，外显子17中的3个碱基缺失并不能在所有具有这种表型的家族中被发现。

2.2.4 镶嵌型NF1

镶嵌型NF1被认为是在胚胎发育期间由体细胞突变引起的。镶嵌型NF1患者不会在所有皮肤区域出现色素病变和神经纤维瘤，尽管他们可能符合NF1的诊断标准。节段型神经纤维瘤病指的就是镶嵌型NF1，其中神经纤维瘤和（或）色素变化仅在单侧的局部区域中发现（图2.5）。根据临床症状，尚不能预测 *NF1* 基因突变是否存在于生殖细胞中，并且已经证明具有节段型NF1的患者可能将突变传递给下一代（Poyhonen 2000；第12章）。这种可能性需要在遗传咨询中考虑。镶嵌型NF1的患病率估计为1/40 000～1/36 000（Ruggieri and Huson 2001），但该数据可能被低估。

2.2.5 Watson综合征

Watson综合征（MIM 193520）是一种极为罕见的常染色体显性遗传综合征，其特征包括咖啡斑、肺动脉狭窄和学习困难。它只在少数几个家庭中被报告过，并且在其中大多数家庭中发现了 *NF1* 突变。

总体而言，本章回顾了NF1在不同年龄段的诊断，因为该疾病的诊断表征在不同的时间上表现的显著程度会不同。尽管NF1在童年时期首次表现出的征象是咖啡斑、丛状神经纤维瘤、视神经胶质瘤、屈曲褶皱区域的雀斑和Lisch结节，但皮肤型神经纤维瘤通常只在青春期开始生长。本章介绍了咖啡斑和具有皮肤肿瘤的综合征的主要鉴别诊断，还讨论了对基因突变的分析在NF1诊断中的作用。

致谢：作者感谢Juha Peltonen教授对手稿的宝贵评论。

（王 薇 译）

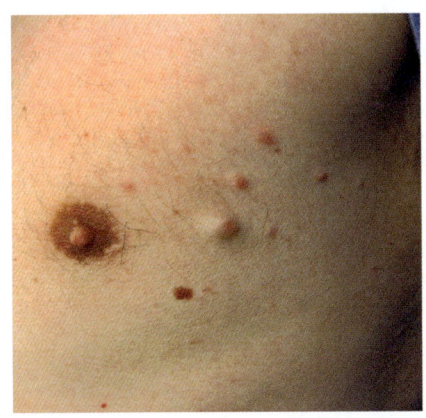

图2.5　1名节段型神经纤维瘤病患者胸部的一组神经纤维瘤

参考文献

[1] Alivuotila L, Hakokari J, Visnapuu V, Korpijaakko-Huuhka AM, Aaltonen O, Happonen RP, Peltonen S, Peltonen J (2010) Speech characteristics in neurofibromatosis type 1. Am J Med Genet A 152A：42－51

[2] Almeida MQ, Stratakis CA (2010) Solid tumors associated with multiple endocrine neoplasias. Cancer Genet Cytogenet 203：30－36

[3] Blumenthal GM, Dennis PA (2008) PTEN hamartoma tumor syndromes. Eur J Hum Genet 16：1289－1300

[4] Brems H, Chmara M, Sahbatou M, Denayer E, Taniguchi K, Kato R, Somers R, Messiaen L, De Schepper S, Fryns JP, Cools J, Marynen P, Thomas G, Yoshimura A, Legius E (2007) Germline loss-of-function mutations in *SPRED1* cause a neurofibromatosis 1-like phenotype. Nat Genet 39：1120－1126

[5] De Raedt T, Brems H, Wolkenstein P, Vidaud D, Pilotti S, Perrone F, Mautner V, Frahm S, Sciot R, Legius E (2003) Elevated risk for MPNST in NF1 microdeletion patients. Am J Hum Genet 72：1288－1292

[6] DeBella K, Szudek J, Friedman JM (2000) Use of the national institutes of health criteria for diagnosis of neurofibromatosis 1 in children. Pediatrics 105：608－614

[7] Descheemaeker MJ, Roelandts K, De Raedt T, Brems H, Fryns JP, Legius E (2004) Intelligence in individuals with a neurofibromatosis type 1 microdeletion. Am J Med Genet A 131：325－326

[8] Digilio MC, Conti E, Sarkozy A, Mingarelli R, Dottorini T, Marino B, Pizzuti A, Dallapiccola B (2002) Grouping of multiple lentigines/LEOPARD and Noonan syndrome on the PTPN11 gene. Am J Hum Genet 71：389－394

[9] Dumitrescu CE, Collins MT (2008) McCune-Albright syndrome. Orphanet J Rare Dis 3：12

[10] Elefteriou F, Kolanczyk M, Schindeler A et al (2009) Skeletal abnormalities in neurofibromatosis type 1：approaches to

therapeutic options. Am J Med Genet A 149A(10): 2327-2338

[11] Evans DG, Baser ME, McGaughran J, Sharif S, Howard E, Moran A (2002) Malignant peripheral nerve sheath tumours in neurofibromatosis 1. J Med Genet 39: 311-314

[12] Ferner RE, Huson SM, Thomas N, Moss C, Willshaw H, Evans GH, Upadhyaya M, Towers R, Gleeson M, Steiger C, Kirby A (2007) Guidelines for the diagnosis and management of individuals with neurofibromatosis 1. J Med Genet 44: 81-88

[13] Friedman JM, Birch PH (1997) Type 1 neurofibromatosis: a descriptive analysis of the disorder in 1,728 patients. Am J Med Genet 70: 138-143

[14] Hyman SL, Arthur Shores E, North KN (2006) Learning disabilities in children with neurofibromatosis type 1: subtypes, cognitive profile, and attention-deficit-hyperactivity disorder. Dev Med Child Neurol 48: 973-977

[15] Juhn E, Khachemoune A (2010) Gardner syndrome: skin manifestations, differential diagnosis and management. Am J Clin Dermatol 11: 117-122

[16] Listernick R, Charrow J, Greenwald M, Mets M (1994) Natural history of optic pathway tumors in children with neurofibromatosis type 1: a longitudinal study. J Pediatr 125: 63-66

[17] Listernick R, Ferner RE, Liu GT, Gutmann DH (2007) Optic pathway gliomas in neurofibromatosis-1: controversies and recommendations. Ann Neurol 61: 189-198

[18] Lodish MB, Stratakis CA (2011) The differential diagnosis of familial lentiginosis syndromes. Fam Cancer 10: 481-490

[19] Messiaen L, Riccardi V, Peltonen J, Maertens O, Callens T, Karvonen SL, Leisti E-L, Koivunen J, Vanderbroucke I, Stephens K, Pöyhönen M (2003) Independent *NF1* mutations in two large families with spinal neurofibromatosis. J Med Genet 40: 122-126

[20] Messiaen L, Vogt J, Bengesser K, Fu C, Mikhail F, Serra E, Garcia-Linares C, Cooper DN, Lazaro C, Kehrer-Sawatzki H (2011) Mosaic type-1 *NF1* microdeletions as a cause of both generalized and segmental neurofibromatosis type-1 (NF1). Hum Mutat 32: 213-219

[21] Nguyen R, Kluwe L, Fuensterer C, Kentsch M, Friedrich RE, Mautner VF (2011) Plexiform neurofibromas in children with neurofibromatosis type 1: frequency and associated clinical deficits. J Pediatr 159: 652-655

[22] Nicolin G, Parkin P, Mabbott D, Hargrave D, Bartels U, Tabori U, Rutka J, Buncic JR, Bouffet E (2009) Natural history and outcome of optic pathway gliomas in children. Pediatr Blood Cancer 53: 1231-1237

[23] Nowak CB (2007) The phakomatoses: dermatologic clues to neurologic anomalies. Semin Pediatr Neurol 14: 140-149

[24] Pasmant E, Sabbagh A, Spurlock G et al (2010) NF1 microdeletions in neurofibromatosis type 1: from genotype to phenotype. Hum Mutat 31: E1506-E1518

[25] Peltonen J, Jaakkola S, Lebwohl M, Renvall S, Risteli L, Virtanen I, Uitto J (1988) Cellular differentiation and expression of matrix genes in type 1 neurofibromatosis. Lab Invest 59: 760-771

[26] Poyhonen M (2000) A clinical assessment of neurofibromatoses in Northern Finland. J Med Genet 37: e43

[27] Raygada M, Arthur DC, Wayne AS, Rennert OM, Toretsky JA, Stratakis CA (2010) Juvenile xanthogranuloma in a child with previously unsuspected neurofibromatosis type 1 and juvenile myelomonocytic leukemia. Pediatr Blood Cancer 54: 173-175

[28] Ruggieri M, Huson SM (2001) The clinical and diagnostic implications of mosaicism in the neurofibromatoses. Neurology 56: 1433-1443

[29] Shah KN (2010) The diagnostic and clinical significance of café-au-lait macules. Pediatr Clin North Am 57: 1131-1153

[30] Stevenson DA, Birch PH, Friedman JM et al (1999) Descriptive analysis of tibial pseudoarthrosis in patients with neurofibromatosis 1. Am J Med Genet 84: 413-419

[31] Stumpf DA, Alksne JF, Anneggers JF et al (1988) Neurofibromatosis. Conference statement. National Institutes of Health Consensus Development Conference. Arch Neurol 45: 575-578

[32] Szudek J, Birch P, Friedman JM et al (2000) Growth in North American white children with neurofibromatosis 1 (NF1). J Med Genet 37: 933-938

[33] Tsang E, Birch P, Friedman JM (2012) Valuing gene testing in children with possible neurofibromatosis 1. Clin Genet 82: 591-593

[34] Upadhyaya M, Huson SM, Davies M, Thomas N, Chuzhanova N, Giovannini S, Evans DG, Howard E, Kerr B, Griffiths S, Consoli C, Side L, Adams D, Pierpont M, Hachen R, Barnicoat A, Li H, Wallace P, Van Biervliet JP, Stevenson D, Viskochil D, Baralle D, Haan E, Riccardi V, Turnpenny P, Lazaro C, Messiaen L (2007) An absence of cutaneous neurofibromas associated with a 3-bp inframe deletion in exon 17 of the *NF1* gene (c. 2970-2972 delAAT): evidence of a clinically significant NF1 genotype-phenotype correlation. Am J Hum Genet 80: 140-151

第3章 "复杂1型神经纤维瘤病"的管理与治疗

Management and Treatment of "Complex Neurofibromatosis 1"

Rosalie E. Ferner and Susan M. Huson

3.1 引言

在英格兰大约有 17 000 名患者患有 1 型神经纤维瘤病(NF1),这是一种遗传肿瘤性疾病,新生儿发病率为 1/3 000~1/2 500,最低患病率为 1/4 000 (Huson et al. 1989)。NF1 对皮肤、神经系统和骨骼有重大影响(1988 年美国国立卫生研究院神经纤维瘤病共识发展会议声明;Huson et al. 1988; Ferner 2007)。该病并发症众多、广泛和多变,即使在同一家庭内也是如此。其范围从认知问题、高血压和胃肠道问题到毁容和包括神经系统肿瘤在内的恶性肿瘤(Huson et al. 1988;Ferner 2007)。许多患者没有与 NF1 相关的严重健康问题,并且在当地临床医师和非专业组织的支持和教育下得到了良好的管理。然而,一些 NF1 患者患有罕见并发症,这些并发症与显著致残率相关,并可能危及生命(Ferner 2011;Huson and Evans 2011)。这些患者的需求最好由一个专业的多学科团队来满足,该团队由熟悉 NF1 罕见症状诊断与管理以及新型疗法进展情况的临床医生和护士组成。

3.2 国家卫生服务委任

英格兰开展了国民保健服务(National Health Service,NHS)的委托工作,以评估人口的需求,并根据他们的需要量身定制保健服务(苏格兰、威尔士和北爱尔兰有不同的调试系统)。选定的卫生服务提供者的职责是提供最佳、安全和有效的以患者为中心的护理。NHS 专科服务部门在全国范围内委托开展高度专业化的服务项目,旨在为英格兰地区受相关病症影响的约 500 人提供卓越的护理及疾病管理服务。其目标是让所有患者都能获得由指定的国家罕见疾病中心提供的资源、专业知识和一系列服务。

3.3 国家委托的"复杂 NF1"服务的发展

NF1 是一种常见的疾病,但受影响的患者有可能出现罕见的"复杂"表现,可能影响多个系统。这包括广泛的、毁容性的且有症状的丛状神经纤维瘤、外周和中枢神经系统并发症、非典型 NF1 表型和骨发育不良(表 3.1)(Ferner et al. 1995,2004;Ferner and Gutmann 2002；Ferner 2007；Ferner and Jackson 2011；Leonard et al. 2007；Listernick et al. 2007；Ferner，Huson and Evans 2011）。复杂NF1的患者不一定只属于某一个医学专科的诊疗范畴，监测和管理往往是分散的，患者必须在不同医院的多个临床科室就诊。

表 3.1　复杂 NF1 的临床表现(Ruggieri and Huson 2001；Ferner，2007)

广泛的、有症状的丛状神经纤维瘤，累及面部、肢体、胸部、腹部或骨盆
颈部神经纤维瘤引起的脊髓压迫
NF1 相关神经病变
非典型神经纤维瘤/恶性周围神经鞘膜瘤
症状性视神经胶质瘤
脑和脊柱胶质瘤
由潜在的结构性病变导致的顽固性癫痫
复杂的神经血管疾病
多发性硬化症
蝶骨大翼发育不良
长骨假关节
非典型表型
节段型 NF1 的产前咨询

1990 年，伦敦盖伊和圣托马斯医院 NHS 信托基金会（Guy's and St. Thomas' Hospitals NHS Foundation Trust London，GSTT）神经内科和中央曼彻斯特大学医院信托基金会（Central Manchester University Hospitals Foundation Trust，CMFT）圣玛丽医院医学遗传学部为伦敦和曼彻斯特地区的 NF1 患者建立了临床服务。作为专业的 NF1 中心，GSTT 和 CMFT 在制订和发布 NF1 诊断和管理的国家共识指南方面发挥了重要作用（Ferner et al. 2007）。这些服务与当地遗传学和神经病学单位、社区儿科医师和神经基金会（非专业 NF 组织）建立了联系。然而，他们发现，英格兰现有的所有当地服务机构都不能满足复杂 NF1 患者的需求。一方面，临床医师和患者均报道了 MPNST 等严重 NF1 并发症的诊断和治疗延误，并将假关节误诊为非意外损伤的病例。另一方面，对无症状的颈部神经纤维瘤进行了不必要的手术干预，对惰性视路胶质瘤进行了化疗。

经过广泛的讨论和向国家专家委托小组提出申请后，国家服务于 2009 年 4 月由 GSTT 和 CMFT 资助并指定，以评估、审查和管理英国复杂 NF1 患者的护理。

无并发症的 NF1 患者继续在现有的临床机构中就诊，进行需要的诊断、遗传咨询、教育、血压、骨骼健康和神经纤维瘤的监测（Ferner et al. 2007）。该诊疗系统需要灵活性，因为一些非复杂疾病的患者在随访过程中会出现复杂 NF1 的临床表现；相反，NF1 的复杂临床表现可能在治疗后消退，患者将转到 GSTT/CMFT 或当地的非复杂 NF1 服务。

3.3.1　国家复杂 NF1 服务的目标

英格兰的国家综合服务中心与临床医师、专职卫生专业人员和神经基金会合作，为 NF1 患者及其家属提供最好的诊断、治疗、教育和支持。

3.4　复杂 NF1 服务的 NF1 相关临床表现：国家委托专家小组的作用(表 3.1)

3.4.1　广泛丛状神经纤维瘤（Huson et al. 1988；Ferner et al. 2007）

广泛丛状神经纤维瘤包括导致面部毁容的、弥漫性累及四肢、胸部、腹部或盆腔的有症状的丛状神经纤维瘤。团队确保患者由擅长神经纤维瘤手术的外科医师诊治；出血、肿瘤再生长、伤口延迟愈合以及神经、呼吸或括约肌障碍的潜在风险需要被讨论。对于有症状的神经纤维瘤，在 $^{18}F-2-氟-2-脱氧-D-葡萄糖正电子发射断层扫描计算机断层扫描$（$^{18}F$-2-fluoro-2-deoxy-D-glucose positron emission tomography computerised tomography，FDG PET CT）上呈阴性的患者，每年监测 2 次，持续 5 年，以确保无恶性改变（见 3.4.4 和 3.4.5）。

3.4.2　颈部丛状神经纤维瘤引起的脊髓压迫（Leonard et al. 2007）

有颈椎神经纤维瘤引起脊髓压迫的神经影像学

证据的 NF1 患者,可以在不手术的情况下长时间保持无症状。患者应由神经科医师和神经外科医师共同进行评估,同时参考经验丰富的神经放射科医师的意见。关于是否需要外科干预的决策必须结合神经功能缺损情况和神经影像学。推荐评估肺功能,因为呼吸功能损害可能由高位脊髓病变引起,并且在显著脊柱侧凸的患者中更为严重。

3.4.3 神经纤维瘤相关神经病变(Ferner et al. 2004; Ferner 2007)

患者表现为神经增粗和呈对称性、长度依赖性轴索神经病。应对所有 NF1 患者进行神经学检查,对非脊神经根、臂丛或腰骶丛疾病引起的运动、感觉或反射改变的患者进行神经传导研究,以排除神经病变的常见病因。由于具有发展为恶性周围神经鞘膜瘤(malignant peripheral nerve sheath tumour, MPNST)的风险,NF1 神经病变需要至少每年监测 1 次。

3.4.4 非典型神经纤维瘤和恶性周围神经鞘膜瘤(Ferner and Gutmann 2002; Ferner 2007)

MPNST 难以诊断和治疗,高级别肿瘤与显著的致残率和病死率相关。非典型神经纤维瘤是多形性和多细胞性肿瘤,但没有有丝分裂的证据,它们可能有恶性潜能,因为非典型神经纤维瘤和 MPNST 都有染色体畸变,且在 FDG PET CT 上有阳性表现(Beert et al. 2011; Ferner et al. 2008)。

丛状神经纤维瘤伴发的持续性疼痛、快速生长、质地坚硬或不明原因的神经功能障碍应立即转诊,并与肉瘤专科单位合作进行评估。

复杂 NF1 服务的职责是通过促使患者快速进入专科肉瘤病房和教育患者有关 MPNST 的知识,来缩短症状出现与诊断 MPNST 之间的时间。目前认为,影响最大的可能是低级别肿瘤,因为高级别肿瘤因快速进展而易被识别。为此,复杂 NF1 诊所与肉瘤单位建立了联席会议,临床专科护士的主要作用是为有症状的神经纤维瘤患者提供电话咨询和分诊。

3.4.5 视神经胶质瘤(Ferner 2007; Listernick et al. 2007)

视神经胶质瘤(optic pathway gliomas, OPG)在 15% 的 NF1 儿童中检测到,但只有 5%~7% 的肿瘤有症状,许多肿瘤不会引起进行性视力退化。在不同的中心,开展化疗的原因各不相同,包括进行性视力丧失、一开始就有严重视力障碍、另一只眼有视力丧失的风险、婴儿无法获得视觉功能以及神经影像学检查显示肿瘤生长。目前,英格兰的儿科肿瘤学家不使用视觉功能作为结局指标,NF1 的结局评估与散发性 OPG 相结合。

与国家儿童肿瘤小组联络,以确保 NF1-OPG 治疗的适应证和方案在所有中心标准化,并系统记录视觉测量结果。复杂 NF1 服务的作用是与儿科眼科医师和视轴矫正师合作,确保就诊的 NF1 儿童至少每年进行 1 次视力检查。鼓励社区儿科医师每年对所有 NF1 儿童进行视觉筛查,建议避免将磁共振成像作为 OPG 的筛查工具,并将 OPG 患者转诊到多学科的复杂 NF1 服务机构。该小组建议已知 OPG 的儿童由儿科肿瘤学家和儿科眼科医师与 NF1 小组合作共同管理。

3.4.6 脑和脊柱神经胶质瘤(Créange et al. 1999; Ferner, 2007)

神经胶质瘤可发生于中枢神经系统的所有部位,并且通常是惰性的,但肿瘤出现在成年期,并且位于视路之外,与较差的预后相关。国家委托服务的作用是与普通神经科医师和神经外科医师联系,强调这些并发症与 NF1 的关联,并在没有临床或神经影像学进展的情况下不鼓励进行临床干预。

3.4.7 结构性病变引起的难治性癫痫(Ferner 2007; Ferner and Jackson 2011)

NF1 使癫痫的终生风险增加约 10 倍:癫痫发作通常是轻微的,局灶性癫痫占主导地位,可能从婴儿期到中年晚期出现。难治性癫痫可能与结构异常有关,包括海马硬化、胶质瘤或胚胎发育不良性神经上皮肿瘤(dysembryoblastic neuro-epithelial tumour, DNET),在某些情况下,神经外科干预有效。复杂

NF1 服务的作用是与癫痫专家联系,强调 NF1 患者认知障碍和骨质疏松症的风险可能增加。监测 25-羟维生素 D 是必要的,因为抗惊厥药物增加了 NF1 中骨质疏松症的风险。开具抗癫痫处方药物时应谨慎,因为这些药物可能会加重认知障碍和情绪障碍。如果在手术前进行神经心理测试,应牢记认知障碍与 NF1 表型相关的可能性。专家小组的职责是通过适当的药物治疗控制癫痫,并在症状归因于其他 NF1 相关问题时对癫痫进行诊断。

3.4.8 多发性硬化症(Ferner et al. 1995; Ferner 2007)

所有形式的多发性硬化症(multiple sclerosis, MS)都可能出现在 NF1 患者中,但与一般人群不同的是,最常见的表现是原发性进行性 MS。由于 NF1 是一种肿瘤抑制相关疾病,理论上,免疫抑制剂治疗会增加恶性肿瘤的风险,在 NF1 患者合并多发性硬化症进行治疗之前,应联系 NF1 专家。患脱髓鞘疾病并出现脊髓病状的患者应进行神经影像学检查,以排除有症状的脊髓神经纤维瘤。

3.4.9 复杂神经血管疾病(Leschziner et al. 2012; Rea et al. 2009; Rosser et al. 2005)

高血压在 NF1 患者中有报道,并增加了神经血管并发症的风险。约 6% 的儿童在神经影像学上发现神经血管紊乱,并与颅内血管的内在异常有关。临床表现从颈内动脉和脑动脉狭窄和(或)闭塞、烟雾病、颅内出血和动脉瘤到放射性血管病变和椎-椎动静脉瘘形成。在一般人群和 NF1 患者中很少报道浅表性铁沉着(Leschziner et al. 2012)。其特征是在脊髓和脑的软膜下层中有含铁血黄素沉积。表现为不可避免的进行性共济失调、耳聋和耳鸣。该病见于既往因高位脊髓病变接受过神经外科手术的患者,也与脑膜膨出、脑肿瘤和创伤相关。

NF1 专家小组应警惕异常神经症状患者(特别是年轻患者)可能患有神经血管疾病,并应促使患者快速被神经血管专家接诊。

3.4.10 长骨假关节(Crawford and Bagamery 1988; Huson et al. 1988; Ferner et al. 2007)

大约 2% 的 NF1 患儿出现长骨弯曲,主要影响胫骨,但也可能累及尺骨、桡骨和腓骨。骨折可能发生在轻微创伤后,愈合延迟,其后果可能是假关节。

复杂 NF1 小组的目的是教育儿科医师确保假关节不被误诊为非意外伤害。需要及时转诊到熟悉这种罕见 NF1 并发症的骨科专科单位。应检查 25-羟维生素 D 水平和骨生物化学,并在必要时予以纠正。

3.4.11 蝶骨翼发育不良(Ferner 2007)

大约 1% 的 NF1 患者有蝶翼缺失,导致颞叶向前推入眼眶,引起搏动性突眼。主要问题在于外观方面,因视力受损而需要进行手术的情况很少见。复杂 NF1 服务的作用是不鼓励对无症状患者进行重大神经外科干预,并确保考虑手术的患者由颅颌面专家团队进行评估。

3.4.12 非典型 NF1 表型(Ferner, Huson and Evans 2011)

在大多数患者中,NF1 的临床诊断简单明了,但大约 2% 转诊到专科 NF 诊所的病例被诊断为非 NF1 的疾病,约 5% 的患者具有 NF1 的部分表现,由 *NF1* 基因或 *RasMapK* 基因的种系或体细胞突变(Legius 综合征)引起(Brems et al. 2007)。复杂 NF1 服务的目的是确保有少见临床表现的患者得到适当的临床评估和基因检测,以促进正确的诊断、咨询和管理。

3.4.13 节段型 NF1 的遗传咨询(Ruggieri and Huson 2001; Maertens et al. 2007; Ferner, Huson and Evans 2011)

在节段型 NF1 中,基因突变发生在受精后,该病的体征和症状仅限于 1 个或多个身体节段。无论受影响的身体部位如何,性腺受累及的风险很小,但确实存在,将全身型 NF1 遗传给孩子。发生这种情况的经验性风险不超过 5%。一些节段型 NF1 患者认为这种风险是不可接受的。CMFT 提供产前遗传咨询和基因检测,首先通过 RNA 血液检测低水平嵌合现象;如果此检测结果正常,则进一步在皮肤活检中培养的黑色素细胞(来自咖啡牛奶斑)或施万细胞(来自神经纤维瘤)中进行突变检测。

3.5 复杂 NF1 的团队(表 3.2)

表 3.2 复杂 NF1 团队成员的角色

团队成员	角色
首席临床医师(神经内科 GSTT;CMFT 遗传学)	领导、协调并代表国家级复杂 NF1 团队 为就诊于复杂 NF1 服务的患者提供临床照护与决策制定
成人神经科医师/儿科神经科医师	诊断、治疗神经系统并发症,与外科团队联络 为年轻人提供的过渡性诊所
遗传学家	诊断、评估复杂 NF1、非典型表型;节段型 NF1 咨询
眼科医师和视轴矫正医师	评估所有复杂 NF1 患儿的视力,监测 OPG 患儿的视力
呼吸内科医师	监测有症状的高位颈/胸神经纤维瘤患者
成人/儿科神经外科医师	神经外科的评估和手术-脊髓压迫,广泛的神经根神经纤维瘤,症状性癫痫,脑胶质瘤,蝶翼发育不良
颅面外科医师	广泛颅面神经纤维瘤的手术评估
肉瘤外科医师	对 MPNST 的评估和处理
肿瘤学家	评估、治疗症状性 OPG 和 MPNST
骨科医师	假关节患者的评估和治疗
整形外科医师	评估、手术治疗广泛丛状神经纤维瘤
PET 医师	对有症状的神经纤维瘤进行恶变评估
神经放射科医师	对神经问题进行神经影像检查
肌肉骨骼放射学	丛状神经纤维瘤、骨发育不良的成像
神经生理学医师	NF1 神经病变的神经传导研究
临床专科护士	NF1 患者的教育、信息和支持电话诊所
成人/儿童心理学家/精神科医师	认知评估,临床心理评估/精神病学评估,治疗

NF1 小组由临床医师、护士、心理学家、协调员和患者代表组成的多学科团队组成。GSTT 和 CMFT 在各个层面上都有密切的联系,定期举行面对面会议、电话会议和视频会议。神经外科、成人和儿童神经内科、颅面外科、肿瘤学和呼吸内科的多学科团队会议有助于对复杂的临床病例做出决策,并确保患者获得适当的专科知识。不同专业之间的联合诊所改善了沟通、教育和管理。全科医师、专科护士和医院临床医师将患者转诊到 GSTT 和 CMFT;来自英格兰南部的患者在伦敦接受评估,来自英格兰北部的患者在曼彻斯特接受评估。目的是在整个英格兰实现复杂 NF1 患者护理的标准化,并制订循证指南以改善临床结果。

国家专家委托团队(National Specialist Commissioning Team,NSCT)每年对每个中心进行 2 次访问,以审核患者数量、服务的地理位置、工作人员招募、接班计划和患者参与服务的情况。预计大多数专科服务需要 5 年时间才能完全发展并能够衡量疾病结局的改善。

3.6 GSTT 2009—2011 年的 NSCT 复杂 NF1 业务

3.6.1 GSTT 患者的人口统计资料

2009—2010 年,重点是招募团队、建立诊所和多学科会议。从 2010 年 4 月至 2011 年 4 月,在 441 个门诊预约中评估了 326 名新患者和随访患者,年龄范围为 1~75 岁(平均年龄为 30 岁,中位年龄为 29 岁,标准差为 15.9 岁)。临床服务正在逐步扩大(2011 年 4 月至 2011 年 10 月患者人数见表 3.3),但一些患者在问题得到治疗后会转到非复杂诊所。

表 3.3 2011 年 4 月至 2011 年 10 月 GSTT 复杂 NF1 门诊患者的人口学统计资料

患者数	2011 年 4 月至 2011 年 10 月
患者总数(新发及随访)	208
男性	102
女性	106

续 表

患 者 数	2011年4月至2011年10月
>50岁的患者	23
>18岁的患者	55
死亡	1

3.6.2　2009年4月至2011年10月GSTT复杂NF1服务的死亡人数

自2009年4月以来,已有7例死亡:4例女性和3例男性(年龄范围为31~66岁;中位年龄为40岁)。死亡原因是MPNST(4例)、脑胶质瘤(1例)、腹膜癌(1例)和多发性硬化症脑干加重(1例)。尽管心血管疾病被认为是NF1的一个重要死亡原因,但在复杂或非复杂服务中,没有患者死于血管疾病(Friedman et al. 2002)。

3.7　复杂NF1的临床表现:2009—2011年GSTT经验

许多严重NF1并发症的患者已经接受了GSTT和CMFT的治疗,但未来的挑战是确定英国所有具有复杂NF1疾病表现的患者。这将需要多种策略的结合,包括查阅基因登记,与专科小组(神经内科医师、儿科医师、眼科医师和肉瘤外科医师)沟通,以及召开教育会议。

3.7.1　广泛丛状神经纤维瘤

GSTT诊所评估了71例患者,年龄范围为4~71岁,有症状性或毁容性神经纤维瘤。18例患者在2009年4月之后被转诊到该诊所,其中17例患者有多个症状性病变。丛状神经纤维瘤位于头颈部(17例)、肢体(17例)、骨盆(8例)和腹部(4例)。20例患者被转诊手术,其中1例患者因顽固性疼痛需要膝上截肢并切断坐骨神经。

3.7.2　颈部神经纤维瘤引起的高脊髓压迫

26例患者年龄为15~67岁,其中22例有手术史。4例患者在2009年4月之后被诊断为脊髓压迫,其中2例需要干预,2例团队未建议手术治疗。1例患者有非器质性功能障碍,另1例患者的症状与神经纤维瘤性神经病变有关,而与颈髓压迫无关。

3.7.3　NF1相关神经病变

19例患者年龄为14~74岁,经临床评估和神经生理学诊断为与NF1相关的轴突神经病变,自2009年4月以来新增6例患者。19人中有4人患有MPNST,1人患有非典型神经纤维瘤。自2009年4月以来,未发现新的恶性肿瘤病例,MPNST患者保持稳定。

3.7.4　非典型纤维神经瘤

20例患者年龄为15~57岁,活检示非典型神经纤维瘤,其中7例在2009年4月之后确诊。8例患者有恶性肿瘤病史,包括视路胶质瘤和恶性周围神经鞘膜瘤。2009年以来发现的病变部位包括腹盆腔(2例)、四肢(3例)、臂丛和颈部(2例)。除1例患者外,其余患者FDG PET CT检查均为阳性,提示有恶性潜能。

3.7.5　恶性周围神经鞘膜瘤

自2000年以来,已有70例疑似NF1和MPNST的GSTT患者,这些患者被诊断为NF1-MPNST(57例)、散发性MPNST(1例)、胃肠道肿瘤(7例)、软组织肉瘤(3例)和骨肉瘤(1例)。有23例患者的MPNST病程超过5年,其中17例患者的病程少于5年,70例患者中有30例死亡。自2009年以来,4例患者分别在确诊后4个月、13个月、19个月和37个月死于转移性病灶。自2009年4月以来,有9例患者被诊断为MPNST,年龄为11~55岁。其中7例为高度恶性肿瘤,2例有MPNST病史,6例有复发或转移性疾病。

3.7.6　视路胶质瘤

GSTT团队治疗了72名NF1相关OPG的儿童和成人,年龄范围为5~43岁,其中8例患者在2009年4月之后被诊断出来。通过视力筛查发现5例OPG,虽然最初无症状,但其中2例最终需要化疗。5例患者先前接受过手术治疗,8例接受过放射治疗,2例随后发展为MPNST,1例发展为脑胶质瘤。72例患者中有15例需要化疗。

3.7.7 脑和脊柱胶质瘤

49例确诊或疑似脑胶质瘤患者,年龄范围为6~56岁,就诊于GSTT诊所。自2009年4月以来,有3例新的胶质瘤被诊断,包括1例颞叶和2例脑干胶质瘤。其中1例患者死于星形细胞瘤引起的进行性神经功能缺损,2例患者因肿瘤生长和神经功能缺损加重而需要手术,并在就诊后10年置入脑室-腹腔分流术治疗进行性脑积水。2例脊髓胶质瘤患者在2009年之前接受了化疗,目前病情稳定。

3.7.8 难治性癫痫

50例GSTT NF1患者,年龄范围为5~75岁,既往或持续有癫痫史,包括13例儿童和37例成人,大多数为不明原因引起的局灶性癫痫。自2009年4月以来,16例患者被诊断为DNET(5例)、胶质瘤(2例)、海马硬化(1例)和颅内分流相关的难治性癫痫(1例)。1例患者在DNET手术后病情好转,多数患者在适当的药物治疗下病情稳定。

3.7.9 复杂的神经血管疾病

6例年龄为3~40岁的患者因复杂的神经血管疾病就诊,包括围产期脑室内出血伴梗阻性脑积水、需要夹闭的大脑中动脉动脉瘤和放射性血管病变。2009年4月以后确诊2例;1例患者主诉耳鸣、头痛、言语障碍、杂音,转诊行神经外科手术治疗,诊断为椎-椎动静脉瘘。1例52岁男性患者因颈髓神经纤维瘤行脊髓减压术后数年出现进行性共济失调和耳聋,并被诊断为表面铁沉积症。他的症状通过听力康复治疗得到改善(Leschziner et al. 2012)。

3.7.10 多发性硬化症

14例患者(年龄为29~69岁;中位年龄为45岁)被评估并诊断为原发性进行性多发性硬化症(4例)、复发缓解型MS(3例)、继发性进行性MS(3例)、未分类MS(1例)和横切性脊髓炎(1例)。2009年4月后诊出6例患者,其中1例死亡与进行性脑干疾病相关。2例患者有脱髓鞘MRI改变,但目前无症状,2例患者需要免疫抑制剂治疗。3例患者已经发展为恶性肿瘤,但诊断是在免疫抑制剂治疗之前,或者患者没有接受针对MS的特异性治疗。

3.7.11 蝶骨翼发育不良

8例患者年龄范围为16~40岁,已被诊断为蝶骨翼发育不良,其中1例在2009年之后接受了新的转诊,并因美容原因接受了眼眶减压术。2例转诊的患者在充分了解拟行手术的范围后选择不接受治疗。

3.7.12 长骨假关节

29例长骨假关节患者年龄为3~48岁,自2009年以来出现3例新病例,其中1例误诊为非意外损伤。主要累及胫骨,但4例有尺骨假关节。

3.7.13 非典型表型(Huson 2011 in Ferner and Jackson 2011)

自2009年在GSTT,共有5名患者,年龄范围为3~24岁,因疑似患NF1而被转诊,随后被诊断为Legius综合征(个人联络Guy Leschziner)、Beckwith-Wiedemann综合征、共济失调毛细血管扩张、Albright病、PTEN-Cowden病(个人联络Dragna Josifova)。

3.7.14 节段型NF1的遗传咨询

节段型NF1遗传咨询的主要专业知识是在CMFT,一对夫妇因男方患有节段型NF1做了产前检测。

3.8 结论

GSTT和CMFT的复杂NF1服务是由国家委任服务团队于2009年4月建立的。由于临床表型的巨大变异性和不可预测性,NF1服务的建立非常复杂。只有确保收集在复杂和非复杂医疗机构之间流动的患者数据,才能确定疾病的自然史。该服务的优势在于为具备诊断和治疗1型神经纤维瘤病专业知识的临床医师和护士提供了坚实的基础设施、标准化的临床治疗和结局指标方案,加上对数据的细致询问,将为评估临床试验提供基线。我们针对 NF1 患者的目标是提供信息,促进社区融合,促进决策的独立性。提高公众对 NF1 的认识至关重要,以便 NF1 患者受到尊重和有尊严的对待,并允许他们在社会中充分发挥其教育、情感、社会和经济潜力。

(顾熠辉 译)

参考文献

[1] Beert E, Brems H, Daniëls B, De Wever I, Van Calenbergh F, Schoenaers J, Debiec-Rychter M, Gevaert O, De Raedt T, Van Den Bruel A, de Ravel T, Cichowski K, Kluwe L, Mautner V, Sciot R, Legius E (2011) Atypical neurofibromas in neurofibromatosis type 1 are premalignant tumors. Genes Chromosomes Cancer 50: 1021-1032

[2] Brems H, Chmara M, Sahbatou M, Denayer E, Taniguchi K, Kato R, Somers R, Messiaen L, De Schepper S, Fryns JP, Cools J, Marynen P, Thomas G, Yoshimura A, Legius E (2007) Germline loss of function mutations in SPRED1 cause a neurofibromatosis 1-like phenotype. Nat Genet 39: 1120-1126

[3] Crawford AH Jr, Bagamery N (1988) Osseous manifestations of neurofibromatosis in childhood. J Pediatr Orthop 6: 72-88

[4] Créange A, Zeller J, Rostaing-Rigattieri S, Brugières P, Degos JD, Revuz J, Wolkenstein P (1999) Neurological complications of neurofibromatosis type 1 in adulthood. Brain 122: 473-481

[5] Ferner RE (2007) Neurofibromatosis 1 and neurofibromatosis 2: a twenty first century perspective. Lancet Neurol 6: 340-351

[6] Ferner RE (2011) Neurofibromatosis 1. In: Ferner RE, Huson SM, Evans DG (eds) Neurofibromatoses in clinical practice, chap 1. Springer, Berlin, pp 1-46

[7] Ferner RE, Gutmann D (2002) International Consensus Group Statement of the management of malignant peripheral nerve sheath tumours in Neurofibromatosis 1. Cancer Res 62: 1573-1577

[8] Ferner RE, Jackson M (2011) Epilepsy in neurofibromatosis 1 and neurofibromatosis 2. In: Shorvon SD, Guerrini R, Andermann F (eds) The causes of epilepsy, chap 25. Cambridge University Press, Cambridge, pp 183-188

[9] Ferner RE, Hughes RAC, Johnson MR (1995) Neurofibromatosis 1 and multiple sclerosis. J Neurol Neurosurg Psychiatry 58: 582-585

[10] Ferner RE, Hughes RA, Hall SM, Upadhyaya M, Johnson MR (2004) Neurofibromatous neuropathy in neurofibromatosis 1 (NF1). J Med Genet 41: 837-841

[11] Ferner RE, Huson SM, Thomas N, Moss C, Willshaw H, Evans DG, Upadhyaya M, Towers R, Gleeson M, Steiger C, Kirby A (2007) Guidelines for the diagnosis and management of individuals with neurofibromatosis 1. J Med Genet 44: 81-88

[12] Ferner RE, Golding JF, Smith M, Calonje E, Jan W, Vijayanathan S, O'Doherty M (2008) [18F] 2-fluoro-2-deoxy-D-glucose positron emission tomography (FDG PET) as a diagnostic tool for neurofibromatosis 1 (NF1) associated malignant peripheral nerve sheath tumours (MPNSTs): a long-term clinical study. Ann Oncol 19: 390-394

[13] Friedman JM, Arbiser J, Epstein JA, Gutmann DH, Huot SJ, Lin AE, McManus B, Korf BR (2002) Cardiovascular disease in neurofibromatosis 1: report of the NF1 Cardiovascular Task Force. Genet Med 4: 105-111

[14] Huson SM (2011) The neurofibromatoses: differential diagnoses and rare subtypes. In: Ferner RE, Huson SM, Evans DG (eds) Neurofibromatoses in clinical practice, chap 3. Springer, Berlin, pp 71-127

[15] Huson SM, Harper PS, Compston DAS (1988) Von Recklinghausen neurofibromatosis: clinical and population study in south east Wales. Brain 111: 55-81

[16] Huson SM, Compston DAS, Clark P, Harper PS (1989) A genetic study of von Recklinghausen neurofibromatosis in south east Wales. 1. Prevalence, fitness, mutation rate, and effect of parental transmission on severity. J Med Genet 26: 704-711

[17] Leonard JR, Ferner RE, Thomas N, Gutmann DH (2007) Cervical cord compression from plexiform neurofibromas in neurofibromatosis 1. J Neurol Neurosurg Psychiatry 78: 1404-1406

[18] Leschziner G, Connor S, Wroe S, Ferner RE (2012) An unusual case of hearing loss in a patient with neurofibromatosis type 1. Clin Neurol Neurosurg 114(6): 735-737

[19] Listernick R, Ferner RE, Liu GT, Gutmann DH (2007) Optic pathway gliomas in neurofibromatosis-1: controversies and recommendations. Ann Neurol 61: 189-198

[20] Maertens O, Schepper SD, Vandesompele J, Brems H, Heyns I, Jansenns S, Speleman F, Legius E, Messiaen L (2007) Molecular dissection of isolated disease features in mosaic neurofibromatosis type one. Am J Hum Genet 81: 243-251

[21] No authors (1988) National Institutes of Health Consensus Development Conference. Statement Neurofibromatosis. Arch Neurol 45: 575-578

[22] Rea D, Brandsema JF, Armstrong D, Parkin PC, deVeber G, MacGregor D, Logan WJ, Askalan R (2009) Cerebral arteriopathy in children with neurofibromatosis type 1. Pediatrics 124: e476-e483

[23] Rosser TL, Vezina G, Packer RT (2005) Cerebrovascular abnormalities in a population of children with neurofibromatosis type 1. Neurology 64: 553-555

[24] Ruggieri M, Huson SM (2001) The clinical and diagnostic implications of mosaicism in the neurofibromatoses. J Neurol 56: 1433-1443

第 4 章 1型神经纤维瘤病死亡率
Mortality in Neurofibromatosis 1
Gareth R. Evans

4.1 引言

部分研究已证实神经纤维瘤病患者的预期寿命普遍缩短。大多数研究报告了 NF1 的死亡率和预期寿命。这类研究主要分为两种类型：队列研究和基于医学死亡证明书研究。这两类研究都显示，NF1 患者的预期寿命相较正常人缩短 8～15 年。

4.2 病死率研究

4.2.1 队列研究

此前已有四项 NF1 相关队列研究。Sorensen 等（1986）曾在丹麦开展了一项全国性队列研究，随访了 212 名 NF1 患者。在长达 42 年的时间里，他们获得了 99% 的患者的随访信息。与当地正常人群相比，NF1 患者亲属的存活率明显下降，先证者的存活率更低，而女性先证患者的存活率最差。45% 的先证 NF1 患者发生恶性肿瘤或良性中枢神经系统肿瘤，相对风险为 4.0（95% CI 2.8～5.6）。与正常人群相比，神经纤维瘤病的男性亲属的肿瘤发病率相同，而女性亲属的肿瘤发病率高于正常人 2 倍（相对风险，1.9；95% CI 1.1～3.1）。其中神经系统肿瘤的比例最高。

Zöller 等（1995）对瑞典哥德堡市的 70 名成年 NF1 患者进行了为期 12 年的跟踪随访。研究者对 NF1 队列患者的预期寿命、死亡率和死亡原因进行了调查，并与瑞典正常人群对比。随访期间，NF1 组中有 22 人死亡，而对比瑞典正常人群中预计死亡人数为 5.1 人（$P<0.001$）。患者死亡时的平均年龄为 61.6 岁，死者中有 12 人（55%）患有恶性肿瘤（3 人为软组织肉瘤，9 人为癌症）。平均死亡年龄比正常人群小 15 岁。

Evans 等（2011）报告了一项英格兰西北部的人群队列研究（McGaughran et al. 1999）。这项研究与前两项队列研究的不同之处在于，它确定了所有 NF1 患者而非仅仅是成年人。因此，该队列人群相对年轻，大多数病例尚未死亡，故该队列偏向于以 MPNST 和胶质瘤为主的年轻群体。即使对比无偏倚的同地区人群，该研究队列也有 26%（34/130）的死亡病例是由 MPNST 引起，而理论上只有 8%～13% 的患者会出现这种并发症（Evans et al. 2002）。尽管如此，Kaplan-Meier 分析法还是减少了偏倚，这是因为该队列中包括了仍然存活的患者。该队列中位生存期大幅提高至 71.5 岁，仅比人口平均生存期少 8 年。这表明，尽管本队列确定的 NF1 患者相对年龄较小，NF1 患者的存活时间比以前的队列研究更接近人群平均存活时间。根据死亡证明，129/

G.R. Evans
Genetic Medicine, Manchester Academic Health Science Centre, St Mary's Hospital, Central Manchester Hospitals Foundation Trust, Manchester M13 9WL, UK
e-mail: gareth.evans@cmft.nhs.uk

130(99%)的病例死因已经确定(表4.1)。如果严格限制生活区域的边界,整体死亡比例为109/1 023 (10%)。最常见的死因是骨髓增生性银屑病[34/130(26%)]。胶质瘤是第二位常见的死因,这也是<20岁的NF1患者最常见的死因(表4.1)。相反,心血管原因死亡并不常见,在年龄<50岁的患者人群中,只有10/80的人死于心血管疾病,其中只有6例有明确的血管来源。值得注意的是,8/10年龄<50岁的心血管原因死亡病例和19/26(73%)心血管原因死亡病例都发生在男性NF1患者中。年龄分别为34岁和44岁的2例死亡病例是由儿童时期放射治疗引起的继发性血管疾病所导致的。与放射治疗无关的血管性死亡最明显的案例是1名20岁男性的胸腔动脉瘤破裂。在该地区队列中,全因死亡的平均年龄和中位年龄分别为43.55岁和44.13岁。

表4.1 曼彻斯特队列中NF1患者按年龄队列划分的死亡原因(updated from Evans et al. 2011)

原因	0~10岁	11~20岁	21~30岁	31~40岁	41~50岁	51~60岁	>60岁	总体	死亡记录含NF诊断
胶质瘤	4	2	3	4	1			14	8/14
恶性周围神经鞘膜瘤		4	11	14	2	3	2	36	21/36
幼年型慢性粒细胞白血病	2							2	1/2
横纹肌肉瘤		1						1	0/1
乳腺癌			1	2	2	3	1	9	1/9
结直肠癌			1		1	1		3	0/3
卵巢癌					1		1	2	0/2
肺癌				1	1	1		3	0/3
淋巴瘤						1		1	0/1
其他肿瘤					1	2		3	0/3
术后良性肿瘤		1		1		1		3	2/3
肿瘤相关	6/7	8/10	16/19	20/28	9/20	10/23	8/31	78/138	35/78
脑血管			1	3	2	4		10	3/10
心肌梗死					2	3	7	12	0/12
心肌病				1	1			2	0/2
肺动脉高压						1		1	0/1
心力衰竭					1	2	1	4	0/4
动脉瘤破裂		1	1	1				3	0/3
心血管相关		1/10	1/19	3/28	7/20	8/23	12/31	32/138	3/32
肺炎	1		1		1			3	2/3

续表

原因	0～10岁	11～20岁	21～30岁	31～40岁	41～50岁	51～60岁	>60岁	总体	死亡记录含NF诊断
四肢瘫痪/脊髓压迫呼吸衰竭				1		1		2	1/2
脊柱后侧突呼吸衰竭					1	1	2	4	3/4
肺纤维化				1		1		2	2/2
慢性阻塞性气道病						1	2	2	1/3
呼吸系统	1/7	0/10	0/19	3/28	1/20	4/23	3/31	12/139	8/12
癫痫		1	1					2	1/2
肝肾综合征				1				1	0/1
败血症						1	1	2	0/2
多器官衰竭							1	1	0/1
肾衰竭				1			1	1	0/2
自杀			1				1	1	0/2
意外事故							2	2	0/2
痴呆							2	2	0/2
小肠绞窄肠系膜梗死						1		1	1/1
其他因素总计	0/7	1/10	2/19	1/28	1/20	2/23	8/31	14/138	2/14
未知					2			2	
总计	7	10	18	29	20	23	31	138	48/136 (36%)

将与NF1相关的死亡人数与英格兰西北部当地正常人口中的死亡人数进行比较，发现男性NF1患者患心血管疾病的比例较当地正常男性高3倍[比例死亡率(proportionate mortality ratio，PMR) 4.1；95% CI 1.4～2.6]。同样，在NF1女性患者中，死因为乳腺癌的病例为正常人群的3.5倍(PMR 3.5；95% CI 1.3～7.7)。此外，NF1女性患者死于脑肿瘤的比例高于正常人群(PMR 29.5；95% CI 12.7～58.1)，但在男性中差异却并不显著(PMR 6.7；95% CI 0.8～24.1)。最值得注意的结果是MPNST导致的死亡：在NF1患者中，MPNST被报告为死因的频率明显高于预期(男性PMR 3 819.6，95% CI 1 971.4～6 672.5；女性PMR 7 788.2，95% CI 4 355.7～12 846.2)。

第四项队列研究来自法国(Duong et al. 2011)。该研究纳入了转诊至法国国家神经纤维瘤转诊中心的NF1患者。1980年至2006年，共有1 895例NF1患者接受了治疗，中位随访时间为6.8年(范围为0.4～20.6年)。其中，1 226例(65%)患者的生存状态已收集：1 159例(94.5%)患者存活，

67例(5.5%)已死亡。NF1组队列的总死亡率明显升高(PMR 2.02；CI 1.6～2.6；$P<10^{-4}$)。超额死亡率发生在10～20岁(PMR 5.2；CI 2.6～9.3；$P<10^{-4}$)和20～40岁(PMR 4.1；CI 2.8～5.8；$P<10^{-4}$)的患者中。同时，男性和女性的死亡率都明显偏高。在10～20岁年龄组中，女性死亡率明显高于男性(分别为 PMR 12.6；CI 5.7～23.9 和 PMR 1.8；CI 0.2～6.4)。58例(86.6%)患者报告了死因，其中最常见的死因为MPNST(60%)。研究发现，与普通人群相比，NF1患者的PMRs明显增加，表明死亡率增高，其中10～40岁NF1患者的总死亡率升高明显，女性往往高于男性。40岁以上的NF1患者死亡率并不高于正常人群，这可能是由于队列中年龄较大的患者人数有限。

4.2.2 死亡证明研究

目前有3项已经发表的NF1死亡证明研究。第一项使用的数据来自1968年至1992年的日本生命统计数据(Imaizumi 1995)。这项研究报告了605例神经纤维瘤病被列为死因的病例，研究病例平均死亡年龄为43岁。不过，作者没有区分NF1和2型神经纤维瘤病(neurofibromatosis 2，NF2)，也没有提供除神经纤维瘤病以外的其他死因数据。此外，由于该研究中只包括了那些将NF1列为基本死因的患者，因此即使是作者也认为神经纤维瘤病的诊断数被低估了(Imaizumi 1995)。该日本死亡证明研究中的平均死亡年龄预计会较正式情况更低，因为NF1不太可能成为老年患者的基础死因。

美国的第二项死亡证明研究(1983—1997)确定了3 770例NF1患者的死因，其平均死亡年龄比正常人群低约15岁(Rasmussen et al. 2001)。NF1男性和女性的平均死亡年龄和中位死亡年龄分别为54.4岁和59岁，对应正常人群死亡年龄分别为70.1岁和74岁。与正常人群相比，NF1患者在死亡证明上列有恶性结缔组织或其他软组织肿瘤的可能性比正常人群高出33倍(PMR 34.3；95% CI 30.8～38.0)。总体而言，该研究中NF1病例死亡证明上列有恶性肿瘤的可能性是预期的1.2倍(PMR 1.21；95% CI 1.14～1.28)，但10～19岁死亡病例的PMR为6.07(95% CI 4.88～7.45)，20～29岁死亡病例的PMR为4.93(95% CI 4.14～5.82)。同样，在<30岁死亡的NF1患者的死因中，心血管疾病也比预期的要多(<10岁 PMR 3.26；95% CI 1.31～6.71；10～19岁 PMR 2.68；95% CI 1.38～4.68；20～29岁 PMR 2.25；95% CI 1.46～3.32)，但在年龄更大的人群中却没有发现该现象。该死亡证明研究病例基于同期全美国32 722 122的死亡病例(1/8 700)。

最新的死亡证明研究来自意大利(Masocco et al. 2011)。作者利用国家死亡率数据库和个体多种死因记录，估算了1995—2006年与NF1相关的死亡率。在研究期间死亡的675.3万人中，有632人被诊断为NF1，但其中只有25%的人根本死亡原因是神经纤维瘤病。NF1相关死亡病例的平均年龄比正常人群低约20岁。进行性别差异分析的结果显示，女性NF1患者可能受到相关并发症的影响更为严重，或者这也可能仅提示在年轻女性的死亡证明中报道NF1的可能性更大。研究发现，结缔组织和其他软组织恶性肿瘤(PMR 22.3；95% CI 15.50～30.95)与脑恶性肿瘤(PMR 4.2；95% CI 2.69～6.15)作为基本死因的比例更高，但其他部位整体恶性肿瘤的比例并不高。他们还发现，在NF1的老年人中，阻塞性慢性支气管炎和肌肉骨骼系统疾病的发病率较高。不过，所有心血管疾病的PMR均低于1.0。

4.3 讨论

综上，目前已有7项对NF1患者死亡率开展的研究。在这些研究中，早期死亡的主要原因是MPNST和胶质瘤。Rasmussen等(2001)关于早期血管疾病因素导致死亡的研究发现得到了Evans等(2011)的支持，即他们发现NF1男性患者心血管死亡的发生率是整体人群的4倍。然而，最近的意大利研究(Masocco et al. 2011)并不支持这一观点。排除MPNST和神经胶质瘤(通常为低级别肿瘤，不被认为是恶性肿瘤)，其他常见肿瘤的恶性风险在NF1患者中可能不会大幅增加。不过，Evans等(2011)发现，有8例NF1患者死于胶质瘤。

虽然死亡证明研究有望克服队列研究的确定性

偏倚,但这些研究依赖于死亡证明上对NF1的准确记录。在Evans等(2011)的研究中,只有35%的NF1患者在死亡证明上将NF1列为诱因。即使是胶质瘤和MPNST等典型NF1的继发肿瘤中,也只有29/48(60%)的患者在死亡证明上记录了NF1或神经纤维瘤病病史。这可能是评估由于常见癌症导致死亡风险的一个典型问题。最近发现的乳腺癌风险增加(Sharif et al. 2006;Walker et al. 2006)就是一个很好的例子。Evans等(2011)发现,NF1患者乳腺癌的PMR增加了3.5(95% CI 1.3~7.7),但只有1/9的死亡证明中记录了NF1。因此,Rasmussen等(2001)和Masocco等(2011)对死亡证明的使用需要评估是否记录了所有与NF1有关的死亡的可能性。Rasmussen等的研究中,8 679例死亡病例中只有1例记录了NF1。在Masocco等(2011)的研究中,这一比例更低,仅为1/10 685。在大多数报告中,NF1的发病率介于1∶2 500和1∶3 000之间(Huson et al. 1989;Lammert et al. 2005;Evans et al. 2010)。如果假定发病率和死亡率保持不变,那么这两项死亡证明研究很可能存在很大偏差,只有23%~35%的NF1预期死亡病例被记录在死亡证明上。NF1死亡人数记录不足也可能导致NF1患者预期寿命缩短的程度被夸大。

一些研究表明,NF1女性患者死于恶性肿瘤比例更高(Sorensen et al. 1986;Rasmussen et al. 2001;Duong et al. 2011)。Evans等(2011)也报告,女性死于恶性肿瘤的人数更多,但并无显著性差异。事实上,这一差异几乎完全可由新发现的NF1与乳腺癌之间的关联来解释(Sharif et al. 2006;Walker et al. 2006)。

几乎所有的研究都表明,NF1患者超常死亡率大多出现在50岁以前,而在50岁之后影响很小。因此,50岁以后没有出现严重NF1并发症的人,预期寿命接近正常。尽管如此,目前还没有一项研究能完全避免此类研究中固有的确认偏倚。理想的研究尚未开展,这需要纳入1个NF1患者队列,对其进行全面评估和跟踪随访,直到每名患者死亡。Sorensen等(1986)所确定的212个全国范围的NF1患者队列已接近成熟,但这显然不是一个完全确定的人群。

4.4 结论

虽然NF1患者在生命最初的40~50年中死于恶性肿瘤的人数明显过多,预期寿命缩短,但整体预期寿命很可能并没有像许多研究中所说的那样缩短15~20年。

致谢:Evans教授得到了曼彻斯特中央基金会生物医学研究中心的支持。

(杨军,魏澄江 译)

参考文献

[1] Duong TA, Sbidian E, Valeyrie-Allanore L, Vialette C, Ferkal S, Hadj-Rabia S, Glorion C, Lyonnet S, Zerah M, Kemlin I, Rodriguez D, Bastuji-Garin S, Wolkenstein P (2011) Mortality associated with neurofibromatosis 1: a cohort study of 1895 patients in 1980 - 2006 in France. Orphanet J Rare Dis 6: 18

[2] Evans DGR, Baser ME, McGaughran J, Sharif S, Donnelly B, Moran A (2002) Malignant peripheral nerve sheath tumours in neurofibromatosis 1. J Med Genet 39: 311 - 314

[3] Evans DG, Howard E, Giblin C, Clancy T, Spencer H, Huson SM, Lalloo F (2010) Birth incidence and prevalence of tumour prone syndromes: estimates from a UK genetic family register service. Am J Med Genet 152A: 327 - 332

[4] Evans DG, Howard E, Wilding A, Ingham SL, Moran A, Scott-Kitching V, Holt F, Huson SM (2011) Mortality in neurofibromatosis 1. Eur J Hum Genet 19: 1187 - 1191

[5] Huson SM, Compston DA, Clark P, Harper PS (1989) A genetic study of von Recklinghausen neurofibromatosis in south east Wales. I. Prevalence, fitness, mutation rate, and effect of parental transmission on severity. J Med Genet 26: 704 - 711

[6] Imaizumi Y (1995) Mortality of neurofibromatosis in Japan, 1968 - 1992. J Dermatol 22: 191 - 195

[7] Lammert M, Friedman JM, Kluwe L, Mautner VF (2005) Prevalence of neurofibromatosis 1 in German children at elementary school enrolment. Arch Dermatol 141: 71 - 74

[8] Masocco M, Kodra Y, Vichi M, Conti S, Kanieff M, Pace M, Frova L, Taruscio D (2011) Mortality associated with neurofibromatosis type 1: a study based on Italian death certificates (1995 - 2006). Orphanet J Rare Dis 6: 11

[9] McGaughran JM, Harris DI, Donnai D et al (1999) A clinical study of type 1 neurofibromatosis in North West England. J Med Genet 36: 192 - 196

[10] Rasmussen SA, Yang Q, Friedman JM (2001) Mortality in neurofibromatosis 1: an analysis using US death certificates. Am J Hum Genet 68: 1110 - 1118

[11] Sharif S, Ferner R, Birch J, Gattamaneni R, Gillespie J, Evans DGR (2006) Second primary tumours in

Neurofibromatosis 1 (NF1) patients treated for optic glioma: substantial risks post radiotherapy. J Clin Oncol 24: 2570 - 2575

[12] Sorensen SA, Mulvihill JJ, Nielsen A (1986) Long term follow up of von Recklinghausen neurofibromatosis: survival and malignant neoplasms. N Engl J Med 314: 1010 - 1015

[13] Walker L, Thompson D, Easton D et al (2006) A prospective study of neurofibromatosis type 1 cancer incidence in the UK. Br J Cancer 95: 233 - 238

[14] Zöller M, Rembeck B, Akesson HO, Angervall L (1995) Life expectancy, mortality and prognostic factors in neurofibromatosis type 1. A twelve-year follow-up of an epidemiological study in Göteborg, Sweden. Acta Derm Venereol 75: 136 - 140

第5章 1型神经纤维瘤病儿童的认知特征：治疗意义

The Cognitive Profile of NF1 Children: Therapeutic Implications

Natalie A. Pride and Kathryn N. North

5.1 NF1患儿的认知学研究

5.1.1 引言

认知障碍是儿童期NF1常见的并发症之一；大约70%的患者存在学习障碍和（或）神经心理缺陷。认知功能障碍会影响患者终身，并且会影响患者的学习成绩、就业机会和整体生命质量。过去15年里，大量的研究都致力于描述NF1的认知表型。尽管NF1患者之间存在显著的差异，但许多核心的神经心理特征已经被确定，这些特征反过来又为疾病机制和治疗靶点的研究提供了基础。本章的目的是总结NF1认知表型的特点以及目前发现的关于相关发病机制和潜在治疗方法的知识。

5.1.2 智力和学习能力

精神发育迟缓曾被认为是NF1的常见症状，早期研究报告称，大约30%的NF1患者存在智力障碍（Samuelsson and Axelsson 1981）。然而，这些报告的研究对象主要是智力受严重影响的患者，且并未使用定量的心理测量评估，从而导致认定偏差，精神发育迟缓的比例被严重高估。基于大量具有一系列身体症状患者的定量数据，目前普遍认为NF1患者中有4%～8%处于智力受损范围（智商<70），而在普通人群中这一比例约为3%（Hyman et al. 2005；North et al. 1997）。通常情况下，患者智商处在平均到低于平均的范围（80～90区间的高位至90～100区间的低位）（Hyman et al. 2005；Levine et al. 2006）。早期研究报告患者拥有更好的语言技能和较差的感知组织技能（Eliason 1986；Legius et al. 1995），后续大多数研究也发现了类似的语言和非语言技能模式（Ferner et al. 1996；Hyman et al. 2005；Moore et al. 2000；North et al. 1995）。一些作者提出了一种特殊的神经心理模型，即非语言学习障碍（non-verbal learning disorder，NVLD），以描述NF1的某些认知表型（Eliason 1986；Wang et al. 2000）。NVLD的特征包括数学能力差；视空间、精细动作和书写缺陷以及语言技能健全背景下的社交问题（Harnadek and Rourke 1994）。尽管数学能力和视空间的缺陷在NF1中极为常见，但随着最近对患者语言、拼写和阅读障碍的研究了解，人们已经不再将NF1概念化为NVLD。诵读困难，一种特殊的

N. A. Pride
Institute for Neuroscience and Muscle Research, The Children's Hospital at Westmead Sydney, Sydney, Australia

K. N. North
University of Sydney, Sydney, Australia
e-mail: kathryn.north@health.nsw.gov.au

M. Upadhyaya and D. N. Cooper (eds.), *Neurofibromatosis Type 1*,
DOI 10.1007/978-3-642-32864-0_5, # Springer-Verlag Berlin Heidelberg 2012

阅读障碍，似乎在 NF1 中很常见（Hofman et al. 1994；Mazzocco et al. 1995）；一项研究发现，约有 50%的患者符合音韵性诵读困难的诊断标准，即非单词阅读受损以及在利用拼写规则来发音阅读方面遇到特殊困难（Watt et al. 2008）。语音处理中的特定损伤，包括音位分割、快速命名、语音记忆、单词识别和解码等也有报道（Cutting and Levine 2010；Mazzocco et al. 1995）。这种缺陷模式与特发性阅读障碍的儿童所见到的缺陷模式相似（Cutting and Levine 2010）。

NF1 中学习障碍（learning disorde，LD）的报告频率因研究而异，估计在 30%~65%（Brewer et al. 1997；Clements-Stephens et al. 2008；Ferner et al. 1996；Huson et al. 1988；Hyman et al. 2006；North et al. 1997）。这种频率的差异是由于不同研究人员使用了不同的 LD 定义。根据当前版本的《精神障碍诊断与统计手册》（Diagnostic and Statistical Manual of Mental Disorders，DSM-Ⅳ TR）（American Psychiatric Association 2000），当某人在阅读、数学或书面表达的标准化测试中取得的成绩远低于预期的年龄、教育程度和智力水平时，就会被诊断为 LD。各种统计方法都可以被用来确定差异是否显著。"远低于"通常被定义为成绩和智商之间的差异超过 2 个标准差（standard deviation，SD）；然而，较小差异（1 个至 2 个 SD 之间）也会被使用，导致研究之间的不一致。在一项涉及 81 名 NF1 患儿（和 49 名未受影响的对照组）的大型队列研究中，Hyman 等（2006）研究了特定学习障碍（specific learning disabilities，SLD）的发生频率，共同标准化测试（WISC Ⅲ 和 WIAT）的成绩和智商之间的差值大于 2 个 SD 即被定义为 SLD。研究发现队列中有 20%表现出 SLD，32%存在一般学习困难（与低智商相符的较差成绩），48%具有与年龄相符的学习能力。研究还指出，SLD 的性别效应显著，这一群体中大部分是男性。这对评估和补救具有重要意义，并表明女性 NF1 患者患 SLD 的风险并不比普通人群高。

5.1.3 视觉空间感

NF1 认知表型的一个显著特征是视空间障碍，表现为难以准确感知和解释视觉信息。线定向判断任务（The Judgement of Line Orientation Task，JLO）是 NF1 有关文献中一贯用于测量视觉空间感的测试，大约 80%的研究记录了 NF1 患儿在这项测试中的缺陷（Dilts et al. 1996；Hofman et al. 1994；Hyman et al. 2005，2007；Levine et al. 2006；Mazzocco et al. 1995；Schrimsher et al. 2003）。其中许多研究称，在他们的 NF1 队列中绝大多数患儿在这一指标上存在受损情况。例如，Hyman 等（2005）将 81 名 NF1 患儿与 49 名未受影响的兄弟姐妹进行比较，发现 56%的 NF1 患儿在 JLO 测试中处于受损范围内（高于一般人口平均值 1 个 SD）。在其他一系列针对视觉空间和视觉感知功能的测试，例如 Beery-Buktenica 视觉-运动整合测试、Rey 复杂图形测试、韦氏智力量表的方块设计子测试以及视觉感知技能测试中，NF1 患儿也表现出了缺陷（Dilts et al. 1996；Hyman et al. 2005）。

5.1.4 注意力

注意力缺陷多动障碍（attention deficit hyperactivity disorder，ADHD）是一种以持续且普遍的注意力缺陷、多动和冲动症状为特征的神经生物学疾病。尽管 NF1 中 ADHD 的确切发病率尚不清楚，但研究队列的估计值从 33%到 49.5%不等（Hofman et al. 1994；Kayl et al. 2000；Koth et al. 2000；Mautner et al. 2002；Payne et al. 2011），远高于一般人群中 ADHD 的估计比例（5%）（Polanczyk et al. 2007）。大多数研究表明，NF1 患儿的 ADHD 更符合以注意缺陷为主的亚型或多动和注意缺陷混合的亚型，不同性别的 ADHD 诊断率通常相等。这与普通人群的情况形成鲜明对比，一般情况下男性 ADHD 的发病率是女性的 2.5~9.0 倍（Durston，2003）。

注意力并非结构单一的机制，而是需要各种神经网络协调运作的多方面的认知过程。它对减少次要信息、选择应对措施和规划最终行动至关重要。NF1 患者在衡量不同方面注意力的测试中所表现的缺陷已有记录。连续执行测试（continuous performance test，CPT）如注意力变量测试（test of variables of attention，TOVA）和 Kiddie's CPT 是常用的评估持续注意力（遗漏错误）的方法，这些测试能够发现 NF1 患儿存在的注意力缺陷。与未受影响的兄弟姐妹（Mazzocco et al. 1995；Sangster et al. 2011）和标准数据（Ferner et al. 1996）相比，NF1 患儿的遗漏错误率较高。相反，也有报告指出 NF1 患儿的 CPT 遗漏错误率处于正常水平（Dilts et al. 1996；Mautner et al. 2002）。尽管这些发现存在不一致性，但使用替代的持续注意力测量方法的其他研究提供了足够的证据，表明 NF1 人群中存在持续注意力缺陷（Hyman et al. 2005）。对选择性注意力等其他类型注意力的研究提供了不一致的结果。Ferner 等（1996）对 98 名 NF1 患儿和 105 名匹配对照进行了 Stroop 任务测试，发现 NF1 患儿表现出持续受损。尽管如此，鉴于这项任务依赖于其他包括反应抑制和单词阅读的认知过程才能成功完成，因此应谨慎看待这一结论。在最近的一项研究中，Payne 等（2011）使用 TEACh 中的 Sky Search 子测试评估选择性注意力，发现 NF1 患者（$n=199$）的表现明显不如未受影响的对照组（$n=55$）。相比之下，Hyman 等（2005）在这项测试中未发现 NF1 患儿（$n=81$）与兄弟姐妹（$n=49$）之间的任何差异。关于选择性注意力缺陷存在与否的研究结果不一致可能是受试者选择和对照组选择（即未受影响的兄弟姐妹与匹配对照）的差异性所致，进一步突显了对具有良好特征的样本和适当对照的需求。然而，注意力缺陷是 NF1 认知表型中常见的表现之一。识别潜在的神经生物学和生化机制可能为 NF1 患儿的 ADHD 最佳靶向治疗以及一般人群中 ADHD 的发病机制提供重要见解。

5.1.5 执行功能

在对 NF1 儿童的早期研究中发现了包括非结构化学习风格、易分心、冲动、计划失败和解决问题能力差在内的多种行为特征；这些特征使人联想到前额叶皮质受损患者的表现（Bawden et al. 1996；Eliason 1986；North et al. 1995）。近年来，研究 NF1 认知表型中执行功能缺陷重要作用的文献显著增加。执行功能是一系列调节和控制其他行为例如解决问题、转移注意力的灵活性、监测和改变行为、在面临新任务和新情况时规划未来行动的能力。执行功能障碍被认为是大脑额叶区域，特别是前额叶皮质和皮质下区域受损的结果。据报道，NF1 存在广泛的执行功能缺陷，包括认知灵活性（Hyman et al. 2005；Joy et al. 1995；Payne et al. 2011；Zoller et al. 1997）、情景转换（Hofman et al. 1994；Mazzocco et al. 1995）、抽象概念形成（Hyman et al. 2005；Payne et al. 2011）、工作记忆（Huijbregts et al. 2010；Rowbotham et al. 2009）、反应抑制（Ferner et al. 1996；Mautner et al. 2002）、分散注意力（Ferner et al. 1996；Payne et al. 2011）和计划（Bawden et al. 1996；Hofman et al. 1994；Hyman et al. 2005；Mazzocco et al. 1995；Payne et al. 2011；Roy et al. 2010）上的功能障碍。对于 NF1 的学龄儿童来说，执行功能障碍可能会导致学习上多方面的问题。僵化的工作方式和认知的不灵活会导致难以在适当的年龄水平适应学校环境，以至于对某些孩子而言，预期的微小偏差都可能导致适应困难和焦虑的产生。执行力不足也会使开始和完成工作、跟踪任务和分配时间变得困难。执行功能障碍与行为障碍、社会功能障碍和生命质量下降相关（Baron 2004；Lezak et al. 2004）。

5.1.6 记忆和学习

"学习"和"记忆"这两个术语经常交换使用——尽管它们代表的是不同的认知过程。学习是指我们如何获取新信息，而记忆是对信息进行编码、存储和稍后检索的过程。海马体位于大脑的内侧颞叶，与学习和记忆功能有关（Kandel et al. 2000）。与这些记忆系统不同的是工作记忆，它与背外侧前额叶皮质密切相关。工作记忆是指在脑海中临时存储和处理信息的能力，被认为是一种执行功能，而非记忆系统的一部分。尽管 NF1 中的工作记忆障碍被很好地记录下来（见 5.1.4），但是否存在学习和记忆缺陷仍有争议。虽然一些研究报告称，NF1 患儿学习和检索新信息的能力完好无损（Hyman et al. 2005；Joy et al. 1995；Moore et al. 1996），但其他研究却并不认同这一点（Ferner et al. 1996；Payne et al. 2012；Ullrich et al. 2010）。用于评估记忆能力的测试往往需要其他认知功能，如语言或视觉空间能力的辅助，因此这些研究大多数都很难确定

NF1患儿是否存在真正的记忆障碍。最近，Payne等（2012）利用一项已被证明能够研究非人类灵长类动物（Taffe et al. 2002）和临床人群（Fowler et al. 2002）海马体功能的测量方式（剑桥神经心理学测试自动组合中的配对关联学习）检测了71名NF1的儿童和29名未受影响的对照者的视觉空间学习能力。他们发现，即使考虑到持续注意力、视觉空间能力和智力，这些缺陷也依然存在，从而为NF1中基于海马体的学习障碍提供了令人信服的证据。

5.1.7 语言

语言可分为两大类：表达性语言和接受性语言。表达性语言障碍是一种言语和书面表达都有困难的沟通障碍。它的特点是难以将口语表达到其发展年龄所期望的水平。如果孩子难以理解别人对他们说的话，即发生了接受性语言障碍。语言缺陷是NF1的学龄儿童的特征。几乎半数对NF1患儿语言进行的研究都发现了该方面的发育延迟（Dilts et al. 1996；Eldridge et al. 1989；Hofman et al. 1994；Hyman et al. 2005；Mazzocco et al. 1995；North et al. 1994）。Dilts等（1996）使用语言基础筛查测试临床评估（clinical evaluation of language fundamentals screening test，CELF）对19名NF1的儿童（6~17岁）进行了广泛的语言能力检查，并将他们在该测试中的表现与匹配的未受影响的兄弟姐妹进行了比较；58%的样本未通过表达性语言筛选测试，这其中又有26%同时表现出接受性语言缺陷。Hyman等（2005）研究了81名NF1患儿的语言表达和接受能力，发现语言发育延迟的程度低于最初的报道。与标准数据相比，NF1组（8~16岁）中分别有15%和2.5%的人表现出接受性和表达性语言延迟。在NF1患儿中还发现了图片命名、语法接受、书面语言和语音处理等测试中的缺陷（Eldridge et al. 1989；Hofman et al. 1994；Hyman et al. 2005；Mazzocco et al. 1995）。最近的证据表明，语言的发育延迟可以在21个月大的儿童中发现。Lorenzo等（2011）使用麦克阿瑟交际发展量表和句子对39名NF1的幼儿（21~30个月）进行家长评估，发现超过70%的幼儿被评为低于年龄预期。在3~5岁的NF1患儿中也发现了语言发育延迟，约37%的儿童表现出语言表达和接受能力的缺陷（Thompson et al. 2010）。这些发现对NF1的儿童管理具有重要意义，它们强调了对2.5岁以下儿童进行语言评估和干预的重要性，从而降低了以后出现文盲问题的风险。

5.2 NF1认知缺陷的神经生物学：人类影像学研究

NF1在行为和生物学上都是一种高度异质性的疾病。NF1患者认知缺陷的高发无疑反映了中枢神经系统功能的紊乱——最近在人类和动物模型中的研究开始深入了解其所涉及的潜在神经解剖学和生物化学机制。

5.2.1 大脑结构异常

结构成像研究提供了大脑发育早期异常的证据，这些异常的出现与NF1认知缺陷的发生（如果不是在这之前就有异常）相重合。

NF1中常见的一个发现是与巨头症相关的大脑体积变大，该发现通过头围和大脑体积的成像测量被记录下来（Greenwood et al. 2005；Moore et al. 1996；Said et al. 1996）。一些研究表明，NF1患儿脑容量的增加似乎主要是由白质的增加（主要在额叶区域和胼胝体）引起的，虽然也有迹象表明后部区域的灰质体积也在增加（Greenwood et al. 2005）。许多研究已经检查了NF1中脑容量和认知功能之间的关系，报告的结果喜忧参半。Moore等报道称，NF1中灰质的增加与智力和学习成绩之间的较大差异有关。相比之下，Said等发现灰质减少与视空间功能差异之间存在关系。

由于神经连通性是NF1的核心问题，胼胝体作为连接两个半球的主要白质结构已经引起了人们的特别关注。许多研究报道了NF1患者的胼胝体增大（Kayl et al. 2000；Moore et al. 2000），其中一些研究发现胼胝体相对于大脑总体积增大（Dubovsky et al. 2001；Pride et al. 2010）。三项研究发现了这种异常与认知之间的相关性。具体而言，较大的胼胝体体积与学习成绩不佳、智力低下、执行功能和视空间障碍有关（Moore et al. 2000；Pride et al.

2010），而胼胝体体积减小与注意力问题有关（Kayl et al. 2000）。

一些其他研究致力于识别大脑中可能导致特定认知障碍的其他区域异常。NF1 患者语言皮质中几个结构，包括颞平面（Billingsley et al. 2002）、额下回和颞横回（Billingsley et al. 2003b）的非典型大小或不对称性，已被记录下来，并被发现与较差的认知或学习表现，特别是语言和学术能力有关。这是一个有趣的发现，因为在诵读困难人群中也有类似的发现。这些关于 NF1 语言皮质对称模式异常的报告可能反映了左半球正常特异化的缺乏；然而，有必要对 NF1 大脑中语言的功能组织做进一步研究。

NF1 中常见的大脑异常之一是脑 MRI 的 T2 加权序列上出现信号增强区域。这些 T2 高信号（T2 hyperintensitie，T2H）发生在 55%～90% 的儿童中，常见于基底节、小脑、丘脑、脑干和皮质下白质。许多研究已经检验了这些病变与认知功能之间的关系。虽然有研究发现智力水平与 T2H 的存在和数量之间存在相关性（Moore et al. 1996；North et al. 1994），但未能发现 T2H 与认知状态之间的关联（Bawden et al. 1996；Ferner et al. 1993；Legius et al. 1995）。最近的研究表明，丘脑或丘脑纹状体区域的 T2H 可能对认知表现产生影响（Chabernaud et al. 2009；Goh et al. 2004；Hyman et al. 2007）。丘脑与几乎所有主要的大脑结构都有相互联系，在信息处理的同步方面尤其令人感兴趣。有人提出，丘脑纹状体区域的 T2H 可能导致皮质-皮质下环路（在执行功能中起主要作用）的改变，导致认知障碍（Chabernaud et al. 2009）。

5.2.2 大脑功能异常

传统 MRI 提供了大脑结构的成像，而功能性 MRI（functional MRI，fMRI）允许对工作中的大脑（即神经活动）进行动态询问，并允许识别 NF1 中异常的认知系统。尽管这项技术的风险和非侵入性都很小，但令人惊讶的是，通过 fMRI 进行的 NF1 研究工作很少。功能性 MRI 已被用于研究 NF1 患者语音处理的神经基础。Billingsley 等（2003a）在书面和听觉押韵测评任务中，研究了 15 名 NF1 患者和 15 名对照者的语音处理能力。与对照组相比，NF1 组的额下区比颞顶叶区表现出明显更多的激活。这种不同的激活模式类似于在普通人群里诵读困难患者中观察到的模式（Shaywitz et al. 1998）；不过 Billingsley 等报告这种激活主要在右半球发生，而非左半球。在书面任务中，与对照组相比，NF1 组表现出相较颞叶和枕叶活动更少的额叶活动（Billingsley et al. 2003a）。作者推测，这种结果模式（额叶活动减少和后部活动增加）可能反映了代偿性神经元募集，即由于额叶功能低下，NF1 患儿利用了比额叶更多的后部区域。考虑到颞顶区白质连接的异常与普通人群里诵读困难个体的阅读能力有关，因此有必要确定 NF1 中是否也发生了白质连接的减少。扩散张量成像应增加关于白质性质的重要信息，以及 NF1 大脑内特定纤维束与阅读障碍间关系的重要信息。

功能性 MRI 也被用于更好地理解 NF1 中介导视觉空间处理的神经系统（Billingsley et al. 2004；Clements-Stephens et al. 2008）。Billingsley 及其同事对 15 名 NF1 患者和 15 名健康受试者进行了 fMRI 检查，结果表明，在视觉空间任务中，与对照组相比，NF1 患者与任务相关的额叶激活到后皮质激活（顶叶、枕叶和颞叶）相对较少。这种模式与他们在 fMRI 任务中的行为表现有关，也与阅读成绩呈正相关。这些数据支持了早期的研究结果，表明 NF1 大脑的额叶区域存在功能异常。在最近的一项功能磁共振成像研究中，Clements-Stephens 等（2008）研究了 13 名 NF1 患儿和 13 名对照组的 JLO 任务的神经基础，发现 NF1 组的右半球激活明显大于左半球。他们将这一发现归因于 NF1 中效率低下的右半球体网络。

背外侧前额叶皮质（prefrontal corte，PFC）对工作记忆和执行功能至关重要。最近对 14 名 NF1 的年轻人和 12 名对照组进行的一项 fMRI 研究显示，在空间工作记忆任务中，NF1 患者的背侧 PFC、顶叶皮质和纹状体的任务相关激活明显少于健康受试者（Shilyansky et al. 2010a）。背外侧 PFC 激活程度与任务表现相关。这些数据表明，额-纹状体通路的异常可能是 NF1 执行功能缺陷的基础。

尽管神经影像学研究为 NF1 中存在的大脑结构和功能异常提供了重要的见解，但更具挑战性的是如何将这些解剖学发现与认知功能形成关联。许多 NF1 的解剖发现和认知之间的研究结论并不一致,这可能是由解剖方法的不敏感性、受试者准入和样本量的多变,或疾病的内在生物学异质性导致的。处于幼儿期的儿童不太可能在未麻醉的情况下保持静止(阻碍获得足够质量的脑成像研究),只能提供有限的机会进行解剖学研究;然而,这恰恰可能是大脑发生影响最深远的变化的时期。另外一个需要考虑的重要问题是,在 NF1 患者中发现的特定认知缺陷是由区域解剖和(或)神经化学异常还是更广泛分布的异常,如连接改变,所引起的。对 NF1 动物模型的研究可能为 NF1 相关认知缺陷的发育时程和神经解剖相关性提供新的见解。

5.3 NF1 认知缺陷的神经生物学:动物研究

NF1 是由编码神经纤维瘤蛋白的 NF1 基因突变引起的。这种蛋白质在大脑和皮肤中高度表达,具有多种生化功能,包括激活 Ras GTP 酶。神经纤维瘤蛋白缺乏导致 Ras 过度活跃,从而引起细胞异常增殖。有人认为,异常的 Ras 信号转导影响了脑内的神经元发育、迁移和凋亡(Billingsley et al. 2003b; North 2000; North et al. 1997)。神经纤维瘤蛋白还增加腺苷酸环化酶/环腺苷酸(AC/cAMP)比值。许多转基因小鼠和苍蝇模型已经被开发出来,以帮助理解 NF1 的认知特征(见第 37 章)。$Nf1$ 基因发生无义突变的杂合小鼠($Nf1^{+/-}$ 小鼠)形成肿瘤的风险增加,并表现出模拟人类 NF1 表型的空间学习、注意力和工作记忆障碍(Costa et al. 2002; Li et al. 2005; Shilyansky et al. 2010a; Silva et al. 1997)。有人提出,这些认知缺陷是 Ras-MAPK 信号级联反应过度激活的结果,这会导致活性依赖的 GABA 释放增加和长时程增强作用(long-term potentiation, LTP)降低,使抑制和兴奋过程失衡(Cui et al. 2008; Li et al. 2005; Shilyansky et al. 2010b; Silva et al. 1997)。Li 及其同事(2005)最近的一项研究发现,用旨在抑制 Ras 功能的治疗干预措施(如药物洛伐他汀)靶向该通路,可降低 $Nf1^{+/-}$ 小鼠的 Ras 活性和 LTP,拯救认知表型。因此,有研究者开展了一项对 24 名 NF1 患儿评估洛伐他汀安全性和耐受性的 I 期研究。结果表明,患儿言语和非言语学习以及记忆的指标有所改善(Acosta et al. 2011)。目前,该药物在 NF1 患儿中的 II 期试验正在进行中。

最近的研究使用具有 $Nf1$ 基因纯合失活的 GFAP 阳性神经胶质细胞的 $Nf1^{+/-}$ 小鼠,发现注意系统功能的行为异常和纹状体中多巴胺水平的降低(Brown et al. 2010a, b)。这些研究还表明,多巴胺摄取抑制剂哌甲酯可以改善这些小鼠的注意力缺陷。总之,这些发现建立了 $Nf1$ 基因表达、注意力和多巴胺能通路之间的机制联系,并为未来的人类临床试验提供了相关启示。迄今为止,只有一项研究调查了哌甲酯对该人群的影响。Mautner 等(2002)在 12 个月的时间里用哌甲酯治疗了 20 名 ADHD 的 NF1 儿童。据报道,这些患儿注意力、社交能力和行为都有所改善。虽然这项研究提供了一些有希望的结果,但这项研究的设计、适当对照组的缺乏以及样本量较小都限制了其解释。此外,作者将他们的研究局限于药物对 ADHD(和 NF1)儿童的影响,而不是针对更广泛的存在注意力缺陷的 NF1 患者。哌甲酯治疗 NF1 注意力缺陷的随机安慰剂对照试验是有必要的。

5.4 评估管理的意义以及未来的方向

从以上对 NF1 认知表型的研究中,我们可以得出几个结论以指导 NF1 患儿的评估和管理。鉴于认知表现的异质性和影响学习成绩的缺陷发生概率,对儿童的认知能力进行全面的神经心理学评估以提供支持是很重要的。评估应该包括对智力、注意力、执行功能、视觉空间能力、语言和学习成绩的测量,且应在入学前进行,以确定课堂安排。最近的证据表明,更严重的认知和学习脆弱性最早在 2.5 岁时就能被发现,突出了在儿童入学前对其进行这些评估的重要性(Lorenzo et al. 2011)。由于 NF1 患儿有患 LD 的风险,因此回顾儿童在学校的发展和深入全面了解 LD 至关重要。儿童在整个学年中都应该得到追踪,此时发现的能力弱点可能出现在对成绩要求增加的较晚年龄段如高中生活中。先前的研究表明,符合 ADHD 标准的 NF1 儿童确实受益于兴奋剂药物治疗(Mautner et al. 2002);因此,应该考虑由儿科医师进行治疗和管理。

目前尚无系统研究阐明发现认知缺陷时的最佳管理方法。通常采取的方法是推荐一系列可以在家里和课堂上实施的策略,这些策略有助于解决特定的认知困难。但这些策略大多数都没有循证依据,目前尚不清楚它们是否被正确实施,或者实施时对该人群是否有效。实施一项评估当前 NF1 认知缺陷管理系统有效性的系统性研究,将极大帮助到参与护理 NF1 患儿的心理学家、教师和家庭。

今天,我们对 NF1 认知障碍的临床方面有了更深入的了解。在理解 NF1 认知功能障碍的遗传和生化缺陷方面也取得了重大进展,并催生了目前正在评估的潜在治疗方法,如洛伐他汀和哌甲酯。改进的 MRI 技术和发展心理神经科学的引入也为我们提供了一些对 NF1 中可能存在的异常大脑发育步骤的洞察。例如,功能性 MRI 和扩散张量成像为 NF1 中的白质连接和神经活动开辟了全新的、有价值的观点,有望为病理生理学提供令人兴奋的见解。然而,终究还是要靠人体和动物研究的结合,以提供有关该疾病所有特征的认知和神经基础以及大脑结构和功能异常的发育神经生物学的精确数据。这些知识将形成对干预的各个阶段的实质性改善,并为开发针对 NF1 认知缺陷的生物靶向干预措施铺平道路。

(李海博,郭子桢 译)

参考文献

[1] Acosta MT, Kardel PG, Walsh KS, Rosenbaum KN, Gioia GA, Packer RJ (2011) Lovastatin as treatment for neurocognitive deficits in neurofibromatosis type 1: phase 1 study. Peadiatr Neurol 45: 241-245

[2] American Psychiatric Association (2000) Diagnostic and statistical manual of mental disorders, 4th edn. American Psychiatric Association, Washington, DC

[3] Baron IS (2004) Neuropsychological evaluation of the child. Oxford University Press, New York Bawden H, Dooley J, Buckley D, Camfield P, Gordon K, Riding M, Llewellyn G (1996) MRI and nonverbal cognitive deficits in children with neurofibromatosis 1. J Clin Exp Neuropsychol 18: 784-792

[4] Billingsley RL, Schrimsher GW, Jackson EF, Slopis JM, Moore B (2002) Significance of planum temporale and planum parietale morphologic features in neurofibromatosis type 1. Arch Neurol 59: 616-622

[5] Billingsley RL, Jackson EF, Slopis JM, Swank PR, Mahankali S, Moore BD 3rd (2003a) Functional magnetic resonance imaging of phonologic processing in neurofibromatosis 1. J Child Neurol 18: 731-740

[6] Billingsley RL, Slopis JM, Swank PR, Jackson EF, Moore B (2003b) Cortical morphology associated with language function in neurofibromatosis type 1. Brain Lang 85: 125-139

[7] Billingsley RL, Jackson EF, Slopis JM, Swank PR, Mahankali S, Moore BD (2004) Functional MRI of visual-spatial processing in neurofibromatosis, type I. Neuropsychologia 42: 395-404

[8] Brewer VR, Moore BD 3rd, Hiscock M (1997) Learning disability subtypes in children with neurofibromatosis. J Learn Disabil 30: 521-533

[9] Brown JA, Emnett RJ, White CR, Yuede CM, Conyers SB, O'Malley KL, Wozniak DF, Gutmann DH (2010a) Reduced striatal dopamine underlies the attention system dysfunction in neurofibromatosis-1 mutant mice. Hum Mol Genet 19: 4515-4528

[10] Brown JA, Gianino SM, Gutmann DA (2010b) Defective cAMP generation underlies the sensitivity of CNS neurons to neurofibromatosis-1 heterozygosity. J Neurosci 30: 5579-5589

[11] Chabernaud C, Sirinelli D, Barbier C, Cottier J-P, Sembely C, Giraudeau B, Deseille-Turlotte G, Lorette G, Barthez M-A, Castelnau P (2009) Thalamo-striatal T2-weighted hyperintensities (unidentified bright objects) correlate with cognitive impairments in neurofibromatosis type 1 during childhood. Dev Neuropsychol 34: 736-748

[12] Clements-Stephens AM, Rimrodt SL, Gaur P, Cutting LE (2008) Visuospatial processing in children with neurofibromatosis type 1. Neuropsychologia 46: 690-697

[13] Costa RM, Federov NB, Kogan JH, Murphy GG, Stern J, Ohno M, Kucherlapati R, Jacks T, Silva AJ (2002) Mechanism for the learning deficits in a mouse model of neurofibromatosis type 1. Nature 415: 526-530

[14] Cui Y, Costa RM, Murphy GG, Elgersma Y, Zhu Y, Gutmann DH, Parada LF, Mody I, Silva AJ (2008) Neurofibromin regulation of ERK signaling modulates GABA release and learning. Cell 135: 549-560

[15] Cutting LE, Levine TM (2010) Cognitive profile of children with neurofibromatosis and reading disabilities. Child Neuropsychol 16: 417-432

[16] Dilts CV, Carey JC, Kircher JC, Hoffman RO, Creel D, Ward K, Clark E, Leonard CO (1996) Children and adolescents with neurofibromatosis 1: a behavioral phenotype. J Dev Behav Pediatr 17: 229-239

[17] Dubovsky EC, Booth TN, Vezina G, Samango-Sprouse SA, Palmer KM, Brasseux CO (2001) MR imaging of the corpus callosum in paediatric patients with neurofibromatosis type 1. Am J Neuroradiol 22: 190-195

[18] Durston S (2003) A review of the biological bases of ADHD: what have we learned from imaging studies? Mental Retard Dev Disabil Res Rev 9: 184-195

[19] Eldridge R, Denckla MB, Bien E, Myers S, Kaiser-Kupfer M, Pikus A, Schlesinger S, Parry D, Dambrosia J, Zasloff M, Mulvihill J (1989) Neurofibromatosis type 1. Am J Dis Child 14: 833-837

[20] Eliason MJ (1986) Neurofibromatosis: implications for learning and behavior. J Dev Behav Pediatr 7: 175-179

[21] Ferner RE, Chaudhuri R, Bingham J, Cox T, Hughes RA (1993) MRI in neurofibromatosis 1. The nature and evolution of increased intensity T2 weighted lesions and their relationship to intellectual impairment. J Neurol Neurosurg Psychiatry 56: 492-495

[22] Ferner RE, Hughes RA, Weinman J (1996) Intellectual impairment in neurofibromatosis 1. J Neurol Sci 138: 125-133

[23] Fowler KS, Saling MM, Conway EL, Semple JM, Louis WJ (2002) Paired associate performance in the early detection of DAT. J Int Neuropsychol Soc 8: 58-71

[24] Goh W, Khong P, Leung C, Wong V (2004) T2-weighted hyperintensities (unidentified bright objects) in children with neurofibromatosis 1: the impact of cognitive function. Neurology 19: 853-858

[25] Greenwood RS, Tupler LA, Whitt JK, Buu A, Dombeck CB, Harp AG, Payne ME, Eastwood JE, Krishnan KR, MacFall JR (2005) Brain morphometry, T2-weighted hyperintensities, and IQ in children with neurofibromatosis type 1. Arch Neurol 62: 1904-1908

[26] Harnadek MCS, Rourke BP (1994) Principal identifying features of the syndrome of non-verbal learning disabilities in children. J Learn Dis 27: 144-154

[27] Hofman KJ, Harris EL, Bryan RN, Denckla MB (1994) Neurofibromatosis type 1: the cognitive phenotype. J Paediatr 124: S1-S8

[28] Huijbregts S, Swaab H, de Sonneville L (2010) Cognitive and motor control in neurofibromatosis type I: influence of maturation and hyperactivity-inattention. Dev Neuropsychol 35: 737-751

[29] Huson SM, Harper PS, Compston DA (1988) Von Recklinghausen neurofibromatosis A clinical and population study in south-east Wales. Brain 111: 1355-1381

[30] Hyman SL, Shores A, North K (2005) The nature and frequency of cognitive deficits in children with neurofibromatosis type 1. Neurology 65: 1037-1044

[31] Hyman SL, Shores EA, North K (2006) Learning disabilities in children with neurofibromatosis type 1: subtypes, cognitive profile, and attention-deficit-hyperactivity disorder. Dev Med Child Neurol 48: 973-977

[32] Hyman SL, Gill DS, Shores EA, Steinberg A, North K (2007) T2 hyperintensities in children with neurofibromatosis type 1 and their relationship to cognitive functioning. J Neurol Neurosurg Psychiatry 78: 1088-1091

[33] Joy P, Roberts C, North K, de Silva M (1995) Neuropsychological function and MRI abnormalities in neurofibromatosis type 1. Dev Med Child Neurol 37: 906-914

[34] Kandel ER, Kupferman I, Iverson S (2000) Learning and memory. In: Kandel ER, Schwartz JH, Jessell TM (eds) Principles of neural science. McGraw-Hill, New York Kayl AE, Moore BD, Slopis JM, Jackson EF, Leeds NE (2000) Quantitative morphology of the corpus callosum in children with neurofibromatosis and attention-deficit hyperactivity disorder. J Child Neurol 15: 90-95

[35] Koth CW, Cutting LE, Denckla MB (2000) The association of neurofibromatosis type 1 and attention deficit hyperactivity disorder. Child Neuropsychol 6: 185-194

[36] Legius EM, Descheemaeker MJ, Steyaert J (1995) Neurofibromatosis type 1 in childhood: correlation of MRI findings with intelligence. Neurology 59: 638-640

[37] Levine TM, Materek A, Abel J, O'Donnell M, Cutting LE (2006) Cognitive profile of neurofibromatosis type 1. Semin Pediatr Neurol 13: 8-20

[38] Lezak MD, Howieson DB, Loring DW (2004) Neuropsychological assessment, 4th edn. Oxford University Press, New York

[39] Li W, Cui Y, Kushner SA, Brown RA, Jentsch JD, Frankland PW, Cannon TD, Silva AJ (2005) The HMG-CoA reductase inhibitor lovastatin reverses the learning and attention deficits in a mouse model of neurofibromatosis type 1. Curr Biol 15: 1961-1967

[40] Lorenzo J, Barton B, Acosta MT, North K (2011) Mental, motor, and language development of toddlers with neurofibromatosis type 1. J Pediatr 158(4): 660-665

[41] Mautner VF, Kluwe L, Thakker SD, Leark RA (2002) Treatment of ADHD in neurofibromatosis type 1. Dev Med Child Neurol 44(3): 164-170

[42] Mazzocco MMM, Turner JE, Denckla MB, Hofman KJ, Scanlon DC, Vellutino FR (1995) Language and reading deficits associated with neurofibromatosis type 1: evidence for a notso-nonverbal learning disability. Dev Neuropsychol 11: 503-522

[43] Moore BD 3rd, Slopis JM, Schomer D, Jackson EF, Levy BM (1996) Neuropsychological significance of areas of high signal intensity on brain MRIs of children with neurofibromatosis. Neurology 46: 1660-1668

[44] Moore BD 3rd, Slopis JM, Jackson EF, De Winter AE, Leeds NE (2000) Brain volume in children with neurofibromatosis type 1: relation to neuropsychological status. Neurology 54: 914-920

[45] North K (2000) Neurofibromatosis type 1. Am J Med Genet 97: 119-127

[46] North K, Joy P, Yuille D, Cocks N, Mobbs E, Hutchins P, McHugh K, de Silva M (1994) Specific learning disability in children with neurofibromatosis type 1: significance of MRI abnormalities. Neurology 44: 878-883

[47] North K, Joy P, Yuille D, Cocks N, Hutchins P (1995) Cognitive function and academic performance in children with neurofibromatosis type 1. Dev Med Child Neurol 37: 427-436

[48] North K, Riccardi V, Samango-Sprouse C, Ferner R, Moore B, Legius E, Ratner N, Denckla MB (1997) Cognitive function and academic performance in neurofibromatosis. 1: consensus statement from the NF1 Cognitive Disorders Task Force. Neurology 48: 1121-1127

[49] Payne JM, Barton B, Shores EA, North KN (2012) Paired associate learning in children with neurofibromatosis type1: implications for clinical trials. J Neurol (Epub ahead of print)

[50] Payne JM, Hyman SL, Shores EA, North K (2011) Assessment of executive function and attention in children with neurofibromatosis type 1: relationships between cognitive measures and realworld behavior. Child Neuropsychol 17(4): 313-329

[51] Polanczyk G, de Lima MS, Horta BL, Biederman J, Rohde LA (2007) The worldwide prevalence of ADHD: a systematic review and metaregression analysis. Am J Psychiatry 164: 942-948

[52] Pride N, Payne JM, Webster R, Shores EA, Rae C, North K (2010) Corpus callosum morphology and its relationship to cognitive function in neurofibromatosis type 1. J Child Neurol 25: 834-841

[53] Rowbotham I, Pit-ten Cate IM, Sonuga-Barke EJS, Huijbregts SCJ (2009) Cognitive control in adolescents with neurofibromatosis type 1. Neuropsychology 23: 50-60

[54] Roy A, Roulin JL, Charbonnier V, Allain P, Fasotti L, Barbarot S, Stalder JF, Terrien A, Le Gall D (2010) Executive dysfunction in children with neurofibromatosis type 1. A study of action planning. J Int Neuropsychol Soc 16:

1056-1063
[55] Said SM, Yeh TL, Greenwood RS, Whitt JK, Tupler LA, Krishnan KR (1996) MRI morphometric analysis and neuropsychological function in patients with neurofibromatosis. Neuroreport 7 (12): 1941-1944
[56] Samuelsson B, Axelsson R (1981) Neurofibromatosis. A clinical and genetic study of 96 cases in Gothenburg, Sweden. Acta Derm Venereol Suppl 95: 67-71
[57] Sangster J, Shores EA, Watt S, North K (2011) The cognitive profile of preschool-aged children with neurofibromatosis type 1. Child Neuropsychol 17(1): 1-16
[58] Schrimsher GW, Billingsley RL, Slopis JM, Moore B (2003) Visual-spatial performance deficits as a diagnostic indicator in children with neurofibromatosis type-1. Am J Med Genet 120A: 326-330
[59] Shaywitz SE, Shaywitz BA, Pugh KR, Fulbright RK, Constable RT, Mencl WE, Shankweiler DP, Liberman AM, Skudlarski P, Fletcher JM (1998) Functional disruption in the organisation of the brain for reading in dyslexia. Proc Natl Acad Sci USA 95: 2636-2641
[60] Shilyansky C, Karlsgodt KH, Cummings DM, Sidiropoulou K, Hardt M, James AS, Ehninger D, Bearden CE, Poirazi P, Jentsch JD, Cannon TD, Levine MS, Silva AJ (2010a) Neurofibromin regulates corticostriatal inhibitory networks during working memory performance. Proc Natl Acad Sci USA 107: 13141-13146
[61] Shilyansky C, Lee YS, Silva AJ (2010b) Molecular and cellular mechanisms of learning disabilities: a focus on NF1. Annu Rev Neurosci 33: 221-243
[62] Silva AJ, Frankland PW, Marowitz Z, Friedman E, Laszlo GS, Cioffi D, Jacks T, Bourtchuladze R (1997) A mouse model for the learning and memory deficits associated with neurofibromatosis type I. Nat Genet 15: 281-284
[63] Taffe MA, Weed MR, Gutierrez T, Davis SA, Gold LH (2002) Differential muscarinic and MD contributions to visor-spatial paired-associate learning in rhesus monkeys. Psychopharmacology (Berl) 160: 253-262
[64] Thompson HL, Viskochil D, Stevemson DA, Chapman KL (2010) Speech-language characteristics of children with neurofibromatosis type 1. J Med Genet 152A: 284-290
[65] Ullrich NJ, Ayr L, Leaffer E, Irons MB, Rey-Casserly C (2010) Pilot study of a novel computerised task to assess spatial learning in children and adolescents with neurofibromatosis type 1. J Child Neurol 2010: 1195-1202
[66] Wang PY, Kaufmann WE, Koth CW, Denckla MB, Barker PB (2000) Thalamic involvement in neurofibromatosis type 1: evaluation with proton MR spectroscopic imaging. Ann Neurol 47: 477-484
[67] Watt SE, Shores A, North K (2008) An examination of lexical and sublexical reading skills in children with neurofibromatosis type 1. Child Neuropsychol 14: 401-418
[68] Zoller ME, Rembeck B, Backman L (1997) Neuropsychological deficits in adults with neurofibromatosis type 1. Acta Neurol Scand 95: 225-232

第6章 单卵双胞胎中1型神经纤维瘤病的临床表现

Clinical Expression of NF1 in Monozygotic Twins

Elizabeth K. Schorry and Emily Sites

6.1 双胞胎研究的历史应用

单卵双胞胎（monozygotic，MZ）指的是受精卵或胚泡分裂成两部分，产生2名基因组（理论上）相同的个体。在所有族群中，单卵双胞胎的自然发生率约为1/260（Machin 2009）。双胞胎研究历来是研究遗传疾病的重要工具。早期的研究假设单卵双胞胎在基因上是完全相同的，任何表型差异都与环境因素有关。因此，通过研究在不同环境下成长的单卵双胞胎，科学家试图理解遗传与环境的相对作用。通过比较单卵双胞胎和双卵双胞胎（dizygotic，DZ）的性状一致性，许多性状的遗传率得以确定。早期研究通常通过胎膜来判断双胞胎的卵性（认为共羊膜囊、共绒毛膜的胎膜代表单卵双胞胎），但后来发现胎膜并不能准确预测双卵性。如今，大多数研究使用高度可变的微卫星标记来确定卵性，若在15个多态性标记中具有相同特征，即可认为单卵性概率超过98%（Frankel et al. 1996）。

6.2 MZ在基因上并非如以前假设的那样完全相同

每个拥有单卵双胞胎的家庭都知道，虽然他们在很多方面表型相似，但总有一些细微差异使得亲近他们的人可以轻松辨别。文献回顾表明，单卵双胞胎之间可能存在显著的表型差异，例如，由于双胎输血综合征或一方获得的干细胞数量多于另一方导致的大小差异。单卵双胞胎常常在重大先天畸形方面存在不一致性，例如先天性心脏病（Machin 2009）。许多具有多因素病因的性状，如神经管缺陷、精神分裂症、双相情感障碍、帕金森病和多发性硬化症，可能在单卵双胞胎中表现为一致或不一致（Bruder et al. 2008；Petronis et al. 2003）。

随着我们对基因组和表观基因组理解的加深，越来越多的证据表明，单卵双胞胎可能在基因和表观基因上存在显著差异。受精后非整倍性分离事件和受精后突变可能导致单卵双胞胎在三倍体或单基因疾病方面的不一致。携带线粒体DNA突变的异

E. K. Schorry
Division of Human Genetics, Cincinnati Children's Hospital Medical Center, Cincinnati, OH, USA
e-mail: elizabeth.schorry@cchmc.org

E. Sites
Children's Memorial Hospital, Chicago, IL, USA

M. Upadhyaya and D. N. Cooper (eds.), *Neurofibromatosis Type 1*,
DOI 10.1007/978-3-642-32864-0_6, # Springer-Verlag Berlin Heidelberg 2012

质性单卵双胞胎可能在线粒体疾病如 Leber 遗传性视神经病方面表现出差异(Biousse et al. 1997)。X 染色体失活和基因印记在单卵双胞胎中也可能存在差异,最著名的例子是单卵双胞胎对 Beckwith - Wiedemann 综合征的差异性表现(Smith et al. 2006)。据估计,多达 10% 的单卵双胞胎在拷贝数变异(copy-number variations,CNV)方面可能存在差异,尽管这一现象的实际意义尚不明确(Bruder et al. 2008)。

6.3 NF1 双胞胎中的研究

双胞胎研究在理解 1 型神经纤维瘤病(NF1)的复杂性方面也具有重要价值。尽管 NF1 基因的突变几乎具有完全的外显率,但其表达却极为多样,从轻度皮肤表现到危及生命的恶性肿瘤并发症不等。NF1 在家族内外均表现出显著的变异性,这使得预测哪些患者有严重并发症的风险以及如何恰当地管理高风险患者变得极为困难。NF1 的基因型-表型相关性有限,目前仅有的例子包括全基因缺失患者表现出的更严重表型(Kayes et al. 1994),以及与第 17 外显子内框缺失相关的不含神经纤维瘤的轻度表型(Upadhyaya et al. 2007)。这种缺乏明确的基因型-表型相关性使得我们意识到,大多数疾病的变异性并不是由特定的 NF1 胚系突变所决定的。

为了解释 NF1 表达的变异性,已提出多种机制,包括胚系修饰基因、二次打击体细胞突变事件、环境因素、表观遗传修饰或受精后突变(Rieley et al. 2011)。多种与 NF1 相关的肿瘤类型中,二次打击事件已被充分证实(Upadhyaya et al. 2009),但对其他特定因素修饰 NF1 表型的证据仍然有限。研究那些具有 NF1 的单卵双胞胎——这些双胞胎的胚系修饰基因和 NF1 突变在理论上应该是相同的——可以成为确定 NF1 特征受 NF1 突变、种系修饰基因或受精后变化影响的重要工具。

至少有 45 篇医学文献是关于 NF1 单卵双胞胎的病例报告(表 6.1)。这些双胞胎的年龄从 6 岁到 43 岁不等,主要为儿童或青年人。Rieley 等(2011)报道的最大系列研究包括 9 对单卵双胞胎和 1 组单卵三胞胎,来自 1 100 名患者群体。他们注意到,这一患者群体中的单卵双胞胎发生率(1/110)显著高于普通人群中的 1/260,并提出 Ras 在早期受精卵中的激活可能增加了单卵双胞胎的发生概率。另一项大型研究由 Easton 等(1993)进行,报告了 6 对双胞胎及 175 名家族成员,并指出随着与探针距离的增加,NF1 特征的变异性也增加,表明修饰基因在 NF1 的表型变异中起到了一定作用。近期的一项研究(Sabbagh et al. 2009)对 750 名 NF1 患者进行了研究,其中包括 6 对单卵双胞胎,也强烈暗示了遗传修饰因子的存在。Harder 等(2010)报告了 8 对 NF1 双胞胎,发现他们在各种特征上存在一致性和不一致性。此外,已报道的 NF1 双胞胎性别比例也表现出偏差,在 31 对报告性别的双胞胎中,女性与男性的比例为 2:1。这与普通人群中单卵双胞胎女性占优的现象相似,可能与女性双胞胎生存率较高或其他尚未确定的因素有关(Machin 2009)。

表 6.1 文献中 41 对 NF1 双胞胎的表型一致性

特 征	一致对数	不一致对数	报 告 者
咖啡牛奶斑数量	24	4	A, F, J, O, P, Q, R
皮肤型神经纤维瘤数量	9	5	A, O, P, R
存在丛状神经纤维瘤	7	13	A, H, I, J, K, O, P, Q, R
MPNST	1	2	J, P, Q
视神经胶质瘤	4	11	A, B, C, D, E, F, G, P, R
学习障碍	7	0	K, M, O, P

续 表

特　　征	一致对数	不一致对数	报　告　者
语言障碍	9	0	P
ADHD	6	0	P, Q
Chiari Ⅰ 畸形	1	0	P
导水管狭窄	1	0	B
Dandy-Walker 畸形	1	0	M
脊柱侧凸	4	8	A, O, P, R
假关节	0	1	N, Q
漏斗胸	4	3	P, Q
癫痫	2	0	A

注：MPNST，恶性周围神经鞘膜瘤；ADHD，注意力缺陷/多动障碍。
作者：A=Easton et al. (1993)，B=Pascual-Castroviejo et al. (1988)，C=Cartwright (1982)，D=Crawford and Buckler (1983)，E=Kelly et al. (1998)，F=Vaughn et al. (1981)，G=Tubridy et al. (2001)，H=Lubinsky (2006)，I=Payne et al. (2003)，J=Akesson et al. (1983)，K=Bauer et al. (1988)，L=M=Koul et al. (2000)，N=Craigen and Clarke (1995)，O=Sabbagh et al. (2009)，P=Rieley et al. (2011)，Q=Melean et al. (2010)，R=Harder et al. (2010)。

除上述 4 项较大的系列研究外，大多数关于 NF1 单卵双胞胎的报告都是个案报告，讨论了双胞胎对 NF1 性状的一致性或不一致性。最极端的例子是那些在临床诊断 NF1 方面表现出表型不一致的单卵双胞胎。有 2 篇报告描述了这种情况，这两对双胞胎的单卵性通过微卫星标记测试得到了确认。Vogt 等(2011)报告了一对不一致的单卵双胞胎，其中受影响的双胞胎在 NF1 中有 30%~40% 的无义突变嵌合，而未受影响的双胞胎未检测到突变；他们推测 NF1 的突变发生在胚泡阶段，也就是双胞胎分裂之后。另外 1 个病例中，1 名被诊断为 NF1 的双胞胎在测试的 3 种细胞类型中均发现了致病性 NF1 突变，而临床上未受影响的双胞胎表现为相同突变的嵌合体(Kaplan et al. 2010)。

尽管在选择发表哪些双胞胎病例时可能存在一定的偏差，但总体来看，这些多组双胞胎的数据可以为我们进一步理解特定 NF1 性状的遗传控制提供见解。

6.3.1　皮肤特征

在多项关于 NF1 双胞胎的研究中，研究者对皮肤特征进行了详细的评估，例如咖啡牛奶斑(café-au-lait, CAL)的数量、皮肤皱褶处的雀斑以及皮肤型神经纤维瘤的存在与否(Rieley et al. 2011；Easton et al. 1993；Sabbagh et al. 2009；Harder et al. 2010)。尽管这些皮肤表现是 NF1 患者中的常见特征，并且与年龄密切相关，但这些研究均发现，双胞胎间咖啡牛奶斑和皮肤型神经纤维瘤的数量总体上保持高度一致，但在具体部位上则没有显著的规律性。相对而言，随着基因距离的增加，兄弟姐妹和其他亲属在这些特征上的一致性显著降低，支持了除 NF1 基因突变外还存在其他强大的遗传成分的假设(Sabbagh et al. 2009)。然而，需谨慎解读皮肤型神经纤维瘤的数量，因为许多研究对象是儿童或年轻人，他们的这类年龄相关特征的数量通常较少。

6.3.2　肿瘤

在 NF1 同卵双胞胎中，肿瘤表现出的共病率显著低于其他特征。由于大多数 NF1 相关的肿瘤需要 NF1 等位基因的"第二次打击"，这种偶发的第二次打击能够解释同卵双胞胎中肿瘤表现的显著差异。丛状神经纤维瘤一般是先天性的,或者在出生后几年显现,其存在与具体部位上的一致性显著较低。然而,目前收集到的关于丛状神经纤维瘤的数据有限。最新研究通过全身 MRI 显示,超过 50% 的 NF1 儿童存在丛状神经纤维瘤,其中许多在外部无法察觉(Nguyen et al. 2011)。现有的双胞胎研究并未对其进行全身 MRI 扫描,因此很多双胞胎对丛状神经纤维瘤的检测不完整,更有可能报道症状性或外部可见的丛状神经纤维瘤。一项研究(Rieley et al. 2011)指出,有双胞胎在脊旁神经纤维瘤的广泛累及方面表现出高度一致,表明可能存在影响多个脊旁肿瘤发生的遗传因素。

视神经通路胶质瘤(optic pathway glioma,OPG)约在 15% 的 NF1 儿童中发生,在大多数病例中无症状。截至目前,文献中报告的 NF1 双胞胎中,有 4 对在视神经胶质瘤的存在上表现出一致性,而 11 对双胞胎仅有 1 人受累(Easton et al. 1993;Cartwright 1982;Crawford and Buckler 1983;Pascual-Castroviejo et al. 1988;Kelly et al. 1998;Harder et al. 2010;Rieley et al. 2011)。尽管可能存在选择性发表的偏倚,但目前看来,OPG 的发生更可能与偶发性或非生殖系修饰因素有关。

6.3.3 恶性肿瘤

恶性周围神经鞘膜瘤(malignant peripheral nerve sheath tumor,MPNST)是 NF1 患者中 8%～13% 会发生的恶性肿瘤,主要来源于丛状神经纤维瘤(Evans et al. 2002)。至今仅有 3 对同卵 NF1 双胞胎被报道过 MPNST,其中 2 对在是否患病上表现出不一致,1 对表现出一致性。Akesson 等(1983)报道了 1 对双胞胎,其中 1 人腿部发展为 MPNST;另外 1 项研究组报道了青春期双胞胎,均有广泛的脊旁神经纤维瘤,但仅有 1 人发展为 MPNST(Rieley et al. 2011)。有趣的是,1 对同卵双胞胎在相似年龄(22 岁和 24 岁)及相同解剖部位(左侧坐骨神经)同时发展为 MPNST(Melean et al. 2010)。上述双胞胎中均未发现 NF1 全基因缺失。由于 NF1 中的恶性肿瘤已知需要 NF1 的双等位基因失活及其他基因(如 TP53、RB1 和 CDKN2A)的共同遗传改变(Spurlock et al. 2010),因此同卵双胞胎在相同身体部位发展出第二次突变的情况确实令人惊讶。研究者推测,丛状神经纤维瘤向 MPNST 转化的过程可能受其他遗传因素影响,而不仅仅是 NF1 突变。

同样,如果存在增加多发性大丛状神经纤维瘤风险的生殖系遗传因素,这些因素也可能直接增加 MPNST 的风险。然而,由于恶性肿瘤的双胞胎样本量仅为 3 对,未来需要进一步收集数据以确定 NF1 同卵双胞胎中恶性肿瘤的共病率。

6.3.4 学习障碍和认知

在大多数报道的双胞胎研究中,均提及了学习障碍和注意力缺陷/多动障碍(attention deficit/hyperactivity disorder,ADHD)等特征。然而,多数情况下并没有正式的神经心理学测试结果。Rieley 等(2011)报告了 10 对双胞胎中,有 4 对在学习障碍(learning disabilities,LD)的存在上表现出一致性,尽管 LD 的类型和影响程度有所不同。另有 4 对年龄较大、适合进行测试的双胞胎表现出一致性,均未出现学习障碍。在 3 对有正式智商测试分数的双胞胎中,没有 1 对的分数差异超过 10 分。

ADHD 的存在与否在 NF1 双胞胎中也表现出高度一致性,没有一对双胞胎在 ADHD 的诊断上存在差异(表 6.1)(Rieley et al. 2011;Melean et al. 2010)。这种在认知和 ADHD 方面的高度一致性,说明这些特征具有强大的遗传成分,这在正常人群中也得到了充分证明。事实上,考虑到双胞胎相关的多种环境因素,包括早产、出生窒息和双胞胎输血综合征的影响,NF1 双胞胎在认知方面表现出如此高的一致性令人意外。

6.3.5 中枢神经系统表现

中枢神经系统的结构性畸形,如 Chiari 畸形、Dandy-Walker 畸形(Dandy-Walker malformation,DWM)和导水管狭窄(aqueductal stenosis,AS),在 NF1 中较为罕见,但其发生率明显高于一般人群。已报道的双胞胎中,有 1 对双胞胎分别出现了这些畸形,且 MRI 显示出的表现非常相似(Rieley et al. 2011;Koul et al. 2000;Pascual-Castroviejo et al. 1988),表明这些畸形受强大的遗传因素影响。这与已知的遗传因素和非NF1人群中这些畸形的家族性病例一致（Schanker et al. 2011；Jalali et al. 2008；Haverkamp et al. 1999）。非综合征性DWM或AS的兄弟姐妹复发风险在一般人群中约为5%（Murray et al. 1985；Burton 1979）。

6.3.6 骨科表现

NF1的骨骼表现是非常有趣的特征，但其潜在的病理生理机制尚未得到充分理解。长骨发育不良发生在3%~5%的NF1患者中，仅有2对同卵双胞胎报道过此现象，且这2对双胞胎在此特征上表现出不一致（Craigen and Clarke 1995；Melean et al. 2010）。考虑到这种病变的罕见性和通常为单侧发生，以及近期数据表明第二次打击在一些假关节组织中有所记录（Stevenson et al. 2006），双胞胎的不一致性进一步支持了长骨发育不良/假关节可能是由偶发的非遗传性事件所触发的观点。

NF1中的脊柱侧凸也很复杂；15%~30%的NF1患者会发生脊柱侧凸，呈现出营养不良型（伴有营养不良的骨骼变化和急剧弯曲的曲线）或非营养不良型（类似于特发性脊柱侧凸的S形曲线）（Crawford and Schorry 1999）。由于一般人群中的特发性脊柱侧凸具有很强的遗传成分（Miller, 2007），可以合理推测NF1中的脊柱侧凸也可能具有遗传成分，并可能受到修饰基因的影响。在同卵双胞胎NF1患者中，已有4对被报告为脊柱侧凸一致，8对表现为不一致（Easton et al. 1993；Sabbagh et al. 2009；Harder et al. 2010；Rieley et al. 2011）。然而，值得注意的是，即使在一致的双胞胎中，曲度、营养不良特征的存在与否以及是否需要手术等方面仍存在差异。这表明在NF1中的脊柱侧凸病程中，既存在遗传性因素，也有非遗传性因素的贡献。可以推测，NF1中的非营养不良性脊柱侧凸可能具有遗传倾向，而发展为营养不良性曲线则可能需要非遗传性事件，如邻近肿瘤或局部骨细胞中的第二次打击遗传事件（Rieley et al. 2011）。

最后一个评估的骨骼特征是胸廓畸形。此特征同样表现出混合的一致性和不一致性，有4对被报道为一致性，3对表现为不一致性（Rieley et al. 2011；Melean et al. 2010）。值得关注的是，有一对同卵双胞胎表现为"镜像对称"，一人患有漏斗胸，另一人则患有鸡胸（Rieley et al. 2011）。胸廓畸形在NF1中的发生率可能被低估了，因为检查显示多达50%的患者可能存在轻度胸壁畸形（Riccardi 1999；Stevenson and Yang 2011）。因此，尽管胸廓畸形的发展受遗传性和非遗传性因素的共同影响，但在经过更仔细的双胞胎胸部检查后，仍需重新评估胸廓畸形的一致性数据。

6.4 新方向

近年来的研究开始探索NF1双胞胎中表观遗传和线粒体差异，以尝试解释其表型差异。Detjen等（2007）通过全线粒体基因组测序，研究了线粒体DNA（mitochondrial DNA，mtDNA）差异是否能解释NF1同卵双胞胎中表现不一致的原因。他们选取了4对在NF1并发症上表现不一致的同卵双胞胎，结果显示，这些双胞胎之间的mtDNA序列差异或异质性并无显著差别，从而排除了mtDNA差异作为双胞胎表型不一致的解释。

另外1种近期提出的可能解释同卵双胞胎之间表型差异的机制是NF1启动子甲基化的差异。已有研究表明，启动子甲基化可以通过荧光素酶实验改变NF1的表达，且甲基化程度与基因表达呈负相关（Zou et al. 2004）。Harder等（2010）提出，启动子甲基化的变化可能调控野生型NF1等位基因的剩余活性，从而影响表型表现。他们在8对同卵双胞胎的淋巴细胞中测量了NF1启动子的甲基化情况，这些双胞胎在NF1特征上的一致性和不一致性有所不同。研究发现，在多个位点上，包括5′UTR，双胞胎间存在显著的甲基化差异。在某个与转录因子结合位点重叠的位点上，甲基化水平的增加与视神经通路胶质瘤（OPG）的发生相关，无论是在双胞胎内部还是双胞胎之间都呈现出一致性。症状性OPG的双胞胎在该区域的甲基化水平高于无OPG的双胞胎。由于样本量较小，无法得出其他疾病表现的统计学显著性结论。因此，需进一步研究包括更多组织类型的数据，以更好地理解NF1启动子甲基化与表型变异之间的关系。

6.5 我们从 NF1 双胞胎中学到了什么

研究 NF1 同卵双胞胎是探索这种复杂疾病的变异表达原因的重要工具。尽管在生殖系 DNA 上是相同的，但同卵双胞胎实际上从来不会真正"完全相同"。其表型差异可能极为显著，例如由于双胞胎形成后发生的体细胞突变，导致 NF1 诊断的完全不一致。多项研究表明，同卵双胞胎在咖啡牛奶斑数量和皮肤型神经纤维瘤等特征上远比同一家族中的其他较远亲属更为相似，这提示生殖系修饰基因在调控这些特征方面起着重要作用。学习障碍、注意力缺陷多动障碍（ADHD）和语言障碍在同卵双胞胎中表现出高度一致性，再次表明生殖系基因在其中发挥了主要作用。

有价值的教训之一来自双胞胎间表型不一致的特征。大多数肿瘤，包括视神经胶质瘤（OPG）和恶性周围神经鞘膜瘤（MPNST），都属于这种情况，这与这些肿瘤中已知发生的偶发性"第二次打击"事件相一致。丛状神经纤维瘤的分析更为复杂，因为并非所有研究都完全检测了这类肿瘤。除少数例外，丛状神经纤维瘤在双胞胎中的一致性通常表现为发生在身体的不同部位。部分双胞胎在丛状神经纤维瘤的部位或肿瘤负担上表现出相似性，这引发了关于遗传修饰因子可能影响总体肿瘤负担的猜测。大多数营养不良性骨骼并发症，如营养不良性脊柱侧凸或胫骨假关节，在双胞胎中表现为不一致，提示非遗传性事件可能起作用；然而，在普通人群中已知的特发性脊柱侧凸和漏斗胸的遗传病因也可能对 NF1 患者中的这些特征产生影响。

双胞胎研究还提出了其他可能导致 NF1 基因表达差异的因素，包括表观遗传差异、NF1 启动子甲基化差异和受精后突变（包括 NF1 或其他基因）。

目前发表的 NF1 双胞胎研究存在一些局限性。首先，可能存在选择性偏倚，即作者更倾向于发表那些特征一致的双胞胎研究，而特征不一致的双胞胎则不太可能被发表。其次，样本量较小，获取大量同卵双胞胎 NF1 病例并不容易。最后，许多 NF1 特征具有年龄依赖性，这导致目前报告的相对年轻患者中未能完全确定某些 NF1 并发症（如肿瘤和恶性肿瘤）的发生。已报道的同卵双胞胎显然是 NF1 研究的宝贵资源，对这些双胞胎进行长期随访以及在这类人群中进行创新性研究，最终可能有助于揭示 NF1 的变异表达机制。

（余　旋　译）

参考文献

[1] Akesson HO, Axelsson R, Samuelsson B (1983) Neurofibromatosis in monozygotic twins: a case report. Acta Genet Med Gemellol 32(3-4): 245-249

[2] Bauer M, Lubs H, Lubs ML (1988) Variable expressivity of neurofibromatosis-1 in identical twins. Neurofibromatosis 1(5-6): 323-329

[3] Biousse V, Brown MD, Newman NJ, Allen JC, Rosenfeld J, Meola G, Wallace DC (1997) De novo 14484 mitochondrial DNA mutation in monozygotic twins discordant for Leber's hereditary optic neuropathy. Neurology 49: 1136-1138

[4] Bruder CE, Piotrowski A, Gijsbers AA, Andersson R, Erickson S, de Stahl TD, Menzel U, Sandgren J, von Tell D, Poplawski A et al (2008) Phenotypically concordant and discordant monozygotic twins display different DNA copy-number-variation profiles. Am J Hum Genet 82(3): 763-771

[5] Burton BK (1979) Recurrence risks for congenital hydrocephalus. Clin Genet 16: 47-53

[6] Cartwright SC (1982) Concordant optic glioma in a pair of monozygotic twins with neurofibromatosis. Clin Pediatr 21(4): 236-238

[7] Craigen MA, Clarke NM (1995) Familial congenital pseudarthrosis of the ulna. J Hand Surg 20(3): 331-332

[8] Crawford MJ, Buckler JM (1983) Optic gliomata affecting twins with neurofibromatosis. Dev Med Child Neurol 25(3): 370-373

[9] Crawford AH, Schorry EK (1999) Neurofibromatosis in children: the role of the orthopaedist. J Am Acad Orthop Surg 7(4): 217-230

[10] Detjen AK, Tinschert S, Kaufmann D, Algermissen B, Nurnberg P, Schuelke M (2007) Analysis of mitochondrial DNA in discordant monozygotic twins with neurofibromatosis type 1. Twin Res Hum Genet 10(3): 486-495

[11] Easton DF, Ponder MA, Huson SM, Ponder BA (1993) An analysis of variation in expression of neurofibromatosis (NF) type 1 (NF1): evidence for modifying genes. Am J Hum Genet 53(2): 305-313

[12] Evans DG, Baser ME, McGaughran J, Sharif S, Howard E, Moran A (2002) Malignant peripheral nerve sheath tumors in neurofibromatosis 1. J Med Genet 39: 311-314

[13] Frankel W, Chan A, Corringham RE, Shepherd S, Reardon A, Wang-Rodriguez J (1996) Detection of chimerism and early engraftment after allogeneic peripheral blood stem cell or bone marrow transplantation by short tandem repeats. Am J Hematol 52: 281-287

[14] Harder A, Titze S, Herbst L, Harder T, Guse K, Tinschert S, Kaufmann D, Rosenbaum T, Mautner VF, Windt E, Wahllander-Danek U, Wimmer K, Mundlos S, Peters H (2010) Monozygotic twins with Neurofibromatosis type 1 (NF1) display differences in methylation of NF1 gene promoter elements, 5′ untranslated region, exon and intron 1. Twin Res Hum Genet 13(6): 582-594

[15] Haverkamp F, Wölfle J, Aretz M, Krämer A, Höhmann B, Fahnenstich H, Zerres K (1999) Congenital hydrocephalus internus and aqueduct stenosis: aetiology and implications for genetic counselling. Eur J Pediatr 158(6): 474-478

[16] Jalali A, Aldinger KA, Chary A, McLone DG, Bowman RM, Le LC, Jardine P, Newbury-Ecob R, Mallick A, Jafari N, Russell EJ, Curran J, Nguyen P, Ouahchi K, Lee C, Dobyns WB, Millen KJ, Pina-Neto JM, Kessler JA, Bassuk AG (2008) Linkage to chromosome 2q36.1 in autosomal dominant Dandy-Walker malformation with occipital cephalocele and evidence for genetic heterogeneity. Hum Genet 123(3): 237-245

[17] Kaplan L, Foster R, Shen Y, Parry DM, McMaster ML, O'Leary MC, Gusella JF (2010) Monozygotic twins discordant for neurofibromatosis 1. Am J Med Genet A 152: 601-606

[18] Kayes LM, Burke W, Riccardi VM, Bennett R, Ehrlich P, Rubenstein A, Stephens K (1994) Deletions spanning the neurofibromatosis 1 gene: Identification and phenotype of five patients. Am J Hum Genet 54: 424-436

[19] Kelly TE, Sproul GT, Huerta MG, Rogol AD (1998) Discordant puberty in monozygotic twin sisters with neurofibromatosis type 1 (NF1). Clin Pediatr 37(5): 301-304

[20] Koul RL, Chacko A, Leven HO (2000) Dandy-Walker syndrome in association with neurofibromatosis in monozygotic twins. Saudi Med J 21(4): 390-392

[21] Lubinsky MS (2006) Non-random associations and vascular fields in neurofibromatosis 1: a pathogenetic hypothesis. Am J Med Genet A 140(19): 2080-2084

[22] Machin G (2009) Non-identical monozygotic twins, intermediate twin types, zygosity testing, and the non-random nature of monozygotic twinning: a review. Am J Med Genet 151C: 110-127

[23] Melean G, Hernandez AM, Valero MC, Hernandez-Imaz E, Martin Y, Hernandez-Chico C (2010) Monozygotic twins with neurofibromatosis type 1, concordant phenotype and synchronous development of MPNST and metastasis. BMC Cancer 10: 407

[24] Miller NH (2007) Genetics of familial idiopathic scoliosis. Clin Orthop Relat Res 462: 6-10

[25] Murray JC, Johnson JA, Bird TD (1985) Dandy-Walker malformation: etiologic heterogeneity and empiric recurrence risks. Clin Genet 28: 272-283

[26] Nguyen R, Kluwe L, Fuensterer C, Kentsch M, Friedrich RE, Mautner VF (2011) Plexiform neurofibromas in children with neurofibromatosis type 1: frequency and associated clinical deficits. J Pediatr 159(4): 652-655

[27] Pascual-Castroviejo I, Verdu A, Roman M, De la Cruz-Medina M, Villarejo F (1988) Optic glioma with progressive occlusion of the aqueduct of Sylvius in monozygotic twins with neurofibromatosis. Brain Dev 10(1): 24-29

[28] Payne MS, Nadell JM, Lacassie Y, Tilton AH (2003) Congenital glaucoma and neurofibromatosis in a monozygotic twin: case report and review of the literature. J Child Neurol 18(7): 504-508

[29] Petronis A, Gottesman II, Kan P, Kennedy JL, Basile VS, Paterson AD, Popendikyte V (2003) Monozygotic twins exhibit numerous epigenetic differences: clues to twin discordance? Schizophr Bull 29(1): 169-178

[30] Riccardi VM (1999) Neurofibromatosis: phenotype, natural history, and pathogenesis. Johns Hopkins University Press, Baltimore, pp ix, 250-ix, 273

[31] Rieley MB, Stevenson DA, Viskochil DH, Tinkle BT, Martin LJ, Schorry EK (2011) Variable expression of neurofibromatosis 1 in monozygotic twins. Am J Med Genet A 155: 478-485

[32] Sabbagh A, Pasmant E, Laurendeau I, Parfait B, Barbarot S, Guillot B, Combemale P, Ferkal S, Vidaud S, Aubourg P, Vidaud D, Wolkenstein P (2009) Unravelling the genetic basis of variable clinical expression in neurofibromatosis 1. Hum Mol Genet 18(15): 2768-2778

[33] Schanker BD, Walcott BP, Nahed BV, Kahle KT, Li YM, Coumans JV (2011) Familial Chiari malformation: case series. Neurosurg Focus 31(3): E1

[34] Spurlock G, Knight SJL, Thomas N, Kiehl T-R, Guha A, Upadhyaya M (2010) Molecular evolution of a neurofibroma to malignant peripheral nerve sheath tumor (MPNST) in an NF1 patient: correlation between histopathological, clinical and molecular findings. J Cancer Res Clin Oncol 136: 1869-1880

[35] Stevenson DA, Yang F-C (2011) The musculoskeletal phenotype of the RASopathies. Am J Med Genet C 157: 90-103

[36] Stevenson DA, Zhou H, Ashrafi S, Messiaen LM, Carey JC, D'Astous JL, Santora SD, Viskochil DH (2006) Double inactivation of NF1 in tibial pseudarthrosis. Am J Hum Genet 79(1): 143-148

[37] Smith AC, Rubin T, Shuman C, Estabrooks L, Aylsworth AS, McDonald MT, Steele L, Ray PN, Weksberg R (2006) New chromosome 11p15 epigenotypes identified in male monozygotic twins with Beckwith-Wiedemann syndrome. Cytogenet Genome Res 113(1-4): 313-317

[38] Tubridy N, Schon F, Moss A, Clarke A, Cox T, Ferner R (2001) Hippocampal involvement in identical twins with neurofibromatosis type 1. J Neurol Neurosurg Psychiatry 71(1): 131-132

[39] Upadhyaya M, Huson SM, Davies M, Thomas N, Chuzhanova N, Giovannini S, Evans DG, Howard E, Kerr B, Griffiths S et al (2007) An absence of cutaneous neurofibromas associated with a 3-bp inframe deletion in exon 17 of the NF1 gene (c.2970-2972 delAAT): evidence of a clinically significant NF1 genotype-phenotype correlation. Am J Hum Genet 80(1): 140-151

[40] Upadhyaya M, Spurlock G, Kluwe L, Chuzhanova N, Bennett E, Thomas N, Guha A, Mautner V (2009) The spectrum of somatic and germline NF1 mutations in NF1 patients with spinal neurofibromas. Neurogenetics 10: 251-263

[41] Vaughn AJ, Bachman D, Sommer A (1981) Neurofibromatosis in monozygotic twins: a case report of spontaneous mutation. Am J Med Genet 8(2): 155-158

[42] Vogt J, Kohlhase J, Morlot S, Kluwe L, Mautner V-F, Cooper DN, Kehrer-Sawatzki H (2011) Monozygotic twins discordant for neurofibromatosis type 1 due to a postzygotic NF1 gene mutation. Hum Mutat 32(6): E2134-E2147

[43] Zou MX, Butcher DT, Sadikovis B, Groves TC, Yee SP, Rodenhiser DI (2004) Characterization of functional elements in the neurofibromatosis (NF1) proximal promoter region. Oncogene 23: 330-339

第 7 章 全身 MRI 对 1 型神经纤维瘤病患者的价值
Value of Whole Body MRI in Patients with NF1
Victor-Felix Mautner

7.1 引言

1 型神经纤维瘤病的特点是几乎所有患者都会出现皮肤型神经纤维瘤,而约 30% 的患者可检测到可见的丛状神经纤维瘤(plexiform neurofibromas, PNF)(Huson et al. 1989)。这两种肿瘤类型都会严重影响患者容貌。皮肤型神经纤维瘤很少引起患者疼痛或功能障碍,而丛状神经纤维瘤则表现为浸润性生长模式,可能会导致 NF1 患者出现功能障碍(Mautner et al. 2006)。

外部 PNF 导致约 10% 的患者出现功能障碍,5% 的患者出现疼痛(Mautner et al. 2006)。然而,PNF 生长有可能发生在体内的任何神经结构上(Tonsgard et al. 1998)。内部丛状神经纤维瘤很少能通过体格检查发现。通过磁共振成像(magnetic resonance imaging, MRI)对单发丛状神经纤维瘤生长模式的分析表明,内部丛状神经纤维瘤是造成大多数患者神经功能障碍、解剖损伤和疼痛的原因(Mautner et al. 2006)。尽管已经开展了一些研究来调查单个 PNF 的自然史,但尚未对其进行过系统的评估(Dombi et al. 2007; Tucker et al. 2009)。

重要的是,PNF 也是恶性前病变,它有可能转化为恶性周围神经鞘膜瘤(malignant peripheral nerve sheath tumors, MPNST),这是造成 NF1 患者死亡的主要原因(Evans et al. 2002; Tucker et al. 2009; Duong et al. 2011)。一些 NF1 患者罹患 MPNST 的风险似乎高于其他患者,但用于区分高风险组和低风险组的危险因素尚未完全明确。

7.2 磁共振成像和估算全身肿瘤体积的方法

在 Mautner 等的研究中,自 2003 年以来一直遵循全身 MRI 方案对 NF1 患者进行临床影像评估。该方案提供了充足的数据,既能准确量化神经鞘瘤患者的肿瘤负荷,又能研究 NF1 肿瘤的内部生长。

全身方案采用了不同的 1.5 T 磁体和序列,使用或不使用静脉造影剂增强均可(Mautner et al. 2008)。受试者以仰卧姿势从头到膝关节,分四或五步成像(头部、胸部、腹部和腿部),这与手术台的最大活动范围和体型有关。使用 T1 和 T2 涡轮自旋回波序列以及带或不带频谱脂肪饱和的 T1 序列对头部进行对比增强成像。在轴向平面使用 T1 梯度回波序列和 T2 STIR(短 T1 反转恢复)技术对身体进行无对比增强成像。切片厚度为 5~10 mm,切片之间无跳跃。

V.-F. Mautner
Department of Neurology, University Medical Centre, Hamburg-Eppendorf, Martinistr. 52, 20246 Hamburg, Germany
e-mail: vmautner@uke.uni-hamburg.de

M. Upadhyaya and D. N. Cooper (eds.), *Neurofibromatosis Type 1*,
DOI 10.1007/978-3-642-32864-0_7, # Springer-Verlag Berlin Heidelberg 2012

磁共振成像分析由受过 NF1 相关肿瘤图像分析培训的医师进行。分析过程中读图者未获取患者的任何其他信息,对所有患者的疾病相关临床信息都不了解。PNF 的体积是用之前 MEDx 软件平台上描述的方法确定的(Dombi et al. 2007)。该方法基于以下信息。

(1) 对比度:即肿瘤(高信号强度)与周围组织(低信号强度)的对比强度。

(2) 强度梯度:定义病变的外部边界(边缘)。

(3) 病变的大小:丛状神经纤维瘤的大小通常很大,小的孤立的高信号强度区域可以忽略,因为它们对 PNF 总体积的影响不大。

这种自动体积分析方法灵敏度高(可检测到小至 10% 的体积变化)、可重复性好(变异系数为 0.6%~5.6%),其结果与人工肿瘤分割相似($R=0.999$)。当无法进行自动肿瘤体积测量时,会记录其原因,并使用 MEDx 软件绘图工具进行手动肿瘤分割以确定肿瘤体积,如前所述(Dombi et al. 2007)。使用这种方法,我们可以较准确地测量最大直径>3 cm 的 PNF。将所有 PNF(最大直径 3 cm)的体积相加,得出全身丛状神经纤维瘤的体积。体积分析忽略了最大直径<3 cm 的病变。

然而,全身 MRI 扫描的分辨率只能对脊柱神经纤维瘤进行有限的评估。当人工追踪可见时,脊柱神经纤维瘤按位置(颈椎、胸椎或腰椎)和大小进行分类。最大直径>3 cm 的脊柱神经纤维瘤的体积会自动计算,并计入 PNF 的总体积中。

7.3 神经纤维瘤病与恶性周围神经鞘膜瘤

NF1 患者罹患 MPNST 的风险比正常人群高出 100 倍(Walker et al. 2006)。据估计,NF1 患者终生罹患 MPNST 的风险为 10%~13%(Evans et al. 2002)。大多数 NF1 患者的 MPNST 都是在青春期或成年早期确诊的。致病基因突变为整个 NF1 基因缺失的 NF1 患者被认为有 16%~25% 的概率罹患 MPNST(DeRaedt et al. 2003)。其他可能与 NF1 患者罹患 MPNST 风险较高有关的因素包括:发生神经纤维瘤性神经病(Drouet et al. 2004; Ferner et al. 2004)、暴露于治疗性放射线(Evans et al. 2002)、以前发生过 MPNST(Ferner et al. 2004; Doorn et al. 1995)以及 NF1 患者的亲属发生过 MPNST(Dales et al. 1983; Poyhonen et al. 1997; Shearer et al. 1994)。

一项针对 464 名 NF1 患者的临床研究发现,MPNST 与皮下神经纤维瘤的存在有关(Tucker et al. 2005)。这一发现得到了 Sbidian 等的证实,他们开发了一种评分方法,可以预测内部肿瘤负荷(Sbidian et al. 2011)。

7.4 相关研究

许多全身 MRI 研究正逐步开展,以探究儿童和成人 PNF 的性质,并调查是否有任何预测方法可识别出有患 MPNST 风险的患者。识别具有恶变高风险的 NF1 患者至关重要,手术切除是目前治疗 MPNST、改善患者预后的唯一方法,若不能尽早诊断 MPNST,会错过手术切除的最佳时机,导致手术无法完全切除恶性病灶,极大地影响患者的生存率。

- NF1 儿童和青少年的全身肿瘤负荷。
- NF1 患者的全身肿瘤负荷。
- *NF1* 基因大片段或微缺失患者的全身肿瘤负荷。

65 名年龄在 1.7 岁至 17.6 岁之间的儿童在常规临床护理中接受了持续、定期的临床检查和全身 MRI 检查。在 65 名儿童中,37 名(57%)儿童共发现了 73 个 PNF,其中 20 名(31%)儿童患有 1 个以上的肿瘤。大多数 PNF 在腿部(23/73),其次是胸部(18/73)和脊柱旁(14/73)。在总共 73 个肿瘤中,18 个 PNF 有症状(25%),且不同身体部位有症状和无症状肿瘤的比例各不相同。头颈部的 11 个肿瘤中有 7 个有症状,而腹部的 11 个肿瘤中却没有 1 个有症状。在 37 名 PNF 儿童患者中,有 17 名(46%)出现了与肿瘤相关的并发症,如运动或神经系统并发症和(或)疼痛。值得注意的是,这些数字可能低于真正的肿瘤负荷,因为直径<3 cm 的病变无法通过 MRI 诊断为 PNF。

在这项针对儿童的试点研究中,PNF 的检出率非常高(57%),从而证实了体内生长的 PNF 是儿童和青少年患者都存在的一个特征。PNF 的儿童有可能发展成神经系统缺陷、器官功能障碍、疼痛和骨骼异常。对儿童进行全身 MRI 检查可以筛查出体内有 PNF 生长的个体,因此需要定期监测肿瘤的生长和发展情况。

肿瘤的大小和位置是预测潜在并发症的重要因素。一方面,较大的 PNF 通常比较小的 PNF 有更高的并发症风险。另一方面,某些身体区域更容易出现并发症,例如睑区。这些身体区域对小肿瘤也很敏感。

PNF 患儿的中位年龄为 11.5 岁。按年龄中位数划分,19 名年龄较小的患儿中有 7 名(37%)出现 PNF 相关症状,18 名年龄较大的患儿中有 10 名(56%)出现 PNF 相关症状。PNF 在年龄较大的儿童中更易导致缺陷,但这一差异在统计学上并不显著($P=0.25$)。

两项针对单个 PNF 生长的研究发现,生长与年龄呈反向相关,但这些研究在方法上存在局限性(Dombi et al. 2007;Tucker et al. 2009)。在首次检查中,约 60% 的患儿有体内肿瘤表现。在对成人和儿童的持续随访中,首次发现 50% 的成人有 PNF,与本文所述研究中 57% 的 NF1 儿童相似。这些数据表明,初次检查时未发现体内肿瘤的患者,日后不太可能出现新的肿瘤。因此,初次就诊时没有内部肿瘤负担的儿童可能属于低风险人群,不会出现与 PNF 相关的缺陷或发展为 MPNST。从这个意义上说,研究结果表明,全身 MRI 有可能成为 NF1 患者终身疾病严重程度的预后标志(Nguyen et al. 2011)。

7.5 肿瘤负担与 MPNST

为了全面评估体内神经纤维瘤与 MPNST 之间的关系,研究人员对 13 名 MPNST 的 NF1 患者和 26 名年龄和性别匹配的 NF1 但无 MPNST 的对照者进行了全身 MRI 检查。

研究显示,MPNST 的 NF1 患者与对照组的皮肤型神经纤维瘤和外部 PNF 数量相似,但 MPNST 的 NF1 患者皮下神经纤维瘤的中位数明显多于对照组。然而,体内 PNF 的存在、可测量的体内 PNF 的中位数,以及全身磁共振成像上内部神经纤维瘤的总体积,在患有多发性骨髓营养不良症的 NF1 患者与未患有多发性骨髓营养不良症的患者之间并无显著差异。

许多罹患 MPNST 的 NF1 患者年龄非常小(Friedrich et al. 2007;Rasmussen et al. 2001):本研究中,罹患 MPNST 的 NF1 患者的中位年龄仅为 30 岁。相比之下,非 NF1 患者确诊 MPNST 的中位年龄为 62 岁(Evans et al. 2002)。NF1 患者的 PNF 快速增长可能发生在儿童身上,但在成人身上并不常见(Friedmann and Riccard 1999;Riccardi 2007),因此我们考虑的是,在全身 MRI 上看到的 PNF 负担是否可能与较年轻的 NF1 患者发生 MPNST 有关。因此,我们将年龄小于本研究中位数(30 岁)、有 MPNST 的 NF1 患者与年龄<30 岁、无 MPNST 的 NF1 对照组进行了比较。所有 6 名年龄<30 岁的有 MPNST 的 NF1 患者都有全身 MRI 显示的体内 PNF,这些患者的中位数和中位体积都明显大于年龄<30 岁的 NF1 对照组。有多发性骨髓营养不良的 NF1 患者与年龄>30 岁的无多发性骨髓营养不良的对照组在全身 MRI 结果上没有明显差异。这可能是由于这组患者中出现 MPNST 的患者仅表现为单个内部 PNF,而后转变为 MPNST,并通过手术切除。

因此,我们发现 NF1 患者皮下神经纤维瘤的中位数与 MPNST 的发生之间存在整体关联。相比之下,我们发现有 MPNST 的 NF1 患者与未有 MPNST 的匹配对照组在皮肤型神经纤维瘤或外部可见 PNF 的中位数上没有差异。我们的研究结果与 Tucker 等(2005)的研究结果相似,他们研究了 476 名法国 NF1 患者,其中 25 人患有 MPNST。他们发现,皮下神经纤维瘤的存在与 MPNST 的发生有关,但与表皮 PNF 的存在或皮肤型神经纤维瘤的数量无关。我们的研究结果也与同一研究者进行的一项队列研究相一致,在该研究中,皮下神经纤维瘤(而非皮肤型神经纤维瘤)与 NF1 成人患者较高的发病风险有关(Khosrotehrani et al. 2005)。

我们观察到的最显著的关联是年龄<30 岁的 NF1 相关 MPNST 患者与内部神经纤维瘤的存在、中位数和中位总体积之间的关联。尽管这一年轻亚

组中的 MPNST 患者人数较少，但这些具有统计学意义关联的出现却非常引人注目。不过，有必要对这些发现进行独立确认（Mautner et al. 2008）。

7.6 微缺失患者的全身磁共振成像

与正常 NF1 患者相比，大片段缺失患者罹患 MPNST 的风险也越来越高。此外，微缺失患者出现外部肿瘤负荷等相关疾病特征的频率增加（De Raedt et al. 2003；Mautner et al. 2010；Pasmant et al. 2010）。因此，我们探讨了内部肿瘤是否会导致大片段缺失 NF1 患者罹患 MPNST 的风险增加。

我们对 30 名大片段缺失的 NF1 患者进行了全身 MRI 检查（Kluwe et al. 2012）（不包括镶嵌型 NF1 缺失患者）。每名患者都与 3 名无大片段缺失的匹配患者（按性别和年龄）进行了比较。30 名缺失患者的肿瘤总体积高于 67 名非缺失患者（中位数：260 mL vs. 168 mL，几何平均数：211 mL vs. 125 mL）。然而，差异并不显著（$P=0.29$，曼-惠特尼 U 检验、双尾非配对 t 检验、假设方差相等）。我们甚至发现，NF1 缺失患者的肿瘤负荷更高的趋势并不明显。我们无法确定这是否是这些缺失患者中 MPNST 发生率较高的原因。与此相反，就个体而言，这可能是真实的，因为几名缺失患者表现出极高的内部肿瘤负荷（4 000～8 000 mL），这在非缺失患者中没有观察到。因此，就个体而言，高内部肿瘤负荷确实是某些缺失患者的特征。然而，作为一个群体，这些患者的内部肿瘤体积并不比没有大缺失的 NF1 患者普遍大。相比之下，镶嵌缺失患者体内肿瘤的频率和体积都很低。这些患者一般不需要进行强化随访检查（Kluwe et al. 2012）。

1 型神经纤维瘤病的特点是症状多样，临床症状的严重程度也各不相同。不同疾病表现的患者需要个性化的治疗策略。然而，迄今为止，NF1 患者微缺失的发生是疾病严重程度的唯一标志，因为这一人群的临床病程明显更严重。本文介绍了全身 MRI 研究的交叉序列数据，以证明这种方法是否可用作 NF1 内部肿瘤表现和发生 MPNST 的疾病严重程度的另一种标志物。

第一，通过全身 MRI 检查，我们可以确定 PNF 的发生频率以及与之相关的儿科临床缺陷。那些自出生起即在体内出现 PNF 的儿童和青少年患者需要定期接受 MRI 监测，以估计肿瘤生长情况和可能出现的并发症。与没有内部肿瘤的儿童相比，这些儿童将来有可能发展为 MPNST。首先，全身随访观察结果表明，无内部肿瘤的儿童在较长的随访期（长达 5 年）内不会出现内部肿瘤表现，但日后仍有罹患 MPNST 的风险。

第二，内部肿瘤负荷与 MPNST 的发生有关，尤其是在 30 岁以下的年龄组。此外，虽然皮肤型神经纤维瘤或外部可见 PNF 的中位数并不能反映 NF1 患者罹患 MPNST 的风险，但 NF1 患者皮下神经纤维瘤的数量与 MPNST 的发生明显相关。因此，出现多个皮下肿瘤的患者更应接受内部肿瘤负荷检查。对这些高危患者进行密切的临床监测和连续定期的 MRI 检查，以了解内部肿瘤的形态或生长变化。此外，PET-CT 可使 MPNST 得到更早的诊断和更有效的治疗。

约 56% 的 NF1 患者在全身 MRI 检查中出现内部肿瘤表现。需要进行随访调查，以确认内部肿瘤是否在年龄较大时停止生长，以及肿瘤的生长（以生长阈值计算）是否意味着从良性 PNF 转变为 MPNST。我们的初步全身随访观察结果表明，没有内部肿瘤的成年人今后不会再长出新的肿瘤，因此不属于这方面的高危患者。

第三，NF1 微缺失患者罹患 MPNST 的风险总体上明显较高；根据全身磁共振成像测量，只有内部肿瘤负荷较高的患者才有较高的"非显著"趋势。这可能是由于本研究调查的微缺失患者人数较少。不过，微缺失和内部肿瘤负荷患者需要更密切的临床和磁共振成像随访检查。

本章讨论的首批全身 MRI 研究目前还不能为在有内部肿瘤的 NF1 患者的常规治疗中使用 MRI 检查提供循证建议。不过，全身 MRI 可用作 NF1 风险组的潜在预后分层指标，以评估内部肿瘤负担和这些肿瘤向 MPNST 恶变的概率。要评估这种方法在临床治疗中的潜在价值，还需要进一步进行纵向研究。

（刘珺，黄景宣　译）

参考文献

[1] Dales RL, McEver VW 3rd, Quispe G, Davies RS (1983) Update on biologic behavior and surgical implications of neurofibromatosis and neurofibrosarcoma. Surg Gynecol Obstet 156(5): 636-640

[2] De Raedt T, Brems H, Wolkenstein P, Vidaud D, Pilotti S, Perrone F, Mautner V, Frahm S, Sciot R, Legius E (2003) Elevated risk for MPNST in NF1 microdeletion patients. Am J Hum Genet 72(5): 1288-1292

[3] Dombi E, Solomon J, Gillespie AJ, Fox E, Balis FM, Patronas N, Korf BR, Babovic-Vuksanovic D, Packer RJ, Belasco J, Goldman S, Jakacki R, Kieran M, Steinberg SM, Widemann BC (2007) NF1 plexiform neurofibroma growth rate by volumetric MRI: relationship to age and body weight. Neurology 68(9): 643-647

[4] Doorn PF, Molenaar WM, Buter J, Hoekstra HJ (1995) Malignant peripheral nerve sheath tumors in patients with and without neurofibromatosis. Eur J Surg Oncol 21(1): 78-82

[5] Drouet A, Wolkenstein P, Lefaucheur JP, Pinson S, Combemale P, Gherardi RK, Brugières P, Salama J, Ehre P, Decq P, Créange A (2004) Neurofibromatosis 1-associated neuropathies: a reappraisal. Brain 127(Pt 9): 1993-2009

[6] Duong TA, Sbidian E, Valeyrie-Allanore L, Vialette C, Ferkal S, Hadj-Rabia S, Glorion C, Lyonnet S, Zerah M, Kemlin I, Rodriguez D, Bastuji-Garin S, Wolkenstein P (2011) Mortality associated with neurofibromatosis 1: a cohort study of 1895 patients in 1980-2006 in France. Orphanet J Rare Dis 6: 18

[7] Evans DG, Baser ME, McGaughran J, Sharif S, Howard E, Moran A (2002) Malignant peripheral nerve sheath tumours in neurofibromatosis 1. J Med Genet 39(5): 311-314

[8] Ferner RE, Hughes RA, Hall SM, Upadhyaya M, Johnson MR (2004) Neurofibromatous neuropathy in neurofibromatosis 1 (NF1). J Med Genet 41(11): 837-841

[9] Friedmann JM, Riccard VM (1999) Clinical and epidemiological features. In: Friedman JM, Gutmann DH, MacCollin M, Riccardi VM (eds) Neurofibromatosis: phenotype, natural history and pathogenesis, 3rd edn. John Hopkins University Press, Baltimore, MD, pp 29-86

[10] Friedrich RE, Hartmann M, Mautner VF (2007) Malignant peripheral nerve sheath tumors (MPNST) in NF1-affected children. Anticancer Res 27(4A): 1957-1960

[11] Huson SM, Compston DA, Harper PS (1989) A genetic study of von Recklinghausen neurofibromatosis in south east Wales. II. Guidelines for genetic counselling. J Med Genet 26(11): 712-721

[12] Khosrotehrani K, Bastuji-Garin S, Riccardi VM, Birch P, Friedman JM, Wolkenstein P (2005) Subcutaneous neurofibromas are associated with mortality in neurofibromatosis 1: a cohort study of 703 patients. Am J Med Genet A 132A(1): 49-53

[13] Kluwe L, Nguyen R, Vogt J, Bengesser K, Mussotter T, Friedrich RE, Jett K, Kehrer-Sawatzki H, Mautner VF (2012) Internal tumor burden in neurofibromatosis type 1 patients with large NF1 deletions. Genes Chromosomes Cancer 51(5): 447-451

[14] Mautner VF, Hartmann M, Kluwe L, Friedrich RE, Fünsterer C (2006) MRI growth patterns of plexiform neurofibromas in patients with neurofibromatosis type 1. Neuroradiology 48(3): 160-165

[15] Mautner VF, Asuagbor FA, Dombi E, Fünsterer C, Kluwe L, Wenzel R, Widemann BC, Friedman JM (2008) Assessment of benign tumor burden by whole-body MRI in patients with neurofibromatosis 1. Neuro Oncol 10(4): 593-598

[16] Mautner VF, Kluwe L, Friedrich RE, Roehl AC, Bammert S, Högel J, Spöri H, Cooper DN, Kehrer-Sawatzki H (2010) Clinical characterisation of 29 neurofibromatosis type-1 patients with molecularly ascertained 1.4 Mb type-1 NF1 deletions. J Med Genet 47: 623-630

[17] Nguyen R, Kluwe L, Fuensterer C, Kentsch M, Friedrich RE, Mautner VF (2011) Plexiform neurofibromas in children with neurofibromatosis type 1: frequency and associated deficits. J Pediatr 159(4): 652. e2

[18] Pasmant E, Sabbagh A, Spurlock G, Laurendeau I, Grillo E, Hamel MJ, Martin L, Barbarot S, Leheup B, Rodriguez D, Lacombe D, Dollfus H, Pasquier L, Isidor B, Ferkal S, Soulier J, Sanson M, Dieux-Coeslier A, Bièche I, Parfait B, Vidaud M, Wolkenstein P, Upadhyaya M, Vidaud D, Members of the NF France Network (2010) NF1 microdeletions in neurofibromatosis type 1: from genotype to phenotype. Hum Mutat 31(6): E1506-E1518

[19] Poyhonen M, Niemela S, Herva R (1997) Risk of malignancy and death in neurofibromatosis. Arch Pathol Lab Med 121(2): 139-143

[20] Rasmussen SA, Yang Q, Friedman JM (2001) Mortality in neurofibromatosis 1: an analysis using U.S. death certificates. Am J Hum Genet 68(5): 1110-1118

[21] Riccardi VM (2007) The genetic predisposition to and histogenesis of neurofibromas and neurofibrosarcoma in neurofibromatosis type 1. Neurosurg Focus 22(6): E3

[22] Sbidian E, Bastuji-Garin S, Valeyrie-Allanore L, Ferkal S, Lefaucheur JP, Drouet A, Brugiere P, Vialette C, Combemale P, Barabarot S, Wolkenstein P (2011) At-risk phenotype of Neurofibromatose-1 patients: a multicentre case-control study. Orphanet J Rare Dis 6: 51

[23] Shearer P, Parham D, Kovnar E, Kun L, Rao B, Lobe T, Pratt C (1994) Neurofibromatosis type I and malignancy: review of 32 pediatric cases treated at a single institution. Med Pediatr Oncol 22(2): 78-83

[24] Tonsgard JH, Kwak SM, Short MP, Dachman AH (1998) CT imaging in adults with neurofibromatosis-1: frequent asymptomatic plexiform lesions. Neurology 50(6): 1755-1760

[25] Tucker T, Wolkenstein P, Revuz J, Zeller J, Friedman JM (2005) Association between benign and malignant peripheral nerve sheath tumors in NF1. Neurology 65(2): 205-211

[26] Tucker T, Friedman JM, Friedrich RE, Wenzel R, Fünsterer C, Mautner VF (2009) Longitudinal study of neurofibromatosis 1 associated plexiform neurofibromas. J Med Genet 46(2): 81-85

[27] Walker L, Thompson D, Easton D, Ponder B, Ponder M, Frayling I, Baralle D (2006) A prospective study of neurofibromatosis type 1 cancer incidence in the UK. Br J Cancer 95(2): 233-238

第8章 1型神经纤维瘤病患者的生命质量
Quality of Life in NF1
Patricia Birch and J. M. Friedman

8.1 引言

生命质量(quality of life，QoL)是每个人特有的对生理、心理和社会方面的个人主观评价(Mandzuk and McMillan 2005)。在一生中，QoL可能随着个人情况和发展阶段而变化(Taylor et al. 2008)。

对于受NF1疾病影响的个人和家庭而言，QoL可能会因疾病的临床影响以及对NF1症状和体征的自我心理反应和社会反应而改变。其他影响NF1患者QoL的因素包括慢性疾病和遗传疾病本身(Mauger et al. 1999)。

NF1的QoL研究已在不同国家和不同年龄的人群中开展。与病情评估相比，健康评估反映了一种更加以患者为中心的全面观点，亦反映了患者对自身健康有独到看法的观点(O'Connor 2004, p.4)。QoL为疾病治疗研究中传统的临床转归评估(Stevenson and Carey 2009；Spuijbroek et al. 2011)或NF1等进展性疾病的病程研究提供了另一种方法。政府或医疗政策的作用也可以通过它们对受疾病影响的个人、家庭和社区的QoL的改变来评估。

对NF1患者QoL的各种研究结果表明，与对照组相比，NF1患者的QoL普遍下降，而且在某些QoL领域存在特定的缺陷和优势。这些研究为采取干预和加强措施来改善QoL提供了方向，也为未来的研究提供了途径。

8.2 QoL的测量

测量与健康相关的QoL使研究人员能够量化病情的影响，并对不同病情进行比较(Spuijbroek et al. 2011)。此外，QoL还可用于病情相同但症状各异的个体间进行比较，这是NF1中常见的情况。重要的是，在疾病不可能治愈或从患者的角度来看治疗措施的影响可能超过其益处时，QoL是一个合适的终点指标。QoL还可用于监测疾病对护理人员的影响，以及衡量社会和家庭支持等更抽象概念的影响。

为了评估与健康相关的QoL，已开发出各种适合不同年龄的量表，但没有一个是专门针对NF1的。最常用的通用量表(O'Connor 2004, p.186)可能是SF-36(Ware and Sherbourne, 1992)，它测量疼痛、社会功能、心理痛苦/幸福、角色限制、精力/疲劳("活力")和一般健康认知等健康概念。该量表的可靠性和有效性已经过广泛测试(O'Connor 2004, pp.186-191)；它有多种语言版本，并且存在不同人群的对照和研究数据，可与有其他特殊疾病（如NF1）的个体进行比较。

除了一般的 QoL 测量方法，一些研究使用了症状特异性 QoL 测量方法。例如，在 NF1 研究中使用了一种皮肤病特异性测量方法，设计初衷是可被观察到的皮肤表现可能会影响个体功能、情绪和身体症状（Page et al. 2006）。此外，Stevenson 和 Carey（2009）评估胫骨发育不良儿童的 QoL 所使用的量表包括了该患者群体的矫形考虑，强调了活动能力和躯体功能等因素。同样，广为认可的 NF1 对语言的影响（Cosyns et al. 2010）促使一个荷兰团队研究与发声相关的 QoL，以及发声障碍对 NF1 患者功能、情感和身体健康的影响（Cosyns et al. 2011）。举例而言，SF-36 等通用 QoL 量表可与针对 NF1 特定症状的量表结合使用（Wolkenstein et al. 2001）。

8.3　成人 NF1 患者的 QoL 研究

Wolkenstein 等（2001）使用通用的 SF-36 量表以及皮肤病 QoL 测量工具 Skindex 经过认证的法语版本，评估疾病严重度和可见度对成人 NF1 患者 QoL 的影响。作者采用 Riccardi 量表（Riccardi 1992）评估严重度，并采用 Ablon 量表（Ablon 1999, p.178）评估可见度。由 128 名 15～73 岁的患者完成了这两份自填问卷。SF-36 结果显示，与来自法国的对照组人群相比，NF1 患者在所有领域的平均 QoL 都较低。在控制年龄和性别变量的情况下，疾病严重度较高的 NF1 患者 SF-36 得分往往较低，尤其是在躯体功能、躯体疼痛、一般健康认知和活力等方面。在情绪、躯体症状和功能这三个领域中，Skindex 得分在疾病可视度较高的 NF1 患者中较低，而与严重度无关。这项研究表明在对 NF1 患者进行评估时，通用的和针对特定症状的 QoL 测量方法都很有价值。此外，通过使用 Skindex，作者还将结果与已发表的其他皮肤病评分进行比较，例如 NF1 皮肤症状的平均影响程度与银屑病相似。

这项研究在罗马大学的一家皮肤病诊所进行了复现，使用的是意大利语版本的 SF-36 和 Skindex（Kodra et al. 2009）。在这项研究中，NF1 对一般 QoL 的影响以及外观对 Skindex 的影响与上述法国研究非常相似。另一项研究（Page et al. 2006）采用了略有差异的研究设计，但使用了英语版本的相同的 QoL 测量方法，在美国人群中复现了法国研究的结果。这些研究共同强调了外观对 NF1 患者 QoL 的重要性，以及美容矫正是改善 NF1 患者 QoL 的重要手段（Kodra et al. 2009）。

大约 2/3 的成年 NF1 患者有某种类型的言语或发声问题，这通常与导致声音频率和强度范围下降的喉部差异有关（Cosyns et al. 2012）。29 名大多来自根特大学医院医学遗传学中心的 NF1 成人患者完成了语音障碍指数测试（Voice Handicap Index，VHI），其中功能分量表用于测量语音障碍对日常活动的影响，情感分量表用于测量患者对语音障碍的感受，身体分量表用于记录喉部不适感。此外，还使用了发声障碍严重程度指数（Dysphonia Severity Index，DSI）和 Riccardi 严重程度量表（Riccardi severity scale），前者是对发声特征进行客观测量，后者是对 NF1 整体严重程度进行测量。

虽然不是正式的 QoL 研究，但 Langenbruch 及其同事（Langenbruch et al. 2011）询问了 132 名接受 NF1 专科医师治疗的成年 NF1 患者和 92 名接受非 NF 专科医师治疗的 NF1 患者，请他们就一些非医疗治疗方面的益处对"医疗质量"进行评分。接受 NF1 专科医师治疗的患者更有可能体验到更多的生活乐趣，也更有可能过上正常的日常生活。然而，两组患者在其他方面，如能否参加正常的休闲活动或能否正常工作等方面并无差异。为了明确接受 NF1 专科医师治疗对提高 NF1 患者 QoL 的重要性，还需要进一步研究。

8.4　儿童 NF1 患者的 QoL 研究

对 NF1 的幼儿、学龄儿童和青少年已有多项研究，这些研究使用了各种健康相关的 QoL 量表，现总结如下，首先是针对年龄最小的儿童患者的研究。

Oostenbrink 等（2007）对荷兰鹿特丹 Erasmus MC-Sophia 儿童医院 NF1 门诊的 34 名 1～6 岁儿童进行了研究，由研究者根据评估皮肤疾病的

Ablon 可见度量表进行评分(Ablon 1999, p. 178)。作者使用婴幼儿 QoL 问卷(Infant Toddler Quality of Life Questionnaire, ITQOL)对这些儿童的 QoL 进行了描述。在一项相关研究中, Spuijbroek 等(2011)将这些 NF1 儿童分别与 4 组其他儿科疾病的儿童以及由 410 名健康荷兰儿童组成的对照组进行了比较。所使用的测量方法包含与儿童躯体功能、生长发育、身体疼痛、情绪、行为、相处和一般健康状况直接相关的分量表。此外,还有 3 个分量表分别测量父母情绪影响、育儿时间影响和家庭凝聚力。最后一个与主量表不同的问题是评估父母对"健康变化"的看法,即目前的健康状况与前一年相比的变化。Oostenbrink 等(2007)报道,NF1 患儿在所有 ITQOL 分量表上的得分都较低,其中在生长发育、一般健康认知和父母情绪影响等分量表达到了具有统计学意义的中度到高度影响。

13 名具有 NF1 主要特征的患儿(其中 6 名患有丛状神经纤维瘤,3 名患有假关节)在所有分量表上的得分都低于没有这些症状的 NF1 患儿,尤其是疼痛分量表。尽管这项研究的规模太小,无法进行广泛的多因素分析,但结果表明入组父母的教育水平和家族遗传性 NF1 这两个因素对数个 ITQOL 分量表具有独立的正面影响,而症状可见度和父母对病情严重程度的感知与数个分量表中较低的分数有关。作者认为,教育水平较高的家庭(代表更好的收入和社会经济地位)可能更有能力满足 NF1 患儿的需求。令人惊讶的发现是,父母一方患有 NF1 对 NF1 患儿的 QoL 有积极影响,这可能与他们对预后的了解和已建立的社会支持有关。然而,该研究并未讨论父母 NF1 病情的严重程度,因此需要进一步研究以确定是否有其他因素,如 NF1 父母的学习障碍影响了他们发现子女的关注点。图 8.1 来自 Spuijbroek 和同事的研究(2011),显示了上述研究中 34 名 NF1 儿童与 410 名荷兰儿童的 ITQOL 情况对比。ITQOL 是典型的量表,可以在特定时间点为儿童及其家庭提供评估。

Krab 等(2009)使用类似方法对 43 名 10 岁及以上的儿童及其父母进行了研究。儿童健康问卷(child health questionnaire, CHQ)有 2 个版本,1 个由家长填写,另一个由儿童填写。CHQ 的分量表

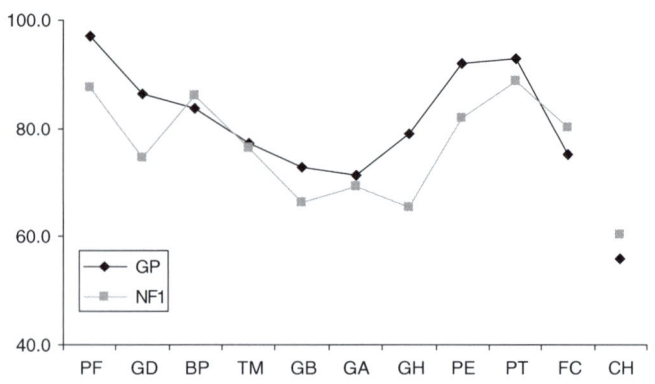

图 8.1 普通人群与 NF1 儿童的 ITQOL 量表得分

GP,普通人群;NF1,1 型神经纤维瘤病。X 轴:ITWOL 分量表;PF,躯体功能;GD,生长发育;BP,躯体疼痛;TM,性格和情绪;GB,一般行为;GA,相处;GH,一般健康状况;PE,父母情绪影响;PT,育儿时间影响;FC,家庭凝聚力。CH,健康变化,是一个单独的项目,用于评估父母对目前的健康状况与前一年相比的看法
[Adapted from Fig. 1, Spuijbroek et al. (2011) Qual Life Res 20: 779–786]

与 ITQOL 的分量表相似但不完全相同。此外,还使用了 Ablon 的可见度量表(Ablon 1999, p. 178)和 Riccardi 严重度量表(Riccardi 1992, p. 286),儿童的行为表现和在校表现则由儿童的老师使用经过验证的荷兰测量方法进行评分。将儿童的自我评分和家长的评分进行比较,图 8.2 显示了儿童和家长评分之间的巨大差异,儿童在一般行为分量表上的得分几乎普遍高于参考样本的平均值,而他们父母的看法则远远低于参考值。尽管家长和儿童的 CHQ 平均分相差很大,但家长和儿童的评分与参考数据的偏差方向一致。作者指出,教师的测量结果显示这些儿童存在大量的行为问题,从而支持了家长的评估,并与儿童自我评估的有效性相抵触。有必要开展进一步研究以确定这种较低的自我意识是否与"在有学习障碍或多动症的儿童身上观察到的更普遍的因素"(Krab et al. 2009)有关,或者是 NF1 所特有的。尽管如此,缺乏准确自我评估的能力可被视为对儿童 QoL 的保护。Krab 等(2009)指出,他们对相对较小的儿童样本进行的探索性回归分析中,CHQ 的几个领域与教师的行为评分之间的关联可能表明改善儿童行为的治疗有可能改善儿童及其家人的 QoL。

Barton 和 North(2006)的研究虽然不是一项 QoL 研究,但也表明 8~16 岁儿童和青少年的自我认知总体上是积极的。如果儿童患有 NF1,无论是

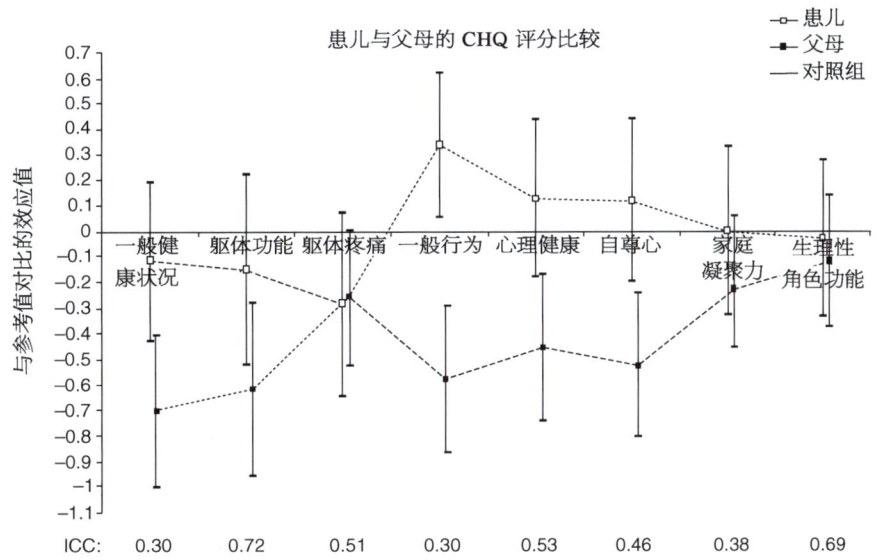

图 8.2 NF1 患儿与父母的 CHQ 评分比较。误差带代表 95% 置信区间 [Reproduced with permission. Krab et al. (2009) J Pediatr 154: 420-425]

否同时患有多动症或学习成绩低下,都会观察到与客观标准相比儿童倾向于高估自己的学习能力。Barton 和 North 认为这可能与 Zoller 和 Rembeck 对 NF1 成人患者的积极自我认知的发现一致,这被认为是一种心理补偿机制 (Zoller and Rembeck 1999)。

有几项研究支持了上述的发现。Vardarinos 及同事(2009)使用 CHQ 家长报告量表评估了 43 名 6~14 岁希腊儿童的 QoL,并与 61 名年龄匹配对照组进行了比较。除躯体功能外,家长对 NF1 患儿所有领域的评分都明显较低。其中,在行为、一般健康和对家庭生活的影响等方面的差异最大。Graf 等(2006)在瑞士进行的一项研究对 46 名 7~16 岁的儿童进行了各种评估:TACQoL(一种通用的 QoL 量表)、儿童行为检查表(Child Behaviour Checklist, CBCL)、家庭关系指数(Family Relationship Index, FRI)、Riccardi 严重度量表(仅躯体部分)、Ablon 可见度量表以及每个家庭社会经济状况的计算。这项研究表明,儿童在运动、认知、社交和情感方面的 QoL 都很低,但儿童的自我评估与家长的评估之间的差异并不显著。与后来 Krab 等(2009)的研究一样,家长和儿童的评估之间的相关性并不高。作者证明了积极的家庭关系与家长报告的较高 TACQoL 分数之间的关系,从而强调了为 NF1 儿童的整个家庭提供支持的必要性。

Wolkenstein 等(2008)使用了一种通用的儿科健康相关 QoL 测量方法 DISABKIDS,该方法可让 8~16 岁的儿童对 QoL 进行自我评估,并由他们的父母代为完成量表。此外,Wolkenstein 等还使用了一种皮肤疾病专用的测量方法,儿童皮肤病 QoL 指数(Children's Dermatology Life Quality Index, CDLQL),类似于之前几项研究中使用的成人皮肤疾病 Skindex 量表。79 名儿童接受了这两份问卷的评估,并将得分与表型测量结果进行了比较。不同于成人的 Skindex 得分,儿童的 CDLQL 得分并没有明显低于对照组,这可能反映了大多数 NF1 儿童的皮肤症状较轻。但有一小部分浅表丛状神经纤维瘤的儿童除外,这也在意料之中。对于大多数儿童患者而言,咖啡牛奶斑或雀斑的存在并不是一个重要的问题。研究表明,平均而言父母在 DISABKIDS 上给孩子的评分比孩子自己的评分更差,特别是在社会包容和排斥项目。此外,与 Spuijbroek 等研究结果一致的是,新发病例父母的平均评分低于/差于有遗传史的病例。NF1 的三个特定方面对 QoL 有显著且独立的负面影响,分别是骨骼病变、学习障碍和丛状神经纤维瘤。作者认为,学习障碍可能是影响 QoL 的主要决定因素之一,因为学习障碍会全面影响儿童在家庭、学校和游戏中的自我形象。这项研究进一步证明了改善儿童功能的重要性以及治疗学习障碍的必要性。Wolkenstein 及其同事还将 NF1 组的一般 QoL 评分与欧洲其他疾病儿童的数据进行了比较,表明 NF1 对一般 QoL 的影响比儿童哮喘更大,与全身性特应性皮炎的影响相似。

Stevenson 和 Carey(2009)展示了一组有和没有胫骨发育不良的 NF1 儿童的初步数据。他们使用儿科结果数据收集工具(Paediatric Outcome Data Collection Instrument,PODCI)证明,这两组儿童在整体功能、转移/移动、运动/躯体功能和疼痛/舒适方面的 QoL 有显著差异。

此外,作者建议使用 QoL 等结果测量方法,从而以一种不同于传统临床结果测量方法的方式量化患者的获益。在胫骨发育不良的病例中,相关研究和临床处理的重点是采取措施促进骨愈合和防止进一步的骨损伤。尽管医学界做出了大量努力,但仍有约 20% 假关节患儿的临床终点是截肢(Stevenson and Carey 2009)。在临床上这种结果可能被视为失败,然而以患者为中心的结果测量可能会产生不同的结果。1 名胫骨发育不良的青少年的家长就很好地阐述了在多次手术矫正失败后截肢对 QoL 的影响:

> 多年来,他的疼痛第一次中止;他可以期待着走到河边,期待着拿到驾照,期待着完成学业和找到工作。这次手术摆脱了一个长期笼罩在我们头上的巨大阴影,他的未来变得更加积极。我和儿子都不后悔尝试了所有可能的选择,但是,如果我们早点意识到试图挽救他的肢体会让我们浪费这么多年的时光、经受长期的身体和精神痛苦、失去自我价值(和朋友)、抑郁等,那么截肢的念头就不再是难以承受和令人沮丧的。事实上,这次手术让他能够回归自己的生活而并不损失什么,除了继续承受的疾病负担。

从临床医师的角度来看,以挽救肢体为目标的胫骨发育不良治疗失败了,但从患者的角度来看,截肢让他的 QoL 得到了显著提高。

8.5 改善 NF1 患者的 QoL

"患者对其疾病和未来的印象与他们的医师、家人、朋友和社会对其病情的看法密切相关"(Ablon 1999, p. 8)。这一研究总结了上述影响 NF1 患者 QoL 的一般和特定因素。

8.5.1 支持团体的作用

支持团体的"关爱社区"提供了一个分享信息、经验和解决方案的社会渠道,同时通过增强个人能力和提高他们有效应对失业或疾病等压力的能力,从而提高 QoL(Reissman 1986,pp. 84-85)。支持小组成员提供交友和社交网络,并充当导师、榜样、教育者和倡导者。

支持团体还能够影响社会和政府态度的改变,从而可能立即或长期改善 QoL。自闭症互助团体的游说活动正是一个例子,在许多国家,这些游说活动已经为早期行为干预筹集了大量专项资金(Autism Society of Canada 2009),并提供了大量额外的研究资金(Wadman 2007)。许多神经纤维瘤病支持团体正努力提高人们对 NF1 的疾病认知,为研究提供资金,并为 NF1 患者家庭提供支持。

8.5.2 政府行动

对遗传病患者的保护措施有可能改善许多 NF1 成人患者的 QoL,如医疗保险的覆盖和平等就业机会的提供。反歧视可以由政府层面主导:在美国,2009 年生效的《遗传信息反歧视法案》(Genetic Information Nondiscrimination Act,GINA)禁止利用遗传信息在就业或获得医疗保险方面施行歧视行为(GinaHelp 2010)。然而,GINA 并不适用于人寿、残疾或长期护理保险。许多 NF1 的成年人,无论其健康状况和风险因素如何,都无法获得人寿或残疾保险以及由此带来的保障。关于 NF1 对死亡率影响的最新数据(如 Evans et al. 2011;Rasmussenet et al. 2001)应取代人寿和健康保险文书中不准确和不完整的信息(如 Williams 2006),使 NF1 患者能够公平地获得保险。

8.5.3 NF1 的 QoL 研究

迄今为止还没有专门用于儿童或成人 NF1 患者的 QoL 测量方法,但其他 QoL 测量方法的组合揭示了未来研究的一些方向。目前没有一项关于 NF1 的研究调查过 NF1 作为一种可遗传疾病对

QoL 的影响程度。在其他遗传病中，研究人员发现患者会产生尴尬、负罪的感觉，并且认为社会会评判那些将一种可以产前诊断的疾病遗传给子女的成年患者（Arnold et al. 2005）。Benjamin 及其同事对 81 名成年人进行的研究包括了有关生育决策的信息，其研究表明约有 1/3 在组建家庭时不知道自己患有 NF1 的人表示，如果他们知道自己患有 NF1，他们的生育计划会因此受到影响。在这项研究中，一些仍考虑生育的患者希望进行产前诊断检测，但其他人则倾向于在孩子出生时进行症状前诊断（Benjamin et al. 1993）。尽管在儿童期进行此类检测的治疗经济学价值无法从直接护理成本的角度得到支持（Tsang et al. 2011），但对于产前诊断检测或新生儿症状前诊断的经济成本尚未得到研究。确诊 NF1 对 QoL 的影响尚未在任何年龄组的患者进行研究。NF1 症状的多样性及其不可预测性使未来的父母在做决定时面临巨大挑战，这也预示着一个 QoL 研究的重要领域。

目前还没有具体的研究对 NF1 成人患者就业和经济困难的影响进行量化，也没有对无法获得保险的压力对 QoL 的影响进行测量。适当的 QoL 研究可能会提供依据，证明缺乏保险和经济拮据给患者带来的压力，从而支持政府介入。其他影响 QoL 的问题包括睡眠障碍、缺乏了解 NF1 的家庭医师、缺乏专门的成人 NF1 诊所，以及 NF1 患者的快速衰老。令人惊讶的是，尽管在其他人群中慢性疼痛被认为是影响 QoL 的一个主要因素，但目前还没有 NF1 慢性疼痛对 QoL 影响的专门研究（Fine 2011）。在儿童患者中，亟待研究的领域是衡量教育和行为干预对儿童及其家长 QoL 的影响。

8.6 结论

使用 QoL 测量方法已经确定了一些通过支持、指导和特定治疗干预措施可能会对 NF1 患者产生积极影响的领域。积极的干预措施如整容手术、语言治疗、儿童期的教育和行为矫正可能对患者及其家人 QoL 产生终身影响。其他领域如睡眠障碍对 QoL 的影响也有待进一步研究。QoL 是一种监测治疗效果，跟踪个体病情进展以及评估医疗保健或社会策略影响的有效手段。NF1 不断进展的生物学特性和治疗手段的缺乏意味着对许多患者来说，QoL 可能是评估治疗成功与否最有效的结果指标，因为改善 QoL 是治疗的出发点也是结果。

（刘丕楠，王博　译）

参考文献

[1] Ablon J (1999) Living with genetic disorder. Auburn House, Westport, CT
[2] Arnold A, McEntagart M, Younger DS (2005) Psychosocial issues that face patients with Charcot-Marie-Tooth disease: the role of genetic counselling. J Genet Counsel 14: 307–318
[3] Autism Society of Canada (2009) Federal Autism Legislation, Bill C-360, a "Step in the right direction". Autism Society of Canada, Ottawa
[4] Barton B, North K (2006) The self-concept of children and adolescents with neurofibromatosis type 1. Child Care Health Dev 33: 401–408
[5] Benjamin CM, Colley A, Donnai D, Kingston H, Harris R, Kerzin-Storrar L (1993) Neurofibromatosis type 1 (NF1): knowledge, experience, and reproductive decisions of affected patients and families. J Med Genet 30: 567–574
[6] Cosyns M, Vandeweghe L, Mortier G, Janssens S, Van Borsel J (2010) Speech disorders in neurofibromatosis type 1: a sample survey. Int J Lang Commun Disord 45: 600–607
[7] Cosyns M, Mortier G, Corthals P, Janssens S, Van Borsel J (2011) Voice characteristics in adults with neurofibromatosis type 1. J Voice 25: 759–764
[8] Cosyns M, Mortier G, Janssens S, Van Borsel J (2012) Voice-related quality of life in adults with neurofibromatosis type 1. J Voice 26(2): e57–e62
[9] Evans DG, O'Hara C, Wilding A, Ingham SL, Howard E, Dawson J et al (2011) Mortality in neurofibromatosis 1: in North West England: an assessment of actuarial survival in a region of the UK since 1989. Eur J Hum Genet 19: 1187–1191
[10] Fine PG (2011) Long-term consequences of chronic pain: mounting evidence for pain as a neurological disease and parallels with other chronic disease states. Pain Med 12: 996–1004
[11] GinaHelp (2010) (Genetic Alliance, the Genetics and Public Policy Center at the Johns Hopkins University, and the National Coalition for Health Professional Education in Genetics). http://www.ginahelp.org. Accessed 13 Dec 2011
[12] Graf A, Landolt MA, Capone Mori A, Boltshauser E (2006) Quality of life and psychological adjustment in children and adolescents with neurofibromatosis type 1. J Pediatr 149: 348–353
[13] Kodra Y, Giustini S, Divona L, Porciello R (2009) Health-related quality of life in patients with neurofibromatosis type 1: a survey of 129 Italian patients. Dermatology 218: 215–220

[14] Krab LC, Oostenbrink R, de Goede-Bolder A, Aarsen FK, Elgersma Y, Moll HA (2009) Health-related quality of life in children with neurofibromatosis type 1: contribution of demographic factors, disease-related factors, and behavior. J Pediatr 154: 420-425

[15] Langenbruch A, Augustin M, Granstrom S, Kluwe L, Mautner V (2011) Clinical and healthcare status of patients with neurofibromatosis type 1. Br J Dermatol 165: 225-227

[16] Mandzuk LL, McMillan DE (2005) A concept analysis of quality of life. J Orthop Nurs 9: 12-18

[17] Mauger D, Zeller J, Revuz J, Wolkenstein P (1999) Retentissement psychologique de la neurofibromatoses de type 1: analyse d'entretiens avec 12 malades en vue d'une évaluation de la qualité de vie. Ann Dermatol Venereol 126: 619-620

[18] O'Connor R (2004) Measuring quality of life in health. Churchill Livingstone, Edinburgh Oostenbrink R, Spong K, de Goede-Bolder A, Landgraf J, Raat H, Moll H (2007) Parental reports of health-related quality of life in young children with neurofibromatosis type 1: Influence of condition-specific determinants. J Pediatr 151: 182-186

[19] Page PZ, Page GP, Ecosse E, Korf BR, Leplege A, Wolkenstein P (2006) Impact of neurofibromatosis 1 on quality of life: a cross-sectional study of 176 American cases. Am J Med Genet A 140(18): 1893-1898

[20] Rasmussen S, Yang Q, Friedman J (2001) Mortality in neurofibromatosis 1: an analysis using U. S. death certificates. Am J Hum Genet 68: 1110-1118

[21] Reissman F (1986) In: Weiss JO, Karkalits JE, Bishop KK, Paul NW (eds) Genetic support groups: volunteers and professional partners. March of Dimes Foundation, White Plains, NY

[22] Riccardi VM (1992) Neurofibromatosis. Phenotype, natural history, and pathogenesis. The Johns Hopkins University Press, Baltimore, MD

[23] Spuijbroek AT, Oostenbrink R, Landgraf JM, Rietveld E, de Goede-Bolder A, van Beeck EF et al (2011) Health-related quality of life in preschool children in five health conditions. Qual Life Res 20: 779-786

[24] Stevenson DA, Carey JC (2009) Health-related quality of life measure in genetic disorders: an outcome variable for consideration in clinical trials. Am J Med Genet C 151C: 255-260

[25] Taylor RM, Gibson F, Franck LS (2008) A concept analysis of health-related quality of life in young people with chronic illness. J Clin Nurs 17: 1823-1833

[26] Tsang E, Birch P, Friedman J (2011) Valuing gene testing in children with possible neurofibromatosis 1. Clin Genet. doi: 10. 1111/j. 1399-0004. 2011. 01801. x

[27] Vardarinos A, Zafeiriou DI, Vargiami E, Pratsidou-Gertsi P, Kontopoulos E, Kanakoudi-Tsakalidou F (2009) Parental reports of health-related qualit of life in Greek children with neurofibromatosis type 1. J Pediatr 155(3): 453

[28] Wadman M (2007) Autism speaks: the United States pays up. Nature 448: 628-629

[29] Ware JJ, Sherbourne C (1992) The MOS 36-item short-form health survey (SF-36). I. Conceptual framework and item selection. Med Care 30: 473-483

[30] Williams DS (2006) Neurofibromatosis. J Insur Med 38: 69-71

[31] Wolkenstein P, Zeller J, Revuz J, Ecosse E, Leplège A (2001) Quality-of-life impairment in neurofibromatosis type 1. A cross-sectional study of 128 cases. Arch Dermatol 137: 1421-1425

[32] Wolkenstein P, Rodriguez D, Ferkal S, Gravier H, Buret V, Algans N et al (2008) Impact of neurofibromatosis 1 upon quality of life in childhood: a cross-sectional study of 79 cases. Br J Dermatol 160: 844-848

[33] Zoller M, Rembeck B (1999) A psychiatric 12-year follow-up of adult patinets wiht neurofibromatosis type 1. J Psychiatr Res 33: 63-68

第9章 NF1 基因：启动子、5′非翻译区和 3′非翻译区
NF1 Gene: Promoter, 5′ UTR, and 3′ UTR

Hua Li and Margaret R. Wallace

9.1 引言

NF1 基因位于人类染色体 17q11.2 上，占据 289 701 bp。NIH NCBI 网站（编号 NG_009018）显示，NF1 的基因组序列从转录起始位点上游 4 951 bp、翻译起始位点（位于 1 号外显子）上游 5 334 bp 开始，而 5′ UTR 长度为 484 bp。NF1 基因具有经典的"CpG 岛"，从近端启动子延伸到 1 号外显子（图 9.1）。脊椎动物的 CpG 岛是富含 C/G 的序列，CG 二核苷酸含量高。CpG 岛会发生胞嘧啶甲基化、影响染色质结构，从而参与基因调控（Deaton and Bird 2011）。CpG 岛的平均大小为 1 kb，大多数通常未甲基化，与活跃的转录事件相关。大多数 CpG 岛位于基因的 5′端。目前，NF1 基因只有 1 个已知的转录起始位点和翻译起始密码子。NF1 基因有 58 个组成型外显子以及 3 个经过充分验证的小型可变剪接外显子[根据原始命名惯例，分别命名为 9a（9brain）、23a 和 48a；根据 NCBI 编号，它们分别位于外显子 11 和 12 之间、25 和 26 之间以及 57 和 58 之间]。有研究还发现外显子 10a 和 10b 之间有另一个可变剪接外显子，称为 10a-2（原始编号系统），该外显子编码 1 个 15 个氨基酸的胞内跨膜结构域（Kaufmann et al. 2002）。这 58 个外显子编码 1 段 2 818 个氨基酸的肽段（mRNA RefSeq 编号 NM_001042492.2），在所有组织中广泛表达。NF1 基因的 3′非翻译区（3′ UTR）长 3 522 bp，包含 2 个多聚腺苷酸化位点，因此在 Northern blot 中会观察到 2 个转录本，分别约为 11 kb 和 13 kb（这部分内容将在 9.3 中进一步介绍）。因此，较大的 NF1 转录本（不含可变剪接外显子）长度为 12 359 bp。目前没有证据显示 NF1 的翻译过程可以从除已知的翻译起始密码子 AUG 以外的其他位置开始。

NF1 基因的部分序列还在其他染色体上存在 7 个重复，主要集中在着丝粒周围区域，并在染色体 2、15 和 21 上的位点发生转录（其中 21 号染色体的表达是睾丸特异性的）（Yu et al. 2005）。这些位点和转录本可能会干扰对 NF1 基因的分子生物学分析。

在另一个 60 kb 的 NF1 内含子（根据传统命名法命名为内含子 27b）内，有 3 个双外显子基因：EVI2B、EVI2A 和 OMG，这些基因在相对 NF1 的反义链上编码，并以相反方向转录。相比于 NF1，这些基因在组织中的表达更有限，但在某些组织中，DNA 的两条链同时转录，这表明它们之间可能存在某种联系。另外，最近的研究对 1 号内含子进行了

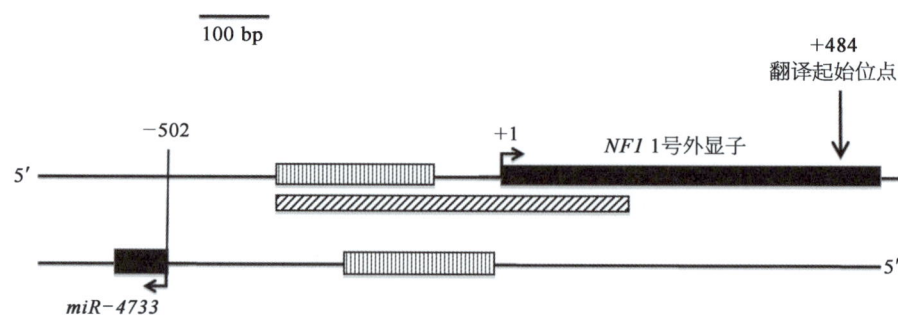

图 9.1 染色体 17q11.2 上 NF1 基因 5′端示意图，按比例绘制。实心黑框代表 NF1 的 1 号外显子和整个 miR-4733 基因，箭头指示它们在每条 DNA 链上的方向。斜线框代表 NF1 5′端的 CpG 岛，与加利福尼亚大学圣克鲁斯分校 genome browser 网站标识一致。竖线框指示 PROSCAN 分析中预测的启动子序列，与其靶基因位于同一链上。NF1 转录起始位点位于 1 号外显子（+1）的起点，miR-4733 的转录起始位点位于 NF1 转录起始点上游 502 bp，位于另一条链上。NF1 的翻译从转录本的 484 bp 开始，5′ UTR 位于 +1 位和 +484 位之间

分析，没有发现代表转录位点的序列，该内含子似乎没有"嵌入"基因(S. Oden and M. Wallace，未发表的数据)。

9.2 启动子

最早的 2 项关于 NF1 启动子的研究显示，人类和啮齿类动物的 NF1 启动子之间存在显著的序列同源性(Bernards et al. 1993；Hajra et al. 1994)。Hajra 等在 1994 年进行了更长的序列研究(翻译起始位点上游约 900 bp)，通过 RNA 酶保护实验，他们在人类和小鼠中找到了 NF1 基因主要的转录起始位点(−484 位)，同时也发现了 2 个次要转录起始位点(−495 位和−483 位)。2 个物种的 NF1 基因中均未发现 TATA 框和 CCAAT 框，但鉴定出了包括 SP1 和 AP2 在内的多个转录因子共有的结合序列，这些序列被包含在 5′ UTR 中。NF1 的 1 号外显子长 544 bp，包含 5′ UTR 以及编码神经纤维瘤蛋白的前 20 个氨基酸，其中主要转录起始点位于−484 位处。根据 UCSC genome browser 定义的 CpG 岛长 472 bp，包含 43 个 CpG 二核苷酸(图 9.1)。1 号外显子的其余部分和 1 号内含子的起始部分也富含 C-G，但 CpG 二核苷酸不如 CpG 岛丰富。

2003 年，Jenne 等对人类和小鼠的 NF1 基因及扩展的侧翼序列进行了比较。这张详细的物理图谱显示，在人类 NF1 基因的 5′端 50 kb 内没有其他基因，最近的 3′端的基因是 KIA1821(RAB11FIP4，约 10 kb 下游)。Mancini 等(1999)发表了启动子(小鼠和人类)5 个区域的甲基化图谱，显示其中 3 个区域(以转录起始位点为+1 时，约−1 000 bp、−3 000 bp 和−4 000 bp 处的几百 bp 区域)始终被甲基化，但在所有检查的组织中，靠近转录起始点(由 SP1 位点扩展)的胞嘧啶(在 CpG 或 CpNpG 中)未被甲基化。而甲基化会影响 SP1 位点和 CREB 结合位点的功能。2004 年，该课题组使用报告基因系统分析了启动子重叠序列的相对启动子活性，发现在 500 bp 片段(以转录起始位点为+1 位，从−270 位到+230 位处)中具有强启动子活性(Zou et al. 2004)。此外，从+230 到翻译起始密码子(+484 位)之间的序列似乎具有转录抑制活性。凝胶迁移实验数据显示，为了维持正常的启动子活性，必须要保证 CREB 位点的完整性。他们还发现，SP1(作为蛋白复合物的一部分)能够结合到−141、+415 和+460 位的 SP1 位点上。这些数据表明，这些转录因子结合位点的甲基化可能影响启动子活性。研究者还提出，从+230 位到+434 位的 4 个 AP2 位点可能部分影响了该区域的抑制活性。另一组研究者利用生物信息学方法(Promoter Inspector、Dragon Promoter Finder、MATCH、MatInspector)，通过比较人类、小鼠、大鼠和河豚(Fugu rubripes)的 NF1 基因，预测了启动子和 1 号内含子前部的调控元件

(Lee and Friedman 2005)。在 NF1 基因 5′ UTR 中，位于翻译起始点上游 310 bp 处的 1 个 24 bp 的序列完全保守，只有在河豚中有 1 个碱基的差异。研究人员还预测了 2 个额外的转录起始点，灵敏度为 80%，靠近翻译起始密码子（以翻译起始点为+1 位时，−116 位和−384 位）。然而，这与 Hajra 等（1994）发现的次要转录起始点并不相同。Yang 等（2005）发现，在髓系祖细胞中，1 种 AML 相关融合蛋白能够结合 NF1 基因启动子并抑制转录，这种蛋白质来自 RUNX1 和 MTG8 基因的染色体易位导致的邻近排列。

NF1 在不同组织中和不同时间上的表达可能由不同的调控系统控制。例如 Huang 等在 2007 年的研究发现，在分化中的髓系细胞中，转录因子 PU.1 结合到复合的 ets/IRF 元件（也被称为 EICE 序列），通过细胞因子信号招募 IRF2 蛋白和 ICSBP 蛋白（也被称为 IRF8）。这种调控系统通常存在于参与炎症反应的基因中。在 NF1 基因中，ets/IRF 调控元件位于−320 位到−336 位（转录起始位点上游），这一近端启动子区域中也存在许多其他关键启动子元件。

几个研究组在 NF1 患者的组织中研究了 NF1 近端启动子/5′ UTR 区域的甲基化事件，认为由甲基化导致的 NF1 转录减少可能与体细胞突变一样能导致"二次打击"。Horan 等（2000）在神经纤维瘤或 MPNST 中没有观察到整体的甲基化水平升高，但他们在肿瘤组织中发现，有些特定位点比正常组织的甲基化频率更高；尽管 Luijten 等在 2000 年的研究中并未发现相同的观察结果，但 Harder 等（2004）和 Fishbein 等（2005）后续也报道了与前人相同的甲基化差异。甲基化大多发生在 CpG 二核苷酸中的胞嘧啶核苷酸上，但 Harder 等在 2004 年的研究中发现了一些非 CpG 的甲基化。值得注意的是，这些位点大多位于预测或已被证明功能的转录因子结合位点内。除了在 5′ UTR 中的小部分外，这些位点大多数位于近端启动子区域内。由于甲基化是受环境影响的动态过程，以上研究以及最近的关于 NF1 单卵双胞胎的研究（Harder et al. 2010）都表明，NF1 启动子（以及 5′ UTR 和内含子）的胞嘧啶甲基化存在个体间的差异。后者的研究中还发现，对患有毛细胞型星形细胞瘤个体的白细胞 DNA 进行分析，发现其甲基化程度更高。然而，根据另一组更早的研究显示，这些星形细胞瘤本身并未显示出甲基化增加（Ebinger et al. 2005）。

2006 年，Ling 等在小鼠研究中发现，母源等位基因的 Igf2/H19 印记控制区（小鼠 7 号染色体）与父源等位基因的 NF1/Wsb1 区域（11 号染色体）在分裂间期细胞核中共定位，而这一现象似乎受 CTCF 转录抑制因子的影响。当这种共定位被破坏时，Igf2、NF1 和 Wsb1 的表达均减少。11 号染色体上 CTCF 的结合位点位于 NF1 基因上游 70 kb、Wsp1 基因下游 20 kb 处。研究人员同样在人类基因组中进行了探究，发现 NF1 和上游 RNF135 之间存在数个 CTCF 结合位点，而在 NF1 基因内部也存在 2 个 CTCF 结合位点（Ling et al. 2011）。这些结果都说明，染色体间的相互作用可能也调控了 NF1 的转录。也有研究证明，一些远离基因甚至几兆碱基的位点也会影响表达（"位置效应"），SOX9 基因及其上游缺失就是其中 1 个例子（e.g., Hill-Harfe et al. 2005）。

我们的研究使用了 PROSCAN（http://www-bimas.cit.nih.gov/molbio/proscan/）和 JASPAR（Bryne et al. 2008）程序，在 NF1 转录起始位点上游 3 kb 内进行了启动子搜索。PROSCAN 预测的启动子序列中得分最高的 1 个启动子（68.33 分，截断值为 53）位于 NF1 转录起始位点上游−362 位到−112 位之间，同时也在反义链上预测到了 1 个新的重叠启动子（77.62 分），位于从−4 位到−254 位（图 9.1）。使用 JASPAR（Bryne et al. 2008）对预测到的新型启动子进行分析，筛选启动子上的调控结合位点，在 NF1 正义链上发现 12 个强阳性位点（得分＞8.0），在反义链上也发现了 12 个阳性位点，但并未发现 CCAAT 框或 TATA 框的信号。NF1 的反义链上存在 1 个与反义启动子转录方向一致的 miRNA（miR-4733, Gene ID：100616266, miRBase ID：MI0017370, http://www.mirbase.org），其转录方向与 NF1 相反（图 9.1）。该 miRNA 在 1 项关于正常人和癌症患者乳腺组织差异的研究中被发现（Persson et al. 2011），但还没有其他研究报道该 miRNA 的重要性。研究者推测，

NF1 启动子上甲基化的改变可能也会影响 miR-4733 的启动子和表达,这使得人们对 *NF1* 启动子甲基化的解读变得更加困难。缺失这一区域后,除了会导致 *NF1* 等位基因的缺失外,还会使这些细胞在 miR-4733 上成为半合子,这可能会产生功能上的影响。

在 *NF1* 启动子或非翻译区域中,人们目前还没有发现任何已被证实具有致病性的 *NF1* 突变。*NF1* 基因具有相对较高的突变率,人类基因突变数据库(http://www.hgmd.org)中录入的 *NF1* 突变有 1 347 个,但在有关"调控"区域的类别中没有被记录的突变位点。研究人员一直在研究这些调控表达的区域,Horan 等(2004)分析了几位 *NF1* 患者的新型启动子/5′ UTR 区域的突变位点(Osborn et al. 2000),发现其中 1 个位点的突变略微改变了荧光素酶报告基因的功能。如果在 *NF1* 患者中发现了 1 个位于新型启动子/5′ UTR 的突变,而患者未患病的生物学父母体内不存在该突变时,就证明了这一突变存在致病性。目前无法简单直接地研究调控区域突变的功能,但如果 1 个突变能够对转录、剪接、翻译或蛋白结合有显著影响的话,就可以间接证明这一突变的功能。任何调控区域的突变都值得关注,因为这些区域在不同物种间具有高度保守性。实际上,尽管 dbSNP 数据库(http://www.ncbi.nlm.nih.gov/snp)中没有报告任何 5′ UTR 多态性,但在翻译起始位点上游的 5 kb 内,已经有 10 个经过验证的单核苷酸多态性(SNP)被报道。

9.3 3′非翻译区(3′ UTR)

1993 年,Bernards 等比较了小鼠 *NF1* cDNA 和人类转录本,发现 UTR 区和编码区都高度保守。1998 年,该研究小组验证了 *NF1* 基因的 2 个多聚腺苷酸化转录本(约 11 kb 和 13 kb),这 2 个转录本的大小差异是由 3′ UTR 长度不同导致的。这 2 个位点与在小鼠 *NF1* 基因中已发现的 2 个多聚腺苷酸化位点一致(Cowley et al. 1998)。所有人类组织中都存在这 2 个转录本,而在睾丸 RNA 的 RNA 印迹(Northern blot)中还显示存在 1 个 9 kb 的转录本。研究者还发现包含完整 3′ UTR 序列的人类 cDNA 很难被克隆。研究者也鉴定出了几种多态性,主要位于小鼠的非保守区域。2000 年,Haeussler 等对 3′ UTR 区域进行了研究,认为 3′ UTR 参与了转录后基因调控,进而影响了 *NF1* 转录本在时间和空间上的数量变化。他们的研究发现了 3′ UTR 上的 5 个似乎能结合蛋白质的区域,并鉴定出其中 1 个区域结合的蛋白质是肿瘤抗原 HuR。HuR 与一个富含 AU 的位点 ARE 结合,而 ARE 被认为是转录本稳定性的负调控因子。这些位点分布在整个 3′ UTR 区域中,而除了 HuR 之外,应该还有其他蛋白质参与了这些位点的调控。这一结果支持了转录后调控影响 *NF1* 转录本水平的假设。

过去 10 年内,人们主要研究的另一个影响转录本稳定性的因素是 miRNA。miRNA 是由较大转录本加工而来的约 22 个核苷酸大小的 RNA。miRNA 能够与转录本 3′ UTR 上的种子序列(8 个核苷酸)结合,当两者序列完全匹配时会导致转录本降解,如果序列不完全匹配,则只会减弱翻译(Calin and Croce 2006)。第一项关于 miRNA 调控 *NF1* 的研究证明了 miR-10b 与能够结合到 3′ UTR 区域,并发现 *NF1* 肿瘤来源的施万细胞中 miR-10b 水平升高(Chai et al. 2010)。进一步研究表明,抑制 miR-10b 会导致 MPNST 细胞增殖、侵袭和迁移能力的下降。尽管 RAS 信号通路水平有所减弱,但神经纤维瘤蛋白的表达并没有显著增加,这表明其他预测的 miR-10b 相关的 RAS 通路靶点可能参与其中,或是 miR-10b 与其他 miRNA 的协同作用导致了肿瘤形成。Subramanian 等在 2010 年还发现 MPNST 中 miR-34a 减少,他们认为这与 p53 失活有关。miR-34a 是 1 种研究较为深入的 miRNA,最近的 1 项研究发现它可以抑制 RAS 信号通路(Kim et al. 2012)。在 miRBase 数据库(http://www.mirbase.org)中对 *NF1* 基因的 3′ UTR 区域进行分析,显示超过 100 个潜在的 miRNA 结合位点。考虑到 3′ UTR 区域的大小,存在这么多位点也是合理的。

尽管目前在 *NF1* 3′ UTR 区域还没有发现致病性的突变位点,但这样的突变是可能存在的。在其他遗传性疾病中,研究者们通过改变 miRNA 结合、隐匿剪接、终止密码子改变或多聚腺苷酸化位点改变等方式发现致病性突变位点，在 NF1 中应该能使用同样的方法。NF1 3′UTR 区域已知存在一些多态性和罕见突变，但它们对 NF1 基因调控的影响尚不清楚。1996 年，Purandare 等报告了首个 3′UTR 区域的突变——位于 mRNA 第 10 647 位的 A 突变为 G。Cowley 等 1998 年报告了 5 个 3′UTR 多态性(3 个常见位点，1 个 5% 杂合性位点，1 个次要等位基因频率小于 1% 的位点)。Upadhyaya 等 1995 年在 1 名轻症 NF1 患者中发现了一个 3′UTR 变异(c. 11715 A>G)，该患者是家族中的首例 NF1 患者，但无法对她的父母是否存在突变进行分析。dbSNP 数据库中列出了 NF1 基因 3′UTR 区域中存在的 12 个经过验证的 SNP，有些是单核苷酸多态性，有些则是插入/缺失突变。未来的研究可以将这些 SNP 的位置以及任何新变异的位置，与潜在的 miRNA 结合位点或其他预测的调控元件进行比对。

9.4 结论

NF1 基因非常庞大，具有 1 个长 3′UTR 区。NF1 编码的神经纤维瘤蛋白的功能仍在不断被发现中，包括其不同亚型的特定功能。NF1 基因启动子的研究尚不充分，但它在所有被研究的组织(包括发育中的组织)中都活跃表达。它有 1 个含经典的 CpG 岛的启动子区域及 5′UTR 区域，但没有 TATA 框或 CCAAT 框。而可变多聚腺苷酸化在 NF1 基因中发挥的作用尚不清楚。NF1 的长 3′UTR 区域可能通过 miRNA 参与了转录后调控，但这方面还未被深入研究。NF1 基因有 1 个主要的转录起始位点，但有证据表明在其他的相邻位点可能存在少量转录活动。在 NF1 的反义链上有 1 个 miRNA 基因，与 NF1 基因呈头对头排列(转录起始位点相隔 502 bp，共享双向启动子)。NF1 的这一特征在文献中尚未被讨论，因为这一元件仅在过去 1 年中才在基因组数据中被发现。目前尚不清楚这 2 个基因是否是协同调控的。人体内的 NF1 基因突变会导致 NF1。尽管 NF1 基因突变率很高，但人们目前还没有在启动子或非翻译区中鉴定出明确的致病突变，这可能是因为在这些区域的突变非常罕见，或是它们的效应不足以导致可识别的表型。一些研究组曾报道过在某些 NF1 相关的肿瘤中，NF1 基因启动子内可能存在适度的特定位点的甲基化，但目前尚无证据表明这种甲基化可以使 NF1 基因沉默。为了更全面地理解 NF1 基因调控区域对其表达的影响，还需要展开更深入地研究。对 NF1 调控区域的研究也将有助于理解突变转录本的可变表达/稳定性，这些突变转录本似乎能逃避常规的无意义介导的衰变(nonsense-mediated decay，NMD)。突变转录本能否产生功能蛋白质尚不清楚，其表现可能因具体的突变类型和环境因素而异。深入理解 NF1 基因的调控区域将有助于开发针对性补偿特定突变的治疗方法。同样，对特定启动子和 UTR 区域更全面的认识对评估这些区域出现的突变或异常甲基化现象非常关键，并且对于制订旨在提高 NF1 基因表达的治疗策略也至关重要。

(章海兵，邢铭烟 译)

参考文献

[1] Bernards A, Snijders AJ, Hannigan GE, Murthy AE, Gusella JF (1993) Mouse neurofibromatosis type 1 cDNA sequence reveals high degree of conservation of both coding and non-coding mRNA segments. Hum Mol Genet 2：645-650

[2] Bryne JC, Valen E, Tang M-H, Marstrand T, Winther O, da Piedade I, Krogh A, Lenhard B, Sandelin A (2008) JASPAR, the open access database of transcription factor-binding profiles：new content and tools in the 2008 update. Nucleic Acids Res 36：D102-D106

[3] Calin GA, Croce CM (2006) MicroRNA signatures in human cancers. Nat Rev Cancer 6：857-866

[4] Chai G, Liu N, Ma J, Li H, Oblinger JL, Prahalad AK, Chang L-S, Wallace MR, Muir D, Guha A, Phipps RJ, Hock JM, Yu X (2010) MicroRNA-10b regulates tumorigenesis in neurofibromatosis type 1. Cancer Sci 101：1997-2004

[5] Cowley GS, Murthy AE, Parry DM, Schneider G, Korf B, Upadhyaya M, Harper P, MacCollin M, Bernards A, Gusella JF (1998) Genetic variation in the 3′ untranslated region of the neurofi-bromatosis 1 gene：application to unequal allelic expression. Somat Cell Mol Genet 24：107-119

[6] Deaton AM, Bird A (2011) CpG islands and the regulation of transcription. Genes Dev 25：1010-1022

[7] Ebinger M, Senf L, Wachowski O, Scheurlen W (2005) No aberrant methylation of neurofibromatosis 1 gene (NF1)

promoter in pilocytic astrocytoma in childhood. Pediatr Hematol Oncol 22: 83-87
[8] Fishbein L, Eady B, Sanek N, Muir D, Wallace MR (2005) Analysis of somatic NF1 promoter methylation in plexiform neurofibromas and Schwann cells. Cancer Genet Cytogenet 157: 181-186
[9] Haeussler J, Haeusler J, Striebel AM, Assum G, Vogel W, Furneaux H, Krone W (2000) Tumor antigen HuR binds specifically to one of five protein-binding segments in the 3' untranslated region of the neurofibromin messenger RNA. Biochem Biophys Res Commun 267: 726-732
[10] Hajra A, Martin-Gallardo A, Tarlé SA, Freedman M, Wilson-Gunn S, Bernards A, Collins FS (1994) DNA sequences in the promoter region of the NF1 gene are highly conserved between human and mouse. Genomics 21: 649-652
[11] Harder A, Rosche M, Reuss DE, Holtkamp N, Uhlmann K, Friedrich R, Mautner VF, von Deimling A (2004) Methylation analysis of the neurofibromatosis type 1 (NF1) promoter in peripheral nerve sheath tumours. Eur J Cancer 40: 2820-2828
[12] Harder A, Titze S, Herbst L, Harder T, Guse K, Tinschert S, Kaufmann D, Rosenbaum T, Mautner VF, Windt E, Wahlländer-Danek U, Wimmer K, Mundlos S, Peters H (2010) Monozygotic twins with neurofibromatosis type 1 (NF1) display differences in methylation of NF1 gene promoter elements, 5' untranslated region, exon and intron 1. Twin Res Hum Genet 13: 582-594
[13] Hill-Harfe K, Kaplan L, Stalker HJ, Zori RT, Pop R, Scherer G, Wallace MR (2005) Fine mapping of chromosome 17 translocation breakpoints 900 kb upstream of SOX9 in acampomelic campomelic dysplasia and a mild, familial skeletal dysplasia. Am J Hum Genet 76: 663-671
[14] Horan MP, Cooper DN, Upadhyaya M (2000) Hypermethylation of the neurofibromatosis type 1 (NF1) gene promoter is not a common event in the inactivation of the NF1 gene in NF1-specific tumours. Hum Genet 107: 33-39
[15] Horan MP, Osborn M, Cooper DN, Upadhyaya M (2004) Functional analysis of polymorphic variation within the promoter and 5' untranslated region of the neurofibromatosis type 1 (NF1) gene. Am J Med Genet A 131: 227-231
[16] Huang W, Horvath E, Eklund EA (2007) PU.1, Interferon regulatory tactor (IRF) 2, and the interferon consensus sequence-binding protein (ICSBP/IRF8) cooperate to activate NF1 transcription in differentiating myeloid cells. J Biol Chem 282: 6629-6643
[17] Jenne DE, Tinschert S, Dorschner MO, Hameister H, Stephens K, Kehrer-Sawatzki H (2003) Complete physical map and gene content of the human NF1 tumor suppressor region in human and mouse. Genes Chromosomes Cancer 37: 111-120
[18] Kaufmann D, Muller R, Kenner O, Leistner W, Hein C, Vogel W, Bartelt B (2002) The N-terminal splice product NF1-10a-2 of the NF1 gene codes for a transmembrane segment. Biochem Biophys Res Commun 294: 496-503
[19] Kim HR, Roe JS, Lee JE, Hwang IY, Cho EJ, Youn HD (2012) A p53-inducible microRNA-34a downregulates Ras signaling by targeting IMPDH. Biochem Biophys Res Commun 418: 682-688
[20] Lee TK, Friedman JM (2005) Analysis of NF1 transcriptional regulatory elements. Am J Med Genet 137A: 130-135
[21] Ling JQ, Li T, Hu JF, Vu TH, Chen HL, Qiu XW, Cherry AM, Hoffman AR (2006) CTCF mediates interchromosomal colocalization between Igf2/H19 and Wsb1/Nf1. Science 312: 269-272
[22] Ling JQ, Hou A, Hoffmann AR (2011) Long-range DNA interactions are specifically altered by locked nucleic acid-targeting of a CTCF binding site. Biochim Biophys Acta 1809: 24-33
[23] Luijten M, Redeker S, van Noesel MM, Troost D, Westerveld A, Hulsebos TJ (2000) Microsatellite instability and promoter methylation as possible causes of NF1 gene inactivation in neurofibromas. Eur J Hum Genet 8: 939-945
[24] Mancini DN, Singh SM, Archer TK, Rodenhiser DI (1999) Site-specific DNA methylation in the neurofibromatosis (NF1) promoter interferes with binding of CREB and SP1 transcription factors. Oncogene 18: 4108-4119
[25] Osborn M, Cooper DN, Upadhyaya M (2000) Molecular analysis of the 5'-flanking region of the neurofibromatosis type 1 (NF1) gene: identification of five sequence variants. Clin Genet 57: 221-224
[26] Persson H, Kvist A, Rego N, Staaf J, Vallon-Christersson J, Luts L, Loman N, Jonsson G, Naya H, Hoglund M, Borg A, Rovira C (2011) Identification of new microRNAs in paired normal and tumor breast tissue suggests a dual role for the ERBB2/Her2 gene. Cancer Res 71: 78-86
[27] Purandare SM, Cawthon R, Nelson LM, Sawada S, Watkins WS, Ward K, Jorde LB, Viskochil DH (1996) Genotyping of PCR-based polymorphisms and linkage-disequilibrium analysis at the NF1 locus. Am J Hum Genet 59: 159-166
[28] Subramanian S, Thayanithy V, West RB, Lee CH, Beck AH, Zhu S, Downs-Kelly E, Montgomery K, Goldblum JR, Hogendoorn PC, Corless CL, Oliveira AM, Dry SM, Nielsen TO, Rubin BP, Fletcher JA, Fletcher CD, van de Rijn M (2010) Genome-wide transcriptome analyses reveal p53 inactivation mediated loss of miR-34a expression in malignant peripheral nerve sheath tumours. J Pathol 220: 58-70
[29] Upadhyaya M, Maynard J, Osborn M, Huson SM, Ponder M, Ponder BA, Harper PS (1995) Characterisation of germline mutations in the neurofibromatosis type 1 (NF1) gene. J Med Genet 32: 706-710
[30] Yang G, Khalaf W, van de Locht L, Jansen JH, Gao M, Thompson MA, van der Reijden BA, Gutmann DH, Delwel R, Clapp DW, Hiebert SW (2005) Transcriptional repression of the Neurofibromatosis-1 tumor suppressor by the t(8;21) fusion protein. Mol Cell Biol 25: 5869-5879
[31] Yu H, Zhao X, Su B, Li D, Xu Y, Luo S, Xiao C, Wang W (2005) Expression of NF1 pseudogenes. Nucleic Acids Res 33: 6445-6458
[32] Zou M-X, Butcher DT, Sadikovic B, Groves TC, Yee S-P, Rodenhiser DI (2004) Characterization of functional elements in the neurofibromatosis (NF1) proximal promoter region. Oncogene 23: 330-339

第10章 1型神经纤维瘤病的胚系突变谱及基因型-表型相关性

The Germline Mutational Spectrum in Neurofibromatosis Type 1 and Genotype – Phenotype Correlations

David N. Cooper and Meena Upadhyaya

10.1 引言

NF1 基因位于染色体 17q11.2 上,长度为 283 kb,包含 61 个外显子,可产生一个 12 kb mRNA 转录本,编码神经纤维瘤蛋白(Upadhyaya 2008)。神经纤维瘤蛋白分子量为 327 kDa,由 2 818 个氨基酸组成,在大多数组织中表达(大脑和中枢神经系统中表达水平最高),并且具有许多亚型(Trovo-Marqui and Tajara 2006)。神经纤维瘤蛋白是一种肿瘤抑制蛋白,作为细胞 Ras 信号通路的关键负性调节因子发挥作用(Bennett et al. 2009)。具体而言,它是一种 Ras 特异性 GTP 酶激活蛋白(GTPase-activating protein, GAP),在结构和序列上与 GAP 超蛋白家族高度同源(Scheffzek et al. 1998)。神经纤维瘤蛋白能够显著增加 Ras 蛋白的内源 GTP 酶活性,加速活性 Ras - GTP 向非活性 Ras - GDP 状态的转换,从而通过 Ras 途径有效减少细胞有丝分裂信号转导。因此,任何导致神经纤维瘤蛋白功能失活的 NF1 基因突变都可能显著增加细胞内活性 Ras - GTP 的水平,从而导致细胞生长失去控制,甚至引发肿瘤形成(Klose et al. 1998; Arun and Gutmann 2004)。

NF1 基因的遗传性突变可导致肿瘤易感综合征 1 型神经纤维瘤病(NF1),影响全球 1/4 000~1/3 000 人。根据 Knudson 的二次命中假说,携带杂合种系 NF1 突变的患者在其第 2 个野生型 NF1 等位基因的体细胞突变后,往往会发生神经纤维瘤。在祖细胞(施万细胞或其前体)中,第 2 个 NF1 等位基因的体细胞缺失以及各种支持细胞中的单倍体功能不足,是肿瘤形成的必要条件(Gutmann et al. 1999; Ingram et al. 2000; Kemkemer et al. 2002; McLaughlin and Jacks 2002; Pemov et al. 2010)。至于 NF1 基因突变率较高的原因,目前尚不清楚,但其突变率是所有人类疾病中报告的高突变率之一(Huson et al. 1989; Kehrer-Sawatzki and Cooper 2008; Evans et al. 2010),并且几乎一半的 NF1 患者的 NF1 突变为新发突变。在此,我们回顾了已知的 NF1 种系突变谱,探讨了不同类型的遗传性 NF1 突变在性质、位置和频率上的差异,并展示了局部 DNA 序列对这些差异产生的重要且可预测的影响。

10.2 NF1 基因的胚系突变谱

截至目前,已有将近 1 300 种 NF1 遗传基因突变被报道,这些突变是导致 NF1 的发病原因(表 10.1)。

D. N. Cooper • M. Upadhyaya
Institute of Medical Genetics, School of Medicine, Cardiff University, Cardiff CF14 4XN, UK
e-mail: Upadhyaya@cardiff.ac.uk

这些突变涉及的片段大小不一，从超过 100 万以上碱基对的大片段缺失，到微小的单碱基对替换，后者改变了编码的氨基酸或剪接位点的功能。下面我们将回顾迄今为止在 NF1 基因中识别出的不同类型的胚系突变。

表 10.1 NF1 基因中不同种系突变摘要[来自人类基因突变数据库的报告（HGMD；http://www.hgmd.org；Stenson et al. 2009），截至 2011 年 11 月]

突变类型	不同突变的数量
错义突变	142
无义突变	167
剪切突变	285
微缺失（≤20 bp）	349
微插入（≤20 bp）	167
插入缺失（≤20 bp）	28
大片段缺失（>20 bp）	129
大片段插入（>20 bp）	12
复杂重排	8
总计	1 287

10.3 错义和无义突变

肿瘤抑制基因特征性地表现出大量的无义突变，NF1 基因也是如此（Mort et al. 2008；Ivanov et al. 2011）。在 NF1 基因编码区域内已知的遗传致病性单碱基对替换中，超过 54% 导致无义突变。许多无义突变位于 CpG 二核苷酸内，这是已知的突变热点。CpG 二核苷酸的高突变性与其在人类基因组中作为胞嘧啶甲基化主要位点有关。胞嘧啶自发脱氨基转化为尿嘧啶，后者被有效识别为非 DNA 碱基，并被尿嘧啶-DNA 糖基化酶清除。然而，5-甲基胞嘧啶的自发脱氨基产生胸腺嘧啶，从而形成 G-T 错配，这种错配由甲基-CpG 结合域蛋白 4（methyl-CpG binding domain protein 4, MBD4）和（或）胸腺嘧啶 DNA 糖基化酶去除，并通过碱基切除修复（base excision repair, BER），该过程效率较低。据估计，在 CpG 二核苷酸内，CG>TG（以及另一条链上的 CG>CA）转换的速率是基础突变率的 5 倍（Krawczak et al. 1998）。在 NF1 基因的背景下，该基因编码区域内 18/23 个 CG>TG/CA 突变均为 CGA>TGA（Arg>Term）；由于此类无义突变平均表型效应更为显著，因此相比错义突变，它们更有可能引起临床关注（Krawczak et al. 1998）。

很明显，胞嘧啶甲基化也发生在哺乳动物基因组中的 CpNpG 位点（其中 N 代表任何核苷酸）（Lister et al. 2009；Lee et al. 2010）。CpNpG 三核苷酸的对称性支持了甲基化模式半保守复制模型（类似于 CpG 二核苷酸）。因此，导致人类遗传性疾病大约 5% 的错义/无义突变可能归因于甲基化介导的 CpHpG 三核苷酸内 5 mC 的脱氨反应（Cooper et al. 2010）。在 NF1 基因中，CpHpG 三核苷酸同样也是突变热点（Rodenhiser et al. 1997）；实际上，目前已知有 24 个 CpHpG>TpHpG/CpHpA 突变的例子，均为 CAG>TAG 的转换（Gln>Term），这与甲基化介导的 5 mC 脱氨基模型一致（见 HGMD）。

NF1 基因中，错义突变簇集现象十分显著。在缺乏明显局部高突变性的情况下，这种现象最可能的原因是临床上对蛋白质功能域失活的筛选。神经纤维瘤蛋白中表征最完善的功能域是由外显子 20-27a 编码的 GTP 酶激活蛋白相关结构域（GAP-related domain, GRD）（Welti et al. 2008）。已有多项研究评估了 GRD 内约 25 个已知自发错义突变体的功能影响（Skinner et al. 1991；Li et al. 1992；Poullet et al. 1994；Morcos et al. 1996；Scheffzek et al. 1997, 1998；Upadhyaya et al. 1997；Klose et al. 1998；Ahmadian et al. 2003）。理论上，对 GRD 内关键残基的生化研究可能揭示了这些残基在 Ras-RasGAP 相互作用中的角色。然而，至今只有 4 种自发 NF1-GRD 突变体（K1423E、R1391K、R1391S 和 R1276P）被进行过功能分析（Ahmadian et al. 2003）。Li 等于 1992 年发现 K1423E 突变导致 GAP 活性降低了 200～300 倍。K1423 残基与 E1437 在 a7/可变环中形成分子内盐桥，从而稳定了 Ras-RasGAP 相互作用；K1423 残基突变破坏这一盐桥，可能产生负电荷，干扰 Ras-RasGAP 相互作用（Klose et al. 1998）。由于 K1423 距离 Ras 活性位点较远，它不太可能直接参与催化过程，但可能决定神经纤维瘤蛋白对 Ras-GTP 的特异性作用（Ahmadian et al. 2003）。在 R1391 残基上的突变已在两种不同的背景下进行了研究，即 R1391K（Skinner et al. 1991）和 R1391S（Upadhyaya et al. 1997）。R1391S 错义突变体 GAP 相关域的活性比野生型 NF1 低约 300 倍（Upadhyaya et al. 1997）。最后，Klose 等（1998）发现，尽管 R1276P 仅导致对 Ras 的结合亲和力略有降低（6.6 倍），但它严重影响了 GTP 水解（大约 8 000 倍）。已知 GAP 结构域的突变会影响微管结合以及 p21-ras 的调节（Xu and Gutmann 1997；Upadyhaya et al. 1997；Klose et al. 1998；Scheffzek et al. 1998）。最近，Thomas 等描述了 10 种 NF1-GRD 变体，这些变体通过遗传学和生物信息学分析以及分子建模被认为是潜在致病的。

第二个结构域由 NF1 基因的外显子 11-17 编码，包括 1 个富含半胱氨酸/丝氨酸的结构域，其中包含 3 个可能与 ATP 结合的半胱氨酸对，以及 3 个潜在的 cAMP 依赖性蛋白激酶（protein kinase，PKA）识别位点，这些位点被 PKA 磷酸化（Fahsold et al. 2000；Mattocks et al. 2004；Welti et al. 2008）。D'Angelo et al.（2006）鉴别出了第三个结构域，包含 1 个 Sec14p 同源片段（残基 1560-1699）和具有 pleckstrin 同源性的区域（残基 1713-1818）。该结构域结合磷脂（Welti et al. 2007），尽管该结构域内的突变会干扰蛋白质整体结构，但似乎不会显著影响其脂质结合功能（Welti et al. 2011）。

10.4 基因转换

基因转换指的是遗传物质从"供体"序列向与之高度同源的"受体"序列的单向转移。人类基因组中存在多个与 NF1 基因同源的不同序列，理论上这些序列有可能通过基因转换机制将突变引入 NF1 基因（Luijten et al. 2001a；Yu et al. 2005）。这些旁系同源序列在多个位置上与原始 NF1 基因发生分化，因此含有大量等位基因，可能通过位点间基因转换而致病（Luijten et al. 2001b）。最近对人类疾病基因的调查中发现，NF1 基因中至少有 9 个已知的错义突变（表 10.2），这些突变可能通过这些 NF1 旁系同源基因之一作为供体进行基因转换而形成（Casola et al. 2012）。

表 10.2 NF1 基因中的单碱基对替换，假定由具有 200 bp 和 92% 序列同源性的 NF1 相关供体序列介导的基因转换（来自 Casola et al. 2012）

HGMD_ID	野生型核苷酸	突变型核苷酸	突变位点	相似度（%）	NF1 同源供体序列的染色体定位	供体起始位点	供体终止位点	CpG
CM000796	A	G	26583996	93.03	15	19399113	19399313	0
CM032012	C	T	26587083	93.03	15	19396329	19396529	0
CM087437	C	T	26551587	94.53	18	14147219	14147419	1
CM087525	A	G	26565668	96.52	2	131671876	131672076	0
CM087525	A	G	26565668	96.52	14	18565252	18565452	0
CM087525	A	G	26565668	96.52	14	19148007	19148207	0
CM087525	A	G	26565668	95.02	22	14725888	14726088	0
CM087526	C	T	26580376	96.02	15	19402801	19403001	1
CM087526	C	T	26580376	95.02	12	36886955	36887154	1

续表

HGMD_ID	野生型核苷酸	突变型核苷酸	突变位点	相似度（%）	NF1同源供体序列的染色体定位	供体起始位点	供体终止位点	CpG
CM087527	A	G	26580422	95.02	15	19402755	19402955	0
CM096910	T	C	26551576	94.03	18	14147230	14147430	0
CM973234	C	G	26584259	93.03	15	19398854	19399050	0

注：在CpG列中，"1"和"0"分别表示突变发生或没有发生在CpG位点。对于CpG二核苷酸中发生的3个C>T转变，应注意的是，通过甲基化介导的5-甲基胞嘧啶脱胺的复发性突变可能是这些病变的另一种原因。

10.5 剪接突变

长期以来，人们已知高比例（至少20%）的NF1基因突变会影响mRNA剪接（Ars et al. 2000；Messiaen et al. 2000）。这很可能与NF1基因的庞大体积及其包含的远超平均水平的内含子（60个）数量有关。然而，NF1基因中与剪接相关的突变数量几乎肯定是被低估的。因此，越来越多的研究开始认识到，那些影响mRNA剪接表型的"深层内含子"突变通常是被忽视的（Raponi et al. 2006；Wimmer et al. 2007；Pros et al. 2008；Cooper 2010）。这些突变可能对临床表型产生不同的影响。例如，Fernández-Rodríguez等于2011年报告了一种"深层内含子"NF1突变（c.3198-314G>A），该突变与相对温和的临床表型相关，部分原因是由于"漏切"现象的存在，一定比例的转录本得以正确剪切，从而可能足以产生接近正常功能水平的神经纤维瘤蛋白。

Wimmer et al.（2007）将NF1剪接相关突变分为5类：由于真实剪接位点突变导致的外显子跳跃（类型Ⅰ）、由深层内含子突变引起的隐性外显子内含（类型Ⅱ）、从头剪接位点的产生导致外显子序列丢失（类型Ⅲ）、真实剪接位点破坏时隐性剪接位点的激活（类型Ⅳ），以及导致外显子跳跃的外显子序列改变（类型Ⅴ）。在类型Ⅴ中，存在破坏外显子剪接增强子的突变（Colapietro et al. 2003；Zatkova et al. 2004；Baralle et al. 2006；Pros et al. 2008），该突变类型在人类遗传疾病中的潜在影响几乎肯定是被低估的。

10.6 调控突变

截至目前，尚未报道NF1基因的调控突变（Zou et al. 2004）。尽管NF1基因的近端启动子区域存在多个功能元件，但在涉及长达987 bp DNA序列（包括基因的启动子和50个侧翼序列）的突变筛查中，并未发现任何致病突变（Osborn et al. 2000；Horan et al. 2004）。

10.7 微缺失、微插入和插入/缺失

微缺失、微插入和插入/缺失分别占NF1基因中所有微病变的31%、15%和2.5%。NF1基因中的大多数微缺失和微插入发生在单核苷酸序列和短正向重复序列内（Rodenhiser et al. 1997）。因此，这些微缺失、微插入和插入/缺失可能是由于滑移诱变机制导致的，涉及单、双或三核苷酸串联重复的一个拷贝的添加或移除（Chuzhanova et al. 2003；Ball et al. 2005）。与这种解释相一致，明显存在几个突变热点，它们同时包含微缺失和微插入；这些热点通常涉及单核苷酸序列中删除或插入1个核苷酸[例如，在密码子76处的$(A)_7$中的A，密码子1 303处的$(T)_4$中的T，以及密码子1 818处的$(C)_5$中的C]。值得注意的是，至少有10个>20 bp、<70 bp的内部外显子缺失也已被报道（详见HGMD）。

10.8 NF1基因的大片段缺失

17q11.2区域中包含NF1基因及其侧翼区域

的大片段缺失是导致 NF1 最常见的复发突变之一。在所有 NF1 患者中，约有 5% 的患者存在 NF1 基因及其侧翼区域的大片段缺失（也称 NF1 微缺失）（Kluwe et al. 2004）。为了完整性，本章将简要讨论这些缺失，但在第 15 章中将对其进行更详细的讨论。

在 NF1 患者的生殖细胞中，已观察到 2 种频发的 NF1 大片段缺失亚型（1 型和 3 型）；这些缺失在大小、相对频率以及各自断裂点的位置上有所不同。最常见的是 1 型缺失，覆盖了 1.4 Mb 的区域，导致包括 NF1 基因在内的 14 个基因丢失。1 型缺失是通过非等位基因同源重组（nonallelic homologous recombination，NAHR）介导的，这种重组发生在 NF1 基因区域两侧的低拷贝重复序列（low-copy repeats，LCR）之间，尤其是 NF1‑REPs A 和 C。在 NF1‑REP 中，已发现有 2 个优先的 NAHR 区域：同源重组位点 PRS2 和 PRS1（Forbes et al. 2004；Raedt et al. 2006）。大多数 1 型缺失的断点位于跨越 PRS2 的 3.4 kb 区域内，而其余的断点则位于跨越 PRS1 的 1.8 kb 区域内。导致 1 型缺失的 NAHR 主要发生在母体减数分裂期间（Upadhyaya et al. 1998；López-Correa et al. 2000）。

3 型 NF1 缺失是由 NF1‑REPs B 和 C 之间的 NAHR 介导，仅涉及 1 Mb 的区域，且发生频率远低于 1 型缺失；实际上，到目前为止仅鉴定出 11 名胚系 3 型缺失的患者。因此，1 型和 3 型缺失均证明了 NF1 基因区域内 LCR 具有较高的重组潜力（Bengesser et al. 2010；Messiaen et al. 2011；Zickler et al. 2012）。

与 1 型和 3 型缺失不同，2 型缺失通常发生在合子后细胞分裂期间，从而导致体细胞镶嵌现象，即正常细胞与携带缺失的细胞共存（Petek et al. 2003；Kehrer-Sawatzki et al. 2004；Steinmann et al. 2007；Roehl et al. 2010）。2 型缺失的断点位于 SUZ12 及其假基因 SUZ12P 内（Petek et al. 2003；Kehrer-Sawatzki et al. 2004；Steinmann et al. 2007；Roehl et al. 2010），发生频率为 9%~20%，低于 1 型 NF1 缺失（Kehrer-Sawatzki et al. 2004；Messiaen et al. 2011；Pasmant et al. 2010）。

与上述由 NAHR 介导的复发性 NF1 缺失不同，已报道了 NF1 基因的多例"非典型"胚系缺失，不一定由同源机制介导，且其断点位置没有明显的复发性（Venturin et al. 2004；Mantripragada et al. 2006）。因此，非典型 NF1 缺失在缺失基因的数量方面可能存在显著差异（Kehrer-Sawatzki et al. 2008 and references therein；Pasmant et al. 2010）。据报道，一例非典型的 1.5 Mb 缺失，在 NF1 基因的 IVS23a 内有 1 个断点是由 Alu 重复序列介导的（Gervasini et al. 2005）。

除了上述涉及整个 NF1 基因的大片段缺失外，还应注意有超过 70 种已知的基因内缺失，这些缺失导致基因内的 1 个或多个外显子被移除（e.g. Wimmer et al. 2006）。多外显子缺失似乎占到了 NF1 基因突变的 2%~7%（De Luca et al. 2007；Orzan et al. 2008）。Wimmer 等（2006）报告了 25 名来自不同家系的 NF1 患者中，其中 2 名患者存在单个或多个外显子缺失，这是由 NF1 基因第 2 外显子的复发性 Alu 序列介导的。

10.9　NF1 基因的大片段复制

Grisart 等（2008）报道了 1 个 1.5 Mb 大小的大片段重复基因，该重复基因包含 NF1 基因和至少 12 个其他基因。这一情况发生在两名兄弟身上，他们均表现出智力缺陷、早发脱发（15 岁）、牙釉质发育不全以及轻微的面部畸形。该重复区域与上述 NF1 微缺失区域完全对应。尽管在 NF1 基因侧翼区域的同源重复序列之间，NAHR 机制预期会产生频率相等的互反产物（即 1 个缺失和 1 个重复），但至今，这仍是唯一一个得到恰当描述的、涉及 NF1 基因复制的案例。

10.10　总体插入

NF1 基因插入导致失活最典型的例子涉及 Alu 元件的反转录转座插入。这些插入发生在 NF1 基因的外显子内（Wimmer et al. 2007；Valero et al. 2011）或内含子内（Wallace et al. 1991），且通常倾向于优先发生在富含 AT 的区域（Wallace et al. 1991）。

Wimmer 等（2011）通过 cDNA 测序筛查 NF1

基因突变发现，在 18 名无亲缘关系的 NF1 患者中存在异常剪接的 *NF1* 转录本，而这些转录本在基因组水平上无法用潜在的微小损伤来解释。进一步的特征分析揭示了致病突变是由 14 个 *Alu* 元件插入、3 个 L1 元件插入以及 1 个约 120 碱基对的 poly(T) 序列插入（可能也是 1 个高度截短的 *Alu* 序列）引起的。这 18 个由 L1 内切酶介导的致病性从头插入，代表了迄今为止在任何人类基因中已发现的数量最多的插入型突变。这些发现表明，反转录转座子插入可能占所有 *NF1* 基因突变的 0.4%。此外，在 1.5 kb 的区域内（*NF1* 外显子 21、22 和 23）发现了 6 个不同的插入位点聚集现象。值得注意的是，3 个不同的整合位点（其中之一位于聚集区域内）分别被重复使用了 2 次，这与反转录转座子在 *NF1* 基因中相对频繁且高度非随机整合的现象相一致。目前尚不清楚这些插入是如何精确干扰 *NF1* 转录本的剪接过程的，但很可能通过多种机制实现，包括简单引入新的剪接位点、破坏外显子剪接增强子，或增加外显子顺式调控元件与其相应剪接位点之间的距离，从而干扰外显子的意义 (Wimmer et al. 2011)。

10.11　*NF1* 基因的其他重排

已有研究报道了 2 例非同源的 t(17;22) 易位，这些易位破坏了 *NF1* 基因 (Viskochil et al. 1990; Kehrer-Sawatzki et al. 1997)。在这 2 例病例中，22q11 的断点位于 1 个回文 AT 富集重复序列 (palindromic AT-rich repeat, PATRR) 内，而 17q11 染色体的断裂点则位于 *NF1* 基因内含子 31 中的 1 个 195 bp PATRR 中心附近 (Kehrer-Sawatzki et al. 1997; Kurahashi et al. 2003)。这些发现与回文序列介导的复发性 t(17;22) 易位机制一致。

此外，还报道了 1 例 (17)(q11.2q25.1) 倒位 (Asamoah et al. 1995)。

10.12　基因型-表型相关性

显然，识别特定的遗传性 *NF1* 基因突变通常无法准确预测受影响个体的疾病潜在严重性或结局。对于许多遗传性疾病，DNA 序列的特定变化与相关疾病特征的最终表现之间，往往存在复杂的时空关系，很难建立准确的相关性。在尝试解释潜在的基因型-表型关系时，必须考虑多种突变和多态性之间的组合效应，包括等位和非等位变异。

在 NF1 的背景下，迄今为止仅报道了 2 个明确的基因型-表型相关性。首先，携带大片段缺失的 NF1 患者往往表现出更为严重的临床表型 (Kayes et al. 1994; Upadhyaya et al. 1998; Spiegel et al. 2005; López-Correa et al. 2001; Mautner et al. 2010; Pasmant et al. 2010)。其次，携带 *NF1* 基因第 17 外显子中 1 个 3 bp 的框内缺失患者 (c.2970-2972 delAAT)，通常不出现皮肤型神经纤维瘤 (Upadhyaya et al. 2007)；目前已知约有 100 名 NF1 患者携带这种 3 bp 缺失，均未出现皮肤型神经纤维瘤。

此外，Upadhyaya 等 (2009) 研究了来自 14 名无亲缘关系的 NF1 患者的 22 个脊髓神经纤维瘤。其中 7 名患者满足 NF1 的诊断标准，而其余 7 名患者仅表现出部分的 NF1 临床特征。后者被定义为家族性脊髓神经纤维瘤病，与经典 NF1 组相比，其携带的常染色体错义和（或）剪接位点突变的数量显著较高 (Kluwe et al. 2003)。

另一种潜在的基因型-表型相关性是，存在视路胶质瘤的 NF1 患者中，5′端 1/3 区域的突变较为常见 (Sharif et al. 2011)。如果这些结果得到证实，可能促使采用更为针对性的方法进行视路胶质瘤的筛查，从而早期识别高风险患者。

已有其他几种尚未充分证实的基因型-表型相关性被提出，其中包括最近发现的几例具有 *NF1* 基因区域 1.4 Mb 重复的非典型 NF1 患者 (Grisart et al. 2008)。其中 2 例患者外表上似乎表现正常。由于普遍存在的家族内表型变异以及迄今为止仅在 1 个家族中报道了 *NF1* 位点重复，所以很难对 *NF1* 重复与表型之间的关系做出结论，显然这一领域需要进一步的研究 (Grisart et al. 2008)。

最近的一项研究描述了 1 个五代人均患有努南综合征和 NF1 的家族，其在基因的第 24 外显子中发现了胚系错义突变（Nyström et al. 2009）。该家族中没有任何患病成员表现出皮肤型神经纤维瘤。作者建议，未来应考虑对努南-NF1家族进行第17外显子 c.2970-2972 delAAT 缺失和第24外显子错义突变的筛查。

最后，NF1基因的非截短型致病突变与NF1患者的肺动脉狭窄之间已经初步确定了基因型-表型相关性（Ben-Sachar et al. 2012）。

在NF1中，基因型与表型之间的相关性很可能受到多种因素的影响，包括NF1基因表达的等位基因特异性差异（Jentarra et al. 2012）、NF1基因甲基化状态的等位基因特异性差异（Harder et al. 2010）、选择性剪接以及未连锁修饰基因的作用（Sabbagh et al. 2009；Pasmant et al. 2011）。

10.13 新突变的亲本起源

NF1基因的新突变率是已知人类遗传疾病中较高的突变率之一（Huson et al. 1989；Takano et al. 1992）。早期研究表明，约90%的自发性NF1基因突变倾向于发生在父源染色体上（Jadayel et al. 1990；Stephens et al. 1992；Lázaro et al. 1996）。然而，这些结论是基于通过连锁分析来确定突变亲本来源的，而非直接检测NF1基因突变。后来研究发现，较大的NF1基因缺失（通过基因内和侧翼的多态性标记简单识别）更倾向于来自母系来源的染色体（Lázaro et al. 1996；Ainsworth et al. 1997；Upadhyaya et al. 1998）。因此，特定NF1基因病变的起源很可能受到其突变类型的影响，其中大片段缺失倾向于在卵子发生过程中出现，而微小病变，如单碱基对替换，则更多发生在精子发生过程中。

10.14 胚系嵌合现象

胚系嵌合现象（Zlotogora 1998）在NF1中似乎较为罕见，因为很少有报道显示健康父母生育了多个患病孩子（Lázaro et al. 1994）。然而，要确认胚系嵌合现象需要对相关个体进行分子分析，因为已有报道表明同一家庭中出现了2个或多个不同的 NF1基因突变的情况（Klose et al. 1999；Upadhyaya et al. 2003）。在染色体嵌合现象源自父系生殖细胞的情况下，据估计有10%~17%的父系精子携带有病理性的NF1基因突变（Lázaro et al. 1994，1995；Bottillo et al. 2010）。

有一案例报告显示，节段型1型神经纤维瘤病（segmental neurofibromatosis type 1，SNF1）的母亲生出了经典型NF1的女儿。SNF1的特点是NF1特征的区域性有限分布，Consoli等（2005）提出，皮肤型嵌合体可能伴随生殖细胞嵌合体（即体细胞和生殖系组织的嵌合体）。这些研究者在患病儿童的淋巴细胞DNA中发现了NF1基因的第31外显子的无义突变（R1947X）。DNA序列分析未能在母亲的外周淋巴细胞、受影响和未受影响皮肤中的角质形成细胞和成纤维细胞中识别此种突变。随后，研究者从每个母体细胞系中克隆了含有NF1基因第31外显子的DNA片段，并使用等位基因特异性PCR对这些克隆进行筛选，R1947X突变在20%的角质形成细胞克隆和8.8%的受影响区域成纤维细胞克隆中被鉴定出来，但在临床上未受影响的组织衍生克隆中未被鉴定出来。这些发现表明，性染色体嵌合现象可在SNF1中发生，这对遗传咨询具有重要意义。

10.15 拷贝数变异（copy-number variation，CNV）

Wong等（2007）研究了95个人类基因组DNA，在5例个体中发现了NF1基因的拷贝数增加，以及在另一例个体中发现了拷贝数缺失（即每190个染色体中有6个CNV）。这些NF1 CNV最初是通过BAC RP11-518B17的异常荧光强度比值检测到的，它跨越了NF1基因的远端部分。随后，Khaja等（2006）通过直接将人类基因组参考序列与Celera组装的基因组参考序列比对，也在NF1基因区域中注意到了这些CNV。由于CNV被认为通过触发NAHR在基因组疾病特征化的区域中产生变异，Steinmann等（2008）为确定NF1基因区域内的CNV是否有可能导致大片段NF1缺失的形成，他们在最常见的大片段缺失类型——1型缺失患者的父母中探究 NF1 基因区域内的 CNV 的频率。然而，结果是阴性的，似乎否定了这些变异介导了 1 型缺失的 NAHR。此外，Steinmann 等（2008）使用多重连接依赖探针扩增（multiplex ligation-dependent probe amplification，MLPA）技术，在来自健康对照组的 167 条染色体中亦未能证实 NF1 位点的 CNV。

10.16 NF1 的分子诊断

大多数 NF1 患者的初步诊断通常依赖于神经纤维瘤病专家的仔细检查，结合临床表现进行判断。NF1 突变的检测与鉴定有助于了解其对 NF1 基因的影响，从而对患者的整体临床评估提供指导（Messiaen and Wimmer 2008；Griffiths et al. 2007）。早期诊断对于患者及其家庭的遗传咨询至关重要，同时也便于对患儿进行定期监测，以预防并发症的发展，如学习障碍、视神经胶质瘤和高血压。然而值得注意的是，NF1 产前诊断的需求有限，这可能是因为识别致病性 NF1 的突变通常难以预测未来患儿在疾病严重程度或进展。尽管如此，仍然需要开发一种更快、更准确且更具成本效益的基于 DNA 的 NF1 检测方法。目前，NF1 基因的常规分子诊断检测平均需要 3～4 周时间。幸运的是，检测较小的 SPRED1 基因仅需 2～3 天（Brems et al. 2007）。对于大多数中等大小的基因，分子检测结果可以在 1 周内生成。在英国，对基因组 DNA 进行的 NF1 检测费用在 700 英镑至 1 000 英镑以上不等，而基于 RNA 的检测费大约为 600 英镑。这是一项昂贵的检测，因为它需要在基因组 DNA 中筛查 57 个外显子。当这项检测实现完全自动化时，成本预计会降低，并伴随灵敏性和特异性的提高，结果报告时间亦大大缩短。

此外，针对 NF1 的适宜胚胎植入前遗传学诊断（preimplantation genetic diagnosis，PGD）方案也已开发出来（Spits et al. 2005），PGD 作为产前诊断的替代方案，可以避免治疗性流产。该诊断在从 3 天龄胚胎中获取的单个细胞上进行；只有那些检测为健康的胚胎才会被植入母亲体内。

10.17 结论

如上所述，NF1 的新突变率是已知的人类遗传性疾病中最高的突变率之一（Huson et al. 1989；Takano et al. 1992）。我们面临的挑战在于如何根据对 NF1 基因胚系突变谱的了解来解释这种高突变率。研究表明，基因的许多不同特征可以影响其突变频率，例如染色体位置、编码序列的长度、内含子的数量和长度、核苷酸组成以及基因内部和侧翼的序列重复性。

尽管如此，NF1 基因的突变谱远未完整；实际上，对 NF1 基因突变的筛查通常只能识别出 80%～95% 的假定存在于 NF1 患者样本中的病理突变（Fahsold et al. 2000；Ars et al. 2000；Messiaen et al. 2000；Mattocks et al. 2004；De Luca et al. 2007），造成这种情况的原因尚不清楚。很可能是由于大量缺失的病变位于远端上游或下游的调控元件中，或者位于内含子的深处。尽管基于 RNA 的突变筛查方法理论上可以检测到后者，但识别前者可能存在巨大困难。不论缺失的病理突变位于何处，NF1 基因种系突变谱的检查使我们得出结论：与许多人类基因一样（Cooper et al. 2011），NF1 基因突变的性质、位置和频率在很大程度上受到局部 DNA 序列环境的影响，并且通常以非常可预测的方式展现出来。

（朱倍瑶 译）

参考文献

[1] Ahmadian MR, Kiel C, Stege P, Scheffzek K (2003) Structural fingerprints of the Ras-GTPase activating proteins neurofibromin and p120GAP. J Mol Biol 329: 699–710

[2] Ainsworth PJ, Chakraborty PK, Weksberg R (1997) Example of somatic mosaicism in a series of de novo neurofibromatosis type 1 cases due to a maternally derived deletion. Hum Mutat 9: 452–457

[3] Ars E, Serra E, García J, Kruyer H, Gaona A, Lázaro C, Estivill X (2000) Mutations affecting mRNA splicing are the most common molecular defects in patients with neurofibromatosis type 1. Hum Mol Genet 9: 237–247

[4] Arun D, Gutmann DH (2004) Recent advances in

[5] Asamoah A, North K, Doran S, Wagstaff J, Ogle R, Collins FS, Korf BR (1995) 17q inversion involving the neurofibromatosis type one locus in a family with neurofibromatosis type one. Am J Med Genet 60: 312-316

[6] Ball EV, Stenson PD, Abeysinghe SS, Krawczak M, Cooper DN, Chuzhanova NA (2005) Microdeletions and microinsertions causing human genetic disease: common mechanisms of mutagenesis and the role of local DNA sequence complexity. Hum Mutat 26: 205-213

[7] Baralle M, Skoko N, Knezevich A, De Conti L, Motti D, Bhuvanagiri M, Baralle D, Buratti E, Baralle FE (2006) NF1 mRNA biogenesis: effect of the genomic milieu in splicing regulation of the NF1 exon 37 region. FEBS Lett 580: 4449-4456

[8] Barron VA, Lou H (2012) Alternative splicing of the neurofibromatosis type 1 pre-mRNA. Biosci Rep 32: 131-138

[9] Bengesser KCD, Steinmann K, Kluwe L, Chuzhanova NA, Wimmer K, Tatagiba M, Tinschert S, Mautner VF, Kehrer-Sawatzki H (2010) A novel third type of recurrent NF1 microdeletion mediated by non-allelic homologous recombination between LRRC37B-containing low-copy repeats in 17q11.2. Hum Mutat 31: 742-751

[10] Bennett E, Thomas N, Upadhyaya M (2009) Neurofibromatosis type 1: its association with the Ras/MAPK pathway syndromes. J Pediatr Neurol 7: 105-115

[11] Ben-Shachar S, Constantini S, Hallevi H, Sach EK, Upadhyaya M, Evans GD, Huson SM (2012) Increased rate of missense/in-frame mutations in individuals with NF1-related pulmonary stenosis: a novel genotype-phenotype correlation. Eur J Hum Genet. doi: 10.1038/ejhg.2012.221

[12] Bottillo I, Torrente I, Lanari V, Pinna V, Giustini S, Divona L, De Luca A, Dallapiccola B (2010) Germline mosaicism in neurofibromatosis type 1 due to a paternally derived multi-exon deletion. Am J Med Genet 152A: 1467-1473

[13] Brems H, Chmara M, Sahbatou M et al (2007) Germline loss-of-function mutations in SPRED1 cause a neurofibromatosis1-like phenotype. Nat Genet 39: 1120-1126

[14] Casola C, Zekonyte U, Phillips AD, Cooper DN, Hahn MW (2012) Interlocus gene conversion events introduce deleterious mutations into at least 1% of human genes associated with inherited disease. Genome Res 22: 429-435

[15] Chuzhanova NA, Anassis EJ, Ball EV, Krawczak M, Cooper DN (2003) Meta-analysis of indels causing human genetic disease: mechanisms of mutagenesis and the role of local DNA sequence complexity. Hum Mutat 21: 28-44

[16] Colapietro P, Gervasini C, Natacci F, Rossi L, Riva P, Larizza L (2003) NF1 exon 7 skipping and sequence alterations in exonic splice enhancers (ESEs) in a neurofibromatosis 1 patient. Hum Genet 113: 551-554

[17] Consoli C, Moss C, Green S, Balderson D, Cooper DN, Upadhyaya M (2005) Gonosomal mosaicism for a nonsense mutation (R1947X) in the NF1 gene in segmental neurofibromatosis type 1. J Invest Dermatol 125: 463-466

[18] Cooper DN (2010) Functional intronic polymorphisms: buried treasure awaiting discovery within our genes. Hum Genomics 4: 284-288

[19] Cooper DN, Mort M, Stenson PD, Ball EV, Chuzhanova NA (2010) Methylation-mediated deamination of 5-methylcytosine appears to give rise to mutations causing human inherited disease in CpNpG trinucleotides, as well as in CpG dinucleotides. Hum Genomics 4: 406-410

[20] Cooper DN, Bacolla A, Férec C, Vasquez KM, Kehrer-Sawatzki H, Chen JM (2011) On the sequence-directed nature of human gene mutation: the role of genomic architecture and the local DNA sequence environment in mediating gene mutations underlying human inherited disease. Hum Mutat 32: 1075-1099

[21] D'Angelo I, Welti S, Bonneau F, Scheffzek K (2006) A novel bipartite phospholipid-binding module in the neurofibromatosis type 1 protein. EMBO Rep 7: 174-179

[22] De Luca A, Bottillo I, Dasdia MC, Morella A, Lanari V, Bernardini L, Divona L, Giustini S, Sinibaldi L, Novelli A, Torrente I, Schirinzi A, Dallapiccola B (2007) Deletions of NF1 gene and exons detected by multiplex ligation-dependent probe amplification. J Med Genet 44: 800-808

[23] Evans DG, Howard E, Giblin C, Clancy T, Spencer H, Huson SM, Lalloo F (2010) Birth incidence and prevalence of tumor-prone syndromes: estimates from a UK family genetic register service. Am J Med Genet 152A: 327-332

[24] Fahsold R, Hoffmeyer S, Mischung C, Gille C, Ehlers C, Kücükceylan N, Abdel-Nour M, Gewies A, Peters H, Kaufmann D, Buske A, Tinschert S, Nürnberg P (2000) Minor lesion mutational spectrum of the entire NF1 gene does not explain its high mutability but points to a functional domain upstream of the GAP-related domain. Am J Hum Genet 66: 790-818

[25] Fernández-Rodríguez J, Castellsagué J, Benito L, Benavente Y, Capellá G, Blanco I, Serra E, Lázaro C (2011) A mild neurofibromatosis type 1 phenotype produced by the combination of the benign nature of a leaky NF1-splice mutation and the presence of a complex mosaicism. Hum Mutat 32: 705-709

[26] Forbes SH, Dorschner MO, Le R, Stephens K (2004) Genomic context of paralogous recombination hotspots mediating recurrent NF1 region microdeletion. Genes Chromosomes Cancer 41: 12-25

[27] Gervasini C, Venturin M, Orzan F, Friso A, Clementi M, Tenconi R, Larizza L, Riva P (2005) Uncommon Alu-mediated NF1 microdeletion with a breakpoint inside the NF1 gene. Genomics 85: 273-279

[28] Griffiths S, Thompson P, Frayling I et al (2007) Molecular diagnosis for NF1: 2 years experience. Fam Cancer 6: 21-34

[29] Grisart B, Rack K, Vidrequin S, Hilbert P, Deltenre P, Verellen-Dumoulin C, Destrée A (2008) NF1 microduplication first clinical report: association with mild mental retardation, early onset of baldness and dental enamel hypoplasia? Eur J Hum Genet 16: 305-311

[30] Gutmann DH, Loehr A, Zhang Y, Kim J, Henkemeyer M, Cashen A (1999) Haploinsufficiency for the neurofibromatosis 1 (NF1) tumor suppressor results in increased astrocyte proliferation. Oncogene 18: 4450-4459

[31] Harder A, Titze S, Herbst L, Harder T, Guse K, Tinschert S, Kaufmann D, Rosenbaum T, Mautner VF, Windt E, Wahlländer-Danek U, Wimmer K, Mundlos S, Peters H (2010) Monozygotic twins with neurofibromatosis type 1 (NF1) display differences in methylation of NF1 gene promoter elements, 5′ untranslated region, exon and intron 1. Twin Res Hum Genet 13: 582-594

[32] Horan MP, Osborn M, Cooper DN, Upadhyaya M (2004) Functional analysis of polymorphic variation within the promoter and 5′ untranslated region of the neurofibromatosis type 1 (NF1) gene. Am J Med Genet 131A: 227-231

[33] Huson SM, Compston DA, Clark P, Harper PS (1989) A genetic study of von Recklinghausen neurofibromatosis in South East Wales. I. Prevalence, fitness, mutation rate, and

effect of parental transmission on severity. J Med Genet 26: 704-711
[34] Ingram DA, Yang FC, Travers JB, Wenning MJ, Hiatt K, New S, Hood A, Shannon K, Williams DA, Clapp DW (2000) Genetic and biochemical evidence that haploinsufficiency of the *Nf1* tumor suppressor gene modulates melanocyte and mast cell fates in vivo. J Exp Med 191: 181-188
[35] Ivanov D, Hamby SE, Stenson PD, Phillips AD, Kehrer-Sawatzki H, Cooper DN, Chuzhanova N (2011) Comparative analysis of germline and somatic microlesion mutational spectra in 17 human tumor suppressor genes. Hum Mutat 32: 620-632
[36] Jadayel D, Fain P, Upadhyaya M, Ponder MA, Huson SM, Carey J, Fryer A, Mathew CG, Barker DF, Ponder BA (1990) Paternal origin of new mutations in von Recklinghausen neurofibromatosis. Nature 343: 558-559
[37] Jentarra GM, Rice SG, Olfers S, Rajan C, Saffen DM, Narayanan V (2012) Skewed allele-specific expression of the *NF1* gene in normal subjects: a possible mechanism for phenotypic variability in neurofibromatosis type 1. J Child Neurol 27(6): 695-702
[38] Kayes LM, Burke W, Riccardi VM, Bennett R, Ehrlich P, Rubenstein A, Stephens K (1994) Deletions spanning the neurofibromatosis 1 gene: identification and phenotype of five patients. Am J Hum Genet 54: 424-436
[39] Kehrer-Sawatzki H, Cooper DN (2008) Mosaicism in sporadic neurofibromatosis type 1: variations on a theme common to other hereditary cancer syndromes? J Med Genet 45: 622-631
[40] Kehrer-Sawatzki H, Häussler J, Krone W, Bode H, Jenne DE, Mehnert KU, Tümmers U, Assum G (1997) The second case of a t(17;22) in a family with neurofibromatosis type 1: sequence analysis of the breakpoint regions. Hum Genet 99: 237-247
[41] Kehrer-Sawatzki H, Kluwe L, Sandig C, Kohn M, Wimmer K, Krammer U, Peyrl A, Jenne DE, Hansmann I, Mautner VF (2004) High frequency of mosaicism among patients with neurofibromatosis type 1 (NF1) with microdeletions caused by somatic recombination of the *JJAZ1* gene. Am J Hum Genet 75: 410-423
[42] Kehrer-Sawatzki H, Schmid E, Fünsterer C, Kluwe L, Mautner VF (2008) Absence of cutaneous neurofibromas in an NF1 patient with an atypical deletion partially overlapping the common 1.4 Mb microdeleted region. Am J Med Genet A 146A: 691-699
[43] Kemkemer R, Schrank S, Vogel W, Gruler H, Kaufmann D (2002) Increased noise as an effect of haploinsufficiency of the tumor-suppressor gene neurofibromatosis type 1 in vitro. Proc Natl Acad Sci USA 99: 13783-13788
[44] Khaja R, Zhang J, Macdonald JR, He Y, Joseph-George AM, Wei J, Rafiq MA, Qian C, Shago M, Pantano L, Aburatani H, Jones K, Redon R, Hurles M, Armengol L, Estivill X, Mural RJ, Lee C, Scherer SW, Feuk L (2006) Genome assembly comparison identifies structural variants in the human genome. Nat Genet 38: 1413-1418
[45] Klose A, Ahmadian MR, Schuelke M, Scheffzek K, Hoffmeyer S, Gewies A, Schmitz F, Kaufmann D, Peters H, Wittinghofer A, Nürnberg P (1998) Selective disactivation of neurofibromin GAP activity in neurofibromatosis type 1. Hum Mol Genet 7: 1261-1268
[46] Klose A, Peters H, Hoffmeyer S, Buske A, Lüder A, Hess D, Lehmann R, Nürnberg P, Tinschert S (1999) Two independent mutations in a family with neurofibromatosis type 1 (NF1). Am J Med Genet 83: 6-12
[47] Kluwe L, Tatagiba M, Fünsterer C, Mautner V (2003) *NF1* mutations and clinical spectrum in patients with spinal neurofibromas. J Med Genet 40: 368-371
[48] Kluwe L, Siebert R, Gesk S, Friedrich RE, Tinschert S, Kehrer-Sawatzki H, Mautner VF (2004) Screening 500 unselected neurofibromatosis 1 patients for deletions of the *NF1* gene. Hum Mutat 23: 111-116
[49] Krawczak M, Ball EV, Cooper DN (1998) Neighboring-nucleotide effects on the rates of germline single-base-pair substitution in human genes. Am J Hum Genet 63: 474-488
[50] Kurahashi H, Shaikh T, Takata M, Toda T, Emanuel BS (2003) The constitutional t(17;22): another translocation mediated by palindromic AT-rich repeats. Am J Hum Genet 72: 733-738
[51] Lázaro C, Ravella A, Gaona A, Volpini V, Estivill X (1994) Neurofibromatosis type 1 due to germ-line mosaicism in a clinically normal father. N Engl J Med 331: 1403-1407
[52] Lázaro C, Gaona A, Lynch M, Kruyer H, Ravella A, Estivill X (1995) Molecular characterization of the breakpoints of a 12-kb deletion in the *NF1* gene in a family showing germ-line mosaicism. Am J Hum Genet 57: 1044-1049
[53] Lázaro C, Gaona A, Ainsworth P, Tenconi R, Vidaud D, Kruyer H, Ars E, Volpini V, Estivill X (1996) Sex differences in mutational rate and mutational mechanism in the *NF1* gene in neurofibromatosis type 1 patients. Hum Genet 98: 696-699
[54] Lee J, Jang SJ, Benoit N, Hoque MO, Califano JA, Trink B, Sidransky D, Mao L, Moon C (2010) Presence of 5-methylcytosine in CpNpG trinucleotides in the human genome. Genomics 96: 67-72
[55] Li Y, Bollag G, Clark R, Stevens J, Conroy L, Fults D, Ward K, Friedman E, Samowitz W, Flobertson M, Bradley P, McCormick F, White R, Cawthon R (1992) Somatic mutations in the neurofibromatosis 1 gene in human tumors. Cell 69: 261-275
[56] Lister R, Pelizzda M, Dowen RH, Hawkins RD, Hon G, Tonti-Filippini J, Nery JR, Lee L, Ye Z, Ngo QM, Edsall L, Antosiewicz-Bourget J, Stewart R, Ruotti V, Millar AH, Thomson JA, Ren B, Ecker JR (2009) Human DNA methylomes at base resolution show widespread epigenomic differences. Nature 462: 315-322
[57] López-Correa C, Brems H, Lazaro C, Marynen P, Legius E (2000) Unequal meiotic crossover: a frequent cause of NF1 microdeletions. Am J Hum Genet 66: 1969-1974
[58] López-Correa C, Dorschner M, Brems H, Lázaro C, Clementi M, Upadhyaya M, Dooijes D, Moog U, Kehrer-Sawatzki H, Rutkowski JL, Fryns JP, Marynen P, Stephens K, Legius E (2001) Recombination hotspot in NF1 microdeletion patients. Hum Mol Genet 10: 1387-1392
[59] Luijten M, Redeker S, Minoshima S, Shimizu N, Westerveld A, Hulsebos TJ (2001a) Duplication and transposition of the *NF1* pseudogene regions on chromosomes 2, 14, and 22. Hum Genet 109: 109-116
[60] Luijten M, Fahsold R, Mischung C, Westerveld A, Nürnberg P, Hulsebos TJ (2001b) Limited contribution of interchromosomal gene conversion to *NF1* gene mutation. J Med Genet 38: 481-485
[61] Mantripragada KK, Thuresson AC, Piotrowski A, Díaz de Ståhl T, Menzel U, Grigelionis G, Ferner RE, Griffiths S, Bolund L, Mautner V, Nordling M, Legius E, Vetrie D, Dahl N, Messiaen L, Upadhyaya M, Bruder CE, Dumanski JP (2006) Identification of novel deletion breakpoints bordered by

[62] Mattocks C, Baralle D, Tarpey P, Ffrench-Constant C, Bobrow M, Whittaker J (2004) Automated comparative sequence analysis identifies mutations in 89% of NF1 patients and confirms a mutation cluster in exons 11-17 distinct from the GAP related domain. J Med Genet 41: e48

[63] Mautner VF, Kluwe L, Friedrich RE, Roehl AC, Bammert S, Högel J, Spöri H, Cooper DN, Kehrer-Sawatzki H (2010) Clinical characterisation of 29 neurofibromatosis type-1 patients with molecularly ascertained 1.4 Mb type-1 NF1 deletions. J Med Genet 47: 623-630

[64] McLaughlin ME, Jacks T (2002) Thinking beyond the tumor cell. NF1 haploinsufficiency in the tumor environment. Cancer Cell 1: 408-410

[65] Messiaen LM, Wimmer K (2008) NF1 mutational spectrum. In: Kaufmann D (ed) Neurofibromatoses. Monographs in human genetics, vol 16. Karger, Basel, pp 63-77

[66] Messiaen LM, Callens T, Mortier G, Beysen D, Vandenbroucke I, Van Roy N, Speleman F, Paepe AD (2000) Exhaustive mutation analysis of the NF1 gene allows identification of 95% of mutations and reveals a high frequency of unusual splicing defects. Hum Mutat 15: 541-555

[67] Messiaen L, Vogt J, Bengesser K, Fu C, Mikhail F, Serra E, Garcia-Linares C, Cooper DN, Lazaro C, Kehrer-Sawatzki H (2011) Mosaic type-1 NF1 microdeletions as a cause of both generalized and segmental neurofibromatosis type-1 (NF1). Hum Mutat 32: 213-219

[68] Morcos P, Thapar N, Tusneem N, Stacey D, Tamanoi F (1996) Identification of neurofibromin mutants that exhibit allele specificity or increased Ras affinity resulting in suppression of activated ras alleles. Mol Cell Biol 16: 2496-2503

[69] Mort M, Ivanov D, Cooper DN, Chuzhanova NA (2008) A meta-analysis of nonsense mutations causing human genetic disease. Hum Mutat 29: 1037-1047

[70] Nyström AM, Ekvall S, Strömberg B, Holmström G, Thuresson AC, Annerén G, Bondeson ML (2009) A severe form of Noonan syndrome and autosomal dominant cafe-au-lait spots—evidence for different genetic origins. Acta Paediatr 98: 693-698

[71] Orzan F, Stroppi M, Venturin M, Valero MC, Hernández C, Riva P (2008) Breakpoint characterization of a novel NF1 multiexonic deletion: a case showing expression of the mutated allele. Neurogenetics 9: 95-100

[72] Osborn M, Cooper DN, Upadhyaya M (2000) Molecular analysis of the 5′-flanking region of the neurofibromatosis type 1 (NF1) gene: identification of five sequence variants. Clin Genet 57: 221-224

[73] Pasmant E, Sabbagh A, Spurlock G, Laurendeau I, Grillo E, Hamel MJ, Martin L, Barbarot S, Leheup B, Rodriguez D, Lacombe D, Dollfus H, Pasquier L, Isidor B, Ferkal S, Soulier J, Sanson M, Dieux-Coeslier A, Bièche I, Parfait B, Vidaud M, Wolkenstein P, Upadhyaya M, Vidaud D, Members of the NF France Network (2010) NF1 microdeletions in neurofibromatosis type 1: from genotype to phenotype. Hum Mutat 31: E1506-E1518

[74] Pasmant E, Sabbagh A, Masliah-Planchon J, Ortonne N, Laurendeau I, Melin L, Ferkal S, Hernandez L, Leroy K, Valeyrie-Allanore L, Parfait B, Vidaud D, Bièche I, Lantieri L, Wolkenstein P, Vidaud M, Members of the NF France Network (2011) Role of noncoding RNA ANRIL in genesis of plexiform neurofibromas in neurofibromatosis type 1. J Natl Cancer Inst 103: 1713-1722

[75] Pemov A, Park C, Reilly KM, Stewart DR (2010) Evidence of perturbations of cell cycle and DNA repair pathways as a consequence of human and murine NF1-haploinsufficiency. BMC Genomics 11: 194

[76] Petek E, Jenne DE, Smolle J, Binder B, Lasinger W, Windpassinger C, Wagner K, Kroisel PM, Kehrer-Sawatzki H (2003) Mitotic recombination mediated by the JJAZF1 (KIAA0160) gene causing somatic mosaicism and a new type of constitutional NF1 microdeletion in two children of a mosaic female with only few manifestations. J Med Genet 40: 520-525

[77] Poullet P, Lin B, Esson K, Tamanoi F (1994) Functional significance of lysine 1423 of neurofibromin and characterization of a second site suppressor which rescues mutations at this residue and suppresses RAS2Val-19-activated phenotypes. Mol Cell Biol 14: 815-821

[78] Pros E, Gómez C, Martín T, Fábregas P, Serra E, Lázaro C (2008) Nature and mRNA effect of 282 different NF1 point mutations: focus on splicing alterations. Hum Mutat 29: E173-E193

[79] Raedt TD, Stephens M, Heyns I, Brems H, Thijs D, Messiaen L, Stephens K, Lazaro C, Wimmer K, Kehrer-Sawatzki H, Vidaud D, Kluwe L, Marynen P, Legius E (2006) Conservation of hotspots for recombination in low-copy repeats associated with the NF1 microdeletion. Nat Genet 38: 1419-1423

[80] Raponi M, Upadhyaya M, Baralle D (2006) Functional splicing assay shows a pathogenic intronic mutation in neurofibromatosis type 1 (NF1) due to intronic sequence exonization. Hum Mutat 27: 294-295

[81] Rodenhiser DI, Andrews JD, Mancini DN, Jung JH, Singh SM (1997) Homonucleotide tracts, short repeats and CpG/CpNpG motifs are frequent sites for heterogeneous mutations in the neurofibromatosis type 1 (NF1) tumour-suppressor gene. Mutat Res 373: 185-195

[82] Roehl AC, Vogt J, Mussotter T, Zickler AN, Spöti H, Högel J, Chuzhanova NA, Wimmer K, Kluwe L, Mautner VF, Cooper DN, Kehrer-Sawatzki H (2010) Intrachromosomal mitotic nonallelic homologous recombination is the major molecular mechanism underlying type-2 NF1 deletions. Hum Mutat 31: 1163-1173

[83] Sabbagh A, Pasmant E, Laurendeau I, Parfait B, Barbarot S, Guillot B, Combemale P, Ferkal S, Vidaud M, Aubourg P, Vidaud D, Wolkenstein P, Members of the NF France Network (2009) Unravelling the genetic basis of variable clinical expression in neurofibromatosis 1. Hum Mol Genet 18: 2768-2778

[84] Scheffzek K, Ahmadian MR, Kabsch W, Wiesmüller L, Lautwein A, Schmitz F, Wittinghofer A (1997) The Ras-RasGAP complex: structural basis for GTPase activation and its loss in oncogenic Ras mutants. Science 277: 333-338

[85] Scheffzek K, Ahmadian MR, Wiesmüller L, Kabsch W, Stege P, Schmitz F, Wittinghofer A (1998) Structural analysis of the GAP-related domain from neurofibromin and its implications. EMBO J 17: 4313-4327

[86] Sharif S, Upadhyaya M, Ferner R, Majounie E, Shenton A, Baser M, Thakker N, Evans DG (2011) A molecular analysis of individuals with neurofibromatosis type 1 (NF1) and optic pathway gliomas (OPGs), and an assessment of genotype-phenotype correlations. J Med Genet 48: 256-260

[87] Skinner RH, Bradley S, Brown AL, Johnson NJE, Rhodes S, Stammers DK, Lowe PN (1991) Use of the Glu-Glu-Phe C-

terminal epitope for rapid purification of the catalytic domain of normal and mutant *ras* GTPase-activating proteins. J Biol Chem 266: 14163-14166

[88] Spiegel M, Oexle K, Horn D, Windt E, Buske A, Albrecht B, Prott EC, Seemanová E, Seidel J, Rosenbaum T, Jenne D, Kehrer-Sawatzki H, Tinschert S (2005) Childhood overgrowth in patients with common *NF1* microdeletions. Eur J Hum Genet 13: 883-888

[89] Spits C, De Rycke M, Van Ranst N et al (2005) Preimplantation genetic diagnosis for neurofibromatosis type 1. Mol Hum Reprod 11: 381-387

[90] Steinmann K, Cooper DN, Kluwe L, Chuzhanova NA, Senger C, Serra E, Lazaro C, Gilaberte M, Wimmer K, Mautner VF, Kehrer-Sawatzki H (2007) Type 2 *NF1* deletions are highly unusual by virtue of the absence of nonallelic homologous recombination hotspots and an apparent preference for female mitotic recombination. Am J Hum Genet 81: 1201-1220

[91] Steinmann K, Kluwe L, Cooper DN, Brems H, De Raedt T, Legius E, Mautner VF, Kehrer-Sawatzki H (2008) Copy number variations in the *NF1* gene region are infrequent and do not predispose to recurrent type-1 deletions. Eur J Hum Genet 16: 572-580

[92] Stenson PD, Mort M, Ball EV, Howells K, Phillips AD, Thomas NS, Cooper DN (2009) The human gene mutation database: 2008 update. Genome Med 1: 13

[93] Stephens K, Kayes L, Riccardi VM, Rising M, Sybert VP, Pagon RA (1992) Preferential mutation of the neurofibromatosis type 1 gene in paternally derived chromosomes. Hum Genet 88: 279-282

[94] Sterne-Weiler T, Howard J, Mort M, Cooper DN, Sanford JR (2011) Loss of exon identity is a common mechanism of human inherited disease. Genome Res 21: 1563-1571

[95] Takano T, Kawashima T, Yamanouchi Y, Kitayama K, Baba T, Ueno K, Hamaguchi H (1992) Genetics of neurofibromatosis 1 in Japan: mutation rate and paternal age effect. Hum Genet 89: 281-286

[96] Thomas L, Richards M, Mort M, Dunlop E, Cooper DN, Upadhyaya M (2012) Assessment of the potential pathogenicity of missense mutations identified in the GTPase-activating protein (GAP)-related domain of the neurofibromatosis type-1 (NF1) gene. Hum Mutat 33: 1687-1696

[97] Trovó-Marqui AB, Tajara EH (2006) Neurofibromin: a general outlook. Clin Genet 70: 1-13

[98] Upadhyaya M (2008) *NF1* gene structure and NF1 genotype/phenotype correlations. In: Kaufmann D (ed) The neurofibromatoses. Karger, Basel, pp 46-62

[99] Upadhyaya M, Osborn MJ, Maynard J, Kim MR, Tamanoi F, Cooper DN (1997) Mutational and functional analysis of the neurofibromatosis type 1 (*NF1*) gene. Hum Genet 99: 88-92

[100] Upadhyaya M, Ruggieri M, Maynard J, Osborn M, Hartog C, Mudd S, Penttinen M, Cordeiro I, Ponder M, Ponder BA, Krawczak M, Cooper DN (1998) Gross deletions of the neurofibromatosis type 1 (*NF1*) gene are predominantly of maternal origin and commonly associated with a learning disability, dysmorphic features and developmental delay. Hum Genet 102: 591-597

[101] Upadhyaya M, Majounie E, Thompson P, Han S, Consoli C, Krawczak M, Cordeiro I, Cooper DN (2003) Three different pathological lesions in the *NF1* gene originating de novo in a family with neurofibromatosis type 1. Hum Genet 112: 12-17

[102] Upadhyaya M, Huson SM, Davies M, Thomas N, Chuzhanova N, Giovannini S, Evans DG, Howard E, Kerr B, Griffiths S, Consoli C, Side L, Adams D, Pierpont M, Hachen R, Barnicoat A, Li H, Wallace P, Van Biervliet JP, Stevenson D, Viskochil D, Baralle D, Haan E, Riccardi V, Turnpenny P, Lazaro C, Messiaen L (2007) An absence of cutaneous neurofibromas associated with a 3-bp inframe deletion in exon 17 of the NF1 gene (c.2970-2972 delAAT): evidence of a clinically significant NF1 genotype-phenotype correlation. Am J Hum Genet 80: 140-151

[103] Upadhyaya M, Spurlock G, Kluwe L, Chuzhanova N, Bennett E, Thomas N, Guha A, Mautner V (2009) The spectrum of somatic and germline *NF1* mutations in NF1 patients with spinal neurofibromas. Neurogenetics 10: 251-263

[104] Valero MC, Martín Y, Hernández-Imaz E, Marina Hernández A, Meleán G, Valero AM, Javier Rodríguez-Álvarez F, Tellería D, Hernández-Chico C (2011) A highly sensitive genetic protocol to detect NF1 mutations. J Mol Diagn 13: 113-122

[105] Venturin M, Gervasini C, Orzan F, Bentivegna A, Corrado L, Colapietro P, Friso A, Tenconi R, Upadhyaya M, Larizza L, Riva P (2004) Evidence for non-homologous end joining and non-allelic homologous recombination in atypical *NF1* microdeletions. Hum Genet 115: 69-80

[106] Viskochil D, Buchberg AM, Xu G, Cawthon RM, Stevens J, Wolff RK, Culver M, Carey JC, Copeland NG, Jenkins NA, White R, O'Connell P (1990) Deletions and a translocation interrupt a cloned gene at the neurofibromatosis type 1 locus. Cell 62: 187-192

[107] Wallace MR, Andersen LB, Saulino AM, Gregory PE, Glover TW, Collins FS (1991) A de novo *Alu* insertion results in neurofibromatosis type 1. Nature 353: 864-866

[108] Welti S, Fraterman S, D'Angelo I, Wilm M, Scheffzek K (2007) The sec14 homology module of neurofibromin binds cellular glycerophospholipids: mass spectrometry and structure of a lipid complex. J Mol Biol 366: 551-562

[109] Welti S, D'Angelo I, Scheffzek K (2008) Structure and function of neurofibromin. In: Neurofibromatoses. Monographs in human genetics, vol 16. Basel, Karger, pp 113-128

[110] Welti S, Kühn S, D'Angelo I, Brügger B, Kaufmann D, Scheffzek K (2011) Structural and biochemical consequences of NF1 associated nontruncating mutations in the Sec14-PH module of neurofibromin. Hum Mutat 32: 191-197

[111] Wimmer K, Yao S, Claes K, Kehrer-Sawatzki H, Tinschert S, De Raedt T, Legius E, Callens T, Beiglböck H, Maertens O, Messiaen L (2006) Spectrum of single- and multiexon *NF1* copy number changes in a cohort of 1,100 unselected NF1 patients. Genes Chromosomes Cancer 45: 265-276

[112] Wimmer K, Roca X, Beiglböck H, Callens T, Etzler J, Rao AR, Krainer AR, Fonatsch C, Messiaen L (2007) Extensive *in silico* analysis of *NF1* splicing defects uncovers determinants for splicing outcome upon 5′ splice-site disruption. Hum Mutat 28: 599-612

[113] Wimmer K, Callens T, Wernstedt A, Messiaen L (2011) The *NF1* gene contains hotspots for L1 endonuclease-dependent de novo insertion. PLoS Genet 7: e1002371

[114] Wong KK, Deleeuw RJ, Dosanjh NS, Kimm LR, Cheng Z, Horsman DE, Macaulay C, Ng RT, Brown CJ, Eichler EE, Lam WL (2007) A comprehensive analysis of common copy-number variations in the human genome. Am J Hum Genet 80: 91-104

[115] Xu H, Gutmann DH (1997) Mutations in the GAP-related domain impair the ability of neurofibromin to associate with microtubules. Brain Res 759: 149-152

[116] Yu H, Zhao X, Su B, Li D, Xu Y, Luo S, Xiao C, Wang W (2005) Expression of NF1 pseudogenes. Hum Mutat 26: 487-488

[117] Zatkova A, Messiaen L, Vandenbroucke I, Wieser R, Fonatsch C, Krainer AR, Wimmer K (2004) Disruption of exonic splicing enhancer elements is the principal cause of exon skipping associated with seven nonsense or missense alleles of NF1. Hum Mutat 24: 491-501

[118] Zickler AM, Hampp S, Messiaen L, Bengesser K, Mussotter T, Roehl AC, Wimmer K, Mautner VF, Kluwe L, Upadhyaya M, Pasmant E, Chuzhanova N, Kestler HA, Högel J, Legius E, Claes K, Cooper DN, Kehrer-Sawatzki H (2012) Characterization of the nonallelic homologous recombination hotspot PRS3 associated with type-3 NF1 deletions. Hum Mutat 33: 372-383

[119] Zlotogora J (1998) Germ line mosaicism. Hum Genet 102: 381-386

[120] Zou MX, Butcher DT, Sadikovic B, Groves TC, Yee SP, Rodenhiser DI (2004) Characterization of functional elements in the neurofibromatosis (NF1) proximal promoter region. Oncogene 23: 330-339

第11章 NF1 基因的剪接机制和突变

Splicing Mechanisms and Mutations in the NF1 Gene

Marco Baralle and Diana Baralle

11.1 引言

前信使 RNA（pre-messenger RNA，pre-mRNA）剪接是指在细胞核内将非编码片段（内含子）从原始转录本中去除，同时将编码片段（外显子）连接起来并输出到细胞质的过程。NF1 的信使 RNA（mRNA）长度为 11～13 kb，其中最常见的编码为神经纤维瘤蛋白（1 种 2818 氨基酸的多肽），就 NF1 的具体情况而言，这意味着要识别 60 个外显子（57 个组成型外显子和 3 个可选择性剪接外显子），这些外显子组成了 NF1 基因的 mRNA 并分布在约 350 kb 的区域内。剪接机制不仅要识别这些外显子，还要将它们正确地连接在一起。

事实上，导致异常 pre-mRNA 剪接缺陷的突变是相当一部分人类遗传疾病的根源，也可能是遗传性疾病最常见的原因，因此了解剪接过程尤为重要（Tazi et al. 2009；Wang et al. 2008）。NF1 基因是已知人类基因中突变率高的基因之一，50% 的 NF1 患者被归类为散发性，它已成为与疾病相关的剪接突变频率的一个广为引用的例子，据估计，这种情况发生的频率为 20%～50%（Ars et al. 2000b；Valero et al. 2011）。事实上，在人类基因突变数据库（Human Gene Mutation Database，HGMD；http://www.hgmd.org）中，NF1 基因所列的 1 300 个突变中有 286 个（22%）被确定为剪接突变。这一数字很可能被低估了，因为许多错义、无义甚至可能是沉默序列变异也可能影响剪接过程（Baralle et al. 2006）。

11.2 Pre-mRNA 剪接概述

内含子的去除由剪接体完成，剪接体是一种动态的多亚基微粒，包含 5 种小型核糖核蛋白 snRNP（U1、U2、U4、U5 和 U6），它们与 200 多种不同的非 snRNP 辅助蛋白共同发挥作用（Nilsen 2003；Wahl et al. 2009）。为了决定剪接，每个内含子的 5' 端都有 1 个 GU 双核苷酸，3' 端有 1 个 AG 双核苷酸，但也有例外（Zhang 1998）。实际上，内含子两端这些近乎 100% 保守的二核苷酸构成了较松散的定义性序列的一部分，分别称为 5' 和 3' 剪接位点（Zhang 1998）。5' 剪接位点是 1 个退化的 8 核苷酸基序，其共识基序为 MAG/GURAGU（其中 M 为 A 或 C，R 为 A 或 G），而全 3' 剪接位点的定义更为松散，由 3

个元素组成：具有共识 CAG 的全 3′剪接位点，其中只有二核苷酸 AG 是普遍保留的；具有分支点（branch point，BP）共识的全 30 剪接位点，其中 1 个 A 核苷酸是普遍保留的；多嘧啶束，通常分布在内含子的最后 40 个核苷酸中，但也可能占据更多空间（图 11.1）。外显子/内含子连接处的最初识别基于 U1 snRNP 与 5′剪接位点、U2 辅助因子（U2AF65/35）与多嘧啶束以及 U2 snRNP 与分支点序列之间的直接相互作用（图 11.1）。在步骤 I 中，分支点序列（branch point sequence，BPS）的腺苷残基对 5′剪接位点进行亲核攻击。这一反应产生了剪接中间产物（游离外显子 1 和套索外显子 2）。在步骤 II 中，外显子 1 攻击 3′剪接位点，生成剪接产物（剪接外显子和套索内含子）。

除了连续识别和连接外显子外，剪接体还能进行可选择性剪接，在这一过程中，剪接体的组装会发生改变，从而以组织特异性和发育方式选择性地使用剪接位点，导致在成熟的 mRNA 中包含或排除替代外显子序列。除了细胞类型、发育阶段和性别特异性调控外，可选择性剪接还可在细胞因子、激素或神经递质等细胞外刺激的作用下进行动态调控，进一步加强对遗传信息流动的控制。然而，在许多情况下，可选择性剪接是如何受这些外部刺激和细胞内信号通路控制的并不清楚（Blaustein et al. 2007）。

以多种不同方式重新连接 RNA 外显子的结果意味着，1 个基因可以产生几种不同的转录本，每种转录本都可能具有不同的功能/特性。这包括改变 mRNA 的稳定性或亚细胞定位，以及添加或删除特定的蛋白质编码序列。蛋白质异构体之间的功能差异包括微妙的调节、开关甚至拮抗作用。典型的可选择性剪接类型有：包含或跳过 1 个或多个外显子（盒式外显子）、通过替代 5′和 3′剪接位点缩短或延长 1 个外显子、2 个或多个外显子相互排斥以及保留内含子（Matlin et al. 2005）。不同的启动子和不同的多腺苷酸化位点可分别指定替代的 5′和 3′末端外显子（Licatalosi and Darnell 2010）（图 11.2）。

如前所述，剪接体识别的顺式作用元件（5′和 3′剪接位点）是高度退化的，这就产生了一个悖论，即剪接这样一个重要而精确的过程，无论是连续剪接还是可选择性剪接，都是由冗余序列决定的（Zhang 1998）。然而，在过去的 10 年中，一个更重要的认识是，尽管这些共识元素是必要的，但绝不足以定义外显子/内含子的边界（Buratti et al. 2006）。剪接体要正确识别 5′剪接位点和 3′剪接位点，还需要其他顺式作用元件的帮助。如果考虑到在 1 个基因中，由于剪接位点（splice sites，ss）的高度退化性，存在着数以百计的假剪接位点，这些假剪接位点与真剪接位点相比，更接近甚至更像共识序列（Sun and Chasin 2000），那么这一点就显得尤为重要。此外，现在已知存在许多辅助剪接顺式作用调控元件，它们可以增强或抑制剪接。

外显子剪接增强子（exon splice enhancers，ESE）最初是在交替剪接的外显子中发现的（Mardon et al.

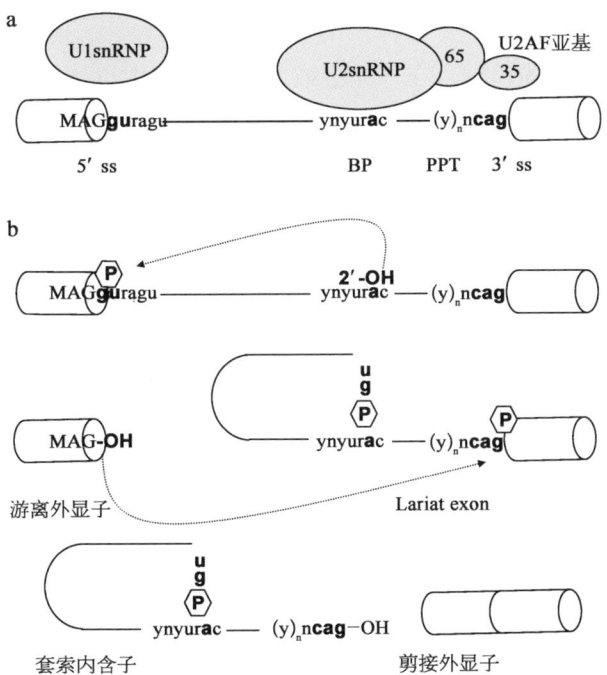

图 11.1 a. 外显子（圆柱）和内含子（黑线）边界周围的保守基序示意图：5′剪接位点、分支点、多嘧啶束和 3′剪接位点，以及识别它们的蛋白质和 snRNA，它们结合后构成剪接体的 E 复合物。只有分别位于外显子-内含子和内含子-外显子交界处的 GU 和 AG 二核苷酸以及分支点上的 A 残基是普遍保守的（用黑色标出）。b. 剪接反应：发生 2 个连续的酯化反应。在步骤 I 中，通常位于分支点内的腺苷残基对 5′剪接位点进行亲核攻击。这一反应生成了剪接中间产物（游离外显子 1 和拉长外显子 2）。在步骤 II 中，外显子 1 对 3′剪接位点进行亲核攻击，生成剪接产物（剪接外显子和长节内含子）

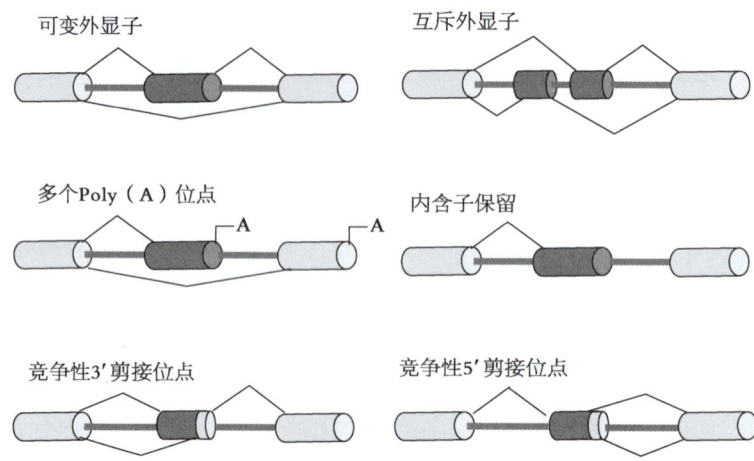

图 11.2 基本的可选择性剪接事件。沿着对角线可以看到可选择性外显子(用深色阴影表示)可能发生的事件。盒式外显子可从 mRNA 中包含或排除。互斥剪接是指从 2 个或多个外显子中只选择 1 个。多个聚(A)位点代表 3′端处理的替代方式。内含子保留是替代剪接的一种形式,内含子保留在 mRNA 中。竞争 3′或 5′剪接位点代表外显子大小发生改变的可选择性剪接事件。这些主题的变体也会出现,从而导致更复杂形式的可选择性剪接

1987),如今也被认为是组成型剪接外显子的常见成分,对刺激外显子剪接十分必要(Pagani and Baralle 2004)。ESE 与先前描述的 E 复合物中的剪接机制成分相互作用,从而协助早期剪接体复合物的形成。这一般是通过丝氨酸/精氨酸内含蛋白(SR 蛋白)来实现的,但并不普遍,SR 蛋白聚集在 ESE 元件上,通过形成相互影响的网络来促进调控剪接和组成剪接(Blencowe 2000)。SR 蛋白具有由 1 个或 2 个 RNA 结合结构域组成的共同结构域,其后是含有重复精氨酸/丝氨酸二肽的 RS 结构域,该结构域可高度磷酸化。这种磷酸化可调节蛋白质与蛋白质之间的相互作用,从而在剪接体中充当跨内含子和跨外显子的 5′和 3′剪接位点之间和(或)增强子与相邻剪接位点之间的桥梁(Long and Caceres 2009)。非线性剪接增强元件(intronic splice enhancer elements, ISE)也存在,并以大致相同的方式发挥作用;例如,它可以通过将 U2AF 募集到上游多嘧啶束来增强 3′剪接位点的识别,也可以通过将 U1 snRNA 募集到 5′剪接位点来增强 5′剪接位点的识别(Izquierdo et al. 2005)。

人们认为,剪接的正向调控是由于蛋白质与蛋白质之间的相互作用加强了对剪接位点的识别,而剪接位点选择的负向调控则往往是由于阻止了对剪接位点的识别。在外显子或内含子序列中也可以发现这些负调控序列,它们分别被称为外显子剪接沉默子(exonic splicing silencers, ESS)和内含子剪接沉默子(intronic splicing silencers, ISS)。hnRNP 是一大类分子,它们与 pre-mRNA 或 hnRNA(异质核 RNA)相关联。目前已确定至少有 20 种 hnRNP,它们被命名为 hnRNP A1 至 hnRNP U (Dreyfuss et al. 2002)。尽管对这些蛋白质的功能还有很多不清楚的地方,但可以认为它们一般是通过立体阻碍来抑制剪接的。例如,hnRNP A1 是研究最多的负剪接调控蛋白,它与 ESE 的位置重叠(Cartegni et al. 2006)被认为阻碍了 SMN2 第 7 外显子中 ESE 的功能。在 ISS 的情况下,hnRNPA1 也有类似的作用模式,即 ISS 元素与分支点之间发生位置重叠,从而阻断 U2 snRNP 的结合(Tange et al. 2001)。

除了与 ESE、ISE、ISS 和 ESS 结合这些更常见的剪接因子外,pre-mRNA 的剪接还可以通过一系列其他剪接因子来控制,这些因子的表达模式更受限制,也更动态。这些因子有可能在组织特异性或发育调控剪接中发挥更大的作用。这些因子的作用机制和影响目前还不十分明确,也不在本文简要概述的范围之内,但读者应该知道,其中可能涉及的因子包括 Nova-1/2、PTB/nPTB、Fox-1/2、 muscleblind-like(MBNL)和 CELF 家族蛋白、Hu 蛋白、TIA1/TIAR，以及可能还有更多尚未确定特性的因子(David and Manley 2008；Li et al. 2007)。

NF1 基因的 pre-mRNA 转录本中组成外显子的处理利用了上述所有类型的剪接调控元件。然而，迄今为止，人们只知道 NF1 基因中存在的部分辅助顺式作用元件(ESE、ESS、ISE 和 ISS)，因为这些元件通常只有在患者体内其中 1 个元件发生突变，导致剪接异常，进而引发 1 型神经纤维瘤病时才会被发现。即便如此，这些病例通常也不会在分子水平上得到全面描述，因为这可能超出了诊断实验室的范围。不过，一些重要病例被进行了详细研究，研究人员对剪接过程提出了有趣的见解。11.4 将讨论这些案例。

11.3 NF1 的选择性剪接

据估计，选择性剪接在人类蛋白质编码基因中的发生率逐年上升，从最初的 5% 到现在几乎无处不在(Wang et al. 2008)，NF1 基因也不例外(表 11.1)。可以认为，NF1 有 3 个不改变阅读框的经典可选择性外显子：9a/9br(Danglot et al. 1995)、23a(Nishi et al. 1991)和 48a(Cawthon et al. 1990)。可选择性外显子 9a/9br 内含物仅限于中枢神经系统，为 NF1 转录本增加了 10 个密码子(Danglot et al. 1995)。可选择性外显子 48a 为 NF1 基因的转录本增加了 18 个密码子，其在心肌和骨骼肌组织中的含量最高(Geist and Gutmann 1996)。虽然在蛋白质水平上也检测到了这些异构体，但在 NF1 转录本中加入任一外显子所导致的 NF1 功能的确切差异尚未完全确定；不过就外显子 48a 而言，它很可能在心脏和骨骼肌的发育和分化中发挥作用(Gutmann et al. 1995)。NF1 外显子 23a 的选择性剪接使蛋白质增加了 21 个氨基酸，这可能是 3 种蛋白质中最有趣的 1 种，因为它位于 GRD 内，而且观察到 2 种蛋白质异构体：跳过外显子的 NF1 Ⅰ型和包含外显子的 NF1 Ⅱ型在下调 Ras 活性能力上相差 10 倍，其中主要在神经元中表达的Ⅰ型异构体(跳过 23a 外显子)在这方面更为活跃(Andersen et al. 1993)。

表 11.1 Ars 等(2000a)、Messiaen 等(1999)、Park 等(1998)和 Vandenbroucke 等(2002a、b)迄今为止深入研究的主要 NF1 可选择性转录本

外 显 子	备 注
9br	插入框内，存在于中枢神经系统
23a	插入框内，主要存在于神经元中
48a	插入框内，存在于心脏和骨骼肌
23a48a	可变外显子，存在于肾上腺、肾脏
7	删除框内
43	删除框内
45	删除框外
29	删除框外
30	删除框外
29/30	删除框外
11(49 种 N-异构体中的大部分)	脑内删除框外
4b	删除框内
37	删除框内

如今，NF1 的选择性剪接情况要复杂得多，还包括其他几种选择性剪接事件(表 11.1)，其中有 1 种被称为 N-异构体的异构体，它不包括外显子 11 和 49 的大部分，在外显子 4a/4b 之间有 1 种潜在的调节性假外显子包含事件，以及在外显子 12b 和 43 中使用选择性剪接位点(Thomson and Wallace 2002；Vandenbroucke et al. 2001，2002a，b)。不过，其中大部分的重要性仍有待鉴定，它们在蛋白质水平上的表达也是如此。

控制这些选择性外显子的组织和发育特异性调控机制大多尚不清楚，唯一的例外是外显子 23a(Barron and Lou 2012；Barron et al. 2010；Zhu et al. 2008)。这就是选择性剪接组合控制的一个完美例子，其中多个不同的调控元件和相关因子对选择性外显子进行细胞类型特异性调控(图 11.3)。由 NF1 基因的外显子 23a 下游富含 UG 的序列组成的 ISE 可通过 TIA-1 和 TIAR 蛋白的结合促进 U1 snRNA 的结合。2 个蛋白质家族(Hu 蛋白和

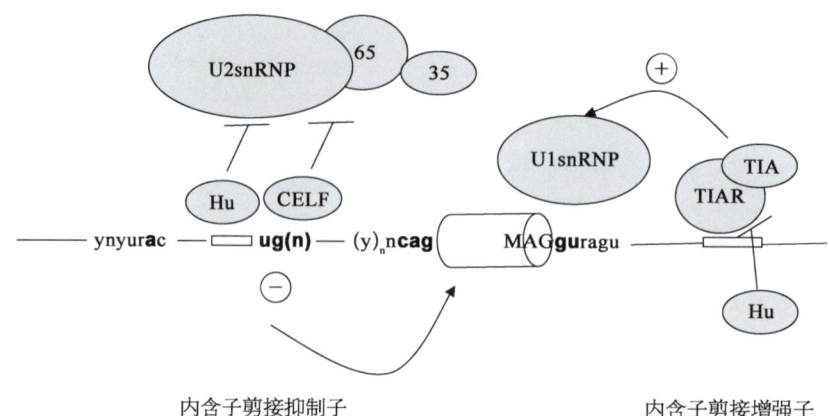

图11.3 外显子23a的可选择性剪接机制示意图(以圆柱体表示)。黑色直线代表内含子,内含子中的小矩形方格是圆圈代表的剪接因子的结合位点。TIAR和TIA的结合有助于U1snRNA与5′剪接位点的结合,从而帮助确定5′剪接位点。Hu蛋白可能会抑制这些因子与内含子剪接增强子的结合。与外显子上游内含子剪接沉默子结合的CELF和Hu蛋白通过阻断U2AF65的结合抑制3′剪接位点的确定

CELF蛋白)是该外显子的负调控因子。Hu蛋白与NF1基因的23a外显子两侧的富含U和AU的序列结合,竞争TIA-1和TIAR蛋白的结合位点,阻止剪接体成分U1和U6与5′剪接位点的结合以及U2AF65与3′剪接位点的结合。CELF蛋白通过与NF1基因外显子23a上游富含UG的元件结合,促进外显子23a的跳接,它们还在那里与U2AF65竞争结合。因此,剪接结果取决于特定细胞类型中哪种因子更丰富。TIA-1和TIAR通常被认为是广泛表达的,而Hu蛋白家族由4个成员组成,其中3个是脑特异性的(Okano and Darnell 1997),CELF蛋白家族由6个成员组成,其中3个是脑特异性蛋白,2个被认为在脑中富集(Dasgupta and Ladd 2012)。大脑中负调控剪接因子水平较高,导致NF1基因的外显子23a的剪接结果出现在该组织中。

11.4 mRNA剪接异常与1型神经纤维瘤病

如上所述,NF1基因是已知人类基因中突变率高的基因之一。虽然其中一些突变不一定会影响蛋白质功能,但由于pre-mRNA中含有负责正确控制剪接的剪接调控元件,如果这些突变发生在剪接调控元件中,则可能会影响剪接功能,从而导致NF1基因转录本的剪接异常和随后的病理变化。这类突变的鉴定一直是临床诊断的焦点。

影响mRNA正确加工的最常见剪接突变形式发生在典型剪接信号中,破坏了剪接供体和受体位点。人类基因突变数据库(HGMD;http://www.hgmd.org)中有222个关于NF1基因剪接突变的报告,其中约78%的突变影响到剪接位点本身。当这些突变发生在5′和3′剪接处100%保守的二核苷酸中时,就像发现约81%影响NF1剪接位点的突变一样,这些突变将导致异常拼接,这是一个不言而喻的事实。然而,要确定所产生的异常剪接类型是外显子跳过、内含子保留、利用隐性剪接位点并包含隐性外显子,还是可选择性剪接,可能比较困难,尽管可以尝试做出相当准确的预测。然而,大量序列变异也属于剪接位点中定义较为松散的区域,预测这些变异是否会导致剪接异常是一项挑战。由于这些变异的广泛性,人们开发了生物信息学程序,试图预测核苷酸变异对剪接的潜在影响。例如MaxEntScan(Yeo and Burge 2004)、NNsplice(Reese et al. 1997)、AST(Carmel et al. 2004)、Spliceport(Dogan et al. 2007)、Spliceview(Rogozin and Milanesi 1997)、HBond(Freund et al. 2003)、ASSA(Nalla and Rogan 2005)、NetGene2(Hebsgaard et al. 1996)和Human Splicing Finder(Hubbard et al. 2007)。这些计算机模拟方法基于核苷酸频率矩阵、

神经网络、氢键形成以及共识中不同位置核苷酸之间的相互依赖关系。显然，由于存在一定程度的不确定性，所以在评估核苷酸变异的影响时需要谨慎。例如，NF1 基因外显子 3 中的内含子+5 G>C 取代被怀疑是 1 个家族中神经纤维瘤病的原因(Baralle et al. 2003)。这一核苷酸变化使剪接位点强度显著下降，但仍高于其他自然使用的剪接位点，例如 NF1 外显子 34 中的剪接位点(使用 NNSplice，NF1 外显子 3 中的突变使该剪接位点的得分从 1 降至 0.83，而 NF1 外显子 34 中剪接位点的得分为 0.41)。然而，使用多个硅学程序有力地表明了这种核苷酸置换是致病的，同时也突出了在评估突变在剪接中可能起的作用时使用尽可能多的预测程序的实用性(例如，MAXENT 预测外显子 37 剪接位点的突变得分从 9.65 分降至 4.99 分，NF1 外显子 34 的 5′剪接位点的得分为 7.13 分)。事实上，利用微型基因系统(Baralle and Baralle 2005)，这已被证明是致病因素。此外，实验还表明，+5 G>C 突变的影响是有特异性的，因为它取决于 5′剪接位点是否存在 G 运行，即使存在该突变，破坏该位点也会导致 MRNA 的正确处理。造成这种情况的功能性原因是，hnRNP H 蛋白与多 G 序列上的 5′剪接位点结合，从而与 U1 碱基配对竞争(Buratti et al. 2004)。这个例子突出表明，包含 5′ss 的不同 RNA 片段既能被共同的蛋白质结合，也能被不同的蛋白质结合，正是这些蛋白质的组合效应决定了 5′ss 是否能被识别。尽管 5′ss 在所有外显子中的作用相同(由 U1snRNA 识别)，但与之结合的蛋白质组合不同，这意味着影响 1 个外显子 5′ss 中剪接位点识别的核苷酸变异在另一个外显子中可能是无害的，这强调了每个 5′ss 都应在各自的序列上下文中进行评估。

另一项评估 NF1 外显子 29 的研究(Raponi et al. 2009)也进一步证明，需要仔细考虑 NF1 基因中每一个潜在的剪接影响突变。如前所述，5′剪接位点强度的预测可能依赖于与 U1snRNP 的互补性；在这项研究中，观察到 U1snRNP 的存在降低了正确识别外显子 29 供体位点的必要性。5′剪接位点内的突变不仅会导致其所在外显子的完全或部分跳过，还可能导致其他形式的异常剪接，如由于使用伪剪接位点或隐性剪接位点而导致隐性外显子包含，NF1 c.7675+1G>A 突变就是这种情况(Wimmer et al. 2007)。通过对几个 5′剪接位点突变的分析，本研究还表明，如果存在 1 个接近真实 5′剪接位点的潜在隐性 5′剪接位点(可使用上述硅学工具进行搜索)，同时该外显子又存在一个强大的 3′剪接位点，则更有可能出现这种结果。

在正常剪接序列不受影响而发生异常剪接的情况下，这些序列变异更有可能影响 ESE。在 HGMD 中，这些变异约占 NF1 剪接突变的 14%。为了能够确定核苷酸变异是否会破坏其中的一个，从而代表一种致病突变，对剪接特别是 ESE 所涉及的顺式作用元件进行了大量的生物信息学预测工作。这些预测程序是通过功能性 SELEX(通过指数富集配体的系统进化)方法"ESE - finder"(Cartegni et al. 2003)、基于 ESE 在外显子中比在内含子中更常见以及在具有弱剪接位点的外显子中更常见的假设，对外显子和内含子之间以及具有弱剪接位点和强剪接位点的外显子之间的六聚体频率差异进行统计分析("ESE 拯救"；Fairbrother et al. 2002)，或者基于从已知调控元件和相应的反式作用因子中得出的共识序列(Paz et al. 2010)。最近，Sroogle 等集成界面已被开发出，可对这些方案的若干产出进行综合分析(Schwartz et al. 2009)。虽然作为研究剪接机制和分析突变的起点非常有用，但序列中存在高分基序并不一定就能确定该序列在其原生上下文中是剪接顺式作用元件，序列的破坏也不一定会导致剪接异常。这一点在 NF1 基因中得到了证明，通过使用迷你基因分析无义、错义、同义和内含变异对高分基序的破坏，明显改变了外显子 29 的包含/排除水平，但在生物信息学程序 29 中并不一定会导致剪接异常(Raponi et al. 2009)。实际情况是，剪接的结果依赖于精细的"力量平衡"，而这种"力量平衡"往往存在于定义外显子边界的各种调控元件之间(Buratti et al. 2006)。

如前所述，NF1 基因中只有少数 ESE 得到了完整的描述，特别是在其作用模式方面。但是，NF1 基因中已知会导致外显子跳越的外显子突变突显了更多 ESE 的存在。另外一个例子存在于 NF1 基因外显子 7 中，在该外显子中存在另外一种转录本（Vandenbroucke et al. 2002b）。ESE-finder（http：//rulai.cshl.edu/cgi-bin/tools/ESE3/esefinder.cgi?process=home）预测的1个同义突变（c.945G>A/Q315Q）破坏了1个ESE，结果显示该突变导致超过70%的外显子跳过，这突出了分析沉默突变对剪接影响的重要性（Bottillo et al. 2007）。事实上，在同一研究中，观察到第二个沉默突变（c.1005T>C/N335N）增加了该外显子在迷你基因系统中的包含率，这强调了应如何研究 NF1 编码序列中的每个核苷酸变化对剪接的潜在影响。尽管外显子7的包含或排除水平的临床意义尚不清楚，但可选择性外显子水平的微小变化最终可能导致病理变化。

对 c.6792C>G（p.Tyr2264X）和 c.6792C>A（p.Tyr2264X）突变所引起的疾病机制的研究，就是1个对 NF1 基因中ESE进行更全面描述的例子，这些突变以前被认为会导致过早终止密码子（premature termination codons，PTC），引起 NF1 外显子37的跳过，但保留了开放阅读框。然而，位于该基因同一区域其他患者的突变，c.6790_6791TTins 和 c.6789_6792TTACdel，都在下游几个碱基对处产生了PTC，但并没有导致该外显子的跳过。通过使用微型基因分析，发现病理突变 c.6792C>G 和 c.6792C>A 实际上破坏了1个A-C rich 剪接调控元件，该元件不仅对 NF1 外显子37的定义很重要，而且对邻近 NF1 外显子36的包含也很重要（Baralle et al. 2006）。随后的 RNA 蛋白复合物研究表明，病理突变 c.6792C>G 突变同时降低了对 YB-1 等阳性剪接因子的亲和力，从而破坏了 ESE，增加了对 hnRNPA1、hnRNPA2 和 DAZAP1 等阴性剪接因子的亲和力，形成了 ESS（Skoko et al. 2008）。在该外显子中存在ESE的内在必要性是为了抵消 NF1 外显子37上的非共识3′剪接位点。我们之所以知道这一点，是因为实验中突变了外显子37的3′剪接位点，使其符合共识，从而消除了对ESE的需要，即使存在这些先前的病理突变，迷你基因也能完全包含该外显子。

位于剪接位点之外的内含子突变是NF1中第三常见的剪接突变，在HGMD中约有5%的剪接突变属于这一类。据观察，深内含子 c.31-279A>G 变异可产生1个剪接位点。在这种特殊情况下，3′剪接位点的使用与 NF1 转录本中已经存在的伪5′剪接位点的激活有关，从而导致内含子序列的外显子化（Raponi et al. 2006）。另外一种情况是产生了1个隐性剪接位点，如3214 del 111突变导致在真实的5′剪接位点上游104 nt处产生了1个隐性5′剪接位点（Ars et al. 2000b）。

11.5　剪接和表型变异性

NF1在肿瘤负荷和疾病严重程度方面表现出很大的临床个体差异，即使在具有相同突变的家庭成员中也是如此。剪接和可选择性剪接的机制受到严格控制，即使是可选择性剪接因子的微小缺陷或替代外显子的反常包含也会导致表型差异（Pagani and Baralle 2004）。据推测，人群中携带相同 NF1 剪接突变的患者之间不同异常转录本的差异，可能是导致该病表型差异的部分原因之一（Ars et al. 2000b）。然而，在这方面对基因型与表型相关性的探讨尚未得出结论性结果（Pros et al. 2006）。由于顺式作用调控元件突变导致的剪接异常程度往往只是部分的，在组织内和个体间可能会有所不同，这是由多种因素造成的，如个体细胞中剪接调控蛋白的差异以及同一个体内不同组织间的差异。例如，剪接有可能在严重脊髓神经纤维瘤的神经表型中发挥作用（Raponi et al. 2006）。在这项研究中，观察到的剪接缺陷涉及结合PTB和nPTB的内含子调控元件，后者仅限于神经元。我们可以假设，这种剪接因子水平的差异可能会导致这种突变的患者出现更严重的脊柱表型。

11.6　基于剪接的治疗方法

Pre-mRNA 剪接和可选择性剪接的失调与大量人类疾病的分子病理学有关。因此，针对 pre-mRNA 的最终治疗策略——剪接疗法——投入了大量精力，可见近期综述（Douglas and Wood 2011；Kole et al. 2012）。所用方法取决于所需的 pre-mRNA 剪接的靶向调节模式以及存在的突变类型。比较有前景的治疗策略之一是使用反义寡核苷酸在

pre-mRNA 剪接过程中剪切特定的突变外显子，从而产生功能性蛋白质。这种方法在杜氏肌肉萎缩症的治疗中尤为成功（Wood et al. 2010）。其他方法则试图包含特定的外显子序列（如 SMN 的情况），以阻止包含假外显子并调节可选择性剪接蛋白同工酶的产生（Kole et al. 2012）。

不幸的是，NF1 没有突变热点，剪接突变的范围之大阻碍了治疗方法的开发。目前，开发一种专门针对剪接突变的疗法投资太大，因为监管要求表明，每种疗法需要针对每种不同的突变分别开发。此外，携带特定突变的患者人数太少，无法进行所需的大规模试验。尽管如此，研究表明，纠正有缺陷的 NF1 的可能性是存在的。治疗性矫正的理想候选突变位于剪接位点之外，不在编码区内，反义吗啉寡聚物（antisense morpholino oligos，AMO）治疗性矫正的可能性已被证明适用于其中 3 个内含子变异（c.288+2025T＞G、c.5749+332A＞G 和 c.7908-321C＞G），每个变异都被观察到创建了 1 个隐性 5′剪接位点，并导致包含 1 个隐性外显子（Pros et al. 2009）。AMO 的设计目的是通过立体阻断剪接机制对新创建的 5′剪接位点的识别，从而迫使使用正确的剪接位点，防止包含隐性外显子。

在存在剪接突变的情况下，另外一种恢复正常转录本剪接的方法是使用能以多种方式影响剪接过程的化学物质；这些物质主要通过阻断组蛋白去乙酰化酶或干扰剪接因子的磷酸化来发挥作用（Sumanasekera et al. 2008）。然而，由于这些药物具有普遍影响，因此必须注意它们对所有转录本剪接的影响，而不仅仅是对 NF1 的影响。就 NF1 的具体情况而言，在 19 个测试的 NF1 剪接突变中，观察到酮素和嘌呤霉素能部分纠正 4 个 NF1 剪接突变（c.910C＞T、c.3113G＞C、c.6724C＞T 和 c.6791dupA）引起的剪接异常，其效果呈剂量依赖性（Pros et al. 2009）。在这项研究中，突变包括无义突变、错义突变和框架转换突变。因此，校正异常剪接仍会产生异常转录本，所以不会产生治疗效果，除非是错义突变。不过，当内含子突变或最终外显子沉默突变产生跳转逆转时，这种方法可能具有治疗意义。

（李悦华，钟民衍　译）

参考文献

[1] Andersen LB, Ballester R, Marchuk DA, Chang E, Gutmann DH, Saulino AM, Camonis J, Wigler M, Collins FS (1993) A conserved alternative splice in the von Recklinghausen neurofibromatosis (NF1) gene produces two neurofibromin isoforms, both of which have GTPase-activating protein activity. Mol Cell Biol 13: 487-495

[2] Ars E, Serra E, de la Luna S, Estivill X, Lazaro C (2000a) Cold shock induces the insertion of a cryptic exon in the neurofibromatosis type 1 (NF1) mRNA. Nucleic Acids Res 28: 1307-1312

[3] Ars E, Serra E, Garcia J, Kruyer H, Gaona A, Lazaro C, Estivill X (2000b) Mutations affecting mRNA splicing are the most common molecular defects in patients with neurofibromatosis type 1. Hum Mol Genet 9: 237-247

[4] Baralle D, Baralle M (2005) Splicing in action: assessing disease causing sequence changes. J Med Genet 42: 737-748

[5] Baralle M, Baralle D, De Conti L, Mattocks C, Whittaker J, Knezevich A, Ffrench-Constant C, Baralle FE (2003) Identification of a mutation that perturbs NF1 gene splicing using genomic DNA samples and a minigene assay. J Med Genet 40: 220-222

[6] Baralle M, Skoko N, Knezevich A, De Conti L, Motti D, Bhuvanagiri M, Baralle D, Buratti E, Baralle FE (2006) NF1 mRNA biogenesis: effect of the genomic milieu in splicing regulation of the NF1 exon 37 region. FEBS Lett 580: 4449-4456

[7] Barron VA, Lou H (2012) Alternative splicing of the neurofibromatosis type I pre-mRNA. Biosci Rep 32: 131-138

[8] Barron VA, Zhu H, Hinman MN, Ladd AN, Lou H (2010) The neurofibromatosis type I pre-mRNA is a novel target of CELF protein-mediated splicing regulation. Nucleic Acids Res 38: 253-264

[9] Blaustein M, Pelisch F, Srebrow A (2007) Signals, pathways and splicing regulation. Int J Biochem Cell Biol 39: 2031-2048

[10] Blencowe BJ (2000) Exonic splicing enhancers: mechanism of action, diversity and role in human genetic diseases. Trends Biochem Sci 25: 106-110

[11] Bottillo I, De Luca A, Schirinzi A, Guida V, Torrente I, Calvieri S, Gervasini C, Larizza L, Pizzuti A, Dallapiccola B (2007) Functional analysis of splicing mutations in exon 7 of NF1 gene. BMC Med Genet 8: 4

[12] Buratti E, Baralle M, De Conti L, Baralle D, Romano M, Ayala YM, Baralle FE (2004) hnRNP H binding at the 5′ splice site correlates with the pathological effect of two intronic mutations in the NF-1 and TSHbeta genes. Nucleic Acids Res 32: 4224-4236

[13] Buratti E, Baralle M, Baralle FE (2006) Defective splicing, disease and therapy: searching for master checkpoints in exon definition. Nucleic Acids Res 34: 3494-3510

[14] Carmel I, Tal S, Vig I, Ast G (2004) Comparative analysis detects dependencies among the 5′ splice-site positions. RNA 10: 828-840

[15] Cartegni L, Wang J, Zhu Z, Zhang MQ, Krainer AR (2003)

ESEfinder: a web resource to identify exonic splicing enhancers. Nucleic Acids Res 31: 3568 - 3571
[16] Cartegni L, Hastings ML, Calarco JA, de Stanchina E, Krainer AR (2006) Determinants of exon 7 splicing in the spinal muscular atrophy genes, SMN1 and SMN2. Am J Hum Genet 78: 63 - 77
[17] Cawthon RM, Weiss R, Xu GF, Viskochil D, Culver M, Stevens J, Robertson M, Dunn D, Gesteland R, O'Connell P et al (1990) A major segment of the neurofibromatosis type 1 gene: cDNA sequence, genomic structure, and point mutations. Cell 62: 193 - 201
[18] Danglot G, Regnier V, Fauvet D, Vassal G, Kujas M, Bernheim A (1995) Neurofibromatosis 1 (NF1) mRNAs expressed in the central nervous system are differentially spliced in the 5' part of the gene. Hum Mol Genet 4: 915 - 920
[19] Dasgupta T, Ladd AN (2012) The importance of CELF control: molecular and biological roles of the CUG-BP, Elav-like family of RNA-binding proteins. Wiley Interdiscip Rev RNA 3: 104 - 121
[20] David CJ, Manley JL (2008) The search for alternative splicing regulators: new approaches offer a path to a splicing code. Genes Dev 22: 279 - 285
[21] Dogan RI, Getoor L, Wilbur WJ, Mount SM (2007) SplicePort—an interactive splice-site analysis tool. Nucleic Acids Res 35: W285 - W291
[22] Douglas AG, Wood MJ (2011) RNA splicing: disease and therapy. Brief Funct Genomics 10: 151 - 164
[23] Dreyfuss G, Kim VN, Kataoka N (2002) Messenger-RNA-binding proteins and the messages they carry. Nat Rev Mol Cell Biol 3: 195 - 205
[24] Fairbrother WG, Yeh RF, Sharp PA, Burge CB (2002) Predictive identification of exonic splicing enhancers in human genes. Science 297: 1007 - 1013
[25] Freund M, Asang C, Kammler S, Konermann C, Krummheuer J, Hipp M, Meyer I, Gierling W, Theiss S, Preuss T et al (2003) A novel approach to describe a U1 snRNA binding site. Nucleic Acids Res 31: 6963 - 6975
[26] Geist RT, Gutmann DH (1996) Expression of a developmentally-regulated neuron-specific iso-form of the neurofibromatosis 1 (NF1) gene. Neurosci Lett 211: 85 - 88
[27] Gutmann DH, Geist RT, Wright DE, Snider WD (1995) Expression of the neurofibromatosis 1 (NF1) isoforms in developing and adult rat tissues. Cell Growth Differ 6: 315 - 323
[28] Hebsgaard SM, Korning PG, Tolstrup N, Engelbrecht J, Rouze P, Brunak S (1996) Splice site prediction in Arabidopsis thaliana pre-mRNA by combining local and global sequence information. Nucleic Acids Res 24: 3439 - 3452
[29] Hubbard TJ, Aken BL, Beal K, Ballester B, Caccamo M, Chen Y, Clarke L, Coates G, Cunningham F, Cutts T et al (2007) Ensembl 2007. Nucleic Acids Res 35: D610 - D617
[30] Izquierdo JM, Majos N, Bonnal S, Martinez C, Castelo R, Guigo R, Bilbao D, Valcarcel J (2005) Regulation of Fas alternative splicing by antagonistic effects of TIA-1 and PTB on exon definition. Mol Cell 19: 475 - 484
[31] Kole R, Krainer AR, Altman S (2012) RNA therapeutics: beyond RNA interference and antisense oligonucleotides. Nat Rev Drug Discov 11: 125 - 140
[32] Lamond AI (1993) The spliceosome. Bioessays 15: 595 - 603
[33] Li Q, Lee JA, Black DL (2007) Neuronal regulation of alternative pre-mRNA splicing. Nat Rev Neurosci 8: 819 - 831
[34] Licatalosi DD, Darnell RB (2010) RNA processing and its regulation: global insights into biological networks. Nat Rev Genet 11: 75 - 87
[35] Long JC, Caceres JF (2009) The SR protein family of splicing factors: master regulators of gene expression. Biochem J 417: 15 - 27
[36] Mardon HJ, Sebastio G, Baralle FE (1987) A role for exon sequences in alternative splicing of the human fibronectin gene. Nucleic Acids Res 15: 7725 - 7733
[37] Matlin AJ, Clark F, Smith CW (2005) Understanding alternative splicing: towards a cellular code. Nat Rev Mol Cell Biol 6: 386 - 398
[38] Messiaen LM, Callens T, Roux KJ, Mortier GR, De Paepe A, Abramowicz M, Pericak-Vance MA, Vance JM, Wallace MR (1999) Exon 10b of the NF1 gene represents a mutational hotspot and harbors a recurrent missense mutation Y489C associated with aberrant splicing. Genet Med 1: 248 - 253
[39] Nalla VK, Rogan PK (2005) Automated splicing mutation analysis by information theory. Hum Mutat 25: 334 - 342
[40] Nilsen TW (2003) The spliceosome: the most complex macromolecular machine in the cell? Bioessays 25: 1147 - 1149
[41] Nishi T, Lee PS, Oka K, Levin VA, Tanase S, Morino Y, Saya H (1991) Differential expression of two types of the neurofibromatosis type 1 (NF1) gene transcripts related to neuronal differentiation. Oncogene 6: 1555 - 1559
[42] Okano HJ, Darnell RB (1997) A hierarchy of Hu RNA binding proteins in developing and adult neurons. J Neurosci 17: 3024 - 3037
[43] Pagani F, Baralle FE (2004) Genomic variants in exons and introns: identifying the splicing spoilers. Nat Rev Genet 5: 389 - 396
[44] Park VM, Kenwright KA, Sturtevant DB, Pivnick EK (1998) Alternative splicing of exons 29 and 30 in the neurofibromatosis type 1 gene. Hum Genet 103: 382 - 385
[45] Paz I, Akerman M, Dror I, Kosti I, Mandel-Gutfreund Y (2010) SFmap: a web server for motif analysis and prediction of splicing factor binding sites. Nucleic Acids Res 38: W281 - W285
[46] Pros E, Larriba S, Lopez E, Ravella A, Gili ML, Kruyer H, Valls J, Serra E, Lazaro C (2006) NF1 mutation rather than individual genetic variability is the main determinant of the NF1-transcriptional profile of mutations affecting splicing. Hum Mutat 27: 1104 - 1114
[47] Pros E, Fernandez-Rodriguez J, Canet B, Benito L, Sanchez A, Benavides A, Ramos FJ, Lopez-Ariztegui MA, Capella G, Blanco I et al (2009) Antisense therapeutics for neurofibromatosis type 1 caused by deep intronic mutations. Hum Mutat 30: 454 - 462
[48] Raponi M, Upadhyaya M, Baralle D (2006) Functional splicing assay shows a pathogenic intronic mutation in neurofibromatosis type 1 (NF1) due to intronic sequence exonization. Hum Mutat 27: 294 - 295
[49] Raponi M, Buratti E, Dassie E, Upadhyaya M, Baralle D (2009) Low U1 snRNP dependence at the NF1 exon 29 donor splice site. FEBS J 276: 2060 - 2073
[50] Reese MG, Eeckman FH, Kulp D, Haussler D (1997) Improved splice site detection in Genie. J Comput Biol 4: 311 - 323
[51] Rogozin IB, Milanesi L (1997) Analysis of donor splice sites in different eukaryotic organisms. J Mol Evol 45: 50 - 59
[52] Schwartz S, Hall E, Ast G (2009) SROOGLE: webserver for integrative, user-friendly visualization of splicing signals. Nucleic Acids Res 37: W189 - W192
[53] Skoko N, Baralle M, Buratti E, Baralle FE (2008) The pathological splicing mutation c. 6792C>G in NF1 exon 37

causes a change of tenancy between antagonistic splicing factors. FEBS Lett 582: 2231-2236

[54] Sumanasekera C, Watt DS, Stamm S (2008) Substances that can change alternative splice-site selection. Biochem Soc Trans 36: 483-490

[55] Sun H, Chasin LA (2000) Multiple splicing defects in an intronic false exon. Mol Cell Biol 20: 6414-6425

[56] Tange TO, Damgaard CK, Guth S, Valcarcel J, Kjems J (2001) The hnRNP A1 protein regulates HIV-1 tat splicing via a novel intron silencer element. EMBO J 20: 5748-5758

[57] Tazi J, Bakkour N, Stamm S (2009) Alternative splicing and disease. Biochim Biophys Acta 1792: 14-26

[58] Thomson SA, Wallace MR (2002) RT-PCR splicing analysis of the NF1 open reading frame. Hum Genet 110: 495-502

[59] Valero MC, Martin Y, Hernandez-Imaz E, Marina Hernandez A, Melean G, Valero AM, Javier Rodriguez-Alvarez F, Telleria D, Hernandez-Chico C (2011) A highly sensitive genetic protocol to detect NF1 mutations. J Mol Diagn 13: 113-122

[60] Vandenbroucke II, Vandesompele J, Paepe AD, Messiaen L (2001) Quantification of splice variants using real-time PCR. Nucleic Acids Res 29: E68-68

[61] Vandenbroucke I, Callens T, De Paepe A, Messiaen L (2002a) Complex splicing pattern generates great diversity in human NF1 transcripts. BMC Genomics 3: 13

[62] Vandenbroucke I, Vandesompele J, De Paepe A, Messiaen L (2002b) Quantification of NF1 transcripts reveals novel highly expressed splice variants. FEBS Lett 522: 71-76

[63] Wahl MC, Will CL, Luhrmann R (2009) The spliceosome: design principles of a dynamic RNP machine. Cell 136: 701-718

[64] Wang ET, Sandberg R, Luo S, Khrebtukova I, Zhang L, Mayr C, Kingsmore SF, Schroth GP, Burge CB (2008) Alternative isoform regulation in human tissue transcriptomes. Nature 456: 470-476

[65] Will CL, Luhrmann R (2011) Spliceosome structure and function. Cold Spring Harb Perspect Biol 3(7): pii: a003707

[66] Wimmer K, Roca X, Beiglbock H, Callens T, Etzler J, Rao AR, Krainer AR, Fonatsch C, Messiaen L (2007) Extensive in silico analysis of NF1 splicing defects uncovers determinants for splicing outcome upon 5′ splice-site disruption. Hum Mutat 28: 599-612

[67] Wood MJ, Gait MJ, Yin H (2010) RNA-targeted splice-correction therapy for neuromuscular disease. Brain 133: 957-972

[68] Yeo G, Burge CB (2004) Maximum entropy modeling of short sequence motifs with applications to RNA splicing signals. J Comput Biol 11: 377-394

[69] Zhang MQ (1998) Statistical features of human exons and their flanking regions. Hum Mol Genet 7: 919-932

[70] Zhu H, Hinman MN, Hasman RA, Mehta P, Lou H (2008) Regulation of neuron-specific alternative splicing of neurofibromatosis type 1 pre-mRNA. Mol Cell Biol 28: 1240-1251

第12章 NF1 基因型和体细胞嵌合现象

NF1 Germline and Somatic Mosaicism

Ludwine Messiaen and Jing Xie

12.1 引言

1 型神经纤维瘤病(neurofibromatosis type 1，NF1，MIM 162200)是一种常见的常染色体显性遗传疾病，全世界约有 1/3 000 的人患病(Huson et al. 1989)。NF1 是一种进行性疾病，随着时间的推移，通常会逐渐出现更多的症状。NF1 具有完全外显率，即使在同一家族内或携带相同突变的单卵双胞胎之间，也会表现出高度的表型变异(Rieley et al. 2011)。患者可能表现出多个咖啡牛奶斑(café-au-lait Macules, CALM)、皮褶雀斑、虹膜 Lisch 结节和神经纤维瘤。神经纤维瘤可分为皮肤型神经纤维瘤和先天性丛状神经纤维瘤。皮肤型神经纤维瘤是一种良性肿瘤，其数量和大小通常会随着年龄增长而增加，但不会发生恶变；先天性丛状神经纤维瘤是一种累及多个神经束的肿瘤，其中约有 5% 的病例可能进展为恶性周围神经鞘膜瘤(malignant peripheral nerve sheath tumor, MPNST)(Korf 1999)。视路神经胶质瘤、蝶骨翼异常、长骨和椎骨的特定骨骼异常也是 NF1 的典型临床表现。此外，NF1 患者常见的表现还有巨头、身材矮小、学习障碍和注意力困难等。NF1 患者发生特定恶性肿瘤的风险也会增加(Brems et al. 2009)。

NF1 是由位于 17 号染色体 q11.2 区域 282 kb 长的 NF1 基因突变引起的，该基因由 57 个常规外显子和至少 3 个可选择性剪接的外显子组成。NF1 转录本的开放阅读框包含 8 454 个核苷酸，编码的神经纤维瘤蛋白可负调控 Ras - GTP 酶(Ballester et al. 1990；Xu et al. 1990)。NF1 作为一个抑瘤基因，其相关的肿瘤，如神经纤维瘤、胃肠道间质瘤、球瘤、幼年型粒单核细胞白血病、星形细胞瘤和嗜铬细胞瘤，都显示携带了 2 个突变的 NF1 拷贝(Brems et al. 2009)。在皮肤型神经纤维瘤和丛状神经纤维瘤中，NF1 基因的 2 个等位基因失活已被证实。然而，额外的遗传改变，包括复杂的核型变化，仅在恶性周围神经鞘膜瘤(MPNST)中被发现。

此外，在胫骨假关节(Stevenson et al. 2006)和咖啡牛奶斑(CALM；De Schepper et al. 2008；Maertens et al. 2007)的组织中也发现了体细胞"二次打击"的 NF1 突变。

双等位基因 NF1 失活遵循 Knudson 的"二次打击假说"。根据这一肿瘤发生模型，1 个等位基因的突变(即"第一次打击"突变)通常是从受累的父母(对于家族病例)或无症状父母的突变生殖细胞中遗传而来的。首次打击突变也可能是由受精卵中的新生突变引起的，或发生在发育早期的胚胎阶段。相对而言，"第二次打击"突变影响的是另一个(野生

L. Messiaen • J. Xie
Medical Genomics Laboratory, Department of Genetics, University of Alabama at Birmingham, 720 20th Street S, Birmingham, AL 35294, USA
e-mail: lmessiaen@uab.edu

M. Upadhyaya and D. N. Cooper (eds.), *Neurofibromatosis Type 1*,
DOI 10.1007/978-3-642-32864-0_12, ♯ Springer-Verlag Berlin Heidelberg 2012

型)等位基因,并且仅特异性地存在于代表肿瘤或咖啡牛奶斑起始细胞的体细胞中。

12.2 嵌合体

无论性别或种族背景如何,NF1 累及约 1/3 000,其中多达 30%～50%的患者为"散发性"或"始发性"病例,即这些患者没有受累的父母,因此不是从父母处遗传该疾病(Friedman 1999;Evans et al. 2010)。由此可见,NF1 基因的新突变率为 $(3.7\sim26)\times10^{-5}$,比大多数其他已知的人类相关基因疾病的突变率高出 10～100 倍(Poyhonen et al. 2000)。这种异常高突变率的原因仍不明确,基因的巨大体积和复杂性可能只是部分因素。Zlotogora 在 1993 年提出,一部分散发性或"始发性"NF1 患者可能是由于受精后体细胞突变导致的。1996 年报道了第一个分子上确认的体细胞嵌合 NF1 患者:1 名 31 岁的患者表现出至少 100 kb 范围内的多外显子缺失(覆盖外显子 4-39),该患者有 7 处咖啡牛奶斑(CALM)、双侧腋窝雀斑和多个小的皮肤型神经纤维瘤(Colman et al. 1996)。

遗传嵌合体是指 2 种或多种遗传上不同的细胞群体,共同存在于同一个个体中,这些细胞群体来源于同一个受精卵。在具有显著皮肤表现的遗传性疾病中,如 1 型神经纤维瘤病,嵌合体现象比在主要影响内部器官的疾病中更容易被观察到。关于 NF1,这里讨论的嵌合体是指患者体内只有一部分细胞群体携带"第一次打击"的 NF1 突变。

以下是几种可能遇到的"第一次打击"NF1 突变的嵌合体类型。当部分生殖细胞(精子或卵子)携带突变时,会发生生殖腺或生殖系嵌合体,这可能导致临床正常的父母生育多个患病的后代。纯生殖腺嵌合体在 NF1 中可能极为罕见,目前仅有 2 个这样的家族被报道(Lázaro et al. 1994;Bottillo et al. 2010)。在胚胎发育早期,即在原肠形成和原始生殖细胞形成与分离之前发生的突变,可能导致生殖腺体细胞嵌合体。在这种情况下,体细胞和生殖细胞都可能是嵌合体。如果突变发生在原始生殖细胞形成并分离之后,患者可能仅表现出体细胞嵌合体,这意味着他们不会将疾病遗传给下一代。Ruggieri 和 Huson(2001)提出了两个术语来描述 NF1 不同的嵌合体类型:嵌合-全身性 NF1 和嵌合-局限性 NF1(或节段性 NF1),以反映突变事件发生的预期时间。嵌合-全身性 NF1 的患者表现出典型的 NF1 相关症状,如色素变化和神经纤维瘤,这些症状并不限于身体的某些部分。对于这种类型的 NF1,单独从临床观察中预测一个散发性患者是否具有先天性 NF1(即所有体细胞中均有 NF1 突变)与嵌合-全身性 NF1,以及在后者的患者中是否涉及生殖腺,可能特别具有挑战性。"嵌合-局限性"(或节段型)NF1 的患者,NF1 相关症状仅局限于身体的某一特定区域。这些受影响的区域可能仅有色素变化、仅有神经纤维瘤,或同时存在色素变化和神经纤维瘤。此外,也可能出现孤立的丛状神经纤维瘤。最近描述的第一个此类患者在这一孤立病变中被证明存在双等位基因 NF1 失活(Beert et al. 2012)。

在节段型 NF1 中,致病突变事件被认为发生在较晚的发育阶段,这解释了为什么临床上观察到的表型仅局限于特定的身体区域。最有可能的是,节段型 NF1 患者的生殖细胞中不携带(第一次打击)NF1 突变。然而,除了突变事件的时间之外,受影响的前体细胞类型、NF1 突变的性质(如低表达型突变或完全的 NF1 基因缺失的突变),以及患者在临床评估时的年龄,都会对患者在特定时间点观察到的表型变异结果产生影响。节段型 NF1 相对较为罕见,其发生频率估计至少比 NF1 低 15 倍,介于 0.001 4% 和 0.002% 之间(Huson and Ruggieri 2000;Wolkenstein et al. 1995;Ingordo et al. 1995;Listernick et al. 2003)。在分子水平上,节段型 NF1 首次通过在 1 名 18 岁男性的色素病变(分布在身体左上象限)中培养的成纤维细胞中发现约 15%～24% 的 NF1 存在缺失,来证明这一疾病确实由后胚层 NF1 突变引起。而在未受影响区域的成纤维细胞中未发现这种微缺失(Tinschert et al. 2000)。然而,随后的一些患者在分子分析和其患病后代出生后的确认中,表现出"嵌合-局限性"或"节段型"NF1 疾病表型,但最终被证实为生殖系嵌合型(Consoli et al. 2005;Callum et al. 2012)。

在临床文献中,已描述了若干节段性 NF1 患者的后代也患有节段型 NF1(Rubenstein et al. 1983;

Huson and Ruggieri 2000；Oguzkan et al. 2004）；这种垂直传播现象很难用父母与子女之间共享突变导致的嵌合现象来解释。这些报道的病例均未进行分子分析，因此其潜在原因仍不清楚。此外，虽然许多临床上被称为"嵌合-局限性"或"节段型"NF1 的病例很可能在受影响的细胞中携带 NF1 突变，但由于未进行分子检测，其确切原因仍未知（Hager et al. 1997；Ruggieri and Huson 2001；Listernick et al. 2003；Morais et al. 2010），文献中还报道了一些患者虽然表现出色素异常等特征，但其特征显然不与 NF1 相关，仍被认为是"节段性"NF1（Castori et al. 2008；Pascual-Castroviejo et al. 2008）。由于这些患者未进行分子水平的分析，无法证明他们是否携带 NF1 突变，所以必须认识到他们的表型可能是由 1 个或多个基因（包括 NF1 基因）的并发缺陷引起的，甚至可能完全是由一个或多个其他基因的缺陷导致，而与 NF1 无关。随着与 NF1 相关的分子工具的广泛应用，临床上报告的"节段型 NF1"病例应附有适当的支持性数据，使用先进的分子遗传分析方法来验证 NF1 的参与，尤其是在患者表现出与 NF1 无关的特征时。

最后，逆转嵌合现象指的是突变的细胞表型在某些体细胞中通过真正的反向点突变、基因转换、非整倍体分离或有丝分裂重组等方式恢复到正常状态。逆转嵌合现象已经在许多涉及皮肤的遗传病中得到了证明，包括大疱性表皮松解症、布卢姆综合征（Bloom syndrome）和范科尼贫血（Fanconi anemia）等（Lai-Cheong et al. 2011），但迄今为止尚未在 NF1 中得到证明。到目前为止，仅有 3 例病例专门针对逆转嵌合现象的存在与否进行了研究：1 名全身表现出 NF1 特征的女性，其皮肤上有几个边界清楚的正常区域，这提示可能存在逆转嵌合现象（Vandenbroucke et al. 2004），另外还有 2 对在 1 型神经纤维瘤病上表现出差异的单卵双胞胎（Kaplan et al. 2010；Vogt et al. 2011）。

截至 2012 年 5 月，所有支持"第一次打击"NF1 突变的嵌合体的分子数据病例总结如下（表 12.1）。这些研究和病例报告的要点如下。

• 在散发性 1 型神经纤维瘤病（NF1）患者中，嵌合现象的发生频率目前仍然在很大程度上未知。一项初步针对携带全基因缺失（total gene deletion，TGD）的患者进行的研究对 146 名携带 TGD 的患者进行了间期 FISH 分析，结果显示有 9.6%（14/146）的患者存在嵌合现象（Messiaen et al. 2011）。在这些患者中，至少 10/14 名患者携带 1.2 Mb 的 NF1 2 型或非典型 TGD 缺失（见第 14 章）。

• 典型的 1.4 Mb 1 型总基因缺失（TGD），以前被认为是由于母体减数分裂期间在同源重组位点（paralogous recombination sites，PRS）1 和 2 之间发生非等位基因同源重组所独有的结果，现在也被证明在罕见情况下可能是由于合子后有丝分裂细胞期间发生的重组所致。这一点已经在 3 名血液中携带嵌合 1 型 TGD 患者中得到证实（Messiaen et al. 2011）。

• 携带 2 型总基因缺失（TGD）的散发性患者中，嵌合现象的发生率非常高，估计至少在 70% 的创始患者中出现（Messiaen et al. 2011）。在这些携带 2 型 TGD 的嵌合创始患者中，女性似乎显著占多数（Kehrer-Sawatzki et al. 2004；Steinmann et al. 2007）。

• 多项研究发现，在携带 2 型（TGD）的情况下，携带 NF1 突变造血细胞的百分比明显高于尿液和口腔上皮细胞或受累及未受累区域成纤维细胞的百分比，这些患者患有广泛性嵌合 NF1（Kehrer-Sawatzki et al. 2004，2012；Vandenbroucke et al. 2004；Steinmann et al. 2007；Kehrer-Sawatzki and Cooper 2008；Roehl et al. 2012）。然而，通过 FISH 分析发现，2 名嵌合患者的血液中所有细胞都携带缺失，而口腔细胞中的携带率较低（Steinmann et al. 2007；Roehl et al. 2012）。这些组织特异性的差异提示，携带 NF1 缺失的造血干细胞可能具有选择性生长优势（Roehl et al. 2012）。

• 携带 2 型总基因缺失（TGD）的嵌合患者疾病表现通常较轻，与携带 1 型 TGD（通常是先天性的）的患者相比，这些患者的外部和内部丛状神经纤维瘤负担显著较低，且没有面部畸形，也没有认知发育迟缓（Kehrer-Sawatzki et al. 2012）。这可能归因于嵌合患者体内存在正常细胞。然而，由于任何存在的丛状病变都有恶性转化的风险，因此仍需进行特殊的临床管理以便早期检测。

表 12.1 所有已发表的分子遗传学研究的患者的突变类型和临床学数据概览

类型	患者编号	表型 年龄	表型 性别	临床特征	分子分析 NF1 首次打击突变	分子分析 方法	分子分析 亲本来源[b]	患病子代	携带突变的细胞的百分比 外周血/培养淋巴细胞	携带突变的细胞的百分比 其他	参考文献
GO	XAT27: I1	—	F	无症状,但有两个患病孩子	Del ivs31–ivs39 及 Ins 30 bp	单倍型分析,BP 克隆,测序,cDNA 分析,qPCR,DNA 印迹	—	突变阴性	N/D	约占精胞 10%	Lázaro 等(1994,1995)
GEN	UF161[a]	31	F	7个 CALM,腋窝雀斑,面部、躯干和四肢有多个小的皮肤型 NF,在第2次妊娠后26岁时首次出现 NF,巨头畸形,发育正常,无节段型分布特征	Del ex4–ivs39 (约 100 kb)	杂合性缺失分析,克隆技术	Mat (UF162)	2个儿子: UF394: 1个 CALM; UF395: 无症状	约 98.5%	在 NF 中是嵌合体	Colman 等(1996)和 Rasmussen 等(1998)
GEN	867	21	F	多个 CALM,腋窝雀斑,多发小 NF,双侧 Lisch 小结节;颅脑 CT 和 MRI 扫描正常	Del ~ivs27–ivs41	单倍型分析	Mat	—	嵌合体	—	Ainsworth 等(1997)
GEN	5b	40.4	F	超过100个皮肤/皮下 NF,智商正常	微缺失	荧光原位杂交	—	女儿 5a: 严重受累	83%	在正常皮肤的成纤维细胞中未检测到(N/D)	Tonsgard 等(1997)
GEN	95–870–P[a]	0.6	F	先天性颈部巨大 PNF 和全身多发性 CALM,面部畸形伴面神经床瘘	微缺失 (约 700 kb)	荧光原位杂交	—	—	77%~84%	在成纤维细胞中未检测到(N/D)	Wu 等(1997)和 Riva 等(2000)
GEN	UF113	10	?	多个 CALM,2个皮肤 NF,腋窝雀斑,无巨头症,发育正常,轻度半侧肥大,双侧感觉神经性听力损失	基因内缺失	杂合性缺失分析,DNA 印迹	Mat	—	小部分	—	Rasmussen 等(1998)

续表

类型	患者编号	表型		临床特征	分子分析				携带突变的细胞百分比			参考文献
		性别	年龄		NF1首次打击突变	方法	亲本来源[b]	患病子代	外周血/培养淋巴细胞	其他		
GEN	—	M	6	严重的NF1：全身分布多个最大达8 cm×5 cm的CALM，腋窝雀斑，生殖器的色素沉着，PNF，生长迟缓，不能爬行，行走、说话，左孔头下和右颈部有皮下NF，面部畸形，严重目早发的精神运动发育迟缓、癫痫，痉挛，小头畸形	微缺失（>1.7 Mb）	荧光原位杂交	—	—	33%	在成纤维细胞中占58%		Streubel等(1999)
GEN	N.R.	M	47	CALM，雀斑，Lisch小结节，NF，巨头症，无PNF	微缺失	荧光原位杂交（位点特异性探针）	—	—	嵌合体	—		Riva等(2000)
SEG	—	M	18	左上象限（颈侧，上躯干，腋窝和左臂）有雀斑和CALM，无NF和Lisch小结节	微缺失	荧光原位杂交	—	—	0~2%	在CALM中的成纤维细胞中有15%~24%，在正常皮肤及毛囊中未检测到(N/D)		Tinschert等(2000)
SEG	—	M	50	左前方，眉间，上眼睑，鼻子和鼻孔有多个柔软的肤色肿瘤。无其他NF1症状	N/D（从NF培养的成纤维细胞未检测到）	蛋白截短测试，酶促突变检测，荧光原位杂交	—	—	未检测到(N/D)	在NFs和正常皮肤中的成纤维细胞中未检测到(N/D)		Schultz等(2002)
GEN	IL39[a]	F	60	大腿和前臂上有4个CALM，左侧腋窝有轻微的雀斑，无皮肤NF或Lisch小结节	微缺失（2型）	荧光原位杂交，BP PCR，单倍型分析	—	2个儿子严重受累	70%	在成纤维细胞中占15%		Petek等(2003) Kehrer-Sawatzki等(2004)和Steinmann等(2007, 2008)
GEN	WB[a]	F	65	超过20个NF，无面部畸形，无智力迟钝	微缺失（2型）	荧光原位杂交，BP克隆，多态性标记分析	—	女儿SB：严重受累	94%	—		Kehrer-Sawatzki等(2004)和Steinmann等(2007, 2008)

续 表

类型	患者编号	表型		分子分析				患病子代	携带突变的细胞		参考文献
		年龄	性别	临床特征	NF1首次打击突变	方法	亲本来源[b]		外周血/淋巴细胞	其他	
GEN	659	47	F	超过1 000个NF,无智力迟钝	微缺失(非典型HKS,个人交流)	荧光原位杂交,BP克隆,多态性标记分析	—	—	96%	在口腔拭子中占52%	Kehrer-Sawatzki等(2004)
GEN	928[a]	35	F	超过6个CALM,雀斑,Lisch小结节,9个皮下NF和20个皮肤NF,1个PNF,无智力迟钝	微缺失(2型)	荧光原位杂交,BP克隆,多态性标记分析	—	—	97.2%~99.8%	在NFs中占80%,在口腔拭子中占55%,在尿液中占61.3%	Kehrer-Sawatzki等(2004, 2012),Steinmann等(2007, 2008)和Roehl等(2012)
GEN	697[a]	11	F	无NF,无面部畸形或智力障碍,写作和阅读能力迟缓	微缺失(2型)	荧光原位杂交,BP克隆,多态性标记分析	Mat	—	95.4%~98.7%	在口腔拭子中占59%,在尿液中占27.6%	Kehrer-Sawatzki等(2004),Steinmann等(2007, 2008)和Roehl等(2012)
GEN	488[a]	33	F	超过6个CALM,雀斑,Lisch小结节,80个皮下NF和140个皮肤NF。1个内部肿瘤和恶性周围神经鞘膜瘤(MPNST),无面部畸形,无智力迟钝	微缺失(2型)	荧光原位杂交,BP克隆,多态性标记分析	—	—	96.8%~100%	在口腔拭子中占56%,在尿液中占46.5%	Kehrer-Sawatzki等(2004),Steinmann等(2007, 2008)和Roehl等(2012)
GEN	938[a]	31	F	超过6个CALM,雀斑,Lisch小结节,1个皮下NF和20个皮肤NF,无面部畸形,无智力迟钝	微缺失(2型)	荧光原位杂交,BP克隆,多态性标记分析	—	—	93.5%~99.6%	在口腔拭子中占80%,在尿液中占23.9%	Kehrer-Sawatzki等(2004),Steinmann等(2007, 2008)和Roehl等(2012)
GEN	KCD[a]	34	F	超过100个NF,无面部畸形,无智力迟钝	微缺失(2型)	荧光原位杂交,BP克隆,多态性标记分析	—	—	92%	在成纤维细胞中占51%	Kehrer-Sawatzki等(2004)和Steinmann等(2007, 2008)
GEN	736[a]	68	F	超过6个CALM,雀斑,Lisch小结节,大约2 000个皮肤NF,无面部畸形,无智力迟钝	微缺失(2型)	荧光原位杂交,BP克隆,多态性标记分析	—	—	93.8%~99.6%	在口腔拭子中占59%,在尿液中占26.7%	Kehrer-Sawatzki等(2004),Steinmann等(2007, 2008)和Roehl等(2012)

续表

类型	患者编号	表型 年龄	表型 性别	临床特征	分子分析 NF1首次打击突变	分子分析 方法	亲本来源[b]	患病子代	携带突变的细胞的百分比 外周血/培养淋巴细胞	携带突变的细胞的百分比 其他	参考文献
GEN	NF296-UHG[a]	38	F	NF1疾病表现及全身，但留有一些边界清晰的皮肤区域未受影响（症状的节段型缺失）。表现为多个CALM，NF、腋窝和腹股沟的雀斑，双侧Lisch小结节，以及右胫骨的先天性假关节	Del ex13–ex28	长距离反转录PCR，荧光原位杂交，qPCR，微卫星分析，多重探针扩增	—（父亲未知，母亲去世）	—	20.5%	在CALMs中的成纤维细胞中占2.4%，在正常皮肤中的成纤维细胞中占0.9%	Vandenbroucke等（2004）和Wimmer等（2006）
SEG/GOSO	—	—	F	雀斑和CALMs集中在左上象限区域，伴有同侧一只眼睛的Lisch小结节	p.Arg1947*	变性高效液相色谱，DNA测序，克隆，等位基因特异性PCR	—	有1个典型NF1的孩子	N/D	在CALMs中的成纤维细胞中约占17.6%，在角质形成细胞中约占40%，在正常皮肤中未检测（N/D）	Consoli等（2005）
SEG	—	40	M	NF病的区域性表现仅限于右侧胸壁	N/D	全面的NF1检测	—	—	N/D		Fortino等（2005）
N/A	NF362-UAB	—	—	—	Del ex10b–ex49	多重连接依赖探针扩增，反转录聚合酶链式反应，微卫星分析	—	—			Wimmer等（2006）
N/A	NF467-UHG	—	—	—	Del ex28–ex40	多重连接依赖探针扩增，反转录聚合酶链式反应，微卫星分析	—	—			Wimmer等（2006）

续 表

类型	患者编号	表型		分子分析				携带突变的细胞的百分比			
		年龄	性别	临床特征	NF1首次打击突变	方法	亲本来源[b]	患病子代	外周血/培养淋巴细胞	其他	参考文献
非典型（镶嵌环状染色体17）	—	9.5	F	轻度脊柱侧弯，步态欠佳。皮肤上有多个CALM，轻度腋窝和腹股沟雀斑，智力迟钝，自闭症特征，认知和语言发育迟缓	嵌合非多余环状17号染色体[17号染色体短臂(17p)上为0.6到2.5兆碱基(Mb)，长臂(17q)上最多约为10兆碱基]	荧光原位杂交，多重连接依赖探针扩增	—	—	12%		Havlovicova等(2007)
SEG	SNF1-1	46	F	仅有NF：多个小型(1～4 mm)的皮肤NF聚集在躯干和颈部的有限身体区域，肠道神经节细胞瘤，右手中指末端的指骨处有1个球形肿瘤	在3个不同的NF中检测到c.2041C＞T(p.Arg681*)	全面的NF1检测，qPCR，荧光原位杂交	—	2个儿子未受累	3.7%	在NF的成纤维细胞中占8%～19.4%，在施万细胞中占41%～47.4%，在毛囊中占1.8%	Maertens等(2007)
SEG	SNF1-2	23	M	仅有色素缺陷：在右腿、臀部和下背部的皮肤中存在多个CALM，背景皮肤有色素沉着，受影响区域有腹股沟雀斑，无NF，Lisch小结节，LD	CALMs和色素沉着皮肤中的非典型微缺失	全面的NF1检测，qPCR，荧光原位杂交	—	—	2%（分析了400个间期细胞）	CALM中的黑色素细胞存在嵌合现象，正常皮肤中未检测到(N/D)	Maertens等(2007)
GEN	SNF1-3	15	F	全身有6个以上的CALM，右手上有几个小的皮肤和皮下NF，位于1个CALM之上，通过全身MRI显示左肩上有1个假定的NF，皮肤皱褶雀斑无LD	多个NF和CALM中存在微缺失(1.84～2.8 Mb)或c.2325+1G＞A	全面的NF1检测，qPCR，荧光原位杂交	—	—	约4% N/D	CALM中的黑色素细胞占54.9%～97.1%，在NF中占67.2%～88.8%，在成纤维细胞占12.3%	Maertens等(2007)

续 表

类型	患者编号	表型		临床特征	分子分析			携带突变的细胞的百分比			参考文献
		年龄	性别		NF1首次打击突变	方法	亲本来源[b]	患病子代	外周血/培养淋巴细胞	其他	
GEN	1630[a]	15	F	6个以上CALM,雀斑,Lisch小结节,无NF,无巨指或巨趾,也无其他常见于大缺损患者的特征	微缺失(2型)	多态性标记分析,断点分析,多重连接依赖探针扩增,阵列比较基因组杂交	—	—	94.1%～98.2%	尿液中占29.3%	Steinmann等(2007, 2008), Kehrer-Sawatzki等(2012), Roehl等(2012)
GEN	1104[a]	36	F	上背部,左肩,右肩,乳房,腰部、腹部右侧有棋盘状分布的色素沉着棕色区域;无腹窝和腹股沟雀斑,Lisch小结节,腹部、大腿前臂有4～6个NF	微缺失(2型)	多态性标记分析,断点分析,多重连接依赖探针扩增,阵列比较基因组杂交	—	—	84%～94%	口腔拭子中占8%,尿液中占15%	Steinmann等(2007, 2008)
GEN	1502[a]	26	F	多个CALM,腋窝和腹股沟雀斑,Lisch小结节,小于10个皮下NF,智商90,脑部和全身MRI未发现任何肿瘤或其他异常	微缺失(2型)	多态性标记分析,断点分析,多重连接依赖探针扩增,阵列比较基因组杂交	—	—	95.9%～99.3%	口腔拭子中占70%,尿液中占54.6%	Steinmann等(2007, 2008), Kehrer-Sawatzki等(2012), Roehl等(2012)
GEN	811-M[a]	—	F	—	微缺失(2型)	多态性标记分析,断点分析,多重连接依赖探针扩增,阵列比较基因组杂交	—	1个女儿受累	93%	—	Steinmann等(2007, 2008)
GEN	HC[a]	—	M	—	微缺失(2型)	多态性标记分析,断点分析,多重连接依赖探针扩增,阵列比较基因组杂交	Mat(PH)	—	100%	在口腔拭子中存在嵌合现象	Steinmann等(2007, 2008)

续表

类型	患者编号	表型			分子分析				携带突变的细胞的百分比			参考文献
		年龄	性别	临床特征	NF1首次打击突变	方法	亲本来源[b]	患病子代	外周血/培养淋巴细胞	其他		
GEN	1860-M[a]	28, 54	M	LD, 发育迟缓, 腋窝和腹股沟雀斑, Lisch小结节, 约1 000个皮肤结节, 皮下NF, 以及臀部和腰部的内部肿瘤	微缺失(2型)	多重连接依赖探针扩增, 单倍型分析, 荧光原位杂交	Mat (1860-MD)	1个儿子患病	94.4%~95.9%	尿液中占50.9%		Steinmann等(2008)和Roehl等(2012)
GO	NF-307: II	—	M	无NF1症状	Del ivs27b-ex30 (c.4773-3622-?_5749+?)	qPCR, 微卫星分析, 多重连接依赖探针扩增, 基于RNA的分析	—	2个女儿和1个孙女患病	N/D	精子细胞中占10%~17%		Bottillo等(2010)
GOSO (患病双胞胎)/？(不一致的同卵双胞胎)	—	57	F	患病的双胞胎: CALM, 皮肤NF, PNF, Lisch小结节, 雀斑。暗示存在性细胞嵌合现象。未患病的双胞胎: 无NF1症状, 有2个正常孩子	p.Arg1968*	测序, 短串联重复标记, 阵列比较基因组杂交	Mat	2个患病孩子, 一个正常孩子 无	存在 存在	存在于成纤维细胞和口腔拭子中 在口腔拭子中存在, 在成纤维细胞中未检测到(N/D)		Kaplan等(2010)
GEN	#3	36	M	9个CALM和巨大症, 双侧腋窝雀斑, 认知正常, 无LD, 无节段性分布, 可能有1个NF	c.2866dupA	单碱基延伸法, 焦磷酸测序法	—	1个患病儿子, 2个正常孩子	24%	—		Muram-Zborovski等(2010)
GEN	—	34	F	20个CALM分布在躯干和上肢, 腋窝和乳房下部雀斑, 轻度脊柱侧弯, 少于50个微小的NF (自18岁起发展), 无Lisch小结节, 无畸形, 无LD	c.3198-314G>A (漏剪接突变)	基于DNA的测序, 单碱基延伸法	—	—	约100%	尿液中约100%, 口腔拭子, 毛发和皮肤中20%~35%		Fernández-Rodríguez等(2011)

续表

类型	患者编号	表型		分子分析				携带突变的细胞的百分比		参考文献
		年龄	性别	临床特征	NF1首次打击突变	方法	亲本来源[b]	患病子代	外周血/培养淋巴细胞	其他
GEN	UAB-r3302	15	M	超过6个CALM,腋窝雀斑,左侧颈部,胸脯和躯干的皮肤NF,左臂上的PNF,右臂上有少数雀斑和CALM,双侧Lisch小结节,无脊柱NF或视神经胶质瘤	微缺失(1型)	多重连接依赖探针扩增,微卫星分析,荧光原位杂交,断点跨越PCR,单核苷酸多态性分析	—	—	约80%	—	Messiaen等(2011)
GEN	UAB-r7332	10	M	超过6个CALM,双侧腋窝和腹股沟雀斑,双侧Lisch小结节,2~6个皮肤NF和2~6个皮肤NF,左侧视神经有症状的视神经胶质瘤,脊柱侧弯	微缺失(根据MLPA结果,可能是1型)	多重连接依赖探针扩增,微卫星分析,荧光原位杂交,断点跨越PCR,单核苷酸多态性分析	—	—	约97%	—	Messiaen等(2011)
GEN	UAB-r3222	27	F	2个CALM,无雀斑,超过100个皮肤NF,无PNF,双侧Lisch小结节,无视神经胶质瘤或骨骼异常,发育正常	微缺失(1型)	多重连接依赖探针扩增,微卫星分析,荧光原位杂交,断点跨越PCR,单核苷酸多态性分析	—	—	50%	—	Messiaen等(2011)
SEG	P067	45	F	约20个小皮肤NF,右上背部和右侧乳房下方有雀斑,腹股沟有雀斑,无CALM或Lisch小结节,无面部畸形,无LD	微缺失(1型)	多重连接依赖探针扩增,微卫星分析,荧光原位杂交,断点跨越PCR,单核苷酸多态性分析	—	—	N/D	存在于NF的施万细胞中	Messiaen等(2011)
SEG	UAB-M1	14	M	3个CALM,左侧大腿上部和左侧腹股沟区有雀斑性高色素沉着,无NF或PNF,无Lisch小结节	微缺失(可能是1型)	多重连接依赖探针扩增,微卫星分析,荧光原位杂交,断点跨越PCR,单核苷酸多态性分析	—	—	N/D	在CALM中的黑色素细胞中存在,在成纤维细胞中未检测到(N/D)	Messiaen等(2011)

续表

类型	患者编号	表型		分子分析			亲本来源[b]	患病子代	携带突变的细胞的百分比		参考文献
		年龄	性别	临床特征	NF1首次打击突变	方法			外周血/培养淋巴细胞	其他	
GEN（表现不一致的单卵双胞胎）	—	3	M	患病的双胞胎：超过6个CALM，腋窝和腹股沟雀斑 未患病的双胞胎：2个CALM	c. 4108C>T(p.Gln1370*)	单核苷酸多态性/等位基因标记分析，单碱基延伸法，克隆技术	Mat	—	30%~40%	口腔拭子中约8%（4%等基因，4%等位基因），尿液中未检测到（N/D）口腔拭子和尿液中未检测到（N/D）	Vogt等（2011）
					N/D			—	N/D		
SEG	—	13	M	在腰骶区域有1个孤立的PNF，无CALM，Lisch小结节及其他NF1特征	首次打击：ins(17;1)(q11.2;p35p36) 二次打击：8.28 Mb del on 17q11.2q12	染色体核型分析，荧光原位杂交，芯片比较基因组杂交	—	—		施万细胞中占61%（通过FISH检测约为21%）通过FISH检测，施万细胞中的比例为13%；通过aCGH检测，比例为15%~20%	Beert等（2012）
GOSO	—	—	M	精子捐献者：仅有4个高色素斑点，位于中线背部，无发育障碍，Lisch小结节，NF	Del ex11 – 23.1	反转录聚合酶链反应，断点克隆，多重连接依赖探针扩增，芯片比较基因组杂交	—	—	存在（通过反转录酶PCR检测到）	在精子细胞中约占20%	Callum等（2012）
GEN	1956[a]	9	M	超过6个CALM，腋窝雀斑，Lisch小结节，脊柱侧弯，发育正常	微缺失（2型）	荧光原位杂交	—	—	96.7%~99.1%	在尿液中占60%	Kehrer-Sawatzki（2012）和Roehl等（2012）
GEN	2442[a]	40	F	超过6个CALM，腋窝雀斑，Lisch小结节，约250个皮肤NF，椎孔肿瘤，正常的脑部、视路和眼窝MRI，脊柱侧弯，身材矮小（<第5百分位）	微缺失（2型）	荧光原位杂交	—	—	98.6%~100%	在尿液中占60%	Kehrer-Sawatzki（2012），Roehl等（2012）

续 表

类型	患者编号	表型			分子分析				携带突变的细胞的百分比		参考文献
		年龄	性别	临床特征	NF1首次打击突变	方法	亲本来源[b]	患病子代	外周血/培养淋巴细胞	其他	
GEN	UC172	—	—	—	微缺失(2型)	荧光原位杂交、微卫星分析、断点克隆	—	—	91.9%～97.9%	在尿液中占64.5%	Roehl 等(2012)
GEN	585	—	—	—	微缺失(2型)	荧光原位杂交、微卫星分析、断点克隆	—	—	94.3%～96.7%	在尿液中占81.9%	Roehl 等(2012)
GEN	3304	47	M	多个CALM,超过1 000个皮肤NF,肌肉张力低,大而柔软的手,漏斗胸,阅读/写作困难,发育迟缓	微缺失(非典型或1型)	荧光原位杂交、微卫星分析、断点克隆	—	女儿患病	16.9%～19.3%	在尿液中占25%	Roehl 等(2012)

注：GO,生殖腺嵌合体；GOSO,性腺体嵌合体；GEN,全身性嵌合体；SEG,节段型嵌合体；NF,神经纤维瘤；PNF,丛状神经纤维瘤；CALM,咖啡牛奶斑；Del,缺失；Ins,插入；N/D,未检测到；M,男性；F,女性；Mat,母源性的；Pat,父源性的；LD,学习障碍；BP,断点。[a] 在多项研究中有所描述的。[b] 嵌合型先证者中携带突变等位基因的亲本来源。

- 广泛性嵌合1型神经纤维瘤病(NF1)与节段型NF1之间的界限可能并没有那么清晰。通常情况下,在血液中难以检测到具有明显节段型表现的患者的突变。然而,在1名成年男性中,性腺嵌合现象被证实,他背部中线有4个色素病变,这是唯一的NF1相关表现(Callum et al. 2012)。这一位于基因内的多外显子缺失,在血液细胞中的存在率≤20%,在精子中的存在率约为20%,是通过反转录PCR优先扩增较短的转录本作为全面NF1检测的一部分而被检测到的(Callum et al. 2012)。低水平的嵌合突变通常会逃避桑格(Sanger)测序、阵列比较基因组杂交(array comparative genome hybridization, aCGH)或多重连接依赖探针扩增(multiplex ligation-dependent probe amplification, MLPA)的检测。

- 来自所有携带嵌合NF1("广泛性"或"节段型")患者的汇总数据清楚地表明,携带NF1"第一次打击"突变的细胞比例通常过低,以至于无法在血液中可靠地检测到(甚至可能不存在),因此可能被遗漏(Tinschert et al. 2000; Consoli et al. 2005; Maertens et al. 2007; Callum et al. 2012)。

- 根据"二次打击"学说,神经纤维瘤中的部分施万细胞亚群携带第2次NF1突变(Serra et al. 2000; Maertens et al. 2006)。在NF1患者的咖啡牛奶斑(CALM)中,黑色素细胞(而非角质形成细胞或成纤维细胞)携带NF1基因的第一次和第二次突变(De Schepper et al. 2008)。Maertens等(2007)证明,准确诊断嵌合性或节段性NF1需要对源自神经嵴的相关细胞(即神经纤维瘤中的施万细胞和咖啡牛奶斑中的黑色素细胞)进行全面的突变分析。在这些特定细胞中,而非在血液、成纤维细胞或角质形成细胞中,可以在节段性NF1患者的不同病变(神经纤维瘤或咖啡牛奶斑)中发现常见的第一次NF1突变。这也解释了为什么在Schultz等(2002)描述的患者的成纤维细胞中没有发现突变。

- 总共有49名患者被报道为在生殖细胞和(或)体细胞中存在合子后"第一次打击"NF1突变的嵌合现象,其中仅6名患者携带影响1个核苷酸的轻微突变,这些突变均导致了提前终止密码子的产生。这可能反映了检测嵌合点突变的技术难题。

- 在这49例患者中,有43例突变为基因内多外显子缺失或大缺失。其中,至少17例缺失跨越1.2 Mb的2型总基因缺失(TGD)。

- 最后,Kaplan等(2010)报道了一对差异双胞胎的病例,其中1名女性在其从B淋巴细胞中培养的EB病毒转化淋巴母细胞和口腔上皮细胞中均携带NF1无义突变,但在她的皮肤成纤维细胞中没有发现该突变,而她在57岁时仍无症状。在另一对差异双胞胎(Vogt et al. 2011)中,患病的3岁双胞胎在血液和口腔细胞中显示出p.Gln1370*无义突变的嵌合现象,而未患病的双胞胎则未发现该突变。这种现象可以解释为合子后突变发生在胚胎生命的第3~4天之后,即双胞胎分裂事件之后。

12.3 NF1的分子诊断

由于NF1基因的体积大、存在多个高度同源的未加工假基因,并且缺乏突变热点,且具有复杂的突变谱(包括显著比例的异常剪接突变,如深内含子剪接突变或影响外显子剪接增强子的突变,以及无义、错义甚至无声突变),NF1的分子诊断极具挑战性(Messiaen and Wimmer 2008)。采用包括基于RNA的中心分析在内的多步骤方法可以获得最高的灵敏性和特异性(Messiaen et al. 2000; Wimmer et al. 2006; Valero et al. 2011)。

随着基因型-表型相关性的逐步揭示,突变分析的临床应用变得越来越重要。例如,大缺失通常会导致更严重的临床表型(Upadhyaya et al. 1998; Riva et al. 2000; Mautner et al. 2010),而外显子17中3 bp框内缺失所导致的1个氨基酸缺失则会产生较轻的表型,不会出现皮肤或浅表丛状神经纤维瘤(Upadhyaya et al. 2007)。此外,通过识别由SPRED1基因突变引起的Legius综合征,发现了有限的遗传异质性(Brems et al. 2007)。Legius综合征患者表现为多个咖啡牛奶斑(CALM),可能伴有或不伴有皮肤皱褶雀斑和巨头症,但不会发展为典型的NF1相关肿瘤(Brems et al. 2012)。对于仅表现为CALM伴有或不伴有雀斑的患者,单凭临床表现很难准确区分先天性NF1、散发性NF1(嵌合体)和Legius综合征。

在95%的"经典NF1"患者中，即具有咖啡牛奶斑（CALM）、皮肤皱褶雀斑和神经纤维瘤的患者，通过综合方法，如RNA测序，可以识别出NF1突变（Messiaen et al. 2009）。然而，即使这些患者表现出CALM、皮肤皱褶雀斑和神经纤维瘤，散发性患者的血液淋巴细胞中NF1突变的检测率也可能较低，这可能是因为某些患者存在嵌合现象，使得NF1突变无法在血液中检测到。

目前报道的大多数广泛性嵌合患者都表现出2型或非典型总基因缺失（TGD），这种缺失在血液淋巴细胞中检测到的比例显著高于尿源或口腔上皮细胞中的比例（Kehrer-Sawatzki et al. 2004，2012；Vandenbroucke et al. 2004；Steinmann et al. 2007；Kehrer-Sawatzki and Cooper 2008；Roehl et al. 2012）。因此，血液是进行分析的1个良好起点样本。为了确定嵌合现象，对于在血液中识别出2型或非典型TGD的散发性患者进行定量测试（如在尿液上皮细胞中的FISH）是合理的。这对于建立嵌合性NF1与先天性NF1的诊断，并为患者和家庭提供关于复发风险的咨询具有重要意义。

在咖啡牛奶斑和神经纤维瘤中的起源细胞，即黑色素细胞（De Schepper et al. 2008）和施万细胞（Serra et al. 2000；Maertens et al. 2006），现在可以用于精确识别节段型NF1患者受累区域中的共同"第一次打击"NF1突变（Maertens et al. 2007）。这对于那些在血液中经过全面测试后无法识别突变的疑似嵌合患者尤为重要。识别这种共同的"第一次打击"突变可以明确诊断节段型或嵌合性NF1。此外，这提供了一个可用于家庭规划的指标（如果需要），因为这种突变可能会遗传给下一代，从而导致先天性NF1（所有体细胞携带遗传的突变）。通过分析精子，可以进一步确定嵌合/节段男性患者的遗传风险，但由于无法筛查卵子，女性患者无法进行类似分析。

在创始患者的诊断方面，未来的进展可能来自深度测序等新技术，这些技术有望提供一种可靠且灵敏的方法来检测低水平的嵌合现象。

（许学文，肖杨 译）

参考文献

[1] Ainsworth P, Chakraborty P, Weksberg R (1997) Example of somatic mosaicism in a series of de novo neurofibromatosis type 1 cases due to a maternally derived deletion. Hum Mutat 9：452-459

[2] Ballester R, Marchuk D, Boguski M, Saulino A, Letcher R, Wigler M, Collins F (1990) The NF1 locus encodes a protein functionally related to mammalian GAP and yeast IRA proteins. Cell 63：851-860

[3] Beert E, Brems H, Renard M, Ferreiro J, Melotte C, Thoelen R, De Wever I, Sciot R, Legius E, Debiec-Rychter M (2012) Biallelic inactivation of NF1 in a sporadic plexiform neurofibroma. Genes Chromosomes Cancer 51：852-857

[4] Bottillo I, Torrente I, Lanari V, Pinna V, Giustini S, Divona L, De Luca A, Dallapiccola B (2010) Germline mosaicism in neurofibromatosis type 1 due to a paternally derived multi-exon deletion. Am J Med Genet A 152A：1467-1540

[5] Brems H, Chmara M, Sahbatou M, Denayer E, Taniguchi K, Kato R, Somers R, Messiaen L, De Schepper S, Fryns J-P, Cools J, Marynen P, Thomas G, Yoshimura A, Legius E (2007) Germline loss-of-function mutations in SPRED1 cause a neurofibromatosis 1-like phenotype. Nat Genet 39：1120-1126

[6] Brems H, Beert E, de Ravel T, Legius E (2009) Mechanisms in the pathogenesis of malignant tumours in neurofibromatosis type 1. Lancet Oncol 10：508-523

[7] Brems H, Pasmant E, Van Minkelen R, Wimmer K, Upadhyaya M, Legius E, Messiaen L (2012) Review and update of SPRED1 mutations causing Legius syndrome. Hum Mutat 33(11)：1538-1546

[8] Callum P, Messiaen L, Bower P, Skovby F, Iger J, Timshel S, Sims C, Falk R (2012) Gonosomal mosaicism for an NF1 deletion in a sperm donor：evidence of the need for coordinated, long-term communication of health information among relevant parties. Hum Reprod 27：1223-1229

[9] Castori M, Majore S, Romanelli F, Didona B, Grammatico P, Zambruno G (2008) Association of segmental neurofibromatosis 1 and oculo-auriculo-vertebral spectrum in a 24-year-old female. Eur J Dermatol 18：22-27

[10] Colman S, Rasmussen S, Ho V, Abernathy C, Wallace M (1996) Somatic mosaicism in a patient with neurofibromatosis type 1. Am J Hum Genet 58：484-574

[11] Consoli C, Moss C, Green S, Balderson D, Cooper DN, Upadhyaya M (2005) Gonosomal mosaicism for a nonsense mutation (R1947X) in the NF1 gene in segmental neurofibromatosis type 1. J Invest Dermatol 125：463-469

[12] De Schepper S, Maertens O, Callens T, Naeyaert J-M, Lambert J, Messiaen L (2008) Somatic mutation analysis in NF1 café au lait spots reveals two NF1 hits in the melanocytes. J Invest Dermatol 128：1050-1053

[13] Evans D, Howard E, Giblin C, Clancy T, Spencer H, Huson S, Lalloo F (2010) Birth incidence and prevalence of tumor-prone syndromes：estimates from a UK family genetic register service. Am J Med Genet A 152A：327-359

[14] Fernández-Rodríguez J, Castellsagué J, Benito L, Benavente Y, Capellá G, Blanco I, Serra E, Lázaro C (2011) A mild neurofibromatosis type 1 phenotype produced by the

combination of the benign nature of a leaky *NF1*-splice mutation and the presence of a complex mosaicism. Hum Mutat 32: 705-714

[15] Fortino S, Andre M, Sudish M, Nicholas MB (2005) Thoracoscopically guided transaxillary resection of adjoining intercostal plexiform neurofibromas: review of mosaicism in neurofi-bromatosis: technical note. Neurosurgery 57 (4 Suppl): E407

[16] Friedman J (1999) Vascular and endocrine abnormalities. In: Friedman JM, Gutmann DH, AmcCollin M, Riccardi VM (eds) Neurofibromatosis. Phenotype, natural history, and pathogenesis. Johns Hopkins University Press, Baltimore, MD, pp 274-296

[17] Hager C, Cohen P, Tschen J (1997) Segmental neurofibromatosis: case reports and review. J Am Acad Dermatol 37: 864-873

[18] Havlovicova M, Novotna D, Kocarek E, Novotna K, Bendova S, Petrak B, Hrdlicka M, Sedlacek Z (2007) A girl with neurofibromatosis type 1, atypical autism and mosaic ring chromosome 17. Am J Med Genet A 143: 76-157

[19] Huson SM, Ruggieri M (2000) The neurofibromatosis. In: Harper J, Oranje JM, Rose M (eds) Textbook of pediatric dermatology, vol 2. Blackwell, Oxford, pp 1204-1224

[20] Huson S, Compston D, Harper P (1989) A genetic study of von Recklinghausen neurofibromatosis in south east Wales II. Guidelines for genetic counselling. J Med Genet 26: 712-733

[21] Ingordo V, D'Andria G, Mendicini S, Grecucci M, Baglivo A (1995) Segmental neurofibromatosis: is it uncommon or underdiagnosed? Arch Dermatol 131: 959-1019

[22] Kaplan L, Foster R, Shen Y, Parry D, McMaster M, O'Leary M, Gusella J (2010) Monozygotic twins discordant for neurofibromatosis 1. Am J Med Genet A 152A: 601-607

[23] Kehrer-Sawatzki H, Cooper DN (2008) Mosaicism in sporadic neurofibromatosis type 1: variations on a theme common to other hereditary cancer syndromes? J Med Genet 45: 622-653

[24] Kehrer-Sawatzki H, Kluwe L, Sandig C, Kohn M, Wimmer K, Krammer U, Peyrl A, Jenne D, Hansmann I, Mautner VF (2004) High frequency of mosaicism among patients with neurofibromatosis type 1 (NF1) with microdeletions caused by somatic recombination of the *JJAZ1* gene. Am J Hum Genet 75: 410-433

[25] Kehrer-Sawatzki H, Vogt J, Mußotter T, Kluwe L, Cooper DN, Mautner V-F (2012) Dissecting the clinical phenotype associated with mosaic type-2 NF1 microdeletions. Neurogenetics 13: 229-236

[26] Korf B (1999) Plexiform neurofibromas. Am J Med Genet 89: 31-38

[27] Lai-Cheong J, McGrath J, Uitto J (2011) Revertant mosaicism in skin: natural gene therapy. Trends Mol Med 17: 140-148

[28] Lázaro C, Gaona A, Lynch M, Kruyer H, Ravella A, Estivill X (1995) Molecular characterization of the breakpoints of a 12-kb deletion in the *NF1* gene in a family showing germ-line mosaicism. Am J Hum Genet 57: 1044-1053

[29] Lázaro C, Ravella A, Gaona A, Volpini V, Estivill X (1994) Neurofibromatosis type 1 due to germ-line mosaicism in a clinically normal father. New Engl J Med 331: 1403-1410

[30] Listernick R, Mancini A, Charrow J (2003) Segmental neurofibromatosis in childhood. Am J Med Genet A 121A: 132-137

[31] Maertens O, Brems H, Vandesompele J, De Raedt T, Heyns I, Rosenbaum T, De Schepper S, De Paepe A, Mortier G, Janssens S, Speleman F, Legius E, Messiaen L (2006) Comprehensive NF1 screening on cultured Schwann cells from neurofibromas. Hum Mutat 27: 1030-1070

[32] Maertens O, De Schepper S, Vandesompele J, Brems H, Heyns I, Janssens S, Speleman F, Legius E, Messiaen L (2007) Molecular dissection of isolated disease features in mosaic neurofibromatosis type 1. Am J Hum Genet 81: 243-294

[33] Mautner VF, Kluwe L, Friedrich RE, Roehl AC, Bammert S, Hogel J, Spori H, Cooper DN, Kehrer-Sawatzki H (2010) Clinical characterization of 29 neurofibromatosis type 1 patients with molecularly ascertained 1.4 Mb type-1 deletions. J Med Genet 47: 623-630

[34] Messiaen L, Callens T, Mortier G, Beysen D, Vandenbroucke I, Van Roy N, Speleman F, Paepe A (2000) Exhaustive mutation analysis of the *NF1* gene allows identification of 95% of mutations and reveals a high frequency of unusual splicing defects. Hum Mutat 15: 541-596

[35] Messiaen L, Wimmer K (2008) NF1 mutational spectrum. In: Kaufmann D (ed) Monographs in human genetics, vol 16. Karger, Basel, pp 63-77

[36] Messiaen L, Yao S, Brems H, Callens T, Sathienkijkanchai A, Denayer E, Spencer E, Arn P, Babovic-Vuksanovic D, Bay C, Bobele G, Cohen B, Escobar L, Eunpu D, Grebe T, Greenstein R, Hachen R, Irons M, Kronn D, Lemire E, Leppig K, Lim C, McDonald M, Narayanan V, Pearn A, Pedersen R, Powell B, Shapiro L, Skidmore D, Tegay D, Thiese H, Zackai E, Vijzelaar R, Taniguchi K, Ayada T, Okamoto F, Yoshimura A, Parret A, Korf B, Legius E (2009) Clinical and mutational spectrum of neurofibromatosis type 1-like syndrome. JAMA 302: 2111-2119

[37] Messiaen L, Vogt J, Bengesser K, Fu C, Mikhail F, Serra E, Garcia-Linares C, Cooper DN, Lazaro C, Kehrer-Sawatzki H (2011) Mosaic type-1 *NF1* microdeletions as a cause of both generalized and segmental neurofibromatosis type-1 (NF1). Hum Mutat 32: 213-222

[38] Morais P, Ferreira O, Bettencourt H, Azevedo F (2010) Segmental neurofibromatosis: a rare variant of a common genodermatosis. Acta Dermatovenerol Alp Panonica Adriat 19: 27-36

[39] Muram-Zborovski T, Vaughn C, Viskochil D, Hanson H, Mao R, Stevenson D (2010) NF1 exon 22 analysis of individuals with the clinical diagnosis of neurofibromatosis type 1. Am J Med Genet A 152A: 1973-1981

[40] Oguzkan S, Cinbis M, Ayter S, Anlar B, Aysun S (2004) Familial segmental neurofibromatosis. J Child Neurol 19: 392-396

[41] Pascual-Castroviejo I, Pascual-Pascual SI, Viaño J (2008) Segmental neurofibromatosis type 1 (NF1) associated with Cobb syndrome: case report. Neuropediatrics 39: 341-343

[42] Petek E, Jenne D, Smolle J, Binder B, Lasinger W, Windpassinger C, Wagner K, Kroisel P, Kehrer-Sawatzki H (2003) Mitotic recombination mediated by the JJAZF1 (KIAA0160) gene causing somatic mosaicism and a new type of constitutional *NF1* microdeletion in two children of a mosaic female with only few manifestations. J Med Genet 40: 520-525

[43] Poyhonen M, Kytölä S, Leisti J (2000) Epidemiology of neurofibromatosis type 1 (NF1) in northern Finland. J Med Genet 37: 632-638

[44] Rasmussen S, Colman S, Ho V, Abernathy C, Arn P, Weiss L, Schwartz C, Saul R, Wallace M (1998) Constitutional and mosaic large *NF1* gene deletions in neurofibromatosis type 1. J Med Genet 35: 468-539

[45] Rieley M, Stevenson D, Viskochil D, Tinkle B, Martin L, Schorry E (2011) Variable expression of neurofibromatosis 1 in monozygotic twins. Am J Med Genet A 155A: 478-563

[46] Riva P, Corrado L, Natacci F, Castorina P, Wu B, Schneider G, Clementi M, Tenconi R, Korf B, Larizza L (2000) NF1 microdeletion syndrome: refined FISH characterization of sporadic and familial deletions with locus-specific probes. Am J Hum Genet 66: 100-109

[47] Roehl A, Mussotter T, Cooper DN, Kluwe L, Wimmer K, Högel J, Zetzmann M, Vogt J, Mautner V-F, Kehrer-Sawatzki H (2012) Tissue-specific differences in the proportion of mosaic large NF1 deletions are suggestive of a selective growth advantage of hematopoietic del(+/−) stem cells. Hum Mutat 33: 541-591

[48] Rubenstein A, Bader J, Aron A, Wallace S (1983) Familial transmission of segmental neurofibromatosis. Neurology 33: 76

[49] Ruggieri M, Huson S (2001) The clinical and diagnostic implications of mosaicism in the neurofibromatoses. Neurology 56: 1433-1476

[50] Schultz E, Kaufmann D, Tinschert S, Schell H, von den Driesch P, Schuler G (2002) Segmental neurofibromatosis. Dermatology 204: 296-303

[51] Serra E, Rosenbaum T, Winner U, Aledo R, Ars E, Estivill X, Lenard H, Lázaro C (2000) Schwann cells harbor the somatic NF1 mutation in neurofibromas: evidence of two different Schwann cell subpopulations. Hum Mol Genet 9: 3055-3119

[52] Steinmann K, Cooper DN, Kluwe L, Chuzhanova N, Senger C, Serra E, Lazaro C, Gilaberte M, Wimmer K, Mautner V-F, Kehrer-Sawatzki H (2007) Type 2 NF1 deletions are highly unusual by virtue of the absence of nonallelic homologous recombination hotspots and an apparent preference for female mitotic recombination. Am J Hum Genet 81: 1201-1221

[53] Steinmann K, Kluwe L, Cooper DN, Brems H, De Raedt T, Legius E, Mautner V-F, Kehrer-Sawatzki H (2008) Copy number variations in the NF1 gene region are infrequent and do not predispose to recurrent type-1 deletions. Eur J Hum Genet 16: 572-652

[54] Stevenson D, Zhou H, Ashrafi S, Messiaen L, Carey J, D'Astous J, Santora S, Viskochil D (2006) Double inactivation of NF1 in tibial pseudarthrosis. Am J Hum Genet 79: 143-151

[55] Streubel B, Latta E, Kehrer-Sawatzki H, Hoffmann G, Fonatsch C, Rehder H (1999) Somatic mosaicism of a greater than 1.7-Mb deletion of genomic DNA involving the entire NF1 gene as verified by FISH: further evidence for a contiguous gene syndrome in 17q11.2. Am J Med Genet 87: 12-18

[56] Tinschert S, Naumann I, Stegmann E, Buske A, Kaufmann D, Thiel G, Jenne D (2000) Segmental neurofibromatosis is caused by somatic mutation of the neurofibromatosis type 1 (NF1) gene. Eur J Hum Genet 8: 455-464

[57] Tonsgard J, Yelavarthi K, Cushner S, Short M, Lindgren V (1997) Do NF1 gene deletions result in a characteristic phenotype? Am J Med Genet 73: 80-86

[58] Upadhyaya M, Ruggieri M, Maynard J, Osborn M, Hartog C, Mudd S, Pentinnen M, Cordeiro I, Ponder M, Ponder BA, Krwaczak M, Cooper DN (1998) Gross deletions of the neurofibromatosis type 1 (NF1) gene are predominantly of maternal origin and commonly associated with a learning disability, dysmorphic features and developmental delay. Hum Genet 102: 591-597

[59] Upadhyaya M, Huson S, Davies M, Thomas N, Chuzhanova N, Giovannini S, Evans D, Howard E, Kerr B, Griffiths S, Consoli C, Side L, Adams D, Pierpont M, Hachen R, Barnicoat A, Li H, Wallace P, Van Biervliet J, Stevenson D, Viskochil D, Baralle D, Haan E, Riccardi V, Turnpenny P, Lazaro C, Messiaen L (2007) An absence of cutaneous neurofibromas associated with a 3-bp inframe deletion in exon 17 of the NF1 gene (c. 2970-2972 delAAT): evidence of a clinically significant NF1 genotype-phenotype correlation. Am J Hum Genet 80: 140-191

[60] Valero MC, Martin Y, Hernandez-Imaz E, Hernandez AM, Melean G, Valero AM, Rodriguez-Alvaraez FJ, Telleria D, Hernandez-Chico C (2011) A highly sensitive genetic protocol to detect NF1 mutations. J Mol Diagn 13: 113-122

[61] Vandenbroucke I, van Doorn R, Callens T, Cobben J, Starink T, Messiaen L (2004) Genetic and clinical mosaicism in a patient with neurofibromatosis type 1. Hum Genet 114: 284-374

[62] Vogt J, Kohlhase J, Morlot S, Kluwe L, Mautner V-F, Cooper D, Kehrer-Sawatzki H (2011) Monozygotic twins discordant for neurofibromatosis type 1 due to a postzygotic NF1 gene mutation. Hum Mutat 32: 47

[63] Wimmer K, Yao S, Claes K, Kehrer-Sawatzki H, Tinschert S, De Raedt T, Legius E, Callens T, Beiglböck H, Maertens O, Messiaen L (2006) Spectrum of single- and multiexon NF1 copy number changes in a cohort of 1,100 unselected NF1 patients. Genes Chromosomes Cancer 45: 265-276

[64] Wolkenstein P, Mahmoudi A, Zeller J, Revuz J (1995) More on the frequency of segmental neurofibromatosis. Arch Dermatol 131: 1465

[65] Wu B, Boles R, Yaari H, Weremowicz S, Schneider G, Korf B (1997) Somatic mosaicism for deletion of the entire NF1 gene identified by FISH. Hum Genet 99: 209-222

[66] Xu G, Lin B, Tanaka K, Dunn D, Wood D, Gesteland R, White R, Weiss R, Tamanoi F (1990) The catalytic domain of the neurofibromatosis type 1 gene product stimulates ras GTPase and complements ira mutants of S. cerevisiae. Cell 63: 835-876

[67] Zlotogora J (1993) Mutations in von Recklinghausen neurofibromatosis: a hypothesis. Am J Med Genet 46: 182-186

第13章 NF1的深部内含子突变以及潜在的治疗干预措施

Deep Intronic *NF1* Mutations and Possible Therapeutic Interventions

Conxi Lázaro, Juana Fernández-Rodríguez, and Eduard Serra

13.1 深部内含子突变：一种特殊类型的剪接突变

剪接是一种复杂且精细调控的细胞机制，包括从前体mRNA转录本中去除内含子并生成成熟信使RNA的过程。这一关键过程需要多个顺式作用元件和反式作用因子参与，在剪接体中完成不同的过程（Hammond and Wood 2011）。正确剪接的关键在于识别内含子-外显子的边界，这些边界由供体或5′端内含子剪接位点（在基因组DNA中为GT）和受体或3′端剪接位点（在基因组DNA中为AG）的高度保守、几乎不变的二核苷酸组成。其他用于剪接位点识别的重要基因组序列包括分支位点和多聚嘧啶区，两者均位于内含子受体位点的上游。其他相关的顺式作用元件位于内含子和外显子区域内，包括剪接位点增强子（SE）和沉默子（SS）的核苷酸基序，它们参与了将反式作用因子——增强子或沉默子招募到剪接机制中。这些元件的DNA序列发生基因组突变，可能改变剪接机制对真正外显子的正确识别，也可能产生1个可以被剪接机制识别的新隐蔽剪接位点。因此，基因突变导致这些元件的DNA序列改变，可能导致剪接过程出错，造成外显子跳跃、部分外显子缺失或内含子区域保留在成熟RNA中。这种情况下，等位基因的突变可能产生框架内或框架外的异常转录本。

经典观点认为，剪接突变仅发生于破坏那些稳定的典型供体和受体剪接位点的DNA序列，因此在突变数据库中只有这些突变被报告为剪接突变〔目前占人类基因突变数据库（HGMD Professional 2011.4；http://www.hgmd.org）中报告的所有点突变的不到10%〕。然而，在过去10年中，大量研究发现其他类型的突变也会影响基因的正确剪接，特别是在使用基于RNA的方法进行组成性突变检测和专注于大基因的遗传分析中（Teraoka et al. 1999；Ars et al. 2000）。这些发现将影响剪接的致病突变组扩展到一系列不同的突变类型（无义突变、错义突变和移码突变等），这些突变会影响对剪接位点识别和mRNA加工很重要的序列。例如，对2 000多名相互无关联的1型神经纤维瘤患者进行的最大规模无偏见综合研究发现,约 30% 的 1 型神经纤维瘤病点突变会影响 mRNA 的正常剪接(L Messiaen, personal communication)。这些突变中的一小部分(约 2%)(Messiaen and Wimmer 2008; Pros et al. 2008; Wimmer et al. 2007)包括位于内含子深处序列中的单核苷酸变化,这些单核苷酸变化会产生新的供体或受体位点,这些位点与附近的隐蔽剪接位点结合,并定义 1 个新的隐蔽外显子,然后剪接体将其整合到成熟的信使 RNA 中。这些突变大多被传统的 DNA 突变检测技术所遗漏,因为它们位于内含子序列深处,且远离内含子-外显子边界,因此在采用这种突变检测方法时不会被扫描到。此外,这些突变中有很大一部分会产生带有过早终止密码子(premature termination codons, PTC)的 mRNA,从而使转录本容易受到无义介导的 mRNA 降解(nonsense-mediated mRNA decay, NMD)机制的降解。因此,为检测深部内含子突变特有的错误剪接效应,最好在提取 RNA 之前使用 NMD 抑制剂(Messiaen et al. 2000)。总之,这些观察结果表明,在大多数研究中,这些突变的频率可能被低估了。

13.2 使用反义寡核苷酸来调控异常剪接

近年来,人们越来越多地在使用反义寡核苷酸(antisense oligonucleotide, AON)介导的疗法,该疗法通过调节不同致病突变中的异常剪接来恢复基因的功能。AON 可以通过与目标的前体 mRNA 的特定序列互补,以遮蔽其剪接基序并纠正被改变的 RNA 剪接,这是一种通过空间位阻抑制剪接机制对该区域识别的疗法。第一个提示 AON 可以用作遗传病治疗药物的报道是来自 β 地中海贫血的研究,他们使用 AON 疗法纠正了因内含子隐蔽位点激活而导致的 β 珠蛋白(betaglobin, *HBB*)基因的异常剪接(Dominski and Kole 1993)。文献中描述了 AON 依赖的剪接调控的不同应用,包括强制跳过 1 个或多个外显子的框移突变以恢复基因的开放阅读框(Aartsma-Rus et al. 2003, 2004),强制选择一个替代剪接位点以阻止致病性转录本的合成(Mercatante and Kole 2002),防止因为深部内含子突变而产生的异常隐蔽外显子插入 mRNA 中(Du et al. 2007; Rincon et al. 2007; Pros et al. 2009; Rodriguez-Pascau et al. 2009; Vega et al. 2009),以及诱导消除含有致病性突变的框架内外显子(Aartsma-Rus et al. 2003, 2004; reviewed in Perez et al. 2010)。

深部内含子突变是 AON 发挥作用的理想靶点,因为它们位于内含子区域,不会影响真正的剪接位点。AON 对新产生的剪接位点进行空间阻断,可以防止剪接机制识别隐蔽外显子,促进正常的剪接。

13.2.1 AON 的类型和递送载体

AON 技术作为一种成功的反义治疗手段,其开发需要克服和面临一系列障碍,包括 AON 的稳定性和细胞传递等若干技术挑战。

为避免 AON 被细胞核酸酶降解,设计 ANO 时采用了不同的类似物,包括磷酰二胺吗啉代寡核苷酸(phosphorodiamidate morpholino oligomers, PMO)(Summerton 1999)、锁核酸(locked nucleic acids, LNA)(Koshkin and Wengel 1998)、肽核酸(peptide nucleic acids, PNA)(Larsen et al. 1999)和 2'-O-甲基硫代磷酸酯(2'-O-methyl phosphorothioate, 2'OMe)(Manoharan 1999)。所有类似物均表现出抗降解稳定性、高度靶亲和力和良好的生物活性(Kurreck 2003)。磷酰二胺吗啉代寡核苷酸(PMO)已经成功用于 1 型神经纤维瘤病的剪接调节(Pros et al. 2009; Fernandez-Rodriguez et al. 2011)。PMO 是寡核苷酸的类似物,其具有的六元吗啉环取代了核糖或脱氧核糖骨架,并具有不带电的磷酸二酰胺亚基间连接。PMO 除了具有高结合特异性、稳定性和抗核酸酶性之外,还表现出高度持久的活性(Summerton and Weller 1997)。因为这些优势特性,PMO 已被用于多种疾病的治疗,包括地中海贫血(Lacerra et al. 2000; Suwanmanee et al. 2002)、杜氏肌营养不良症(McClorey et al. 2006)、Hutchinson - Gilford 早衰综合征(Scaffidi and Misteli 2005)、共济失调毛细血管扩张症(Du et al. 2007)以及丙酸和甲基丙二酸血症(Rincon et al. 2007)。

AON 技术的另外一个重要挑战是将反义寡聚体递送到靶细胞中。最初，人们开发了不同的技术来转染体外细胞培养物，包括电穿孔、脂质体、阳离子聚合物和其他内体转运试剂(Thierry et al. 2003；Merdan et al. 2002)。然而，对于 AON 的体内递送，这些技术都表现出效率低下和毒性明显的特点。在这种情况下，修饰 AON 末端相比未修饰的 AON 是更有效的促进细胞递送的方案。两个很有前景的例子是与细胞穿透肽连接的吗啉代寡核苷酸(Morpholino oligos linked to cell-penetrating peptide，PPMO)和 Vivo-Morpholinos(Moulton and Jiang 2009)。PPMO 是与吗啉代寡核苷酸连接的富含精氨酸的细胞穿透肽。与未经修饰的吗啉代寡核苷酸相比，细胞穿透肽具有两个优势：增强内体吸收和增强内体转运(Abes et al. 2008)。Vivo-Morpholinos 通过其树枝状分子骨架上的 8 个胍基基团与吗啉代寡核苷酸相连(Li and Morcos 2008)，可有效递送至大多数小鼠组织(Morcos et al. 2008)，Vivo-Morpholinos 已成功被用作不同动物模型的治疗药物(Osorio et al. 2011)。

13.3 使用反义寡核苷酸逆转 1 型神经纤维瘤病深部内含子突变的影响

正如之前所述，约 2% 的 1 型神经纤维瘤病的胚系突变是深部内含子核苷酸改变，这些改变可以激活或者产生新的剪接位点，并导致 mRNA 出现致病的隐蔽外显子(Messiaen and Wimmer 2008；Pros et al. 2008)(总结于表 13.1)。这些突变是反义疗法的理想靶点，因为真正的剪接位点仍保持完好，且保留了其正常剪接的潜力。接下来，我们总结了迄今为止使用 AON 逆转 1 型神经纤维瘤病深部内含子突变效应的研究结果(Pros et al. 2009；Fernandez-Rodriguez et al. 2011)，重点介绍不同突变和细胞类型特异性之间的差异、AON 作用所需的剂量和持续时间(在我们的研究中为 PMO)、作用方式以及对神经纤维瘤蛋白功能的影响。

表 13.1　文献报道的 1 型神经纤维瘤病深部内含子突变情况

突　　变	内含子	mRNA 效应	本研究的患者	参　考　文　献
c.288+2025T>G[a]	3	r.288_289ins288+1917_288+2024	1	Pros 等(2008)
c.889-942G>T	6	r.888_889ins889-931_889-873	—	Pros 等(2008)
c.1393-592A>G	10a	r.1392_1393ins1393-673_1393-597	—	Pros 等(2008)
c.1527+1159C>T	10b	r.1527_1528ins1527+1103_1527+1157	—	Spits 等(2005)，Wimmer 等(2007)和 Pros 等(2008)
c.1642-449A>G	10c	未描述	—	Jeong 等(2006)
c.3198-314G>A[a]	19a	r.3197-3198ins3198-214-3198-312, r.3197-3198ins3198-245-3198-312	7	Fernandez-Rodriguez 等(2011)
c.5749+332A>G[a]	30	r.5749_5750ins5749+155_5749+331	2,3	Perrin 等(1996)，Ars 等(2000)和 Wimmer 等(2007)
c.5750-2792A>G	30	r.5749_5750ins5750-278_5750-108	—	Raponi 等(2006)
c.7908-321C>G[a]	45	r.7907_7908ins7908-322_7908-391	4[b],5[b],6[b]	Pros 等(2008)

注：在 cDNA 水平上描述了序列变化(用"c"表示)。+1 核苷酸表示对应参考序列 NM_000267.2 中 ATG 翻译起始密码子的 A。[a] 已进行了 PMO 治疗的突变。[b] 来自同一家族的患者。

13.3.1 PMO 的作用依赖于突变且在不同细胞类型之间存在差异

为了测试 PMO 将致病突变逆转成正常剪接的疗效,我们从 7 名具有 4 个独立深部内含子胚系突变的 1 型神经纤维瘤病患者身上获取了样本(表 13.1、图 13.1)。从这些患者身上收获原代淋巴细胞和成纤维细胞系,并设计了特定的 PMO 来阻断导致 NF1 基因中出现隐蔽外显子突变的效应。研究中的 3 个突变产生了隐蔽的供体剪接位点(c.288+2025T>G,c.5749+332A>G 和 c.7908-321C>G),第 4 个突变产生了隐蔽的受体位点(c.3198-314G>A)。所有的突变都在其对应的野生型基因的成熟 mRNA 中插入隐蔽外显子(图 13.1),这种情况要么产生易被 NMD 机制降解的框架外转录本,要么产生截短形式的神经纤维瘤蛋白。所有

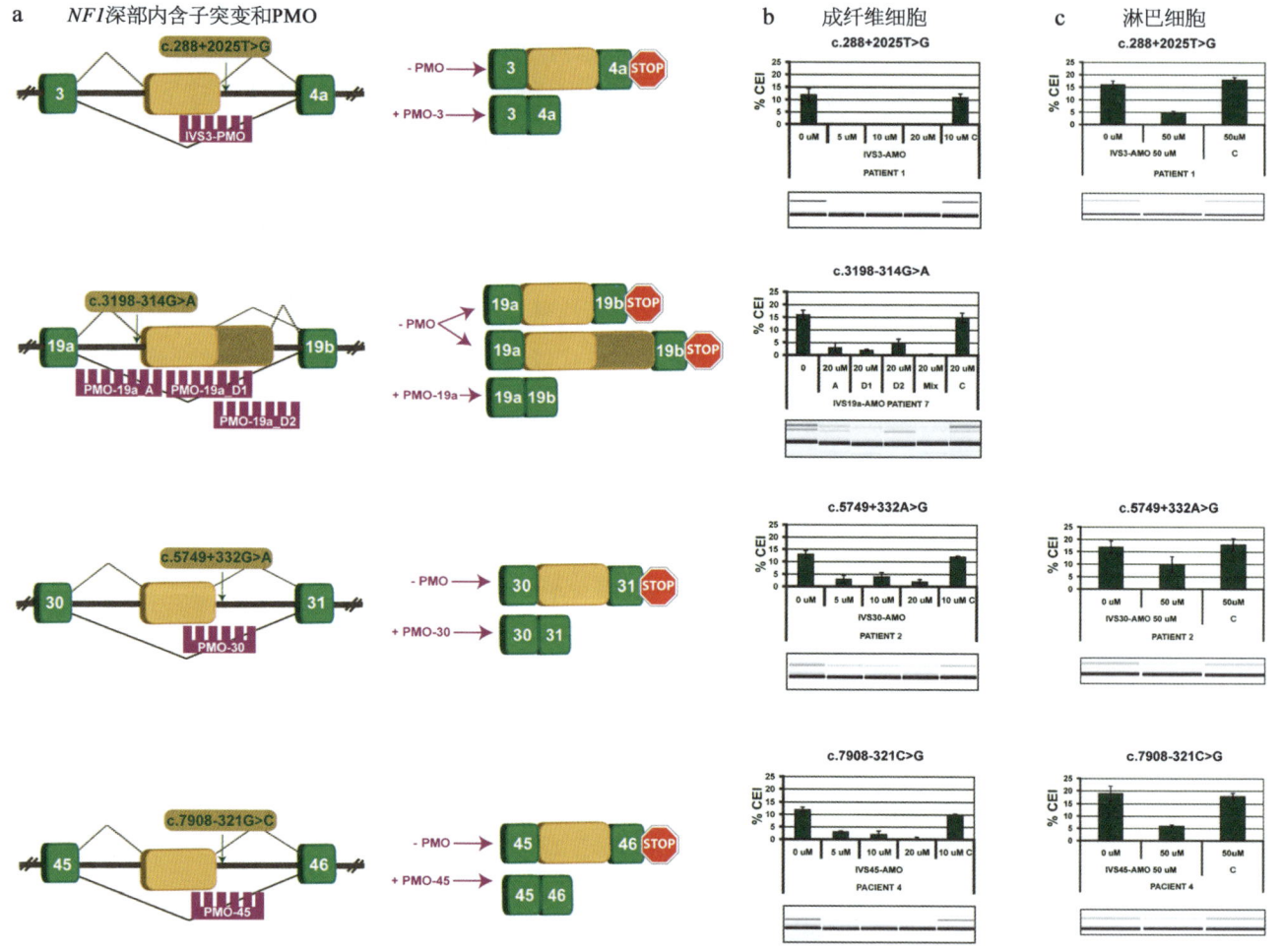

图 13.1 a. 本研究中检测的 4 种突变以及设计用于治疗这些突变的反义吗啉代寡核苷酸的示意图。b. 通过 PMO 处理成纤维细胞培养物以纠正异常剪接。使用特异性引物对总 RNA 进行 RT-PCR 检测,以分析 2 种转录本(野生型和含有隐蔽外显子的转录本)。每个图的 y 轴显示含有隐蔽外显子的转录本与总数的比例。数据由来自至少 3 个独立实验的平均值±标准差组成的条形图表示。对应的安捷伦电泳凝胶显示在每个图下方。对于第 3、30 和 45 内含子中的突变,显示了使用不同 PMO 浓度(5 mM、10 mM 和 20 mM)处理 24 小时后的剂量反应。针对特异性 PMO(C) 的对照如下:IVS30-PMO、IVS45-PMO 和 IVS3-PMO 分别针对 c.288+2025T>G、c.5749+332A>G 和 c.7908-321C>G 突变。对于突变 c.3198-314G>A(内含子 19a),设计了 3 种不同的反义寡核苷酸并同时使用这 3 条来治疗。在所有实验中都观察到校正效果,并且当使用 3 种混合物时得到完全校正。CEI 为包含隐蔽外显子,WT 为野生型。c. EBV 转化淋巴细胞系中针对突变 c.288+2025T>G、c.5749+332A>G 和 c.7908-321C>G 的 PMO 处理。EBV 转化淋巴细胞在 72 小时后用 50 mM PMO 处理。针对特异性 PMO(C) 的对照如下:IVS30-PMO、IVS45-PMO 和 IVS3-PMO,分别用于 c.288+2025T>G、c.5749+332A>G 和 c.7908-321C>G 突变。CEI 为包含隐蔽外显子,WT 为野生型

PMO 均由 Gene Tools 公司（Philomath，OR）设计、合成和纯化。对于其中 1 个突变（c.3198-314G＞A），还设计了 PMO 用于阻止对用作隐蔽外显子插入供体位点的 2 个野生型对应基因组序列的识别（图 13.1）。PMO 治疗的最佳条件在成纤维细胞上确定，并在可能的情况下，随后使用 EBV 转化的淋巴细胞进行了 PMO 治疗的研究。

为了确定 PMO 不同浓度校正异常剪接的效果，对不同突变进行了剂量-反应实验，包括用 3 种不同的 PMO 浓度（5 mM、10 mM 和 20 mM）处理成纤维细胞 24 小时（图 13.1）。在没有 PMO 的情况下，异常剪接转录本（包含隐蔽外显子）的百分比占 NF1 总 mRNA（野生型＋异常剪接转录本）的 10%～15%。正如所想的那样，含有隐蔽外显子的 NF1 mRNA 的百分比较低，这是因为 NMD 机制降解了部分异常转录本，以及由于剪接机制识别了部分突变等位基因中真正的内含子-外显子边界并产生野生型转录本的结果。当用专门设计的 PMO 处理细胞时，可以观察到异常剪接的完全校正或剂量依赖性校正，效果取决于突变本身。对于大多数测试的突变，PMO 的最佳浓度是 20 mM，因此这个浓度也被用于其余的突变和实验（图 13.1）。PMO 的疗效显然是和突变本身有关的。相比之下，对于携带相同 NF1 突变（例如，c.5749＋332A＞G 和 c.7908-321C＞G）的不同患者细胞，在添加 PMO 后表现出相似的效果（Pros et al. 2009）。

为了评估时间对吗啉代寡核苷酸治疗后突变校正的影响，我们对 3 种携带突变的成纤维细胞系进行了时间进程分析（Pros et al. 2009）。一般来说，在成纤维细胞中 PMO 处理 24 小时后，不同突变的 NF1 剪接校正效率从 87% 到 100% 不等。

有多种因素可以解释所研究突变之间的 PMO 效果差异，例如，隐蔽受体/供体剪接位点强度的差异或 PMO 进入前 mRNA 二级结构的不同。可以采用不同的策略来提高 PMO 恢复这些突变的正常剪接的效果，包括：设计不同的 PMO 来阻断突变位点；使用吗啉代寡核苷酸组合，其中一个针对特定的突变位点，另一个阻断对应的野生型隐蔽位点；或者只使用吗啉代寡核苷酸针对后者；设计吗啉代寡核苷酸针对外显子的剪接增强子（exon splicing enhancer, ESE）元件。有研究表明 PMO 在一些情况下可能对某个隐蔽剪接位点的校正效果比对其他位点更有效（Du et al. 2007）。从这个意义上讲，我们对突变 c.3198-314G＞A 的研究结果（其中设计了 3 个 PMO 来阻断所有使用的隐蔽剪接位点）表明，尽管每个 PMO 都能够降低突变转录本的水平，但只有当 3 个 PMO 组合使用时才能观察到完全的纠正效果（图 13.1），这在其他遗传疾病中也有描述（Gurvich et al. 2008）。

为了深入了解吗啉代寡核苷酸治疗的细胞类型特异性，除了成纤维细胞外，研究还分析了来自同一患者的转化淋巴细胞。EBV 转化淋巴细胞系接受 50 mM PMO 治疗后，在 72 小时正常剪接的恢复程度最高（尽管恢复不完全）（图 13.1）。同时测试了较低浓度的吗啉代寡核苷酸，但发现其效果比较差。一般来说，在转化淋巴细胞系中观察到的异常剪接校正效果较差（30%～70%，具体取决于突变），需要更高浓度的吗啉代寡核苷酸和更长的暴露时间才能产生与成纤维细胞中相似的效果。在成纤维细胞和淋巴细胞中观察到的疗效不同，可能是因为淋巴细胞系转染本身比较困难（Galletti et al. 2007；Seiffert et al. 2007）。在另外一项比较研究中，作者利用电穿孔方法将吗啉代寡核苷酸递送到细胞中，从而在真皮成纤维细胞和 B 淋巴细胞系中获得了相似的转染效率。但是这两种类型的细胞需要不同的电穿孔方案。结果表明，需要更多的电穿孔循环次数和更高的吗啉代寡核苷酸浓度才能在淋巴细胞中达到与成纤维细胞相同的递送效率（Scaffidi and Misteli 2005）。这两种细胞类型所需的不同条件与其他研究小组在淋巴细胞（Du et al. 2007）和成纤维细胞（Rincon et al. 2007）中使用相同传递系统得到的结果一致。

13.3.2 PMO 持久和特异的疗效及其对神经纤维瘤蛋白功能的影响

通过在所有研究中同时应用不同的对照 PMO，突变特异性 PMO 的特异性得以揭示（图 13.1）。只有突变特异性 PMO 在所有实验中都表现出对异常剪接具有校正作用，这表明 PMO 的疗效是具有序列特异性的。研究人员也在原代成纤维细胞培养物中评估了 PMO 对异常剪接校正疗效的稳定性和持续时间。尽管观察到疗效在不同突变之间具有差异,但在所有研究条件下,在应用 PMO 治疗后,异常剪接在 20 天内维持近乎完全的校正(Pros et al. 2009)。

我们还研究了吗啉代寡核苷酸对 *NF1* 突变的作用模式。为了排除 PMO 治疗后 NMD 通路增强导致异常转录本水平下降的可能性,在有或无 PMO 的情况下,来自不同患者的成纤维细胞接受了嘌呤霉素(1 种 NMD 抑制剂)的处理。在嘌呤霉素存在的情况下,PMO 处理后异常剪接完全或显著得到纠正(具体取决于突变),这表明 PMO 直接作用于 *NF1* 的剪接,并与 NMD 机制无关(Pros et al. 2009)。此外,在 PMO 处理后观察到野生型转录本水平(相对于对照基因)增加,这也证实了 PMO 通过阻断对突变产生的新剪接位点的识别来诱导正确剪接(Pros et al. 2009)。综上所述,这些结果表明 PMO 以序列特异性的方式通过阻止剪接机制识别 *NF1* 基因中新产生的异常剪接位点来发挥作用。

最后,因为无法直接评估神经纤维瘤蛋白的功能,所以对其进行了间接的功能分析以确认 PMO 治疗也能在功能水平上纠正异常剪接。神经纤维瘤蛋白是已报道的 Ras 蛋白负调节因子,因此可以检测患者来源的原代成纤维细胞培养物中的 Ras-GTP 水平。研究对携带 4 种不同深部内含子突变的成纤维细胞进行了评估,并比较特定 PMO 处理前后的 Ras-GTP 水平。制备细胞裂解物,并进行 Ras 活化实验(图 13.2)。所有未经处理的患者来源的成纤维细胞培养物中的活性 Ras-GTP 水平均高于野生型对照成纤维细胞,这与突变型成纤维细胞中神经纤维瘤蛋白活性较低的观察结果一致。然而,携带突变的成纤维细胞的 Ras-GTP 水平在 PMO 处理后显著下降,降到与野生型对照成纤维细胞相似的水平。这一结果表明 PMO 治疗不仅纠正了异常剪接,而且这种纠正还恢复了野生型神经纤维瘤蛋白的功能,提高了对 Ras 蛋白的总体 GAP 活性。

13.4　AON 治疗:从实验室到临床

目前尚未就 AON 技术针对 1 型神经纤维瘤病患者在临床上治疗深部内含子突变的适用性得出明确结论;迄今为止,还没有在 1 型神经纤维瘤病的临床前动物模型或临床试验中应用这种反义技术。然而,最近在杜氏肌营养不良症(Duchenne muscular dystrophy, DMD)患者中使用 AON 介导的第 51 外显子跳跃疗法的临床试验取得了成功,这让人们对这种疗法的最终成功产生了合理的预期(试验目前正在扩展到其他外显子)(reviewed in Muntoni and Wood 2011; van Putten and Aartsma-Rus 2011)。就像所有治疗人类疾病的药物一样,AON 技术从实验室到临床的过程也需要逐步满足一些要求。这些步骤包括体外概念验证,然后是一系列临床试验。DMD 是 AON 技术作为治疗策略的最佳例子。首先,利用健康和源自患者的原代人类成肌细胞的培养物获得了原理验证(Aartsma-Rus et al. 2002, 2003, 2004)。使用不同的 AON 化合物对 DMD 小鼠模型 mdx 小鼠进行了临床前体内试验(Goyenvalle et al. 2010; Heemskerk et al. 2009;

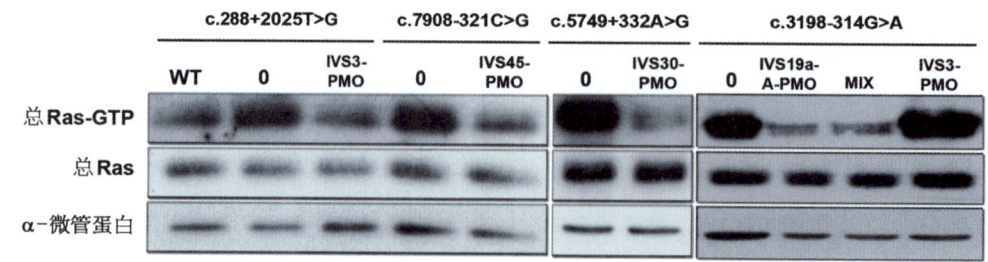

图 13.2　PM 治疗后患者的成纤维细胞 Ras-GTP 水平降低。通过量化细胞裂解物中的 Ras-GTP 水平间接评估神经纤维瘤蛋白 GTPase 活性。在所有实验中,针对特定突变的 PMO 治疗将 Ras 活性降低到与 WT 对照成纤维细胞相似的水平,这可能是通过恢复神经纤维瘤蛋白功能实现的。针对 g.3198-314G>A 突变设计的非特异性 PMO(IVS45-PMO 20 mM)的使用对 Ras-GTP 水平没有影响

Wu et al. 2008；Yin et al. 2009）。使用 AON 进行了两项探索性临床试验，目的是校正编码截短形式的肌营养不良蛋白的 mRNA 阅读框架，并产生与贝克尔肌营养不良症（一种较轻的疾病）患者类似的转录本。两项临床试验的方法都是强制跳过 *DMD* 基因的第 51 外显子。一项试验使用了 2OMePS（PRO051）（van Deutekom et al. 2007），另一项试验使用了吗啉寡聚体（AVI – 4658）（Kinali et al. 2009）。在这两项试验中，将 AON 直接注射到肌肉都能显著纠正肌营养不良蛋白的表达水平，这证明了该技术的可行性，而且不会产生临床上严重的副作用。在最近的一项 I 至 IIa 期临床试验中，通过皮下注射 PRO051 进行全身给药可以纠正肌营养不良蛋白的表达，且没有严重的不良反应，并且接受治疗的患者的行走能力略有改善，但患者之间的疗效存在相当大的差异（Goemans et al. 2011）。应用 PMO 治疗的首个系统性临床试验也显示治疗后肌营养不良蛋白的恢复水平令人满意（Cirak et al. 2011）。目前，更多针对 DMD 的临床试验正在进行中，其中包括 III 期临床试验和一些涉及其他 *DMD* 基因外显子的研究（Muntoni 2010；van Putten and Aartsma-Rus 2011）。对于其他肌营养不良症和其他疾病，AON 治疗仍处于从实验室到临床的不同阶段（Muntoni 2010；van Putten and Aartsma-Rus 2011）。

AON 疗法的开发仍面临一些挑战（Goyenvalle et al. 2010），例如如何确保 AON 有效递送至所有需要治疗的组织，甚至特异地靶向治疗组织。因为较差的细胞摄取率和相对较快的循环清除率，第一种 AON 化合物在临床试验中需要反复给药。不过，最近使用与 PMO（PPMO）或 Vivo-Morpholinos 结合的细胞穿透肽的研发成果解决了大部分递送方面的问题，向前迈出了一大步，并揭示了一种可能被证明是有效的策略，尽管这种方法仍有改进空间（Moulton and Jiang 2009；Muntoni 2010）。

出于监管限制和安全考虑，AON 疗法的开发存在一定的局限性。来自第一个 DMD 临床试验收集的数据是振奋人心的，但是参与的患者数量很少，最终的给药方案也需要合理制订，而且必须提供超过 1 年以上治疗时间的数据。目前尚未证实 AON 的长期治疗是否安全并最终能改善 DMD 患者的生命质量，因此目前应持谨慎态度。鉴于每个 AON 都是针对特定的突变（或在强制跳过的情况下是针对特定的外显子），使用该技术的临床试验需要注意的事项之一是可以招募的患者数量较少，因为多数疾病都需要个性化的 AON 方案。根据现行法规，每个 AON 都被视为一种新药，因此每个针对不同外显子或突变的 AON 都必须经历许多不同的临床开发步骤，并承担此过程所需的所有费用（Muntoni 2010）。为了克服这一困难，而且由于同一化学类别的 AON 通常表现出更多的相似性而不是差异，同一类型的化学上相似的 AON 应该被视为同一药物类别，而不管其涉及的突变或外显子如何。这样做有助于积累足够的临床数据来促进技术的研发，从而为深部内含子突变和其他 RNA 错误剪接疾病带来有效疗法。

还有许多问题要在 1 型神经纤维瘤病中解决，首先是临床前动物模型。如果动物造模成功，DMD 的 AON 疗法提供的研究基础可以加快 1 型神经纤维瘤病患者的临床试验，从而可能为深部内含子突变导致错误剪接的 1 型神经纤维瘤病患者，以及其他 AON 可治疗的 *NF1* 突变患者提供有据可依的治疗机会。

13.5 结论

一些 1 型神经纤维瘤病致病突变位于 *NF1* 基因的内含子区域内。这些深部内含子突变导致 *NF1* mRNA 中出现隐蔽外显子，最终产生异常的神经纤维瘤蛋白。我们回顾了大量研究结果，这些结果证明 PMO 能够有效纠正这些 1 型神经纤维瘤病基因突变产生的异常剪接。我们对来自 7 名 1 型神经纤维瘤病患者的淋巴细胞和成纤维细胞原代培养物进行了测试，这些患者一共携带了 4 种不同的 *NF1* 突变。在所有实验中，PMO 都恢复了基因的正确剪接和神经纤维瘤蛋白功能（通过间接评估其下调 Ras – GTPase 的能力）。总之，这些结果证明了 PMO 在体外具有纠正 *NF1* 致病突变的能力。目前使用 AON 技术治疗 DMD 患者的临床试验取得了成功，这将会促进 1 型神经纤维瘤病临床前动物模型的发展。深部内含子突变约占迄今为止报告的所有1型神经纤维瘤病胚系突变的2%。AON技术可应用于携带此类突变的患者,或许还可应用于能产生异常转录本的其他类型突变的1型神经纤维瘤病患者。

致谢：我们感谢参与本研究的患者,感谢他们在所有实验中的贡献与合作。我们感谢Josep Biayna对手稿提出的重要建议和修改,并感谢ICO-IMPPC神经纤维瘤病工作组的所有成员。作者特别感谢西班牙神经纤维瘤病协会（Asociación Española de Afectados de Neurofibromatosis）的资助和在研究过程中给予的大力支持。我们还要感谢西班牙抗癌协会（Asociación Española Contra el Cáncer）,该协会将我们的研究小组评为2010年稳定的癌症研究小组之一。研究基金赞助者：西班牙健康研究基金；卡洛斯三世健康研究所；加泰罗尼亚健康研究所和加泰罗尼亚自治政府。研究基金编号：ISCIIIRIC（RD06/0020/1051、RD06/0020/1050、2009SGR290、PI10/01422、CA08/00248）。

（易成刚,罗蒙　译）

参考文献

[1] Aartsma-Rus A, Bremmer-Bout M, Janson AA, den Dunnen JT, van Ommen GJ, van Deutekom JC (2002) Targeted exon skipping as a potential gene correction therapy for Duchenne muscular dystrophy. Neuromuscul Disord 12(Suppl 1)：S71 - S77

[2] Aartsma-Rus A, Janson AA, Kaman WE, Bremmer-Bout M, den Dunnen JT, Baas F, van Ommen GJ, van Deutekom JC (2003) Therapeutic antisense-induced exon skipping in cultured muscle cells from six different DMD patients. Hum Mol Genet 12(8)：907 - 914

[3] Aartsma-Rus A, Janson AA, Kaman WE, Bremmer-Bout M, van Ommen GJ, den Dunnen JT, van Deutekom JC (2004) Antisense-induced multiexon skipping for Duchenne muscular dystrophy makes more sense. Am J Hum Genet 74(1)：83 - 92

[4] Abes R, Moulton HM, Clair P, Yang ST, Abes S, Melikov K, Prevot P, Youngblood DS, Iversen PL, Chernomordik LV et al (2008) Delivery of steric block morpholino oligomers by (R-X-R)4 peptides：structure-activity studies. Nucleic Acids Res 36(20)：6343 - 6354

[5] Ars E, Serra E, Garcia J, Kruyer H, Gaona A, Lazaro C, Estivill X (2000) Mutations affecting mRNA splicing are the most common molecular defects in patients with neurofibromatosis type 1. Hum Mol Genet 9(2)：237 - 247 [published erratum appears in Hum Mol Genet 2000 9(4)：659]

[6] Cirak S, Arechavala-Gomeza V, Guglieri M, Feng L, Torelli S, Anthony K, Abbs S, Garralda ME, Bourke J, Wells DJ et al (2011) Exon skipping and dystrophin restoration in patients with Duchenne muscular dystrophy after systemic phosphorodiamidate morpholino oligomer treatment：an open-label, phase 2, dose-escalation study. Lancet 378(9791)：595 - 605

[7] Dominski Z, Kole R (1993) Restoration of correct splicing in thalassemic pre-mRNA by antisense oligonucleotides. Proc Natl Acad Sci USA 90(18)：8673 - 8677

[8] Du L, Pollard JM, Gatti RA (2007) Correction of prototypic ATM splicing mutations and aberrant ATM function with antisense morpholino oligonucleotides. Proc Natl Acad Sci USA 104(14)：6007 - 6012

[9] Fernandez-Rodriguez J, Castellsague J, Benito L, Benavente Y, Capella G, Blanco I, Serra E, Lazaro C (2011) A mild neurofibromatosis type 1 phenotype produced by the combination of the benign nature of a leaky NF1-splice mutation and the presence of a complex mosaicism. Hum Mutat 32(7)：705 - 709

[10] Galletti R, Masciarelli S, Conti C, Matusali G, Di Renzo L, Meschini S, Arancia G, Mancini C, Mattia E (2007) Inhibition of Epstein Barr Virus LMP1 gene expression in B lymphocytes by antisense oligonucleotides：uptake and efficacy of lipid-based and receptor-mediated delivery systems. Antiviral Res 74(2)：102 - 110

[11] Goemans NM, Tulinius M, van den Akker JT, Burm BE, Ekhart PF, Heuvelmans N, Holling T, Janson AA, Platenburg GJ, Sipkens JA et al (2011) Systemic administration of PRO051 in Duchenne's muscular dystrophy. N Engl J Med 364(16)：1513 - 1522

[12] Goyenvalle A, Babbs A, Powell D, Kole R, Fletcher S, Wilton SD, Davies KE (2010) Prevention of dystrophic pathology in severely affected dystrophin/utrophin-deficient mice by morpholino-oligomer-mediated exon-skipping. Mol Ther 18(1)：198 - 205

[13] Gurvich OL, Tuohy TM, Howard MT, Finkel RS, Medne L, Anderson CB, Weiss RB, Wilton SD, Flanigan KM (2008) DMD pseudoexon mutations：splicing efficiency, phenotype, and potential therapy. Ann Neurol 63(1)：81 - 89

[14] Hammond SM, Wood MJ (2011) Genetic therapies for RNA mis-splicing diseases. Trends Genet 27(5)：196 - 205

[15] Heemskerk H, de Winter CL, van Ommen GJ, van Deutekom JC, Aartsma-Rus A (2009) Development of antisense-mediated exon skipping as a treatment for Duchenne muscular dystrophy. Ann N Y Acad Sci 1175：71 - 79

[16] Jeong SY, Park SJ, Kim HJ (2006) The spectrum of NF1 mutations in Korean patients with neurofibromatosis type 1. J Korean Med Sci 21(1)：107 - 112

[17] Kinali M, Arechavala-Gomeza V, Feng L, Cirak S, Hunt D, Adkin C, Guglieri M, Ashton E, Abbs S, Nihoyannopoulos P et al (2009) Local restoration of dystrophin expression with the morpholino oligomer AVI-4658 in Duchenne muscular dystrophy：a single-blind, placebocontrolled, dose-escalation, proof-of-concept study. Lancet Neurol 8(10)：918 - 928

[18] Koshkin AA, Wengel J (1998) Synthesis of novel 2′,3′-linked bicyclic thymine ribonucleosides. J Org Chem 63(8)：2778 - 2781

[19] Kurreck J (2003) Nucleic acids chemistry and biology. Angew Chem Int Ed Engl 42(44)：5384 - 5385

[20] Lacerra G, Sierakowska H, Carestia C, Fucharoen S, Summerton J, Weller D, Kole R (2000) Restoration of hemoglobin A synthesis in erythroid cells from peripheral blood of thalassemic patients. Proc Natl Acad Sci USA 97(17): 9591–9596

[21] Larsen HJ, Bentin T, Nielsen PE (1999) Antisense properties of peptide nucleic acid. Biochim Biophys Acta 1489(1): 159–166

[22] Li YF, Morcos PA (2008) Design and synthesis of dendritic molecular transporter that achieves efficient in vivo delivery of morpholino antisense oligo. Bioconjug Chem 19(7): 1464–1470

[23] Manoharan M (1999) 2′-carbohydrate modifications in antisense oligonucleotide therapy: importance of conformation, configuration and conjugation. Biochim Biophys Acta 1489(1): 117–130

[24] McClorey G, Fall AM, Moulton HM, Iversen PL, Rasko JE, Ryan M, Fletcher S, Wilton SD (2006) Induced dystrophin exon skipping in human muscle explants. Neuromuscul Disord 16(9–10): 583–590

[25] Mercatante DR, Kole R (2002) Control of alternative splicing by antisense oligonucleotides as a potential chemotherapy: effects on gene expression. Biochim Biophys Acta 1587(2–3): 126–132

[26] Merdan T, Kopecek J, Kissel T (2002) Prospects for cationic polymers in gene and oligonucleotide therapy against cancer. Adv Drug Deliv Rev 54(5): 715–758

[27] Messiaen L, Wimmer K (2008) NF1 mutational spectrum. In: Kaufmann D (ed) Neurofibromatoses, Monographs in human genetics. Karger, Basel, pp 63–77

[28] Messiaen LM, Callens T, Mortier G, Beysen D, Vandenbroucke I, Van Roy N, Speleman F, Paepe AD (2000) Exhaustive mutation analysis of the NF1 gene allows identification of 95% of mutations and reveals a high frequency of unusual splicing defects. Hum Mutat 15(6): 541–555

[29] Morcos PA, Li Y, Jiang S (2008) Vivo-Morpholinos: a non-peptide transporter delivers Morpholinos into a wide array of mouse tissues. Biotechniques 45(6): 613–614, 616, 618 passim

[30] Moulton JD, Jiang S (2009) Gene knockdowns in adult animals: PPMOs and vivo-morpholinos. Molecules 14(3): 1304–1323

[31] Muntoni F (2010) The development of antisense oligonucleotide therapies for Duchenne muscular dystrophy: report on a TREAT-NMD workshop hosted by the European Medicines Agency (EMA), on September 25th 2009. Neuromuscul Disord 20(5): 355–362

[32] Muntoni F, Wood MJ (2011) Targeting RNA to treat neuromuscular disease. Nat Rev Drug Discov 10(8): 621–637

[33] Osorio FG, Navarro CL, Cadinanos J, Lopez-Mejia IC, Quiros PM, Bartoli C, Rivera J, Tazi J, Guzman G, Varela I et al (2011) Splicing-directed therapy in a new mouse model of human accelerated aging. Sci Transl Med 3(106): 106ra107

[34] Perez B, Rodriguez-Pascau L, Vilageliu L, Grinberg D, Ugarte M, Desviat LR (2010) Present and future of antisense therapy for splicing modulation in inherited metabolic disease. J Inherit Metab Dis 33(4): 397–403

[35] Perrin G, Morris MA, Antonarakis SE, Boltshauser E, Hutter P (1996) Two novel mutations affecting mRNA splicing of the neurofibromatosis type 1 (NF1) gene. Hum Mutat 7(2): 172–175

[36] Pros E, Fernandez-Rodriguez J, Canet B, Benito L, Sanchez A, Benavides A, Ramos FJ, Lopez-Ariztegui MA, Capella G, Blanco I et al (2009) Antisense therapeutics for neurofibromatosis type 1 caused by deep intronic mutations. Hum Mutat 30(3): 454–462

[37] Pros E, Gomez C, Martin T, Fabregas P, Serra E, Lazaro C (2008) Nature and mRNA effect of 282 different NF1 point mutations: focus on splicing alterations. Hum Mutat 29(9): E173–E193

[38] Raponi M, Upadhyaya M, Baralle D (2006) Functional splicing assay shows a pathogenic intronic mutation in neurofibromatosis type 1 (NF1) due to intronic sequence exonization. Hum Mutat 27(3): 294–295

[39] Rincon A, Ugarte M, Aguado C, Desviat LR, Sanchez-Alcudia R, Perez B (2007) Propionic and methylmalonic acidemia: antisense therapeutics for intronic variations causing aberrantly spliced messenger RNA. Am J Hum Genet 81(6)

[40] Rodriguez-Pascau L, Coll MJ, Vilageliu L, Grinberg D (2009) Antisense oligonucleotide treatment for a pseudoexon-generating mutation in the NPC1 gene causing Niemann-Pick type C disease. Hum Mutat 30(11): E993–E1001

[41] Scaffidi P, Misteli T (2005) Reversal of the cellular phenotype in the premature aging disease Hutchinson-Gilford progeria syndrome. Nat Med 11(4): 440–445

[42] Seiffert M, Stilgenbauer S, Dohner H, Lichter P (2007) Efficient nucleofection of primary human B cells and B-CLL cells induces apoptosis, which depends on the microenvironment and on the structure of transfected nucleic acids. Leukemia 21(9): 1977–1983

[43] Spits C, De Rycke M, Van Ranst N, Joris H, Verpoest W, Lissens W, Devroey P, Van Steirteghem A, Liebaers I, Sermon K (2005) Preimplantation genetic diagnosis for neurofibromatosis type 1. Mol Hum Reprod 11(5): 381–387

[44] Summerton J (1999) Morpholino antisense oligomers: the case for an RNase H-independent structural type. Biochim Biophys Acta 1489(1): 141–158

[45] Summerton J, Weller D (1997) Morpholino antisense oligomers: design, preparation, and properties. Antisense Nucleic Acid Drug Dev 7(3): 187–195

[46] Suwanmanee T, Sierakowska H, Fucharoen S, Kole R (2002) Repair of a splicing defect in erythroid cells from patients with beta-thalassemia/HbE disorder. Mol Ther 6(6): 718–726

[47] Teraoka SN, Telatar M, Becker-Catania S, Liang T, Onengut S, Tolun A, Chessa L, Sanal O, Bernatowska E, Gatti RA et al (1999) Splicing defects in the ataxia-telangiectasia gene, ATM: underlying mutations and consequences. Am J Hum Genet 64(6): 1617–1631

[48] Thierry AR, Vives E, Richard JP, Prevot P, Martinand-Mari C, Robbins I, Lebleu B (2003) Cellular uptake and intracellular fate of antisense oligonucleotides. Curr Opin Mol Ther 5(2): 133–138

[49] van Deutekom JC, Janson AA, Ginjaar IB, Frankhuizen WS, Aartsma-Rus A, Bremmer-Bout M, den Dunnen JT, Koop K, van der Kooi AJ, Goemans NM et al (2007) Local dystrophin restoration with antisense oligonucleotide PRO051. N Engl J Med 357(26): 2677–2686

[50] van Putten M, Aartsma-Rus A (2011) Opportunities and challenges for the development of antisense treatment in neuromuscular disorders. Expert Opin Biol Ther 11(8): 1025–1037

[51] Vega AI, Perez-Cerda C, Desviat LR, Matthijs G, Ugarte M, Perez B (2009) Functional analysis of three splicing mutations identified in the PMM2 gene: toward a new therapy for congenital disorder of glycosylation type Ia. Hum Mutat 30(5): 795–803

[52] Wimmer K, Roca X, Beiglbock H, Callens T, Etzler J, Rao

AR, Krainer AR, Fonatsch C, Messiaen L (2007) Extensive *in silico* analysis of *NF1* splicing defects uncovers determinants for splicing outcome upon 5′ splice-site disruption. Hum Mutat 28(6): 599-612

[53] Wu B, Moulton HM, Iversen PL, Jiang J, Li J, Li J, Spurney CF, Sali A, Guerron AD, Nagaraju K et al (2008) Effective rescue of dystrophin improves cardiac function in dystrophin-deficient mice by a modified morpholino oligomer. Proc Natl Acad Sci USA 105(39): 14814-14819

[54] Yin H, Moulton HM, Betts C, Seow Y, Boutilier J, Iverson PL, Wood MJ (2009) A fusion peptide directs enhanced systemic dystrophin exon skipping and functional restoration in dystrophindeficient *mdx* mice. Hum Mol Genet 18(22): 4405-4414

第14章 NF1 微缺失及其突变机制
NF1 Microdeletions and Their Underlying Mutational Mechanisms

Hildegard Kehrer-Sawatzki and David N. Cooper

14.1 NF1 微缺失的类型及其估计频率

最常见的复发性 NF1 微缺失类型是跨越 1.4 Mb 的 1 型 NF1 缺失。1 型缺失的断点位于 LCR 内,称为 NF1-REPa 和 NF1-REPc(Dorschner et al. 2000;Jenne et al. 2001;López-Correa et al. 2001)。1 型缺失与 14 个蛋白质编码基因的丢失有关,包括 NF1 和 2 个 miRNA 基因(MIR 365-2 和 MIR 193 a)(图 14.1)。大多数 1 型 NF1 微缺失是母系遗传的生殖系缺失(Upadhyaya et al. 1998;López-Correa-Correa et al. 2000;Steinmann et al. 2008),其断裂点通常位于减数分裂非等位基因同源重组的 2 个热点区域内(Jenne et al. 2001;López-Correa et al. 2001;Forbes et al. 2004;De Raedt et al. 2006)。据估计,在 NF1 患者的大型队列研究中,所有 NF1 微缺失中有 70%~80% 为 1 型(Messiaen et al. 2011;Passiaen et al. 2010)。

2 型 NF1 微缺失包括 1.2 Mb,与包括 NF1 在内的 13 个基因的丢失相关。它们的断裂点位于 SUZ12 基因及其假基因 SUZ12P 内,紧邻 NF1-REP 的侧翼(图 14.1)。2 型 NF1 缺失的发生频率低于 1 型 NF1 缺失,所有 NF1 微缺失中仅有 10%~20% 为 2 型(Kehrer-Sawatzki et al. 2004;Messiaen et al. 2011)。2 型和 1 型 NF1 缺失都被认为是重复性的,因为无关联患者中缺失的断点位于高度同源的序列内。在 2 型缺失的情况下,这些断裂点位于 SUZ12 基因及其衍生的假基因内,而 1 型 NF1 微缺失的断裂点位于 NF1-REPa 和 NF1-REPc 内。

3 型 NF1 微缺失同样是多发的,其特征在于位于 NF1-REPb 和 NF1-REPc 内的断点(Bengesser et al. 2010;Pasvessel et al. 2010;Zickler et al. 2012)。3 型缺失跨越 1.0 Mb,包含 9 个蛋白质编码基因(图 14.1)。与 1 型和 2 型缺失相比,3 型缺失发生频率低得多。事实上,3 型 NF1 微缺失仅占所有大型 NF1 缺失的 1.4%~4%(Messiaen et al. 2011;Pasmant et al. 2010)。

除了 3 种基本类型的多发性 NF1 微缺失外,还有一些少见的非典型 NF1 缺失断点。延伸的序列同源性在这些缺失的断点处不明显。实际上,非典型 NF1 微缺失在其大小、断点位置和位于缺失区域内的基因数量方面是异质的(Mantripragada et al. 2006;Kehrer-Sawatzki et al. 2008 and references

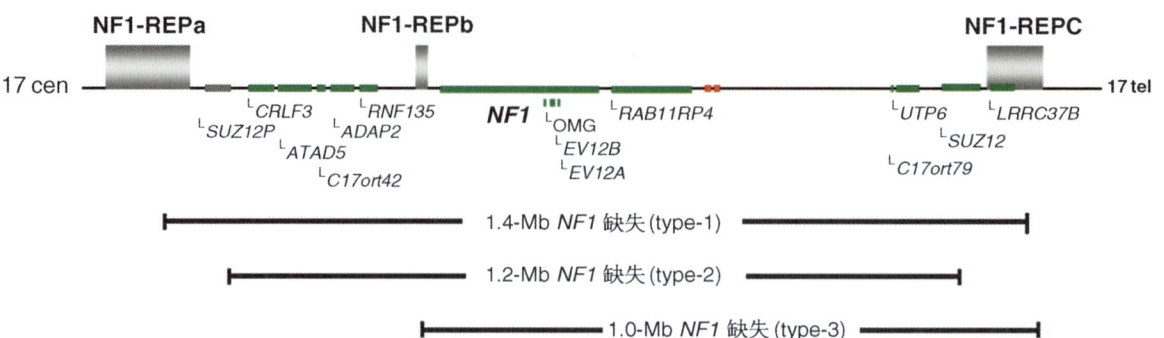

图 14.1 NF1 基因区域示意图显示了 3 个 NF1-REP 的相对位置，以及位于该区域内的蛋白质编码基因（绿色条）和 2 个 miRNA 基因（*MIR 365-2* 和 *MIR 193a*），红色条带。还显示了 1 型、2 型和 3 型 NF1 微缺失的相对程度

therein；Pasmant et al. 2008, 2010）。据估计，所有 *NF1* 微缺失中有 8%～10% 为非典型缺失（Messiaen et al. 2011；Passiaen et al. 2010）。

14.2 嵌合现象和 *NF1* 微缺失

合子后发生的突变导致与正常细胞的嵌合现象，可影响疾病的临床表现以及传播风险（Erickson 2010；Gottlieb et al. 2001；Kehrer-Sawatzki and Cooper 2008；Youssoufian and Pyeritz 2002）。在至少 10% 携带 *NF1* 微缺失的患者中观察到与正常细胞的嵌合现象（Messiaen et al. 2011）。关于 *NF1* 微缺失的类型和镶嵌现象的频率，已经注意到了一定的偏差。因此，在具有 2 型 *NF1* 缺失的个体中，经常观察到与正常细胞的嵌合现象（Petek et al. 2003；Kehrer-Sawatzkietal. 2004；Roehl et al. 2010 2012；Steinmann et al. 2007），这意味着这些 2 型缺失一定发生在合子后。至少 44% 的 2 型 *NF1* 缺失患者表现出体细胞嵌合现象（Messiaen et al. 2011），尽管在实践中，嵌合型 2 型 *NF1* 缺失患者的比例可能相当高（Kehrer-Sawatzki et al. 2004）。显然，2 型缺失患者血液样本中携带缺失的细胞比例非常高，在大多数情况下超过 90%（Kehrer-Sawatzki et al. 2004；Roehl et al. 2010；Steinmann et al. 2007）。在尿源性和颊上皮细胞中观察到 2 型 *NF1* 微缺失的细胞比例显著较低（Roehl et al. 2012）。因此，在早期发育阶段，似乎携带 *NF1* 微缺失的造血干细胞表现出优于无缺失的正常细胞的选择性生长优势，导致受影响患者外周血中具有高比例缺失的细胞（Roehl et al. 2012）。

与 2 型缺失形成鲜明对比的是，所有新发 1 型 *NF1* 微缺失患者中仅 2%～4% 表现出嵌合现象（Messiaen et al. 2011）。体细胞嵌合现象（表明 3 型 *NF1* 缺失为合子后起源）的频率目前尚不清楚，事实上这种现象是否会发生也不得而知。迄今为止，仅分析了 11 例具有该缺失类型的患者，并且未发现其中任何 1 名患者表现出与正常细胞的嵌合现象（Zickler et al. 2012）。

14.3 *NF1* 微缺失的机制

14.3.1 NAHR 和重复性 *NF1* 微缺失

非等位基因同源重组（nonallelic homologous recombination，NAHR）是导致 1 型、2 型和 3 型 *NF1* 微缺失的主要机制。NAHR 是导致人类基因组中多态性和疾病相关拷贝数变体（copy number variant，CNV）的主要机制之一（Conrad et al. 2010；Kidd et al. 2010；Mills et al. 2011；Neumann et al. 2010；Stankiewicz and Lupski 2010）。假设 NAHR 的分子过程和决定簇与减数分裂等位基因同源重组（allelic homologous recombination，AHR）相似，但 NAHR 采用的是非常相似但非等位基因的模板来修复起始双链断裂（double-strand break，DSB），而不是等位基因同源模板（reviewed by Sasaki et al. 2010）。在减数分裂和有丝分裂期间，同源重组代表了 DNA 损伤（如 DSB）的非常精确的修复机制（Mao et al. 2008）。因此，在使用等位或非等位模板通过同源重组修复的断点连接处，是无

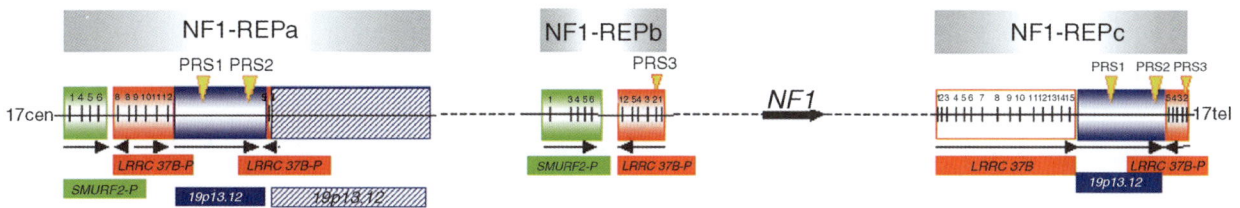

图 14.2　NF1-REP 的序列组成，其中包含不同的片段重复（亚基），以不同的颜色突出显示。NF1-REPa、NF1-REPb 和 NF1-REPc 中的 *LRRC37B-P* 序列标记为红色。功能性 *LRRC37B* 基因位于 NF1-REPc 的着丝粒部分内，并且包含 15 个外显子。与染色体 19p13.2 同源的序列以蓝色表示。位于 NF1-REP 内的 NAHR 热点 PRS1、PRS2 和 PRS3 的相对位置由黄色箭头指示

法检测到小的额外畸变的，例如几个核苷酸的插入。含有多个重复序列的染色体区域，如 NF1 基因区域，本质上容易发生反复的 NAHR 介导的重排。在位于 *NF1* 基因区域内的重复序列中，有称为 NF1-REP 的低拷贝重复序列，它揭示了不同重复亚基或旁系同源序列的模块结构（图 14.2）。NF1-REPa 跨越 130 kb，位于 *NF1* 基因的 370 kb 着丝粒，而 NF1-REPc 长度为 75 kb，位于 *NF1* 基因的 640 kb 端粒。NF1-REPb 位于 *NF1* 的 44 kb 处，是 3 个 LCR 中最短的，跨度仅为 43 kb。NF1-REPs a 和 c 含有与位于 19p13.12 序列高度相似的旁系同源序列（Jenne et al. 2003；Forbes et al. 2004；De Raedt et al. 2004）。这些旁系同源序列来源于位于 19p13.12 的亲脂蛋白-1 前体基因（latrophilin-1 precursor gene，*LPHN1*）（Forbes et al. 2004）。相比之下，在 NF1-REPb 中不存在与 19p13.12 同源的序列，如图 14.2 所示。位于 NF1-REP 内的另一组旁系同源序列是功能性 *LRRC37B* 基因的假基因拷贝，其位于 NF1-REPc 内。*LRRC37B* 假基因片段存在于所有 3 种 NF1-REP 中（图 14.2；Jenne et al. 2003；Forbes et al. 2004；De Raedt et al. 2004）。

除 *LRRC37B* 序列外，NF1-REPs a 和 b 还含有 *SMURF2*（SMAD 特异性 E3 泛素蛋白连接酶 2）基因的假基因片段，这些片段在 NF1-REPc 中不存在（图 14.2）。总之，NF1-REP 包含形成每个 NF1-REP 的特征性结构的不同旁系同源序列块。重要的是，这些旁系同源序列中的一些之间的序列同源性 95% 远超过 9 kb。这种高度的同源性以及 LCR 之间的距离似乎允许旁系同源序列的异位配对，并可能引起它们之间的 NAHR。

人们普遍认为，NAHR 最好通过双链断裂（DSB）修复模型来解释，该模型首先在酵母中描述（Szostak et al. 1983）。根据这个模型，重组事件（等位基因的或非等位基因的）是在减数分裂 I 的前期由 DSB 启动的（图 14.3a）。然后产生可迁移的异源双链 DNA 结构，并将其转化为双霍利迪连接，随后将其分离。根据这种分离是否与交换有关，观察到 NAHR 或非等位基因转化（NAHGC；图 14.3）。因此，NAHGC 和 NAHR 代表了可供选择的过程，但只有 NAHR 会产生重排，如缺失或重复。NAHR 可发生在染色体之间（染色体间 NAHR）或 1 条染色体或染色单体内（染色体内 NAHR）。1 型 *NF1* 缺失已被证明是由母体减数分裂 I 期间的染色体间 NAHR 引起的（López-Correa et al. 2000；Steinmann et al. 2008）。相比之下，嵌合型 2 型 *NF1* 缺失总是由染色体内 NAHR 引起，未观察到母系或父系染色体的优势；在考虑到这些缺失的合子后起源的情况下，这并不意外（Roehl et al. 2010）。NF1-REPa 和 NF1-REPc 之间染色体间 NAHR 在母体减数分裂中的优势可能与长网丝期有关，这是雌性减数分裂 I 的一个独特特征。网丝期在双线期之后，双线期是雌性和雄性减数分裂前期 I 所共有的。在双线期，同源染色体之间的联会复合体降解，同源染色体彼此轻微分离，但仍在交叉处（发生交换的区域）保持紧密结合。同源染色体之间的交叉一直持续到它们在后期 I 分离。在人类胚胎卵子发生中，所有卵母细胞在进入网丝期之前都发育到这个阶段。雌性减数分裂停滞在网丝期许多年，直到青春期后减数分裂继续（Vogel and Motulsky 1996）。相比之下，在雄性减数分裂 I 期间没有观察到这种在网丝期阶段的延长停滞，其仅

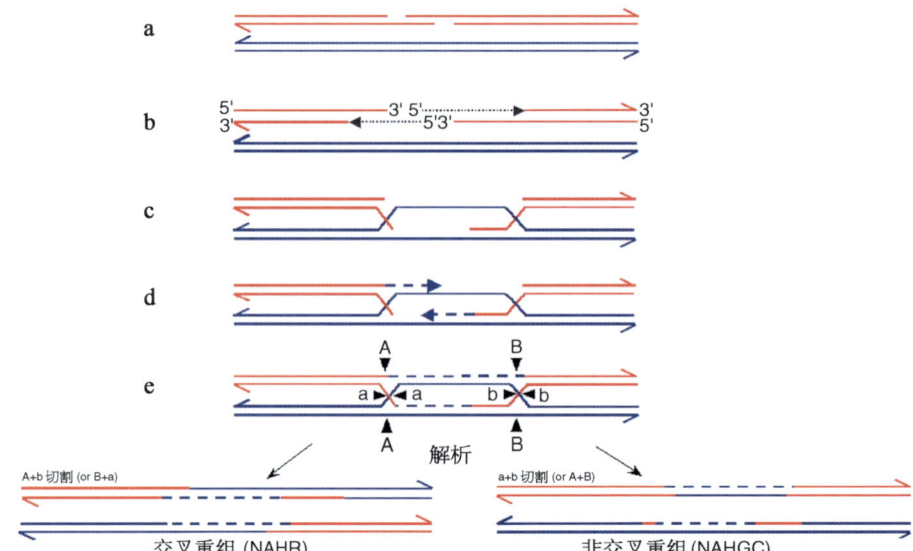

图 14.3 根据 Szostak 等(1983)为等位基因同源重组所概述的双链断裂修复模型,高度同源序列(如 NF 1 - REP)之间的非等位基因同源重组(NAHR)。a. 参与重组事件的旁系同源序列用红线和蓝线表示。用红色表示的并行同源物经历双链断裂(DSB),其启动重组。b. 起始端在 $5'→3'$ 的方向被进一步切除。c. 断裂的双链侵入未断裂的双链导致异源双链 DNA 的形成。d. DNA 合成和第二末端捕获导致双霍利迪连接(dHJ)的形成。e. 在两个位置切割 DNA 链的酶可分解 dHJ。根据切割哪条链,染色单体的交换发生或不发生。交叉分辨率与一条染色体上的缺失和另一条染色体上的重复相关。非交换的消除以及随后的序列错配的修复导致非等位基因同源基因转化(NAHGC),其可通过旁系同源序列变体(PSV)的非互惠转移来检测。PSV 是各 LCR 特异性的非多态性位点。在重组过程中,特异于 1 个 LCR 的 PSV 可以转移到其旁系同源物,导致在受体 LCR 的旁系同源物位置引入 SNP

持续几天(Vogel and Motulsky 1996)。女性减数分裂期间延长的网丝期阶段可能与 NF1 - REPa 和 NF1 - REPc 之间染色体间 NAHR 的优势有关,这种重组导致了 1 型 *NF1* 微缺失的发生。尽管 NF1 - REP 之间的异位配对在雄性和雌性减数分裂中可能以相似的频率发生,但触发 NAHR 的 DSB 更可能发生在卵母细胞延长的网丝期阶段。另一种解释在雌性减数分裂期间 NF1 - REPa 和 NF1 REPc 之间优先发生染色体间 NAHR 的假设是,卵母细胞特异性 DNA 序列和(或)组蛋白修饰可以触发 NAHR。也可能是携带 1 型 *NF1* 缺失的精子存活率较低或参与受精的频率较低;这可以解释为什么父系遗传的 1 型 *NF1* 缺失比母系遗传的缺失少得多。

到目前为止,对起源于染色体的 NAHR 事件导致的 3 型 *NF1* 缺失还了解不足。这是因为迄今为止仅确定了 11 例 3 型缺失患者,并且无法进行使用微卫星标记确定缺失是否通过染色体间或染色体内重组发生的家族研究(Zickler et al. 2012)。在这 11 例 3 型 *NF1* 缺失中的 5 例鉴定了亲本来源。其中 4 人的缺失发生在父亲的 17 号染色体上。由于在这些患者中与正常细胞的嵌合现象不明显,所以假定 3 型缺失发生在父本减数分裂期间(Zickler et al. 2012)。然而,减数分裂前有丝分裂细胞周期中发生的这些 3 型缺失尚不能明确排除。与 3 型缺失相反,大多数 1 型 *NF1* 缺失是母系遗传的(López-Correa et al. 2000;Steinmann et al. 2008)。

14.3.2 *NF1* 微缺失和 *NAHR* 热点

对多发性 1 型和 3 型 *NF1* 微缺失的分析,以及对几种其他已知 NAHR 介导的重排分析,揭示了相应的断点通常发生在几百个碱基对的热点内(Lindsay et al. 2006;Reiter et al. 1996,1998;Turner et al. 2008;Visser et al. 2005)。1 型 *NF1* 微缺失的断点聚集在 NAHR 热点内,称为旁系同源重组位点(paralogous recombination site, PRS)1 和 2(De Raedt et al. 2006;Forbes et al. 2004;

Jenne et al. 2001；López-Correa et al. 2001）。PRS1 和 PRS2 位于与染色体 19p13.12 同源的 NF1-REPa 和 NF1-REPc 区域内（图 14.2）。大多数 1 型 NF1 缺失（67%）的断点位于 PRS2 NAHR 热点内，而只有 22% 的 1 型缺失断点聚集在 PRS1 内（De Raedt et al. 2006）。

3 型 NF1 微缺失断点也聚集在 NAHR 热点内。到目前为止，已经鉴定了 11 名具有 3 型缺失的患者，并且这 11 名患者中 10 名的断裂点位于这个称为 PRS3 的 1 kb 热点内（Bengesser et al. 2010；Zickler et al. 2012）。PRS3 位于 NF1-REPb 和 NF1-REPc 低拷贝重复序列的 *LRRC37B* 假基因内。后者在 9.2 kb 区域内显示出 97.8% 的序列同一性，并且定位于直接方向（图 14.2）。*LRRC37B-P* 旁系同源物是位于 NF1-REPc 近端部分的功能性 *LRRC37B* 基因的假基因，尽管与 *LRRC37B* 假基因相比是反向的。*LRRC37B-P* 旁系同源物，以及与位于 NF1-REP 内的 19 号染色体同源的序列，在猩猩基因组中是容易鉴定的，因此，它们的扩增肯定先于猩猩谱系与其他猿类共同祖先的分歧 12～16 Mya。在 NF1-REPc 中，PRS3 位于 PRS2 的 12 kb 端粒和 PRS1 的 31 kb 端粒。*LRRC37B* 基因还含有 1 个与 PRS3 同源的区域，与 NF1-REPb 和 NF1-REPc 的序列同源性 >98%。与 PRS3 同源的 *LRRC37B* 内的区域包括内含子 1 和外显子 2 的部分（Zickler et al. 2012）。

目前，还不完全清楚是什么样的序列特征决定了 NAHR 热点的位置和活性。在减数分裂期间，NAHR 和 AHR 相关的交换都聚集在 500 bp 至 2 kb 的狭窄热点区域内（Jeffreys et al. 2001；Crawford et al. 2004；McVean et al. 2004；Coop et al. 2008；Webb et al. 2008）。因此，特定基因组区域内断点的聚集似乎是减数分裂同源重组的一般特征，并且有理由假设 AHR 和 NAHR 是相关的过程。因此，关于 NAHR 序列特征的结论也可以从 AHR 热点的详细分析中推导出来。已经鉴定了激活 AHR 热点的顺式和反式作用因子或序列（Jeffreys and Neumann 2002，2005；Peters 2008；Ubeda and Wilkins 2011；Zheng et al. 2010）。其中最好表征的是 13-mer 简并序列基序（CCNCCNTNNCCNC），其

被认为在募集交叉事件至所有 AHR 热点的 40% 中起关键作用（Myers et al. 2008）。组蛋白甲基转移酶 PRDM9 通过其锌指阵列与该 13 聚体基序结合，并在 AHR 热点处反式充当重组起始因子（Baudat et al. 2010；Berg et al. 2010；Parvanov et al. 2010）。*PRDM9* 基因在人类中具有高度多态性，尤其是在其编码的锌指阵列结构域方面，这种遗传变异可影响 AHR 热点活性（Baudat et al. 2010；Berg et al. 2010；Parvanov et al. 2010）的报告。然而，*PRDM9* 变异体本身仅占热点利用率群体变异的 18%（Baudat et al. 2010）。因此，必须存在 AHR 热点活性的额外调节剂。

PRDM9 基因座的遗传变异也影响 NAHR 活性，如 17p11.2-p12 中 CMT 1A-REP 介导的复制和缺失所示（Berg et al. 2010）。在 PRDM9A 等位基因纯合的健康供体的精子中，观察到 CMT1A-REP 之间的从头重排发生频率比非 A 等位基因纯合的个体高 20 倍以上（Berg et al. 2010）。此外，在总共 5 个不同的充分表征的 NAHR 热点（包括负责 1 型 NF1 缺失的 PRS2）中发现了 13-mer 序列基序 CCNCNTNNCCNC（Myers et al. 2008）。然而，这个 13-mer 基序 CCNCCNTNNCCNC 在 PRS1 和 PRS3 中都不存在。从 1 型和 3 型缺失的相对频率估计，其中断点位于其各自的热点中，PRS2 代表比 PRS1 或 PRS3 强烈得多的热点。因此，13-mer 基序的存在或缺失可以在一定程度上决定 NAHR 热点强度。然而，13 聚体基序不太可能是 NAHR 热点活性的唯一决定因素。可能存在影响 NAHR 频率和断裂点定位的其他未知序列或结合因子。

介导 *NF1* 微缺失的 PRS 1、2 和 3 热点不仅可以通过这些热点内发生的 NAHR 事件的频率来区分，还可以通过其变异模式（通过每 kb 的 SNP 数量来测量）来区分（De Raedt et al. 2006；Zickler et al. 2012）。在 NAHR 热点以及 AHR 热点内，基因转化通常增加（Baudat and de Massy 2007）。重要的是，由没有交换的同源重组引起的基因转化似乎比与交换相关的重组更频繁。事实上，等位基因转化事件被认为比与交换相关的 AHR 事件发生的频率高 4～15 倍（Jeffreys and May 2004）。频繁基因转换的结果是 SNP 数量的增加，因为在重组过程

中,所涉及的LCR之间的序列差异被交换了(图14.3)。通过这些方法,将旁系同源序列变体转化为SNP。在NF1-REPa和NF1-REPc内的PRS1和PRS2热点中,已经观察到5~11个SNP/kb的SNP频率,其指示频繁的非等位基因同源基因转化(NAHGC)(De Raedt et al. 2006)。在NF1-REPc的PRS3中也观察到了高数量的SNP(7个SNP/kb);这表示与基因组平均值相比,SNP密度增加了7倍(Sachidanandam et al. 2001; Frazer et al. 2007)。相比之下,NF1-REPb和LRRC37B中PRS3内SNP频率要低得多(2SNPs/kb)(Zickler et al. 2012)。位于NF1-REPb中的PRS3与位于NF1-REPc中的PRS3所观察到的SNP密度,可能可以根据所涉及的基因转化事件的极性来解释。在NF1-REPb到NF1-REPc的重组过程中可能发生单向序列转移,导致NF1-REPc中的SNP密度较高,但NF1-REPb中没有。根据这一假设,NF1-REPc在重组过程中应不成比例地成为受体(Zickler et al. 2012)。如图14.2所示,重组起始双链断裂发生在受体序列(即NF1-REPc)上,其在同源重组期间接受来自用作DSB修复模板的完整供体序列(即NF1-REPb)的DNA"补丁",而没有交叉。从NF1-REPb到NF1 REPc的单向序列转移的结果将是受体序列(NF1-REPc)比未断裂的供体链(NF1-REPb)包含更多数量的SNP,如所观察到的。相比之下,NAHGC期间的双向序列转移意味着在另一条链入侵之前,两个LCR以相等的概率参与DSB诱导。因此,在NAHGC过程中,两条链预期以相似的速率获得SNP,导致两个重组LCR中的高SNP频率。因此,双向基因转化事件最有可能解释在NF1-REPa和NF1-REPc的PRS1和PRS2内观察到的SNP频率升高(De Raedt et al. 2006)。

除了与PRS3相比PRS1和PRS2内基因转换事件方向性的差异之外,已经注意到这些热点之间的进一步差异,这些差异可能已经影响了与其祖先基因座正在进行的序列交换。NF1-REPa和NF1-REPc内的PRS1和PRS2不参与与位于染色体19上的其祖先基因座的序列交换(De Raedt et al. 2006)。相比之下,这些携带PRS3的LRRC37B假基因的起源序列,LRRC37B基因,在NF1-REPc内与PRS3积极参与NAHGC(Zickler et al. 2012)。因此,与其祖先基因座的序列交换和单向序列转移可以解释NF1-REPc内PRS3的异常变异模式。此外,接近两个活跃的NAHR热点可能影响了NF1-REPc内PRS3的出现(图14.2)。NF1-REPc中PRS3与PRS1和PRS2的空间接近性(但NF1-REPb中没有)可能促进了该NAHR热点PRS3的最近出现以及其多态性变异水平增加的特征(Zickler et al. 2012)。

如上所述,假设AHR和NAHR在机制上非常相似,那么,我们有理由认为,NAHR活动增加的区域也会经历频繁的AHR。与该预测一致,PRS1和PRS2热点以及位于CMT1A-REP内的NAHR热点与预先存在的AHR热点重叠(De Raedt et al. 2006; Lindsay et al. 2006)。PRS1和PRS2位于与染色体19p13.12同源区域内的NF1-REPa和NF1-REPc内(图14.2)。这些序列的祖先基因座被称为REP 19,在与NAHR热点PRS1和PRS2旁系同源的区域内含有强AHR热点(De Raedt et al. 2006)。此外,NAHR热点PRS1和PRS2本身位于NF1-REPa和NF1-REPc内,并与弱AHR热点重叠。这些发现为旁系同源序列内重组热点模式的保守性提供了很好的证据(De Raedt et al. 2006)。然而,NAHR热点也可以重新出现,而不是总是起源于预先存在的AHR断点区域内。支持这一假设的是观察到介导3型NF1微缺失的PRS3 NAHR热点未在预先存在的AHR热点上发展(Zickler et al. 2012)。PRS3代表了一个弱的,可能是进化上相当年轻的NAHR热点,具有不同于PRS1和PRS2的独特序列特性。

两者合计,分析经常性NF1微缺失的断点产生了生物学重要的新信息和不同强度减数分裂NAHR热点的序列特征。

14.3.3 有丝分裂和减数分裂NAHR介导的NF1微缺失

1型和3型NF1微缺失大多起源于减数分裂,而2型缺失大多发生在胚胎发育早期(原肠胚形成前),并由有丝分裂NAHR介导(Roehl et al. 2010,

2012)。有趣的是,在嵌合2型缺失患者中观察到明显的女性优势,这与其他类型 NF1 微缺失的平等性别分布形成对比。女性占优势的原因尚不清楚。

分析 NF1 微缺失多发的机制有可能表明 NF1 基因区有丝分裂和减数分裂 NAHR 之间的差异和相似性。最显著的区别似乎是2型 NF1 微缺失的有丝分裂 NAHR 断裂点不聚集在仅几百个碱基对的狭窄区域内,这将被清楚地识别为 NAHR 热点。相比之下,1型和3型缺失的断点明确地聚集在 NAHR 活性的热点中(López-Correa et al. 2001; De Raedt et al. 2006; Zickler et al. 2012)。受精后发生基因突变导致1型 NF1 的微缺失的情况非常少见。据估计,只有2%的1型 NF1 缺失发生在合子后 NAHR,断裂点位于 PRS2 和 PRS1 热点内(Messiaen et al. 2011)。人类基因组中的其他 NAHR 热点已被证明仅在减数分裂期间起作用,而在有丝分裂期间根本不起作用(Turner et al. 2008)。

尽管2型 NF1 缺失断点不聚集在独特的热点内,但它们是非随机分布的。在2型缺失的重组区(recombination region,RR)内观察到能够形成非 B DNA 的短序列数量不成比例(Roehl et al. 2010)。这些重复序列很可能促进了 DSB 的形成,DSB 触发了 NAHR 事件,最终导致了2型 NF1 微缺失。此外,在染色体内 NAHR 介导的60% 2型缺失的断点处观察到 Alu 元件(Roehl et al. 2010)。Alu 元件是众所周知的重组序列(reviewed by Konkel and Batzer 2010),因此可能有助于局部 DSB 形成和随后的2型缺失基础 NAHR。

对减数分裂和有丝分裂 NAHR 引起的 NF1 微缺失所涉及序列的详细分析表明,这些序列的 GC 含量和 DNA 双链体稳定性存在差异。与之相对地位于 NF1-REPa 和 NF1-REPb 内的减数分裂 NAHR 断裂点侧翼的序列特征在于高 GC 含量和高 DNA 双链体稳定性,与有丝分裂 NAHR 事件相关的2型缺失断裂点位于 GC 含量和 DNA 稳定性显著较低的区域内(Roehl et al. 2010)。

2型和1型 NF1 微缺失的染色体机制似乎也有很大的不同。1型缺失由染色体间 NAHR 引起,而2型缺失发生在17号染色体内,或者由1个染色单体内的染色体内 NAHR 引起,或者由姐妹染色单体196H 之间的 NAHR 引起(Roehl et al. 2010)。我们可以假设,染色体配对和染色质结构的差异与染色体内合子后 NAHR 的优先发生,是导致2型 NF1 微缺失的原因。与减数分裂联会复合体中同源染色体紧密稳定配对相反,有丝分裂细胞周期中同源染色体的配对在性质上不同,可能不太稳定(reviewed by Meaburn and Misteli 2007)。尽管如此,减数分裂和有丝分裂重组的过程可能至少有一些机制上的相似性。在酵母中,有丝分裂期间的同源重组由接头分子中间体介导,其链组成和大小与减数分裂双霍利迪接头的链组成和大小相同(Bzymek et al. 2010)。在有丝分裂 DSB 修复期间,优先在酵母姐妹染色单体之间形成双霍利迪连接,而在减数分裂期间,同源物间重组的优先性是明显的(Bzymek et al. 2010)。这些观察结果与 NF1 微缺失的染色体机制差异相似:染色体内 NAHR 是导致合子后起源的2型 NF1 缺失的主要机制,而母体减数分裂期间的染色体间 NAHR 负责生殖系1型 NF1 微缺失(López-Correa et al. 2000; Roehl et al. 2010)。

有丝分裂 NAHR 潜在的2型 NF1 微缺失可能发生在胚泡阶段,甚至更早,当然在胚胎第12天和原肠胚形成开始之前。这一结论可以从以下观察结果得出:在2型 NF1 微缺失患者中,在所有3个生殖细胞层的衍生物中均可检测到携带缺失的细胞,内胚层(泌尿系统上皮细胞)、中胚层(血细胞)和外胚层(皮肤成纤维细胞、神经纤维瘤衍生细胞和颊上皮)(Roehl et al. 2012)。然而,有丝分裂 NAHR 引起的 NF1 微缺失也可能在生命后期体细胞中发生,从而导致肿瘤发生。在来自具有生殖系基因内 NF1 突变患者的皮肤型神经纤维瘤中,已经确定了由于体细胞2型缺失导致的野生型 NF1 等位基因的丢失(Garcia-Linares et al. 2011)。然而,对更大系列的皮肤以及丛状神经纤维瘤的分析表明,NAHR 介导的 NF1 微缺失导致的 NF1 基因体细胞失活并不是导致杂合性丢失的常见事件(GarciaLinares et al. 2011; Steinmann et al. 2009)。

SUZ12 序列而不是侧翼 NF1-REP 是 NAHR 在受精后细胞周期中导致 NF1 微缺失的首选靶点

的原因尚未阐明。NF1-REPa 和 NF1-REPc 共有的最大高同源性序列块(97.5%)延伸超过 51 kb (Forbes et al. 2004)。*SUZ12* 和 *SUZ12P* 之间的序列同源性超过 45 kb,达到 96% (Roehl et al. 2010)。同源区长度或序列同源性平均程度的这些相对较小的差异似乎不太可能是观察到的 *NF1* 基因区减数分裂与有丝分裂 NAHR 断裂点位置偏好的原因。其他未知的功能被认为是导致断点本地化差异的原因。

14.3.4 非典型 *NF1* 微缺失及其致病机制

与 NAHR 介导的突变机制相比,非典型 *NF1* 微缺失与非复发性断点的突变机制不太清楚。迄今为止,在文献中已报道了 41 个非典型 *NF1* 微缺失(Cnossen et al. 1997; Dorschner et al. 2000; Jenne et al. 2001; Kayes et al. 1992, 1994; Kehrer-Sawatzki et al. 2003, 2005, 2008; Mantripragada et al. 2006; Pasmant et al. 2008, 2009, 2010; Riva et al. 2000; Venturin et al. 2004a, 2004b; Upadhyaya et al. 1996)。然而,在这 41 个缺失中,只有 6 个缺失的断点在碱基对水平上被表征(表 14.1)。在这 6 个缺失的着丝粒和端粒断裂点的序列没有表现出超过几百个碱基对的延伸序列同源性,这一发现似乎排除了同源重组作为这些缺失的基础机制的可能。此外,在相应的缺失断点处未观察到少量碱基对的小插入或其他重排,如倒位。因此,可以合理地假设非同源末端连接(nonhomologous end joining,NHEJ)介导了这 6 种非典型 *NF1* 缺失。然而,由于到目前为止仅分析了 6 个具有非复发性断点的 *NF1* 微缺失,所以不能排除基于复制的机制,如"分叉停滞和模板转换"(fork stalling and template switching,FoSteS)或复制起点的异常激发也可以解释非典型 *NF1* 微缺失的发生。事实上,基于复制的错误已被认为是与各种疾病相关的其他非复发性基因组重排的原因(Ankala et al. 2012; Bauters et al. 2008; Lee et al. 2007; Liu et al. 2011; Vissers et al. 2009; Zhang et al. 2009a, b, 2010)。需要对大量非典型 *NF1* 微缺失的断点进行详细分析,以阐明基于复制的错误作为这些缺失的假定机制的作用。

表 14.1 迄今为止在 6 个非典型 *NF1* 微缺失断点处检测到的序列

患 者	着丝粒断点	端粒断裂点	缺失的长度	突变机制	参考文献
6[a]	位于 *BLMH*(白霉素水解酶)基因内含子 1 的独特序列内	位于 *ACCN1*(阿米洛利敏感阳离子通道 1)基因内含子 1 内的独特序列内	3 Mb	NHEJ	Venturin 等(2004a)
442	位于 *EFCAB5*(EF-手形钙结合结构域 5)基因的内含子部分 LINE 元件内	位于 *SUZ12*(zeste12 的抑制基因)内含子 15 的独特序列内	2 Mb	NHEJ	Kehrer-Sawatzki 等(2005)
552	位于 *NF1* 基因内含子 21 内的独特序列内	位于 *ACCN1*(阿米洛利敏感阳离子通道 1,神经元)基因内含子 1 内的独特序列内	2.7 Mb	NHEJ	Kehrer-Sawatzki 等(2008)
DUB	位于 *PIPOX*(哌啶酸氧化酶)基因内含子 4 内的 305-bp 的 NSx 内	位于 *GGNBP2*(配子生成素结合蛋白 2)基因内含子 5 内的 47 bp MIRB(全染色体散布重复类型 B)内	7.6 Mb	NHEJ	Pasmant 等(2008)
NF00028	位于 NF 1-REPa 内 LRRC 37 B 假基因内含子 1 内的 116 bp LINE 元件内	位于 *RAB11FIP4*(RAB11 家族相互作用蛋白 4)基因内含子 1 的 96 bp 内	837 kb	NHEJ	Pasmant 等(2009)
NF00358[a]	位于 *BLMH* 基因内含子 1 的独特序列内	位于 *RAB11FIP4* 基因内含子 3 的 307 bp 内	1.2 Mb	NHEJ	Pasmant 等(2009)

注:[a] 这两个患者的着丝粒断裂点不同。

14.4 基因型/表型相关性和 *NF1* 微缺失

NF1 微缺失的分析不仅在潜在突变机制的背景下，而且在 NF1 的基因型/表型相关性方面都很有意义。许多研究表明，与基因内 *NF1* 突变患者相比，*NF1* 微缺失患者的临床表型更为严重（De Raedt et al. 2003；Descheemaeker et al. 2004；Kluwe et al. 2003；Mautner et al. 2010；Mensink et al. 2006；Pasmant et al. 2010；Upadhyaya et al. 1998；Venturin et al. 2004b；Wu et al. 1995，1999）。虽然作为一个群体，具有 *NF1* 微缺失的患者似乎较具有基因内 *NF1* 突变的患者表现出更严重的 *NF1* 形式，但在一些具有大的 *NF1* 缺失的个体患者之间观察到了临床变异性（Tonsgard et al. 1997）。

Descheemaeker 等（2004）分析了 11 例 1 型 *NF1* 微缺失患者，确定其平均全量表智商（full scale IQ，FSIQ）为 76.0。相比之下，在 106 个表现出基因内 *NF1* 突变的 NF1 个体中，平均 FSIQ 为 88.5。因此，具有 1 型 *NF1* 微缺失患者的平均 FSIQ 显著低于没有这种缺失的 NF1 患者的平均 FSIQ。尽管 1 型 *NF1* 缺失患者组的平均智力通常低于无 *NF1* 微缺失患者组，但已注意到两组之间存在大量重叠（Descheemaeker et al. 2004）。对另外 21 例分子上确定的 1 型 *NF1* 微缺失患者的研究也表明，与一般 NF1 人群相比，1 型 *NF1* 微缺失与认知发育延迟和（或）学习障碍不成比例相关（Mautner et al. 2010）。此外，在这 21 例 1 型缺失的 NF1 患者中，有 8 例（38%）观察到精神发育迟滞（IQ<70）（Mautner et al. 2010）。与无此类缺失的 NF1 个体相比，在 1 型 *NF1* 微缺失患者中不成比例发生的其他特征为畸形面部特征、高大身材、大头畸形、大手和大脚、关节过度灵活性和恶性周围神经鞘膜瘤（malignant peripheral nerve sheath tumour，MPNST）（Mautner et al. 2010）。尽管所有 NF1 个体中 MPNST 的终生风险为 8%~13%（Evans et al. 2002；Ingham et al. 2011），但据估计，*NF1* 微缺失患者的 MPNST 终生风险为 16%~26%（De Raedt et al. 2003；Mautner et al. 2010；Passimme et al. 2010）。由于 MPNST（和神经胶质瘤）是 NF1 患者预期寿命缩短的两个最常见原因（Evans et al. 2011），所以 *NF1* 微缺失患者需要加强临床护理和监督。

对 *NF1* 微缺失患者的基因型/表型相关性研究也表明，这些患者患有高负荷的真皮神经纤维瘤和外部可见的丛状神经纤维瘤（Kayes et al. 1994；Dorschner et al. 2000；Mautner et al. 2010）。在 *NF1* 微缺失患者中通过全身 MRI 测定的内部肿瘤负荷体积评估表明，作为一个组，*NF1* 微缺失患者的内部肿瘤负荷并不高于无 *NF1* 微缺失患者（Kluwe et al. 2012）。然而，在单个患者水平上，极高的肿瘤负荷（>3 000 mL 的总肿瘤体积）在非嵌合性 *NF1* 微缺失患者中比在无 *NF1* 微缺失 NF1 患者中显著更常见。

据报道，在 *NF1* 大缺失的患者中，尤其是在 2~6 岁的学龄前儿童中，身高增长和腕骨骨龄加速是最明显的（Spiegel et al. 2005）。相比之下，生长迟缓和身材矮小在一般 NF1 人群中很常见（Riccardi 1992，1999；Huson and Hughes 1994）。位于 1 型 *NF1* 微缺失区间的 RING 指蛋白 135（RNF 135）基因很可能是一个很好的候选修饰基因，该基因负责在 *NF1* 微缺失患者中观察到的过度生长。这一论断源于观察到 5 名无 NF1 但有与面部畸形相关的过度生长综合征和不同程度学习障碍的患者，他们的 *RNF135* 基因内存在突变（Douglas et al. 2007）。这 5 个突变包括 4 个不同的 *RNF135* 无义突变和 1 个 *RNF135* 错义突变。Douglas 等（2007）鉴定了第 6 名过度生长综合征的患者，该患者缺失了整个 *RNF135* 基因及其侧翼序列，这是由 NF1-REPa 和 NF1-REPb 之间的异常重组介导的，导致整个 *RNF135* 基因以及位于 *NF1* 基因附近的其他基因（但不是 *NF1* 基因本身）的缺失。这些发现表明，*RNF135* 单倍不足也可能是在 *NF1* 微缺失患者中观察到过度生长的原因（Douglas et al. 2007）。重要的是，在 6 例 *RNF135* 突变患者中观察到的畸形面部特征与在 *NF1* 微缺失患者中观察到的特征相似（Douglas et al. 2007）。*RNF135* 广泛表达，但其功能尚未完全表征。编码的蛋白质在其N-末端具有RING指结构域,在其C-末端具有B30.2/SPRY结构域。通过其RING指结构域,*RNF135*与视黄酸诱导基因-Ⅰ(retinoic acid-inducible gene-Ⅰ,RIG-Ⅰ)结合,RIG-Ⅰ是一种细胞质RNA解旋酶,其与线粒体外膜上的蛋白质相互作用,以发出病毒衍生RNA存在的信号。*RNF135*通过泛素化RIG-Ⅰ促进RIG-Ⅰ介导的Ⅰ型干扰素诱导,从而调节RIG-Ⅰ对病毒RNA最小拷贝的应答(Oshiumi et al. 2009)。到目前为止,还不清楚*RNF135*单倍不足如何导致在*NF1*微缺失患者和基因内*RNF135*突变患者中观察到的过度生长表型。在来自MPNST活检的施万细胞和MPNST细胞系中,发现*RNF135*和也位于*NF1*微缺失区间内的centaurin-alpha 2(*CENTA2*)均下调(Passim met al. 2011)。因此,Passimme等(2011)认为,这2种基因可能与*NF1*微缺失患者中观察到的恶性肿瘤风险增加有关。

很容易推测,位于*NF1*微缺失区域内的*MIR193a* miRNA基因单倍不足也可能导致大*NF1*缺失患者的肿瘤风险增加。miR-193a通过直接靶向致癌基因(如K-Ras)的30个非翻译区抑制细胞转化,miR-193a过表达抑制不同类型癌细胞的致瘤性(Iliopoulos et al. 2011)。此外,miR-193a抑制原癌基因c-kit的表达(Gao et al. 2011)。然而,与真皮神经纤维瘤相比,丛状神经纤维瘤和MPNST中miR193-a的表达水平似乎未发生变化(Passim met al. 2011)。然而,不能以任何程度的确定性排除miR-193a不参与NF1的恶性转化,因为miR-193a表达受CpG甲基化调节,CpG甲基化很可能在恶性转化期间短暂发生。

我们可以假设,*NF1*微缺失的大小有相关的临床表型的影响。由于不同类型的*NF1*微缺失在缺失区域中包含的基因数量方面是可区分的,因此缺失类型对于疾病的临床表达很重要。然而,大多数已经研究过相关临床表型的患者都有1型*NF1*缺失。这可能是因为1型*NF1*微缺失是迄今为止最常见的*NF1*微缺失类型。临床上,仅有2种非嵌合型*NF1*微缺失被详细研究过(Vogt et al. 2011)。这些患者表现出临床特征(如高肿瘤负荷、学习障碍、大手和大脚、关节过度灵活和大头畸形),据报道,这些临床特征也经常发生在生殖系1型*NF1*缺失的患者中。因此,经常观察到的与1型*NF1*微缺失相关的严重临床表现可能延伸到2型*NF1*缺失。然而,要证实这一论断,对大量非嵌合型2型*NF1*微缺失患者的进一步研究将是必要的。

14.5 结论

许多NF1微缺失断点的详细分析表明,NAHR是NF1微缺失多发的主要机制,而那些具有非复发性断点的缺失似乎经常由NHEJ引起。然而,*NF1*微缺失的全部机制和这些机制的具体特征远未被完全理解。例如,目前尚不清楚为什么减数分裂NAHR断裂点聚集在NF1-REP内,以及为什么有丝分裂NAHR事件的断裂点优先位于*SUZ12*序列内。此外,目前还不清楚在何种程度上复制为基础的错误有助于非典型非复发性NF1缺失的发生。也不知道是否存在特定的多态性结构变异体,这些变异可能会增加*NF1*微缺失的发生风险。最后,需要更详细地研究修饰基因的影响及其在*NF1*微缺失患者中观察到的更严重临床表型的潜力。

(张松 译)

参考文献

[1] Ankala A, Kohn JN, Hegde A, Meka A, Ephrem CL, Askree SH, Bhide S, Hegde MR (2012) Aberrant firing of replication origins potentially explains intragenic nonrecurrent rearrangements within genes, including the human DMD gene. Genome Res 22: 25-34

[2] Baudat F, de Massy B (2007) Regulating double-stranded DNA break repair towards crossover or non-crossover during mammalian meiosis. Chromosome Res 15: 565-577

[3] Baudat F, Buard J, Grey C, Fledel-Alon A, Ober C, Przeworski M, Coop G, de Massy B (2010) PRDM9 is a major determinant of meiotic recombination hotspots in humans and mice. Science 327: 836-840

[4] Bauters M, Van Esch H, Friez MJ, Boespflug-Tanguy O, Zenker M, Vianna-Morgante AM, Rosenberg C, Ignatius J, Raynaud M, Hollanders K, Govaerts K, Vandenreijt K, Niel F, Blanc P, Stevenson RE, Fryns JP, Marynen P, Schwartz CE, Froyen G (2008) Nonrecurrent *MECP2* duplications mediated by genomic architecture-driven DNA breaks and

break-induced replication repair. Genome Res 18: 847-858

[5] Bengesser K, Cooper DN, Steinmann K, Kluwe L, Chuzhanova NA, Wimmer K, Tatagiba M, Tinschert S, Mautner VF, Kehrer-Sawatzki H (2010) A novel third type of recurrent *NF1* microdeletion mediated by non-allelic homologous recombination between *LRRC37B*-containing low-copy repeats in 17q11. 2. Hum Mutat 31: 742-751

[6] Berg IL, Neumann R, Lam KW, Sarbajna S, Odenthal-Hesse L, May CA, Jeffreys AJ (2010) *PRDM9* variation strongly influences recombination hot-spot activity and meiotic instability in humans. Nat Genet 42: 859-863

[7] Bzymek M, Thayer NH, Oh SD, Kleckner N, Hunter N (2010) Double Holliday junctions are intermediates of DNA break repair. Nature 464: 937-941

[8] Cnossen MH, van der Est MN, Breuning MH, van Asperen CJ, Breslau-Siderius EJ, van der Ploeg AT, de Goede-Bolder A, van den Ouweland AM, Halley DJ, Niermeijer MF (1997) Deletions spanning the neurofibromatosis type 1 gene: implications for genotype-phenotype correlations in neurofibromatosis type 1? Hum Mutat 9: 458-464

[9] Conrad DF, Bird C, Blackburne B, Lindsay S, Mamanova L, Lee C, Turner DJ, Hurles ME (2010) Mutation spectrum revealed by breakpoint sequencing of human germline CNVs. Nat Genet 42: 385-391

[10] Coop G, Wen X, Ober C, Pritchard JK, Przeworski M (2008) High-resolution mapping of crossovers reveals extensive variation in fine-scale recombination patterns among humans. Science 319: 1395-1398

[11] Crawford DC, Bhangale T, Li N, Hellenthal G, Rieder MJ, Nickerson DA, Stephens M (2004) Evidence for substantial fine-scale variation in recombination rates across the human genome. Nat Genet 36: 700-706

[12] De Raedt T, Brems H, Wolkenstein P, Vidaud D, Pilotti S, Perrone F, Mautner V, Frahm S, Sciot R, Legius E (2003) Elevated risk for MPNST in *NF1* microdeletion patients. Am J Hum Genet 72: 1288-1292

[13] De Raedt T, Brems H, Lopez-Correa C, Vermeesch JR, Marynen P, Legius E (2004) Genomic organization and evolution of the *NF1* microdeletion region. Genomics 84: 346-360

[14] De Raedt T, Stephens M, Heyns I, Brems H, Thijs D, Messiaen L, Stephens K, Lazaro C, Wimmer K, Kehrer-Sawatzki H, Vidaud D, Kluwe L, Marynen P, Legius E (2006) Conservation of hotspots for recombination in low-copy repeats associated with the *NF1* microdeletion. Nat Genet 38: 1419-1423

[15] Descheemaeker MJ, Roelandts K, De Raedt T, Brems H, Fryns JP, Legius E (2004) Intelligence in individuals with a neurofibromatosis type 1 microdeletion. Am J Med Genet A 131: 325-326

[16] Dorschner MO, Sybert VP, Weaver M, Pletcher BA, Stephens K (2000) *NF1* microdeletion breakpoints are clustered at flanking repetitive sequences. Hum Mol Genet 9: 35-46

[17] Douglas J, Cilliers D, Coleman K, Tatton-Brown K, Barker K, Bernhard B, Burn J, Huson S, Josifova D, Lacombe D, Malik M, Mansour S, Reid E, Cormier-Daire V, Cole T, Childhood Overgrowth Collaboration, Rahman N (2007) Mutations in *RNF135*, a gene within the *NF1* microdeletion region, cause phenotypic abnormalities including overgrowth. Nat Genet 39: 963-965

[18] Erickson RP (2010) Somatic gene mutation and human disease other than cancer: an update. Mutat Res 705: 96-106

[19] Evans DG, Baser ME, McGaughran J, Sharif S, Howard E, Moran A (2002) Malignant peripheral nerve sheath tumours in neurofibromatosis 1. J Med Genet 39: 311-314

[20] Evans DG, O'Hara C, Wilding A, Ingham SL, Howard E, Dawson J, Moran A, Scott-Kitching V, Holt F, Huson SM (2011) Mortality in neurofibromatosis 1: in North West England: an assessment of actuarial survival in a region of the UK since 1989. Eur J Hum Genet 19: 1187-1191

[21] Forbes SH, Dorschner MO, Le R, Stephens K (2004) Genomic context of paralogous recombination hotspots mediating recurrent *NF1* region microdeletion. Genes Chrom Cancer 41: 12-25

[22] Frazer KA, Ballinger DG, Cox DR, Hinds DA, Stuve LL, Gibbs RA, Belmont JW, Boudreau A, Hardenbol P, Leal SM, Pasternak S, Wheeler DA, Willis TD, Yu F, Yang H, Zeng C, Gao Y, Hu H, Hu W, Li C, Lin W, Liu S, Pan H, Tang X, Wang J, Wang W, Yu J, Zhang B, Zhang Q, Zhao H, Zhao H, Zhou J, Gabriel SB, Barry R, Blumenstiel B, Camargo A, Defelice M, Faggart M, Goyette M, Gupta S, Moore J, Nguyen H, Onofrio RC, Parkin M, Roy J, Stahl E, Winchester E, Ziaugra L, Altshuler D, Shen Y, Yao Z, Huang W, Chu X, He Y, Jin L, Liu Y, Shen Y, Sun W, Wang H, Wang Y, Wang Y, Xiong X, Xu L, Waye MM, Tsui SK, Xue H, Wong JT, Galver LM, Fan JB, Gunderson K, Murray SS, Oliphant AR, Chee MS, Montpetit A, Chagnon F, Ferretti V, Leboeuf M, Olivier JF, Phillips MS, Roumy S, Sallée C, Verner A, Hudson TJ, Kwok PY, Cai D, Koboldt DC, Miller RD, Pawlikowska L, Taillon-Miller P, Xiao M, Tsui LC, Mak W, Song YQ, Tam PK, Nakamura Y, Kawaguchi T, Kitamoto T, Morizono T, Nagashima A, Ohnishi Y, Sekine A, Tanaka T, Tsunoda T, Deloukas P, Bird CP, Delgado M, Dermitzakis ET, Gwilliam R, Hunt S, Morrison J, Powell D, Stranger BE, Whittaker P, Bentley DR, Daly MJ, de Bakker PI, Barrett J, Chretien YR, Maller J, McCarroll S, Patterson N, Pe'er I, Price A, Purcell S, Richter DJ, Sabeti P, Saxena R, Schaffner SF, Sham PC, Varilly P, Altshuler D, Stein LD, Krishnan L, Smith AV, Tello-Ruiz MK, Thorisson GA, Chakravarti A, Chen PE, Cutler DJ, Kashuk CS, Lin S, Abecasis GR, Guan W, Li Y, Munro HM, Qin ZS, Thomas DJ, McVean G, Auton A, Bottolo L, Cardin N, Eyheramendy S, Freeman C, Marchini J, Myers S, Spencer C, Stephens M, Donnelly P, Cardon LR, Clarke G, Evans DM, Morris AP, Weir BS, Tsunoda T, Mullikin JC, Sherry ST, Feolo M, Skol A, Zhang H, Zeng C, Zhao H, Matsuda I, Fukushima Y, Macer DR, Suda E, Rotimi CN, Adebamowo CA, Ajayi I, Aniagwu T, Marshall PA, Nkwodimmah C, Royal CD, Leppert MF, Dixon M, Peiffer A, Qiu R, Kent A, Kato K, Niikawa N, Adewole IF, Knoppers BM, Foster MW, Clayton EW, Watkin J, Gibbs RA, Belmont JW, Muzny D, Nazareth L, Sodergren E, Weinstock GM, Wheeler DA, Yakub I, Gabriel SB, Onofrio RC, Richter DJ, Ziaugra L, Birren BW, Daly MJ, Altshuler D, Wilson RK, Fulton LL, Rogers J, Burton J, Carter NP, Clee CM, Griffiths M, Jones MC, McLay K, Plumb RW, Ross MT, Sims SK, Willey DL, Chen Z, Han H, Kang L, Godbout M, Wallenburg JC, L'Archevêque P, Bellemare G, Saeki K, Wang H, An D, Fu H, Li Q, Wang Z, Wang R, Holden AL, Brooks LD, McEwen JE, Guyer MS, Wang VO, Peterson JL, Shi M, Spiegel J, Sung LM, Zacharia LF, Collins FS, Kennedy K, Jamieson R, Stewart J, International HapMap Consortium (2007) A second generation human haplotype map of over 3.1 million SNPs. Nature 449: 851-861

[23] Gao XN, Lin J, Li YH, Gao L, Wang XR, Wang W, Kang HY, Yan GT, Wang LL, Yu L (2011) MicroRNA-193a represses c-kit expression and functions as a methylation-silenced tumor suppressor in acute myeloid leukemia. Oncogene 30: 3416-3428

[24] Garcia-Linares C, Fernández-Rodríguez J, Terribas E, Mercadé J, Pros E, Benito L, Benavente Y, Capellà G, Ravella A, Blanco I, Kehrer-Sawatzki H, Lázaro C, Serra E (2011) Dissecting loss of heterozygosity (LOH) in neurofibromatosis type 1-associated neurofibromas: importance of copy neutral LOH. Hum Mutat 32: 78-90

[25] Gottlieb B, Beitel LK, Trifiro MA (2001) Somatic mosaicism and variable expressivity. Trends Genet 17: 79-82

[26] Huson SM, Hughes RAC (eds) (1994) The neurofibromatosis—a pathogenetic and clinical overview. Chapman & Hall, London, p 169

[27] Iliopoulos D, Rotem A, Struhl K (2011) Inhibition of miR-193a expression by Max and RXRa activates K-Ras and PLAU to mediate distinct aspects of cellular transformation. Cancer Res 71: 5144-5153

[28] Ingham S, Huson SM, Moran A, Wylie J, Leahy M, Evans DG (2011) Malignant peripheral nerve sheath tumours in NF1: improved survival in women and in recent years. Eur J Cancer 47: 2723-2728

[29] Jeffreys AJ, May CA (2004) Intense and highly localized gene conversion activity in human meiotic crossover hot spots. Nat Genet 36: 151-156

[30] Jeffreys AJ, Neumann R (2002) Reciprocal crossover asymmetry and meiotic drive in a human recombination hot spot. Nat Genet 31: 267-271

[31] Jeffreys AJ, Neumann R (2005) Factors influencing recombination frequency and distribution in a human meiotic crossover hotspot. Hum Mol Genet 14: 2277-2287

[32] Jeffreys AJ, Kauppi L, Neumann R (2001) Intensely punctate meiotic recombination in the class II region of the major histocompatibility complex. Nat Genet 29: 217-222

[33] Jenne DE, Tinschert S, Reimann H, Lasinger W, Thiel G, Hameister H, Kehrer-Sawatzki H (2001) Molecular characterization and gene content of breakpoint boundaries in patients with neuro-fibromatosis type 1 with 17q11.2 microdeletions. Am J Hum Genet 69: 516-527

[34] Jenne DE, Tinschert S, Dorschner MO, Hameister H, Stephens K, Kehrer-Sawatzki H (2003) Complete physical map and gene content of the human *NF1* tumor suppressor region in human and mouse. Genes Chromosomes Cancer 37: 111-120

[35] Kayes LM, Riccardi VM, Burke W, Bennett RL, Stephens K (1992) Large *de novo* DNA deletion in a patient with sporadic neurofibromatosis 1, mental retardation, and dysmorphism. J Med Genet 29: 686-690

[36] Kayes LM, Burke W, Riccardi VM, Benett R, Ehrlich P, Rubinstein A, Stephens K (1994) Deletions spanning the neurofibromatosis I gene: identification and phenotype of five patients. Am J Hum Genet 54: 424-436

[37] Kehrer-Sawatzki H, Cooper DN (2008) Mosaicism in sporadic neurofibromatosis type 1: variations on a theme common to other hereditary cancer syndromes? J Med Genet 45: 622-631

[38] Kehrer-Sawatzki H, Tinschert S, Jenne DE (2003) Heterogeneity of breakpoints in non-LCR-mediated large constitutional deletions of the 17q11.2 NF1 tumour suppressor region. J Med Genet 40: E116

[39] Kehrer-Sawatzki H, Kluwe L, Sandig C, Kohn M, Wimmer K, Krammer U, Peyrl A, Jenne DE, Hansmann I, Mautner VF (2004) High frequency of mosaicism among patients with neurofi-bromatosis type 1 (NF1) with microdeletions caused by somatic recombination of the *JJAZ1* gene. Am J Hum Genet 75: 410-423

[40] Kehrer-Sawatzki H, Kluwe L, Fünsterer C, Mautner VF (2005) Extensively high load of internal tumors determined by whole body MRI scanning in a patient with neurofibromatosis type 1 and a non-LCR-mediated 2-Mb deletion in 17q11.2. Hum Genet 116: 466-475

[41] Kehrer-Sawatzki H, Schmid E, Fünsterer C, Kluwe L, Mautner VF (2008) Absence of cutaneous neurofibromas in an NF1 patient with an atypical deletion partially overlapping the common 1.4 Mb microdeleted region. Am J Med Genet A 146A: 691-699

[42] Kidd JM, Graves T, Newman TL, Fulton R, Hayden HS, Malig M, Kallicki J, Kaul R, Wilson RK, Eichler EE (2010) A human genome structural variation sequencing resource reveals insights into mutational mechanisms. Cell 143: 837-847

[43] Kluwe L, Friedrich RE, Peiper M, Friedman J, Mautner VF (2003) Constitutional *NF1* mutations in neurofibromatosis 1 patients with malignant peripheral nerve sheath tumors. Hum Mutat 22: 420

[44] Kluwe L, Nguyen R, Vogt J, Bengesser K, Mussotter T, Friedrich RE, Jett K, Kehrer-Sawatzki H, Mautner V-F (2012) Internal tumour burden in neurofibromatosis 1 patients with large *NF1* deletions. Genes Chrom Cancer 51: 447-451

[45] Konkel MK, Batzer MA (2010) A mobile threat to genome stability: the impact of non-LTR retrotransposons upon the human genome. Semin Cancer Biol 20: 211-221

[46] Lee JA, Carvalho CMB, Lupski JR (2007) A DNA replication mechanism for generating nonre-current rearrangements associated with genomic disorders. Cell 131: 1235-1247

[47] Lindsay SJ, Khajavi M, Lupski JR, Hurles ME (2006) A chromosomal rearrangement hotspot can be identified from population genetic variation and is coincident with a hotspot for allelic recombination. Am J Hum Genet 79: 890-902

[48] Liu P, Erez A, Nagamani SC, Dhar SU, Kołodziejska KE, Dharmadhikari AV, Cooper ML, Wiszniewska J, Zhang F, Withers MA, Bacino CA, Campos-Acevedo LD, Delgado MR, Freedenberg D, Garnica A, Grebe TA, Hernández-Almaguer D, Immken L, Lalani SR, McLean SD, Northrup H, Scaglia F, Strathearn L, Trapane P, Kang SH, Patel A, Cheung SW, Hastings PJ, Stankiewicz P, Lupski JR, Bi W (2011) Chromosome catastrophes involve replication mechanisms generating complex genomic rearrangements. Cell 146: 889-903

[49] López-Correa C, Brems H, Lazaro C, Marynen P, Legius E (2000) Unequal meiotic crossover: a frequent cause of *NF1* microdeletions. Am J Hum Genet 66: 1969-1974

[50] López-Correa C, Dorschner M, Brems H, Lazaro C, Clementi M, Upadhyaya M, Dooijes D, Moog U, Kehrer-Sawatzki H, Rutkowski JL, Fryns JP, Marynen P, Stephens K, Legius E (2001) Recombination hotspot in NF1 microdeletion patients. Hum Mol Genet 10: 1387-1392

[51] Mantripragada KK, Thuresson AC, Piotrowski A, Díaz de Ståhl T, Menzel U, Grigelionis G, Ferner RE, Griffiths S, Bolund L, Mautner V, Nordling M, Legius E, Vetrie D, Dahl N, Messiaen L, Upadhyaya M, Bruder CE, Dumanski JP (2006) Identification of novel deletion breakpoints bordered by segmental duplications in the *NF1* locus using high resolution array-CGH. J Med Genet 43: 28-38

[52] Mao Z, Bozzella M, Seluanov A, Gorbunova V (2008) DNA

[53] Mautner VF, Kluwe L, Friedrich RE, Roehl AC, Bammert S, Högel J, Spöri H, Cooper DN, Kehrer-Sawatzki H (2010) Clinical characterisation of 29 neurofibromatosis type-1 patients with molecularly ascertained 1.4 Mb type-1 *NF1* deletions. J Med Genet 47: 623-630

[54] McVean GA, Myers SR, Hunt S, Deloukas P, Bentley DR, Donnelly P (2004) The fine-scale structure of recombination rate variation in the human genome. Science 304: 581-584

[55] Meaburn KJ, Misteli T (2007) Cell biology: chromosome territories. Nature 445: 379-781

[56] Mensink KA, Ketterling RP, Flynn HC, Knudson RA, Lindor NM, Heese BA, Spinner RJ, Babovic-Vuksanovic D (2006) Connective tissue dysplasia in five new patients with *NF1* microdeletions: further expansion of phenotype and review of the literature. J Med Genet 43: e8

[57] Messiaen L, Vogt J, Bengesser K, Fu C, Mikhail F, Serra E, Garcia-Linares C, Cooper DN, Lazaro C, Kehrer-Sawatzki H (2011) Mosaic type-1 *NF1* microdeletions as a cause of both generalized and segmental neurofibromatosis type-1 (NF1). Hum Mutat 32: 213-219

[58] Mills RE, Walter K, Stewart C, Handsaker RE, Chen K, Alkan C, Abyzov A, Yoon SC, Ye K, Cheetham RK, Chinwalla A, Conrad DF, Fu Y, Grubert F, Hajirasouliha I, Hormozdiari F, Iakoucheva LM, Iqbal Z, Kang S, Kidd JM, Konkel MK, Korn J, Khurana E, Kural D, Lam HY, Leng J, Li R, Li Y, Lin CY, Luo R, Mu XJ, Nemesh J, Peckham HE, Rausch T, Scally A, Shi X, Stromberg MP, Stütz AM, Urban AE, Walker JA, Wu J, Zhang Y, Zhang ZD, Batzer MA, Ding L, Marth GT, McVean G, Sebat J, Snyder M, Wang J, Ye K, Eichler EE, Gerstein MB, Hurles ME, Lee C, McCarroll SA, Korbel JO, 1000 Genomes Project (2011) Mapping copy number variation by population-scale genome sequencing. Nature 470: 59-65

[59] Myers S, Freeman C, Auton A, Donnelly P, McVean G (2008) A common sequence motif associated with recombination hot spots and genome instability in humans. Nat Genet 40: 1124-1129

[60] Neumann R, Lawson VE, Jeffreys AJ (2010) Dynamics and processes of copy number instability in human gamma-globin genes. Proc Natl Acad Sci USA 107: 8304-8309

[61] Oshiumi H, Matsumoto M, Hatakeyama S, Seya T (2009) Riplet/RNF135, a RING finger protein, ubiquitinates RIG-I to promote interferon-beta induction during the early phase of viral infection. J Biol Chem 284: 807-817

[62] Parvanov ED, Petkov PM, Paigen K (2010) Prdm9 controls activation of mammalian recombination hotspots. Science 327: 835

[63] Pasmant E, de Saint-Trivier A, Laurendeau I, Dieux-Coeslier A, Parfait B, Vidaud M, Vidaud D, Bièche I (2008) Characterization of a 7.6-Mb germline deletion encompassing the *NF1* locus and about a hundred genes in an NF1 contiguous gene syndrome patient. Eur J Hum Genet 16: 1459-1466

[64] Pasmant E, Sabbagh A, Masliah-Planchon J, Haddad V, Hamel MJ, Laurendeau I, Soulier J, Parfait B, Wolkenstein P, Bièche I, Vidaud M, Vidaud D (2009) Detection and characterization of *NF1* microdeletions by custom high resolution array CGH. J Mol Diagn 11: 524-529

[65] Pasmant E, Sabbagh A, Spurlock G, Laurendeau I, Grillo E, Hamel MJ, Martin L, Barbarot S, Leheup B, Rodriguez D, Lacombe D, Dollfus H, Pasquier L, Isidor B, Ferkal S, Soulier J, Sanson M, Dieux-Coeslier A, Bièche I, Parfait B, Vidaud M, Wolkenstein P, Upadhyaya M, Vidaud D, Members of the NF France Network (2010) *NF1* microdeletions in neurofibromatosis type 1: from genotype to phenotype. Hum Mutat 31: E1506-E1518

[66] Pasmant E, Masliah-Planchon J, Lévy P, Laurendeau I, Ortonne N, Parfait B, Valeyrie-Allanore L, Leroy K, Wolkenstein P, Vidaud M, Vidaud D, Bièche I (2011) Identification of genes potentially involved in the increased risk of malignancy in *NF1*-microdeleted patients. Mol Med 17: 79-87

[67] Petek E, Jenne DE, Smolle J, Binder B, Lasinger W, Windpassinger C, Wagner K, Kroisel PM, Kehrer-Sawatzki H (2003) Mitotic recombination mediated by the JJAZF1 (KIAA0160) gene causing somatic mosaicism and a new type of constitutional *NF1* microdeletion in two children of a mosaic female with only few manifestations. J Med Genet 40: 520-525

[68] Peters AD (2008) A combination of *cis* and *trans* control can solve the hotspot conversion paradox. Genetics 178: 1579-1593

[69] Reiter LT, Murakami T, Koeuth T, Pentao L, Muzny DM, Gibbs RA, Lupski JR (1996) A recombination hotspot responsible for two inherited peripheral neuropathies is located near a mariner transposon-like element. Nat Genet 12: 288-297

[70] Reiter LT, Hastings PJ, Nelis E, De Jonghe P, van Broeckhoven C, Lupski JR (1998) Human meiotic recombination products revealed by sequencing a hotspot for homologous strand exchange in multiple HNPP deletion patients. Am J Hum Genet 62: 1023-1033

[71] Riccardi VM (1992) Neurofibromatosis: phenotype, natural history and pathogenesis, 2nd edn. Johns Hopkins University Press, Baltimore, pp 142-153

[72] Riccardi VM (1999) Skeletal system. In: Friedman J, Gutmann D, MacCollin M, Riccardi VM (eds) Neurofibromatosis: phenotype, natural history and pathogenesis, 3rd edn. Johns Hopkins University Press, Baltimore, pp 250-255

[73] Riva P, Corrado L, Natacci F, Castorina P, Wu BL, Schneider GH, Clementi M, Tenconi R, Korf BR, Larizza L (2000) *NF1* microdeletion syndrome: refined FISH characterization of sporadic and familial deletions with locus-specific probes. Am J Hum Genet 66: 100-109

[74] Roehl AC, Vogt J, Mussotter T, Zickler AN, Spöri H, Högel J, Chuzhanova NA, Wimmer K, Kluwe L, Mautner VF, Cooper DN, Kehrer-Sawatzki H (2010) Intrachromosomal mitotic nonallelic homologous recombination is the major molecular mechanism underlying type-2 *NF1* deletions. Hum Mutat 31: 1163-1173

[75] Roehl AC, Mussotter T, Cooper DN, Kluwe L, Wimmer K, Högel J, Zetzmann M, Vogt J, Mautner VF, Kehrer-Sawatzki H (2012) Tissue-specific differences in the proportion of mosaic large *NF1* deletions are suggestive of a selective growth advantage of hematopoietic del(+/−) stem cells. Hum Mutat 33: 541-550

[76] Sachidanandam R, Weissman D, Schmidt SC, Kakol JM, Stein LD, Marth G, Sherry S, Mullikin JC, Mortimore BJ, Willey DL, Hunt SE, Cole CG, Coggill PC, Rice CM, Ning Z, Rogers J, Bentley DR, Kwok PY, Mardis ER, Yeh RT, Schultz B, Cook L, Davenport R, Dante M, Fulton L, Hillier L, Waterston RH, McPherson JD, Gilman B, Schaffner S,

Van Etten WJ, Reich D, Higgins J, Daly MJ, Blumenstiel B, Baldwin J, Stange-Thomann N, Zody MC, Linton L, Lander ES, Altshuler D, International SNP, Group MW (2001) A map of human genome sequence variation containing 1.42 million single nucleotide polymorphisms. Nature 409: 928–933

[77] Sasaki M, Lange J, Keeney S (2010) Genome destabilization by homologous recombination in the germ line. Nat Rev Mol Cell Biol 11: 182–195

[78] Spiegel M, Oexle K, Horn D, Windt E, Buske A, Albrecht B, Prott EC, Seemanova E, Seidel J, Rosenbaum T, Jenne D, Kehrer-Sawatzki H, Tinschert S (2005) Childhood overgrowth in patients with common NF1 microdeletions. Eur J Hum Genet 13: 883–888

[79] Stankiewicz P, Lupski JR (2010) Structural variation in the human genome and its role in disease. Ann Rev Med 61: 437–455

[80] Steinmann K, Cooper DN, Kluwe L, Chuzhanova NA, Senger C, Serra E, Lazaro C, Gilaberte M, Wimmer K, Mautner VF, Kehrer-Sawatzki H (2007) Type 2 NF1 deletions are highly unusual by virtue of the absence of nonallelic homologous recombination hotspots and an apparent preference for female mitotic recombination. Am J Hum Genet 81: 1201–1220

[81] Steinmann K, Kluwe L, Cooper DN, Brems H, De Raedt T, Legius E, Mautner VF, Kehrer-Sawatzki H (2008) Copy number variations in the NF1 gene region are infrequent and do not predispose to recurrent type-1 deletions. Eur J Hum Genet 16: 572–580

[82] Steinmann K, Kluwe L, Friedrich RE, Mautner VF, Cooper DN, Kehrer-Sawatzki H (2009) Mechanisms of loss of heterozygosity in neurofibromatosis type 1-associated plexiform neurofibromas. J Invest Dermatol 129: 615–621

[83] Szostak JW, Orr-Weaver TL, Rothstein RJ, Stahl FW (1983) The double-strand-break repair model for recombination. Cell 33: 25–35

[84] Tonsgard JH, Yelavarthi KK, Cushner S, Short MP, Lindgren V (1997) Do NF1 gene deletions result in a characteristic phenotype? Am J Med Genet 73: 80–86

[85] Turner DJ, Miretti M, Rajan D, Fiegler H, Carter NP, Blayney ML, Beck S, Hurles ME (2008) Germline rates of de novo meiotic deletions and duplications causing several genomic disorders. Nat Genet 40: 90–95

[86] Ubeda F, Wilkins JF (2011) The Red Queen theory of recombination hotspots. J Evol Biol 24: 541–553

[87] Upadhyaya M, Roberts SH, Maynard J, Sorour E, Thompson PW, Vaughan M, Wilkie AO, Hughes HE (1996) A cytogenetic deletion, del(17)(q11.22q21.1), in a patient with sporadic neurofibromatosis type 1 (NF1) associated with dysmorphism and developmental delay. J Med Genet 33: 148–152

[88] Upadhyaya M, Ruggieri M, Maynard J, Osborn M, Hartog C, Mudd S, Penttinen M, Cordeiro I, Ponder M, Ponder BA, Krawczak M, Cooper DN (1998) Gross deletions of the neurofibromatosis type 1 (NF1) gene are predominantly of maternal origin and commonly associated with a learning disability, dysmorphic features and developmental delay. Hum Genet 102: 591–597

[89] Venturin M, Gervasini C, Orzan F, Bentivegna A, Corrado L, Colapietro P, Friso A, Tenconi R, Upadhyaya M, Larizza L, Riva P (2004a) Evidence for non-homologous end joining and nonallelic homologous recombination in atypical NF1 microdeletions. Hum Genet 115: 69–680

[90] Venturin M, Guarnieri P, Natacci F, Stabile M, Tenconi R, Clementi M, Hernandez C, Thompson P, Upadhyaya M, Larizza L, Riva P (2004b) Mental retardation and cardiovascular malformations in NF1 microdeleted patients point to candidate genes in 17q11.2. J Med Genet 41: 35–41

[91] Visser R, Shimokawa O, Harada N, Kinoshita A, Ohta T, Niikawa N, Matsumoto N (2005) Identification of a 3.0-kb major recombination hotspot in patients with Sotos syndrome who carry a common 1.9-Mb microdeletion. Am J Hum Genet 76: 52–67

[92] Vissers LE, Bhatt SS, Janssen IM, Xia Z, Lalani SR, Pfundt R, Derwinska K, deVries BB, Gilissen C, Hoischen A, Nesteruk M, Wisniowiecka-Kowalnik B, Smyk M, Brunner HG, Cheung SW, van Kessel AG, Veltman JA, Stankiewicz P (2009) Rare pathogenic microdeletions and tandem duplications are microhomology-mediated and stimulated by local genomic architecture. Hum Mol Genet 18: 3579–3593

[93] Vogel F, Motulsky AG (1996) Human genetics: problems and approaches. Springer, Berlin Vogt J, Nguyen R, Kluwe L, Roehl AC, Mussotter T, Cooper DN, Mautner VF, Kehrer-Sawatzki H, Schuhmann M (2011) Delineation of the clinical phenotype associated with non-mosaic type-2 NF1 deletions: two case reports. J Med Case Rep 5: 577

[94] Webb AJ, Berg IL, Jeffreys A (2008) Sperm cross-over activity in regions of the human genome showing extreme breakdown of marker association. Proc Natl Acad Sci USA 105: 10471–10476

[95] Wu BL, Austin MA, Schneider GH, Boles RG, Korf BR (1995) Deletion of the entire NF1 gene detected by the FISH: four deletion patients associated with severe manifestations. Am J Med Genet 59: 528–535

[96] Wu R, López-Correa C, Rutkowski JL, Baumbach LL, Glover TW, Legius E (1999) Germline mutations in NF1 patients with malignancies. Genes Chromosomes Cancer 26: 376–380

[97] Youssoufian H, Pyeritz RE (2002) Mechanisms and consequences of somatic mosaicism in humans. Nat Rev Genet 3: 748–758

[98] Zhang F, Khajavi M, Connolly AM, Towne CF, Batish SD, Lupski JR (2009a) The DNA replication FoSTeS/MMBIR mechanism can generate genomic, genic and exonic complex rearrangements in humans. Nat Genet 41: 849–853

[99] Zhang F, Carvalho CM, Lupski JR (2009b) Complex human chromosomal and genomic rearrangements. Trends Genet 25: 298–307

[100] Zhang F, Seeman P, Liu P, Weterman MA, Gonzaga-Jauregui C, Towne CF, Batish SD, De Vriendt E, De Jonghe P, Rautenstrauss B, Krause KH, Khajavi M, Posadka J, Vandenberghe A, Palau F, Van Maldergem L, Baas F, Timmerman V, Lupski JR (2010) Mechanisms for nonrecurrent genomic rearrangements associated with CMT1A or HNPP: rare CNVs as a cause for missing heritability. Am J Hum Genet 86: 892–903

[101] Zheng J, Khil PP, Camerini-Otero RD, Przytycka TM (2010) Detecting sequence polymorphisms associated with meiotic recombination hotspots in the human genome. Genome Biol 11: R103

[102] Zickler AM, Hampp S, Messiaen L, Bengesser K, Mussotter T, Roehl AC, Wimmer K, Mautner VF, Kluwe L, Upadhyaya M, Pasmant E, Chuzhanova N, Kestler HA, Högel J, Legius E, Claes K, Cooper DN, Kehrer-Sawatzki H (2012) Characterization of the nonallelic homologous recombination hotspot PRS3 associated with type-3 NF1 deletions. Hum Mutat 33: 372–383

第15章 NF1 基因的体细胞突变谱
The Somatic Mutational Spectrum of the NF1 Gene

Meena Upadhyaya, Nadia Chuzhanova, and David N. Cooper

15.1 引言

1型神经纤维瘤病（neurofibromatosis type 1，NF1）是一种常见并具有多种肿瘤易感性的常染色体显性遗传综合征，在全球范围内，每3 000人至4 000人中就有1人患病（Huson et al. 1988；Lammert et al. 2005）。NF1的临床症状多样，典型临床特征包括皮肤的异常色素沉着（如咖啡牛奶斑和腹股沟或腋窝雀斑）、虹膜错构瘤（Lisch结节）以及位于皮肤的良性周围神经鞘膜瘤（神经纤维瘤）。神经纤维瘤呈现出多种不同的亚型，并与各种不同的临床并发症相关。几乎所有NF1成年患者身上都会出现皮肤型神经纤维瘤（Upadhyaya et al. 2007）。另外，30%～50%的NF1患者会进展为一种弥漫性更强的肿瘤——丛状神经纤维瘤（plexiform neurofibroma，PNF），然而这些良性的肿瘤中有10%～15%会向恶性周围神经鞘膜瘤（malignant peripheral nerve sheath tumour，MPNST）转归，这也是NF1患者主要的疾病负担来源（Walker et al. 2006；Bennett et al. 2009；Upadhyaya 2011）。

癌症的形成标志着细胞从正常受到严格控制的增长转变为失去严格调控的状态，从而使得癌细胞增殖不受控制甚至发生转移。这种在细胞调控上的巨大变化是遗传和表观遗传共同调控的结果。激活的癌基因会因"功能增益"的突变而促进细胞生长，而肿瘤抑癌基因（tumour suppressor gene，TSG）则是通过"功能缺失"的突变促使细胞增殖。这些抑癌基因通常负责编码蛋白质，并进一步参与癌细胞的生长调节、凋亡启动、细胞黏附和DNA修复。根据Knudson的"二次打击"学说，1个抑癌基因的2个等位基因必须同时失活，细胞才会发生转化（Knudson 1971；Stratton 2011；Pao and Girard 2011）。一般来说，患者会遗传1个带有抑癌基因突变的等位基因；随后，受精后会发生体细胞第二次突变，导致剩余的正常等位基因失活。因此，与抑癌基因失活相关的癌症中，体细胞突变十分关键。通过全面分析肿瘤基因组，我们可以发现许多体细胞基因突变和表观遗传变化。但值得注意的是，并非每个肿瘤中的所有体细胞突变都与肿瘤形成有关，只有一部分真正起到了促进作用。反复出现的突变更可能直接导致癌症（驱动突变），而与之相反，癌症基

Some of the unpublished mutations in Supplementary Table 2 of Laycock-van Spyk et al. (2011) have now been published by Thomas et al. (2012a, b).

M. Upadhyaya (*) • D. N. Cooper
Institute of Medical Genetics, School of Medicine, Cardiff University, Cardiff, UK
e-mail: upadhyaya@cardiff.ac.uk

N. Chuzhanova
School of Science and Technology, Nottingham Trent University, Nottingham, UK

M. Upadhyaya and D. N. Cooper (eds.), *Neurofibromatosis Type 1*,
DOI 10.1007/978-3-642-32864-0_15, # Springer-Verlag Berlin Heidelberg 2012

因组中的大部分体细胞出现的突变（"过客"突变）可能并没有重要的病理意义（Ivanov et al. 2011；Stratton 2011；Pao and Girard 2011）。

1型神经纤维瘤病基因（NF1）位于17q11.2染色体上（Ballester et al. 1990），横跨283 kb的基因组DNA，并包含61个外显子（Upadhyaya et al. 2007；Upadhyaya 2008）。NF1基因的产物，神经纤维瘤蛋白，是活化的信号通路Ras及其相关Ras促分裂原活化激酶（Ras/MAPK）的负调控因子。NF1是一种抑癌基因，这意味着由它引起的任何肿瘤都必须经历第二次的体细胞突变，这次突变使得正常的NF1等位基因失活，导致神经纤维瘤蛋白的功能完全缺失。因此，这种双重突变（$NF1^{-/-}$）对NF1肿瘤形成是至关重要的（Sawada et al. 1996）。与NF1相关的肿瘤包括多种良性和恶性肿瘤，它们很可能都源自神经嵴细胞的肿瘤发生（Carroll and Ratner 2008）。几种小鼠模型成功地再现了NF1在人类中的多种临床表型，并证实NF1确实是一种典型的抑癌基因（Cichowski et al. 1999；Cichowski and Jacks 2001）。然而，为何只有少部分良性肿瘤最终会演变为恶性肿瘤，这个问题仍然是未知的。与此同时，最近的癌症基因组测序研究显示，体细胞NF1基因的突变不仅发生在NF1相关的肿瘤中，还出现在很多不与NF1相关的常见肿瘤中（Parsons et al. 2008；Ding et al. 2008；Sangha et al. 2008；Brennan et al. 2009；McGillicuddy et al. 2009；Haferlach et al. 2010；Holzel et al. 2010）。

在NF1疾病中，很少能发现明确的基因型与表型之间的相关性，常见的是在家族中不同成员之间的临床表现差异很大（Easton et al. 1993；Upadhyaya 2010）。这种家庭内部成员间的表型差异突显了第二次基因突变的重要性，因为体细胞NF1突变的类型和发生时间的不同，可能有助于解释患者出现不同表型的原因（Kehrer-Sawatzki and Cooper 2008）。因此，对NF1相关肿瘤中体细胞突变谱系的认识，是理解其涉及分子途径的关键所在，这对于改进临床治疗方案和开发新的治疗方法至关重要。在此，我们将回顾迄今为止在NF1相关肿瘤中报道的体细胞NF1突变情况，以评估这些突变如何促进肿瘤生长，以及是否能够找到任何与基因型表型相关的联系。

15.2 NF1相关肿瘤

15.2.1 皮肤型神经纤维瘤

周围良性神经鞘膜瘤（即神经纤维瘤）是NF1的典型临床表现之一。这些起源于皮肤感觉神经的肿瘤被称为真皮神经纤维瘤或皮肤型神经纤维瘤，它们通常表现为与单一神经末梢相关的单个瘤体。皮肤型神经纤维瘤内表现出广泛的细胞异质性，包含了增殖活跃的施万细胞（Schwann cells，SC）、成纤维细胞、肥大细胞和周围神经细胞。施万细胞被认为是神经纤维瘤中的初始细胞类型，并且NF1基因的双等位基因失活仅在这些细胞中发生。施万细胞还是已知能刺激神经纤维瘤形成和生长的多种生长因子的靶细胞。

皮肤型神经纤维瘤的形成可能来源于皮肤前体细胞（Le et al. 2009），这些细胞具备类似神经嵴的特征，并且很可能受到激素的调控，因为大部分此类肿瘤主要在青春期开始发展（McLaughlin and Jacks 2003）。此外，妊娠期间肿瘤的大小和数量有所增加，也有证据表明在产后肿瘤的大小会有所减小（Dugoff and Sujansky 1996；Roth et al. 2008）。

20%~50%的皮肤型神经纤维瘤在NF1基因位置表现出杂合性缺失（loss of heterozygosity，LOH），而这些病变中的大部分是由于细胞分裂时的遗传重组所致（Eisenbarth et al. 2000；Serra et al. 2001；Wiest et al. 2003；Upadhyaya et al. 2004；Spurlock et al. 2007；Thomas et al. 2010；Garcia-Linares et al. 2011）。研究人员发现，将皮肤型神经纤维瘤中体细胞NF1突变的不同类型进行比较，与之前报告的胚系对应基因突变的相对频率存在显著差异（$P=0.001$）（Thomas et al. 2012a）。更详细的内容可以参见第26章。

15.2.2 丛状神经纤维瘤

与皮肤内较大神经相连的肿瘤可能会在真皮层内扩散，形成弥漫性肿块。丛状神经纤维瘤（plexiform

neurofibromas，PNF)是体积较大的肿瘤,通常与主干神经和神经丛有关;其生长速度缓慢,可位于体内或体外器官,并导致严重毁容。30%~50%的NF1患者会出现PNF,尽管PNF通常是良性的,但其生长可能导致神经损伤的发生。10%~15%的PNF可能转变成为恶性肿瘤(Evans et al. 2002)。

虽然神经纤维瘤的遗传基础尚未完全明确,但由于所有肿瘤细胞都同时存在体细胞 NF1 基因突变,所以双等位基因 NF1 失活可能是必要条件(Upadhyaya 2010)。丛状神经纤维瘤的细胞组成与皮肤型神经纤维瘤相似。大约70%的丛状神经纤维瘤在 NF1 位点被报道存在 LOH(John et al. 2000；Upadhyaya et al. 2008b)。然而,NF1 患者胚系 NF1 基因突变的类型或位置,与其肿瘤中体细胞相对应的基因突变类型或位点的表现形式上并无明显的关联(Upadhyaya et al. 2008b)。尽管施万细胞中的 NF1 基因出现失活的情况,但非肿瘤细胞仍然参与肿瘤的发展。在丛状神经纤维瘤的小鼠模型中,NF1 单倍体不足的肥大细胞会促进炎症并加速肿瘤的形成和生长(Staser et al. 2012)。因此,阐明在双等位基因失活的 NF1 基因初始细胞类型中,单倍体不足的情况下,肿瘤微环境的具体分子间的作用机制,是理解神经纤维瘤形成的关键所在。

丛状神经纤维瘤产生于施万细胞分化的确切阶段仍有争议。目前认为丛状神经纤维瘤是先天性的,因此,神经嵴干细胞或其他祖细胞可能在胚胎发育过程中导致这些肿瘤,尽管有研究指出,有 NF1 缺陷的胎儿神经嵴干细胞无法直接形成丛状神经纤维瘤(Joseph et al. 2008；Carroll and Ratner 2008)。不同小鼠肿瘤模型的研究表明,分化的胶质细胞包括成熟的非髓鞘施万细胞(即 Remak 束)可能是肿瘤的起源细胞(Zheng et al. 2008；Yang et al. 2008；Zhu et al. 2002；Joseph et al. 2008；reviewed by Staser et al. 2012)。Wu 等(2008)的研究表明,在胚胎发育大约第12.5天,即使在微环境中存在野生型细胞,通过 NF1(flox/flox);DhhCre 小鼠模型驱动的胶质前体细胞的广泛缺失,也能导致丛状神经纤维瘤的发生。

一个有趣但无法解释的现象是,一些轻型 NF1 患者从未出现任何皮肤或丛状神经纤维瘤,但他们却携带相同的胚系 NF1 突变(c. 2970-2972delAAT),即丧失一个甲硫氨酸残基的框内3个碱基缺失(Upadhyaya et al. 2007)(详见第36章)。

15.2.3 恶性周围神经鞘膜瘤

10%~15%的丛状神经纤维瘤细胞最终可能会恶变为恶性周围神经鞘膜瘤(MPNST)。MPNST是一种侵袭性很强的软组织肉瘤,在 NF1 患者中的年发病率为0.16%,而正常人群中仅为0.001%(Ducatman et al. 1986),NF1 患者的终生发病风险为8%~13%(Evans et al. 2002；McCaughan et al. 2007；由 Upadhyaya 2011 综述)。这种恶性肿瘤是 NF1 患者主要的发病和死亡原因。这种恶变通常起源于已有的丛状神经纤维瘤或非典型神经纤维瘤(Spurlock et al. 2010；Beert et al. 2011)。通过非侵入性^{18}F-2-氟-2-脱氧-D-葡萄糖正电子发射断层扫描(^{18}F-2-fluoro-2-deoxy-D-glucose positron emission tomography，FDG-PET)可以较准确地鉴别良性 PNF 和 MPNST,且具有一定灵敏性(Benz et al. 2010),这证明 FDG-PET 非侵入性成像在未来诊断中的潜在作用。非典型神经纤维瘤的症状包括高密度细胞组成的周围神经鞘膜瘤,是由缺乏有丝分裂的高染色质细胞核的细胞组成。Beert 等(2011)最近的一项研究显示,非典型神经纤维瘤是癌前病变肿瘤,CDKN2A/2B 缺失是其向 MPNST 发展的第一步。作者在一个瘤体组织中观察到从良性-非典型神经纤维瘤向中度级别 MPNST 的明确转变,并在组织病理学和阵列 CGH 分析中验证这一转变。导致这种恶性转化的异常分子途径在很大程度上仍不清楚,研究人员正在努力探究其中涉及的分子缺陷。

携带大片段(通常为1.4 Mb)基因组缺失的 NF1 患者(该缺失不仅删除了整个 NF1 基因,还包括若干侧翼基因)在某些群体中更易发展为 MPNST(De Raedt et al. 2003；Upadhyaya et al. 2006)。事实上,超过90%的 MPNST 被发现有大片段 NF1 体细胞缺失(Upadhyaya et al. 2008a)。最近的研究还指出,已确证携带的1型1.4 Mb NF1 缺失的患者,其丛状神经纤维瘤、皮下神经纤维瘤、脊柱神经纤维瘤和 MPNST 的发生率显著高于普通 NF1 人群（Mautner et al. 2010）。与 MPNST 相关的缺失断点，并未发现涉及大多数体系 NF1 缺失的同源重复序列（Kehrer-Sawatzki 2008）。然而，体细胞缺失最小的共同重叠区域却在约 2.2 Mb 的区间内，该区间包含了大部分在复发性 NF1 常染色体缺失中被删除的基因（Pasmant et al. 2010）。

虽然双等位 NF1 基因失活是肿瘤转化的必要条件，但单靠 NF1 位点的突变不足以解释肿瘤发生的过程，因为大多数良性神经纤维瘤也有这种双等位 NF1 失活。其他位点参与的最佳证据与 TP53 基因有关，该基因的多种不同突变已在恶性周围神经鞘膜瘤（MPNST）中发现，但在良性神经纤维瘤中尚未发现类似突变（Menon et al. 1990; Legius et al. 1994; Upadhyaya et al. 2008a; Upadhyaya 2011）。携带 Nf1 和 Tp53 基因杂合突变的小鼠会向恶性肿瘤转归（Cichowski et al. 1999; Vogel et al. 1999），这可能表明 Tp53 的缺失是转化的关键。编码 p16INK4A 和 p14ARF 的 CDKN2A 基因纯合缺失也与 NF1 相关的恶性肿瘤有关（Kourea et al. 1999; Mantripragada et al. 2008; Nielsen et al. 1999）。PTEN 基因的拷贝数变化和（或）PI3K/AKT 通路的激活可能是 NF1 恶性转化的限制性条件（Gregorian et al. 2009）。然而，目前尚未确定与 MPNST 发展相关的特异性基因表达特征，尽管多个细胞周期和信号调控基因（CDKN2A、TP53、RB1、EGFR、CD44、PDGFRA、HGF、MET 和 SOX9）经常表现出失调。

这些恶性肿瘤中的突变异质性增加了发病机制的探索难度。我们选取了 10 名无亲属关系 NF1 患者中 10 个 MPNST 切片，分析 NF1、TP53、RB1、PTEN 和 CDKN2A 基因杂合性丧失（loss of heterozygosity, LOH）的分子异质性（Thomas et al. 2012b; Gerlinger et al. 2012）。结果显示，TP53 基因的 LOH 数据与同一肿瘤切片中的 p53 免疫组织化学分析结果相关（Thomas et al. 2012b）。此外，大约 70% 的 MPNST 显示出肿瘤内的分子异质性，同一肿瘤样本不同切片之间 LOH 水平的差异证实了这一结果（Thomas et al. 2012a, b）。这项研究首次系统分析了 NF1 患者的 MPNST 内分子异质性。因此，了解 NF1 相关肿瘤中存在的分子异质性，不仅对体细胞突变检测的优化很关键，而且对理解 NF1 肿瘤发生的机制也很重要，这是开发特异性靶向癌症治疗药物的前提条件（详见第 29 章和第 38 章）。

15.2.4 脊柱神经纤维瘤

大约 40% 的 NF1 患者会出现脊神经的肿瘤。这在家族性脊柱神经纤维瘤（familial spinal neurofibromatosis, FSNF）的患者中尤为明显，涉及多个脊神经根的双侧肿瘤往往是这些 NF1 患者的唯一表现。一部分 NF1 患者有 FSNF，表现为多发性双侧脊柱肿瘤，但其他临床特征少见，这是 NF1 特有的变异形式（Pulst et al. 1991; Poyhonen et al. 1997; Ars et al. 1998）。与经典 NF1 患者相比，FSNF 患者更有可能携带胚系错义或剪接位点突变（Upadhyaya et al. 2009）。最近的一项研究发现，对 22 个脊柱肿瘤进行分析，其中 8 个出现 LOH，大多数（75%）是由于有丝分裂重组而非基因组缺失（Upadhyaya et al. 2009）。

15.2.5 低级别毛细胞型星形细胞瘤

大约 15% 的儿童 NF1 患者会出现低级别毛细胞型星形细胞瘤（Listernick et al. 1994）。这些良性肿瘤累及视觉通路（视神经胶质瘤）或大脑的其他区域，并伴有神经纤维瘤蛋白的完全丧失（Gutmann et al. 2003）。NF1 相关的视神经胶质瘤（optic pathway gliomas, OPG）主要发生在幼儿期。然而，仅有约 5% 的患者有症状。关于视觉筛查在检测 NF1 相关视神经胶质瘤中的作用和性质尚存争议，而认知障碍的存在常常使儿童在视觉测试中难以配合。从临床和放射学角度都很难确定哪些肿瘤会更具侵袭性，因此需要进行干预。在最近的一项研究中，Sharif 等（2011）确诊了 80 名 NF1 OPG 患者，并对其中的 29 名患者进行了分子分析。结果显示，NF1 基因 5′端 1/3 区域有病理性突变的簇集。作者将这些结果结合另外两个 NF1 OPG 队列的结果，总体上发现了相同的趋势。因此，与未患视神经胶质瘤（OPG）的 NF1 患者相比，OPG 的 NF1 患者的突变显然更集中于 NF1 基因的 5′端，这似乎是

NF1 患者中突变的一个真实特征(基因 5′1/3 处的突变,$OR=6.05$,$P=0.003$)。

NF1 表达缺失是 NF1 相关毛细胞型星形细胞瘤发病机制中的一个重要原发性遗传事件。LOH 和 NF1 失活在早发和晚发的 NF1 相关毛细胞型星形细胞瘤中均被发现(Gutmann et al. 2000;2003)(详见第 22 章)。

15.2.6 胃肠道间质瘤

胃肠道间质瘤(gastrointestinal stromal tumour,GIST)是胃肠道中最常见的间叶性肿瘤。尽管大多数 GIST 携带 KIT 和 PDGFRA 的活化体细胞突变,但 NF1 相关 GIST(NF1‐associated GIST,NF1‐GIST)中未检测到此类突变可能表明其具有不同的致病机制。在 NF1 患者中,大多数(60%)GIST 发生在小肠,而散发性非 NF1 GIST 通常发生在胃部(Miettinen et al. 2006)。

在胃肠道的间质细胞(interstitial cells of Cajal,ICC)以及缺乏 KIT 或 PDGRA 突变的 NF1‐GIST 中已鉴定出体细胞 NF1 突变。与散发性 GIST 不同,NF1‐GIST 中 Ras/MAPK 通路的信号转导增加。这表明,在 c‐KIT 和 PDGFRA 表达水平正常的情况下,神经纤维瘤蛋白水平的下降会导致肿瘤形成。这也表明 NF1 单倍体不足是 ICC 增生所必需的,再次证明尽管体细胞 NF1 突变是肿瘤发生的必要条件,但它本身不足以导致肿瘤,还需要额外的遗传因素。这些观察结果与 Knudson 的"二次打击"学说一致。通过基因缺失、基因内缺失以及通过有丝分裂重组的 LOH 导致的 NF1 基因体细胞失活也有报道(Maertens et al. 2006;Stewart et al. 2007b)。

15.2.7 胃癌

胃类癌肿瘤与多发性内分泌肿瘤、萎缩性胃炎和恶性贫血相关,但在 NF1 患者中非常罕见。在 1 例来自 NF1 患者的胃类癌肿瘤中已检测到 NF1 位点的 LOH(Stewart et al. 2007a)。

15.2.8 幼年型粒单核细胞白血病

年轻的 NF1 特别容易患上幼年型粒单核细胞白血病(juvenile myelomonocytic leukaemia,JMML)(Stiller et al. 1994),这是一种克隆性造血疾病,其特征是对粒细胞-巨噬细胞集落刺激因子(granulocyte-macrophage colony-stimulating factor,GM‐CSF)的高度敏感性(至少在体外)。此外,15%~20% 的 JMML 患者携带体细胞 NF1 失活,尽管大多数患者没有表现出其他 NF1 症状(Flotho et al. 2007)。患者还可能携带其他基因的失活突变,最近的一项研究发现 70%~80% 的突变涉及 Ras/MAPK 通路中的基因,包括 PTPN11、NRAS 和 KRAS 以及 NF1(Yoshimi et al. 2010)。此外,CBL 和 ASXL1 中也有体细胞突变的报道(Sugimoto et al. 2009)。在大多数情况下,NF1 基因通过 LOH 或复合杂合微缺失(Steinemann et al. 2010)出现缺失,导致神经纤维瘤蛋白的完全丧失和 Ras/MAPK 通路信号转导的过度活跃。LOH 可能通过低拷贝数重复(low copy number repeat,LCR)元件介导的 1.2~1.4 Mb 间质缺失发生,这些元件位于 NF1 基因的两侧(Chen et al. 2010)。也有报道称,在一个未知的启动细胞中,通过双重有丝分裂重组导致 17 号染色体单亲间质异位(50~52.7 Mb),从而出现 LOH(Steinemann et al. 2010)。这种罕见的现象可能表明,$NF1^{-/-}$ 细胞具有选择性优势,这可以解释为什么 NF1 患者有患白血病的倾向(Stephens et al. 2006)。不同组织中镶嵌型大型 NF1 第 2 缺失比例,提示造血 $del^{(+/-)}$ 干细胞有选择性生长优势(Roehl et al. 2012)(详见第 30 章)。

15.2.9 神经母细胞瘤

神经母细胞瘤是一种起源于交感神经系统中神经嵴细胞的神经内分泌肿瘤。大多数此类肿瘤发生在腹部。神经母细胞瘤与 NF1 的关联非常罕见(Kushner et al. 1985)。在神经母细胞瘤细胞系和原发性肿瘤中已经发现了 NF1 基因的体细胞突变,但这并不会导致 Ras‐GTP 的表达水平提高(The et al. 1993;Hölzel et al. 2010)。

15.2.10 嗜铬细胞瘤

嗜铬细胞瘤(phaeochromocytomas,PC)是极为罕见的肿瘤,每百万个体中仅观察到 1~6 例。

PC由神经嵴衍生的嗜铬细胞发展而来，肿瘤细胞产生并释放儿茶酚胺，导致高血压和潮红。这些肿瘤位于肾上腺髓质，主要与 *RET*、*VHL*、*SDHB*、*SDHC* 和 *SDHD* 基因的突变相关，尽管在 *NF1* 区域（以及 17q 和 17p 上的其他位点）也发现了 LOH。大约 3% 的 NF1 患者会发生嗜铬细胞瘤。已经有报道指出几例 NF1 相关嗜铬细胞瘤中有神经纤维瘤蛋白表达缺失和 LOH（Gutmann et al. 1994, 1995; Bausch et al. 2007）。在另一项研究中，NF1 相关嗜铬细胞瘤中已报告了 LOH 和拷贝数中性 LOH（Burnichon et al. 2011）。这些肿瘤中 *NF1* 位点周围的频繁 LOH 和神经纤维瘤蛋白表达缺失表明 *NF1* 基因突变促成了 NF1 患者肾上腺肿瘤的发展（详见第 25 章）。

15.2.11 血管球瘤

血管球瘤是体积较小（<5 mm）的良性肿瘤，但通常非常痛，特异性地在每个指端的高度神经支配的球状体内发展。这些肿瘤似乎是由双等位基因 *NF1* 失活的 α-平滑肌肌动蛋白阳性细胞发展而来，导致 Ras/MAPK 活性增加（Brems et al. 2009）。血管球瘤中的体细胞 *NF1* 突变常常各不相同，表明存在高度特异性的致瘤事件。Brems et al. (2009) 建议，尽管血管球瘤罕见，但现在应将其视为 NF1 疾病谱系的一个组成部分（详见第 24 章）。

15.2.12 横纹肌肉瘤

横纹肌肉瘤发生在儿童期，是儿童中最常见的软组织肉瘤。与 NF1 相关的横纹肌肉瘤发病率约为普通人群的 20 倍（0.02%～0.03%）（Friedman et al. 2002）。在 NF1 儿童中，横纹肌肉瘤往往发生在膀胱和前列腺（Sung et al. 2004; Bien et al. 2007）。目前尚无关于横纹肌肉瘤中 *NF1* 体细胞突变的数据。

15.2.13 乳腺癌

有报告称女性 NF1 患者的乳腺癌风险增加（Sharif et al. 2007）。50 岁以下 NF1 女性患乳腺癌的终生风险为 8.4%，约为普通人群累积风险的 4 倍。在一项基于芯片的研究中，Lee 等（2010）报告了乳腺恶性叶状肿瘤中 *NF1* 位点的拷贝数丢失。然而，迄今为止尚未在 NF1 相关的乳腺癌中发现 *NF1* 体细胞突变，除了在 1 例 NF1 相关的乳腺肿瘤中观察到了 LOH（Upadhyaya et al. 未发表）。

15.3 与 DNA 错配修复缺陷有关的 NF1 样特征

在少数具有 DNA 错配修复（mismatch repair, MMR）缺陷的家庭中，有一些罕见的受影响个体，这些个体具有涉及 *MLH1*、*MSH2*、*MSH6* 或 *PMS2* 基因的双等位（纯合或复合杂合）MMR 突变或更复杂的杂合 MMR 突变组合，可能具有若干 NF1 样特征，通常表现为咖啡牛奶斑和皮肤皱褶雀斑，有时偶尔会有少数皮肤型神经纤维瘤。这些个体及其具有相同双等位基因错配修复基因突变的受累兄弟姐妹，通常有未受影响的父母，并可能出现一些满足 NF1 诊断标准的大面积牛奶咖啡斑，尽管迄今尚未报告任何生殖系 *NF1* 基因突变（Wimmer and Etzler 2008; Bandipalliam 2005）。

15.4 NF1 相关肿瘤的体细胞突变谱

为了更好地理解 NF1 肿瘤的发生，对所有已发表和许多未发表（来自我们自己实验室）的与 NF1 肿瘤相关的体细胞 *NF1* 变异进行了荟萃分析（Laycock-van Spyk et al. 2011）。截至 2011 年 11 月，在不同的 NF1 相关肿瘤中报告了大约 600 种不同的体细胞 *NF1* 基因变化，其中超过一半与 LOH 相呼应（Laycock-van Spyk et al. 2011）。检测到的 LOH 水平在皮肤型神经纤维瘤、PNF 和 MPNST 中分别为 40%、79% 和 85%（表 15.1）。78%（28/36）的皮肤型神经纤维瘤、44%（11/25）的 PNF 和 16%（5/31）的 MPNST 表现出由有丝分裂重组引起的 LOH。79%（15/19）表现出 LOH 的 JMML 样本似乎通过有丝分裂重组，导致整个 17q 臂丢失，这表明可能与这种肿瘤类型存在显著的相关性。

表 15.1　(a) 不同 NF1 相关肿瘤中体细胞 *NF1* 微缺失的类型。(b) 不同 NF1 相关肿瘤中体细胞 *NF1* 微缺失的百分比分布

(a)

肿瘤类型	突变类型							
	缺失	插入	插入缺失	无义突变	剪接位点	错义突变	截短	总和
皮肤型神经纤维瘤	82	15	2	59	32	21	158	211
丛状神经纤维瘤	6	1	—	7	2	2	14	18
脊柱神经纤维瘤	—	—	—	—	2	1	0	3
恶性周围神经鞘膜瘤	7	1	1	1	—		10	10
胃肠道间质瘤	1	—		3	1		4	5
幼年型粒单核细胞白血病	a	a	a	1		a	1	1
血管球瘤	2	1		1	2		4	6
总和	98	18	3	72	39	24	191	254

(b)

肿瘤类型	突变类型(%)							
	缺失	插入	插入缺失	无义突变	剪接位点	错义突变	截短	总和
皮肤型神经纤维瘤	38.9	7.1	0.9	28.0	15.2	10.0	75	211
丛状神经纤维瘤	33.3	5.5	—	38.9	11.1	11.1	78	18
脊柱神经纤维瘤	—	—	—	—	66.6	33.3	0	3
恶性周围神经鞘膜瘤	70	10	10	10	—		100	10
胃肠道间质瘤	20	—		60	20		80	5
幼年型粒单核细胞白血病	a	a	a	100	a	a	100	1
血管球瘤	33.3	16.7	—	16.7	33.3	—	67	6

注：ª在几种幼年型粒单核细胞白血病肿瘤中存在 *NF1* 复合杂合性突变(无法区分是来源胚系还是体系突变)(参见 Laycock-van Spyk et al. 2011)。

本章主要关注 NF1 的体细胞微缺失。关于 LOH 研究的详细信息，请参考最近发表的综述文章(Laycock-van Spyk et al. 2011)。肿瘤 DNA 分析还鉴定了 254 个体细胞 *NF1* 基因变异，包括无义突变、错义突变、剪接位点突变、微缺失、微插入和 <20 bp 的插入-缺失事件(indels)以及 >20 bp 的缺失/插入(表 15.1)。还确定了所有微缺失和微插入对 *NF1* 阅读框的影响。在 NF1 肿瘤中检测到的体细胞 *NF1* 突变中，大约 75%(191/254)预计会导致截短蛋白的突变。在这 191 个发生突变的个体中，只有 18 个是由碱基的插入或重复引起的；其余 173 个截短是由微缺失、无义突变或其他移码事件引起的(表 15.1a)。剪接位点突变占突变谱的相当一部分(39/254；15.4%)，而错义变化仅占检测到的体细胞 *NF1* 突变的 9.4%(24/254)。

由于缺乏体细胞突变数据，尤其是罕见肿瘤的体

细胞突变数据，在现阶段尝试对各种肿瘤类型进行直接比较是不明智的。尽管如此，表 15.1 尝试总结现有数据。数据中的固有偏移是显而易见的，其中 211/254（83%）的突变变化来源于皮肤型神经纤维瘤 DNA 分析。因此，皮肤型神经纤维瘤中各种突变类型的相对频率基本与总体突变谱相当，皮肤型神经纤维瘤中无义突变、剪接位点突变和错义突变的频率分别为 28%（59/211）、15%（32/211）和 10%（21/211）（表 15.1a）。然而，表 15.1a 和表 15.2 强调了在所有肿瘤类型中，尤其是皮肤型神经纤维瘤，NF1 基因体细胞失活的截断突变比例高达 191/254（约 75%）。

表 15.2 LOH 和 NF1 微缺失在不同类型的 NF1 相关肿瘤中对体细胞 NF1 突变谱的影响

肿瘤类型	LOH	点突变	总和
皮肤型神经纤维瘤	144(40%)	211(60%)	355(100%)
丛状神经纤维瘤	67(79%)	18(21%)	85(100%)
脊柱神经纤维瘤	7(70%)	3(30%)	10(100%)
恶性周围神经鞘膜瘤	55(85%)	10(15%)	65(100%)
低级别毛细胞型星型细胞瘤	18(100%)	0(0%)	18(100%)
胃肠道间质瘤	3(38%)	5(62%)	8(100%)
幼年型粒单核细胞白血病	18(95%)	1[a](5%)	19(100%)
嗜铬细胞瘤	10(100%)	0(0%)	10(100%)
血管球瘤	1(14%)	6(86%)	7(100%)
总和	323(55%)	254(44%)	577(100%)

注：[a] 复合杂合性 NF1 突变在 5 个造血肿瘤中被发现。由于没有分析其他组织，因此无法区分这些突变是生殖系还是体细胞 NF1 点突变。

表 15.2 进一步比较了体细胞微缺失和 LOH 的频率分布。皮肤型神经纤维瘤、PNF 和 MPNST 在 LOH 上表现出显著差异。部分原因可能是由于每种肿瘤类型中的分子重排程度不同；例如，MPNST 预计会比良性皮肤型神经纤维瘤表现出更多的遗传异常。然而，所进行的分析方案也会直接影响得出的结论，因为在某些研究中可能没有筛查微缺失或 LOH。

总之，更严重的 MPNST 表现出比其他肿瘤类型更高程度的遗传异常，LOH 在这些肿瘤中更为常见。由于目前可供分析的突变数据相对有限，所以无法在较罕见的肿瘤类型内部和其他肿瘤之间进行进一步比较。

15.5 已知体细胞 NF1 基因的突变机制

NF1 基因的体细胞失活可能涉及由不同突变机制导致的基因内突变，以及 LOH 和启动子区域的表观遗传学修饰。在 Laycock-van Spyk 等（2011）列出的 254 个体细胞 NF1 微缺失中，有 72 个是无义突变，其中 36 个位于不同肿瘤的 15 个密码子中（密码子 192、304、426、440、816、1241、1306、1362、1513、1569、1604、1748、1939、1976、2429）。这 15 种不同的重复性无义突变中的 10 种涉及 CpG 二核苷酸内的 C>T 或 G>A 转变，因此与 5-甲基胞嘧啶（5-methylcytosine，5mC）甲基化介导的脱氨反应这一内源性突变机制相符。在这 72 个无义突变中，有 28 个已被报道为 NF1 患者的胚系突变[Human Gene Mutation Database (HGMD); http://www.hgmd.org; Stenson et al. 2008]，表明相同的突变机制在体细胞和胚系中都起了作用。在 15 个反复出现的体细胞无义突变中，有 12 个在胚系中也有独立报道（密码子 192、304、426、440、816、1241、1306、1362、1513、1569、1748 和 2429），这证明了这种突变机制的重要性。在这 15 个无义突变中，有 10 个对应于 CpG 二核苷酸内的 C>T 或 G>A 转变，因此我们可以推测突变的胞嘧啶在体细胞和胚系中都必须被甲基化，从而解释了这些位点在两个细胞系中都容易发生甲基化介导的脱氨基作用。

此外，在 Laycock-van Spyk 等（2011）列出的体细胞 NF1 突变中，有 21 种不同的错义突变。其中有 2 种（位于密码子 519 和 776）在不同的肿瘤或研究领域中被多次报道，但它们都不符合 5mC 甲基化介导的脱氨基机制。那么在这 21 种错义突变中，只有 1 种（位于密码子 176）也在胚系中被报告（参见 HGMD）。由于这种 Asp176Glu 突变在 NF1 相关的肿瘤中也被多次报告,因此,这种氨基酸残基可能对体细胞和胚系中神经纤维瘤蛋白的功能都很重要。这种残基在包括果蝇和河豚在内的多种不同物种中的进化是保守的,在 250 个无关的正常个体中也未发现该残基的多态性。

然而,无义突变并不是唯一在体细胞中反复出现的 NF1 突变类型。在 Laycock-van Spyk 等(2011)列出的体细胞 NF1 微缺失中,其中 6 个在不同肿瘤中多次被报告(c. 1888delG、c. 2033delC、c. 3058delG、c. 4374_4375delCC 和 c. 5731delT)。这 4 个微缺失发生在单核苷酸重复区域(分别为 G4、C5、C7 和 T3),提示在 DNA 复制分叉处可能存在滑移错配模式。重要的是,c. 2033delC 也在胚系中被报告(见 HGMD),这表明 C 五核苷酸序列在胚系和体细胞中都是突变的热点。1 个微小插入(c. 1733insT,位于 T6 序列内)也被报道反复出现在体细胞中,但迄今为止尚未在胚系中被报告。有兴趣深入比较人类肿瘤抑制基因中胚系和体细胞突变的读者请参考 Ivanov 等的报道(2011)。

近期有报道指出,NF1 基因的 LOH 是由体细胞 NF1 突变引起的,并且在 NF1 相关肿瘤中被报道(Laycock-van Spyk et al. 2011)。导致 LOH 的机制多种多样,包括缺失、染色体不分离导致的染色体丢失(可能伴随或不伴随重复)、基因转换、点突变、表观遗传失活和有丝分裂重组。其中,有丝分裂重组通过拷贝中性杂合性丧失(loss of heterozygosity, LOH)导致抑瘤基因失活具有重要意义。表 15.3 归纳了在不同 NF1 肿瘤中观察到的有丝分裂重组现象。研究显示,这种现象在皮肤型神经纤维瘤和 JMML 中更为常见(Serra et al. 2001;Stewart et al. 2007a, b, 2012;Steinmann et al. 2010;Upadhyaya et al. 2008b, 2009;Garcia-Linares et al. 2011;Laycock-van Spyk et al. 2011)。

表 15.3 不同 NF1 相关肿瘤中 NF1 基因相关 LOH 的机制基础

肿瘤类型	染色体重排	基因组缺失
皮肤型神经纤维瘤	28	8
丛状神经纤维瘤	11	14

续 表

肿瘤类型	染色体重排	基因组缺失
脊柱神经纤维瘤	7	1
恶性周围神经鞘膜瘤	5	26
低级别毛细胞型星型细胞瘤	0	2
胃肠道间质瘤	1	1
幼年型粒单核细胞白血病	15	4
嗜铬细胞瘤	0	0
血管球瘤	2	0

注:信息仅适用于被明确鉴定 LOH 具体机制的病例(参见 Laycock-van Spyk et al. 2011)。

15.6 胚系与体细胞 NF1 突变谱的比较

通过组合分析同一肿瘤中观察到的体细胞突变和胚系突变(表 15.4),肿瘤中出现的体细胞突变类型与同一肿瘤中出现的胚系突变类型没有关联($P=0.366$)。仅比较了体细胞中的错义突变、无义/移码突变和剪接位点突变与生殖系中的长缺失和无义/移码突变,结果发现,内含子、错义、无义突变、微缺失和微插入突变在体细胞和胚系之间的比例没有显著差异($P=0.498$)。进一步比较体细胞和胚系突变频率(数据来源于 HGMD;Stenson et al. 2008),发现体细胞中的错义突变、无义突变、微缺失/微插入和剪接突变与胚系突变之间存在显著差异(Fisher 精确检验,$P=0.000\ 14$)。体细胞中无义突变的比例(25%)高于胚系(15%),而剪接位点突变的比例(15%)低于胚系(26%)。此外,33%的体细胞错义/无义突变是 CpG 和 CpHpG 寡核苷酸(H 可以是 A、T 或 C)中的 C>T 和 G>A 改变。与胚系突变相比,这些寡核苷酸中的体细胞突变比例显著偏高($P=0.007$)。在 NF1 基因内含子区域中,体细胞和胚系突变的位置没有显著差异(Fisher 精确检验,$P=0.334$);只有少量突变发生在外显子/内含子和内含子/外显子连接处两侧的 ±15 bp

区域之外。研究还报道了,在 NF1 基因内含子区,所有体细胞突变(只有 1 个例外)分别发生在外显子/内含子和内含子/外显子交界区的 +6 bp 和 −12 bp 范围内,而在正常人群中观察到的所有内含子变化都发生在这些区域之外(未发表数据)。

表 15.4　特定类型体细胞突变与同一肿瘤中识别的胚系突变类型的相对发生频率

胚系突变类型	体细胞突变类型				总和
	错义突变	无义突变	大片段缺失	剪接位点突变	
大片段缺失	3	41	4	3	51
错义突变	1	8	0	1	10
无义突变	14	78	3	14	109
剪接位点突变	1	11	0	2	14
总和	19	138	7	20	184

15.7　非 NF1 相关肿瘤中的 NF1 基因体细胞突变

多项研究在非 NF1 相关的肿瘤中发现了体细胞 NF1 基因突变。例如,体细胞 NF1 异常已在多发胶质母细胞瘤(glioblastoma multiforme, GBM)、肺腺癌、恶性乳腺肿瘤、白血病、卵巢浆液性癌(ovarian serous carcinomas, OSC)和神经母细胞瘤中被鉴定出来(Ding et al. 2008; Parsons et al. 2008; Sangha et al. 2008; McGillicuddy et al. 2009; Haferlach et al. 2010; Hölzel et al. 2010; Lee et al. 2010)。这些肿瘤中一些 NF1 基因的变化较为常见,因此可能成为特定的预后和诊断标志。例如,23% 的散发性 GBM 含有失活的 NF1 体细胞突变,这可能使这些 GBM 肿瘤分化为间充质分子亚类(Brennan et al. 2009)。同样,在 22%(9/41)的原发性 OSC 中检测到 NF1 突变,其中 6 个表现出双等位基因失活(Sangha et al. 2008)。有趣的是,所有 9 个 OSC 样本也都含有 TP53 突变,这表明 TP53 在 OSC 发病机制中可能起到重要作用(Sangha et al. 2008)。

鉴于神经纤维瘤蛋白在多种细胞信号通路中扮演着重要角色,因此它的缺失会影响不同癌症中的不同分子亚型也就不足为奇了。实际上,未来肿瘤治疗的效果很大程度上将依赖于我们能否成功识别这些肿瘤的分子亚型。

15.8　结论

我们在本章报告了 NF1 基因的体细胞突变谱。我们旨在研究体细胞 NF1 病变与胚系突变的相互作用,并探讨如何才能更好地理解肿瘤发生的病理生理机制。关于 NF1 肿瘤的拷贝数变化详见第 27 章。

NF1 基因的双等位基因失活导致功能性神经纤维瘤蛋白的完全缺失,从而启动致病过程并最终形成神经鞘膜瘤。NF1 基因失活可能通过影响几个 DNA 碱基出现微缺失,或者可能影响大染色体区域甚至整个第 17 号染色体的重大基因组发生变化。在 MPNST 中,不同基因位点上的其他突变也参与了肿瘤的进展。

在突变发生的分子机制方面,5-甲基胞嘧啶的甲基化介导脱氨作用和多核苷酸重复区内的滑移错配似乎是导致胚系和体细胞中出现共享突变热点的主要原因。对于某些类型的肿瘤,胚系和体细胞之间可能存在相互作用,即胚系突变的位置可以影响后续体细胞突变的性质、频率和位置(Lamlum et al. 1999; Dworkin et al. 2010)。然而,目前尚无证据表明这种现象在 NF1 肿瘤发生过程中存在。

尽管我们对 NF1 基因在肿瘤发生中作用的了解在不断加深,但恶性转化的明确标志物仍未被发现。小鼠和其他动物模型,包括斑马鱼(Padmanabhan et al. 2009),为研究带来了新的视角,通过各种基因敲除和诱变方法促进了功能研究。很明显,为了明确 NF1 基因在 NF1 相关肿瘤中的作用,我们必须进一步了解体细胞(二次突变)突变的意义。我们对各种 NF1 相关肿瘤类型中已知的体细胞 NF1 突变进行的荟萃分析,却未能发现任何具体的基因型相关性。由于突变数据集规模有限,暂时难以得出可靠的结论,所以需要更大和更明确的患者群体来进行更可靠的比较。此外,也迫切需要找到预后标志,这些标志能可靠地区分可能进展为恶性肿瘤和不太可能进展为恶性肿瘤的良性神经纤维瘤。

然而,我们的综述强调了 NF1 是一个高度个性化的临床群体,在患者内部和患者之间都表现出极端的体细胞突变异质性。这些突变最终引起肿瘤形成的分子变化。如果我们能够理解这些变化如何引起肿瘤发生,不仅可以更好地提供遗传咨询,还能在探索开发新药物疗法方面取得更大进展。

突变分析结合功能分析能够加深我们对癌症生物学基础的了解,并有助于识别体细胞如何改变基因影响的生物通路,从而开发新的治疗策略。由于 MPNST 的固有异质性,需要更大规模的研究才能获得统计上有意义的结果。随着测序能力的快速提升和成本的不断下降,基因组范围的分析可能很快就能应用于大多数 NF1 相关肿瘤。整合结构和功能数据有望让我们更好地理解体细胞 NF1 变化是如何编程肿瘤的发生、维持和进展的。

未来的发展应集中在肿瘤样本的准确临床信息收集、影像学技术的改进。除此以外,在解释结果时应考虑肿瘤遗传异质性,以及这种异质性对肿瘤生物学和治疗反应的影响。对于具有复杂核型的实体肿瘤研究,出现的系统性方法匮乏的问题,我们正在通过全基因组测序来解决,不久将提供 NF1 肿瘤基因组的最全面特征描述,包括大规模的染色体重排。

致谢:我们衷心感谢所有 NF1 患者及其家属的支持。

(胡杏 译)

参考文献

[1] Ars E, Kruyer H, Gaona A, Casquero P et al (1998) A clinical variant of neurofibromatosis type 1: familial spinal neurofibromatosis with a frameshift mutation in the NF1 gene. Am J Hum Genet 62: 834-841

[2] Ballester R, Marchuk D, Boguski M, Saulino A et al (1990) The NF1 locus encodes a protein functionally related to mammalian GAP and yeast IRA proteins. Cell 63: 851-859

[3] Bandipalliam P (2005) Syndrome of early onset colon cancers, hematologic malignancies & features of neurofibromatosis in HNPCC families with homozygous mismatch repair gene mutations. Fam Cancer 4: 323-333

[4] Bausch B, Borozdin W, Mautner VF, Hoffmann MM et al (2007) Germline NF1 mutational spectra and loss-of-heterozygosity analyses in patients with pheochromocytoma and neurofi-bromatosis type 1. J Clin Endocrinol Metab 92: 2784-2792

[5] Beert E, Brems H, Daniëls B, De Wever I, Van Calenbergh F, Schoenaers J, Debiec-Rychter M, Gevaert O, De Raedt T, Van Den Bruel A, de Ravel T, Cichowski K, Kluwe L, Mautner V, Sciot R, Legius E (2011) Atypical neurofibromas in neurofibromatosis type 1 are premalignant tumors. Genes Chromosomes Cancer 50: 1021-1032

[6] Bennett E, Thomas N, Upadhyaya M (2009) Neurofibromatosis type 1: its association with the Ras/MAPK pathway syndromes. J Paediatr Neurol 7: 105-115

[7] Benz MR, Czernin J, Dry SM, Tap WD et al (2010) Quantitative F18-fluorodeoxyglucose positron emission tomography accurately characterizes peripheral nerve sheath tumors as malignant or benign. Cancer 116: 451-458

[8] Bien E, Stachowicz-Stencel T, Sierota D, Polczynska K, Szolkiewicz A, Stefanowicz J, Adamkiewicz-Drozynska E, Czauderna P, Kosiak W, Dubaniewicz-Wybieralska M, Izycka Swieszewska E, Balcerska A (2007) Sarcomas in children with neurofibromatosis type 1-poor prognosis despite aggressive combined therapy in four patients treated in a single oncological institution. Childs Nerv Syst 23: 1147-1153

[9] Brems H, Park C, Maertens O, Pemov A et al (2009) Glomus tumors in neurofibromatosis type 1: genetic functional, and clinical evidence of a novel association. Cancer Res 69: 7393-7401

[10] Brennan C, Momota H, Hambardzumyan D, Ozawa T et al (2009) Glioblastoma subclasses can be defined by activity among signal transduction pathways and associated genomic alterations. PLoS One 4: e7752

[11] Burnichon N, Vescovo L, Amar L, Libé R, de Reynies A, Venisse A, Jouanno E, Laurendeau I, Parfait B, Bertherat J, Plouin PF, Jeunemaitre X, Favier J, Gimenez-Roqueplo AP (2011) Integrative genomic analysis reveals somatic mutations in pheochromocytoma and paraganglioma. Hum Mol Genet 20: 3974-3985

[12] Carroll SL, Ratner N (2008) How does the Schwann cell lineage form tumors in NF1? Glia 56(14): 1590-1605

[13] Chen JM, Cooper DN, Ferec C, Kehrer-Sawatzki H et al (2010) Genomic rearrangements in inherited disease and cancer. Semin Cancer Biol 20: 222-233

[14] Cichowski K, Jacks T (2001) NF1 tumor suppressor gene function: narrowing the GAP. Cell 104: 593-604

[15] Cichowski K, Shih T, Schmitt E, Santiago S et al (1999) Mouse models of tumor development in neurofibromatosis type 1. Science 286: 2172-2176

[16] De Raedt T, Brems H, Wolkenstein P, Vidaud D et al (2003) Elevated risk for MPNST in NF1 microdeletion patients. Am J Hum Genet 72: 1288-1292

[17] Ding L, Getz G, Wheeler D, Mardis E et al (2008) Somatic mutations affect key pathways in lung adenocarcinoma. Nature 455: 1069-1075

[18] Ducatman B, Scheithauer B, Piepgras D, Reiman H et al (1986) Malignant peripheral nerve sheath tumors. A clinicopathologic study of 120 cases. Cancer 57: 2006-2021

[19] Dugoff L, Sujansky E (1996) Neurofibromatosis type 1 and

pregnancy. Am J Med Genet 66: 7-10
[20] Dworkin AM, Ridd K, Bautista D, Allain DC et al (2010) Germline variation controls the architecture of somatic alterations in tumors. PLoS Genet 6: e1001136
[21] Easton DF, Ponder MA, Huson SM, Ponder BA (1993) An analysis of variation in expression of neurofibromatosis (NF) type 1 (NF1): evidence for modifying genes. Am J Hum Genet 53: 305-313
[22] Eisenbarth I, Beyer K, Krone W, Assum G (2000) Toward a survey of somatic mutation of the NF1 gene in benign neurofibromas of patients with neurofibromatosis type 1. Am J Hum Genet 66: 393-401
[23] Evans D, Baser M, McGaughran J, Sharif S et al (2002) Malignant peripheral nerve sheath tumours in neurofibromatosis 1. J Med Genet 39: 311-314
[24] Flotho C, Steinemann D, Mullighan C, Neale G et al (2007) Genome-wide single-nucleotide polymorphism analysis in juvenile myelomonocytic leukemia identifies uniparental disomy surrounding the NF1 locus in cases associated with neurofibromatosis but not in cases with mutant RAS or PTPN11. Oncogene 26: 5816-5821
[25] Friedman JM, Arbiser J, Epstein JA, Gutmann DH, Huot SJ, Lin AE, McManus B, Korf BR (2002) Cardiovascular disease in neurofibromatosis 1: report of the NF1 Cardiovascular Task Force. Genet Med 4: 105-111
[26] Garcia-Linares C, Fernandez-Rodriguez J, Terribas E, Mercade J et al (2011) Dissecting loss of heterozygosity (LOH) in neurofibromatosis type 1-associated neurofibromas: importance of copy neutral LOH. Hum Mutat 32: 78-90
[27] Gerlinger M, Rowan AJ, Horswell S, Math M, Larkin J, Endesfelder D et al (2012) Intratumour heterogeneity and branched evolution revealed by multiregion sequencing. N Engl J Med 366: 883-892
[28] Gregorian C, Nakashima J, Dry S, Nghiemphu P et al (2009) PTEN dosage is essential for neurofibroma development and malignant transformation. Proc Natl Acad Sci USA 106: 19479-19484
[29] Gutmann DH, Cole JL, Stone WJ, Ponder BA, Collins FS (1994) Loss of neurofibromin in adrenal gland tumors from patients with neurofibromatosis type I. Genes Chromosomes Cancer 10: 55-58
[30] Gutmann DH, Geist RT, Rose K, Wallin G, Moley JF (1995) Loss of neurofibromatosis type I (NF1) gene expression in pheochromocytomas from patients without NF1. Genes Chromosomes Cancer 13(2): 104-109
[31] Gutmann D, Donahoe J, Brown T, James C et al (2000) Loss of neurofibromatosis 1 (NF1) gene expression in NF1-associated pilocytic astrocytomas. Neuropathol Appl Neurobiol 26: 361-367
[32] Gutmann D, James C, Poyhonen M, Louis D et al (2003) Molecular analysis of astrocytomas presenting after age 10 in individuals with NF1. Neurology 61: 1397-1400
[33] Haferlach C, Dicker F, Kohlmann A, Schindela S et al (2010) AML with CBFB-MYH11 rearrangement demonstrate RAS pathway alterations in 92% of all cases including a high frequency of NF1 deletions. Leukemia 24: 1065-1069
[34] Hölzel M, Huang S, Koster J, Ora I et al (2010) NF1 is a tumor suppressor in neuroblastoma that determines retinoic acid response and disease outcome. Cell 142: 218-229
[35] Huson S, Harper P, Compston D (1988) von Recklinghausen neurofibromatosis. A clinical and population study in south-east Wales. Brain 111(Pt 6): 1355-1381
[36] Ivanov D, Hamby SE, Stenson PD, Phillips AD et al (2011) Comparative analysis of germline and somatic microlesion mutational spectra in 17 human tumor suppressor genes. Hum Mutat 32: 620-632
[37] John A, Ruggieri M, Ferner R, Upadhyaya M (2000) A search for evidence of somatic mutations in the NF1 gene. J Med Genet 37: 44-49
[38] Joseph N, Mosher J, Buchstaller J, Snider P et al (2008) The loss of Nf1 transiently promotes self-renewal but not tumorigenesis by neural crest stem cells. Cancer Cell 13: 129-140
[39] Kehrer-Sawatzki H (2008) Structure of the NF1 gene region and mechanisms underlying gross NF1 deletions. In: Kaufmann D (ed) Neurofibromatoses. Karger, Basel, pp 46-62
[40] Kehrer-Sawatzki H, Cooper DN (2008) Mosaicism in sporadic neurofibromatosis type 1: variations on a theme common to other hereditary cancer syndromes? J Med Genet 45: 622-631
[41] Knudson AJ (1971) Mutation and cancer: statistical study of retinoblastoma. Proc Natl Acad Sci USA 68: 820-823
[42] Kourea H, Orlow I, Scheithauer B, Cordon-Cardo C et al (1999) Deletions of the INK4A gene occur in malignant peripheral nerve sheath tumors but not in neurofibromas. Am J Pathol 155: 1855-1860
[43] Kushner BH, Hajdu SI, Helson L (1985) Synchronous neuroblastoma and von Recklinghausen's disease: a review of the literature. J Clin Oncol 3: 117-120
[44] Lamlum H, Ilyas M, Rowan A, Clark S et al (1999) The type of somatic mutation at APC in familial adenomatous polyposis is determined by the site of the germline mutation: a new facet to Knudson's 'two-hit' hypothesis. Nat Med 5: 1071-1075
[45] Lammert M, Friedman JM, Kluwe L, Mautner VF (2005) Prevalence of neurofibromatosis 1 in German children at elementary school enrollment. Arch Dermatol 141: 71-74
[46] Laycock-van Spyk S, Thomas N, Cooper DN, Upadhyaya M (2011) Neurofibromatosis type 1-associated tumours: their somatic mutational spectrum and pathogenesis. Hum Genomics 5: 623-690
[47] Le L, Shipman T, Burns D, Parada L (2009) Cell of origin and microenvironment contribution for NF1-associated dermal neurofibromas. Cell Stem Cell 4: 453-463
[48] Lee J, Wang J, Torbenson M, Lu Y et al (2010) Loss of SDHB and NF1 genes in a malignant phyllodes tumor of the breast as detected by oligo-array comparative genomic hybridization. Cancer Genet Cytogenet 196: 179-183
[49] Legius E, Dierick H, Wu R, Hall B et al (1994) TP53 mutations are frequent in malignant NF1 tumors. Genes Chromosomes Cancer 10: 250-255
[50] Listernick R, Charrow J, Greenwald M, Mets M (1994) Natural history of optic pathway tumors in children with neurofibromatosis type 1: a longitudinal study. J Pediatr 125: 63-66
[51] Maertens O, Prenen H, Debiec-Rychter M, Wozniak A et al (2006) Molecular pathogenesis of multiple gastrointestinal stromal tumors in NF1 patients. Hum Mol Genet 15: 1015-1023
[52] Mantripragada K, Spurlock G, Kluwe L, Chuzhanova N et al (2008) High-resolution DNA copy number profiling of malignant peripheral nerve sheath tumors using targeted microarray-based comparative genomic hybridization. Clin Cancer Res 14: 1015-1024
[53] Mautner VF, Kluwe L, Friedrich RE, Roehl AC et al (2010) Clinical characterisation of 29 neurofibromatosis type-1 patients with molecularly ascertained 1.4 Mb type-1 NF1

[54] McCaughan J, Holloway S, Davidson R, Lam W (2007) Further evidence of the increased risk for malignant peripheral nerve sheath tumour from a Scottish cohort of patients with neurofibro-matosis type 1. J Med Genet 44: 463-466

[55] McGillicuddy LT, Fromm JA, Hollstein PE, Kubek S et al (2009) Proteasomal and genetic inactivation of the NF1 tumor suppressor in gliomagenesis. Cancer Cell 16: 44-54

[56] McLaughlin ME, Jacks T (2003) Progesterone receptor expression in neurofibromas. Cancer Res 63: 752-755

[57] Menon A, Anderson K, Riccardi V, Chung R et al (1990) Chromosome 17p deletions and p53 gene mutations associated with the formation of malignant neurofibrosarcomas in von Recklinghausen neurofibromatosis. Proc Natl Acad Sci USA 87: 5435-5439

[58] Miettinen M, Fetsch J, Sobin L, Lasota J (2006) Gastrointestinal stromal tumors in patients with neurofibromatosis 1: a clinicopathologic and molecular genetic study of 45 cases. Am J Surg Pathol 30: 90-96

[59] Nielsen G, Stemmer-Rachamimov A, Ino Y, Moller M et al (1999) Malignant transformation of neurofibromas in neurofibromatosis 1 is associated with CDKN2A/p16 inactivation. Am J Pathol 155: 1879-1884

[60] Padmanabhan A, Lee JS, Ismat FA, Lu MM, Lawson ND, Kanki JP, Look AT, Epstein JA (2009) Cardiac and vascular functions of the zebrafish orthologues of the type I neurofibromatosis gene NF1. Proc Natl Acad Sci USA 106: 22305-22310

[61] Pao W, Girard N (2011) New driver mutations in non-small-cell lung cancer. Lancet Oncol 12: 175-180

[62] Parsons DW, Jones S, Zhang X, Lin JC et al (2008) An integrated genomic analysis of human glioblastoma multiforme. Science 321: 1807-1812

[63] Pasmant E, Vidaud D, Harrison M, Upadhyaya M (2010) Different sized somatic NF1 locus rearrangements in neurofibromatosis 1-associated malignant peripheral nerve sheath tumors. J Neurooncol 102: 341-346

[64] Poyhonen M, Leisti E, Kytölä S, Leisti J (1997) Hereditary spinal neurofibromatosis: a rare form of NF1? J Med Genet 34: 184-187

[65] Pulst SM, Riccardi VM, Fain P, Korenberg JR (1991) Familial spinal neurofibromatosis: clinical and DNA linkage analysis. Neurology 41: 1923-1927

[66] Roehl AC, Mussotter T, Cooper DN, Kluwe L, Wimmer K, Högel J, Zetzmann M, Vogt J, Mautner VF, Kehrer-Sawatzki H (2012) Tissue-specific differences in the proportion of mosaic large NF1 deletions are suggestive of a selective growth advantage of hematopoietic del(+/-) stem cells. Hum Mutat 33: 541-550

[67] Roth T, Ramamurthy P, Muir D, Wallace M et al (2008) Influence of hormones and hormone metabolites on the growth of Schwann cells derived from embryonic stem cells and on tumor cell lines expressing variable levels of neurofibromin. Dev Dyn 237: 513-524

[68] Sangha N, Wu R, Kuick R, Powers S et al (2008) Neurofibromin 1 (NF1) defects are common in human ovarian serous carcinomas and co-occur with TP53 mutations. Neoplasia 10: 1362-1372

[69] Sawada S, Florell S, Purandare S, Ota M et al (1996) Identification of NF1 mutations in both alleles of a dermal neurofibroma. Nat Genet 14: 110-112

[70] Serra E, Rosenbaum T, Winner U, Aledo R et al (2000) Schwann cells harbor the somatic NF1 mutation in neurofibromas: evidence of two different Schwann cell subpopulations. Hum Mol Genet 9: 3055-3064

[71] Serra E, Rosenbaum T, Nadal M, Winner U et al (2001) Mitotic recombination effects homozy-gosity for NF1 germline mutations in neurofibromas. Nat Genet 28: 294-296

[72] Sharif S, Moran A, Huson SM, Iddenden R, Shenton A, Howard E, Evans DG (2007) Women with neurofibromatosis 1 are at a moderately increased risk of developing breast cancer and should be considered for early screening. J Med Genet 44: 481-484

[73] Sharif S, Upadhyaya M, Ferner R, Majounie E, Shenton A, Baser M, Thakker N, Evans DG (2011) A molecular analysis of individuals with neurofibromatosis type 1 (NF1) and optic pathway gliomas (OPGs), and an assessment of genotype-phenotype correlations. J Med Genet 48: 256-260

[74] Spurlock G, Griffiths S, Uff J, Upadhyaya M (2007) Somatic alterations of the NF1 gene in an NF1 individual with multiple benign tumours (internal and external) and malignant tumour types. Fam Cancer 6: 463-471

[75] Spurlock G, Knight SJ, Thomas N, Kiehl TR, Guha A, Upadhyaya M (2010) Molecular evolution of a neurofibroma to malignant peripheral nerve sheath tumor (MPNST) in an NF1 patient: correlation between histopathological, clinical and molecular findings. J Cancer Res Clin Oncol 136: 1869-1880

[76] Staser K, Yang FC, Clapp DW (2012) Pathogenesis of plexiform neurofibroma: tumor-stromal/hematopoietic interactions in tumor progression. Annu Rev Pathol 7: 469-495

[77] Steinemann D, Arning L, Praulich I, Stuhrmann M et al (2010) Mitotic recombination and compound-heterozygous mutations are predominant NF1-inactivating mechanisms in children with juvenile myelomonocytic leukemia and neurofibromatosis type 1. Haematologica 95: 320-323

[78] Stenson PD, Ball E, Howells K, Phillips A et al (2008) Human Gene Mutation Database: towards a comprehensive central mutation database. J Med Genet 45: 124-126

[79] Stephens K, Weaver M, Leppig K, Maruyama K et al (2006) Interstitial uniparental isodisomy at clustered breakpoint intervals is a frequent mechanism of NF1 inactivation in myeloid malignancies. Blood 108: 1684-1689

[80] Stewart W, Traynor JP, Cooke A, Griffiths S et al (2007a) Gastric carcinoid: germline and somatic mutation of the neurofibromatosis type 1 gene. Fam Cancer 6: 147-152

[81] Stewart D, Corless C, Rubin B, Heinrich M et al (2007b) Mitotic recombination as evidence of alternative pathogenesis of gastrointestinal stromal tumours in neurofibromatosis type 1. J Med Genet 44: e61

[82] Stewart DR, Pemov A, Van Loo P, Beert E, Brems H, Sciot R, Claes K, Pak E, Dutra A, Richard Lee CC, Legius E (2012) Mitotic recombination of chromosome arm 17q as a cause of loss of heterozygosity of NF1 in neurofibromatosis type 1-associated glomus tumors. Genes Chromosomes Cancer 51: 429-437

[83] Stiller C, Chessells J, Fitchett M (1994) Neurofibromatosis and childhood leukaemia/lymphoma: a population-based UKCCSG study. Br J Cancer 70: 969-972

[84] Stratton MR (2011) Exploring the genomes of cancer cells: progress and promise. Science 331: 1553-1558

[85] Sugimoto Y, Muramatsu H, Makishima H, Prince C et al (2009) Spectrum of molecular defects in juvenile myelomonocytic leukaemia includes ASXL1 mutations. Br J Haematol 150: 83-87

[86] Sung L, Anderson JR, Arndt C, Raney RB, Meyer WH, Pappo AS (2004) Neurofibromatosis in children with

[87] The I, Murthy AE, Hannigan GE, Jacoby LB, Menon AG, Gusella JF, Bernards A (1993) Neurofibromatosis type 1 gene mutations in neuroblastoma. Nat Genet 3: 62-66

[88] Thomas L, Kluwe L, Chuzhanova N, Mautner V et al (2010) Analysis of NF1 somatic mutations in cutaneous neurofibromas from patients with high tumor burden. Neurogenetics 11: 391-400

[89] Thomas L, Spurlock G, Eudall C, Thomas NS, Mort M, Hamby SE, Chuzhanova N, Brems H, Legius E, Cooper DN, Upadhyaya M (2012a) Exploring the somatic NF1 mutational spectrum associated with NF1 cutaneous neurofibromas. Eur J Hum Genet 20(4): 411-419

[90] Thomas L, Mautner VF, Cooper D, Upadhyaya M (2012) Molecular heterogeneity in malignant peripheral nerve sheath tumors (MPNSTs) associated with neurofibromatosis type 1 (NF1). Hum Genomics 6: 18

[91] Upadhyaya M (2008) NF1 gene structure and NF1 genotype/phenotype correlations. In: Kaufmann D (ed) Neurofibromatoses. Karger, Basel, pp 46-62

[92] Upadhyaya M (2010) Neurofibromatosis type 1 (NF1): diagnosis and recent advances. Expert Opin Med Genet 4: 307-322

[93] Upadhyaya M (2011) Genetic basis of tumorigenesis in NF1 malignant peripheral nerve sheath tumors. Front Biosci 16: 937-951

[94] Upadhyaya M, Han S, Consoli C et al (2004) Characterization of the somatic mutational spectrum of the neurofibromatosis type 1 (NF1) gene in neurofibromatosis patients with benign and malignant tumors. Hum Mutat 23: 134-146

[95] Upadhyaya M, Spurlock G, Majounie E, Griffiths S et al (2006) The heterogeneous nature of germline mutations in NF1 patients with malignant peripheral serve sheath tumours (MPNSTs). Hum Mutat 27: 716

[96] Upadhyaya M, Huson S, Davies M, Thomas N et al (2007) An absence of cutaneous neurofibromas associated with a 3-bp inframe deletion in exon 17 of the NF1 gene (c. 2970-2972 delAAT): evidence of a clinically significant NF1 genotype-phenotype correlation. Am J Hum Genet 80: 140-151

[97] Upadhyaya M, Kluwe L, Spurlock G, Monem B et al (2008a) Germline and somatic NF1 gene mutation spectrum in NF1-associated malignant peripheral nerve sheath tumors (MPNSTs). Hum Mutat 29: 74-82

[98] Upadhyaya M, Spurlock G, Monem B, Thomas N et al (2008b) Germline and somatic NF1 gene mutations in plexiform neurofibromas. Hum Mutat 29: E103-E111

[99] Upadhyaya M, Spurlock G, Kluwe L, Chuzhanova N et al (2009) The spectrum of somatic and germline NF1 mutations in NF1 patients with spinal neurofibromas. Neurogenetics 10: 251-263

[100] Upadhyaya M, Spurlock G, Thomas L, Thomas NS, Richards M, Mautner VF, Cooper DN, Guha A, Yan J (2012) Microarray-based copy number analysis of neurofibromatosis type-1 (NF1)-associated malignant peripheral nerve sheath tumours (MPNSTs) reveals a role for Rho-GTPase pathway genes in NF1 tumorigenesis. Hum Mutat. 33: 763-776

[101] Vogel K, Klesse L, Velasco-Miguel S, Meyers K et al (1999) Mouse tumor model for neurofibro-matosis type 1. Science 286: 2176-2179

[102] Walker L, Thompson D, Easton D, Ponder B, Ponder M, Frayling I, Baralle D (2006) A prospective study of neurofibromatosis type1 cancer incidence in the UK. Br J Cancer 95: 233-238

[103] Wiest V, Eisenbarth I, Schmegner C, Krone W et al (2003) Somatic NF1 mutation spectra in a family with neurofibromatosis type 1: toward a theory of genetic modifiers. Hum Mutat 22: 423-427

[104] Wimmer K, Etzler J (2008) Constitutional mismatch repair-deficiency syndrome: have we so far seen only the tip of an iceberg? Hum Genet 124: 105-122

[105] Wu J, Williams J, Rizvi T, Kordich J et al (2008) Plexiform and dermal neurofibromas and pigmentation are caused by Nf1 loss in desert hedgehog-expressing cells. Cancer Cell 13: 105-116

[106] Yang FC, Ingram DA, Chen S, Zhu Y et al (2008) Nf1-dependent tumors require a microenvironment containing $Nf1^{+/-}$ and c-kit-dependent bone marrow. Cell 135: 437-448

[107] Yoshimi A, Kojima S, Hirano N (2010) Juvenile myelomonocytic leukemia: epidemiology etiopathogenesis, diagnosis, and management considerations. Paediatr Drugs 12: 11-21

[108] Zheng H, Chang L, Patel N, Yang J, Lowe L et al (2008) Induction of abnormal proliferation by nonmyelinating Schwann cells triggers neurofibroma formation. Cancer Cell 13: 117-128

[109] Zhu Y, Ghosh P, Charnay P, Burns D et al (2002) Neurofibromas in NF1: Schwann cell origin and role of tumor environment. Science 296: 920-922

第16章 1型神经纤维瘤病与构成性错配修复缺陷之间的关系

Relationship Between NF1 and Constitutive Mismatch Repair Deficiency

Katharina Wimmer

16.1 引言：DNA错配修复体系

基因组DNA不断受到内源性和外源性损伤。如不能修复这种损伤会导致DNA突变、重排，以及其他可能导致细胞转化的有害事件。因此，所有生物体都进化出了有效的DNA修复途径以保护其基因组。高度保守的错配修复（mismatch repair，MMR）系统是保持基因组完整性的关键。它可纠正因DNA聚合酶引起的复制错误，并在校对时跳过（Jiricny 2006a）。在人类中，5个MMR基因（MSH2、MSH6、MSH3、MLH1和PMS2）在这一过程中发挥着至关重要的作用。碱基-碱基不匹配和小的插入-删除环（insertion-deletion loop，IDL）可由异二聚体MSH2·MSH6（MutSα）或MSH2·MSH3（MutSβ）检测出。MutSα丰度更高，参与修复碱基-碱基错配和1～2个核苷酸的错位，而MutSβ识别较大的IDL。错配结合的MutSα（或MutSβ）募集第二个异二聚体MLH1·PMS2（MutLα）。MutLα在PMS2亚基中具有核酸内切酶活性，可跨越不匹配，在远端位点引入随机缺口（Kadyrov et al. 2006）。随后在错配的 5′ 侧加载 EXO1激活其 5′-3′ 核酸外切酶活性，从而去除含有错误的DNA片段。修复过程通过聚合酶 δ 及其辅因子的增殖细胞核抗原（proliferation cell nuclear antigen，PCNA）和复制因子 C（replication factor C，RFC）填充单链间隙来完成。然后连接酶 I 封闭剩余的缺口（在Jiricny 2006b中综述）。

在没有MMR的情况下，碱基-碱基错配和IDL未能得到校正将导致表型突变。包含1～2个或几个以上核苷酸单元的重复序列基序，即微卫星，是聚合酶滑动错误的常见靶点。在这些位点，未校正的IDL可导致微卫星的缩短和延长。因此，来源于克隆性增殖MMR缺陷细胞的组织表现出微卫星不稳定性（microsatellite instability，MSI），这很容易通过一组微卫星标记的PCR扩增和片段分析来检测（Boland et al. 1998）。

除了DNA修复外，MMR系统还参与细胞的许多活动。它参与细胞对多种DNA损伤剂的凋亡反应。MMR缺乏的细胞对甲基化试剂诱导的死亡抗性比MMR充足的细胞高出100倍（reviewed in Stojic et al. 2004）。此外，MMR系统还涉及免疫球蛋白的种类转换重组和免疫球蛋白基因可变区的体细胞超突变（Durandy 2009）。

K. Wimmer
Division of Human Genetics, Medical University Innsbruck, Innsbruck, Austria
e-mail: Katharina.wimmer@i-med.ac.at

16.2 构成性错配修复缺陷综合征

近20年来,错配修复缺陷(mismatch repair,MMR)对人类癌症发展的贡献已得到公认[for a recent review, see Peltomaki (2003)]。MMR 基因 *MSH2*、*MSH6*、*MLH1* 和 *PMS2* 的胚系杂合(单等位基因)突变与常染色体显性遗传性疾病林奇综合征有关(Aaltonen 等,1993)。该综合征主要易患结直肠癌和子宫内膜癌,但也易患其他类型的癌症,包括尿路、胃、小肠、卵巢和脑肿瘤(Lynch 和 de la Chapelle 2003;Lynch 等,2009)。患者通常在40~50岁发病。在林奇综合征相关肿瘤中,MMR 缺乏是由于体细胞突变或杂合性缺失导致野生型 MMR 等位基因缺失所致。

1999年,两份报告描述了林奇综合征家族近亲结婚的后代表型,他们携带 *MLH1* 纯合胚系突变(Ricciardone et al. 1999;Wang et al. 1999)。这些人在儿童早期(年龄在14个月至6岁之间)患上了血液系统恶性肿瘤(其中1人患髓母细胞瘤)。值得注意的是,他们还表现出1型神经纤维瘤病(NF1)的临床特征。此后,据报道,超过100名儿童和年轻成人患者携带林奇综合征的4个MMR基因的双等位基因(纯合或复合杂合)突变。OMIM 为这种独特的儿童癌症综合征指定了一个编号(♯276300),其获得了不同的名称,例如错配修复癌症综合征(OMIM)和错配修复缺陷综合征(Scott et al. 2007b)。我们采用了后一个名称,并且将其扩展到构成性错配修复缺陷(constitutional mismatch repair deficiency,CMMR‐D)(Wimmer and Etzler 2008),以避免与林奇综合征患者的肿瘤(以及表现出 MLH1 高甲基化的散发性肿瘤)中所见的体细胞错配修复缺陷(mismatch repair deficiency,MMR‐D)混淆。

我自己对 CMMR‐D 临床表型的了解主要来源于医学文献(截至2012年1月,56篇文章报道了114名患者)和14例迄今未发表的病例(其中大多数病例的突变分析主要针对 PMS2 基因,主要在我们机构进行);因此,在解释这些数据时,必须牢记潜在的偏倚。

CMMR‐D 患者的肿瘤谱非常广泛,主要分为4个类型:① 以淋巴瘤为主的血液系统恶性肿瘤,即非霍奇金淋巴瘤(non-Hodgkin's lymphoma,NHL),特别是 T 系 NHL 和 T 及 B 系急性淋巴细胞白血病,但也包括髓系白血病(reviewed by Ripperger et al. 2010);② 脑(中枢神经系统)肿瘤,包括胶质母细胞瘤和其他高级别星形细胞瘤、髓母细胞瘤以及幕上原始神经外胚层肿瘤(reviewed by Johannesma et al. 2011);③ 林奇综合征相关癌主要发生在结直肠,但也可发生在小肠、子宫内膜、卵巢、上尿路和膀胱,以及多发性肠息肉(reviewed by Durno et al. 2010 and Herkert et al. 2011);④ 胚胎肿瘤和其他恶性肿瘤,包括横纹肌肉瘤。表16.1总结了从80个家系128名患者中推断出的完整肿瘤谱。

表16.1 CMMR‐D 综合征的肿瘤谱(2012年1月更新)

恶性肿瘤	例数	诊断时中位年龄	范围
血液系统恶性肿瘤			
非霍奇金淋巴瘤和其他淋巴瘤	28	6	0.4~17
急性淋巴细胞白血病	7	6	2~21
AML	3	9	6~10
不典型 CML	1	1	
非特定白血病	1	n.r.	
总计	40	6	0.4~17
脑瘤			
胶质母细胞瘤和其他星形细胞瘤	51	9	2~35
幕上原始神经外胚层肿瘤(SPNET)	7	8	4~14
髓母细胞瘤	4	7	6~7
脑血管肉瘤	1	12	
总计	68	9	2~35
HNPCC 相关肿瘤			
结直肠癌	45	16	8~48
十二指肠/空肠/回肠癌	13	17	11~41

续表

恶性肿瘤	例数	诊断时中位年龄	范围
子宫内膜癌	5	24	23~35
输尿管/肾盂癌	3	19	
膀胱乳头状移行细胞癌	1	21	
卵巢癌	1	17	
总计	68	17	8~48
其他			
神经母细胞瘤	1	13	
Wilms 瘤	1	4	
卵巢神经外胚层肿瘤	1	21	
婴儿型肌纤维瘤病	1	1	
横纹肌肉瘤	1	4	
基底细胞癌	1	n.r.	
腮腺黏液表皮样癌	1	11	
总计	7		

MMR 基因突变在双等位基因患者中的分布与林奇综合征不同。*MLH1* 和 *MSH2* 杂合突变占林奇综合征病例的绝大多数（约 90%）（de la Chapelle 2004；Liu et al. 1996；Peltomaki 2003），而 *MSH6* 的突变约占 10%（Berends et al. 2002；Hendriks et al. 2004；Plaschke et al. 2004）。*PMS2* 突变在林奇综合征中的占比似乎很小。相比之下，CMMR-D 患者约 62%（79/128）携带 *PMS2* 双等位基因突变，约 17%（22/128）携带 *MSH6* 突变，仅约 21%（27/128）携带 *MLH1* 或 *MSH2* 突变。造成这种差异的原因可能有如下几个：① *PMS2* 单等位基因突变的外显率似乎低于其他 MMR 基因。这可能部分解释了林奇综合征中 PMS2 杂合突变携带者的发病率较低。这些患者经常使用修订的 Bethesda 标准（Umar et al. 2004）来进行筛选，并且往往缺乏明确的携带 *PMS2* 双等位基因突变的家族史。② 比较 *MLH/MSH2* 和 *MSH6/PMS2* 双等位基因突变携带者的肿瘤谱与恶性肿瘤的发病年龄（表 16.2）也显示出基因型-表型相关的趋势。携带 *MLH1/MSH2* 双等位基因突变的 CMMR-D 患者往往比 *MSH6/PMS2* 突变携带者更早发展为恶性肿瘤和癌前病变（首次诊断肿瘤的平均年龄为 4.5 岁 vs. 9 岁）。*MLH1/MSH2* 双等位基因突变携带者血液系统恶性肿瘤的发病率更高，而 *MSH6/PMS2* 突变携带者脑肿瘤和林奇综合征相关肿瘤的发病率似乎更高。因此，*MSH6/PMS2* 双等位基因突变的 CMMR-D 患者经常表现出特科特综合征（曾被认为是林奇综合征的一种亚型）的表型。与 *MLH/MSH2* 携带相比，*MSH6/PMS2* 双等位基因突变的患者更有可能在第一个肿瘤中存活下来而后发生第二肿瘤（28% vs. 40%）。这些因素可能有助于在 *MSH6* 和 *PMS2* 突变患者中诊断 CMMR-D。③ 除了可能的调查偏倚外，可以推测某些 *MLH1* 和 *MSH2* 的纯合突变是不可存活的，但 *PMS2* 和 *MSH6* 突变则不太可能是这种情况。

在大多数 CMMR-D 患者中都可发现类似 NF1 的临床症状，下文将对此进行讨论（见 16.3）。另外一个反复报道的皮肤特征（在至少 9 名 CMMR-D 患者中）是区域皮肤色素沉着不足（灰叶斑、白癜风）。对 *PMS2* 和 *MSH6* 双等位基因突变患者（分别为 3 名和 8 名）的分析表明，MMR 基因的构成性缺陷可导致免疫球蛋白（immunoglobulin, Ig）种类转换重组受损，其特征是 IgG2、IgG4 和 IgA 的减少或缺失伴随（特别是在年轻患者中）IgM 水平的增加，即高 IgM 综合征（Gardes et al. 2012；Péron et al. 2008）。在一名 *MSH2* 纯合突变的患者中也观察到表明体液缺陷的这种 IgA 缺乏（Whiteside et al. 2002）。Gardes 等（2012）报道，与 *MSH6* 缺乏相比，*PMS2* 缺乏会导致更严重的 Ig 种类转换重组缺陷，并可能导致感染的易感性。2 名患者发展为红斑狼疮（Plaschke et al. 2006；Rahner et al. 2008）。在 4 名 CMMR-D 患者中观察到胼胝体发育不全（Baas et al. 2012 and Gururangan et al. 2008）。到目前为止，其他先天性畸形仅在个别患者中描述：1 名患者先天性无脾、左侧异构和室间隔缺损（Herkert et al. 2011），1 名肾皮质囊肿（Durno et al. 2012；Gallinger et al. 2004）以及 2 名血管瘤（Leenen et al. 2011；Baas et al. 2012）。

表16.2 MLH1/MSH2 和 MSH6/PMS2 双等位基因突变携带者之间总体肿瘤谱和恶性肿瘤发病年龄的差异

基因	患者（家庭）数	肿瘤类型											初诊肿瘤时中位年龄（范围）（岁）	患大于1种恶性肿瘤的患者数（%）
		血液系统		脑		LS相关		其他		胃肠道和肝脏的癌前肿瘤[a]			
		患者数（%）	诊断时中位年龄（范围）（岁）	患者数（%）	诊断时中位年龄（范围）（岁）	患者数（%）	诊断时中位年龄（范围）（岁）	患者数（%）	诊断时中位年龄（范围）（岁）	患者数（%）	诊断时中位年龄（范围）（岁）		
MLH1	16(10)	6(37)	2.6(1~6)	7(44)	4.5(3~14)	5(31)	12(9~22)	1(6)	4	2(12)	9.5(9~10)	4.5(1~22)	4(25)
MSH2	12(6)	5(42)	3(0.4~2.5)	3(25)	13(3~14)	5(42)	14(11~39)	0	—	6(50)	13(6~46)	7(0.4~39)	4(33)
MLH1/MSH2	28(16)	11(39)	2(0.4~6)	10(36)	6(3~14)	10(36)	13(9~39)	1(3.5)	4	8(29)	11.5(6~46)	4.5(0.4~39)	8(29)
MSH6	22(14)	8(36)	8.5(5~11)	11(50)	9(2~17)	9(41)	13(8~31)	0	—	5(23)	11(9~17)	9(2~31)	9(41)
PMS2	78(49)	19(24)	7.5(2~21)	46(59)	9(2~35)	35(45)	16(9~32)	6(8)	11(1~21)	27(35)	15(7~24)	9.5(1~28)	31(40)
MSH6/PMS2	100(63)	27(27)	7(2~21)	57(57)	9(2~35)	44(44)	16(8~32)	6(6)	11(1~21)	32(32)	13.5(7~24)	9(1~31)	40(40)

注：[a] 到目前为止，仅有2例报告为肝腺瘤。LS，林奇综合征。

16.3 CMMR-D 和 NF1 的临床重叠

据报道，表 16.1 中列出的 128 名 CMMR-D 患者中有 83 人存在 NF1 相关特征。只有 3 名患者（Kets et al. 2009；Rahner et al. 2008；Sjursen et al. 2009）缺乏 NF1 的征象。83 名患者均出现 1 个以上的咖啡牛奶斑（café-au-lait macule，CALM）。但并不是所有的患者都达到了 NF1 诊断所需的 6 个咖啡斑的标准。在一些患者中，已经报道了 CALM 的半身或节段分布（Auclair et al. 2007；Wang et al. 1999）（图 16.1a、b 显示了 1 名 MSH6 复合杂合突变的患者 CALM 和 freckling 的节段分布）。此外，一些报告强调 CMMR-D 患者的 CALM 色素沉着程度不同，边缘不规则，因此与 NF1 患者不同（De Vos et al. 2006；Kruger et al. 2008；Scott et al. 2007a；Tan et al. 2008）。然而，这些细微的差异可能只有经验丰富的临床医师才能识别，而它们也可能并非在所有患者中都能显现出来（图 16.1c 显示了 1 名 PMS2 复合杂合突变患者仅有的 2 个 CALM）。其他与 NF1 相关的体征出现频率较低。Lisch 结节和神经纤维瘤各报道了 4 名患者（Auclair et al. 2007；Gallinger et al. 2004；Ricciardone et al. 1999；Wang et al. 1999）。胫骨假关节（Wang et al. 1999）和单侧蝶翼骨发育不良（Dr. Shenkmann, personal communication）各报告了 1 名患者。然而，就其皮肤表现而言，只有少数患者真正符合美国国立卫生研究院（NIH）的 NF1 标准。总之，CALM 和 NF1 的表现是 CMMR-D 的标志，应作为诊断标准（见 16.5）。

由于 CMMR-D 与 NF1 的临床重叠，许多 CMMR-D 患者过去曾被误诊为 NF1。这不仅混淆了这些患者及其家族的正确诊断，也可能影响了我们对 NF1 及其与罕见肿瘤关系的了解。

NF1 患儿的脑肿瘤多为低级别，分类为 WHO Ⅰ级的毛细胞星形细胞瘤，它们通常不会发展为恶性肿瘤。然而，一些病例报告（Distelmaier et al. 2007；Glover et al. 1991；Uyttebroeck et al. 1995）和一项回顾性的临床病理研究（Huttner et al. 2010）为儿童胶质母细胞瘤和 NF1 的相关性提供了证据。高级别星形细胞肿瘤，主要为 WHO Ⅳ级胶质母细胞瘤，是 CMMR-D 患者中发现的最常见肿瘤（到目前为止＞50 名患者），这一事实至少对一些患者的 NF1 诊断提出了挑战。因此，作为易患高级别星形细胞瘤和 NF1 体征的潜在疾病，儿童患者须明确排除 CMMR-D。NF1 与儿童高级别星形细胞瘤的关系仍有待进一步研究及重新评估。

在解释胚胎性肿瘤患者的数据时，CMMR-D 和 NF1 临床表现中的重叠也应牢记。特别是据报道，儿童最常见的软组织肉瘤——横纹肌肉瘤（rhabdomyosarcoma，RMS）与 NF1 有关（Sung et al. 2004）。到目前为止，在 3 名 CMMR-D 患者中报告了横纹肌肉瘤（Kratz et al. 2009；Wang et al. 1999），其中 2 名患者推测有 PMS2 和 MLH1 基因突变，但未经证实，因此这 2 名患者不包括在表 16.1 中。在 CMMR-D 患者中发现的其他胚胎肿瘤包括神经母细胞瘤（De Rosa et al. 2000）和 Wilms 瘤（Poley et al. 2007；Wagner et al. 2003），它们与 NF1 的关联仍在争论中。

NF1 儿童患幼年性粒单核细胞白血病（juvenile myelomonocytic leukemia，JMML）的风险增加已得到充分证实（见第 30 章）。到目前为止，还没有 CMMR-D 患者患 JMML 的报道。NF1 儿童也可患单体 7 型骨髓增生异常综合征（myelodysplastic

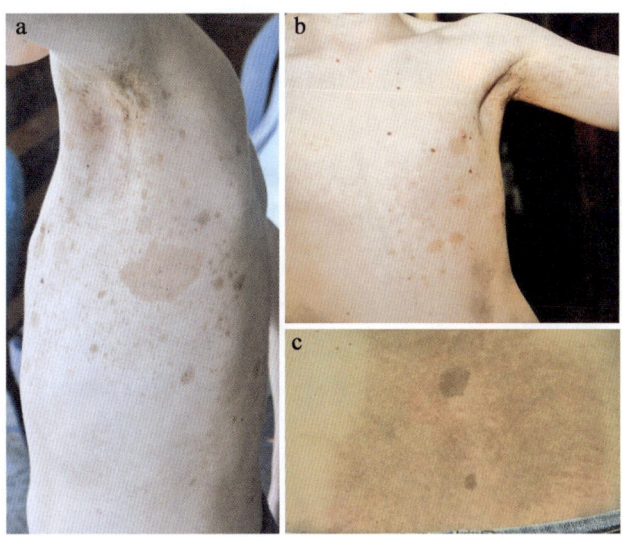

图 16.1 2 名 CMMR-D 患者的色素表现。注意第 1 名携带 MSH6 复合杂合突变患者（a、b）的节段分布。第 2 名患者（c）为 PMS2 复合杂合突变，下背部只有 2 个咖啡牛奶斑

syndromes，MDS)(Shannon et al. 1992)。在 2 项报告中报道了 5 例因治疗继发的单体 7 型 MDS 与 NF1 相关。这 5 名患者存在不同的原发恶性肿瘤，并且临床上表现为 NF1(Maris et al. 1997；Perilongo et al. 1993)。在这些患者中，没有 1 例在肿瘤细胞的 NF1 基因座发现 LOH，尽管这是髓系恶性肿瘤中 NF1 失活最常见的二次打击机制(Stephens et al. 2006)。这 5 例患者的原发恶性肿瘤包括高级别星形细胞瘤、淋巴细胞白血病和 Wilms 瘤，这些恶性肿瘤也在 CMMR-D 患者中观察到(表 16.1)。此外，MDS/AML 也是 2 名 CMMR-D 患者的第二种恶性肿瘤(Etzler et al. 2008；Scott et al. 2007b)，其中至少有 1 名患者因 t(2;7)易位而导致染色体 7q 部分缺失。综合来看，可以想到至少报道中的一些患继发性单体 7 型 MDS 的患者，实际应为 CMMR-D 而非 NF1。

为了避免将被误诊为 NF1 的 CMMR-D 患者纳入前瞻性研究和未来的病例报告，所有表现出 NF1 特征的儿童恶性肿瘤患者，如果父母无 NF1，也无明显与 NF1 相关的恶性肿瘤(如 MPNST 或 JMML)，则应排除 MMR 缺陷。

16.4　*NF1* 基因是 MMR-D 的靶标之一

尽管绝大多数 CMMR-D 患者表现出 CALM，并且在某些情况下还表现出 NF1 的其他迹象，但大多数患者经检测并没有发现潜在的 *NF1* 胚系突变(即使经过综合突变分析时也是如此)(Auclair et al. 2007；Etzler et al. 2008；Hegde et al. 2005；Menko et al. 2004；Ostergaard et al. 2005；Trimbath et al. 2001)。有人提出 CMMR-D 患者的 NF1 表现是由合子后 NF1 突变引起的，由于构成性 DNA 修复缺陷，这些患者发育早期 *NF1* 突变频率增加，但由于其镶嵌状态，这种突变通常在血细胞中检测不到(见第 12 章)。在几个 CMMR-D 患者中观察到的 NF1 特征为半身或节段分布支持了这一观点。到目前为止，仅在 Ricciardone 等(1999)最初描述的 1 名患者中发现了有害的 *NF1* 突变(Alotaibi et al. 2008)。由于在患者的血细胞中(没有镶嵌现象的证据)发现 CpG 二核苷酸处的重现性 C 到 T 转变(C.3721C>T)，并且该转变为杂合状态，作者推测，这是发生在胚胎细胞中的一种非常早期的体细胞突变。此外，他们假设由 *MLH1* 纯合突变引起的 MMR 缺陷协同 *NF1* 杂合突变可能导致在该患者中观察到的表型，即>10 个腹部 CALM、12 个月大时出现 2 个皮肤纤维瘤和 1 种非典型髓细胞白血病。这一假设得到了小鼠模型的支持——Mlh1 缺乏加速了 *Nf1* 杂合子小鼠的髓系白血病发生(Gutmann et al. 2003)。

Wang 及其同事的一项研究也证明 *NF1* 基因是 MMR 缺乏的 1 个靶点(Wang et al. 2003)。在显示 MSI 的 4/10 肿瘤细胞系中，对 *NF1* 突变的筛选成功地鉴定了 7 种 *NF1* 改变(其中 1 个已鉴定的突变 p.D176E 是已知的 *NF1* 多态性，因此，此处未考虑携带这种突变的细胞系)，而在 5 种 MMR 充足的肿瘤细胞系中均未发现 NF1 突变。这项研究在显示 MSI 的 5 个原发肿瘤中发现了 2 种 *NF1* 突变，亚克隆分析揭示 Mlh1 缺陷的小鼠胚胎成纤维细胞系中的 Nf1 镶嵌突变。10 个 *NF1* 突变中有 5 个是移码突变，其中 4 个位于 *NF1* 编码序列中的单核苷酸重复序列。这反映了 MMR 缺陷的典型突变足迹，因此支持 MMR 缺陷细胞中 *NF1* 突变率加速的观点。此外可以推测，神经纤维瘤蛋白失活可能致瘤，这导致林奇综合征相关肿瘤的发生和肿瘤细胞系中携带 *NF1* 突变细胞的克隆扩增(Bertholon et al. 2006)。

尽管强有力的证据表明 *NF1* 突变是 CMMR-D 患者 NF1 临床特征的根本原因，但这些患者的 CALM 和雀斑以及非 NF1 相关的皮肤特征(如皮肤色素沉着)也可能代表"孤立"的皮肤表现，而不是镶嵌或节段性 NF1 的临床特征。事实上，CALM 也存在于其他遗传综合征(如 Legius 综合征、LEOPARD 综合征、尼梅亨断裂综合征和范科尼贫血)中。因此可以想象，其他基因的体细胞突变也可能解释在 CMMR-D 患者中观察到的皮肤表现。

16.5　CMMR-D 患者的诊断策略

鉴于 CMMR-D 的肿瘤谱广泛，所有表现出多个 CALM 的儿童恶性肿瘤患者都应怀疑 CMMR-D 综合征。由于 CMMR-D 患者的 NF1 体征不是由 NF1 胚系突变引起的，所以 CMMR-D 患者的父母通常不会表现出 NF1 症状。然而同样患病的兄弟姐妹可能出现 NF1 的相关特征，因此，如果有兄弟姐妹患病，那么存在＞6 个 CALM 或雀斑的 CMMR-D 患者可能满足 NF1 临床诊断的第二个 NIH 标准。鉴于这一潜在陷阱，有人建议将 NF1 的 NIH 诊断标准措辞从"一级亲属"（包括兄弟姐妹）改为"父母或后代"（Huson 2008）。

在超过 50% 的家庭中，儿童患者携带 MMR 基因纯合突变时表明父母有血缘关系（在大多数患者中）或存在创始人突变（De Vos et al. 2006）。

由于错配修复基因中的单等位基因突变导致林奇综合征，CMMR-D 患者通常会有患林奇综合征相关癌症的亲属。然而必须记住，*MSH6* 单等位基因（特别是 *PMS2*）突变的外显率低，因此，在 *MSH6* 或 *PMS2* 双等位基因突变携带者中可能无可疑的家族史。

综上所述，有人认为儿童恶性肿瘤患者表现出以下一种或多种特征时，需要高度怀疑 CMMR-D 综合征：

- 咖啡斑或 NF1 的其他症状，色素减退的皮肤病变。
- 父母为近亲婚配。
- 林奇综合征相关肿瘤家族史。
- 患第二肿瘤或兄弟姐妹患恶性肿瘤。

CMMR-D 综合征的诊断流程在很大程度上遵循林奇综合征的方案。第一步通常为分析肿瘤组织的 MSI 和评估致病性 MMR 基因的丢失。MSI 分析根据当前方案为使用一组 5-6 二核苷酸（Umar et al. 2004）或单核苷酸（Goel et al. 2010）来重复标记。该方法是诊断 CMMR-D 患者胃肠道肿瘤 MMR 缺乏的可靠工具。然而该分析可能无法显示脑肿瘤中的 MSI（Leenen et al. 2011；Wimmer and Etzler 2008）。为解释 CMMR-D 患者脑肿瘤中 MSI 缺失而提出的一个假设是脑组织中的 MMR-D 可能通过与复制后 DNA 修复不同的机制来导致肿瘤发生（Bougeard et al. 2003；Poley et al. 2007）。此外，胃肠道肿瘤和脑肿瘤的 MSI 程度和模式可能不同，这使得常规用于林奇综合征相关肿瘤的 MSI 分析技术对脑肿瘤的可靠性较低（Giunti et al. 2009）。免疫组织化学（immunohistochemistry，IHC）在 CMMR-D 患者的所有实体瘤中都得到了有效的应用，并可指导 4 种 MMR 基因的后续突变分析。*PMS2* 或 *MSH6* 的截断突变通常会导致这些蛋白质的单独丢失，而 *MLH1* 或 *MSH2* 的突变将分别导致 MLH1/PMS2 或 MSH2/MSH6 的同时缺失，因为 MLH1 和 MSH2 是 MLH1/PMS2 和 MSH2/MSH6 异二聚体形成的必要条件。值得注意的是，在错义突变的情况下 IHC 可能显示突变 MMR 基因的正常表达。IHC 可检测出 CMMR-D 患者的肿瘤和非肿瘤组织中 1 个（或 2 个）MMR 基因的表达缺失，这一点与林奇综合征不同，后者仅在肿瘤细胞中检测到表达缺失。MMR 基因的表达缺失也可以在 CMMR-D 患者的血液淋巴细胞中检测，例如通过蛋白质印迹法（Péron et al. 2008）。同样，通过分析每次 PCR 反应稀释至 1~3 个基因组当量的 DNA 样本，可以在 CMMR-D 患者的正常非瘤组织中检测 MSI（Agostini et al. 2005；Felton et al. 2007）。然而迄今为止，尚未开发出检测 CMMR-D 患者非肿瘤组织中 MMR 表达缺失和 MSI 的标准化程序。CMMR-D 的诊断应通过基因的特异性突变分析来确认。现在对所有 MMR 基因（包括历史上困难的 *PMS2* 基因）都有可靠和稳健的综合分析方法（Etzler et al. 2008；van der Klift et al. 2010；Vaughn et al. 2011；Wernstedt et al. 2012）。

16.6 CMMR-D 患者及其亲属的咨询、随访和治疗

CMMR-D 综合征儿童患者的确诊对其家族也有重要意义。因此在患儿检测前应向父母提供遗传咨询，告知其有潜在的 25% 的遗传风险和父母双方均存在杂合突变的可能。一旦发现突变，应按照既定的跨学科咨询指南，向所有可能为杂合突变携带者的家庭成员提供检测。杂合突变携带者应按照林奇综合征指南进行随访（Vasen et al. 2007）。由于与 *MLH1* 和 *MSH2* 突变相比，*PMS2* 单等位基因突变的外显率可能会降低，因此在这种情况下，标准指南可能会有所放宽。Senter 等（2008）提出 *PMS2* 突变携带者可能应该遵循中间的筛查方案，例如从

30岁开始每1～2年进行1次结肠镜检查（正如对 MSH6 突变个体所建议的方案）（Bonadona et al. 2011；Lindor et al. 2006）。通过未来的研究，了解到更多关于其癌症风险和癌症谱系的信息，针对 PMS2 杂合突变个体的咨询和随访建议可能会被进一步修改。

由于 CMMR-D 癌症风险显著，且与之相关的恶性肿瘤种类繁多，因此制订患者的治疗和随访建议仍然是一项挑战。最近 Durno 等（2012）提出了一种筛查方案，重点是检测 CMMR-D 患者的脑肿瘤、白血病、淋巴瘤和胃肠道恶性肿瘤。该方案包括（从出生开始）每4个月1次的全血细胞计数、红细胞沉降率和乳酸脱氢酶，以及出生时的脑超声，之后每6个月1次 MRI 检查。根据他们的建议，结肠镜和食管胃十二指肠镜（视频胶囊内镜）应从3岁或诊断时开始每年进行1次。Herkert 等（2011）建议从6岁开始每年进行结肠镜检查，从8岁开始进行视频胶囊内镜检查。Durno 和同事们补充了林奇综合征患者成年后的一般建议，包括妇科和泌尿道筛查（Bonadona et al. 2011；Lindor et al. 2006）。目前还没有关于这些患者恶性肿瘤的最佳治疗建议。然而应该提到的是，几份报告强调 MMR 缺陷细胞对替莫唑胺等 O^6 甲基化物的细胞毒性具有很强的抵抗力（Allan and Travis 2005；Fedier and Fink 2004）。这表明 O^6 甲基化物可能对 MMR-D 综合征患者具有高度诱变性和无效性，使用它们可能会增加肿瘤复发或发生第二肿瘤的风险（Scott et al. 2007a，b）。

16.7 结论

CMMR-D 综合征是所有存在咖啡牛奶斑的恶性肿瘤患儿的重要鉴别诊断，这些患儿可能有或没有 NF1 的其他体征，并且患非 NF1 相关（如 MPNST 或 JMML）的恶性肿瘤。识别这种癌症综合征的儿童患者很重要，因为它对更广泛的家族有深远的影响。

CMMR-D 和 NF1 的重叠表现可能导致过去对 CMMR-D 患者的误诊。如 NF1 患者发生罕见肿瘤，重新评估诊断可能是可取的。

有强烈的迹象表明，CMMR-D 患者的 NF1 表现是由于受精后 NF1 基因突变引起。由于固有的 MMR 缺陷，这些患者 NF1 突变的频率可能更高。然而这一发现并不排除 CMMR-D 患者有其他的遗传变异从而导致色素变化的可能。

据推测，NF1 杂合和 MMR 双等位基因突变共同促进了 CMMR-D 患者的肿瘤发生。NF1 基因是 MMR 缺陷的靶点，这一发现也可能引发人们的猜测，即 MMR 能力的个体间差异可能在改变 NF1 的表型方面发挥作用，例如通过影响 NF1 二次打击后突变的发生率。

（陈森敏　译）

参考文献

[1] Aaltonen LA, Peltomaki P, Leach FS, Sistonen P, Pylkkanen L, Mecklin JP, Jarvinen H, Powell SM, Jen J, Hamilton SR et al (1993) Clues to the pathogenesis of familial colorectal cancer. Science 260：812-816

[2] Agostini M, Tibiletti MG, Lucci-Cordisco E, Chiaravalli A, Morreau H, Furlan D, Boccuto L, Pucciarelli S, Capella C, Boiocchi M, Viel A (2005) Two PMS2 mutations in a Turcot syndrome family with small bowel cancers. Am J Gastroenterol 100：1886-1891

[3] Allan JM, Travis LB (2005) Mechanisms of therapy-related carcinogenesis. Nat Rev Cancer 5：943-955

[4] Alotaibi H, Ricciardone MD, Ozturk M (2008) Homozygosity at variant MLH1 can lead to secondary mutation in NF1, neurofibromatosis type I and early onset leukemia. Mutat Res 637：209-214

[5] Auclair J, Leroux D, Desseigne F, Lasset C, Saurin JC, Joly MO, Pinson S, Xu XL, Montmain G, Ruano E, Navarro C, Puisieux A, Wang Q (2007) Novel biallelic mutations in MSH6 and PMS2 genes：gene conversion as a likely cause of PMS2 gene inactivation. Hum Mutat 28：1084-1090

[6] Baas AF, Gabbett M, Rimac M, Kansikas M, Raphael M, Nievelstein RA, Nicholls W, Offerhaus J, Bodmer D, Wernstedt A, Krabichler B, Strasser U, Nyström M, Zschocke J, Robertson SP, van Haelst MM, Wimmer K (2012) Agenesis of the corpus callosum and gray matter heterotopia in three patients with constitutional mismatch repair deficiency syndrome. Eur J Hum Genet (in press)

[7] Berends MJ, Wu Y, Sijmons RH, Mensink RG, van der Sluis T, Hordijk-Hos JM, de Vries EG, Hollema H, Karrenbeld A, Buys CH, van der Zee AG, Hofstra RM, Kleibeuker JH (2002) Molecular and clinical characteristics of MSH6 variants：an analysis of 25 index carriers of a germline variant. Am J Hum Genet 70：26-37

[8] Bertholon J, Wang Q, Galmarini CM, Puisieux A (2006)

Mutational targets in colorectal cancer cells with microsatellite instability. Fam Cancer 5: 29-34

[9] Boland CR, Thibodeau SN, Hamilton SR, Sidransky D, Eshleman JR, Burt RW, Meltzer SJ, Rodriguez-Bigas MA, Fodde R, Ranzani GN, Srivastava S (1998) A National Cancer Institute Workshop on Microsatellite Instability for cancer detection and familial predisposition: devel-opment of international criteria for the determination of microsatellite instability in colorectal cancer. Cancer Res 58: 5248-5257

[10] Bonadona V, Bonaiti B, Olschwang S, Grandjouan S, Huiart L, Longy M, Guimbaud R, Buecher B, Bignon YJ, Caron O, Colas C, Nogues C, Lejeune-Dumoulin S, Olivier-Faivre L, Polycarpe-Osaer F, Nguyen TD, Desseigne F, Saurin JC, Berthet P, Leroux D, Duffour J, Manouvrier S, Frebourg T, Sobol H, Lasset C, Bonaiti-Pellie C (2011) Cancer risks associated with germline mutations in MLH1, MSH2, and MSH6 genes in Lynch syndrome. JAMA 305: 2304-2310

[11] Bougeard G, Charbonnier F, Moerman A, Martin C, Ruchoux MM, Drouot N, Frebourg T (2003) Early onset brain tumor and lymphoma in MSH2-deficient children. Am J Hum Genet 72: 213-216

[12] de la Chapelle A (2004) Genetic predisposition to colorectal cancer. Nat Rev Cancer 4: 769-780

[13] De Rosa M, Fasano C, Panariello L, Scarano MI, Belli G, Iannelli A, Ciciliano F, Izzo P (2000) Evidence for a recessive inheritance of Turcot's syndrome caused by compound heterozygous mutations within the PMS2 gene. Oncogene 19: 1719-1723

[14] De Vos M, Hayward BE, Charlton R, Taylor GR, Glaser AW, Picton S, Cole TR, Maher ER, McKeown CM, Mann JR, Yates JR, Baralle D, Rankin J, Bonthron DT, Sheridan E (2006) PMS2 mutations in childhood cancer. J Natl Cancer Inst 98: 358-361

[15] Distelmaier F, Fahsold R, Reifenberger G, Messing-Juenger M, Schaper J, Schneider DT, Gobel U, Mayatepek E, Rosenbaum T (2007) Fatal glioblastoma multiforme in a patient with neurofibromatosis type I: the dilemma of systematic medical follow-up. Childs Nerv Syst 23: 343-347

[16] Durandy A (2009) Immunoglobulin class switch recombination: study through human natural mutants. Philos Trans R Soc Lond B Biol Sci 364: 577-582

[17] Durno CA, Holter S, Sherman PM, Gallinger S (2010) The gastrointestinal phenotype of germline biallelic mismatch repair gene mutations. Am J Gastroenterol 105: 2449-2456

[18] Durno CA, Aronson M, Tabori U, Malkin D, Gallinger S, Chan HS (2012) Oncologic surveillance for subjects with biallelic mismatch repair gene mutations: 10 year follow-up of a kindred. Pediatr Blood Cancer 59: 652-656

[19] Etzler J, Peyrl A, Zatkova A, Schildhaus HU, Ficek A, Merkelbach-Bruse S, Kratz CP, Attarbaschi A, Hainfellner JA, Yao S, Messiaen L, Slavc I, Wimmer K (2008) RNA-based mutation analysis identifies an unusual MSH6 splicing defect and circumvents PMS2 pseudogene interference. Hum Mutat 29: 299-305

[20] Fedier A, Fink D (2004) Mutations in DNA mismatch repair genes: implications for DNA damage signaling and drug sensitivity (review). Int J Oncol 24: 1039-1047

[21] Felton KE, Gilchrist DM, Andrew SE (2007) Constitutive deficiency in DNA mismatch repair. Clin Genet 71: 483-498

[22] Gallinger S, Aronson M, Shayan K, Ratcliffe EM, Gerstle JT, Parkin PC, Rothenmund H, Croitoru M, Baumann E, Durie PR, Weksberg R, Pollett A, Riddell RH, Ngan BY, Cutz E, Lagarde AE, Chan HS (2004) Gastrointestinal cancers and neurofibromatosis type 1 features in children with a germline homozygous MLH1 mutation. Gastroenterology 126: 576-585

[23] Gardes P, Forveille M, Alyanakian MA, Aucouturier P, Ilencikova D, Leroux D, Rahner N, Mazerolles F, Fischer A, Kracker S, Durandy A (2012) Human MSH6 deficiency Is associated with impaired antibody maturation. J Immunol 188: 2023-2029

[24] Giunti L, Cetica V, Ricci U, Giglio S, Sardi I, Paglierani M, Andreucci E, Sanzo M, Forni M, Buccoliero AM, Genitori L, Genuardi M (2009) Type A microsatellite instability in pediatric gliomas as an indicator of Turcot syndrome. Eur J Hum Genet 17: 919-927

[25] Glover TW, Stein CK, Legius E, Andersen LB, Brereton A, Johnson S (1991) Molecular and cytogenetic analysis of tumors in von Recklinghausen neurofibromatosis. Genes Chrom Cancer 3: 62-70

[26] Goel A, Nagasaka T, Hamelin R, Boland CR (2010) An optimized pentaplex PCR for detecting DNA mismatch repair-deficient colorectal cancers. PLoS One 5: e9393

[27] Gururangan S, Frankel W, Broaddus R, Clendenning M, Senter L, McDonald M, Eastwood J, Reardon D, Vredenburgh J, Quinn J, Friedman HS (2008) Multifocal anaplastic astrocytoma in a patient with hereditary colorectal cancer, transcobalamin II deficiency, agenesis of the corpus callosum, mental retardation, and inherited PMS2 mutation. Neuro Oncol 10: 93-97

[28] Gutmann DH, Winkeler E, Kabbarah O, Hedrick N, Dudley S, Goodfellow PJ, Liskay RM (2003) Mlh1 deficiency accelerates myeloid leukemogenesis in neurofibromatosis 1 (Nf1) heterozygous mice. Oncogene 22: 4581-4585

[29] Hegde MR, Chong B, Blazo ME, Chin LH, Ward PA, Chintagumpala MM, Kim JY, Plon SE, Richards CS (2005) A homozygous mutation in MSH6 causes Turcot syndrome. Clin Cancer Res 11: 4689-4693

[30] Hendriks YM, Wagner A, Morreau H, Menko F, Stormorken A, Quehenberger F, Sandkuijl L, Moller P, Genuardi M, Van Houwelingen H, Tops C, Van Puijenbroek M, Verkuijlen P, Kenter G, Van Mil A, Meijers-Heijboer H, Tan GB, Breuning MH, Fodde R, Wijnen JT, Brocker-Vriends AH, Vasen H (2004) Cancer risk in hereditary nonpolyposis colorectal cancer due to MSH6 mutations: impact on counseling and surveillance. Gastroenterology 127: 17-25

[31] Herkert JC, Niessen RC, Olderode-Berends MJ, Veenstra-Knol HE, Vos YJ, van der Klift HM, Scheenstra R, Tops CM, Karrenbeld A, Peters FT, Hofstra RM, Kleibeuker JH, Sijmons RH (2011) Paediatric intestinal cancer and polyposis due to bi-allelic PMS2 mutations: case series, review and follow-up guidelines. Eur J Cancer 47: 965-982

[32] Huson SM (2008) The neurofibromatoses: classification, clinical features and genetic counselling. In: Kaufmann D (ed) Neurofibromatoses, vol 16, Monographs in human genetics. Karger, Basel, pp 1-20

[33] Huttner AJ, Kieran MW, Yao X, Cruz L, Ladner J, Quayle K, Goumnerova LC, Irons MB, Ullrich NJ (2010) Clinicopathologic study of glioblastoma in children with neurofibromatosis type 1. Pediatr Blood Cancer 54: 890-896

[34] Jiricny J (2006a) The multifaceted mismatch-repair system. Nat Rev Mol Cell Biol 7: 335-346

[35] Jiricny J (2006b) MutLalpha: at the cutting edge of mismatch repair. Cell 126: 239-241

[36] Johannesma P, van der Klift H, van Grieken N, Troost D, Te

Riele H, Jacobs M, Postma T, Heideman D, Tops C, Wijnen J, Menko F (2011) Childhood brain tumours due to germline bi-allelic mismatch repair gene mutations. Clin Genet 80: 243-255

[37] Kadyrov FA, Dzantiev L, Constantin N, Modrich P (2006) Endonucleolytic function of MutLalpha in human mismatch repair. Cell 126: 297-308

[38] Kets CM, Hoogerbrugge N, van Krieken JH, Goossens M, Brunner HG, Ligtenberg MJ (2009) Compound heterozygosity for two MSH2 mutations suggests mild consequences of the initiation codon variant c. 1A>G of MSH2. Eur J Hum Genet 17: 159-164

[39] Kratz CP, Holter S, Etzler J, Lauten M, Pollett A, Niemeyer CM, Gallinger S, Wimmer K (2009) Rhabdomyosarcoma in patients with constitutional mismatch-repair-deficiency syndrome. J Med Genet 46: 418-420

[40] Kruger S, Kinzel M, Walldorf C, Gottschling S, Bier A, Tinschert S, von Stackelberg A, Henn W, Gorgens H, Boue S, Kolble K, Buttner R, Schackert HK (2008) Homozygous PMS2 germline mutations in two families with early-onset haematological malignancy, brain tumours, HNPCC-associated tumours, and signs of neurofibromatosis type 1. Eur J Hum Genet 16: 62-72

[41] Leenen C, Geurts-Giele W, Dubbink H, Reddingius R, van den Ouweland A, Tops C, van de Klift H, Kuipers E, van Leerdam M, Dinjens W, Wagner A (2011) Pitfalls in molecular analysis for mismatch repair deficiency in a family with biallelic pms2 germline mutations. Clin Genet 80: 558-565

[42] Lindor NM, Petersen GM, Hadley DW, Kinney AY, Miesfeldt S, Lu KH, Lynch P, Burke W, Press N (2006) Recommendations for the care of individuals with an inherited predisposition to Lynch syndrome: a systematic review. JAMA 296: 1507-1517

[43] Liu B, Parsons R, Papadopoulos N, Nicolaides NC, Lynch HT, Watson P, Jass JR, Dunlop M, Wyllie A, Peltomaki P, de la Chapelle A, Hamilton SR, Vogelstein B, Kinzler KW (1996) Analysis of mismatch repair genes in hereditary non-polyposis colorectal cancer patients. Nat Med 2: 169-174

[44] Lynch HT, de la Chapelle A (2003) Hereditary colorectal cancer. N Engl J Med 348: 919-932

[45] Lynch HT, Lynch JF, Attard TA (2009) Diagnosis and management of hereditary colorectal cancer syndromes: Lynch syndrome as a model. CMAJ 181: 273-280

[46] Maris JM, Wiersma SR, Mahgoub N, Thompson P, Geyer RJ, Hurwitz CG, Lange BJ, Shannon KM (1997) Monosomy 7 myelodysplastic syndrome and other second malignant neoplasms in children with neurofibromatosis type 1. Cancer 79: 1438-1446

[47] Menko FH, Kaspers GL, Meijer GA, Claes K, van Hagen JM, Gille JJ (2004) A homozygous MSH6 mutation in a child with café-au-lait spots, oligodendroglioma and rectal cancer. Fam Cancer 3: 123-127

[48] Ostergaard JR, Sunde L, Okkels H (2005) Neurofibromatosis von Recklinghausen type 1 phenotype and early onset of cancers in siblings compound heterozygous for mutations in MSH6. Am J Med Genet A 139: 96-105, discussion 196

[49] Peltomaki P (2003) Role of DNA mismatch repair defects in the pathogenesis of human cancer. J Clin Oncol 21: 1174-1179

[50] Perilongo G, Felix CA, Meadows AT, Nowell P, Biegel J, Lange BJ (1993) Sequential development of Wilms tumor, T-cell acute lymphoblastic leukemia, medulloblastoma and myeloid leukemia in a child with type 1 neurofibromatosis: a clinical and cytogenetic case report. Leukemia 7: 912-915

[51] Péron S, Metin A, Gardes P, Alyanakian MA, Sheridan E, Kratz CP, Fischer A, Durandy A (2008) Human PMS2 deficiency is associated with impaired immunoglobulin class switch recombination. J Exp Med 205: 2465-2472

[52] Plaschke J, Engel C, Kruger S, Holinski-Feder E, Pagenstecher C, Mangold E, Moeslein G, Schulmann K, Gebert J, von Knebel Doeberitz M, Ruschoff J, Loeffler M, Schackert HK (2004) Lower incidence of colorectal cancer and later age of disease onset in 27 families with pathogenic MSH6 germline mutations compared with families with MLH1 or MSH2 mutations: the German Hereditary Nonpolyposis Colorectal Cancer Consortium. J Clin Oncol 22: 4486-4494

[53] Plaschke J, Linnebacher M, Kloor M, Gebert J, Cremer FW, Tinschert S, Aust DE, von Knebel DM, Schackert HK (2006) Compound heterozygosity for two MSH6 mutations in a patient with early onset of HNPCC-associated cancers, but without hematological malignancy and brain tumor. Eur J Hum Genet 14: 561-566

[54] Poley JW, Wagner A, Hoogmans MM, Menko FH, Tops C, Kros JM, Reddingius RE, Meijers-Heijboer H, Kuipers EJ, Dinjens WN (2007) Biallelic germline mutations of mismatch-repair genes: a possible cause for multiple pediatric malignancies. Cancer 109: 2349-2356

[55] Rahner N, Hoefler G, Hogenauer C, Lackner C, Steinke V, Sengteller M, Friedl W, Aretz S, Propping P, Mangold E, Walldorf C (2008) Compound heterozygosity for two MSH6 mutations in a patient with early onset colorectal cancer, vitiligo and systemic lupus erythematosus. Am J Med Genet A 146A: 1314-1319

[56] Ricciardone MD, Ozcelik T, Cevher B, Ozdag H, Tuncer M, Gurgey A, Uzunalimoglu O, Cetinkaya H, Tanyeli A, Erken E, Ozturk M (1999) Human MLH1 deficiency predisposes to hematological malignancy and neurofibromatosis type 1. Cancer Res 59: 290-293

[57] Ripperger T, Beger C, Rahner N, Sykora KW, Bockmeyer CL, Lehmann U, Kreipe HH, Schlegelberger B (2010) Constitutional mismatch repair deficiency and childhood leukemia/lymphoma-report on a novel biallelic MSH6 mutation. Haematologica 95: 841-844

[58] Scott RH, Homfray T, Huxter NL, Mitton SG, Nash R, Potter MN, Lancaster D, Rahman N (2007a) Familial T-cell non-Hodgkin lymphoma caused by biallelic MSH2 mutations. J Med Genet 44: e83

[59] Scott RH, Mansour S, Pritchard-Jones K, Kumar D, MacSweeney F, Rahman N (2007b) Medulloblastoma, acute myelocytic leukemia and colonic carcinomas in a child with biallelic MSH6 mutations. Nat Clin Pract Oncol 4: 130-134

[60] Senter L, Clendenning M, Sotamaa K, Hampel H, Green J, Potter JD, Lindblom A, Lagerstedt K, Thibodeau SN, Lindor NM, Young J, Winship I, Dowty JG, White DM, Hopper JL, Baglietto L, Jenkins MA, de la Chapelle A (2008) The clinical phenotype of Lynch syndrome due to germ-line PMS2 mutations. Gastroenterology 135: 419-428

[61] Shannon KM, Watterson J, Johnson P, O'Connell P, Lange B, Shah N, Steinherz P, Kan YW, Priest JR (1992) Monosomy 7 myeloproliferative disease in children with neurofibromatosis, type 1: epidemiology and molecular analysis. Blood 79: 1311-1318

[62] Sjursen W, Bjornevoll I, Engebretsen LF, Fjelland K, Halvorsen T, Myrvold HE (2009) A homozygote splice site PMS2 mutation as cause of Turcot syndrome gives rise to two different abnormal transcripts. Fam Cancer 8: 179-186

[63] Stephens K, Weaver M, Leppig KA, Maruyama K, Emanuel PD, Le Beau MM, Shannon KM (2006) Interstitial uniparental isodisomy at clustered breakpoint intervals is a frequent mechanism of NF1 inactivation in myeloid malignancies. Blood 108: 1684-1689

[64] Stojic L, Brun R, Jiricny J (2004) Mismatch repair and DNA damage signalling. DNA Repair (Amst) 3: 1091-1101

[65] Sung L, Anderson JR, Arndt C, Raney RB, Meyer WH, Pappo AS (2004) Neurofibromatosis in children with Rhabdomyosarcoma: a report from the Intergroup Rhabdomyosarcoma study IV. J Pediatr 144: 666-668

[66] Tan TY, Orme LM, Lynch E, Croxford MA, Dow C, Dewan PA, Lipton L (2008) Biallelic PMS2 mutations and a distinctive childhood cancer syndrome. J Pediatr Hematol Oncol 30: 254-257

[67] Trimbath JD, Petersen GM, Erdman SH, Ferre M, Luce MC, Giardiello FM (2001) Café-au-lait spots and early onset colorectal neoplasia: a variant of HNPCC? Fam Cancer 1: 101-105

[68] Umar A, Boland CR, Terdiman JP, Syngal S, de la Chapelle A, Ruschoff J, Fishel R, Lindor NM, Burgart LJ, Hamelin R, Hamilton SR, Hiatt RA, Jass J, Lindblom A, Lynch HT, Peltomaki P, Ramsey SD, Rodriguez-Bigas MA, Vasen HF, Hawk ET, Barrett JC, Freedman AN, Srivastava S (2004) Revised Bethesda Guidelines for hereditary nonpolyposis colorectal cancer (Lynch syndrome) and microsatellite instability. J Natl Cancer Inst 96: 261-268

[69] Uyttebroeck A, Legius E, Brock P, Van de Cassey W, Casaer P, Casteels-Van Daele M (1995) Consecutive glioblastoma and B cell non-Hodgkin's lymphoma in a young child with von Recklinghausen's neurofibromatosis. Med Pediatr Oncol 24: 46-49

[70] van der Klift HM, Tops CM, Bik EC, Boogaard MW, Borgstein AM, Hansson KB, Ausems MG, Gomez Garcia E, Green A, Hes FJ, Izatt L, van Hest LP, Alonso AM, Vriends AH, Wagner A, van Zelst-Stams WA, Vasen HF, Morreau H, Devilee P, Wijnen JT (2010) Quantification of sequence exchange events between PMS2 and PMS2CL provides a basis for improved mutation scanning of Lynch syndrome patients. Hum Mutat 31: 578-587

[71] Vasen HF, Moslein G, Alonso A, Bernstein I, Bertario L, Blanco I, Burn J, Capella G, Engel C, Frayling I, Friedl W, Hes FJ, Hodgson S, Mecklin JP, Moller P, Nagengast F, Parc Y, Renkonen-Sinisalo L, Sampson JR, Stormorken A, Wijnen J (2007) Guidelines for the clinical management of Lynch syndrome (hereditary non-polyposis cancer). J Med Genet 44: 353-362

[72] Vaughn CP, Hart KJ, Samowitz WS, Swensen JJ (2011) Avoidance of pseudogene interference in the detection of 3′ deletions in PMS2. Hum Mutat 32: 1063-1071

[73] Wagner A, Reddingius RE, Kros JM, Dinjens WN, Sleddens H, Hoogmans MM, v. d. Velde A, Tops C, Wijnen J, Meijers-Heijboer H, Menko F (2003) Wilms tumor and glioblastoma in a child with a double MLH1 germline mutation. Fam Cancer 2(Suppl 1): 57

[74] Wang Q, Lasset C, Desseigne F, Frappaz D, Bergeron C, Navarro C, Ruano E, Puisieux A (1999) Neurofibromatosis and early onset of cancers in hMLH1-deficient children. Cancer Res 59: 294-297

[75] Wang Q, Montmain G, Ruano E, Upadhyaya M, Dudley S, Liskay RM, Thibodeau SN, Puisieux A (2003) Neurofibromatosis type 1 gene as a mutational target in a mismatch repair-deficient cell type. Hum Genet 112: 117-123

[76] Wernstedt A, Valtorta E, Armelao F, Togni R, Girlando S, Baudis M, Heinimann K, Messiaen L, Staehli N, Zschocke J, Marra G, Wimmer K (2012) Improved multiplex ligation-dependent probe amplification analysis identifies a deleterious PMS2 allele generated by recombination with crossover between PMS2 and PMS2CL. Genes Chromosomes Cancer 51: 819-831

[77] Whiteside D, McLeod R, Graham G, Steckley JL, Booth K, Somerville MJ, Andrew SE (2002) A homozygous germ-line mutation in the human MSH2 gene predisposes to hematological malignancy and multiple café-au-lait spots. Cancer Res 62: 359-362

[78] Wimmer K, Etzler J (2008) Constitutional mismatch repair-deficiency syndrome: have we so far seen only the tip of an iceberg? Hum Genet 124: 105-122

第17章 NF1 基因的进化论
Insights into NF1 from Evolution

Britta Bartelt-Kirbach and Dieter Kaufmann

17.1 引言

NF1 基因编码的神经纤维瘤蛋白的主要亚型包含 2 818 个氨基酸，其分子量大约为 320 kDa。它包含 1 个位于中心的与 GAP 相关的结构域，使其成为 Ras GTP 酶活化蛋白超家族的成员。GAP 相关结构域（GAP-related domain，GRD）覆盖了蛋白质序列的第 1 172 至 1 538 个氨基酸。这个大型蛋白质最近被发现还有 2 个额外的结构域（D'Angelo et al. 2006）。氨基酸残基 1560-1698 包含 1 个 Sec14 同源域，而在 1715-1816 处发现了 1 个类似磷脂酰肌醇结合蛋白同源域（简称 PH 结构域）。总的来说，这 3 个结构域仅覆盖了整个蛋白质的大约 20%。

即使在今天，剩余蛋白质的功能仍然不甚清楚。然而，聚焦进化的保守性可以让我们了解神经纤维瘤蛋白的功能相关区域。

17.2 NF1 编码区的进化

17.2.1 NF1 基因的起源

确定 NF1 基因序列后，对其进行与其他已知基因序列的比较，以识别其功能域。最初它与哺乳动物 Ras GTP 酶活化蛋白（GTPase-activating protein，GAP）（Gutman et al. 1991）的同源性被验证，但这个"GAP 相关结构域"只占整个神经纤维瘤蛋白的 10%。在寻找蛋白质的其他重要部分时，研究者还分析了来自其他物种的同源序列。与其他 GTP 酶活化蛋白的比较显示，人类的神经纤维瘤蛋白与酿酒酵母蛋白中的 IRA1 和 IRA2 蛋白（Ballester et al. 1990）有更广泛的同源性。神经纤维瘤蛋白、IRA1、IRA2 和 GAP 的 N-末端彼此之间没有共同之处。有趣的是，在这些蛋白质的其余部分中，NF1 基因编码的神经纤维瘤蛋白与 2 种 IRA 蛋白之间发现了 16~17 个同源区块，这些区块集中于 1 个中心区域（区块 1 至 10）和 1 个 C 末端区域（区块 11 至 17）。然而，GAP 序列仅在催化域内第 223 至 232 个氨基酸残基（第 7 至 10 区块）处与 NF1 和 IRA 蛋白显示出有限的同源性。Ballester 等（1990）因此得出结论，NF1 与酵母菌中的 IRA 蛋白的联系比 GAP 蛋白更为密切，特别是在 C 末端域，它与 IRA2 最为接近。2006 年，Klaus Scheffzek 研究团队鉴定了位于 GRD 下游的 NF1 基因的两个新域，这些域位于 Ballester 等发现的 C

B. Bartelt-Kirbach
Institute of Anatomy and Cell Biology, University of Ulm, Albert-Einstein-Allee 11, 89081 Ulm, Germany
e-mail: britta.bartelt@uni-ulm.de

D. Kaufmann
Institute of Human Genetics, University of Ulm, Albert-Einstein-Allee 11, 89081 Ulm, Germany
e-mail: dieter.h.kaufmann@uni-ulm.de

M. Upadhyaya and D. N. Cooper (eds.), *Neurofibromatosis Type 1*,
DOI 10.1007/978-3-642-32864-0_17, # Springer-Verlag Berlin Heidelberg 2012

末端域中（D'Angelo et al. 2006）。Sec14 同源域和 PH 样域在人类 *NF1*、果蝇 *Nf1*、粗糙脉孢菌（*Neurospora crassa*）*Nf1* 同源物（与人类序列大约有 21% 的残基一致性）、黏菌（*Dictyosteliumdiscoideum*）*Nf1* 同源物以及酿酒酵母（*Saccharomyces cerevisiae*）*IRA1* 和 *IRA2* 之间显示出高度同源性（D'Angelo et al. 2006）。

Golovnina 等（2006）系统探讨了 *NF1* 起源和进化的问题。他们使用人类和小鼠 *Nf1* 序列在不同数据库中进行了基本局部比对搜索（basic local alignment search tool，BLAST），识别了来自后口动物（脊椎动物、棘皮动物、被囊动物）、节肢动物（昆虫、蟹类）和扁形动物（扁虫、绦虫）的 22 个 *Nf1* 样序列。此外，他们还在真菌中发现了 4 个相似性较弱的 *NF1* 同源蛋白。综合以上发现得出结论，*NF1* 同源物分布在所有主要的后口动物和真菌中。有趣的是，在圆虫（秀丽隐杆线虫、布氏隐杆线虫、雷曼隐杆线虫、马来布鲁氏丝虫）和软体动物［光滑拟酵母（*B. glabrata*）］等前口动物中并未发现 *NF1* 同源序列。这可以解释为 *NF1* 基因是在大约 5.8 亿年前双侧动物群进化之后（双侧动物进化为后口动物和前口动物）才出现的，另一解释是 *NF1* 基因可能在圆虫和软体动物的进化中丢失。节肢动物门（包括可以确定拥有 *NF1* 基因的昆虫）与线虫动物门（圆虫）同属于前口动物的同一分支，而软体动物则属于另一分支。因此，*NF1* 基因更可能是在圆虫和软体动物的进化中丢失。

随着对各个生物谱系完整基因组测序的不断深入，Golovnina 等（2006）发现的 4 个真菌中假定 *NF1* 同源蛋白值得更加关注。其中 2 个蛋白质与神经纤维瘤蛋白的同源性非常低。另 2 个蛋白质与人类神经纤维瘤蛋白的 2 005 个氨基酸［粗糙脉孢菌（*Neurospora crassa*）的类神经纤维瘤蛋白］和 2 452 个氨基酸［新生隐球菌（*Cryptococcus neoformans*）假定蛋白 CNBF2880］非常相似，包括 GRD、Sec14 同源域和 PH 样域。

BLAST 比对（Stephen et al. 1997，2005）显示，与神经纤维瘤蛋白有关的粗糙脉孢菌蛋白（Q8WZX6，2 735 个氨基酸）与人类神经纤维瘤蛋白（2 818 个氨基酸同种型）之间存在 3 个同源区块。第一区块覆盖人类神经纤维瘤蛋白的第 185 至 413 个氨基酸，并且显示出 24% 的一致性。第二区块也是最大的区块（氨基酸残基 683 - 2419），有 29% 的一致性，包括 GRD、Sec14 同源域和 PH 样域。第三区块位于氨基酸 2672 和 2713 之间，显示出 27% 的一致性。新生隐球菌（*C. neoformans*）假定蛋白 CNBF2880（XP_774608）在氨基酸残基 123 到 2468 之间与人类神经纤维瘤蛋白显示出主要同源区块，一致性为 27%，还有一个小的同源区块，一致性为 22%（氨基酸残基 2635 - 2742）。

针对当前 85 个真菌基因组数据库（2012 年 5 月 22 日版本）对人类神经纤维瘤蛋白（2 818 个氨基酸的同种型）进行新的 BLAST 搜索，得到了 134 个匹配项，其中大部分对应 Ras GTP 酶激活蛋白。这些匹配项中的 31 个覆盖了≥60% 以上的神经纤维瘤蛋白查询序列，其一致性范围从 22% 到 31%（图 17.1）。另 36 个仅对应神经纤维瘤蛋白序列的 6%，位于 GRD 范围内，并且在这个区域的一致性为 32%～35%。列表中 2 个蛋白质，来自尖镰刀菌（*Fusarium oxysporum*）的假设蛋白 FOXB_00813 和来自里氏木霉（*Trichoderma reesei*）的 Ras GTP 酶激活蛋白，覆盖了人类神经纤维瘤蛋白序列的 79%，并且具有 27% 的一致性。4 个蛋白质已经被标注为神经纤维瘤蛋白（表 17.1a），分别是异刺棒束霉菌（*Metarhizium anisopliae*）和蝗虫刺棒束霉菌（*Metarhizium acridum*）（Gao et al. 2011）的假定神经纤维瘤蛋白，谢菲尔糖酵母（*Scheffersomyces stipitis*）（Jeffries et al. 2007）的 Ras GTP 酶激活蛋白 RasGAP/神经纤维瘤蛋白，以及巴西束孢子酵母（*Spathaspora passalidarum*）的 Ras GTP 酶激活蛋白 RasGAP/神经纤维瘤蛋白（Wohlbach et al. 2011）。上述酿酒酵母蛋白质 IRA1 和 IRA2 分别显示出 52% 和 49% 的覆盖率，并且分别具有 23% 和 21% 的一致性。

此外，将人类神经纤维瘤蛋白与 39 个当前原生动物数据库进行 BLAST 比对，除了许多其他匹配项外，还发现了几个注释过的神经纤维瘤蛋白同源物，它们甚至具有更高的覆盖率（表 17.1b）。所有这些同源物都包含 GRD、Sec14 同源域和 PH 样域。

搜索植物数据库的结果表明，植物中并没有发现与人类神经纤维瘤蛋白具有同源性的序列。

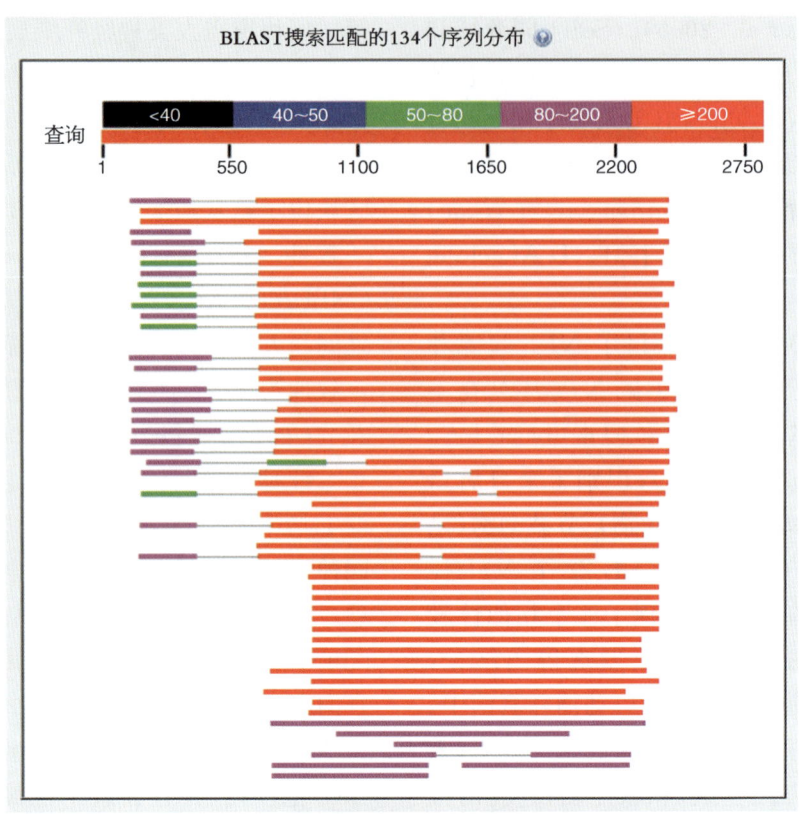

图 17.1 使用人类神经纤维瘤蛋白(2 818 个氨基酸)作为查询序列对真菌基因组数据库进行 BLAST 搜索。每一行代表一个同源的真菌蛋白质

表 17.1 神经纤维瘤蛋白的最早同源体包括：(a) 真菌中的人类神经纤维瘤蛋白同源体；(b) 原生生物中的人类神经纤维瘤蛋白同源体

蛋 白 质	种	登 录 号	覆盖度(%)	一致度(%)
(a)				
FOXB_00813	尖镰孢菌(Fusarium oxysporum)	EGU88669	79	27
Ras GTP 酶激活蛋白	里氏木霉(Trichoderma reesei)	EGR44283	79	27
CNBF2880	新型隐球菌(Cryptococcus neoformans)	XP_774608	70	29
假定的神经纤维瘤蛋白	绿僵菌(Metarhizium anisopliae)	EFY99233	69	28
假定的神经纤维瘤蛋白	蝗虫绿僵菌(Metarhizium acridum)	EFY84834	66	28
与神经纤维瘤蛋白相关的蛋白质	粗糙链孢霉(Neurospora crassa)	Q8WZX6	60	29
Ras GTP 酶激活蛋白 RasGAP/神经纤维瘤蛋白	帕萨达拉木霉(Spathaspora passalidarum)	EGW32510	54	21
IRA1	酿酒酵母(Saccharomyces cerevisiae)	EDV11970	52	23
IRA2p	酿酒酵母(Saccharomyces cerevisiae)	NP_014560	49	21
Ras GTP 酶激活蛋白 RasGAP/神经纤维瘤蛋白	树干毕赤酵母(Scheffersomyces stipitis)	XP_001386919	47	22

续表

蛋 白 质	种	登 录 号	覆盖度(%)	一致度(%)
(b)				
神经纤维瘤蛋白	苍白多节孢子虫(*Polysphondylium pallidum*)	EGG19811	91	31
神经纤维瘤蛋白	束状黏菌(*Dictyostelium fasciculatum*)	EFA82125	91	30
Nf1	奥氏囊孢子虫(*Capsaspora owczarzaki*)	EFW43762	84	44
类神经纤维瘤蛋白	苍白多节孢子虫(*Polysphondylium pallidum*)	EFA86557	56	46

因此,*NF1* 基因的起源确实可以追溯到早期生物,如酵母和其他真菌。植物、真菌和动物的共同祖先大约生活在 12 亿年前(Feng et al. 1997)(图 17.2),这表明 *NF1* 是一个极为古老且必不可少的基因。有趣的是,真菌与人类的神经纤维瘤蛋白不仅在 GRD(GTP 酶调节域)、Sec14 和 PH 样结构域上显示出同源性,而且这种相似性可能扩展到这些结构域之外。因此,这个区域可能存在尚未揭示的神经纤维瘤蛋白的功能。

17.2.2 *NF1* 基因的结构在漫长的进化过程中保持了高度的保守性

昆虫(节肢动物门)具有一个明显可识别的 *Nf1* 基因,该基因的编码区域大小与人类的相应基因几乎相同。1997 年,Bernards 研究小组成功鉴定了果蝇中的 *Nf1* 基因同源物(The et al. 1997)。该基因由 17 个构成性外显子和两个可变剪接外显子组成,由此编码的 2 种蛋白质分别包含 2 764 和 2 802 个氨基酸,与人类的神经纤维瘤蛋白具有 60% 的序列相似性。人类的 *NF1* 基因包含 60 个外显子,包括 3 个可变剪接的外显子,其主要同工型由 2 818 个氨基酸组成。显著的是,整个序列长度上均观察到了序列的相似性。人类与果蝇 *NF1* 基因的主要区别在于外显子的数量,尽管两者编码的蛋白质大小几乎相同。

在生命进化树上向上至脊椎动物,被详细研究的下一个 *NF1* 基因同源体是弓头鱼,也称为河豚。它之所以独特是因为其基因组非常紧凑,大约只有 400 Mb 碱基对,而人类基因组则大约有 3 000 Mb 碱基对。这种紧凑性归因于内含子和基因间序列的缩减,以及重复序列的缺乏。Kehrer-Sawatzki 团队于 1998 年发现,由于基因组紧凑的特性,河豚的 *Nf1* 基因大小仅为人类同源基因的约 1/13。他们对基因结构进行详细分析后发现,该基因由 57 个外显子构成,其中 51 个外显子的大小与人类相应的外显子一致。内含子与外显子的边界在绝大多数情况下与人类基因完全一致,仅第 16 个外显子是个例外。河豚的 *Nf1* 基因缺少了第 12b 外显子,以及另外 2 个可变剪接的外显子 9br 和 48a。氨基酸序列的比较结果表明,河豚与人类的神经纤维瘤蛋白在整体上具有 91.5% 的相似度和 88.5% 的一致度。特别是在 GAP 相关结构域的最小催化片段(包含 230 个氨基酸)中,相似度达到了 93.5%,一致度为 90.9%。这一高同源性区域不仅包括 GRD,还扩展到了 Sec14 结构域。

值得注意的是,基因结构在辐鳍鱼纲(河豚所属的类群)和肉鳍鱼纲(陆生脊椎动物所属的类群)之间已经相同,这两个类群大约在 4.2 亿年前就已经分离(图 17.2)。

17.2.3 *NF1* 基因的编码序列几乎没有观察到进一步的变化

小鼠神经纤维瘤蛋白由 2 841 个氨基酸组成,与人类的同源蛋白在序列上高度相似(98.5%),仅在 45 个氨基酸位置上存在差异,这 45 个差异中的 22 个集中在氨基酸序列的 625 至 900 号区域,该区域紧邻 IRA 相关片段(氨基酸 900 至 2350)。因此,这个区域可能作为连接不同功能域的链节。

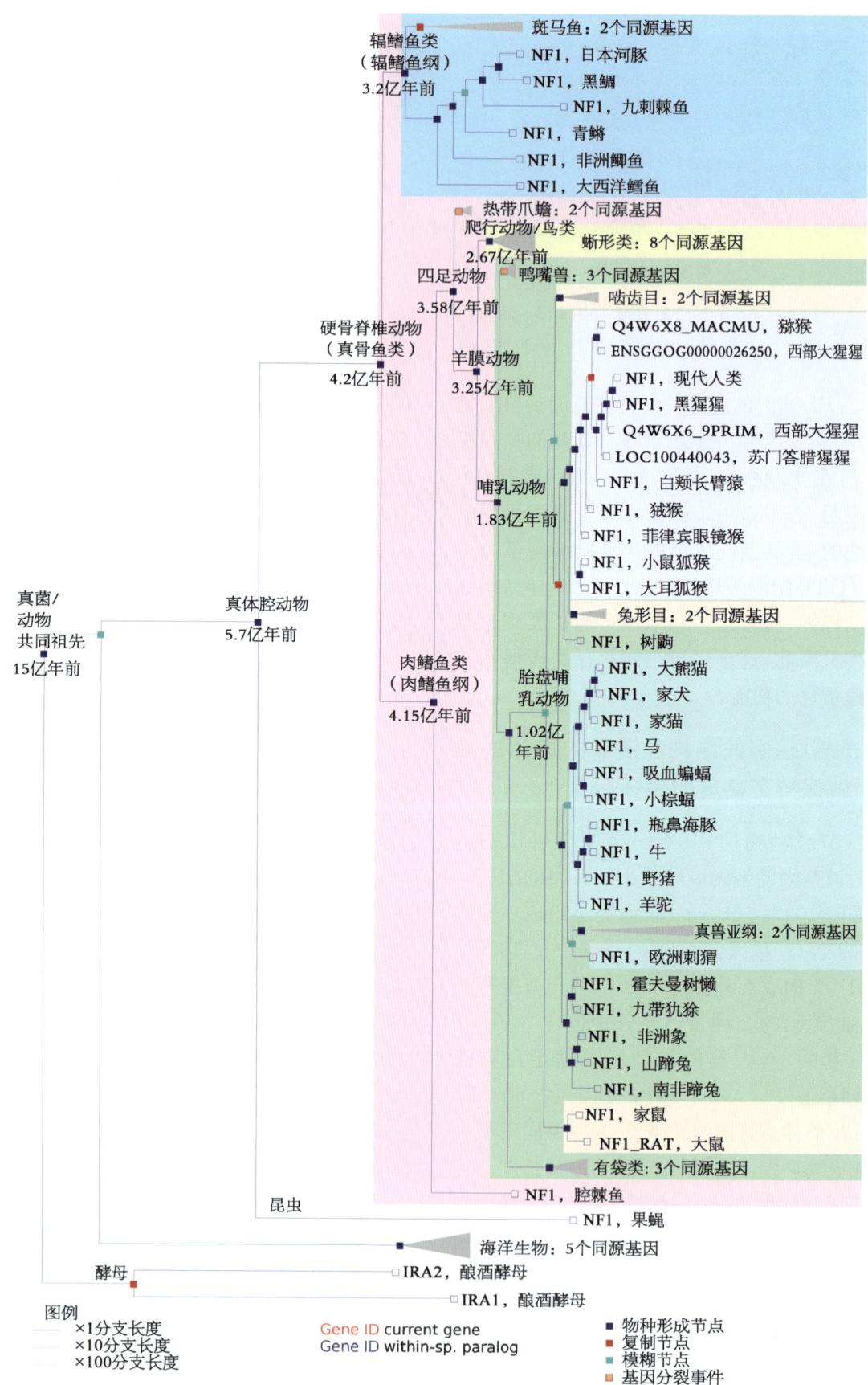

图 17.2　*NF1* 基因的进化树（Ensembl）

人类（2839 AA）与黑猩猩（2939 AA）的神经纤维瘤蛋白在氨基酸序列上具有100%的一致性，这反映出在灵长类动物中，该蛋白质在功能和结构上受到了严格的限制（Assum and Schmegner 2008）。据推测，人类与这些灵长类动物的分化发生在大约600万年前。人类的神经纤维瘤蛋白与大猩猩（*Gorilla gorilla*）、猩猩（*Pongo abelii*）以及白颊长臂猿（*Nomascus leucogenys*）中的相应同源蛋白具有完全相同的序列，显示出100%的序列同一性。在不同种类的灵长类动物中，神经纤维瘤蛋白的氨基酸序列与人类的同一性存在差异：猕猴（*Macaca mulatta*）的序列与人类有96%的相似性，包含2690个氨基酸；狨猴（*Callithrix jacchus*）的序列与人类完全相同，即100%的相似性；而鼠狐猴（*Microcebus murinus*）的序列与人类的相似性则为83%（Ensembl数据库）（图17.2）。

17.3 基因组中 *NF1* 区域的变异情况

NF1 基因的进化显示出明显的选择性压力，以维持神经纤维瘤蛋白的功能。这种压力不仅在灵长类动物的 *NF1* 基因区域及其周边区域的近期演化中有所体现，同样也在人类群体的遗传多样性中观察到。

17.3.1 灵长类进化中 *NF1* 区域的重排

在灵长类动物进化中，NF1 基因区域附近经历了染色体结构的重排，这种变化引起了基因排列顺序的改变（表17.2）。在猕猴的第16号染色体上，位于 NF1 基因上游的 *GOSR1* 与 *WSB1* 之间约3 Mb 的区域。这一区域在小鼠的第11号染色体和狗的第9号染色体上呈现为倒置状态（Assum and Schmegner 2008）。猕猴的基因顺序与黑猩猩及人类在染色体17的 NF1 区域有所不同，这种差异是由三次染色体倒位事件造成的。这些事件包括 *NF1* 与 *SUZ12* 之间700 kb 区域以及 *CLRF3* 与 *RNF135* 之间200 kb 区域的交换，共同促成了一系列复杂的染色体重排。

表 17.2 *NF1* 的直接基因组邻域

A	*GOSR1*	*WSB1*	*NF1*	*SUZ12*	*CLRF3*	*RNF135*	*RHOT1*
B	*WSB1*	*GOSR1*	*NF1*	*SUZ12*	*CLRF3*	*RNF135*	*RHOT1*
C	*WSB1*	*GOSR1*	*CLRF3*	*RNF135*	*NF1*	*SUZ12*	*RHOT1*

注：A，小鼠（第11号染色体）/狗（第9号染色体）；B，猕猴（第16号染色体）；C，人类（第17号染色体）/黑猩猩（第17号染色体）（Assum and Schmegner 2008）。

17.3.2 灵长类进化中 *NF1* 回文式富 AT 序列的保守性

回文序列分散在人类基因组中可能导致染色体易位。在人类中，在 NF1 基因的第40个内含子中检测到了一种回文式 AT 富集重复序列（17PATRR）（Kehrer-Sawatzki et al. 1997；Kurahashi et al. 2003）。对黑猩猩和大猩猩中17PATRR 的分析显示，它们的 17PATRR 与人类中的几乎完全相同（Inagaki et al. 2005）。在旧大陆猴中观察到了相似的短倒置重复序列，但在小鼠、大鼠、狗和新大陆猴的相应区域中并未检测到回文序列。Inagaki 等于2005年提出，17PATRR 最初在灵长类动物的进化过程中偶然形成一种小型倒置重复序列，随后在类人猿的演化中逐渐发展成为较大的 PATRR 结构。根据这一观点，回文序列在大约2500万年前形成。真核生物基因组中的长回文序列往往不稳定，倾向于采取二级结构，并且易于发生缺失（Farah et al. 2002；Cunningham et al. 2003）。17PATRR 在人类和大型猿类中的保守性是出乎意料的。Inagaki 团队认为，这种回文序列对于灵长类动物中 *NF1* 基因的特有功能至关重要，而狗和啮齿类动物并未发现类似的结构。

17.3.3 *NF1* 区域的特征是 GC 含量低

人类基因组的 GC 含量在不同区域呈现差异。存在一些长度为几百千碱基的 DNA 片段，这些片段 GC 含量相对一致，称为等位基因组。等位基因组与基因重组等基本生物学特性密切相关（Bernardi 2000；Costantini et al. 2006；Schmegner et al. 2007）。等位基因组的结构在哺乳动物的演化中保持了保守性，正如 Schmegner 等在2005年的研究中指出的 NF1 区域就是一个例证。无论是在人类、小鼠还是狗的基因组中，NF1 基因的全长 GC 含量都较低，不足 40%。在这些物种中，NF1 基因下游区域的 GC 含量升高至 45%，而在 NF1 基因的直接上游区域，GC 含量则迅速超过了 50%。相邻的等位基因组通过一个仅 5 kb 长度的碱基分隔（Assum and Schmegner 2008）。

17.3.4　NF1 基因区域的高度连锁不平衡

连锁不平衡（linkage disequilibrium，LD）是指 2 个或多个位点上等位基因的非随机关联，其在人类基因组中的分布是不均一的。LD 在人类基因组中的分布是不均匀的。在 2000 年，Eisenbarth 发现整个 NF1 基因位于一个大约 300 kb 的区域内，该区域具有持续的高连锁不平衡（Eisenbarth et al. 2000）。连锁不平衡在向染色体的着丝粒方向延伸，在 NF1 基因与 RNF135 基因之间 87 kb 的基因间区域内结束；而在端粒方向，连锁不平衡的边界则位于 NF1 基因与 RAB11FIP4 基因间的基因间区域。除了 NF1 基因本身，还有 3 个基因——EVI2A（细胞浆病毒整合位点 2A）、EVI2B（细胞浆病毒整合位点 2B）和 OMG（少突胶质细胞髓鞘糖蛋白），它们都嵌入在 NF1 基因的第 27b 内含子中，同样位于连锁不平衡程度高的区域。这些区域的界限与 DNA 序列 GC 含量的变化相吻合，这表明连锁不平衡的模式与等位基因组的结构有关联（Schmegner et al. 2005a）。

17.3.5　人类 NF1 基因单核苷酸多态性

人类 NF1 基因编码区域的单核苷酸多态性（SNP）分析揭示了明显的连锁不平衡现象。目前已知 NF1 基因中至少存在 32 个同义 SNP 和 8 个非同义 SNP，这些 SNP 的分布频率已经得到确认（NCBI，dbSNP database）。在研究的人类群体中，非同义 SNP 的等位基因频率均低于 1%，具体包括：rs112306990（0.005%）、rs145891889（0.005%）、rs17881753（0.001%）、rs9907627（0.014%）、rs140523180（0.001%）、rs17884349（0.022%）、rs2230850（0.007%）和 rs148154172（0.001%）。NF1 基因的编码区域显示出极低的重组频率，而其周围的序列则展现出与整个基因组平均值相近的重组频率（Assum and Schmegner 2008）。这些数据揭示了人类中神经纤维瘤蛋白的功能维持受到重要的自然选择影响。

17.3.6　欧洲人群中的两种 NF1 基因单倍型

2005 年，基于 Schmegner 等（2005b）的研究，从 NF1 基因中得到的遗传变异数据被用来推断欧洲地区解剖学现代人类的人口演化历史。欧洲人群的单倍型结构研究未发现在解剖学现代人类近期演化中 NF1 基因受到正向选择的证据。系统发育树中显示两个亚群为两个古老且明显分离的分支，具有较小的变异性。德国基因库中的单倍群 1 序列表现出极低的群内变异，这通常见于经历过严重瓶颈事件后快速扩张的种群。而单倍群 2 序列则展现出更深层次的分支，形成多个亚群，占分析染色体的 33%，这符合一个长期稳定规模的种群的典型模式。因此 Schmegner 等（2005b）提出单倍群 2 是两个古老亚种群的混合体。这个种群最近经历了一次瓶颈事件，之后在大约 13 万至 15 万年前开始人口数量的增长（Assum and Schmegner 2008）。基因库的主要部分，即单倍群 1，可能代表了新石器时代农民的较晚移民潮和种群扩张；其余的基因可能来源于现代人类在欧洲的早期定居者。欧洲人群的 NF1 基因单倍型是两个古老非洲人群基因混合的结果。非洲拥有更丰富的单倍型多样性，并且欧洲人群两个亚群的最古老单倍型仅在非洲有记录（Assum and Schmegner 2008）。

17.4　NF1 基因内部包含的基因及其起源

人类 NF1 基因的第 37 个内含子中存在 1 个经过剪接的假基因，该假基因来源于腺苷酸激酶同工酶 3（adenylate kinase isozyme 3，AK3）（Xu et al. 1992）。这个假基因仅有 3 处不影响氨基酸序列的碱基变化，暗示它在进化上相对年轻。这一推断得到了支持，因为在河豚的 Nf1 基因内含子序列中并未发现这一假基因（Kehrer-Sawatzki et al. 1998）。

NF1 基因第 27b 内含子反向链上含有 3 个额

外的基因：*OMG*、*EVI2A* 和 *EVI2B*（Cawthon et al. 1990，1991；O'Connell et al. 1990；Viskochil et al. 1991），这些基因由于其古老的特性，应当受到更多的关注。

17.4.1 *OMG*

OMG 是一种在中枢神经系统（CNS）髓鞘化过程中，在胶质细胞中表达的含有 440 个氨基酸的细胞表面蛋白。紧密髓鞘是随着脊椎动物的演化而发展出的一种神经组织结构（Waehneldt 1990）。这使得大约 4.4 亿年前，在软骨鱼类（鲨鱼和鳐鱼）的类群中首次出现了细长轴突的形成（Saavedra et al. 1989；Yoshida and Colman 1996）。

Vourc'h 等（2003）对来自 7 个不同目中 12 种真兽亚纲哺乳动物的 OMG 基因进行了测序，并将其编码的蛋白质序列与小鼠和人类的相应序列进行了比较分析（Mikol et al. 1990，1993）。所有物种的蛋白质大小均为 440 个氨基酸，并且包含 5 个结构域。在 14 种哺乳动物物种中，序列一致性达到了 71%。

Ensembl 数据库（http://www.ensembl.org，2012 年 5 月第 67 版）记录了 37 个 *OMG* 基因，这些基因均属于约 4.2 亿年历史的硬骨脊椎动物（Euteleostomi）类群。*OMG* 基因在以下类群中被发现：辐鳍鱼类（Actinopterygii），包括河豚和斑马鱼；肉鳍鱼类（Sarcopterygii），以腔棘鱼（*Latimeria chalumnae*）为代表；四足动物，例如两栖动物爪蟾（*Xenopus tropicalis*）；以及爬行动物、鸟类和哺乳动物。

因此，*OMG* 基因的起源与有髓鞘轴突的形成时间相吻合。

17.4.2 *EV12A*

人类 *EVI2A* 基因（之前称为 *EVI2*）在对 *NF1* 基因的搜索过程中被发现（Cawthon et al. 1990；O'Connell et al. 1990）。此前，小鼠中的相应基因已被认为与小鼠骨髓性白血病的发病有关（Buchberg et al. 1990）。*EVI2A* 基因编码的是一种由 236 个氨基酸组成的跨膜蛋白。

Ensembl 数据库记录显示，37 个基因在羊膜动物类群（包括爬行动物、鸟类和哺乳动物）中占主导地位。此外，两栖动物爪蟾（*Xenopus tropicalis*）和肉鳍鱼类腔棘鱼（*Latimeria chalumnae*）也具有 *EVI2A* 基因的同源基因。然而，辐鳍鱼类如河豚（Fugu）和斑马鱼（Zebrafish）并未发现此类同源基因。这表明 *EVI2A* 基因可能起源于约 4.15 亿年前的肉鳍鱼类类群，该类群也是陆地脊椎动物的起源。

17.4.3 *EVI2B*

EVI2B 基因于 1991 年由 Cawthon 等（Cawthon et al. 1991）首次描述，该基因编码的蛋白质由 448 个氨基酸组成，并包含 1 个跨膜结构域。

Ensembl 数据库记录了 32 个 *EVI2B* 基因，这些基因仅在哺乳动物中发现。在这些数据中，鸭嘴兽（*Ornithorhynchus anatinus*）拥有最古老的 *EVI2B* 基因同源体，其与人类 *EVI2B* 蛋白的同源性大约为 40%。依据数据库的资料，*EVI2B* 基因约有 1.83 亿年的历史。

17.4.4 以上 3 个基因在 *NF1* 基因的内含子中首次出现的确切时间

河豚的 *Nf1* 基因第 27b 内含子并未显示出与 *EVI2A* 或 *OMG* 序列的相似性，这暗示了这些基因可能在大约 4 亿年前硬骨鱼和哺乳动物的谱系分化之后才插入该内含子区域。Kehrer-Sawatzki 团队在该内含子的反向链上发现了 1 种单外显子基因，该基因具有 1 095 个碱基对的开放阅读框和 1 个含有 365 个氨基酸的假定蛋白质。这个蛋白质与人类 *EVI2B* 蛋白中的 302 个氨基酸具有 42.7% 的相似性和 27% 的序列一致性。研究表明河豚的 *EVI2B* 基因在肝脏和肾脏中有表达活性，而在大脑中则未检测到其表达。尽管如此，该河豚 *EVI2B* 基因的同源序列并未被记录在 Ensembl 数据库之中。通过使用 BLAST 工具对比人类 *EVI2B* 蛋白序列与核苷酸数据库，我们能够检测到 1 个具有 24% 覆盖度和 33% 一致性的序列。此外，在鸟类中，仅在鸡（*Gallus gallus*）中发现了另一个同源序列，具有 20% 的覆盖度和 44% 的一致性。而在哺乳动物中，*EVI2B* 基因的覆盖度几乎达到了 100%。鉴于此，河豚 *EVI2B* 基因同源序列的功能仍然是一个未解之谜。

通过查阅 Ensembl 数据库中各物种 NF1 基因组区域的记录，可以明显发现这 3 个基因似乎在首次出现后不久即被嵌入 NF1 基因的内含子区域（表 17.3）。OMG 基因在河豚以及其他几种辐鳍鱼的 Nf1 基因内含子中并未发现，但在斑马鱼（Danio rerio）中却有这一基因的存在。EVI2A 基因则在腔棘鱼（Latimeria）的 Nf1 基因内部被检测到。而根据 Ensembl 数据库的记录，EVI2B 基因首次在袋鼠的 Nf1 基因内含子中被识别。

表 17.3 OMG、EVI2A 和 EVI2B 存在于 NF1 基因内含子中

组	物 种	OMG	EVI2A	EVI2B
胎盘哺乳动物	人类（智人）	+	+	+
	长臂猿（白颊长臂猿）	+	+	+
	大猩猩（西部大猩猩）	−	+	+
	猕猴（猕猴属猕猴）	+	+	+
	狨猴（狨属普通狨猴）	+	+	+
	鼠狐猴（小鼠狐猴）	+	+	+
	羊驼（小羊驼）	+	+	+
	象（非洲象）	+	+	+
	牛（欧洲牛）	+	+	+
	马（马属）	+	+	+
	海豚（普通瓶鼻海豚）	+	+	+
	猪（欧亚野猪）	+	+	+
	狗（家犬）	+	−	+
	猫（家猫）	−	−	+
	大熊猫（大熊猫属大熊猫）	+	+	+
	小鼠（小家鼠）	+	+	+
	豚鼠（普通豚鼠）	+	−	+
	鼠兔（高原鼠兔）	(+)	+	−
	鼠（褐家鼠）	+	+	+
	袋鼠（小袋鼠）	+	+	+
	大型蝙蝠（马来大狐蝠）	+	+	+
	小蝙蝠（小棕蝠）	+	+	+
	眼镜猴（菲律宾眼镜猴）		+	−
	兔子（家兔）	+	+	+

续 表

组	物 种	OMG	EVI2A	EVI2B
胎盘哺乳动物	豚鼠(豚鼠科)	＋	＋	＋
	刺猬(欧洲刺猬)	－	－	－
	小刺猬鼩(马达加斯加小刺猬鼩)	－	＋	(＋)
	蹄兔(南非蹄兔)	(＋)	(＋)	(＋)
	树鼩(贝氏树鼩)	＋	＋	＋
	婴猴(加氏婴猴)	－	－	－
	树懒(霍氏树懒)	－	－	－
	犰狳(九带犰狳)	－	＋	－
有袋类动物	袋獾(塔斯马尼亚袋獾)	＋	＋	＋
	负鼠(小美洲负鼠)	－	＋	－
	沙袋鼠(红颈袋鼠)	＋	(＋)	＋
鸟类	鸡(家鸡)	＋	＋	o
	火鸡(普通火鸡)	＋	＋	o
	斑胸草雀(斑纹草雀)	＋	＋	o
肉鳍鱼类	腔棘鱼(矛尾鱼)	＋	＋	o
两栖动物	非洲爪蟾	＋	＋	o
辐鳍鱼类	斑马鱼	＋	o	o
	青鳉(日本青鳉)	－	o	o
	棘背鱼(九刺棘背鱼)	－	o	o
	黑鲷	－	o	o
	河豚(红鳍东方鲀)	－	o	＋?
	尼罗罗非鱼	－	o	o
	鳕鱼(大西洋鳕鱼)	－	o	o
昆虫	果蝇(黑腹果蝇)	o	o	o

注：＋，基因存在于 $NF1$ 内含子中；－，基因存在但不在 $NF1$ 内含子中；(＋)，假基因基因内含子中；o，基因在基因组中不存在；＋?，关于基因存在于 $NF1$ 内含子中的数据不一致。

尽管这 3 个基因已经嵌入 $Nf1$ 基因中，但它们在不同物种间表现出显著的变异性。在某些物种里，1 个或多个基因可能从 $NF1$ 内含子中再次丢失，或者转变为假基因（表 17.3）。鉴于 $NF1$ 基因本身在长时间跨度内变化甚微，这种现象确实引人注目。

17.5 总结

NF1 基因非常古老,其同源序列甚至在真菌中也有发现,而这些真菌大约在 12 亿年前就与动物界分离。从真菌到哺乳动物,神经纤维瘤蛋白的氨基酸序列比较反映出高度的结构和功能保守性。尽管在哺乳动物的不同物种中,NF1 基因区域在进化过程中经历了多次重排,但其位点的等位基因结构仍然保持不变。此外,在现代人类的进化历程中,并未观察到 NF1 基因受到正选择的影响。神经纤维瘤蛋白保持正确结构和功能所面临的强烈自然选择压力,反映在不同人类群体中单核苷酸多态性(SNP)的稀缺性上。OMG、EVI2A 和 EVI2B 这 3 个基因在首次出现不久后被整合进了 NF1 基因的内含子区域。尽管如此,与 NF1 基因的其他区域相比,这些基因所在的区域显示出了更高的遗传多样性。

(倪鑫,王生才 译)

使用软件

BLAST

Altschul SF, Madden TL, Schäffer AA, Zhang J, Zhang Z, Miller W, Lipman DJ (1997) Gapped BLAST and PSI-BLAST: a new generation of protein database search programs. Nucleic Acids Res 25(17): 3389-3402

Altschul SF, Wootton JC, Gertz EM, Agarwala R, Morgulis A, Schäffer AA, Yu YK (2005) Protein database searches using compositionally adjusted substitution matrices. FEBS J 272 (20): 5101-5109

EnsEmbl

Flicek P, Amode MR, Barrell D, Beal K, Brent S, Carvalho-Silva D, Clapham P, Coates G, Fairley S, Fitzgerald S, Gil L, Gordon L, Hendrix M, Hourlier T, Johnson N, Kähäri AK, Keefe D, Keenan S, Kinsella R, Komorowska M, Koscielny G, Kulesha E, Larsson P, Longden I, McLaren W, Muffato M, Overduin B, Pignatelli M, Pritchard B, Riat HS, Ritchie GR, Ruffier M, Schuster M, Sobral D, Tang YA, Taylor K, Trevanion S, Vandrovcova J, White S, Wilson M, Wilder SP, Aken BL, Birney E, Cunningham F, Dunham I, Durbin R, Fernández-Suarez XM, Harrow J, Herrero J, Hubbard TJ, Parker A, Proctor G, Spudich G, Vogel J, Yates A, Zadissa A, Searle SM (2012) Ensembl 2012. Nucleic Acids Res 40 (database issue): D84-D90

EnsEmbl GeneTree

Vilella AJ, Severin J, Ureta-Vidal A, Durbin A, Heng L, Birney E (2009) EnsemblCompara GeneTrees: Analysis of complete, duplication-aware phylogenetic trees in vertebrates. Genome Res 19: 327-335

dbSNP NCBI

Sherry ST, Ward MH, Kholodov M, Baker J, Phan L, Smigielski EM, Sirotkin K (2001) dbSNP: the NCBI database of genetic variation. Nucleic Acids Res 29(1): 308-311

参考文献

[1] Assum G, Schmegner C (2008) NF1 gene in evolution. In: Kaufmann D (ed) Neurofibromatoses, vol 16, Monographs in human genetics. Karger, Basel, pp 103-112

[2] Ballester R, Marchuk D, Boguski M, Saulino A, Letcher R, Wigler M, Collins F (1990) The NF1 locus encodes a protein functionally related to mammalian GAP and yeast IRA proteins. Cell 63(4): 851-859

[3] Bernardi G (2000) Isochores and the evolutionary genomics of vertebrates. Gene 241: 3-17

[4] Bernards A, Snijders AJ, Hannigan GE, Murthy AE, Gusella JF (1993) Mouse neurofibromatosis type 1 cDNA sequence reveals high degree of conservation of both coding and noncoding mRNA segments. Hum Mol Genet 2(6): 645-650

[5] Buchberg AM, Bedigian HG, Jenkins NA, Copeland NG (1990) Evi-2, a common integration site involved in murine myeloid leukemogenesis. Mol Cell Biol 10(9): 4658-4666

[6] Cawthon RM, O'Connell P, Buchberg AM, Viskochil D, Weiss RB, Culver M, Stevens J, Jenkins NA, Copeland NG, White R (1990) Identification and characterization of transcripts from the neurofibromatosis 1 region: the sequence and genomic structure of EVI2 and mapping of other transcripts. Genomics 7(4): 555-565

[7] Cawthon RM, Andersen LB, Buchberg AM, Xu GF, O'Connell P, Viskochil D, Weiss RB, Wallace MR, Marchuk DA, Culver M et al (1991) cDNA sequence and genomic structure of EV12B, a gene lying within an intron of the neurofibromatosis type 1 gene. Genomics 9(3): 446-460

[8] Costantini M, Clay O, Auletta F, Bernardi G (2006) An isochore map of human chromosomes. Genome Res 16: 536-541

[9] Cunningham LA, Coté AG, Cam-Ozdemir C, Lewis SM (2003) Rapid, stabilizing palindrome rearrangements in somatic cells by the center-break mechanism. Mol Cell Biol 23: 8740-8750

[10] D'Angelo I, Welti S, Bonneau F, Scheffzek K (2006) A novel bipartite phospholipid-binding module in the neurofibromatosis type 1 protein. EMBO Rep 7(2): 174-179

[11] Eisenbarth I, Vogel G, Krone W, Vogel W, Assum G (2000) An isochore transition in the NF1 gene region coincides with a switch in the extent of linkage disequilibrium. Am J Hum Genet 67: 873-880

[12] Farah JA, Hartsuiker E, Mizuno K, Ohta K, Smith GR

(2002) A 160-bp palindromic is a Rad50 Rad32-dependent mitotic recombination hotspot in *Schizosaccharomyces pombe*. Genetics 161: 461–468

[13] Feng DF, Cho G, Doolittle RF (1997) Determining divergence times with a protein clock: update and reevaluation. Proc Natl Acad Sci USA 94(24): 13028–13033

[14] Gao Q, Jin K, Ying SH, Zhang Y, Xiao G, Shang Y, Duan Z, Hu X, Xie XQ, Zhou G, Peng G, Luo Z, Huang W, Wang B, Fang W, Wang S, Zhong Y, Ma LJ, St Leger RJ, Zhao GP, Pei Y, Feng MG, Xia Y, Wang C (2011) Genome sequencing and comparative transcriptomics of the model entomopathogenic fungi *Metarhizium anisopliae* and *M. acridum*. PLoS Genet 7(1): e1001264

[15] Gutmann DH, Wood DL, Collins FS (1991) Identification of the neurofibromatosis type 1 gene product. Proc Natl Acad Sci USA 88(21): 9658–9662

[16] Golovnina K, Blinov A, Chang LS (2006) Evolution and origin of neurofibromin, the product of the neurofibromatosis type 1 (*NF1*) tumor-suppressor gene. BGRS 3(5): 142–146

[17] Inagaki H, Ohye T, Kogo H, Yamada K, Kowa H, Shaikh TH, Emanuel BS, Kurahashi H (2005) Palindromic AT-rich repeat in the *NF1* gene is hypervariable in humans and evolutionarily conserved in primates. Hum Mutat 26(4): 332–342

[18] Jeffries TW, Grigoriev IV, Grimwood J, Laplaza JM, Aerts A, Salamov A, Schmutz J, Lindquist E, Dehal P, Shapiro H, Jin YS, Passoth V, Richardson PM (2007) Genome sequence of the lignocellulose-bioconverting and xylose-fermenting yeast *Pichia stipitis*. Nat Biotechnol 25(3): 319–326

[19] Kehrer-Sawatzki H, Haussler J, Krone W, Bode H, Jenne DE, Mehnert KU, Tummers U, Assum G (1997) The second case of a t(17;22) in a family with neurofibromatosis type 1: sequence analysis of the breakpoint regions. Hum Genet 99: 237–247

[20] Kehrer-Sawatzki H, Maier C, Moschgath E, Elgar G, Krone W (1998) Genomic characterization of the neurofibromatosis type 1 gene of *Fugu rubripes*. Gene 222(1): 145–153

[21] Kurahashi H, Shaikh T, Takata M, Toda T, Emanuel BS (2003) The constitutional t(17;22): another translocation mediated by palindromic AT-rich repeats. Am J Hum Genet 72: 733–738

[22] Mikol DD, Alexakos MJ, Bayley CA, Lemons RS, Le Beau MM, Stefansson K (1990) Structure and chromosomal localization of the gene for the oligodendrocyte-myelin glycoprotein. J Cell Biol 111(6 Pt 1): 2673–2679

[23] Mikol DD, Rongnoparut P, Allwardt BA, Marton LS, Stefansson K (1993) The oligodendrocyte-myelin glycoprotein of mouse: primary structure and gene structure. Genomics 17(3): 604–610

[24] O'Connell P, Viskochil D, Buchberg AM, Fountain J, Cawthon RM, Culver M, Stevens J, Rich DC, Ledbetter DH, Wallace M et al (1990) The human homolog of murine Evi-2 lies between two von Recklinghausen neurofibromatosis translocations. Genomics 7(4): 547–554

[25] Saavedra RA, Fors L, Aebersold RH, Arden B, Horvath S, Sanders J, Hood L (1989) The myelin proteins of the shark brain are similar to the myelin proteins of the mammalian peripheral nervous system. J Mol Evol 29(2): 149–156

[26] Schmegner C, Berger A, Vogel W, Hameister H, Assum G (2005a) An isochore transition zone in the *NF1* gene region is a conserved landmark of chromosome structure and function. Genomics 86: 439–445

[27] Schmegner C, Hoegel J, Vogel W, Assum G (2005b) Genetic variability in a genomic region with long-range linkage disequilibrium reveals traces of a bottleneck in the history of the European population. Hum Genet 118: 276–286

[28] Schmegner C, Hameister H, Vogel W, Assum G (2007) Isochores and replication time zones: a perfect match. Cytogenet Genome Res 116: 167–172

[29] The I, Hannigan GE, Cowley GS, Reginald S, Zhong Y, Gusella JF, Hariharan IK, Bernards A (1997) Rescue of a *Drosophila* NF1 mutant phenotype by protein kinase A. Science 276(5313): 791–794

[30] Viskochil D, Cawthon R, O'Connell P, Xu GF, Stevens J, Culver M, Carey J, White R (1991) The gene encoding the oligodendrocyte-myelin glycoprotein is embedded within the neurofibro-matosis type 1 gene. Mol Cell Biol 11(2): 906–912

[31] Vourc'h P, Moreau T, Arbion F, Marouillat-Védrine S, Müh JP, Andres C (2003) Oligodendrocyte myelin glycoprotein growth inhibition function requires its conserved leucine-rich repeat domain, not its glycosylphosphatidyl-inositol anchor. J Neurochem 85(4): 889–897

[32] Waehneldt TV (1990) Phylogeny of myelin proteins. Ann N Y Acad Sci 605: 15–28

[33] Wohlbach DJ, Kuo A, Sato TK, Potts KM, Salamov AA, Labutti KM, Sun H, Clum A, Pangilinan JL, Lindquist EA, Lucas S, Lapidus A, Jin M, Gunawan C, Balan V, Dale BE, Jeffries TW, Zinkel R, Barry KW, Grigoriev IV, Gasch AP (2011) Comparative genomics of xylose-fermenting fungi for enhanced biofuel production. Proc Natl Acad Sci USA 108(32): 13212–13217

[34] Xu G, O'Connell P, Stevens J, White R (1992) Characterization of human adenylate kinase 3 (AK3) cDNA and mapping of the AK3 pseudogene to an intron of the NF1 gene. Genomics 13(3): 537–542

[35] Yoshida M, Colman DR (1996) Parallel evolution and coexpression of the proteolipid proteins and protein zero in vertebrate myelin. Neuron 16(6): 1115–1126

第18章 1型神经纤维瘤病修饰基因
Modifier Genes in NF1

Eric Pasmant, Dominique Vidaud, and Pierre Wolkenstein

18.1 引言

虽然1型神经纤维瘤病（NF1）是一种常见的常染色体显性遗传病，但其临床表现具有高度变异性和不可预测性。许多NF1患者已被基因分型，但基因型与表型之间相关性的证据却很少。由于NF1表型的复杂性、其对年龄的强依赖性、许多临床特征的非独立性，以及致病性NF1突变巨大的等位基因异质性，可能存在重要的NF1基因型-表型相关性尚未被挖掘。然而，具有相同突变NF1患者的疾病表型可能非常严重，也可能非常轻。导致表型变异（包括家系内的变异性）的原因包括非连锁基因（修饰基因）和环境效应（包括偶然事件）。家系研究首先表明，在大多数NF1家系中观察到的表达变异可能是由于修饰基因的影响。NF1中存在修饰基因的第一个证据来自大规模家系研究。NF1小鼠模型强化了这些假设。最近的靶向基因策略已经能够帮助识别相关的候选基因，基因组革命可能会带来该领域的巨大进展。

18.2 表型研究：NF1修饰基因的首次证据

NF1临床表型变异的机制仍不清楚，可能是由于复杂的病理生理学机制以及多种因素的参与。该病的主要临床特征包括多个咖啡牛奶（café-au-lait，CAL）斑、腋窝雀斑、Lisch结节和神经纤维瘤，其发生和数量因人而异，甚至在同一家系内也存在差异。此外，约1/3的患者会出现一种或多种并发症。这些并发症几乎可以影响任何器官，并且有极大的不可预测性。恶性周围神经鞘膜瘤（MPNST）的发生是NF1严重的并发症之一。

历史上，NF1被描述为一种非常可变的疾病。人们很快就清楚了NF1突变的性质并不是唯一的变异来源，因为NF1在同一家系成员之间的表达也表现出相当大的差异。Carey等（Carey et al. 1986）观察到3/4的NF1家系个体间的严重程度表现出明显的差异。影响表型变异的其余因素可能是由于修饰基因、环境因素或它们的组合。这里使用术语

E. Pasmant · D. Vidaud
UMR745 INSERM, Université Paris Descartes, Sorbonne Paris Cité, Faculté des Sciences Pharmaceutiques et Biologiques, Paris 75006, France

Service de Biochimie et de Génétique Moléculaire, Hôpital Cochin, AP-HP, 75014, Paris, France
e-mail: eric.pasmant@gmail.com

P. Wolkenstein
Département of Dermatologie, Centre de référence des neurofibromatoses, Hôpital Henri-Mondor, AP-HP and EA 4393 LIC, Université Paris Est Créteil (UPEC), 94000, Créteil, France

M. Upadhyaya and D. N. Cooper (eds.), *Neurofibromatosis Type 1*,
DOI 10.1007/978-3-642-32864-0_18, # Springer-Verlag Berlin Heidelberg 2012

"修饰基因"来表示任何与 NF1 基因座不连锁的基因,其基因型调节 NF1 表型的一个或几个特征。原则上,NF1 表型的变异可以由单个修饰基因位点决定,也可能存在多个相互作用的修饰基因。然而,除了修饰基因以外的其他因素,如环境因素,也可能解释疾病表达的变异性。因此,在探索修饰基因之前,重要的是验证这些其他因素并不能解释疾病表达的所有变异,并评估临床表型受遗传因素控制的证据。为此,第一步是通过比较相关和非相关 NF1 患者临床表型的相关性来揭示家系因素的作用。通过考察不同类型亲属之间的表型相关性,可以确定遗传因素是否对每个 NF1 表型的总体表型变异有显著贡献。因此,如果表达变异主要由 NF1 突变决定,那么同一家系内不同个体的表型相关性在近亲之间和远亲之间应该是相同的。相比之下,如果表型变异主要由与 NF1 位点不连锁的基因中的等位基因(修饰基因)决定,那么表型相关性会随着亲缘关系的变远而降低。近亲之间的相关性高于远亲之间的相关性也可能是共同环境效应的结果。这种可能性可以通过比较同卵双生子和同胞的表型相关性来具体检验。

18.2.1 第一条线索:NF1 同卵双生子的研究以及 NF1 临床特征之间的关联

双生子研究在历史上一直是研究遗传病的一个非常有价值的工具。收集双生子数据对于估算与临床表型相关的遗传力十分有帮助。遗传力定义为由遗传方差引起的表型变异所占的比例(Vineis and Pearce 2010, 2011)。双生子通常被认为共享相同的环境。如果同卵(monozygotic, MZ)双生子在临床表型上比异卵双生子更相似,就应该用修饰基因对临床表型的影响来解释。因此,作为研究 NF1 中可变表达的遗传成分的一种手段,NF1 的 MZ 双生子被广泛研究。文献中至少有 30 例 MZ 双生子合并 NF1 的病例报道。大部分 NF1 双生子文献都集中于案例报道。在许多 NF1 的 MZ 双生子中观察到临床症状高度一致(咖啡斑、腋窝及腹股沟雀斑、Lisch 结节、癫痫、非发育不良性脊柱侧弯、肾血管性高血压、单侧上睑下垂、皮肤型神经纤维瘤),表明遗传因素对家系间和家系内的表型变异性有重要影响(Easton et al. 1993;Sabbagh et al. 2009;Melean et al. 2010)。原则上,这种一致性是很容易解释的,不仅由于在 MZ 双生子中存在相同的 NF1 突变,还由于 MZ 双生子基因组遗传学上几乎一致,以及它们在围产期前和围产期环境中都有极为相似的经历。也有报道少数 MZ 双生子合并 NF1 的病例在疾病的临床表现方面有明显差异(Rieley et al. 2011),证明了其潜在的生物学复杂性。然而,在这类病例中,致病的 NF1 突变并不都被鉴定出来,导致这些 MZ 双生子临床症状不一致的本质因素仍然是谜。有趣的是,最近的一项研究报道了 1 对 NF1 表型不一致的 MZ 双生子,其中突变分析揭示,在受影响的个体中发生了合子后的 NF1 基因突变,导致 NF1 突变的体细胞嵌合体(Vogt et al. 2011)。在一些报道中,NF1 双生子中的肿瘤显示出明显低于其他特征的一致性。由于许多与 NF1 相关的肿瘤需要在另外一个 NF1 等位基因中发生二次打击,所以二次打击事件的散发性被认为可以解释双生子中肿瘤的差异。或者,可能存在其他影响肿瘤出现和生长的非遗传因素,如表观遗传学改变、其他肿瘤相关基因的体细胞突变或环境事件等。相反,最近的一篇报道描述了 1 对受 NF1 影响的 MZ 双生子,这对双生子的 NF1 从头突变导致左侧坐骨神经丛状神经纤维瘤,在相似的年龄演变成 MPNST,并在相同的年龄发生肺转移(Melean et al. 2010)。来自 MZ 双生子的数据虽然宝贵,但由于几个限制因素,应该予以谨慎考虑。首先,MZ 双生子的样本容量总是较小的(最大的研究中为 10 对)。此外,NF1 的某些并发症可能尚未被完全确定,需要进行常规影像学检查(如丛状神经纤维瘤)。最后,双生子往往年龄较小,因此不清楚未来会出现哪些额外的 NF1 并发症。

通过研究 NF1 症状之间的关联,也获得了 NF1 中存在修饰基因的线索。个体临床特征的发生之间存在几个具有统计学意义的关联。Szudek 等在受影响的亲子对中发现 Lisch 结节、视路胶质瘤、学习障碍、巨颅畸形和身材矮小的发生之间有显著关联,但这项研究没有试图调整来自同一家系的多个亲属对的非独立性或个体中临床特征之间的关联(Szudek et al. 2000)。接下来的研究拓展分析了不同类别亲属之间 NF1 特征的相关性。通过比较观察到的相关性发现，NF1 遗传变异的来源通常是重要的，并因不同的临床特征而有所不同（Szudek et al. 2002）。

18.2.2　NF1 中可变表达的遗传成分的评估

为了评估遗传因素对 NF1 表型变异的贡献，几项研究在一系列多病例 NF1 家系中检测了许多与 NF1 相关的特征。由于可变表达的模式是微妙的，所以需要非常多的患者和（或）非常大的家系数据来确定影响 NF1 表型的修饰基因。事实上，NF1 家系分析中最重要的混杂因素是年龄。考虑到许多 NF1 疾病特征的进行性发展和年龄对分析的潜在混杂影响，数据必须能够代表所有年龄组。许多疾病特征在年龄较大的 NF1 患者中更为普遍（Cnossen et al. 1998），如果不加以控制，可能会使年龄相近的患病亲属（同胞）之间产生相关性，或者使年龄差异较大的亲属（父母和子女）之间的相关性变得模糊。嵌合体是另外一个必须考虑的因素。新发 NF1 病例中的体细胞嵌合体必须考虑，因为它可能导致较轻或不典型的 NF1 表型（Kehrer-Sawatzki and Cooper 2008；Messiaen et al. 2011）。

通过考察不同类型亲属之间的表型相关性，提供了 NF1 中强遗传成分的证据，并提示非连锁修饰基因参与了疾病的可变表达。迄今为止，仅有 3 项研究在 NF1 家系大队列中评估了 NF1 中可变表达的遗传成分（Easton et al. 1993；Szudek et al. 2002；Sabbagh et al. 2009）。

在 1993 年发表的一项研究中，Easton 等研究了来自 48 个家系的 175 个 NF1 个体，其中包括 6 对 MZ 双生子、76 对同胞、60 对亲子对、54 对二级亲属对和 43 对三级亲属对（Easton et al. 1993）。对 8 个 NF1 临床特征进行评分：3 个数量性状（咖啡牛奶斑、皮肤型神经纤维瘤的数量和头围）以及 5 个二元性状（有无丛状神经纤维瘤、有无视路胶质瘤、有无脊柱侧弯、有无癫痫以及有无认知障碍）。3 个定量变量——咖啡牛奶斑、皮肤型神经纤维瘤数和头围之间存在显著的家系内相关性：MZ 双生子之间的相关性最高，一级亲属之间的相关性较低，而较远的亲属之间的相关性更低。MZ 双生子之间的高相关性表明在表达变异中具有很强的遗传成分，但远亲之间的低相关性表明 NF1 位点的突变类型本身只起到次要作用。Easton 等认为 NF1 的表达在很大程度上由其他修饰位点的基因型决定，并且这些修饰基因具有性状特异性。

在 Easton 等的研究大约 10 年后，发表了第二个大家系表型相关性研究（Szudek et al. 2002）。Szudek 等研究了 373 个有 2 个或 2 个以上 NF1 成员的家系（346/373 为核心家系，包括 1 个受影响的父母和 1 个及以上受影响的子女或 2 个及以上受影响的同胞）中 904 个患病个体的 NF1 特征的家系聚集性。该样本量是 Easton 等研究的 5 倍，并考察了（咖啡牛奶斑、皮肤褶皱部位雀斑、Lisch 结节、皮肤型神经纤维瘤、皮下神经纤维瘤、丛状神经纤维瘤、癫痫、脊柱侧弯、视路胶质瘤和其他肿瘤等）10 个临床特征。所有表型性状均被视为二元变量。与 Easton 等的研究不同，咖啡牛奶斑和皮肤型神经纤维瘤未被计数。使用多元回归来评估 NF1 的 10 个临床特征中每个临床特征在不同亲属类别之间的关联，同时调整相关特征、年龄和性别等协变量。正如 Easton 等所描述的，研究表明非连锁修饰基因和正常的 NF1 等位基因可能都参与了 NF1 特定临床特征的发展，但不同特征中的相对贡献不同。Szudek 等认为大多数 NF1 临床特征具有重要的遗传成分，但不止一个遗传因素可能参与其中，并且各种遗传和非遗传效应的相对重要性可能因不同的特征而异。

这两个研究都是至关重要的，因为它们共同证明了 NF1 表达变异中强大的遗传成分。然而，也必须考虑到一定的局限性。Easton 等的研究调查的患者数量有限，而 Szudek 等的研究虽然调查了更多的患者，但由于大家系的数量较少，无法调查到更多的远亲。此外，本研究没有将咖啡牛奶斑和皮肤型神经纤维瘤（NF1 的主要表现）作为定量变量进行分析，而是将这些特征作为二元性状处理。在第三个大型家系表型研究中，Sabbagh 等使用基于最大似然法的方差成分分析来估计可归因于遗传效应的表型变异比例（Sabbagh et al. 2009），对 12 个 NF1 相关的临床特征进行家系相关性分析，包括 5 个数量性状（小和大咖啡斑的数量，以及皮肤、皮下和丛状神经纤维瘤的数量）和 7 个二元性状，对来自 275

个家系的 750 例 NF1 患者的这些表型性状进行了评分。除肿瘤外，所研究的所有临床特征在校正年龄和性别后均表现出显著的家系聚集性。对大多数患者而言，这种家系相关性模式表明有很强的遗传成分，而 NF1 组成型突变并没有显著影响。与 Szudek 和 Easton 的研究结果一致，NF1 临床特征之间的几个关联具有统计学意义，表明一些 NF1 特征可能由共同的遗传因素决定。这些结果表明，某些性状的组合可能存在共同的遗传修饰。

这 3 个大型研究探索了 NF1 家系中的表型相关性，表明与 NF1 非连锁的遗传修饰解释了 NF1 的可变表达（Easton et al. 1993；Szudek et al. 2002；Sabbagh et al. 2009）。这一假设在 NF1 基因被鉴定后建立的 NF1 小鼠模型中得到了证实。

18.3 NF1 小鼠模型的建立：证实修饰基因存在

人类是典型的自然种群，比实验室动物表现出更大的遗传多样性和更广泛的环境多样性，因此人类的基因型-表型相关性远不如实验室小鼠清晰。在实验动物中，修饰效应通常源于遗传背景（以单基因或多基因方式遗传）。小鼠的遗传背景指除感兴趣的突变基因以外的遗传构成（所有位点上的所有等位基因）。修饰基因的证据可能来自不同血缘品系背景之间出现的不能由致病基因或环境因素（在实验室小鼠中得到控制）解释的一系列表型。

NF1 基因的鉴定使得构建 Nf1 无效突变的小鼠模型成为可能，这些小鼠有望重现人类 NF1 的临床特征，包括神经纤维瘤和 MPNST（Carroll and Ratner 2008；Parrinello and Lloyd 2009；Staser et al. 2012）。由于 NF1 患者遗传了 NF1 基因的一个缺陷拷贝，所以第一种方法是构建携带 1 个 Nf1 基因靶向破坏的小鼠。Nf1 "敲除" 突变杂合子小鼠（$Nf1^{+/-}$）与对应的人类一样，具有生存能力、生育能力和肿瘤易感性。然而，令人失望的是，在这些小鼠中仅发现了在人类 NF1 患者中观察到的部分表型（Jacks et al. 1994）。这些动物没有表现人类疾病的一些标志性特征，包括神经纤维瘤和 MPNST。这些观察结果表明，$Nf1^{+/-}$ 小鼠没有形成神经纤维瘤，因为在小鼠施万细胞中剩余的功能性 Nf1 等位基因失活发生的频率很低。因此，二次打击突变被认为是关键事件。鉴于第二个 Nf1 等位基因的突变似乎是肿瘤形成中的一个关键步骤，该事件在相关细胞类型中发生的频率可能不足以启动小鼠神经纤维瘤和 MPNST 的发生。这种假说在人类中也被提出，因为错配修复基因（mismatch repair genes，MMR）被认为是 NF1 相关肿瘤发生的潜在修饰基因（见下文）。有趣的是，另外一种动物模型已经指出 MMR 基因在神经纤维瘤形成中的作用（Feitsma et al. 2008）：在斑马鱼 3 个主要 MMR 基因（mlh1、msh2 和 msh6）的敲除突变体中观察到神经纤维瘤发生的频率很低。

18.3.1 小鼠遗传背景与 NF1 相关肿瘤易感性

NF1 小鼠模型的发展为深入了解 NF1 相关肿瘤的发生和发展提供了关键的机会。已有研究探索了小鼠遗传背景与 NF1 相关肿瘤易感性之间的关联（Reilly et al 2000，2004，2006）。这方面内容在本书的另外一个章节中展开。小鼠模型在不同程度上重现了人类 NF1 的对应表型。然而，必须强调小鼠模型在模拟完整的人类 NF1 表型方面存在局限性。例如，缺乏 Nf1 可变剪接外显子 23a 的小鼠表现出特异性学习障碍（Costa et al. 2001），而在人类中，外显子 23a 在中枢神经系统神经元中被特异性跳过。这些观察结果支持用特定的人类遗传学方法来鉴定人类中的 NF1 修饰基因。

18.4 遗传学方法：首次通过靶向策略证明 NF1 中存在修饰基因以及全基因组技术的前景

大样本的表型研究表明 NF1 基因的突变类型并不能解释表型变异。NF1 基因型-表型相关性的研究验证了这些观察结果。

18.4.1 NF1 基因型-表型相关性：NF1 突变类型无影响

NF1 表型变异可能是由于存在修饰基因，但

NF1突变的等位基因异质性也可能是解释疾病变异的因素之一。几乎一半的NF1病例是由散发突变引起的，并且已经报道了大量不同的NF1致病性突变。这种极端的变异性使得挖掘基因型-表型相关性变得更加困难。在不同的致病性突变中，5%～10%为包含整个NF1基因座和邻近基因的17q11大片段缺失。自1992年首次报道以来，许多研究报道了携带基因组NF1缺失的患者比基因内NF1突变的患者具有更严重的临床表型。这种"邻近基因综合征"似乎包括容貌畸形、学习障碍、心血管畸形、儿童期过度生长、更高的肿瘤负荷和更早的良性神经纤维瘤的发生，并且MPNST的发生率可能更高(Castle et al. 2003；Mautner et al. 2010；Pasmant et al. 2010)。有研究表明，其他几个基因的共同缺失应该是导致这种更严重表型的原因。OMG和RNF135单倍型不足可能与学习障碍有关，RNF135基因可能与面神经发育异常有关，SUZ12和CENTA2基因可能与心血管畸形有关。研究推测，恶性肿瘤风险增加可能是由于同样位于NF1缺失区间内的一个或多个基因(抑癌基因而非原癌基因)的表达变化所致(Bartelt-Kirbach et al. 2009；Pasmant et al. 2011a)。

另外一方面，对于NF1基因内突变(>90%的病例)的患者，迄今为止，除了NF1基因第17外显子的3bp框内缺失(c.2970-2972delAAT)与以无皮肤型神经纤维瘤为特征的特殊临床表型相关外，尚未建立明确的基因型-表型相关性(Upadhyaya et al. 2007)。其他研究试图在非典型NF1表型和(或)突变类型的背景下明确更多的基因型-表型相关性。有多发性脊柱肿瘤但几乎没有NF1其他临床症状的患者已被报道，这表明NF1有一个亚类或一种独特的遗传形式，称为脊柱神经纤维瘤病，与较轻度的NF1突变或其他遗传改变有关(Kaufmann et al. 2001；Wimmer et al. 2002；Kluwe et al. 2003)。然而，一些研究表明，脊柱肿瘤患者可出现多种NF1症状和NF1突变。最近，一篇文章观察到在视路胶质瘤患者中NF1基因的致病性突变趋向于聚集在NF1基因5′端的1/3部位(Sharif et al. 2011)。然而，这些发现仍然需要进一步的证据来证实。其他潜在的基因型-表型相关性仍有待发现。尽管如此，由于同一个NF1家系的不同患病成员即使具有相同的NF1突变，疾病表型也往往截然不同，正如表型研究所揭示的那样，NF1等位基因突变本身并不能解释所有的疾病变异性。

18.4.2 正常(未突变)NF1等位基因无影响

通过比较不同类型亲属之间的表型相关性，大量家系研究为NF1可变表达中的强遗传成分提供了证据，并表明非连锁的修饰基因，可能还有正常的NF1等位基因，参与了疾病的可变表达。NF1表型变异实际上可能是由于NF1正常等位基因的另外一个变异体的影响，该变异体位于原发突变的相对位置。最近的一项研究通过基于家系的关联研究，探究了正常NF1等位基因在NF1可变表达中的作用(Sabbagh et al. 2009)。在313个NF1家系的1 132个个体中对NF1基因的9个单核苷酸多态性(single-nucleotide polymorphisms，SNP)标签进行了基因分型。基于单个标记或单倍型分析，在所检测的12个临床特征中，没有发现任何1个NF1变异体对患病后代的传播有显著的偏差。本研究提供的证据表明，在大多数NF1临床特征中存在很强的遗传成分，而NF1基因对疾病变异没有显著的影响，因为组成型NF1突变和正常的NF1等位基因似乎对每个性状的总体表型变异都没有显著贡献，这也证实了之前表型探究的发现。

18.4.3 遗传方法鉴定修饰基因的策略

用于探究遗传因素在表型表达中作用的策略通常根据可用的数据类型分为两类：连锁研究和关联研究。如果有家系数据，可以考虑通过跟踪临床表型和标记在家系中的分离来进行连锁分析。连锁分析通常用贯穿整个基因组的随机标记系统地进行。它最初是作为一种在遗传异质性存在的情况下检验连锁关系的方法而提出的，但也可以用于确定修饰基因在孟德尔疾病中的作用。连锁的另外一种策略是在携带与疾病相关的原发性突变的个体样本中检测与临床表型的关联。对于定性临床表型，在有临床表型和无临床表型的患者中比较标记基因型的分布，并检测有显著差异的标记。这些基因可能与表型表达有关或与表型表达相关的基因座有关。对于定量临床表型，不同基因型的表型平均值可以用 ANOVA 或 t 检验进行比较（Génin et al. 2008）。已经提出了新的方法来计算和校正关联中的人口分层。然而，这些方法成本较大，因此在探索修饰基因时可能难以应用。另外一种策略是基于"病例-父母"三人组设计的基于家系的关联检验和传递不平衡检验（transmission disequilibrium test，TDT）。这种方法的优点是既检验了连锁，又检验了关联，从而保证了任何显著的结果都并非由群体混合导致（Ott et al. 2011）。这些测试的基本思想是比较父母传递以及不传递给他们受影响的孩子的等位基因。因此，寻找修饰基因必须根据患病儿童的表型类别，考察是否存在亲代传递的差异。

策略还可以基于方法区分，可以是扫描整个基因组的系统性方法，也可以是对候选基因或候选通路有选择性的更聚焦的方法（Génin et al. 2008）。

18.4.3.1 假设驱动法：生物学驱动的候选基因

与在全基因组范围内盲目搜索修饰基因不同，识别修饰基因的另外一个可接受的策略是关注有限的、精心选择的基因，即所谓的候选基因。候选基因根据感兴趣的表型不同而不同。候选基因法可定义为研究遗传因素对某一复杂性状的影响，通过：① 提出假说并确定可能在疾病病因中发挥作用的候选基因；② 识别这些基因内或附近的变异（SNP）；③ 对人群中的变异进行基因分型；并利用统计学方法（连锁或关联）来判断这些变异与表型之间是否存在相关性（Tabor et al. 2002）。从精心选择的候选基因中测试变异体是有一定优势的，有几个原因：测试的变异体数量一般较少，从而避免了统计分析时多重比较带来的误差。对候选基因产物及其变异体的详细理解将有助于掌握更多机制，并促进评估修饰效应的实验性研究。

有许多不同的方法可以用来选择候选基因。首先可以着眼于与该疾病所涉及的主要突变在相同通路上的基因，或者也可关注位于其他通路中的间接影响该疾病的基因。基于动物模型的方法也得到了应用。对神经纤维瘤蛋白生化功能的进一步了解，可能有助于发现对特定表型特征的发展至关重要的相互作用蛋白和上下游效应因子。通过这种生物学驱动的方法，已经提出了几种 NF1 相关肿瘤发生的修饰基因。在人类和小鼠中，肿瘤的发展是由不同细胞谱系中普遍存在的 *NF1* 杂合性和不可预测的 *NF1* 杂合性丢失所共同导致的（Staser et al. 2010）。已经从不同的神经纤维瘤中分离出具有 *NF1* 突变等位基因（$NF1^{-/-}$）的神经纤维瘤衍生的施万细胞，有丝分裂重组是这种杂合性丢失最可能的机制（Serra et al. 2001）。由于有丝分裂重组表现出个体间变异，控制这一现象的基因被认为通过影响体细胞突变率参与调节 NF1 患者神经纤维瘤数量的广泛变异性。一些研究者还推测 *MMR* 基因的变异可以改变 NF1 相关神经纤维瘤的体细胞突变率。

18.4.3.2 错配修复基因假说

NF1 相关神经纤维瘤的数量在 NF1 患者中差异很大，可能是由于体细胞 *NF1* 基因突变的累积量不同。二次打击和杂合性丢失事件在几种 NF1 肿瘤类型（Upadhyaya et al. 2008a，b；Thomas et al. 2010）甚至胫骨发育不良（Stevenson et al. 2007）中都已被报道，但这不太可能解释 NF1 特征的全部变异性。两个研究小组阐述了 DNA MMR 在 NF1 神经纤维瘤发生、发展中的作用。两者都提供了证据表明 MMR 抑制会导致神经纤维瘤中 *NF1* 基因的高突变率（Wiest et al. 2003；Wang et al. 2003）。从这些发现中，我们推测 NF1 患者 *MMR* 基因的早期或组成性突变可能导致 *NF1* 中二次打击的积累（*MMR* 基因是人类基因中突变率较高的基因之一）。然而，除了一个单独报道外，在 NF1 患者中并未检测到人类 *MMR* 基因的组成性突变（Alotaibi et al. 2008）。Alotaibi 等描述了组成性 *NF1* 胚系突变和组成性 *MLH1* 纯合缺陷的独特共现。迄今为止，所有其他携带 *MMR* 基因突变并具有 NF1 特征的病例均未发现携带 *NF1* 胚系突变。因此，在高肿瘤负荷的 NF1 患者中，甲基化被推测是导致 MMR 活性降低的一种机制，因为 *MMR* 基因的组成性突变似乎非常罕见。在这个假说中，通过甲基化下调 *MMR* 基因启动子区域将是 NF1 表型严重程度的重要修饰因子。最近的一项研究分析了 NF1 中肿瘤负荷（以皮肤型神经纤维瘤的数量来定义)的增加是否与 MMR 基因的甲基化有关(Titze et al. 2010)。Titze 等对 NF1 患者白细胞中最常涉及人类癌症的 MMR 基因启动子(MLH1、MSH6、PMS2 和 MSH2)进行甲基化特异性聚合酶链反应(methylation-specific PCR，MSP)。然而，他们仅在部分 NF1 患者血液白细胞中发现 MSH2 启动子甲基化增强的证据。

一些研究还提出了其他可能调节 NF1 表型表达的候选修饰基因。最近关于人类基因组功能结构的报道表明，转录差异也可以解释疾病表达的变异性，基因的转录结构域可能远远超出通常的调控序列。这些观点与 NF1 小鼠模型观察到的结果一致，即在具有特定表型的小鼠品系背景中，NF1 表达水平不同。然而，NF1 转录水平的决定因素，可视为相关的 NF1 修饰基因，仍有待发现。

选择特定 NF1 表型性状的候选修饰基因的另外一种策略是使用"无先验"的遗传学方法。

18.4.4 NF1 中一个修饰基因的首次鉴定：概念的证明

在最近的一项研究中，Pasmant 等(Pasmant et al. 2011b)在 NF1 相关丛状神经纤维瘤中使用全基因组高分辨率阵列比较基因组杂交鉴定 NF1 中肿瘤发展的候选修饰基因。首次发现 9p21.3 缺失是 NF1 相关丛状神经纤维瘤中唯一的复发性体细胞改变。9p21.3 中最小的共同缺失区域包括 CDKN2A - CDKN2B - ARF 基因簇和 ANRIL 基因(1 个大的非编码 RNA)。然后利用位于 9p21.3 区域的 SNP 标签对来自 306 个家系的 1 105 名受试者进行了基于家系的关联研究。发现 SNP rs2151280(位于 ANRIL)的等位基因 T 与丛状神经纤维瘤的较高数量有较强的相关性。这种关联只在丛状神经纤维瘤中观察到，而在真皮神经纤维瘤中不存在，表明 SNP rs2151280 对丛状神经纤维瘤的发生具有特异性作用，而对真皮神经纤维瘤没有作用。为了确认 rs2151280、CDKN2A、CDKN2B、ARF 和 ANRIL 的功能，在 124 例 NF1 患者外周血中进行表达分析。rs2151280(和其他 SNP 标签相比与更高数量的丛状神经纤维瘤相关)的等位基因 T 与 ANRIL 转录水平降低显著相关。第一个与丛状神经纤维瘤数量相关的 NF1 修饰基因的发现为该疾病尤其是神经纤维瘤发生的分子机制开辟了新的视角。本研究揭示了全基因组特征对于鉴定参与丛状神经纤维瘤发生的候选修饰基因的意义。因此，NF1 表型性状的候选修饰基因研究获得了概念的证明。靶向策略为鉴定导致 NF1 遗传特征和并发症的新变异体带来了巨大的希望。然而，这种候选基因方法受到了质疑，因结果缺乏可重复性，且因其具有无法包括所有可能的致病基因和多态性的局限性(Tabor et al. 2002)。随着新的全基因组技术的应用，目前出现了一种替代策略。

18.4.5 从遗传学到基因组学：NF1 全基因组关联研究和下一代测序的前景

低成本的基因分型阵列使得研究人员不必基于候选基因进行关联研究，而可以以无偏倚的方式进行全基因组关联研究(genome-wide association studies，GWAS)。GWAS 可以搜寻到数百万个与人类复杂性状相关联的常见 SNP(Hindorff et al. 2009；Manolio 2010)。常见人类 DNA 序列变异库目前已经可以访问，覆盖了人类基因组的所有常见变异。截至 2011 年，变异位点(dbSNP 135)公共目录包含大约 5 200 万个 SNP。结构变异数据库(例如 dbVAR)提供了大基因组变异位置的索引。人类基因组单体型图计划(The International HapMap Project)对几个群体中等位基因频率和附近变异体之间的相关模式(一种被称为连锁不平衡的现象)进行了编目。千人基因组计划(The 1000 Genomes Project)于 2008 年启动，其目标是为在每个群体中等位基因频率至少为 1% 的 DNA 多态性创建一个公共参考数据库。

GWAS 方法在探究强大的遗传关联方面已被证明非常有用。随着超大批量基因分型平台(每个样品有 10 万～100 万个基因型)的问世，人们对在 NF1 中进行 GWAS 鉴定修饰基因的可能性越来越感兴趣。一个广泛的共识是，现在启动此类研究的时机已经成熟，特别是多阶段抽样的研究设计使效率显著提高，可通过使用高密度全基因组技术仅测试一部分受试者，然后在初始扫描确定的区域测试其他受试者和(或)其他 SNP。在通过 GWAS 识别出一个疾病相关区域后,需要对该区域的序列变异进行全面的研究,以识别出可能解释关联信号的全部变异。因为 GWAS 不能完全捕获每个区域的 DNA 变异,所以有假设提出,与 GWAS 使用的标签 SNP 相比,部分被连锁不平衡捕获的因果变异可能显示出与表型更强的相关性。因此,GWAS 之后的一个重要步骤是收集相关区域中存在的更完整的变异目录(包括频率较低的变异),并测试其与感兴趣的表型的相关性。随着下一代测序技术的进展和千人基因组计划(2010)数据的揭示,研究者必须选择(或组合)多种策略来提出并测试可能的多态性位点,尤其包括下一代测序(Lander 2011)。下一代测序技术支持高通量测序,并已将成本降低到每个基因组测序只需 5 000 美元,据估计,这些成本将进一步下降,可能在 1 年内降至 1 000 美元的水平。研究罕见变异将需要对基因中的蛋白质编码(或其他)区域进行测序,以确定那些在病例中罕见变异的出现频率高于对照组的区域。罕见变异是否会揭示修饰基因必须等待下一代测序的结果。因此,使用这些全基因组方法在 NF1 中鉴定修饰基因似乎颇具前景。

GWAS 中测试的标记数量巨大,需要用多个测试进行校正,并使用非常严格的标准来得出显著的关联。因此,有必要对表型良好的 NF1 患者进行大规模队列研究,从而发现效应较弱的遗传修饰因子。临床文件中记录的信息质量往往不尽如人意,临床医师已经开始构建以电子格式存储的非常庞大、高质量的临床数据库。基于从详尽的临床档案中检索到的高质量数据的研究势必变得越来越重要。标准化是这些项目取得成功的根本要素。未来这一领域的成果需要治疗 NF1 患者的临床医师、研究其全球负担的流行病学家、对了解其可变性感兴趣的遗传学家、设计研究以更好地了解这种变异性质的临床研究人员,以及研究目前知之甚少的 NF1 个体间差异机制的基础科学家共同努力。

18.5 结论

队列研究表明,NF1 的表型表达在近亲中趋于相似,但不幸的是,这种相似性的程度远远达不到可对临床严重程度进行有用的预测所需的程度。为了提供更精确的预测,将需要鉴定更多相关的修饰基因。NF1 基因座变异的贡献相对较小,这表明精确的 NF1 突变的信息通常是无益的。修饰基因的概念是通过鉴定一个影响丛状神经纤维瘤数量的修饰基因来证明的(Pasmant et al. 2011a, b)。修饰基因研究中的第一个也可能是最重要的步骤仍然是确定所要探究的修饰基因相关的临床表型,以及选择研究人群。修饰基因通常至少有两个等位基因,分别被认为是"促进疾病"和"抑制疾病"。这些抑制疾病的修饰基因改变了性状表达的表型阈值,导致更少的携带者个体受到影响。新的疾病治疗方法可以基于模仿并可能增强自然发生的修饰基因的效应。了解疾病表型可变性的一般机制,特别是与抑制疾病相关的机制,可能有助于 NF1 并发症的预测、治疗甚至预防(Nadeau 2001)。

阐明 NF1 表型表达变异的原因可能为疾病的分子生物学机制提供重要线索,也可能通过改变这些效应提供替代治疗方法。由于已知遗传修饰可以改变疾病的病程,它们的蛋白质产物将成为治疗干预的直接靶点。

(郑婷婷 译)

参考文献

[1] 1000 Genomes Project Consortium (2010) A map of human genome variation from population-scale sequencing. Nature 467:1061-1073

[2] Alotaibi H, Ricciardone MD, Ozturk M (2008) Homozygosity at variant MLH1 can lead to secondary mutation in NF1, neurofibromatosis type 1 and early onset leukemia. Mutat Res 637:209-214

[3] Altshuler D, Daly MJ, Lander ES (2008) Genetic mapping in human disease. Science 322:881-888

[4] Bartelt-Kirbach B, Wuepping M, Dodrimont-Lattke M, Kaufmann D (2009) Expression analysis of genes lying in the NF1 microdeletion interval points to four candidate modifiers for neurofibroma formation. Neurogenetics 10:79-85

[5] Carey JC, Baty BJ, Johnson JP, Morrison T, Skolnick M, Kivlin J (1986) The genetic aspects of neurofibromatosis. Ann NY Acad Sci 486:45-56

[6] Carroll SL, Ratner N (2008) How does the Schwann cell lineage form tumors in NF1? Glia 56:1590-1605

[7] Castle B, Baser ME, Huson SM, Cooper DN, Upadhyaya M (2003) Evaluation of genotype-phenotype correlations in neurofibromatosis type 1. J Med Genet 40: e109

[8] Cnossen M, de Goede-Bolder A, van den Broek K, Waasdorp C, Oranje A, Stroink H, Simonsz H, van den Ouweland A, Halley D, Niermeijer M (1998) A prospective 10 year follow up study of patients with neurofibromatosis type 1. Arch Dis Child 78: 408-412

[9] Costa RM, Yang T, Huynh DP, Pulst SM, Viskochil DH, Silva AJ, Brannan CI (2001) Learning deficits, but normal development and tumor predisposition, in mice lacking exon 23a of Nf1. Nat Genet 27: 399-405

[10] Easton DF, Ponder MA, Huson SM, Ponder BA (1993) An analysis of variation in expression of neurofibromatosis (NF) type 1 (NF1): evidence for modifying genes. Am J Hum Genet 53: 305-313

[11] Feitsma H, Kuiper RV, Korving J, Nijman IJ, Cuppen E (2008) Zebrafish with mutations in mismatch repair genes develop neurofibromas and other tumors. Cancer Res 68: 5059-5066

[12] Génin E, Feingold J, Clerget-Darpoux F (2008) Identifying modifier genes of monogenic disease: strategies and difficulties. Hum Genet 124: 357-368

[13] Hindorff LA, Sethupathy P, Junkins HA et al (2009) Potential etiologic and functional implications of genome-wide association loci for human diseases and traits. Proc Natl Acad Sci USA 106: 9362-9367

[14] Jacks T, Shih TS, Schmitt EM, Bronson RT, Bernards A, Weinberg RA (1994) Tumour predispo-sition in mice heterozygous for a targeted mutation in Nf1. Nat Genet 7: 353-361

[15] Kaufmann D, Müller R, Bartelt B, Wolf M, Kunzi-Rapp K, Hanemann CO, Fahsold R, Hein C, Vogel W, Assum G (2001) Spinal neurofibromatosis without café-au-lait macules in two families with null mutations of the NF1 gene. Am J Hum Genet 69: 1395-1400

[16] Kehrer-Sawatzki H, Cooper DN (2008) Mosaicism in sporadic neurofibromatosis type 1: variations on a theme common to other hereditary cancer syndromes? J Med Genet 45: 622-631

[17] Kluwe L, Tatagiba M, Fünsterer C, Mautner V (2003) NF1 mutations and clinical spectrum in patients with spinal neurofibromas. J Med Genet 40: 368-371

[18] Lander ES (2011) Initial impact of the sequencing of the human genome. Nature 470: 187-197

[19] Manolio TA (2010) Genomewide association studies and assessment of the risk of disease. N Engl J Med 363: 166-176

[20] Mautner VF, Kluwe L, Friedrich RE, Roehl AC, Bammert S, Högel J, Spöri H, Cooper DN, Kehrer-Sawatzki H (2010) Clinical characterisation of 29 neurofibromatosis type-1 patients with molecularly ascertained 1.4 Mb type-1 NF1 deletions. J Med Genet 47: 623-630

[21] Melean G, Hernandez AM, Valero MC, Hernandez Imaz E, Martin Y, Hernandez-Chico C (2010) Monozygotic twins with neurofibromatosis type 1, concordant phenotype and synchronous development of MPNST and metastasis. BMC Cancer 10: 407

[22] Messiaen L, Vogt J, Bengesser K, Fu C, Mikhail F, Serra E, Garcia-Linares C, Cooper DN, Lazaro C, Kehrer-Sawatzki H (2011) Mosaic type-1 NF1 microdeletions as a cause of both generalized and segmental neurofibromatosis type-1 (NF1). Hum Mutat 32: 213-219

[23] Nadeau JH (2001) Modifier genes in mice and humans. Nat Rev Genet 2: 165-174

[24] Ott J, Kamatani Y, Lathrop M (2011) Family-based designs for genome-wide association studies. Nat Rev Genet 12: 465-474

[25] Parrinello S, Lloyd AC (2009) Neurofibroma development in NF1-insights into tumour initiation. Trends Cell Biol 19: 395-403

[26] Pasmant E, Sabbagh A, Spurlock G, Laurendeau I, Grillo E, Hamel MJ, Martin L, Barbarot S, Leheup B, Rodriguez D, Lacombe D, Pasquier L, Isidor B, Ferkal S, Soulier J, Sanson M, Dieux-Coeslier A, Bièche I, Parfait B, Vidaud M, Wolkenstein P, Upadhyaya M, Vidaud D, Members of the NF France Network (2010) NF1 microdeletions in neurofibromatosis type 1: from genotype to phenotype. Hum Mutat 31: E1506-1518

[27] Pasmant E, Masliah-Planchon J, Lévy P, Laurendeau I, Ortonne N, Parfait B, Valeyrie-Allanore L, Leroy K, Wolkenstein P, Vidaud M, Vidaud D, Bièche I (2011a) Identification of genes potentially involved in the increased risk of malignancy in NF1-microdeleted patients. Mol Med 17: 79-87

[28] Pasmant E, Sabbagh A, Masliah-Planchon J, Ortonne N, Laurendeau I, Melin L, Ferkal S, Hernandez L, Leroy K, Valeyrie-Allanore L, Parfait B, Vidaud D, Bièche I, Lantieri L, Wolkenstein P, Vidaud M, the members of the NF France Network (2011b) Role of noncoding RNA ANRIL in genesis of plexiform neurofibromas in neurofibromatosis type 1. J Natl Cancer Inst 103: 1713-1722

[29] Reilly KM, Loisel DA, Bronson RT, McLaughlin ME, Jacks T (2000) Nf1; Trp53 mutant mice develop glioblastoma with evidence of strain-specific effects. Nat Genet 26: 109-113

[30] Reilly KM, Tuskan RG, Christy E, Loisel DA, Ledger J, Bronson RT, Smith CD, Tsang S, Munroe DJ, Jacks T (2004) Susceptibility to astrocytoma in mice mutant for Nf1 and Trp53 is linked to chromosome 11 and subject to epigenetic effects. Proc Natl Acad Sci USA 101: 13008-13013

[31] Reilly KM, Broman KW, Bronson RT, Tsang S, Loisel DA, Christy ES, Sun Z, Diehl J, Munroe DJ, Tuskan RG (2006) An imprinted locus epistatically influences Nstr1 and Nstr2 to control resistance to nerve sheath tumors in a neurofibromatosis type 1 mouse model. Cancer Res 66: 62-68

[32] Rieley MB, Stevenson DA, Viskochil DH, Tinkle BT, Martin LJ, Schorry EK (2011) Variable expression of neurofibromatosis 1 in monozygotic twins. Am J Med Genet A 155A: 478-485

[33] Sabbagh A, Pasmant E, Laurendeau I, Parfait B, Barbarot S, Guillot B, Combemale P, Ferkal S, Vidaud M, Aubourg P, Vidaud D, Wolkenstein P, Members of the NF France Network (2009) Unravelling the genetic basis of variable clinical expression in neurofibromatosis 1. Hum Mol Genet 18: 2768-2778

[34] Serra E, Rosenbaum T, Nadal M, Winner U, Ars E, Estivill X, Lázaro C (2001) Mitotic recombination effects homozygosity for NF1 germline mutations in neurofibromas. Nat Genet 28: 294-296

[35] Sharif S, Upadhyaya M, Ferner R, Majounie E, Shenton A, Baser M, Thakker N, Evans DG (2011) A molecular analysis of individuals with neurofibromatosis type 1 (NF1) and optic pathway gliomas (OPGs), and an assessment of genotype-phenotype correlations. J Med Genet 48: 256-260

[36] Staser K, Yang FC, Clapp DW (2010) Plexiform neurofibroma genesis: questions of Nf1 gene dose and hyperactive mast cells. Curr Opin Hematol 17: 287-293

[37] Staser K, Yang FC, Clapp DW (2012) Pathogenesis of

plexiform neurofibroma: tumor-stromal/hematopoietic interactions in tumor progression. Annu Rev Pathol 7: 469-495

[38] Stevenson DA, Moyer-Mileur LJ, Murray M, Slater H, Sheng X, Carey JC, Dube B, Viskochil DH (2007) Bone mineral density in children and adolescents with neurofibromatosis type 1. J Pediatr 150: 83-88

[39] Szudek J, Birch P, Riccardi VM, Evans DG, Friedman JM (2000) Associations of clinical features in neurofibromatosis 1 (NF1). Genet Epidemiol 19: 429-439

[40] Szudek J, Joe H, Friedman JM (2002) Analysis of intrafamilial phenotypic variation in neurofi-bromatosis 1 (NF1). Genet Epidemiol 23: 150-164

[41] Tabor HK, Risch NJ, Myers RM (2002) Candidate-gene approaches for studying complex genetic traits: practical considerations. Nat Rev Genet 3: 391-397

[42] Thomas L, Kluwe L, Chuzhanova N, Mautner V, Upadhyaya M (2010) Analysis of *NF1* somatic mutations in cutaneous neurofibromas from patients with high tumor burden. Neurogenetics 11: 391-400

[43] Titze S, Peters H, Wahrisch S, Harder T, Guse K, Buske A, Tinschert S, Harder A (2010) Differential *MSH2* promoter methylation in blood cells of neurofibromatosis type 1 (NF1) patients. Eur J Hum Genet 18: 81-87

[44] Upadhyaya M, Huson SM, Davies M, Thomas N, Chuzhanova N, Giovannini S, Evans DG, Howard E, Kerr B, Griffiths S, Consoli C, Side L, Adams D, Pierpont M, Hachen R, Barnicoat A, Li H, Wallace P, Van Biervliet JP, Stevenson D, Viskochil D, Baralle D, Haan E, Riccardi V, Turnpenny P, Lazaro C, Messiaen L (2007) An absence of cutaneous neurofibromas associated with a 3-bp inframe deletion in exon 17 of the *NF1* gene (c. 2970-2972 delAAT): evidence of a clinically significant NF1 genotype-phenotype correlation. Am J Hum Genet 80: 140-151

[45] Upadhyaya M, Spurlock G, Monem B, Thomas N, Friedrich RE, Kluwe L, Mautner V (2008a) Germline and somatic *NF1* gene mutations in plexiform neurofibromas. Hum Mutat 29: E103-11

[46] Upadhyaya M, Kluwe L, Spurlock G, Monem B, Majounie E, Mantripragada K, Ruggieri M, Chuzhanova N, Evans DG, Ferner R, Thomas N, Guha A, Mautner V (2008b) Germline and somatic *NF1* gene mutation spectrum in NF1-associated malignant peripheral nerve sheath tumors (MPNSTs). Hum Mutat 29: 74-82

[47] Vineis P, Pearce N (2010) Missing heritability in genome-wide association study research. Nat Rev Genet 11: 589

[48] Vineis P, Pearce E (2011) Genome-wide association studies may be misinterpreted: genes versus heritability. Carcinogenesis 32: 1295-1298

[49] Vogt J, Kohlhase J, Morlot S, Kluwe L, Mautner VF, Cooper DN, Kehrer-Sawatzki H (2011) Monozygotic twins discordant for neurofibromatosis type 1 due to a postzygotic *NF1* gene mutation. Hum Mutat 32: E2134-2147

[50] Wang Q, Montmain G, Ruano E, Upadhyaya M, Dudley S, Liskay RM, Thibodeau SN, Puisieux A (2003) Neurofibromatosis type 1 gene as a mutational target in a mismatch repair-deficient cell type. Hum Genet 112: 117-123

[51] Wiest V, Eisenbarth I, Schmegner C, Krone W, Assum G (2003) Somatic *NF1* mutation spectra in a family with neurofibromatosis type 1: toward a theory of genetic modifiers. Hum Mutat 22: 423-427

[52] Wimmer K, Mühlbauer M, Eckart M, Callens T, Rehder H, Birkner T, Leroy JG, Fonatsch C, Messiaen L (2002) A patient severely affected by spinal neurofibromas carries a recurrent splice site mutation in the *NF1* gene. Eur J Hum Genet 10: 334-338

第19章 使用小鼠模型剖析影响 1 型神经纤维瘤病易感性的遗传和表观遗传的复杂相互作用

Dissection of Complex Genetic and Epigenetic Interactions Underlying NF1 Cancer Susceptibility Using Mouse Models

Georgette N. Jones and Karlyne M. Reilly

19.1 引言

NF1 在疾病中的可变表现度是值得关注的。虽然 NF1 基因是完全外显的,但该病的患者表现出一系列的表型。这给患者及医师带来了一个难题:难以预测每个患者会出现哪些疾病并发症。确定与疾病相关的表型变异的来源引起了广泛的兴趣。遗传因素、环境因素和饮食均可影响包括 NF1 在内的多种疾病的表型变异和差异易感性。患者家族间和家族内表型变异的比较揭示了独立于 NF1 等位基因遗传的可遗传因素以及环境因素。在本章中,我们将重点关注已知能在人类和小鼠模型中影响 NF1 可变表现度的可遗传因素。一旦这些因素被表征,即可被用于预测 NF1 病程的发展。

尽管我们对 NF1 的肿瘤发生和发展机制有了越来越多的了解,但 NF1 患者表现出不同肿瘤发展易感性的原因尚不明确。小鼠模型是解决这个问题的有力工具。在本章中,我们将总结小鼠模型是如何促进我们对 NF1 中遗传复杂性和上位性相互作用的理解。基于 NF1 恶性肿瘤小鼠模型的研究表明,与 NF1 无关的修饰基因,包括个体的性别和来自母亲或父亲的疾病遗传,影响发生不同类型肿瘤的风险。综上所述,这些数据表明,NF1 患者遗传和表观遗传背景的细微差异会对发生 NF1 相关肿瘤的风险产生深远的影响。

19.2 NF1 的表型变异

19.2.1 患者的表现度差异

因为 NF1 具有高度的多效性,研究其表现度需要深入了解其个体或集体表型之间的关联。例如,色素沉着特征(例如咖啡斑、皮褶雀斑和 Lisch 结节)的表现度彼此高度相关,如果个体大量表现出某一种特征,其可能会患有更多的相关特征(Szudek et al. 2003)。所有 3 种形式的神经纤维瘤(皮肤、皮下和丛状)的发生率和严重程度也高度相关,皮下神经纤维瘤在一定程度上可能与色素沉着表型组相关(Szudek et al. 2003)。在三方群组中,视路胶质瘤(optic pathway glioma, OPG)、大头畸形和其他肿瘤也相互关联(Szudek et al. 2003)。这些关联的家系研究显示,受影响的一级亲属比受影响的二级亲属具有更大的色素沉着特征相关表现度,表明其受到遗传或环境/饮食效应相似性增加的作用,而非遗传性 NF1 突变的影响(Szudek et al. 2002)。受累一级亲属的色素沉着和神经纤维瘤特征在兄弟姐妹中的表达相关性高于亲子之间的相关性,有趣的是,父亲和孩子之间的神经纤维瘤和 Lisch 结节表达相关性(父系遗传)高于母亲和孩子之间的相关性(母系遗传),表明除了遗传以外,表观遗传修饰因子也可以影响表型(Szudek et al. 2002)。在一个独立的患者队列中,控制了年龄和性别变量后,观察到非肿瘤特征(包括神经纤维瘤)在家族内的高度相关性,但家族间表现度不受 NF1 突变类型的影响(Sabbagh et al. 2009)。尽管最初认为家族间变异与 NF1 基因中发现的许多突变有关,但总的来说,这些家族相关性研究提示特定突变似乎在影响表现度方面发挥的作用很小。实际上很少有 NF1 突变与表型相关,这表明表现度的可变性主要是由与 NF1 无关的遗传因素或环境/饮食因素引起的。

19.2.2 NF1 小鼠模型和品系依赖性效应

患者的遗传修饰因子可以通过全基因组关联研究(genome-wide association studies,GWAS)或通过在病例对照研究中测试候选修饰因子确定。这些研究需要检验非常大的队列,以排除人群的固有异质性。由于 NF1 表型的可变表达度,必须通过更多的患者来研究给定的表型(如肿瘤数量)。NF1 的小鼠模型可以用来培育大量低异质性的研究个体,使得研究人员能够控制环境、饮食、性别、父母遗传和遗传背景等因素,从而就这些不同的因素如何影响 NF1 的变异性提出重点问题。

通过各种实验设计,对观察到的表型和全基因组基因型之间关联进行统计分析,从而识别小鼠中的候选修饰基因[see Reilly (2009) for additional review]。这种连锁分析可以确定基因组中引起品系表型特异性差异的可变区域。在这些区域内,自然遗传变异,如单核苷酸多态性(single nucleotide polymorphism,SNP),可通过改变蛋白质序列、影响转录水平或稳定性、改变 mRNA 剪接或改变可广泛影响基因表达的 miRNA 的序列来影响修饰蛋白的功能。除了对基因的潜在影响,自然发生的遗传变异可能通过表观遗传机制导致表型变异,例如通过改变印记标记、DNA 甲基化位点或染色质调节因子的结合位点。尽管这些自然发生的变异在种群进化过程中可能是可以耐受的,但在个体中,这些遗传或染色体修饰可能在 NF1 突变的背景下对肿瘤产生更大的影响。通过确定在小鼠模型中导致表型变异性的基因组区域,并研究引起这些效应的分子机制,研究者可以提出可验证的假设,并在患者群体中进一步研究以解释 NF1 的差异表现度。

目前已经开发了大量的 NF1 小鼠模型用于更好地理解肿瘤起始的机制、微环境的作用,并研究参与 NF1 肿瘤发生的信号网络。但由于遗传背景的异质性(不易消除),以及共同培育多个突变小鼠品系以获得所需表型的要求,许多模型对于研究品系特异性对肿瘤易感性的影响作用有限。这使得通过大型动物队列进行育种以确定修饰因子这一过程变得非常昂贵且时间漫长。能够体现疾病各方面特征的更简单的小鼠模型对于建立交叉设计来确定修饰因子更为有效。

19.2.2.1 NF1 的 $Nf1^{+/-}$、$Nf1^{-/-}$ 小鼠模型

$Nf1^{+/-}$ 小鼠在近交系 129S4/SvJae 背景以及 129S4/SvJae;C57BL/6J 杂交背景上进行工程化。这些动物不具有 NF1 的诊断性神经纤维瘤或色素沉着特征,但确实发生了神经纤维肉瘤、白血病和嗜铬细胞瘤(Jacks et al. 1994)。虽然 F1 杂交 (129S4/SvJae x C57BL/6J)- $Nf1^{+/-}$ 小鼠发生嗜铬细胞瘤,但近交系 129S4/SvJae - $Nf1^{+/-}$ 动物从未发生这些肾上腺肿瘤(Tischler et al. 1995)。这有力地表明,$Nf1$ 突变小鼠受到品系特异性表型变异性的影响。然而,由于 NF1 相关表型的潜伏期长和外显率低,该模型在 NF1 修饰因子研究中的应用有限。来自 $Nf1^{-/-}$ 129S4/SvJae 嵌合体小鼠的胚胎干细胞注射到 C57BL/6J 囊胚中,导致神经纤维瘤的发生,这与嵌合体的程度相关(Cichowski et al. 1999),但尚未在该模型中检查品系特异性效应。此外,需要通过显微注射每个囊胚来创建单个小鼠模型,这使得该模型对于繁育映射修饰因子所需的大量动物不切实际。最后,在各种神经系统区室中 $Nf1$ 组织特异性敲除产生了研究 NF1 相关肿瘤生

物学的稳健模型(Bajenaru et al. 2003；Wu et al. 2008；Zhu et al. 2002)。因为这些条件性 $Nf1^{-/-}$ 模型涉及结合最少 3 个突变等位基因，所以还没有进行研究来比较品系背景对表型的影响，这些模型将难以适用于修饰因子映射研究。

19.2.2.2　NF1 的 *NPcis* 小鼠模型

由于 $Nf1^{+/-}$ 小鼠不会发生与 NF1 相关的常见病变，并且组织特异性敲除小鼠需要至少 3 个等位基因突变来启动肿瘤发生，所以在小鼠中进行的 NF1 修饰因子研究主要使用 NF1 相关恶性肿瘤的 *NPcis* 模型。*NPcis* 小鼠被改造为传递 *Nf1* 和 *Trp53* 的单个等位基因突变。*TP53* 肿瘤抑制基因的突变曾被描述为人类 NF1 MPNST 进展中常见的二次打击(Menon et al. 1990)。此外，*TP53* 缺失常见于自发性星形细胞瘤(van Meyel et al. 1994；Watanabe et al. 1997)。$Nf1^{+/-}$ 和 $Trp53^{+/-}$ 小鼠杂交产生 $Nf1^{+/-}$；$Trp53^{+/-}$ 反式(*NPtrans*) 小鼠对 MPNST 的易感性增加(Cichowski et al. 1999)。然而，*NPtrans* 小鼠与野生型动物杂交，减数分裂重组将两个突变等位基因连接到同一染色体上，产生具有 $Nf1^{+/-}$；$Trp53^{+/-}$ cis(*NPcis*)的后代，这种易感性进一步增加(Cichowski et al. 1999)。在小鼠中，*Nf1* 和 *Trp53* 在 11 号染色体上彼此相距约 5 cM(Buchberg et al. 1992)。鉴于它们非常接近，两个突变的顺式等位基因共同遗传而它们之间不发生减数分裂重组的可能性是相当高的，LOH 事件通常导致 *Nf1* 和 *Trp53* 的野生型等位基因丢失，从而在该模型中启动肿瘤发生(Cichowski et al. 1999；Reilly et al. 2000)(图 19.1)。

NPcis 小鼠会发生与人类 NF1 综合征相关的自发性癌症。最常见的是发生 MPNST 或脑星形细胞瘤，较小可能发生脊髓星形细胞瘤、嗜铬细胞瘤、组织细胞肉瘤和淋巴瘤(Reilly et al. 2000，2004)。从 5 月龄左右开始，高达 80% 的 *NPcis* 小鼠发生 MPNST(Cichowski et al. 1999 年)，尽管如下所述，这些肿瘤的发生率取决于小鼠品系背景和突变等位基因的亲本遗传(Cichowski et al. 1999；Reilly et al. 2006)。这些肿瘤通常起源于四肢和躯干的周围神经，它们表现出与人类肿瘤相似的组织学特征，如梭形细胞、有丝分裂象以及 S100 和 p75 免疫反应性(Reilly et al. 2006)。与 MPNST 一样，星形细胞瘤的发生率取决于品系和遗传；然而，根据研究，高达 70%~100% 的 *NPcis* 小鼠在 6 月龄时可发生星形细胞瘤(Reilly et al. 2000，2004)。世界卫生组织(World Health Organization，WHO) 描述了人类 4 级星形细胞瘤(Ⅰ至Ⅳ)，其组织学的不同提示了肿瘤的严重程度(Kleihues et al. 1993)。*NPcis* 小鼠发生的肿瘤类似 WHO Ⅱ至Ⅳ级的星形细胞瘤(Reilly et al. 2004)，边界弥散，核分裂象数量增多，胶质细胞核细长。在极少数情况下，*NPcis* 星形细胞瘤还表现出区域坏死、新生血管形成和多核巨细胞，表明低级病变进展为恶性 WHO Ⅳ级肿瘤，也称为多形性胶质母细胞瘤(glioblastoma multiforme，GBM)(Reilly et al. 2000)。除大脑外，在 *NPcis* 小鼠脊髓中还观察到星形细胞瘤。与 WHO Ⅱ级和Ⅲ级脑肿瘤相似，这些脊髓肿瘤呈弥漫性浸润，并表现出大量有丝分裂象(Amlin-Van Schaick et al. 2012c)。低级别脊髓星形细胞瘤可进展表现为 GBM 样病理，有时会扩

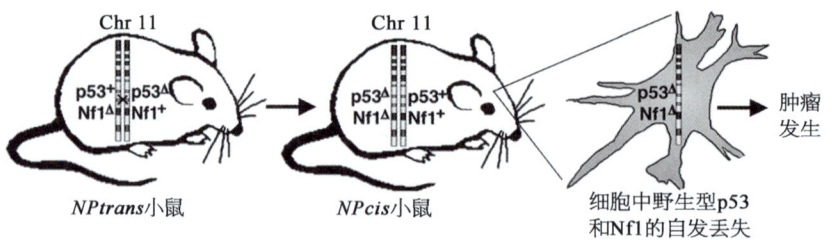

图 19.1　*NPcis* 小鼠模型最初是通过 *NPtrans* 小鼠中 *Nf1* 基因和 *Trp53*(*tp53*) 基因之间罕见的重组事件(左)而构建，使得 *Nf1* 的突变(*Nf1D*)和 *Trp53* 的突变(*p53D*)在顺式(中)11 号染色体的相同拷贝上连接。随着小鼠年龄的增长，*Nf1*(*Nf1*$^+$)和 *Trp53*(*p53*$^+$)的野生型拷贝可以在细胞中自发丢失，导致肿瘤发生

散到脑内形成继发性肿瘤（Amlin-Van Schaick et al. 2012c）。

19.3 表型变异的原因

用于研究的 *NPcis* 模型的优势不仅在于遗传机制的简单性、多种肿瘤类型的高外显率以及与人类状况的相似性。重要的是，*Nf1* 等位基因状态、性别、品系特异性和亲代遗传都可以在 *NPcis* 小鼠中进行独立测试，并在决定肿瘤发生易感性方面发挥不同的作用。结合人类研究数据和 *NPcis* 模型可以阐明这些不同的遗传因素如何导致 NF1 的可变表达。

19.3.1 *NF1* 基因突变和等位基因

在数百个已确定的 *NF1* 突变中，迄今为止已有 2 个在患者中表现出基因型-表型相关性。一种突变涉及 *NF1* 等位基因的大量缺失（通常是母系遗传），导致 *NF1* 微缺失综合征，患者表现出严重的学习缺陷和生长畸形（Mensink et al. 2006; Riva et al. 2000; Spiegel et al. 2005; Upadhyaya et al. 1998; Venturin et al. 2004）。另一种突变是框内 17 号外显子 3 个碱基对的缺失，称为 delAAT，是一种导致皮肤型神经纤维瘤的完全缺失（Upadhyaya et al. 2007）。由于其他 *NF1* 突变通常与明确定义的表型无关，且 NF1 患者的易感因素不会增加未受影响的家庭成员的总体患癌风险（Airewele et al. 2001），这导致了一种假设，即非连锁修饰因子和野生型 *NF1* 等位基因的细微改变都可以影响表型，尽管每个因素的影响可能取决于特定的临床特征（Szudek et al. 2002）。

在人类和小鼠中已经观察到了正常 *NF1* 的内源性表达水平的差异，并且有可能改变 NF1 表型。一项研究发现，大约 30% 未受影响的个体表现出 *NF1* 等位基因表达比例偏离正常的 50∶50（母系∶父系）(Jentarra et al. 2011）。健康个体在这两种等位基因之间的自然表达差异可能高达 25%，这可能会根据 NF1 个体中野生型 *NF1* 基因拷贝的固有表达改变而潜在地改变表现度（Jentarra et al. 2011）。另一项研究表明，疾病表型不一致的同卵双胞胎表现出不同水平的 *NF1* 启动子、5-0-UTR 和外显子 1 甲基化（Harder et al. 2010），这表明 *NF1* 基因表达可能在遗传和表观遗传水平上受到调节。在肿瘤形成前，野生型和 *NPcis* 小鼠在不同品系背景下表现出 *Nf1* 的表达差异。C57BL/6J 背景下，*Nf1* 在大脑和坐骨神经中的表达水平高于 129S4/SvJae 背景（Hawes et al. 2007; Tuskan et al. 2008）。不同品系中 *Nf1* 表达水平的差异与组织特异性肿瘤易感性无关。在中枢神经系统中，与 129S4/SvJae 品系相比，C57BL/6J 品系更容易发生星形细胞瘤，并且在大脑中表达更高水平的 *Nf1*。然而，在周围神经系统中，C57BL/6J 和 129S4/SvJae 对 MPNST 同样易感，但正常神经中 C57BL/6J *Nf1* 的表达水平仍高于 129S4/SvJae（Hawes et al. 2007）。在患者中，SNP 分析显示野生型 *NF1* 等位基因与表现度无关，进一步支持了独立于 *NF1* 位点的修饰因子的作用（Sabbagh et al. 2009）。当比较 NPcis 突变小鼠中表现出可变表型的品系时，小鼠在 *Nf1* 中显示出相对较少的异质 SNP。总的来说，这些研究表明，虽然个体之间存在 *NF1* 表达的差异，但其在疾病的可变表现度中的作用仍有待研究。这种作用可能是由可变的交互作用因素引起的，并非与 *NF1* 直接相关。

除了 *NF1* 表达水平的差异外，神经纤维瘤蛋白异构体表达的差异可能会影响 *NF1* 的可变表现度。例如，一些研究小组已经表明，*NF1* 转录物的 RNA 加工可能会影响表现度，其中某些点突变会导致选择性剪接的变化，从而导致基因产物功能的改变（Skuse et al. 1997）。虽然已知 CELF、Hu 和 TIA-1 都可以调节 *NF1* 剪接，但并没有报道这些基因本身在 NF1 肿瘤发生中的改变（Barron et al. 2012）。结果表明，这些剪接因子的未命名调节因子可能负责影响 *NF1* 剪接从而导致该疾病的可变表现度。与 *NF1* 表达水平的变化一样，*NF1* 剪接的变化可能是由于可变的反式作用因子的作用，而与 *NF1* 基因无关。

由于许多 NF1 表型的出现需要 *NF1* 野生型等位基因的失活或丢失，所以野生型等位基因丢失的变异性可能会潜在地影响表型变异。一项研究发现，NF1 患者的每个神经纤维瘤可能是由不同体细胞受到 NF1 的二次打击引起的,影响这些突变率的因素(可能是细胞修复损伤的能力)都是致瘤性的潜在修饰因子——然而,仍然没有确定的修饰因子(Wiest et al. 2003)。染色体的不稳定性也与肿瘤修饰有关,最显著的是与 NF1 野生型拷贝的丢失有关(Bartelt-Kirbach et al. 2009;Kehrer-Sawatzki et al. 2008;Stephens et al. 2006)。虽然已经假设了几个特定的候选基因(主要基于肿瘤中的表达变化),但需要对候选基因进行进一步分析(Bartelt-Kirbach et al. 2009;Kehrer-Sawatzki et al. 2008)。在 NPcis 小鼠中,我们的研究发现,肿瘤发生的差异是基于突变染色体是遗传自母亲还是父亲(见下文)。初步数据表明,这是由于母系和父系等位基因上 Nf1 和 Trp53 的野生型拷贝丢失的不同机制造成的(K. M. Reilly unpublished data)。需要进一步的研究来确定 NF1 基因突变频率的变化对 NF1 疾病的可变表现度的重要性。

19.3.2 个体的性别

NF1 表型变异明显的遗传来源之一是个体的性别。已知神经纤维瘤在青春期和妊娠期间发生率增加(Huson and Hughes 1994),并且在小鼠模型中对类固醇激素有不同程度的反应(Li et al. 2010),突出了性激素在 NF1 中的作用。与男性相比,女性一生中患至少 1 种侵袭性恶性肿瘤或脑肿瘤的风险明显增加(Airewele et al. 2001)。相比之下,女性 NF1 患者比男性 NF1 患者存活时间更长(Evans et al. 2011;Ingham et al. 2011)。然而,普通人群中女性的存活时间比男性长,男性和女性 NF1 患者的生存时间都比无 NF1 人群短。因此,与无 NF1 人群相比,女性 NF1 患者比男性更容易受到 NF1 所致存活率降低的影响(Airewele et al. 2001;Masocco et al. 2011;Rasmussen et al. 2001)。

在 NPcis 小鼠中,性别与肿瘤易感性之间也存在类似的复杂关系。根据交叉设计,男性发生星形细胞瘤的频率更高,但星形细胞瘤的级别低于女性(Reilly 2010)。这已被证明取决于品系背景和来自母亲或父亲的疾病遗传(Amlin-Van Schaick et al. 2012b)。在 MPNST 的情况下,同样根据交叉设计,雄性比雌性发生更多的 MPNST,生存时间更短,并且雄性和雌性受到品系背景的不同影响(Walrath et al. 2009)。此外,我们的初步数据表明,与男性相比,女性中神经纤维瘤表型的修饰机制存在很大差异(G. N. Jones and K. M. Reilly, unpublished data)。

19.3.3 与 NF1 无关的基因

表现度的家族间和家族内变异研究(Carey et al. 1979;Easton et al. 1993;Sabbagh et al. 2009;Szudek et al. 2002)支持与 NF1 无关的修饰基因的作用。在一份报告中,近 75% 的研究家庭表现出家族内表型变异(Carey et al. 1979)。在家族中,同卵双胞胎在表现度上的相似性最高,当将这些先证与一级亲属(即其他兄弟姐妹或父母)相比时,这种相似性降低,而与二级亲属(例如,表兄弟姐妹,阿姨/叔叔或祖父母)相比,这种相似性甚至更高(Easton et al. 1993)。考虑到 NF1 突变在一个给定的家庭中是固定的,家庭环境是相对统一的,这些数据表明,环境之外的遗传改变和特定的 NF1 突变是表型变异的原因。

如上所述,通过对照育种实验,小鼠模型可用于解析遗传效应。在 NPcis 小鼠中,特定肿瘤的发病率、潜伏期和大小以及总体肿瘤谱都与品系背景进行了比较(Amlin-Van Schaick et al. 2012a, b;Reilly et al. 2000,2004,2006;Walrath et al. 2009)。在 C57BL/6J - NPcis 和 129S4/svzai - npcis 近交系之间观察到星形细胞瘤易感性的差异最大,其中近 75% 的 C57BL/6J - NPcis 小鼠和约 20% 的 129S4/svzai - npcis 小鼠发生脑病变(Reilly et al. 2004)。在 C57BL/6J - NPcis 和 129S4/svzai - npcis 动物的脊髓星形细胞瘤中也观察到同样的趋势(Amlin-Van Schaick et al. 2012c)。此外,C57BL/6J 与 129S4/SvJae 杂交的 F1 代背景下的 NPcis 小鼠对星形细胞瘤的易感性不同取决于 C57BL/6J 和 129S4/SvJae 品系从亲本引入的方式(Reilly et al. 2004)。且其发生星形细胞瘤的频率比两种品系的亲本近交系更高(Amlin-Van Schaick et al. 2012b)。这些数据表明,对星形细胞瘤的易感性并不是一种简单的孟德尔特征,而是由基因组中具有复杂上位相互作用的许多基因控制的。

与星形细胞瘤一样，NPcis 小鼠的 MPNST 发生率也受到品系的影响，C57BL/6J 品系高度易感 (Reilly et al. 2006)。重要的是，改变星形细胞瘤发病率的品系与改变 MPNST 发病率的品系并不相同 (Reilly et al. 2004，2006)，这表明修饰机制可能针对不同的组织类型（例如外周和中枢神经系统）。C57BL/6J 和 A/J 品系的 F1 杂交品系对 MPNST 具有抗性(Reilly et al. 2006)，这表明 MPNST 的优势修饰因子是由 A/J 品系携带的。这些 C57BL/6J 与 A/J 杂交的 F1 代 NPcis 小鼠比 C57BL/6J - NPcis 小鼠更容易发生星形细胞瘤；然而，由于 MPNST 比星形细胞瘤更容易在更小的年龄出现，这种肿瘤谱的转变可能是由于小鼠在没有 MPNST 的情况下存活的时间更长，从而在未来发展为星形细胞瘤。由于患者的许多 NF1 表型出现在生命的特定时期（例如，幼儿的视神经胶质瘤，青春期的神经纤维瘤和成人的 MPNST），重要的是要考虑影响一种表型的修饰剂可能更直接地作用于更早期的表型。小鼠模型的研究强调了遗传多态性对 NF1 表型变异的复杂相互作用。

19.3.4　NF1 的母系或父系遗传

患者数据表明，NF1 的表型差异取决于该疾病是遗传自母亲还是父亲。这些数据的很大一部分可归因于减数分裂期间雄性和雌性生殖系突变机制的差异，从而导致不同类型的新生 NF1 突变(Lazaro et al. 1996；Steinmann et al. 2007)。包括 NF1 在内的大缺失更有可能出现在母体胚系中，并与更严重的疾病相关，如 NF1 微缺失综合征。如上所述，当 NF1 突变遗传自父亲时，与遗传自母亲时相比，神经纤维瘤和 Lisch 结节在父亲和孩子之间的相关性更高(Szudek et al. 2002)。

NPcis 小鼠显示亲代遗传对肿瘤表型有很强的影响。从母亲那里遗传突变的 NPcis 小鼠 (NPcis^{mat}) 与从父亲那里遗传突变的 NPcis 小鼠 (NPcis^{pat}) 相比，对 MPNST 发育的易感性显著降低，但对星形细胞瘤的易感性更高(Reilly 2009，2010；Reilly et al. 2006)。在近交系中，两组小鼠之间的唯一区别是突变等位基因的遗传，从而可以进行比较。这些数据表明，这种表型变异的原因与 Nf1 和 Trp53 突变所在的小鼠 11 号染色体直接相关，而不是比如线粒体变异或者其他染色体上的印迹基因等其他可变的遗传因素。此外，亲本遗传的这种影响与品系背景无关，因此可以在各种自交系和 F1 杂交背景中观察到(Reilly et al. 2004，2006)。由于小鼠可以以可控的方式杂交在一起，所以可以研究亲代遗传和遗传变异对肿瘤变异的相对贡献，并鉴定候选修饰基因。

19.4　已被证实的 NF1 修饰因子

到目前为止，只有少数特定的 NF1 候选修饰位点或基因已被证实。尽管需要进一步研究来完全阐明它们的作用机制，但现有证据已经可以支持它们作为调节因子的作用。在 NF1 家系研究中，GDNF 单核苷酸多态性（SNP）变体的父系遗传与 NF1 的母系遗传相互作用，增加了肠梗阻（一种与 NF1 相关的胃肠道特征表现）的易感性(Bahuau et al. 2001)。同样，ANRIL 作为非编码 RNA 中的单等位基因变体与 NF1 患者的神经纤维瘤发生率相关 (Pasmant et al. 2011)。在另一项研究中，错配修复基因 MSH2 启动子的甲基化在患者间存在差异，并与神经纤维瘤负荷呈正相关(Titze et al. 2010)。启动子的甲基化增加会导致 MSH2 的表达降低，进而可能导致 DNA 损伤修复缺陷，增加肿瘤发生的风险。

在 NPcis 小鼠模型中对修饰因子进行定位分析，已经鉴定出几个与恶性周围神经鞘膜瘤（MPNST）和星形细胞瘤易感性相关的位点。相对于 C57BL/6J 品系，A/J 品系在 NPcis 小鼠中表现出对 MPNST 的显著抗性(Reilly et al. 2006)。通过在回交群体中对修饰位点的定位分析，鉴定出两个与神经鞘肿瘤抗性(Nerve sheath tumor resistance，Nstr)相关的位点：一个位于 19 号染色体的着丝点附近 (Nstr1，LOD=3.0)，是 NPcis^{pat} 小鼠易感性的特异性位点；另一个位于 15 号染色体近端(Nstr2，LOD=2.6)，是 NPcis^{mat} 小鼠所特有的(Reilly et al. 2006)。对于这两个 Nstr 修饰位点，A/J 标志物与更强的抗性表型相关，而 B6 标志物与更高的

MPNST 易感性相关。Nstr1 在 19 号染色体上的定位已通过染色体替换品系（其 19 号染色体来自 A/J 品系，其余基因组来自 C57BL/6J 品系）得到独立证实（Walrath et al. 2009）。*Nstr1* 位于人类 11q13-12 区域，该区域在人类恶性周围神经鞘膜瘤（MPNST）中存在易位（Jhanwar et al. 1994；Mertens et al. 1995，2000）。*Nstr2* 位于人类 5p13-15 和 8q22-24 区域。人类 8q22-23 区域在 MPNST 中扩增，并且也发生了易位（Mertens et al. 2000；Rey et al. 1993；Schmidt et al. 2001）。有趣的是，*Nstr2* 与小鼠 15 号染色体和人类 5 号染色体上的 *GDNF* 基因发生了重叠（图 19.2）。由于 *Nstr1* 和 *Nstr2* 分别在 *NPcis*^{pat} 和 *NPcis*^{mat} 小鼠中显示连锁特异性，这表明这些修饰因子与从母亲或父亲继承的突变的 11 号染色体发生了上位效应。一旦确定这两个修饰位点的调节基因，在患者中验证这些候选基因时，就必须考虑这种上位效应。

在 *NPcis* 小鼠的星形细胞瘤中，129S4/SvJae 品系表现出整体抗性，而 C57BL/6J 品系则表现为易感。然而，C57BL/6J 和 129S4/SvJae 的 F1 杂交体可能比任何亲本纯合品系更易发生星形细胞瘤（Amlin-Van Schaick et al. 2012b），这表明隐性的抗性修饰因子在星形细胞瘤表型中也发挥作用。C57BL/6J 和 129S4/SvJae 小鼠的杂交研究表明，在 *Nf1* 和 *Trp53* 周围 30 Mb 区域存在一个修饰因子，称为 *Mastr1*。这一修饰因子可能直接与 C57BL/6J 和 129S4/SvJae 中 *Nf1* 的差异表达有关（见 19.3.1），或者可能改变星形细胞瘤表型区域的另一个连锁基因。为了在全基因组范围内研究星形细胞瘤的修饰因子，从而进行 C57BL/6J 和 129S4/SvJae 品系之间的回交定位分析。到目前为止，已经成功证实了两个修饰位点，其显示出性别特异性或组织定位特异性（Amlin-Van Schaick et al. 2012a，b）。

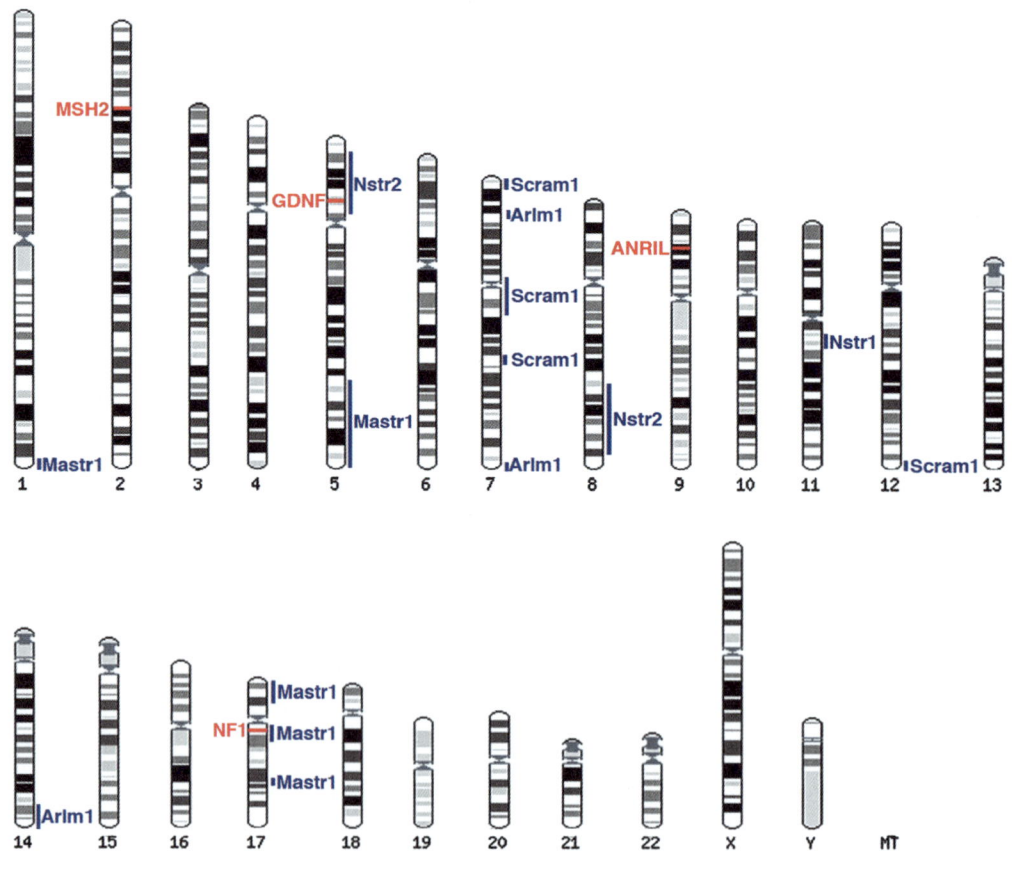

图 19.2　在人类基因组中探索的 NF1 修饰因子。被确定为潜在 NF1 修饰因子的人类基因以红色显示在人染色体左侧。小鼠修饰位点以蓝色显示在人染色体右侧，并映射到人基因组的同源区域。由于修饰位点代表基因组的广泛区域，所以通常会映射到多个人染色体。跨物种的比较可能有助于将来缩小这些位点区域

在 C57BL/6J 和 129S4/SvJae 品系之间的 $NPcis^{pat}$ 回交研究中,证实了一个修饰因子修饰位点位于 12 号染色体远端,在雄性中与星形细胞瘤相连锁,但在雌性中并不存在此联系(Amlin-Van Schaick et al. 2012b)。这个修饰位点被称为雄性星形细胞瘤抗性修饰位点 1(Arlm1),在 C57BL/6J 品系中表现出隐性抗性。尽管 Arlm1 修饰位点区域很大,涉及 503 个基因,但通过比较小鼠和人类正常大脑与脑瘤数据,将该区域的候选修饰基因缩小至不到 15 个。Arlm1 与人类 7p15-21、7q36 和 14q32 区域具有同源性,这些区域在人类胶质瘤中发生扩增或缺失,该区域内的候选基因与男性胶质瘤患者的生存时间显著相关,但与女性胶质瘤患者的生存时间无关。除了 Arlm1 与个体性别的交互作用外,回交研究还表明 Arlm1 与 Y 染色体具有多态性的交互作用。在携带 Y 染色体 129S4/SvJae 等位基因的回交雄性中,Arlm1 与星形细胞瘤的发病率连锁。相比之下,在携带 Y 染色体 C57BL/6J 等位基因的回交雄性中,与 Arlm1 与星形细胞瘤不存在连锁关系,类似于雌性(K. M. Reilly, unpublished data)。这些数据说明,决定星形细胞瘤整体易感性的是品系、性别和疾病亲本遗传之间的上位效应。

NPcis 小鼠在大脑和脊髓中均会发生星形细胞瘤。目前还不清楚脊髓星形细胞瘤是起源于脊髓,还是肿瘤细胞从大脑的起始区域扩散而来。在极少数情况下,仅在小鼠脊髓中观察到星形细胞瘤,这提示脊髓可能是肿瘤发生的原发部位。为了更好地了解中枢神经系统中星形细胞瘤位置的定位机制,在 C57BL/6J 和 129S4/SvJae 的回交中对脊髓星形细胞瘤的修饰因子进行了定位。在 $NPcis^{mat}$ 回交小鼠的 5 号染色体远端,发现一个脊髓对星形细胞瘤的抗性调节因子 1(Spinal cord resistance to astrocytoma modifier 1,Scram1)(LOD 评分 > 5.0)(Amlin-Van Schaick et al. 2012c)。与 Arlm1 修饰位点类似,C57BL/6J 等位基因与对脊髓星形细胞瘤的抗性相关,尽管 C57BL/6J 品系对星形细胞瘤总体上来说更为易感。Scram1 的等位基因 129S4/SvJae 的纯合子小鼠会在较短时间内发生更多脊髓星形细胞瘤,而对大脑星形细胞瘤的发生几乎没有影响。Scram1 修饰位点与人类 12q24、7p11、7q22-21 和 7p22 染色体区域同源,这些区域在人类星形细胞瘤中都存在扩增或缺失,尽管是否在脊髓肿瘤中存在特异性还不太清楚(Amlin-Van Schaick et al. 2012c)。由于人类脊髓星形细胞瘤极为罕见,对其的了解十分有限,所以在小鼠模型中研究这些肿瘤对于建立可验证的假设至关重要,以便进一步检查少数可用的患者样本。

旨在探索小鼠 NF1 相关肿瘤修饰因子的研究突出了遗传背景、性别和亲代遗传之间相互作用的复杂性。迄今为止,在 NPcis 小鼠模型中探索的所有多态性修饰因子都是特异存在于 $NPcis^{mat}$ 或 $NPcis^{pat}$ 小鼠的,这表明肿瘤发生的机制可能因小鼠 11 号染色体的遗传方式而存在根本性差异。此外,不同类型的肿瘤(星形细胞瘤或恶性周围神经鞘膜瘤)受不同位点和不同品系背景所修饰,这表明易感性(或抗性)机制是特异于组织类型的。最后,对于特定的肿瘤类型,雌性和雄性小鼠表现出不同位点的连锁作用,突出了需要分别分析雌性和雄性的必要性,并且表明肿瘤发生在两性之间可能存在根本性差异。图 19.2 总结了在人类中探索的修饰因子位点以及在小鼠中探索的与人类基因组相关的修饰位点。

19.5 在小鼠中模拟人类多样性:协作交叉研究

尽管在过去几十年中,使用小鼠进行的癌症研究取得了诸多进展,但这些模型在修饰因子研究中的主要限制在于其近亲繁殖的特性。稳定的近交系小鼠可以作为识别数量性状位点(quantitiative trait loci, QTLs)的有力工具,但它们限制了我们对人类多样性如何影响癌症风险的理解。尽管实验室中有许多小鼠品系可供使用,但在不同品系之间,基因组的许多大区域基本没有变化,这导致即使在涉及 2 个或 3 个品系的混合背景下,整体的遗传多样性仍然不足。为了解决这些问题,我们正在开发 1 个约 500 条重组近交(recombinant inbred, RI)小鼠系组成的遗传参考种群,这些小鼠系代表了高度多样化的基因组,可以用于严格的修饰因子研究（Collaborative Cross Consortium 2012；Threadgill and Churchill 2012a，b）。

协同杂交（Collaborative Cross，CC）起源于复杂性状联盟（Complex Trait Consortium），其理念是小鼠研究将从使用高度多样化和高度可重复的重组近交系（RI）中受益，这些品系可用于系统生物学和复杂性状的鉴定，如NF1修饰因子（Churchill et al. 2004；Threadgill et al. 2002）。当前的连锁图谱绘制通常识别出具有数百个可能候选基因的数量性状位点（QTL），而在CC小鼠系中进行的QTL图谱绘制将更加精确，并且由于在CC小鼠中控制了长距离连锁不平衡，因此会映射出更少的假阳性位点（Collaborative Cross Consortium 2012）。对如此大规模的小鼠群体进行比较，将会划定参与表型变异的更狭窄的基因组区间，减少候选修饰因子的数量，而这些修饰因子更有可能在修饰表型中发挥重要作用。

为了在小鼠中建立受控的遗传多样性，协同杂交（Collaborative Cross）项目使用了8个近交小鼠品系。这些创始品系中有5个（A/J、C57BL/6J、129S1/SvImJ、NOD/LtJ和NZO/HlLtJ）是实验室衍生的近交品系，另外3个（CAST/EiJ、PWK/PhJ和WSB/EiJ）是野生的近交小鼠；通过结合，它们携带的遗传多样性均匀地分布在整个基因组中。通过系统地对这8个创始品系杂交两代，然后至少进行20代随机兄妹近交，已经建立了大约500条重组近交系（RI）用于测试。预计在每只小鼠中将发生超过100次重组事件，从而提供每个创始品系的大量基因组组合。总体而言，整个小鼠群体可能会经历超过100 000次重组事件，每个谱系都将进行全面的基因分型，并公开提供用于研究（Churchill et al. 2004；Threadgill et al. 2002）。迄今为止，已有多个团队承担了开发这些谱系的艰巨任务，创始品系在重组近交（RI）小鼠群体中的分布结果表明，所有8个创始品系在每个协同交叉（CC）谱系中以不同的数量存在，并且每个谱系之间表现出高度的多样性（Aylor et al. 2012；Durrant et al. 2011；Philip et al. 2011）。早期的复杂性状鉴定研究表明，CC小鼠中的QTL可以映射到小至0.5～1 Mb的区域（Aylor et al. 2012；Durrant et al. 2011）。这种精确的映射几乎无法通过两品系方法实现，因为两品系方法通常最多只能得到几兆碱基大小的QTL。这些交叉谱系提供的资源对于旨在识别肿瘤发生候选修饰因子的研究极其宝贵，而这些研究成果可以应用于进行中的NF1研究。

19.6 总结

迄今为止，在确定肿瘤起始和进展的各种机制方面已取得了显著进展，但对肿瘤发生的遗传易感性知之甚少。尽管在人类研究中已经取得了一些进展，但由于内在多样性，识别修饰基因和通路变得复杂。通过使用最先进的小鼠遗传学方法，我们能够识别可能影响癌症风险的相关区域和基因。将各种近交小鼠模型的研究结果与人类患者进行关联变得越来越可行，这为寻找NF1修饰因子提供了有力的工具。

（韩岩，陈犹白 译）

参考文献

[1] Airewele GE, Sigurdson AJ, Wiley KJ, Frieden BE, Caldarera LW, Riccardi VM, Lewis RA, Chintagumpala MM, Ater JL, Plon SE, Bondy ML (2001) Neoplasms in neurofibromatosis 1 are related to gender but not to family history of cancer. Genet Epidemiol 20：75-86

[2] Amlin-Van Schaick J, Kim S, Broman KW, Reilly KM (2012a) Scram1 is a modifier of spinal cord resistance for astrocytoma on mouse Chr 5. Mamm Genome 23：277-285

[3] Amlin-Van Schaick JC, Kim S, DiFabio C, Lee MH, Broman KW, Reilly KM (2012b) *Arlm1* is a male-specific modifier of astrocytoma resistance on mouse Chr 12. Neuro Oncol 14：160-174

[4] Amlin-Van Schaick J, Kim S, Broman KW, Reilly KM (2012c) Scram1 is a modifier of spinal cord resistance for astrocytoma on mouse Chr 5. Mamm Genome 23(3-4)：277-285

[5] Aylor DL, Valdar W, Foulds-Mathes W, Buus RJ, Verdugo RA, Baric RS, Ferris MT, Frelinger JA, Heise M, Frieman MB et al (2012) Genetic analysis of complex traits in the emerging Collaborative Cross. Genome Res 21：1213-1222

[6] Bahuau M, Pelet A, Vidaud D, Lamireau T, LeBail B, Munnich A, Vidaud M, Lyonnet S, Lacombe D (2001) GDNF as a candidate modifier in a type 1 neurofibromatosis (NF1) enteric phenotype. J Med Genet 38：638-643

[7] Bajenaru ML, Hernandez MR, Perry A, Zhu Y, Parada LF, Garbow JR, Gutmann DH (2003) Optic nerve glioma in mice requires astrocyte *Nf1* gene inactivation and *Nf1* brain heterozygosity. Cancer Res 63: 8573-8577

[8] Barron VA, Lou H (2012) Alternative splicing of the neurofibromatosis type I pre-mRNA. Biosci Rep 32: 131-138

[9] Bartelt-Kirbach B, Wuepping M, Dodrimont-Lattke M, Kaufmann D (2009) Expression analysis of genes lying in the NF1 microdeletion interval points to four candidate modifiers for neurofibroma formation. Neurogenetics 10: 79-85

[10] Buchberg AM, Buckwalter MS, Camper SA (1992) Mouse chromosome 11. Mamm Genome 3 (Spec No): S162-S181

[11] Carey JC, Laub JM, Hall BD (1979) Penetrance and variability in neurofibromatosis: a genetic study of 60 families. Birth Defects Orig Artic Ser 15: 271-281

[12] Churchill GA, Airey DC, Allayee H, Angel JM, Attie AD, Beatty J, Beavis WD, Belknap JK, Bennett B, Berrettini W et al (2004) The Collaborative Cross, a community resource for the genetic analysis of complex traits. Nat Genet 36: 1133-1137

[13] Cichowski K, Shih TS, Schmitt E, Santiago S, Reilly K, McLaughlin ME, Bronson RT, Jacks T (1999) Mouse models of tumor development in neurofibromatosis type 1. Science 286: 2172-2176

[14] Collaborative Cross Consortium (2012) The genome architecture of the Collaborative Cross mouse genetic reference population. Genetics 190: 389-401

[15] Durrant C, Tayem H, Yalcin B, Cleak J, Goodstadt L, de Villena FP, Mott R, Iraqi FA (2011) Collaborative Cross mice and their power to map host susceptibility to *Aspergillus fumigatus* infection. Genome Res 21: 1239-1248

[16] Easton DF, Ponder MA, Huson SM, Ponder BA (1993) An analysis of variation in expression of neurofibromatosis (NF) type 1 (NF1): evidence for modifying genes. Am J Hum Genet 53: 305-313

[17] Evans DG, O'Hara C, Wilding A, Ingham SL, Howard E, Dawson J, Moran A, Scott-Kitching V, Holt F, Huson SM (2011) Mortality in neurofibromatosis 1: in North West England: an assessment of actuarial survival in a region of the UK since 1989. Eur J Hum Genet 19: 1187-1191

[18] Harder A, Titze S, Herbst L, Harder T, Guse K, Tinschert S, Kaufmann D, Rosenbaum T, Mautner VF, Windt E et al (2010) Monozygotic twins with neurofibromatosis type 1 (NF1) display differences in methylation of *NF1* gene promoter elements, 5′ untranslated region, exon and intron 1. Twin Res Hum Genet 13: 582-594

[19] Hawes JJ, Tuskan RG, Reilly KM (2007) *Nf1* expression is dependent on strain background: implications for tumor suppressor haploinsufficiency studies. Neurogenetics 8: 121-130

[20] Huson SM, Hughes RAC (1994) The neurofibromatoses: a pathogenetic and clinical overview, 1st edn. Chapman & Hall Medical, London Ingham S, Huson SM, Moran A, Wylie J, Leahy M, Evans DG (2011) Malignant peripheral nerve sheath tumours in NF1: improved survival in women and in recent years. Eur J Cancer 47: 2723-2728

[21] Jacks T, Shih TS, Schmitt EM, Bronson RT, Bernards A, Weinberg RA (1994) Tumour predisposition in mice heterozygous for a targeted mutation in Nf1. Nat Genet 7: 353-361

[22] Jentarra GM, Rice SG, Olfers S, Rajan C, Saffen DM, Narayanan V (2012) Skewed allele-specific expression of the NF1 gene in normal subjects: a possible mechanism for phenotypic variability in neurofibromatosis type 1. J Child Neurol 27: 695-702

[23] Jhanwar SC, Chen Q, Li FP, Brennan MF, Woodruff JM (1994) Cytogenetic analysis of soft tissue sarcomas. Recurrent chromosome abnormalities in malignant peripheral nerve sheath tumors (MPNST). Cancer Genet Cytogenet 78: 138-144

[24] Kehrer-Sawatzki H, Schmid E, Funsterer C, Kluwe L, Mautner VF (2008) Absence of cutaneous neurofibromas in an NF1 patient with an atypical deletion partially overlapping the common 1.4 Mb microdeleted region. Am J Med Genet A 146A: 691-699

[25] Kleihues P, Burger PC, Scheithauer BW (1993) The new WHO classification of brain tumours. Brain Pathol 3: 255-268

[26] Lazaro C, Gaona A, Ainsworth P, Tenconi R, Vidaud D, Kruyer H, Ars E, Volpini V, Estivill X (1996) Sex differences in mutational rate and mutational mechanism in the *NF1* gene in neurofibromatosis type 1 patients. Hum Genet 98: 696-699

[27] Li H, Zhang X, Fishbein L, Kweh F, Campbell-Thompson M, Perrin GQ, Muir D, Wallace M (2010) Analysis of steroid hormone effects on xenografted human NF1 tumor schwann cells. Cancer Biol Ther 10: 758-764

[28] Masocco M, Kodra Y, Vichi M, Conti S, Kanieff M, Pace M, Frova L, Taruscio D (2011) Mortality associated with neurofibromatosis type 1: a study based on Italian death certificates (1995-2006). Orphanet J Rare Dis 6: 11

[29] Menon AG, Anderson KM, Riccardi VM, Chung RY, Whaley JM, Yandell DW, Farmer GE, Freiman RN, Lee JK, Li FP et al (1990) Chromosome 17p deletions and p53 gene mutations associated with the formation of malignant neurofibrosarcomas in von Recklinghausen neuro-fibromatosis. Proc Natl Acad Sci USA 87: 5435-5439

[30] Mensink KA, Ketterling RP, Flynn HC, Knudson RA, Lindor NM, Heese BA, Spinner RJ, Babovic-Vuksanovic D (2006) Connective tissue dysplasia in five new patients with NF1 microdeletions: further expansion of phenotype and review of the literature. J Med Genet 43: e8

[31] Mertens F, Rydholm A, Bauer HF, Limon J, Nedoszytko B, Szadowska A, Willen H, Heim S, Mitelman F, Mandahl N (1995) Cytogenetic findings in malignant peripheral nerve sheath tumors. Int J Cancer 61: 793-798

[32] Mertens F, Dal Cin P, De Wever I, Fletcher CD, Mandahl N, Mitelman F, Rosai J, Rydholm A, Sciot R, Tallini G et al (2000) Cytogenetic characterization of peripheral nerve sheath tumours: a report of the CHAMP study group. J Pathol 190: 31-38

[33] Pasmant E, Sabbagh A, Masliah-Planchon J, Ortonne N, Laurendeau I, Melin L, Ferkal S, Hernandez L, Leroy K, Valeyrie-Allanore L et al (2011) Role of noncoding RNA *ANRIL* in genesis of plexiform neurofibromas in neurofibromatosis type 1. J Natl Cancer Inst 103: 1713-1722

[34] Philip VM, Sokoloff G, Ackert-Bicknell CL, Striz M, Branstetter L, Beckmann MA, Spence JS, Jackson BL, Galloway LD, Barker P et al (2011) Genetic analysis in the Collaborative Cross breeding population. Genome Res 21: 1223-1238

[35] Rasmussen SA, Yang Q, Friedman JM (2001) Mortality in neurofibromatosis 1: an analysis using U.S. death certificates. Am J Hum Genet 68: 1110-1118

[36] Reilly KM (2009) Brain tumor susceptibility: the role of genetic factors and uses of mouse models to unravel risk. Brain

Pathol 19: 121-131

[37] Reilly KM (2010) The $Nf1 -/+$; $Trp53 -/+$ cis mouse model of anaplastic astrocytoma and secondary glioblastoma: dissecting genetic susceptibility to brain cancer. In: Van Meir EG (ed) CNS cancer: models, markers, prognostic factors, targets, and therapeutic approaches. Springer, Berlin

[38] Reilly KM, Loisel DA, Bronson RT, McLaughlin ME, Jacks T (2000) Nf1;Trp53 mutant mice develop glioblastoma with evidence of strain-specific effects. Nat Genet 26: 109-113

[39] Reilly KM, Tuskan RG, Christy E, Loisel DA, Ledger J, Bronson RT, Smith CD, Tsang S, Munroe DJ, Jacks T (2004) Susceptibility to astrocytoma in mice mutant for Nf1 and Trp53 is linked to chromosome 11 and subject to epigenetic effects. Proc Natl Acad Sci USA 101: 13008-13013

[40] Reilly KM, Broman KW, Bronson RT, Tsang S, Loisel DA, Christy ES, Sun Z, Diehl J, Munroe DJ, Tuskan RG (2006) An imprinted locus epistatically influences Nstr1 and Nstr2 to control resistance to nerve sheath tumors in a neurofibromatosis type 1 mouse model. Cancer Res 66: 62-68

[41] Rey JA, Bello MJ, Kusak ME, de Campos JM, Pestana A (1993) Involvement of 22q12 in a neurofibrosarcoma in neurofibromatosis type 1. Cancer Genet Cytogenet 66: 28-32

[42] Riva P, Corrado L, Natacci F, Castorina P, Wu BL, Schneider GH, Clementi M, Tenconi R, Korf BR, Larizza L (2000) NF1 microdeletion syndrome: refined FISH characterization of sporadic and familial deletions with locus-specific probes. Am J Hum Genet 66: 100-109

[43] Sabbagh A, Pasmant E, Laurendeau I, Parfait B, Barbarot S, Guillot B, Combemale P, Ferkal S, Vidaud M, Aubourg P et al (2009) Unravelling the genetic basis of variable clinical expression in neurofibromatosis 1. Hum Mol Genet 18: 2768-2778

[44] Schmidt H, Taubert H, Wurl P, Bache M, Bartel F, Holzhausen HJ, Hinze R (2001) Cytogenetic characterization of six malignant peripheral nerve sheath tumors: comparison of karyotyping and comparative genomic hybridization. Cancer Genet Cytogenet 128: 14-23

[45] Skuse GR, Cappione AJ (1997) RNA processing and clinical variability in neurofibromatosis type I (NF1). Hum Mol Genet 6: 1707-1712

[46] Spiegel M, Oexle K, Horn D, Windt E, Buske A, Albrecht B, Prott EC, Seemanova E, Seidel J, Rosenbaum T et al (2005) Childhood overgrowth in patients with common NF1 microdeletions. Eur J Hum Genet 13: 883-888

[47] Steinmann K, Cooper DN, Kluwe L, Chuzhanova NA, Senger C, Serra E, Lazaro C, Gilaberte M, Wimmer K, Mautner VF, Kehrer-Sawatzki H (2007) Type 2 NF1 deletions are highly unusual by virtue of the absence of nonallelic homologous recombination hotspots and an apparent preference for female mitotic recombination. Am J Hum Genet 81: 1201-1220

[48] Stephens K, Weaver M, Leppig KA, Maruyama K, Emanuel PD, Le Beau MM, Shannon KM (2006) Interstitial uniparental isodisomy at clustered breakpoint intervals is a frequent mechanism of NF1 inactivation in myeloid malignancies. Blood 108: 1684-1689

[49] Szudek J, Joe H, Friedman JM (2002) Analysis of intrafamilial phenotypic variation in neurofi-bromatosis 1 (NF1). Genet Epidemiol 23: 150-164

[50] Szudek J, Evans DG, Friedman JM (2003) Patterns of associations of clinical features in neurofi-bromatosis 1 (NF1). Hum Genet 112: 289-297

[51] Threadgill DW, Churchill GA (2012a) Ten years of the Collaborative Cross. Genetics 190: 291-294

[52] Threadgill DW, Churchill GA (2012b) Ten years of the collaborative cross. G3 (Bethesda) 2: 153-156

[53] Threadgill DW, Hunter KW, Williams RW (2002) Genetic dissection of complex and quantitative traits: from fantasy to reality via a community effort. Mamm Genome 13: 175-178

[54] Tischler AS, Shih TS, Williams BO, Jacks T (1995) Characterization of pheochromocytomas in a mouse strain with a targeted disruptive mutation of the neurofibromatosis gene $Nf1$. Endocr Pathol 6: 323-335

[55] Titze S, Peters H, Wahrisch S, Harder T, Guse K, Buske A, Tinschert S, Harder A (2010) Differential $MSH2$ promoter methylation in blood cells of Neurofibromatosis type 1 (NF1) patients. Eur J Hum Genet 18: 81-87

[56] Tuskan RG, Tsang S, Sun Z, Baer J, Rozenblum E, Wu X, Munroe DJ, Reilly KM (2008) Realtime PCR analysis of candidate imprinted genes on mouse chromosome 11 shows balanced expression from the maternal and paternal chromosomes and strain-specific variation in expression levels. Epigenetics 3: 43-50

[57] Upadhyaya M, Ruggieri M, Maynard J, Osborn M, Hartog C, Mudd S, Penttinen M, Cordeiro I, Ponder M, Ponder BA et al (1998) Gross deletions of the neurofibromatosis type 1 ($NF1$) gene are predominantly of maternal origin and commonly associated with a learning disability, dysmorphic features and developmental delay. Hum Genet 102: 591-597

[58] Upadhyaya M, Huson SM, Davies M, Thomas N, Chuzhanova N, Giovannini S, Evans DG, Howard E, Kerr B, Griffiths S et al (2007) An absence of cutaneous neurofibromas associated with a 3-bp inframe deletion in exon 17 of the NF1 gene (c.2970-2972 delAAT): evidence of a clinically significant NF1 genotype-phenotype correlation. Am J Hum Genet 80: 140-151

[59] van Meyel DJ, Ramsay DA, Casson AG, Keeney M, Chambers AF, Cairncross JG (1994) p53 mutation, expression, and DNA ploidy in evolving gliomas: evidence for two pathways of progression. J Natl Cancer Inst 86: 1011-1017

[60] Venturin M, Guarnieri P, Natacci F, Stabile M, Tenconi R, Clementi M, Hernandez C, Thompson P, Upadhyaya M, Larizza L, Riva P (2004) Mental retardation and cardiovascular malformations in NF1 microdeleted patients point to candidate genes in 17q11.2. J Med Genet 41: 35-41

[61] Walrath JC, Fox K, Truffer E, Gregory Alvord W, Quinones OA, Reilly KM (2009) Chr 19 (A/J) modifies tumor resistance in a sex- and parent-of-origin-specific manner. Mamm Genome 20: 214-223

[62] Watanabe K, Sato K, Biernat W, Tachibana O, von Ammon K, Ogata N, Yonekawa Y, Kleihues P, Ohgaki H (1997) Incidence and timing of p53 mutations during astrocytoma progression in patients with multiple biopsies. Clin Cancer Res 3: 523-530

[63] Wiest V, Eisenbarth I, Schmegner C, Krone W, Assum G (2003) Somatic $NF1$ mutation spectra in a family with neurofibromatosis type 1: toward a theory of genetic modifiers. Hum Mutat 22: 423-427

[64] Wu J, Williams JP, Rizvi TA, Kordich JJ, Witte D, Meijer D, Stemmer-Rachamimov AO, Cancelas JA, Ratner N (2008) Plexiform and dermal neurofibromas and pigmentation are caused by $Nf1$ loss in desert hedgehog-expressing cells. Cancer Cell 13: 105-116

[65] Zhu Y, Ghosh P, Charnay P, Burns DK, Parada LF (2002) Neurofibromas in NF1: Schwann cell origin and role of tumor environment. Science 296: 920-922

第20章 神经纤维瘤蛋白：蛋白质结构域及其功能特点

Neurofibromin: Protein Domains and Functional Characteristics

Klaus Scheffzek and Stefan Welti

20.1 引言

肿瘤抑制基因 NF1 能够编码一种巨细胞蛋白即神经纤维瘤蛋白(320 kDa)(DeClue et al. 1991；Gutmann et al. 1991)。但由于基因改变，NF1 的患者中这一基因无功能(Viskochil et al. 1990；Cawthon et al. 1990；Wallace et al. 1990)。神经纤维瘤蛋白在发育过程中广泛表达(Daston and Ratner 1992)，尤其在成人神经元、施万细胞和少突胶质细胞中的表达水平最高(Daston et al. 1992)。通过免疫染色/标记以及电镜技术，神经纤维瘤蛋白在不同组织以及细胞中的分布已经得到了研究(reviewed by Sherman et al. 1998)。但神经纤维瘤蛋白或其片段定位于细胞核的观察意义目前尚不清楚(Vandenbroucke et al. 2004；Leondaritis et al. 2009；Li et al. 2001；Godin et al. 2012)。

神经纤维瘤蛋白(Trovo-Marqui and Tajara 2006)编码一种 RasGTP 酶激活蛋白(Ras-specific GTPase activating protein, RasGAP)(Ballester et al. 1990；Martin et al. 1990；Xu et al. 1990a)。通过加速 Ras 结合 GTP 的水解，即 Ras 的信号激活形式，来下调小鸟苷酸结合蛋白(guanine nucleotide binding protein, GNBP) Ras 的生物活性。Ras 调节的生理作用非常重要，是因为我们一直认为在诸多人类恶性肿瘤中都存在 Ras 的突变，各种突变皆能导致 GTP 的水解速度降低，最终不足以终止下游信号且对 GAP 不敏感(Trahey and McCormick 1987；Bos et al. 1987；Prior et al. 2012；Pylayeva-Gupta et al. 2011)。与之相反的是，一些 NF1 缺陷的肿瘤类型表现出了激活 Ras 水平的升高，这就提示神经纤维瘤蛋白在各自的细胞类型中是一种主要的 RasGAP(Basu et al. 1992；Bollag et al. 1996b；DeClue et al. 1992；Feldkamp et al. 1999；Guha et al. 1996；Kim et al. 1995；Lau et al. 2000；Sherman et al. 2000)。除了能够对 NF1 患者产生一系列病理生理影响之外，NF1 基因还被发现与多种高侵袭性的恶性肿瘤相关，诸如胶质母细胞瘤(McLendon et al. 2008；Parsons et al. 2008)、腺癌(Ding et al. 2008)，以及卵巢癌(Bell et al. 2011；Sangha et al. 2008)。这就体现了其对细胞生长控制的根本性影响。神经纤维瘤蛋白能够与主要的 Ras 亚型 H-、K-和 N-Ras 有效地相互作用(Ahmadian et al. 1997a)，但与致癌/转化的 Ras 突变体交互作用不强(Bollag and McCormick 1991)。

与神经纤维瘤蛋白在 Ras/MAPK 通路中的调

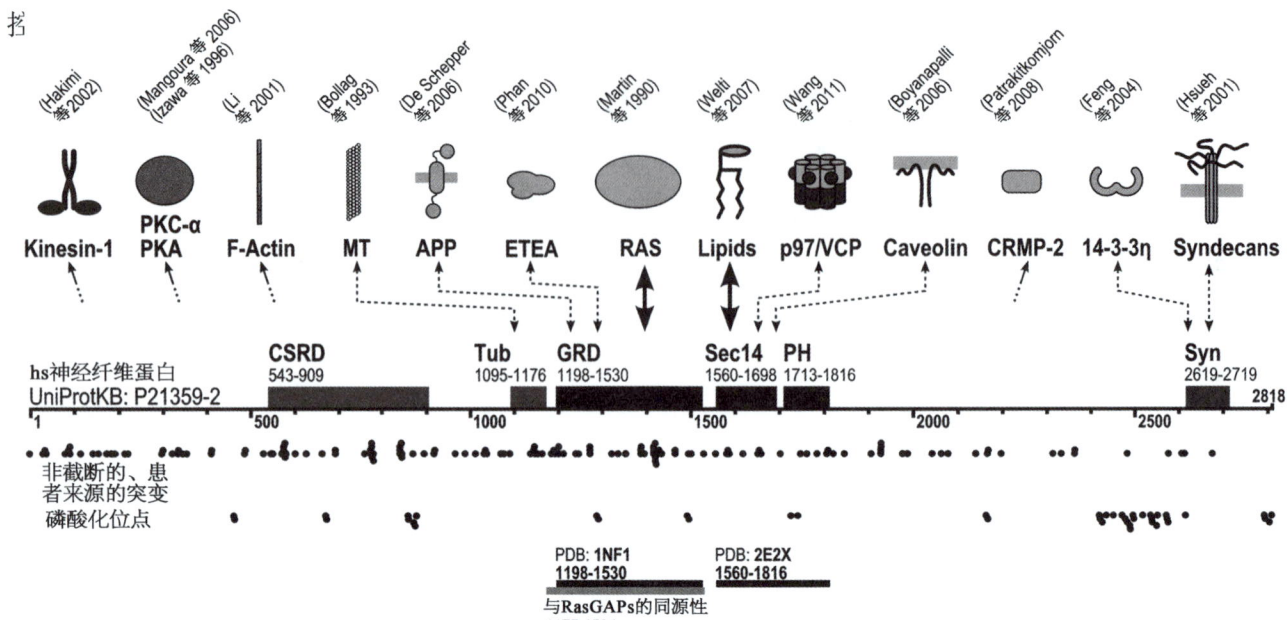

图 20.1 人神经纤维瘤蛋白的结构域,包括已报告的相互作用伙伴。直箭头表示图中底部所概述结构数据的可用性。非截断的、患者来源的突变近似位置(表 20.1 和表 20.2)(Bausch et al. 2007;Brinckmann et al. 2007;Boyanapalli et al. 2006;Cai et al. 2005;DeLuca et al. 2003;Hudson et al. 1997;Kaufmann et al. 2001;Kluwe et al. 2003a,b;Messiaen et al. 2000;Pascual-Castroviejo et al. 2007;Upadhyaya et al. 2008;Wimmer et al. 2007),实验验证的磷酸化位点(Phosphosite Plus——http://www.phosphosite.org)在标记的结构域下方用黑点表示。结构域边界的编号以氨基酸的形式给出

作用一致,NF1 缺陷影响着细胞生长控制(Bollag and McCormick 1991)、神经发育(Hegedus et al. 2007;Romero et al. 2007)、认知(Ferner et al. 1996;Shilyansky et al. 2010)以及其他的细胞/生物过程。

神经纤维瘤蛋白在脊椎动物中高度保守,其序列一致性通常 > 90%(Bernards et al. 1993;Bernards 2003)。在早期进化的红河豚中也同样如此(Kehrer-Sawatzki et al. 1998)。在黑腹果蝇中已经发现了 1 种神经纤维瘤蛋白同源物(The et al. 1997),其与脊椎动物神经纤维瘤蛋白的序列一致性约为 60%。它的删除/截断与生长、逃避行为的缺陷相关(The et al. 1997)。除了在历史性的 IRA1/IRA2 样本以外(Buchberg et al. 1990),神经纤维瘤蛋白的同源物也在其他低等真核生物中被发现,特别是在包括盘基网柄菌在内的真菌(Zhang et al. 2008)、粗脉孢菌(Galagan et al. 2003)以及嗜热毛壳菌(Amlacher et al. 2011)中。

催化 RasGAP 活性位于神经纤维瘤蛋白的中心部分,即 GAP 相关结构域(GRD),它被定义为与前 120 个 GAP 密切同源的区域(图 20.1)。利用结构生物学手段,我们已经确定了 1 个由 Sec14 样脂质结合域组成的二分结构模块(Aravind et al. 1999)、1 个 pleckstrin 同源性(pleckstrin homology,PH)结构域,但其具体的生理功能目前尚不清楚(D'Angelo et al. 2006;Welti et al. 2007)(图 20.1)。尽管通过生物信息学分析推测神经纤维瘤蛋白在很大程度上是有序且高度螺旋状的,但神经纤维瘤蛋白剩余部分的编码情况仍旧不甚明确。因而许多区域在操作上只能被定义为"域"(Izawa et al. 1996)。对于一个结构的实体意义,这种定义肯定是值得怀疑的,因此就需要进一步的分析研究,来使这些结构得到确定。

据报道,除了 Ras 家族以外,许多其他蛋白也能与神经纤维瘤蛋白相互作用。其中包括蛋白激酶 A(protein kinase A,PKA)(Izawa et al. 1996)、蛋白激酶 C(protein kinase C,PKC)(Mangoura et al. 2006;Leondaritis et al. 2009)、小窝蛋白-1(Boyanapalli et al. 2006;Patrakitkomjorn et al. 2008;Lin and Hsueh 2008)、黏附激酶(Kweh et al.

2009)、微管蛋白（Bollag et al. 1993）、淀粉样前体蛋白（DeSchepper et al. 2006）、跨膜蛋白聚糖（Hsueh et al. 2001）、驱动蛋白-1（Hakimi et al. 2002）、核 PML-小体（Godin et al. 2012）、UBX-UBD 蛋白 ETEA（Phan et al. 2010）以及 p97/VCP（Wang et al. 2011）。尽管其中一些蛋白研究支持神经纤维瘤蛋白参与调节细胞骨架结构，但其各自相互作用的生理意义在很大程度上仍旧不甚明确，还需要进一步的深入研究。

20.2　GAP 相关域：核心功能模块

催化 GAP 结构域，通常被称为 GAP 相关结构域（GAP-related domain，GRD），包括 1 个最初被发现与 p120GAP 的催化结构域同源的中心片段（Ballester et al. 1990；Martin et al. 1990；Xu et al. 1990b）。在 1095-1577 之间的片段通常被认为是"GAP"，但其催化活性最小可以缩小到 229 个氨基酸片段（残基 1248-1477）（Ahmadian et al. 1996）。GRD 的结构呈现为 1 种细长的蛋白质分子，主要由螺旋元素组成（Scheffzek et al. 1998a）（图 20.2）。它由 1 个与最小中心催化域（GAPc）一致的中心部分（Ahmadian et al. 1996）和 1 个额外的结构域（GAPex）组成，分别由 N 端和 C 端约 50 个残基的螺旋排列形成。GAPc 表面的 1 个浅口袋由保守的残基排列形成了 Ras 结合区（Scheffzek et al. 1998a）。其结构与 p120GAP 的催化结构域非常类似（Scheffzek et al. 1996），通过与 Ras 共结晶阐明了致癌 Ras 突变体中 GTPase 激活及其缺失的结构基础（Scheffzek et al. 1997）。Ras-RasGAP 复合物显示 Ras 与上述 GAPc 中的口袋结合（图 20.2）。正如预期的那样，GTP/GDP 感受开关 I 和开关 II 区域以及核苷酸结合袋区域形成了 Ras-RasGAP 界面的主要成分，这主要由极性相互作用主导（Scheffzek et al. 1997）。活性位点与 GDP-AlF$_3$ 结合，这是一种假定的过渡态模拟磷转移反应，其中平面 AlF$_3$ 部分被认为是模仿末端转移到水解水分子或由此衍生的亲核基团（Wittinghofer 1997）。有研究发现，只有在 GRD 存在的情况下，Ras 才能与 GDP-AlFx 形成复合物，单独的 Ras 是无法形成的。这一发现表明了 RasGAP（以及其他一些普通的 GAP）是通过稳定了 GTP 结合的 Ras 的活性位点来发挥作用的，该稳定作用由 Ras 和 GRD 形成的异二聚体蛋白复合物介导（Mittal et al. 1996；Scheffzek et al. 1998b）。在 Ras-RasGAP 复合物中，化学排列的稳定与间隙域具有高度保守的精氨酸残基（神经纤维瘤蛋白 Arg1276），也称为精氨酸"手指"，与假设 GDP-AlFx 过渡状态和额外的残留部分来自 FLR 指纹图案稳定催化重要开关 I/II 地区（Scheffzek et al. 1997）。催化过程中的一个关键成分是高度保守的 Gln61，它可以稳定水解水分子。其构象由 Arg1391 和开关 II 来稳定（图 20.2）。突变分析证实了 Arg1276 和 Arg1391 在 GAP 催化中的重要性，导致 GAP 活性分别降低了 2 000 次和 50 倍（Ahmadian et al. 1997b；Sermon et al. 1998）。重要的是，在伴有部分严重症状的 NF1 患者中都发现了突变（Upadhyaya et al. 1997b；Klose et al. 1998）（见下文）。

研究发现 RasGAP 提供了 1 个精氨酸残基来补充 Ras 原本相当低效的活性位点。这一发现支持了小分子可以被设计出来以帮助恢复致癌 Ras 的 GTPase 活性的观点（Scheffzek et al. 1998b；Wittinghofer et al. 1997）。虽然目前还没有这样的化合物，但指环（携带催化精氨酸）和 Ras 之间的接触主要涉及主链接触仍旧值得关注（Scheffzek et al. 1997）。因此，想要设计一种专门模拟某一特定指环并配有一个相关精氨酸的多肽是相当困难的。

20.3　患者来源的 GRD 突变

GAP 活性对神经纤维瘤蛋白细胞功能具有重要作用。针对患者的研究发现在 GRD 中有两处成簇的非截断性突变，其中之一同样与神经纤维瘤蛋白的细胞功能密切相关（Fahsold et al. 2000）。如图 20.2 所示，来自 GRD 和 Ras 的不同环和基序是有效的 GTP 水解所必需的，并且在所有这些区域都发现了导致 GAP 活性受损的突变。

关于神经纤维瘤蛋白，精氨酸手指 Arg1276 的突变对 GAP 活性的影响同样重要。其中最突出的

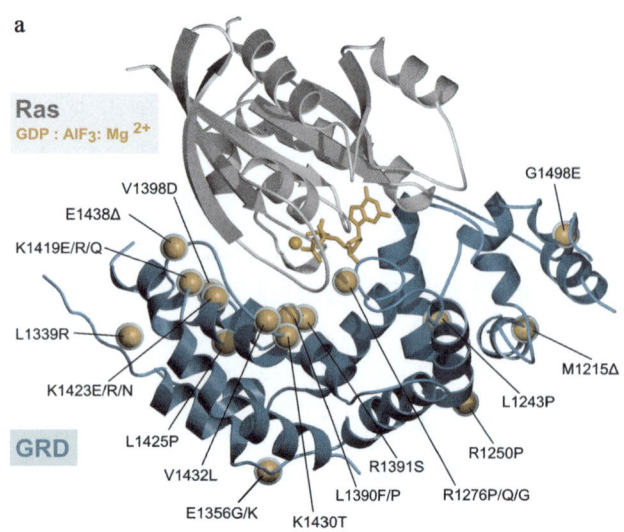

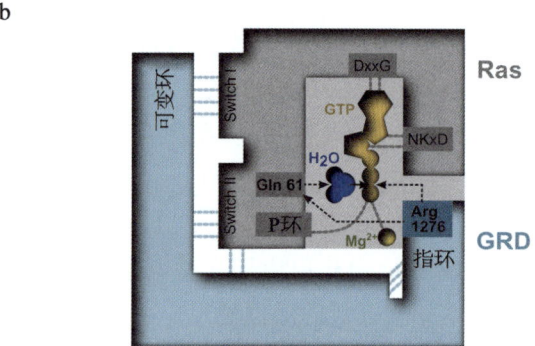

图 20.2 GRD-Ras 复合物的模型和 GAP 机制。a. GRD 与 Ras 的结构带表示。GRD(PDB：1NF1) 与 Ras：RasGAP 复合物 (PDB：1WQ1) 中的 p120GAP 组分叠加。GDP、AlF$_3$ 和 Mg^{2+} 表示为黄色的棒状模型。非截断的、患者来源的突变的位置表示为黄色的球体。b. GRD 通过 Ras 明显加速了 GTP 向 GDP+P 的水解过程。P-Loop、Mg^{2+}、NKxD 和 DxxG 基序稳定结合的 GTPin 对水解反应有利。该反应本身是由一个由 Ras-Gln61 定位的水分子引发的。只有在与 GRD 结合后，反应才能有效进行。GRD 稳定了 Ras 的开关 I 和开关 II 区域，并与 Arg1276 补充了 Ras 活性位点。Arg1276 通过中和产生的负电荷来稳定反应的过渡状态，并帮助定位 Ras-Gln61(Bos et al. 2007; Scheffzek and Ahmadian 2005; Sondek et al. 1994)

是 Arg1276Pro，体外研究发现在 Ras 结合亲和力不受影响的情况下，GTP 水解速率降低了 8 000 倍。这一突变是在 1 例严重的恶性神经鞘瘤患者中发现的，进一步的遗传分析证实，GAP 活性的丧失足以导致 NF1 的发生 (Klose et al. 1998)。因此，指环的稳定也很重要，FLR 基序中的 Arg1391->Ser 突变能够导致 GTPase 活性降低 300 倍 (Upadhyaya et al. 1997b)。这种突变近期也在胶质母细胞瘤的癌症基因组分析中被发现，突显了神经纤维瘤蛋白在 Ras 调控中的整体作用。

在 GRD 的 Ras 结合槽中还发现许多其他的突变，这些突变可能造成了 GRD 结合界面的改变，进而导致 GRD 对 Ras 的亲和力降低。此外，Ras 开关 I、II 区域的稳定是 GTP 有效水解的另一先决条件，这种突变也可能对此造成损害。例如，Lys1423->Glu 突变导致 GRD 分子内盐桥的破坏，进而阻止所有结合的进行 (Ahmadian et al. 2003; Li et al. 1992)。

其他突变并不直接影响图 20.2 突出显示的蛋白质基序。但这类邻近区域的突变可能会产生诸如 Leu1339->Arg 的间接影响 (Fahsold et al. 2000)。而最后一组突变影响 GAP 活性的概率较低，这表明与空间邻近域相关的神经纤维瘤蛋白的其他功能可能受到了影响 (表 20.1)。

20.4 Sec14-PH 模块

在探索 NF1 基因的编码序列其他结构域的过程中，我们发现了另一个可以结晶的可溶性片段 (Bonneau et al. 2004)。该片段的晶体结构定义为一段 Sec14 同源样区域 (Aravind et al. 1999)，其后是一段 plecstrin 同源性(PH)结构域 (D'Angelo et al. 2006)。前者已经通过生物信息学手段进行了预测 (Aravind et al. 1999)，但后者仅仅是通过各自片段的晶体结构测定进行了检测。这两个域的结构排列定义了一种具有调节特征的二分模块 (图 20.3)。

Sec14 结构域的特征是一种笼状的脂质结合袋，覆盖有一个能够限制配体进入内部的螺旋盖段 (Bankaitis et al. 2010)(图 20.3)。它们以独立蛋白的形式在各种样本中被发现，诸如 Sec14p(Sha et al. 1998)、α-生育酚结合蛋白 (Meier et al. 2003; Min et al. 2003) 以及上清蛋白因子 (Stocker 2004)。sec14 样结构域也可以作为信号调节因子的模块，如 RhoGEF、RhoGAPs、PTPases (Phillips et al. 2006)，以及神经纤维瘤蛋白 (Aravind et al. 1999; D'Angelo et al. 2006)。它们通常与脂质配体结合，但这些相关的脂质结合物的具体成分目前

表 20.1 GRD 区域的患者来源的非截断突变

突　变	位　置	潜在或已证明的影响	参　考　资　料
R1204G/W	GAPex	在该结构中不可见。引起更高的灵活度(G)或庞大残基(W)。可能会影响域折叠	Ars 等(2003), Krkljus 等(1998)
ΔM1215 L1243P	GAPex 核心	破坏结构域折叠 可能会破坏螺旋被破坏,影响结构域折叠,影响 Arg 手指稳定性	Fahsold 等 (2000), Ferner 等 (2004)
R1250P	表面、远离的 Ras 结合槽	结构域折叠受损,影响指环稳定性	Fahsold 等(2000)
R1276G/P/Q	Arg 手指,活性部位残基	Ras 进行 GAP 辅助 GTP 水解降低 500~8 000 倍	Mattocks 等 (2004), Klose 等 (1998)
R1325G	邻近 Ras-结合沟	在该结构中不可见。影响结构域折叠	Fahsold 等 (2000), Lee 等 (2006)
L1339R	核心,邻近 Ras 结合沟	Ras 结合界面引入正电荷,可能会影响结构域折叠,造成 Ras 结合界面的不稳定	Fahsold 等(2000)
E1356G/K	表面,远离 Ras 结合沟	最终影响其他神经纤维瘤蛋白结构域	Upadhyaya 等(2009), Trovó 等(2004)
L1390F/P	FLR 修饰	影响指环稳定性,Ras 进行 GAP 辅助 GTP 水解降低	Nystrom 等 (2009), Lee 等 (2006)
R1391S	FLR 修饰	Ras 水解指环稳定受损,Ras 进行 GAP 辅助 GTP 水解降低	Upadhyaya 等(1997b)
V1398D	Ras 结合沟	可能导致 Ras 结合接触界面显著改变	Upadhyaya 等(1998)
K1419E/Q/R	Ras 结合沟	可能导致 Ras 结合接触界面显著改变,可能是离子作用导致 Ras-Glu37 受损	Mattocks 等(2004), Upadhyaya 等(1997b), Purandare 等(1994)
K1423E/N/R	Ras 结合沟	无法稳定 Ras 的开关Ⅱ区域,Ras 进行 GAP 辅助 GTP 水解降低 200~400 倍	Li 等 (1992), De Luca 等 (2003), Han 等(2001)
L1425P	Ras 结合沟	螺旋受损,可能导致 Ras 结合接触界面的较大改变	Peters 等(1999)
K1430T	可变环	影响 Ras 开关Ⅰ区域稳定性,可能会影响 Arg 手指	De Luca 等(2005)
K1430T	可变环	影响 Ras 开关Ⅰ区域稳定性,可能会影响 Arg 手指	De Luca 等(2005)
V1432L	可变环	影响 Ras 开关Ⅰ区域稳定性,可能会影响 Arg 手指	De Luca 等(2005)
ΔE1438	可变环	Ras 开关Ⅰ区域不稳定,Ras 结合不正确	Ars 等(2003)
S1468G	远离 Ras 结合沟	在结构中不可见。最终影响其他神经纤维瘤蛋白结构域。不太可能影响 GTP 的水解	Li 等(1992)

续表

突　变	位　　置	潜在或已证明的影响	参 考 资 料
G1498E	远离 Ras 结合沟	在结构中不可见。最终影响到其他神经纤维瘤蛋白结构域。不太可能影响 GTP 的水解	Ars 等（2003）
N1504S	表面、远离 Ras 结合沟	在结构中不可见。最终影响到其他神经纤维瘤蛋白结构域。不太可能影响 GTP 的水解	Fahsold 等（2000）

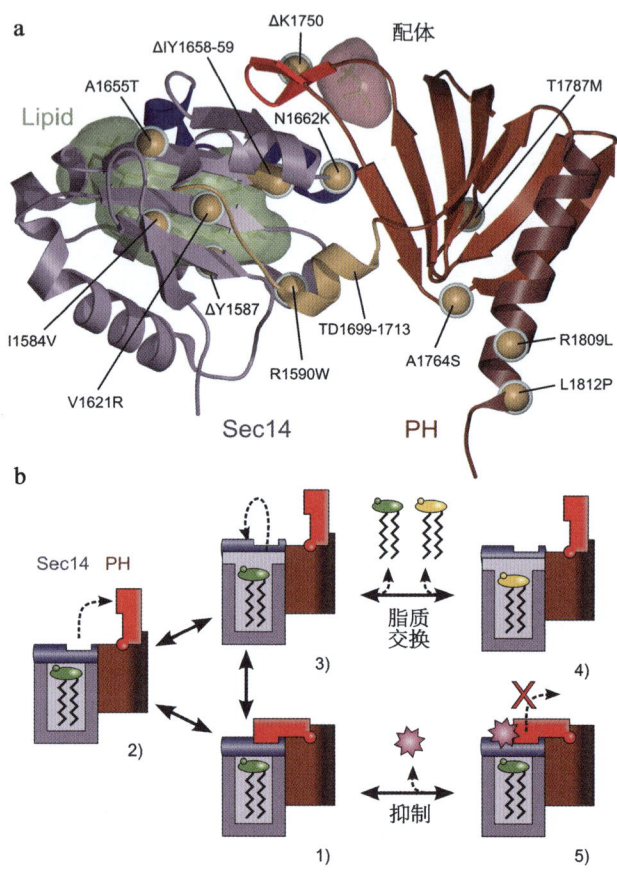

图 20.3　Sec14 - PH 模块和脂质交换的机制模型。a. 神经纤维瘤蛋白 Sec14 - PH 模块的 Ribbon 表示（PDB：2e2x）。PH 结构域为红色/棕色，Sec14 结构域为蓝色/紫色。患者来源的非截断突变位置用黄色球体表示。绿色的脂质和调节配体（紫色）都显示为条带状和棒状。b. 脂质交换的机制模型。（1 至 3）PH 衍生的突出物"锁"（红色）和 Sec14"盖"螺旋（蓝色）关闭 Sec14 脂质结合笼，能够改变它们的构象，允许脂质交换（4）。（5）在盖锁界面对接的调节绑定或相互作用伙伴可以防止脂质交换反应（D'Angelo et al. 2006；Welti et al. 2007，2011）

尚不清楚。同样，在各类 sec14 的样本中，其生理/生化功能仍有待进一步研究阐明。在 RhoGAP、Dbs 和 PTP - MEG2 中，Sec14 样结构域影响该蛋白质的定位，但其机制尚不清楚（Sirokmany et al. 2005；Kostenko et al. 2004；Huynh et al. 2003）。Sec14 模块在高等真核生物极其重要，目前研究已经发现一系列疾病的发生与该基因位点的改变相关。包括 Cayman 小脑共济失调（Bomar et al. 2003）、共济失调伴维生素 E 缺乏症（Ouahchi et al. 1995）、与视网膜结合蛋白缺失相关的视网膜变性综合征（Maw et al. 1997；Fishman et al. 2004），以及 Bothnia 营养不良（He et al. 2009）。在 1 例 Bothnia 营养不良患者 CRALBP 基因中检测到的氨酸突变结构生化分析表明，突变残基部分堵塞了脂质结合袋，继而引起了视网膜结合减少，这是该改变致病的主要原因（He et al. 2009）。

在不使用洗涤剂的情况下，纯化结晶的 Sec14 - PH 蛋白结构显示存在一种与 Sec14 部分内部结合的甘油磷脂，其可能是从细菌表达宿主的脂质池中获取的（D'Angelo et al. 2006）。进一步的生化和晶体学研究以及质谱研究确定了磷脂酰甘油（phosphatidylglycerol，PG）和磷脂酰乙醇胺（phosphatidylethanolamine，PE）是 Sec14 - PH 模块的主要结合物（Welti et al. 2007）。由于 PE 在含有神经纤维瘤蛋白的细胞中含量丰富，而 PG 几乎不存在，所以 PE 被认为是 Sec14 部分的主要候选生理脂质配体（Welti et al. 2007）。

脂质结合在包括神经纤维瘤蛋白在内的一系列信号调节蛋白 Sec14 模块中的准确功能仍有待确定。尽管有假说提出其具有感知脂质环境的作用，但从蛋白质结构来看，这一感知机制并不显著，因为结合的脂质基本上受到了膜环境的完全屏蔽。

二分模块的 PH 部分与许多参与信号转导而功能不同的蛋白质结构域共享其折叠。包括磷酸酪氨酸结合（phosphotyrosine binding，PTB）结构域、磷脂结合 PH 结构域、多脯氨酸结合支持的 Vasp 同源结构域和 PH 样模块，都已经被证实参与蛋白质-蛋白质相互作用（Lemmon and Ferguson 2000；Lemmon 2004；Peterson and Volkman 2009）。神经纤维瘤蛋白 PH 样部分最显著的特征是一个连接 PH 核心种两个 b 链的突起，从域核心延伸到 Sec14 部分的螺旋盖并与之相互作用，它覆盖了推测的脂质结合腔入口（D'Angelo et al. 2006）。

尽管 Sec14 - PH 模块的确切功能目前尚不清楚，但其结构表明这两者之间存在相互调节作用。前文所述的 b - 突起能够影响 Sec14 螺旋盖的构象，从而控制脂质结合笼的配体通路。

20.5 患者来源的 Sec14 - PH 模块突变

虽然对 Sec14 - PH 模块的功能研究显示了蛋白质交互界面的存在，但该模块的确切功能仍不清楚（D'Angelo et al. 2006；Welti et al. 2007，2011）。因此，从患者中发现的位于该神经纤维瘤蛋白域的突变可能会为该模块潜在新功能位置及性质研究提供有价值的信息。然而这类研究需要验证该遗传改变仅仅影响特定的蛋白质功能，但不能影响蛋白质的翻译，也不会引起不溶或聚合。根据这一推理路线，可以证实携带 ΔK1750 和 I1584V 突变的全长神经纤维瘤蛋白在培养的患者外周血细胞中正常存在。尽管 I1584V 的结构分析没有显示出明变化，但 K1750 缺失能够导致局部重排，影响体外调节配体的结合。这两种突变似乎都指向了 Sec14 - PH 模块中的一项新功能（Welti et al. 2011）。据报道，另外一种缺失突变（ΔY1587）能够干扰神经纤维瘤蛋白与 p97/VCP 之间的相互作用（Wang et al. 2011）。有趣的是，缺失的残基并不像预期的那样位于蛋白质的表面，而是位于 Sec14 结构域的脂质结合笼内，与周围环境所隔绝。其位于一个大的 b 片的中心位置，说明在去除 Y1587 后，同一 b 链中的邻近残基将被翻转 180°。这将导致整个 Sec14 结构域的大量重排，参与蛋白质-蛋白质相互作用的表面片也会发生显著的改变。有研究报道一种串联重复（TD1699 - 1712）（Tassabehji et al. 1993），连接 Sec14 和 PH 样结构域的连接体螺旋肽本质上是重复的。这种改变的晶体结构显示，两个域相对的折叠和方向都保持不变时，重复的连接区域在晶体中似乎是可变的（Welti et al. 2011）。插入的残基可能会遮挡蛋白质交互界面，也可能会与周围的神经纤维瘤蛋白结构域发生空间冲突。据推测，其他一些突变可能会引入干扰模块折叠的变化，又或者影响邻近的非 Sec14 - PH 模块神经纤维瘤蛋白结构域（表 20.2）。

表 20.2　Sec14 - PH 区患者来源的非截断突变

突　变	位　置	潜在或已证明的影响	参　考　资　料
I1584V（PDB 3P7Z）	Sec14 - 笼背侧，核心	结构几乎没有变化 邻近表面贴片灵活性增加 患者细胞样本中正常数量蛋白的改变	Fahsold 等（2000）
ΔY1587	Sec14 笼内	据报道是与 p97/VCP 交互所必需的 导致了许多 b 链残基的翻转、主要蛋白质核心和脂质结合 笼的重构	Wang 等（2011）
R1590W	Sec14 界面，表面	大量残基进入结构域界面影响域间相互作用	Upadhyaya 等（1997a）
V1621R	Sec14 笼背侧，核心	将带电残基引入核心影响的 Sec14 笼结构	Jeong 等（2006）
A1655T	Sec14 笼背侧，表面	体积增加，表面改变或影响 Sec14 笼结构	Wang 等（2011）
ΔIY1658/5	Sec14 背侧，核心	b 链缩短，影响 Sec14 笼结构	Wu 等（1999）
N1662K	Sec14 界面，核心	影响域交互	Wu 等（1999）

续 表

突　变	位　置	潜在或已证明的影响	参考资料
TD1699-1712 (PDB 3PEG)	Sec14-PH 连接	结构类似，连接区域可变，体积明显增加并可能会影响其他结构域或阻碍蛋白质结合	Tassabehji 等（1993）
ΔK1750 (PDB 3PG7)	PH-b 突起/锁	盖-锁区域的局部改变 结合调节配体能力降低 患者细胞样本中正常数量的蛋白质改变	Fahsold 等（2000）
A1764S	PH-核心	影响 PH 折叠	Han 等（2001）
T1787M	PH-表面	最终影响其他神经纤维瘤蛋白结构域	Lee 等（2006）
R1809L	PH-表面	最终影响其他神经纤维瘤蛋白结构域	Griffiths 等（2007）
L1812P	PH 表面	最终影响其他神经纤维瘤蛋白结构域	Griffiths 等（2007）

20.6　功能特征

据报道，神经纤维瘤蛋白参与了多种细胞过程，但其引起某些反应的序列目前尚不清楚。鉴于神经纤维瘤蛋白在 Ras 调控中的普遍作用，Ras 信号能够引起许多生物或细胞层面的特征性改变也是显而易见的，包括多种细胞增殖表型（see reviews Cichowski and Jacks 2001；Zhu and Parada 2001，2002；Harrisingh and Lloyd 2004；Trovo-Marqui and Tajara 2006；Grewal et al. 2011）。但也有人提出神经纤维瘤蛋白可能具有独立于 RasGAP 的肿瘤抑制功能（Johnson et al. 1993）。除了经典的 Ras 信号级联，研究发现 mTOR 通路以 Ras/PI3K 依赖的方式受到神经纤维瘤蛋白的严格调控，在一些 NF1 缺陷肿瘤或者细胞培养中也可以观察到这种激活（Johannessen et al. 2005；Dasgupta and Gutmann 2003）。这些发现表明 mTOR 通路是一个有望治疗神经纤维瘤蛋白缺陷肿瘤的药物靶点（Johannessen et al. 2005；Dasgupta and Gutmann 2003）。

学习障碍在 NF1 青少年中出现的比例很高（North 2000；Ozonoff 1999；Acosta et al. 2006；Ferner et al. 1996）。对 $NF1^{+/-}$ 小鼠动物模型的研究发现，差异剪接的 23a 外显子对学习非常关键（Costa et al. 2001）。而通过遗传药物抑制 Ras 活性，能够恢复小鼠在 Morris 水迷宫实验中的空间学习能力（Costa et al. 2002）。外显子 23a 编码了一段 21 个残基肽段（Nishi et al. 1991；Andersen et al. 1993）插入 GRD 的螺旋段（Scheffzek et al. 1998a），这与 GAP 活性降低约 10 倍有关（Uchida et al. 1992）。尽管 GRD 的结构并不能显示插入物影响 GAP 活性的直接机制，但在全长神经纤维瘤蛋白中，也必须考虑其可能通过分子内途径或其他间接途径对 Ras-GRD 相互作用产生调节作用（Scheffzek et al. 1998a）。还有研究观察到，学习表型可以通过多种干预手段来恢复，例如通过基因或药物手段降低 Ras 活性（Costa et al. 2002）能够证实神经纤维瘤蛋白介导的 Ras 调节在学习过程中的突出作用。NF1 对认知缺陷的影响体现在 Ras 信号通路对学习相关过程的作用（Weeber and Sweatt 2002）。详细的分子及细胞学研究已经发现，神经纤维瘤蛋白介导的 ERK/突触蛋白 I 信号通路能够调节小鼠 GABA 释放、突触可塑性和学习行为（Cui et al. 2008）。考虑到 Ras 信号通路参与了认知过程（Weeber and Sweatt 2002），神经纤维瘤蛋白能够影响神经元的发育也并不令人意外（Hegedus et al. 2007；Lush et al. 2008；Romero et al. 2007；Zhu et al. 2001；Yunoue et al. 2003）。

据报道，神经纤维瘤蛋白在细胞骨架结构调控中的作用涉及 Rho-Rock-LIMK2-cofilin 通路，这一过程有赖于 GAP 活性（Ozawa et al. 2005），但也可能通过 GAP 以外的机制完成（Starinsky-Elbaz et al. 2009）。神经纤维瘤蛋白也被发现与微管相关（Gregory et al. 1993），当其在昆虫细胞中过表达时会与微管蛋白共纯化（Bollag et al. 1996a）。微管蛋白结合区域与 GRD 重叠，在 GRD 外核的 N 端需要 80 个额外的残基（残基 1095 – 1569）（Bollag et al. 1996a）。GRD 核心中的一些错义突变阻断了与微管蛋白的相互作用，而其他突变则不干扰微管蛋白的结合，作者认为这显示了其在差异定位中的作用（Xu and Gutmann 1997）。

有文献报道神经纤维瘤蛋白与小窝蛋白-1 的相互作用（Boyanapalli et al. 2006）参与调节 ras、Akt 以及黏着斑激酶（focal adhesion kinase，FAK），其 N 端区域已被证实能够直接与神经纤维瘤蛋白的 C 端片段相互作用（Kweh et al. 2009）。推测的小泡蛋白结合基序能够与 Sec14 – PH 模块部分重叠（D'Angelo et al. 2006）。然而这一基序的结构与位置构建很难合理地形成蛋白质-蛋白质界面。还有研究证实神经纤维瘤蛋白能够调节 cAMP 信号通路，但其分子细节尚不清楚（Tong et al. 2002）。在果蝇中，这一途径对控制体型和学习都有重要作用（The et al. 1997；Guo et al. 2000；Ho et al. 2007）。

20.7 监管方面

神经纤维瘤蛋白的活性受到多种因素的影响。据报道，脂质对 RasGAP 依赖的 Ras 下调具有抑制作用（Bollag and McCormick 1991；Han et al. 1991），但其结果及解读尚存在一些争议（Sermon et al. 1996）。所观察到抑制作用的意义也尚未在体内实验中得到确认。

差异剪接是调节蛋白细胞活性的常见机制。对于 NF1 – pre – mRNA，已经有 4 种不同剪接变异的文献报道（Barron and Lou 2012）。尤其重要的是 GRD 内的替代剪接变体，包括 GRD 内的 23a 外显子（Nishi et al. 1991；Andersen et al. 1993）（见上文）。对这两种变体的生化分析表明，包括外显子 23a 在内的 2 型转录物编码变体的 GAP 活性比 1 型变体低 10 倍（Uchida et al. 1992）。尽管目前尚不明确这种生化差异在多大程度上能够转化为相应的生理表现，但有趣的是，包含 23a 外显子在内的变体能够恢复其他 NF1$^{+/-}$ 小鼠的学习缺陷（Costa et al. 2001）。

神经纤维瘤蛋白可以在 C 端被 PKA S/T 磷酸化，这一修饰对于与 14 – 3 – 3 蛋白的相互作用非常重要，但这一发现的相关性目前尚不清楚（Izawa et al. 1996；Feng et al. 2004）。除此之外，PKCa 已被证实可以使神经纤维瘤蛋白磷酸化，从而增强 RasGAP 的活性，并与肌动蛋白细胞骨架产生相互作用（Mangoura et al. 2006；Leondaritis et al. 2009）。全细胞蛋白质组学研究已经确认了一些来自神经纤维瘤蛋白的磷酸肽（http://www.phosphosite.org 及其中的参考文献）。然而，个体修饰的生物学相关性仍有待明确。

有研究证实，生长因子刺激之后泛素/蛋白酶体途径的蛋白水解能够在程度和时间上动态调节 Ras 信号（Cichowski et al. 2003）。降解的启动需要扩展的 GRD 残基（Martin et al. 1990），包括对微管蛋白结合极其重要的 N 端区域（Cichowski et al. 2003；Bollag et al. 1993）。通过下拉实验进行的蛋白质组学研究发现，UBX – UBD 蛋白 ETEA 能够直接作用于 GRD，其中 UBX 结构域对于介导神经纤维瘤蛋白的泛素化至关重要（Phan et al. 2010），例如下调 Ras 信号（Cichowski et al. 2003）。

综上所述，我们可以通过多种手段来控制神经纤维瘤蛋白的细胞活性。鉴于神经纤维瘤蛋白在调节 Ras 信号通路和 Ras 亚型区室组织中的关键作用（Rocks et al. 2005，2006），可能存在差异定位机制以确保定位的准确。

20.8 总结

神经纤维瘤蛋白是 NF1 的主要参与者，其由基因改变引起的一系列功能障碍正是 NF1 的病因。了解该蛋白质的生化和生理功能对于理解 NF1 至关重要。此外，还要了解该蛋白质的结构以及其与结合伙伴的相互作用。根据当前已知的 GRD、Sec14 和 PH 样结构域结构，经验证的结构片段覆盖了整个蛋白质的 25%。与细胞中翻译蛋白兼容的非截断突变在分析高序列分辨率方面的功能中是无价的。根据结构,如果它们位于显著的机制影响区域,就可以评估它们的作用,还有助于验证其衍生的功能机制。未来的工作将要集中于神经纤维瘤蛋白未知区域的结构分析,以及验证现已报道的各种相互作用伙伴的意义,以期尽可能详细地定义神经纤维瘤蛋白的完整功能谱。

校样中新增的说明: 自本章接受发表以来,Thomas 等(2012)报告了对 15 种 NF1 体细胞错义突变(11 种新发现突变和 4 种先前报告但未明确功能性表征的突变)在 NF1-GRD 区域的潜在致病性的功能评估。这些突变包括 p. R1204G、p. R1204W、p. R1276Q、p. L1301R、p. I1307V、p. T1324N、p. E1327G、p. Q1336R、p. E1356G、p. R1391G、p. V1398D、p. K1409E、p. P1412R、p. K1436Q、p. S1463F。与野生型 NF1 蛋白相比,10 种 NF1-GRD 变体被认为可能具有致病性,因为这些变体表现出显著升高的活性 GTP 结合型 Ras 水平。其余 5 种 NF1-GRD 变体则由于其活性 Ras 水平与野生型蛋白相似,被认为不太可能具有病理意义。这些结论与生物信息学分析和分子模型数据一致。

致谢: 我们感谢同事们分享意见和讨论,并因篇幅限制未能提供全面的参考文献而致歉。我们实验室的工作得到了美国国防部、德国联邦教育和研究部、巴登-符腾堡基金会(德国)以及彼得和特劳德尔·恩格尔霍恩基金会(德国彭茨贝格)的资助。

(张文川,吴祎炜 译)

参考文献

[1] Acosta MT, Gioia GA, Silva AJ (2006) Neurofibromatosis type 1: new insights into neurocognitive issues. Curr Neurol Neurosci Rep 6(2): 136-143

[2] Ahmadian MR, Wiesmuller L, Lautwein A et al (1996) Structural differences in the minimal catalytic domains of the GTPase-activating proteins p120GAP and neurofibromin. J Biol Chem 271(27): 16409-16415

[3] Ahmadian MR, Hoffmann U, Goody RS et al (1997a) Individual rate constants for the interaction of Ras proteins with GTPase-activating proteins determined by fluorescence spectroscopy. Biochemistry (Mosc) 36(15): 4535-4541

[4] Ahmadian MR, Stege P, Scheffzek K et al (1997b) Confirmation of the arginine-finger hypothesis for the GAP-stimulated GTP-hydrolysis reaction of Ras. Nat Struct Biol 4(9): 686-689

[5] Ahmadian MR, Kiel C, Stege P et al (2003) Structural fingerprints of the Ras-GTPase activating proteins neurofibromin and p120GAP. J Mol Biol 329(4): 699-710

[6] Amlacher S, Sarges P, Flemming D et al (2011) Insight into structure and assembly of the nuclear pore complex by utilizing the genome of a eukaryotic thermophile. Cell 146(2): 277-289

[7] Andersen LB, Ballester R, Marchuk DA et al (1993) A conserved alternative splice in the von Recklinghausen neurofibromatosis (NF1) gene produces two neurofibromin isoforms, both of which have GTPase-activating protein activity. Mol Cell Biol 13(1): 487-495

[8] Aravind L, Neuwald AF, Ponting CP (1999) Sec14p-like domains in NF1 and Dbl-like proteins indicate lipid regulation of Ras and Rho signaling [letter]. Curr Biol 9(6): R195-R197

[9] Ars E, Kruyer H, Morell M et al (2003) Recurrent mutations in the NF1 gene are common among neurofibromatosis type 1 patients. J Med Genet 40(6): e82

[10] Ballester R, Marchuk D, Boguski M et al (1990) The NF1 locus encodes a protein functionally related to mammalian GAP and yeast IRA proteins. Cell 63(4): 851-859

[11] Bankaitis VA, Mousley CJ, Schaaf G (2010) The Sec14 superfamily and mechanisms for crosstalk between lipid metabolism and lipid signaling. Trends Biochem Sci 35(3): 150-160

[12] Barron VA, Lou H (2012) Alternative splicing of the neurofibromatosis type I pre-mRNA. Biosci Rep 32(2): 131-138

[13] Basu TN, Gutmann DH, Fletcher JA et al (1992) Aberrant regulation of ras proteins in malignant tumour cells from type 1 neurofibromatosis patients [see comments]. Nature 356(6371): 713-715

[14] Bausch B, Borozdin W, Mautner VF et al (2007) Germline NF1 mutational spectra and loss-of-heterozygosity analyses in patients with pheochromocytoma and neurofibromatosis type 1. J Clin Endocrinol Metab 92(7): 2784-2792

[15] Bell D, Berchuck A, Birrer M et al (2011) Integrated genomic analyses of ovarian carcinoma. Nature 474(7353): 609-615

[16] Bernards A (2003) GAPs galore! A survey of putative Ras superfamily GTPase activating proteins in man and Drosophila. Biochim Biophys Acta 1603(2): 47-82

[17] Bernards A, Snijders AJ, Hannigan GE et al (1993) Mouse neurofibromatosis type 1 cDNA sequence reveals high degree of conservation of both coding and non-coding mRNA segments. Hum Mol Genet 2(6): 645-650

[18] Bollag G, McCormick F (1991) Differential regulation of rasGAP and neurofibromatosis gene product activities. Nature 351(6327): 576-579

[19] Bollag G, McCormick F, Clark R (1993) Characterization of full-length neurofibromin: tubulin inhibits Ras GAP activity. EMBO J 12(5): 1923-1927

[20] Bollag G, Adler F, elMasry N et al (1996a) Biochemical characterization of a novel KRAS insertion mutation from a human leukemia. J Biol Chem 271(51): 32491-32494

[21] Bollag G, Clapp DW, Shih S et al (1996b) Loss of NF1 results in activation of the Ras signaling pathway and leads to

[22] Bomar JM, Benke PJ, Slattery EL et al (2003) Mutations in a novel gene encoding a CRAL-TRIO domain cause human Cayman ataxia and ataxia/dystonia in the jittery mouse. Nat Genet 35(3): 264-269

aberrant growth in haematopoietic cells. Nat Genet 12(2): 144-148

[23] Bonneau F, D'Angelo I, Welti S et al (2004) Expression, purification and preliminary crystallo-graphic characterization of a novel segment from the neurofibromatosis type 1 protein. Acta Crystallogr D Biol Crystallogr 60(Pt 12 Pt 2): 2364-2367

[24] Bos JL, Fearon ER, Hamilton SR et al (1987) Prevalence of ras gene mutations in human colorectal cancers. Nature 327(6120): 293-297

[25] Bos JL, Rehmann H, Wittinghofer A (2007) GEFs and GAPs: critical elements in the control of small G proteins. Cell 129(5): 865-877

[26] Boyanapalli M, Lahoud OB, Messiaen L et al (2006) Neurofibromin binds to caveolin-1 and regulates ras, FAK, and Akt. Biochem Biophys Res Commun 340(4): 1200-1208

[27] Brinckmann A, Mischung C, Bassmann I et al (2007) Detection of novel NF1 mutations and rapid mutation prescreening with pyrosequencing. Electrophoresis 28(23): 4295-4301

[28] Buchberg AM, Cleveland LS, Jenkins NA et al (1990) Sequence homology shared by neurofibro-matosis type-1 gene and IRA-1 and IRA-2 negative regulators of the RAS cyclic AMP pathway. Nature 347(6290): 291-294

[29] Cai Y, Fan Z, Liu Q et al (2005) Two novel mutations of the NF1 gene in Chinese Han families with type 1 neurofibromatosis. J Dermatol Sci 39(2): 125-127

[30] Cawthon RM, Weiss R, Xu GF et al (1990) A major segment of the neurofibromatosis type 1 gene: cDNA sequence, genomic structure, and point mutations. Cell 62(1): 193-201

[31] Cichowski K, Jacks T (2001) NF1 tumor suppressor gene function: narrowing the GAP. Cell 104(4): 593-604

[32] Cichowski K, Santiago S, Jardim M et al (2003) Dynamic regulation of the Ras pathway via proteolysis of the NF1 tumor suppressor. Genes Dev 17(4): 449-454

[33] Costa RM, Yang T, Huynh DP et al (2001) Learning deficits, but normal development and tumor predisposition, in mice lacking exon 23a of Nf1. Nat Genet 27(4): 399-405

[34] Costa RM, Federov NB, Kogan JH et al (2002) Mechanism for the learning deficits in a mouse model of neurofibromatosis type 1. Nature 415(6871): 526-530

[35] Cui Y, Costa RM, Murphy GG et al (2008) Neurofibromin regulation of ERK signaling modulates GABA release and learning. Cell 135(3): 549-560

[36] D'Angelo I, Welti S, Bonneau F et al (2006) A novel bipartite phospholipid-binding module in the neurofibromatosis type 1 protein. EMBO Rep 7(2): 174-179

[37] Dasgupta B, Gutmann DH (2003) Neurofibromatosis 1: closing the GAP between mice and men. Curr Opin Genet Dev 13(1): 20-27

[38] Daston MM, Ratner N (1992) Neurofibromin, a predominantly neuronal GTPase activating protein in the adult, is ubiquitously expressed during development. Dev Dyn 195(3): 216-226

[39] Daston MM, Scrable H, Nordlund M et al (1992) The protein product of the neurofibromatosis type 1 gene is expressed at highest abundance in neurons, Schwann cells, and oligoden-drocytes. Neuron 8(3): 415-428

[40] De Luca A, Buccino A, Gianni D et al (2003) NF1 gene analysis based on DHPLC. Hum Mutat 21(2): 171-172

[41] De Luca A, Bottillo I, Sarkozy A et al (2005) NF1 gene mutations represent the major molecular event underlying neurofibromatosis-Noonan syndrome. Am J Hum Genet 77(6): 1092-1101

[42] De Schepper S, Boucneau JM, Westbroek W et al (2006) Neurofibromatosis type 1 protein and amyloid precursor protein interact in normal human melanocytes and colocalize with melanosomes. J Invest Dermatol 126(3): 653-659

[43] DeClue JE, Cohen BD, Lowy DR (1991) Identification and characterization of the neurofibromatosis type 1 protein product. Proc Natl Acad Sci USA 88(22): 9914-9918

[44] DeClue JE, Papageorge AG, Fletcher JA et al (1992) Abnormal regulation of mammalian p21ras contributes to malignant tumor growth in von Recklinghausen (type 1) neurofibromatosis. Cell 69(2): 265-273

[45] Ding L, Getz G, Wheeler DA et al (2008) Somatic mutations affect key pathways in lung adenocarcinoma. Nature 455(7216): 1069-1075

[46] Fahsold R, Hoffmeyer S, Mischung C et al (2000) Minor lesion mutational spectrum of the entire NF1 gene does not explain its high mutability but points to a functional domain upstream of the GAP-related domain. Am J Hum Genet 66(3): 790-818

[47] Feldkamp MM, Angelov L, Guha A (1999) Neurofibromatosis type 1 peripheral nerve tumors: aberrant activation of the Ras pathway. Surg Neurol 51(2): 211-218

[48] Feng L, Yunoue S, Tokuo H et al (2004) PKA phosphorylation and 14-3-3 interaction regulate the function of neurofibromatosis type I tumor suppressor, neurofibromin. FEBS Lett 557(1-3): 275-282

[49] Ferner RE, Hughes RA, Weinman J (1996) Intellectual impairment in neurofibromatosis 1. J Neurol Sci 138(1-2): 125-133

[50] Ferner RE, Hughes RA, Hall SM et al (2004) Neurofibromatous neuropathy in neurofibromatosis 1 (NF1). J Med Genet 41(11): 837-841

[51] Fishman GA, Roberts MF, Derlacki DJ et al (2004) Novel mutations in the cellular retinaldehyde-binding protein gene (RLBP1) associated with retinitis punctata albescens: evidence of inter-familial genetic heterogeneity and fundus changes in heterozygotes. Arch Ophthalmol 122(1): 70-75

[52] Galagan JE, Calvo SE, Borkovich KA et al (2003) The genome sequence of the filamentous fungus Neurospora crassa. Nature 422(6934): 859-868

[53] Godin F, Villette S, Vallee B et al (2012) A fraction of neurofibromin interacts with PML bodies in the nucleus of the CCF astrocytoma cell line. Biochem Biophys Res Commun 418(4): 689-694

[54] Gregory PE, Gutmann DH, Mitchell A et al (1993) Neurofibromatosis type 1 gene product (neurofibromin) associates with microtubules. Somat Cell Mol Genet 19(3): 265-274

[55] Grewal T, Koese M, Tebar F et al (2011) Differential regulation of RasGAPs in cancer. Genes Cancer 2(3): 288-297

[56] Griffiths S, Thompson P, Frayling I et al (2007) Molecular diagnosis of neurofibromatosis type 1: 2 years experience. Fam Cancer 6(1): 21-34

[57] Guha A, Lau N, Huvar I et al (1996) Ras-GTP levels are elevated in human NF1 peripheral nerve tumors. Oncogene 12(3): 507-513

[58] Guo HF, Tong J, Hannan F et al (2000) A

neurofibromatosis-1-regulated pathway is required for learning in Drosophila [see comments]. Nature 403(6772): 895-898

[59] Gutmann DH, Wood DL, Collins FS (1991) Identification of the neurofibromatosis type 1 gene product. Proc Natl Acad Sci USA 88(21): 9658-9662

[60] Hakimi MA, Speicher DW, Shiekhattar R (2002) The motor protein kinesin-1 links neurofibromin and merlin in a common cellular pathway of neurofibromatosis. J Biol Chem 277(40): 36909-36912

[61] Han JW, McCormick F, Macara IG (1991) Regulation of Ras-GAP and the neurofibromatosis-1 gene product by eicosanoids. Science 252(5005): 576-579

[62] Han SS, Cooper DN, Upadhyaya MN (2001) Evaluation of denaturing high performance liquid chromatography (DHPLC) for the mutational analysis of the neurofibromatosis type 1 (NF1) gene. Hum Genet 109(5): 487-497

[63] Harrisingh MC, Lloyd AC (2004) Ras/Raf/ERK signalling and NF1. Cell Cycle 3(10): 1255-1258

[64] He X, Lobsiger J, Stocker A (2009) Bothnia dystrophy is caused by domino-like rearrangements in cellular retinaldehyde-binding protein mutant R234W. Proc Natl Acad Sci USA 106(44): 18545-18550

[65] Hegedus B, Dasgupta B, Shin JE et al (2007) Neurofibromatosis-1 regulates neuronal and glial cell differentiation from neuroglial progenitors in vivo by both cAMP- and Ras-dependent mechanisms. Cell Stem Cell 1(4): 443-457

[66] Ho IS, Hannan F, Guo HF et al (2007) Distinct functional domains of neurofibromatosis type 1 regulate immediate versus long-term memory formation. J Neurosci 27(25): 6852-6857

[67] Hsueh YP, Roberts AM, Volta M et al (2001) Bipartite interaction between neurofibromatosis type I protein (neurofibromin) and syndecan transmembrane heparan sulfate proteoglycans. J Neurosci 21(11): 3764-3770

[68] Hudson J, Wu CL, Tassabehji M et al (1997) Novel and recurrent mutations in the neurofibromatosis type 1 (NF1) gene. Hum Mutat 9(4): 366-367

[69] Huynh H, Wang X, Li W et al (2003) Homotypic secretory vesicle fusion induced by the protein tyrosine phosphatase MEG2 depends on polyphosphoinositides in T cells. J Immunol 171(12): 6661-6671

[70] Izawa I, Tamaki N, Saya H (1996) Phosphorylation of neurofibromatosis type 1 gene product (neurofibromin) by cAMP-dependent protein kinase. FEBS Lett 382(1-2): 53-59

[71] Jeong SY, Park SJ, Kim HJ (2006) The spectrum of NF1 mutations in Korean patients with neurofibromatosis type 1. J Korean Med Sci 21(1): 107-112

[72] Johannessen CM, Reczek EE, James MF et al (2005) The NF1 tumor suppressor critically regulates TSC2 and mTOR. Proc Natl Acad Sci USA 102(24): 8573-8578

[73] Johnson MR, Look AT, DeClue JE et al (1993) Inactivation of the NF1 gene in human melanoma and neuroblastoma cell lines without impaired regulation of GTP.Ras. Proc Natl Acad Sci USA 90(12): 5539-5543

[74] Kaufmann D, Muller R, Bartelt B et al (2001) Spinal neurofibromatosis without cafe-au-lait macules in two families with null mutations of the NF1 gene. Am J Hum Genet 69(6): 1395-1400

[75] Kehrer-Sawatzki H, Maier C, Moschgath E et al (1998) Genomic characterization of the neurofi-bromatosis type 1 gene of Fugu rubripes. Gene 222(1): 145-153

[76] Kim HA, Rosenbaum T, Marchionni MA et al (1995) Schwann cells from neurofibromin deficient mice exhibit activation of p21ras, inhibition of cell proliferation and morphological changes. Oncogene 11(2): 325-335

[77] Klose A, Ahmadian MR, Schuelke M et al (1998) Selective disactivation of neurofibromin GAP activity in neurofibromatosis type 1. Hum Mol Genet 7(8): 1261-1268

[78] Kluwe L, Friedrich RE, Peiper M et al (2003a) Constitutional NF1 mutations in neurofibromatosis 1 patients with malignant peripheral nerve sheath tumors. Hum Mutat 22(5): 420

[79] Kluwe L, Tatagiba M, Funsterer C et al (2003b) NF1 mutations and clinical spectrum in patients with spinal neurofibromas. J Med Genet 40(5): 368-371

[80] Kostenko EV, Mahon GM, Cheng L et al (2004) The Sec14 homology domain regulates the cellular distribution and transforming activity of the Rho-specific guanine nucleotide exchange factor, Dbs. J Biol Chem 280(4): 2807-2817

[81] Krkljus S, Abernathy CR, Johnson JS et al (1998) Analysis of CpG C-to-T mutations in neurofi-bromatosis type 1. Mutations in brief no. 129. Online. Hum Mutat 11(5): 411

[82] Kweh F, Zheng M, Kurenova E et al (2009) Neurofibromin physically interacts with the N-terminal domain of focal adhesion kinase. Mol Carcinog 48(11): 1005-1017

[83] Lau N, Feldkamp MM, Roncari L et al (2000) Loss of neurofibromin is associated with activation of RAS/MAPK and PI3-K/AKT signaling in a neurofibromatosis 1 astrocytoma. J Neuropathol Exp Neurol 59(9): 759-767

[84] Lee MJ, Su YN, You HL et al (2006) Identification of forty-five novel and twenty-three known NF1 mutations in Chinese patients with neurofibromatosis type 1. Hum Mutat 27(8): 832

[85] Lemmon MA (2004) Pleckstrin homology domains: not just for phosphoinositides. Biochem Soc Trans 32(Pt 5): 707-711

[86] Lemmon MA, Ferguson KM (2000) Signal-dependent membrane targeting by pleckstrin homology (PH) domains. Biochem J 350(Pt 1): 1-18

[87] Leondaritis G, Petrikkos L, Mangoura D (2009) Regulation of the Ras-GTPase activating protein neurofibromin by C-tail phosphorylation: implications for protein kinase C/Ras/extracellular signal-regulated kinase 1/2 pathway signaling and neuronal differentiation. J Neurochem 109(2): 573-583

[88] Li Y, Bollag G, Clark R et al (1992) Somatic mutations in the neurofibromatosis 1 gene in human tumors. Cell 69(2): 275-281

[89] Li C, Cheng Y, Gutmann DA et al (2001) Differential localization of the neurofibromatosis 1 (NF1) gene product, neurofibromin, with the F-actin or microtubule cytoskeleton during differentiation of telencephalic neurons. Brain Res Dev Brain Res 130(2): 231-248

[90] Lin YL, Hsueh YP (2008) Neurofibromin interacts with CRMP-2 and CRMP-4 in rat brain. Biochem Biophys Res Commun 369(2): 747-752

[91] Lush ME, Li Y, Kwon CH et al (2008) Neurofibromin is required for barrel formation in the mouse somatosensory cortex. J Neurosci 28(7): 1580-1587

[92] Mangoura D, Sun Y, Li C et al (2006) Phosphorylation of neurofibromin by PKC is a possible molecular switch in EGF receptor signaling in neural cells. Oncogene 25(5): 735-745

[93] Martin GA, Viskochil D, Bollag G et al (1990) The GAP-related domain of the neurofibromatosis type 1 gene product interacts with ras p21. Cell 63(4): 843-849

[94] Mattocks C, Baralle D, Tarpey P et al (2004) Automated comparative sequence analysis identifies mutations in 89% of NF1 patients and confirms a mutation cluster in exons 11-17

distinct from the GAP related domain. J Med Genet 41(4): e48

[95] Maw MA, Kennedy B, Knight A et al (1997) Mutation of the gene encoding cellular retinaldehyde-binding protein in autosomal recessive retinitis pigmentosa. Nat Genet 17(2): 198-200

[96] McLendon R, Friedman A, Bigner D et al (2008) Comprehensive genomic characterization defines human glioblastoma genes and core pathways. Nature 455(7216): 1061-1068

[97] Meier R, Tomizaki T, Schulze-Briese C et al (2003) The molecular basis of vitamin E retention: structure of human alpha-tocopherol transfer protein. J Mol Biol 331(3): 725-734

[98] Messiaen LM, Callens T, Mortier G et al (2000) Exhaustive mutation analysis of the NF1 gene allows identification of 95% of mutations and reveals a high frequency of unusual splicing defects. Hum Mutat 15(6): 541-555

[99] Min KC, Kovall RA, Hendrickson WA (2003) Crystal structure of human alpha-tocopherol transfer protein bound to its ligand: implications for ataxia with vitamin E deficiency. Proc Natl Acad Sci USA 100(25): 14713-14718

[100] Mittal R, Ahmadian MR, Goody RS et al (1996) Formation of a transition-state analog of the Ras GTPase reaction by Ras-GDP, tetrafluoroaluminate, and GTPase-activating proteins. Science 273(5271): 115-117

[101] Nishi T, Lee PS, Oka K et al (1991) Differential expression of two types of the neurofibromatosis type 1 (NF1) gene transcripts related to neuronal differentiation. Oncogene 6(9): 1555-1559

[102] North K (2000) Neurofibromatosis type 1. Am J Med Genet 97(2): 119-127

[103] Nystrom AM, Ekvall S, Allanson J et al (2009) Noonan syndrome and neurofibromatosis type I in a family with a novel mutation in NF1. Clin Genet 76(6): 524-534

[104] Ouahchi K, Arita M, Kayden H et al (1995) Ataxia with isolated vitamin E deficiency is caused by mutations in the alpha-tocopherol transfer protein. Nat Genet 9(2): 141-145

[105] Ozawa T, Araki N, Yunoue S et al (2005) The neurofibromatosis type 1 gene product neurofibromin enhances cell motility by regulating actin filament dynamics via the Rho-ROCK-LIMK2-cofilin pathway. J Biol Chem 280(47): 39524-39533

[106] Ozonoff S (1999) Cognitive impairment in neurofibromatosis type 1. Am J Med Genet 89(1): 45-52

[107] Parsons DW, Jones S, Zhang X et al (2008) An integrated genomic analysis of human glioblastoma multiforme. Science 321(5897): 1807-1812

[108] Pascual-Castroviejo I, Pascual-Pascual SI, Velazquez-Fragua R et al (2007) Familial spinal neurofibromatosis. Neuropediatrics 38(2): 105-108

[109] Patrakitkomjorn S, Kobayashi D, Morikawa T et al (2008) Neurofibromatosis type 1 (NF1) tumor suppressor, neurofibromin, regulates the neuronal differentiation of PC12 cells via its associating protein, CRMP-2. J Biol Chem 283(14): 9399-9413

[110] Peters H, Hess D, Fahsold R et al (1999) A novel mutation L1425P in the GAP-region of the NF1 gene detected by temperature gradient gel electrophoresis (TGGE). Mutation in brief no. 230. Online. Hum Mutat 13(4): 337

[111] Peterson FC, Volkman BF (2009) Diversity of polyproline recognition by EVH1 domains. Front Biosci 14: 833-846

[112] Phan VT, Ding VW, Li F et al (2010) The RasGAP proteins Ira2 and neurofibromin are negatively regulated by Gpb1 in yeast and ETEA in humans. Mol Cell Biol 30(9): 2264-2279

[113] Phillips SE, Vincent P, Rizzieri KE et al (2006) The diverse biological functions of phosphatidy-linositol transfer proteins in eukaryotes. Crit Rev Biochem Mol Biol 41(1): 21-49

[114] Prior IA, Lewis PD, Mattos C (2012) A comprehensive survey of ras mutations in cancer. Cancer Res 72(10): 2457-2467

[115] Purandare SM, Lanyon WG, Connor JM (1994) Characterisation of inherited and sporadic mutations in neurofibromatosis type-1. Hum Mol Genet 3(7): 1109-1115

[116] Pylayeva-Gupta Y, Grabocka E, Bar-Sagi D (2011) RAS oncogenes: weaving a tumorigenic web. Nat Rev Cancer 11(11): 761-774

[117] Rocks O, Peyker A, Kahms M et al (2005) An acylation cycle regulates localization and activity of palmitoylated Ras isoforms. Science 307(5716): 1746-1752

[118] Rocks O, Peyker A, Bastiaens PI (2006) Spatio-temporal segregation of Ras signals: one ship, three anchors, many harbors. Curr Opin Cell Biol 18(4): 351-357

[119] Romero MI, Lin L, Lush ME et al (2007) Deletion of Nf1 in neurons induces increased axon collateral branching after dorsal root injury. J Neurosci 27(8): 2124-2134

[120] Sangha N, Wu R, Kuick R et al (2008) Neurofibromin 1 (NF1) defects are common in human ovarian serous carcinomas and co-occur with TP53 mutations. Neoplasia 10(12): 1362-1372

[121] Scheffzek K, Ahmadian MR (2005) GTPase activating proteins: structural and functional insights 18 years after discovery. Cell Mol Life Sci 62(24): 3014-3038

[122] Scheffzek K, Lautwein A, Kabsch W et al (1996) Crystal structure of the GTPase-activating domain of human p120GAP and implications for the interaction with Ras. Nature 384(6609): 591-596

[123] Scheffzek K, Ahmadian MR, Kabsch W et al (1997) The Ras-RasGAP complex: structural basis for GTPase activation and its loss in oncogenic Ras mutants. Science 277(5324): 333-338

[124] Scheffzek K, Ahmadian MR, Wiesmuller L et al (1998a) Structural analysis of the GAP-related domain from neurofibromin and its implications. EMBO J 17(15): 4313-4327

[125] Scheffzek K, Ahmadian MR, Wittinghofer A (1998b) GTPase-activating proteins: helping hands to complement an active site. Trends Biochem Sci 23(7): 257-262

[126] Sermon BA, Eccleston JF, Skinner RH et al (1996) Mechanism of inhibition by arachidonic acid of the catalytic activity of Ras GTPase-activating proteins. J Biol Chem 271(3): 1566-1572

[127] Sermon BA, Lowe PN, Strom M et al (1998) The importance of two conserved arginine residues for catalysis by the ras GTPase-activating protein, neurofibromin. J Biol Chem 273(16): 9480-9485

[128] Sha B, Phillips SE, Bankaitis VA et al (1998) Crystal structure of the *Saccharomyces cerevisiae* phosphatidylinositol-transfer protein. Nature 391(6666): 506-510

[129] Sherman L, Daston M, Ratner N (1998) Neurofibromin: distribution, cell biology and role in neurofibromatosis type 1. In: Upadhyaya M, Cooper DN (eds) Neurofibromatosis type 1—form genotype to phenotype. BIOS Scientific, Oxford, pp 113-131

[130] Sherman LS, Atit R, Rosenbaum T et al (2000) Single cell

Ras-GTP analysis reveals altered Ras activity in a subpopulation of neurofibroma Schwann cells but not fibroblasts. J Biol Chem 275 (39): 30740-30745

[131] Shilyansky C, Lee YS, Silva AJ (2010) Molecular and cellular mechanisms of learning disabilities: a focus on NF1. Annu Rev Neurosci 33: 221-243

[132] Sirokmany G, Szidonya L, Kaldi K et al (2005) Sec14 homology domain targets p50RhoGAP to endosomes and provides a link between Rab- and Rho GTPases. J Biol Chem 281(9): 6096-6105

[133] Sondek J, Lambright DG, Noel JP et al (1994) GTPase mechanism of G proteins from the 1.7-A crystal structure of transducin alpha-GDP-AIF-4. Nature 372(6503): 276-279

[134] Starinsky-Elbaz S, Faigenbloom L, Friedman E et al (2009) The pre-GAP-related domain of neurofibromin regulates cell migration through the LIM kinase/cofilin pathway. Mol Cell Neurosci 42(4): 278-287

[135] Stocker A (2004) Molecular mechanisms of vitamin E transport. Ann NY Acad Sci 1031: 44-59

[136] Tassabehji M, Strachan T, Sharland M et al (1993) Tandem duplication within a neurofibromatosis type 1 (NF1) gene exon in a family with features of Watson syndrome and Noonan syndrome. Am J Hum Genet 53(1): 90-95

[137] The I, Hannigan GE, Cowley GS et al (1997) Rescue of a Drosophila NF1 mutant phenotype by protein kinase A. Science 276(5313): 791-794

[138] Thomas L, Richards M, Mort M, Dunlop E, Cooper DN, Upadhayaya M. (2012) Assessment of the potential pathogenicity of missense mutations identified in the GTPase-activating protein (GAP)-related domain of the neurofibromatosis type-1 (NF1) gene. Hum. Mutat. 33: 1687-1696

[139] Tong J, Hannan F, Zhu Y et al (2002) Neurofibromin regulates G protein-stimulated adenylyl cyclase activity. Nat Neurosci 5(2): 95-96

[140] Trahey M, McCormick F (1987) A cytoplasmic protein stimulates normal N-ras p21 GTPase, but does not affect oncogenic mutants. Science 238(4826): 542-545

[141] Trovó AB, Goloni-Bertollo EM, Mancini UM et al (2004) Mutational analysis of the GAP-related domain of the neurofibromatosis type 1 gene in Brazilian NF1 patients. Genet Mol Biol 27(3): 326-330

[142] Trovo-Marqui AB, Tajara EH (2006) Neurofibromin: a general outlook. Clin Genet 70(1): 1-13

[143] Uchida T, Matozaki T, Suzuki T et al (1992) Expression of two types of neurofibromatosis type 1 gene transcripts in gastric cancers and comparison of GAP activities. Biochem Biophys Res Commun 187(1): 332-339

[144] Upadhyaya M, Maynard J, Osborn M et al (1997a) Six novel mutations in the neurofibromatosis type 1 (NF1) gene. Hum Mutat 10(3): 248-250

[145] Upadhyaya M, Osborn MJ, Maynard J et al (1997b) Mutational and functional analysis of the neurofibromatosis type 1 (NF1) gene. Hum Genet 99(1): 88-92

[146] Upadhyaya M, Ruggieri M, Maynard J et al (1998) Gross deletions of the neurofibromatosis type 1 (NF1) gene are predominantly of maternal origin and commonly associated with a learning disability, dysmorphic features and developmental delay. Hum Genet 102(5): 591-597

[147] Upadhyaya M, Spurlock G, Monem B et al (2008) Germline and somatic NF1 gene mutations in plexiform neurofibromas. Hum Mutat 29(8): E103-E111. doi: 10.1002/humu.20793

[148] Upadhyaya M, Spurlock G, Kluwe L et al (2009) The spectrum of somatic and germline NF1 mutations in NF1 patients with spinal neurofibromas. Neurogenetics 10(3): 251-263. doi: 10.1007/s10048-009-0178-0

[149] Vandenbroucke I, Van Oostveldt P, Coene E et al (2004) Neurofibromin is actively transported to the nucleus. FEBS Lett 560(1-3): 98-102

[150] Viskochil D, Buchberg AM, Xu G et al (1990) Deletions and a translocation interrupt a cloned gene at the neurofibromatosis type 1 locus. Cell 62(1): 187-192

[151] Wallace MR, Marchuk DA, Andersen LB et al (1990) Type 1 neurofibromatosis gene: identification of a large transcript disrupted in three NF1 patients. Science 249(4965): 181-186

[152] Wang HF, Shih YT, Chen CY et al (2011) Valosin-containing protein and neurofibromin interact to regulate dendritic spine density. J Clin Invest 121(12): 4820-4837. doi: 10.1172/JCI45677 [doi] 45677 [pii]

[153] Weeber EJ, Sweatt JD (2002) Molecular neurobiology of human cognition. Neuron 33(6): 845-848. doi: S0896627302006347 [pii]

[154] Welti S, Fraterman S, D'Angelo I et al (2007) The sec14 homology module of neurofibromin binds cellular glycerophospholipids: mass spectrometry and structure of a lipid complex. J Mol Biol 366(2): 551-562

[155] Welti S, Kuhn S, D'Angelo I et al (2011) Structural and biochemical consequences of NF1 associated nontruncating mutations in the Sec14-PH module of neurofibromin. Hum Mutat 32(2): 191-197. doi: 10.1002/humu.21405

[156] Wimmer K, Roca X, Beiglbock H et al (2007) Extensive in silico analysis of NF1 splicing defects uncovers determinants for splicing outcome upon 5' splice-site disruption. Hum Mutat 28(6): 599-612. doi: 10.1002/humu.20493

[157] Wittinghofer A (1997) Signaling mechanisms: aluminum fluoride for molecule of the year. Curr Biol 7(11): R682-R685

[158] Wittinghofer A, Scheffzek K, Ahmadian MR (1997) The interaction of Ras with GTPase-activating proteins. FEBS Lett 410(1): 63-67

[159] Wu R, Lopez-Correa C, Rutkowski JL et al (1999) Germline mutations in NF1 patients with malignancies. Genes Chromosomes Cancer 26(4): 376-380. doi: 10.1002/(SICI)1098-2264(199912)26: 4<376: AID-GCC13>3.0.CO;2-O [pii]

[160] Xu H, Gutmann DH (1997) Mutations in the GAP-related domain impair the ability of neurofibromin to associate with microtubules. Brain Res 759(1): 149-152

[161] Xu GF, Lin B, Tanaka K et al (1990a) The catalytic domain of the neurofibromatosis type 1 gene product stimulates ras GTPase and complements ira mutants of S. cerevisiae. Cell 63(4): 835-841

[162] Xu GF, O'Connell P, Viskochil D et al (1990b) The neurofibromatosis type 1 gene encodes a protein related to GAP. Cell 62(3): 599-608

[163] Yunoue S, Tokuo H, Fukunaga K et al (2003) Neurofibromatosis type I tumor suppressor neurofibromin regulates neuronal differentiation via its GTPase-activating protein function toward Ras. J Biol Chem 278(29): 26958-26969

[164] Zhang S, Charest PG, Firtel RA (2008) Spatiotemporal regulation of Ras activity provides directional sensing. Curr Biol 18(20): 1587-1593. doi: 10.1016/j.cub.2008.08.069 [doi] S0960-9822(08)01244-X [pii]

[165] Zhu Y, Parada LF (2001) Neurofibromin, a tumor suppressor in the nervous system. Exp Cell Res 264(1): 19-28

[166] Zhu Y, Parada LF (2002) The molecular and genetic basis of neurological tumours. Nat Rev Cancer 2(8): 616-626. doi: 10.1038/nrc866 [doi] nrc866 [pii]

[167] Zhu Y, Romero MI, Ghosh P et al (2001) Ablation of NF1 function in neurons induces abnormal development of cerebral cortex and reactive gliosis in the brain. Genes Dev 15(7): 859-876. doi: 10.1101/gad.862101

第21章 1型神经纤维瘤病骨骼异常的分子基础
Molecular Basis of Bone Abnormalities in NF1

David A. Stevenson and Florent Elefteriou

21.1 引言

1型神经纤维瘤病（NF1）由 NF1 基因的失活突变导致 RAS 信号增强，进而影响骨细胞及其前体细胞的增殖、分化和功能。尽管 NF1 的神经及皮肤表现最受关注，但骨骼系统在 NF1 中的受累也不容忽视。NF1 骨骼系统异常发病率高，随着动物模型的完善，以及对复杂骨骼异常机制的理解不断深入，NF1 中的骨骼系统异常近年来逐渐受到关注。近年来，人体和动物模型的相关研究更好地阐明了 NF1 中骨骼相关问题的分子机制。神经纤维瘤蛋白功能丧失对骨骼影响的分子机制在人体中尚未阐明，目前所知的大部分研究均以动物模型为基础。本章节中，我们将回顾 NF1 骨骼系统的临床表型、分子和细胞研究，以及相关动物模型的开发。

21.2 临床骨骼系统表型

NF1 的骨骼异常早已为人所知，且已有多篇文献阐述（Elefteriou et al. 2009；Stevenson and Yang 2011；Alwan et al. 2005；Crawford and Schorry 1999；Vitale et al. 2002；Ruggieri et al. 1999）。胫骨假关节和蝶骨翼发育不良在 NF1 中相对特有，这些改变最初被认为是 NF1 的一种特征性骨病变，且作为 NF1 的诊断标准之一（Gutmann et al. 1997）。NF1 相关骨骼异常包括长骨弯曲（图 21.1）和假关节（特别是胫骨）、萎缩型和非萎缩型脊柱侧弯、脊柱后凸、蝶骨翼发育不良、骨质减少、成人高骨折率、骨囊肿、骨过度生长、前胸壁异常和身材矮小（Crawford and Schorry 1999；Vitale et al. 2002；Elefteriou et al. 2009；Friedman and Birch 1997；Ruggieri et al. 1999；Stevenson et al. 1999, 2005, 2007a；Illes et al. 2001；Kuorilehto et al. 2005；Yilmaz et al. 2007；Lammert et al. 2005；Dulai et al. 2007；Brunetti-Pierri et al. 2008；Tucker et al. 2009；Caffarelli et al. 2010；Seitz et al. 2010）。然而，一些骨骼系统问题可能部分是由于关节、肌肉和韧带的异常，而不是骨细胞发育的缺陷所致（例如扁平足、非萎缩型脊柱侧弯、脊柱后凸、前胸壁异常）（Johnson et al. 2010；Kossler et al. 2011；Souza et al. 2009）。这些多样的骨骼系统异常可能是由于 RAS 信号通路增强对多个器官系统多种细胞类型的异常影响的综合效应所致。尽管存在多种多样

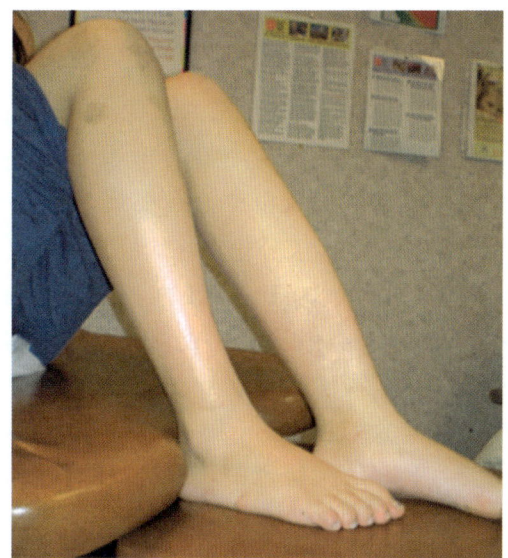

图 21.1　NF1 患者左腿前外侧弯曲不伴有假关节

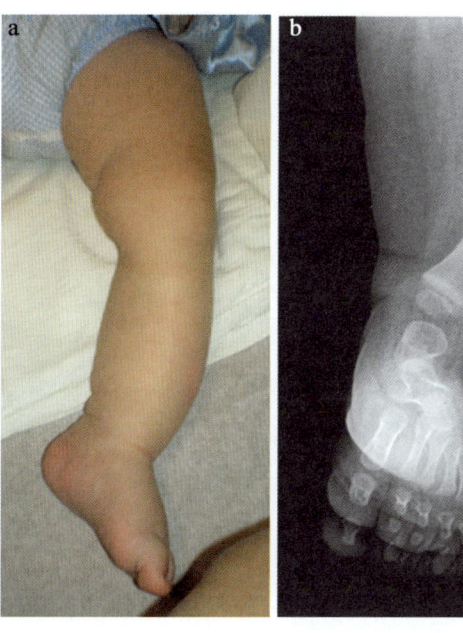

图 21.2　a. 伴有左腿前外侧弯曲的 NF1 患儿照片。b. 腿部 X 线片显示胫骨前外侧弯曲，无假关节，但腓骨假关节

的骨科表现，但本章将重点讨论一些明显与骨相关的典型骨骼发现。

21.2.1　长骨发育不良

长骨发育不良或骨病最常影响胫骨，尽管其他长骨也可能受累。典型的胫骨发育不良影像学表现包括前外侧弯曲伴有髓腔狭窄和弯曲顶点的皮质增厚（Stevenson et al. 2007b）。当胫骨受累时，腓骨通常也会受累（Stevenson et al. 1999）（图 21.2）。我们假设在一些情况下，腓骨的伴随弯曲部分是由于胫骨弯曲的机械效应。然而，弯曲的腓骨也可能出现假关节，就像没有胫骨受累的孤立性腓骨假关节一样。这种胫骨和腓骨发育不良的关联可能是机械效应与局部微环境共同作用的结果。长骨弯曲和假关节并不是 NF1 的普遍表现，约发生在 3%～5% 的 NF1 患者中（Friedman and Birch 1997）。此外，这一表型通常是单侧的。观察到的长骨弯曲及随后发生的假关节形成与 NF1 高度相关。这些发现表明，NF1 单倍体失活促进了长骨弯曲和假关节的发生，但可能需要额外的修饰因子，例如 NF1 的双重失活。

在 2 例伴有胫骨假关节的 NF1 患者的假关节组织中，发现 NF1 的杂合性丢失，并且在其中 1 名患者的假关节组织中确认了保留等位基因突变的 NF1 双重失活（Stevenson et al. 2006）。然而，在其他病例中并未观察到杂合性丢失（Sakamoto et al. 2007），这表明可能存在混合的细胞群、具有 NF1 双重失活的其他组织或细胞谱系，或者更有可能的是存在其他修饰因子。

在胫骨骨折远端和近端骨段之间发现的组织，通常被描述为"假关节组织"，但其特性一直难以界定。这是一种高度细胞化的组织，并且已有多种描述（例如，"纤维性错构瘤""纤维瘤样组织"）（Mariaud-Schmidt et al. 2005；Cho et al. 2008；Ippolito et al. 2000）。在组织学上，这种增生组织具有相当均匀的致密纤维软骨外观，并且 S100 表达阴性（Stevenson et al. 2006；Sakamoto et al. 2007；Briner and Yunis 1973）。Mariaud-Schmidt 等（2005）对 2 名患者的假关节部位进行检测，发现该组织由纤维细胞组成，提出"错构瘤样"组织是由一种未分化的膜性组织形成的。Blauth 等（1984）对 10 例假关节进行了组织学和电子显微镜检查，发现其表面是一种具有纺锤形细胞核的长形细胞组成的细胞性纤维组织。Cho 等（2008）对 7 例 NF1 患者的"纤维错构瘤"组织进行培养，发现这些细胞具有高度破骨细胞生成能力，并保持了间充质谱系免疫表型（即 $CD44^+/CD105^+/CD45^-/CD14^-$）。这些细胞似乎处于成骨分化的不同阶段，且具有较低的成骨性（Cho et al. 2008）。然而，假关节的解剖部位不仅由这种增生的纤维组织组成，因为仍然存在近端和远端骨碎片、骨膜以及其他细胞的混合。Sakamoto 等（2007）报告称，假关节区域的骨小梁外观上与骨纤维性发育不良相似，具有明显的成骨细胞边缘。Heervä 等（2010）分析了 3 名 NF1 患者假关节区域组织样本，显示存在大量与骨和骨凹陷接触的多核抗酒石酸磷酸酶（tartrateresistant acid phosphatase，TRACP）阳性破骨细胞，但也注意到许多（约 50%）破骨细胞位于远离骨表面的纤维假关节组织中。在假关节部位的各种骨细胞功能中，可能存在各种细胞成分之间复杂的相互作用。值得注意的是，组织学分析通常是在已形成假关节并发生骨折的区域进行的，根据 NF1 小鼠模型的临床表型，这些涉及的骨和骨髓的组织异常很可能在骨折和假关节形成之前已经存在。

21.2.2　脊柱侧凸

脊柱侧弯是 NF1 患者较常见的骨骼异常之一，尽管不同报告中的脊柱侧弯发生率差异很大（Young et al. 2002）。这种差异可能直接反映了所谓的脊柱侧弯本身固有的变异性。脊柱侧弯指的是基于前后位 X 线片的脊柱弯曲，但脊柱是多维的，且由多个骨性结构组成。在侧位上，脊柱存在正常的后凸和前凸，而在前后位上的轻微弯曲（即 9°至 20°之间）可能在临床上不易识别。在 NF1 中，脊柱侧弯通常被分类为"萎缩型"或"非萎缩型"。Durrani 等（2000）尝试将 NF1 中的"萎缩型"脊柱侧弯定义为存在特定影像学特征的脊柱侧弯（例如肋骨铅笔征、椎骨凹陷、横突细长改变）。在尝试理解 NF1 对骨性结构的直接影响的背景下，萎缩型脊柱侧弯确实是需要考虑的一种脊柱侧弯类型，尽管 Durrani 等（2000）列出的一些影像学特征并不一定是原发性的骨发育不良（Alwan 等 2005）。邻近神经纤维瘤的机械应力或肿瘤分泌因子可能会影响脊柱侧弯的发展和进展。尽管非萎缩型脊柱侧弯可能不是原发性骨病，但它的发生可能是由于椎骨存在的一种在 X 线片上无法观察到的骨稳态紊乱。

Brunetti-Pierri 等（2008）回顾了 3 例 NF1 患者的椎骨样本，这些患者骨量减少并正在接受脊柱侧弯手术，并将这些样本与尸检对照样本以及 1 例成骨不全患者的样本进行了比较。NF1 椎骨样本显示骨小梁的数量和厚度减少，但是存在正常的骨黏合线和存活的骨细胞，骨的矿化程度与对照组相似。电子显微镜下矿物质含量严重减少。在骨表面，观察到大量衬细胞取代了分化良好的成骨细胞。与成骨不全患者的骨样本相比，NF1 椎骨中的衬细胞分化不良，几乎没有类似于活性成骨细胞的细胞质结构。报道中并未描述这些患者的脊柱侧弯类型是否为萎缩型或非萎缩型，也未说明分析的椎骨是否外观发育异常。在后续研究中，比较非萎缩型与萎缩型脊柱侧弯患者的椎骨，或在萎缩型短节段脊柱侧弯的个体中比较不同区域的椎骨结构，将有助于理解 NF1 伴脊柱侧弯的形成机制。

21.2.3　蝶骨翼发育不良

蝶骨翼发育不良的病因尚不清楚。蝶骨翼发育不良的严重程度不同，轻微的发育不良可能不容易被识别。严重蝶骨翼发育不良的患者可能会出现眼科并发症和明显的面部不对称，引起美容问题。在许多情况下，蝶骨翼的发育不良往往伴随着一个面部邻近区域的丛状神经纤维瘤。蝶骨翼发育不良的发生率、单侧性及家族内外变异性与长骨发育不良相似，这再次表明 NF1 一些骨科相关表型的发生需要二次打击和其他修饰因子。

21.2.4　骨质疏松症/骨量减少

许多研究报告了 NF1 儿童和成人的骨密度（bone mineral density，BMD）下降（Illes et al. 2001；Kuorilehto et al. 2005；Lammert et al. 2005；Stevenson et al. 2005，2007a；Dulai et al. 2007；Yilmaz et al. 2007；Brunetti-Pierri et al. 2008；Tucker et al. 2009；Caffarelli et al. 2010；Seitz et al. 2010）。与临床表现提示体细胞事件或修饰效应的长骨发育不良、蝶骨翼发育不良和萎缩型脊柱侧弯不同，NF1 中广泛且更常见的骨质减少和骨质疏松表明，NF1 单倍体不足本身就可能影响骨细胞功能。

尽管来自多个国家的大量独立研究通过双能 X 线吸收法测量证实了骨密度（BMD）的下降，但在临床上解读面积骨密度(areal BMD)存在问题,特别是在生长中的个体,尤其是身高较矮且可能骨骼较小的个体。NF1 中骨密度下降的临床影响尚存争议,尤其是在表面上没有发育异常的骨骼中。有些人可能会认为骨密度与骨骼的形状和大小是相称的。Stevenson 等(2009)使用外周定量计算机断层扫描评估了腿部的体积参数,结果显示胫骨的强度应变指数下降,提示其易于骨折。此外,Tucker 等(2009)报告称 NF1 成人的骨折率增加。

骨吸收标志物可以提供一些证据表明 NF1 患者骨吸收更为活跃。一些研究表明,NF1 个体的骨吸收标志物增加(Stevenson et al. 2008;Tucker et al. 2009),而在另一个队列研究中并未发现此现象(Duman et al. 2008)。Stevenson 等(2011a)使用尿吡啶交联物作为骨吸收标志物测定其他 RAS 病(即 Noonan 综合征、Costello 综合征和心面皮肤综合征)也显示出类似的增加,这进一步证实了 RAS 信号转导通路激活导致骨吸收增加的观点。

多位研究者对来自造血系的人类骨细胞进行体外测定,进一步证实了体内骨吸收标志物增加的结果(Yang et al. 2006;Heervä et al. 2010;Stevenson et al. 2011a、b)。Yang 等(2006)在少数 NF1 个体培养的成骨前体细胞上应用了在相关的 NF1 小鼠模型中进行的方法,显示了增加的多个破骨细胞功能,这一结果后续在更大的 NF1 患者队列中得到了证实(Stevenson et al. 2011a、b)。来自 NF1 个体中培养的单核细胞显示出破骨细胞形成增加、破骨细胞迁移增加以及基于凹坑吸收测定的活性增加。Heerva 等(2010)在人类体外研究中显示了类似的发现,并且还记录了在血清剥夺条件下,来自 NF1 患者的单核细胞与健康对照组相比存活率更高。因此,NF1 单倍体不足至少影响了破骨细胞的功能。但这些研究是在体外培养细胞暴露于各种生长因子下进行的,对于 $NF1^{+/-}$ 破骨细胞在体内的具体影响目前暂无定论。

Seitz 等(2010)对 14 名 NF1 患者进行了髂骨嵴骨活检,并与年龄和性别匹配的尸检对照进行了组织学和组织形态计量学分析。他们观察到成骨细胞和破骨细胞数量的增加,提示骨转换增加。其他发现包括小梁厚度减少和骨基质矿化缺陷,同时伴有未矿化骨基质体积和厚度的增加。这些发现提示可能存在骨软化症,而这些患者来自德国的一个队列,该地区的 NF1 患者一直被报道维生素 D 缺乏(Lammert et al. 2005;Tucker et al. 2009)。因此,除了 NF1 对骨细胞功能的直接影响外,其他因素也可能导致 NF1 中观察到的骨质减少和骨质疏松(如维生素 D 缺乏、激素失衡、不活动、肌张力低)。

尽管对临床骨骼表型的了解以及一些人体细胞体外研究在某些方面揭示了部分 NF1 中骨骼异常的分子基础,但仍有许多疑问尚未阐明。最近,NF1 中骨骼的动物模型的建立为 NF1 骨骼机制的研究提供了更多的便利。

21.3 动物模型

动物模型对于理解 NF1 在骨重塑和修复生物学中的作用,以及鉴定那些能够靶向预防或治疗 NF1 骨骼表现的关键分子或机制至关重要。这些遗传模型也可以作为临床前模型,用于评估选定和靶向药物方法的有效性,但这些模型具有局限性,并且与真实的人体环境相差甚远。

21.3.1 小鼠模型中 Nf1 单倍体不足的影响

神经纤维瘤蛋白在骨髓间质系和造血谱系中表达,因此其功能丧失可以通过多种机制共同影响骨重塑和修复。神经纤维瘤蛋白在成骨前体细胞、软骨细胞、成骨细胞和破骨细胞中表达,1 个或 2 个 Nf1 拷贝的丢失会引发这些细胞中 RAS 和 ERK1/2 的持续激活(Yu et al. 2005;Kuorilehto et al. 2004;Elefteriou et al. 2006;Wu et al. 2006;Yang et al. 2006;Kolanczyk et al. 2007;Wang et al. 2011)。

$Nf1^{-/-}$ 小鼠在胚胎期致死,但 Nf1 杂合子($Nf1^{+/-}$)小鼠是可存活的(Brannan et al. 1994;Lakkis and Epstein 1998)。$Nf1^{+/-}$ 小鼠在正常条件下并不会表现出骨质减少,但在卵巢切除后相对于野生型小鼠会丢失更多的骨量。这至少部分是由于破骨细胞介导的骨吸收增加所致(Yang et al. 2006)。从这些小鼠中提取的 $Nf1^{+/-}$ 成骨细胞在体外表现出增殖增加和分化受损,并分泌更多的骨桥蛋白，这是一种已知促进破骨细胞生成和破骨细胞迁移的基质蛋白。另外，$Nf1^{+/-}$ 破骨细胞前体在细胞黏附、迁移、分化和活性上表现出依赖于 RAC1 和 PI3K 的细胞自主缺陷（Yan et al. 2008；Yang et al. 2006）。这些数据表明，NF1 单倍体不足会导致 NF1 患者中观察到的骨量减少。但是为什么需要通过卵巢切除才能在 $Nf1^{+/-}$ 小鼠中观察到相关骨表型仍不清楚。同样不清楚的是，其他骨细胞或组织中的 Nf1 单倍体不足在何种程度上导致了这种骨表型。

$Nf1^{+/-}$ 小鼠已被用作 NF1 胫骨远端骨折后骨愈合的临床前模型。众所周知，小鼠具有强大的骨愈合能力，因此 $Nf1^{+/-}$ 小鼠并未出现假关节形成，但表现出延迟的骨痂形成和愈合、延迟的软骨去除、纤维侵入、新骨合成不足以及过度的分解代谢（Schindeler et al. 2008a，b）。这项研究表明，NF1 单倍体不足至少是 NF1 假关节形成的部分原因。

21.3.2　Nf1 功能丧失对小鼠的影响

最严重的 NF1 表现具有局灶性和单侧性，加上发育过程中 NF1 缺乏所导致的致死性，这些都证实了以下假设：体细胞 NF1 功能丧失可能是这些骨缺陷的根本原因。因此，基于 Parada 团队（Zhu et al. 2001）生成的 floxed Nf1 小鼠和 cre 转基因小鼠的各种条件性突变小鼠模型被构建，在骨组织和细胞中使用特定的启动子驱动 cre 重组（因此 Nf1 缺失），生成了多种条件性突变小鼠模型。

第一个生成的条件性模型是以成熟成骨细胞中 Nf1 功能丧失为特征，使用 2.3 kb Ⅰ型胶原启动子-cre 小鼠（Dacquin et al. 2002）。该模型对骨最具特异性，但由于 Nf1 重组仅限于成熟成骨细胞，早期成骨祖细胞的承诺或分化中 Nf1 缺失的影响未能反映出来。尽管如此，$Nf1^{ob-/-}$ 小鼠表现出几种椎骨骨异常，包括由于胶原生产增加和矿化延迟导致的矿化不良的骨基质生成，以及破骨细胞形成的增加（Elefteriou et al. 2006）。这些发现也在具有胫骨假关节的 NF1 患者的胫骨活检中观察到（Wang et al. 2011），表明 Nf1 调节成骨细胞功能，即骨基质生产和矿化，以及对破骨细胞生成的支持。$Nf1^{ob-/-}$ 小鼠还表现出椎骨皮质和松质骨密度降低，以及较野生型小鼠更弱的骨力学性能（Zhang et al. 2011），但在长骨中（至少在年轻小鼠中）骨密度没有显著变化（Wu et al. 2011）。$Nf1^{ob-/-}$ 小鼠在经受胫骨远端骨折后，与 $Nf1^{+/-}$ 小鼠一样，未显示假关节，但表现出延迟愈合和桥接、高皮质孔隙率和过度骨质形成，伴随机械性能减弱。也未观察到纤维错构瘤（Wang et al. 2010）。

将 $Nf1^{ob-/-}$ 小鼠转移到 $Nf1^{+/-}$ 杂合子环境下并未显著改变这些骨参数，但与 $Nf1^{ob-/-}$ 小鼠相比，其导致脊柱椎管面积增加和成骨细胞数量减少（Zhang et al. 2011）。

第二个生成的 NF1 小鼠模型是基于使用 Prx 启动子-cre 小鼠，该模型允许在间充质谱系中早期丧失 Nf1 功能。与 $Nf1^{ob-/-}$ 小鼠相反，在这个模型中可以评估 Nf1 缺失在细胞承诺和分化中的影响，但由于 floxed Nf1 等位基因在软骨细胞、肌肉和内皮细胞中也发生了重组，导致观察到的骨骼表型的解释变得复杂。此外，Prx 启动子仅在肢体中驱动 cre 表达，因此无法在这个模型中评估 Nf1 在中轴骨和脊柱侧弯发展中的作用。尽管存在这些复杂性，该模型复现了许多 NF1 的骨骼表型，包括骨量减少、骨质疏松和胫骨弯曲。$Nf1^{prx-/-}$ 小鼠的严重体型减小源于生长板发育缺陷，这可能与 NF1 患者相对身材矮小无关。同时 $Nf1^{prx-/-}$ 模型中的骨愈合能力也有受损。使用皮质损伤和膜内骨修复模型，Kolanczyk 等（2007，2008）在这些损伤中复现了 NF1 假关节的许多特征，包括愈合延迟、纤维软骨组织的持续存在和骨细胞外基质矿化受损。

$Nf1^{col2-/-}$ 模型是基于Ⅱ型胶原蛋白启动子-Cre 小鼠，与 $Nf1^{prx-/-}$ 模型相似（Wang et al. 2011）。尽管这些小鼠主要用于研究软骨发育，但它们在胚胎发育期间软骨膜中的成骨软骨前体细胞中重组基因，而这些前体细胞在后期会发育成成骨细胞。与 $Nf1^{prx-/-}$ 模型相比，Cre 在 $Nf1^{col2-/-}$ 模型中表达于中轴骨。该基因型小鼠表现出胫骨弯曲、巨颅畸形、萎缩型脊柱侧弯、脊柱后凸、骨质疏松、骨皮质孔隙度增加、骨矿化障碍以及破骨细胞生成增加，所有这些都是 NF1 的特征。这些小鼠的骨骼在机械结构上也较弱。然而，它们存在严重生长不足（类似于 $Nf1^{prx-/-}$ 小鼠，由于软骨细胞中缺乏 $Nf1$），且其中很大比例的小鼠在断奶后不久就会死亡。该模型还表现出椎间盘形成缺陷，这一缺陷对观察到的脊柱侧弯的贡献尚不清楚。

Periostin Cre 小鼠也被用来在骨内膜表面上失活 $Nf1$。令人惊讶的是，PeriCre+；$Nf1^{flox/-}$ 小鼠而非 PeriCre+；$Nf1^{flox/flox}$ 小鼠显示出骨量、骨密度和成骨细胞数量的减少，这表明在这一模型中观察到的骨骼表型需要单倍体不足的造血微环境。与 WT HSC 相比，经 γ 辐照的移植了 $Nf1^{-/-}$ 造血干细胞（hematopoietic stem cells，HSC）小鼠的 PeriCre+；$Nf1^{flox/flox}$ 胫骨的骨体积和骨密度减少，这再次表明 $Nf1^{+/-}$ 微环境会影响骨折骨中的骨细胞分化或功能（Wu et al. 2011）。该模型中骨愈合本身是否受损还有待通过力学检测和定量骨愈合测量来验证。

另外一种在骨细胞中实现 $Nf1$ 功能失活的方法是局部递送 Cre 腺病毒。Dr. Schindeler 和 Dr. Little 的研究团队使用这种方法成功地模拟出 NF1 假关节病（El-Hoss et al. 2011）。这种策略的优势在于不需要进行大量繁殖，从而节省了大量时间。与其他基于 Cre 过表达的模型不同，这种方法非常局部，可以靶向多个骨元素。该方法已被应用于 NF1 假关节的疾病模型，并且理论上可以用作萎缩型脊柱侧弯的模型。通过放射学评估，无论 $Nf1^{flox/flox}$ 小鼠是否具有 $Nf1^{+/-}$ 背景，使用这种 Cre-腺病毒方法进行局部 Nf1 失活会降低胫骨骨折愈合能力。该模型中还观察到了与人类假关节活检中类似的"纤维错构瘤"，以及巨大的多核 TRAP 阳性破骨细胞，其中许多未衬在骨表面（El-Hoss et al. 2011）。

21.4 分子靶点和治疗

在 $Nf1^{+/-}$ 和 $Nf1^{-/-}$ 细胞（包括成骨细胞）中 RAS 和 ERK 的特征性激活，促使研究人员在以骨愈合延迟为特征的 NF1 小鼠模型中尝试使用洛伐他汀。洛伐他汀通过抑制甲羟戊酸途径，进而抑制 RAS 的棕榈酰化和活性，尽管其对 RAS 抑制的选择性不高，但仍被认为是治疗 NF1 表现的合理选择。在 $Nf1^{prx-/-}$ 和 $Nf1^{ob-/-}$ 小鼠模型中，口服高剂量洛伐他汀和通过缓释微粒在骨折部位局部递送低剂量洛伐他汀，都对骨愈合和骨痂的机械性能具有益处（Kolanczyk et al. 2008；Wang et al. 2010）。

然而，由于洛伐他汀尚未被批准用于治疗骨疾病，研究人员还测试了其他获批但靶向性较低的药物，包括骨形态发生蛋白-2（bone morphogenetic protein-2，BMP-2）和双膦酸盐。在使用 $Nf1^{+/-}$ 小鼠进行的开放性骨折愈合研究中，Schindeler 等（2011）发现，仅使用 BMP-2 作为促生长刺激并不能改善骨愈合。相反，BMP-2 与唑来膦酸联合使用，可能通过限制 BMP-2 诱导的破骨细胞生成增加，从而改善骨愈合（Schindeler et al. 2011）。

21.5 结论

人类 NF1 表型和相关实验模型均表明神经纤维瘤蛋白在骨细胞功能中起关键作用。NF1 中的骨骼异常并不可忽视，它们有着较高的发病率，且缺乏干预措施。尽管目前可用的小鼠模型未能完全复现 NF1 骨骼并发症的自然病史和表型，但它们提供了一个坚实的理论框架，使我们能够更好地理解 NF1 中骨异常的分子基础，并测试治疗方法。尽管他汀类药物、双膦酸盐和 BMP 在 NF1 假关节实验模型中的有益效果令人鼓舞，但这些药物也存在局限性，未来可能需要测试和开发新的治疗靶点或组合治疗方法。虽然还有很多需要了解的内容，但我们正处于将已知信息转化为临床试验的前沿（Elefteriou et al. 2009），需要协调多中心和多学科的努力来设计预防或治疗 NF1 骨骼系统异常的策略。

致谢：感谢儿童肿瘤基金会及其国际骨科联盟成员在 NF1 相关骨异常的分子基础研究的概念和思路开发中所提供的帮助。

（邱勇，乔军　译）

参考文献

[1] Alwan S, Tredwell SJ, Friedman JM (2005) Is osseous dysplasia a primary feature of neurofibro-matosis 1 (NF1)? Clin Genet 67: 378-390

[2] Blauth M, Harms D, Schmidt D, Blauth W (1984) Light- and electron-microscopic studies in congenital pseudarthrosis. Arch Orthop Trauma Surg 103: 269-277

[3] Brannan CI, Perkins AS, Vogel KS, Ratner N, Nordlund ML, Reid SW, Buchberg AM, Jenkins NA, Parada LF, Copeland NG (1994) Targeted disruption of the neurofibromatosis type-1 gene leads to developmental abnormalities in heart and various neural crest-derived tissues. Genes Dev 8: 1019-1029

[4] Briner J, Yunis E (1973) Ultrastructure of congenital pseudarthrosis of the tibia. Arch Pathol 95: 97-99

[5] Brunetti-Pierri N, Doty SB, Hicks J, Phan K, Mendoza-Londono R, Blazo M, Tran A, Carter S, Lewis RA, Plon SE, Phillips WA, O'Brian Smith E, Ellis KJ, Lee B (2008) Generalized metabolic bone disease in Neurofibromatosis type 1. Mol Genet Metab 94: 105-111

[6] Caffarelli C, Gonnelli S, Tanzilli L, Vivarelli R, Tamburello S, Balestri P, Nuti R (2010) Quantitative ultrasound and dual energy x-ray absorptiometry in children and adolescents with neurofibromatosis of type 1. J Clin Densitom 13: 77-83

[7] Cho TJ, Seo JB, Lee HR, Yoo WJ, Chung CY, Choi IH (2008) Biologic characteristics of fibrous hamartoma from congenital pseudarthrosis of the tibia associated with neurofibromatosis type 1. J Bone Joint Surg Am 90: 2735-2744

[8] Crawford AH, Schorry EK (1999) Neurofibromatosis in children: the role of the orthopaedist. J Am Acad Orthop Surg 7: 217-230

[9] Dacquin R, Starbuck M, Schinke T, Karsenty G (2002) Mouse alpha1 (I)-collagen promoter is the best known promoter to drive efficient Cre recombinase expression in osteoblast. Dev Dyn 224: 245-251

[10] Dulai S, Briody J, Schindeler A, North KN, Cowell CT, Little DG (2007) Decreased bone mineral density in neurofibromatosis type 1: results from a pediatric cohort. J Pediatr Orthop 27: 472-475

[11] Durrani AA, Crawford AH, Chouhdry SN, Saifuddin A, Morley TR (2000) Modulation of spinal deformities in patients with neurofibromatosis type 1. Spine 25: 69-75

[12] Duman O, Ozdem S, Turkkahraman D, Olgac ND, Gungor F, Haspolat S (2008) Bone metabolism markers and bone mineral density in children with neurofibromatosis type-1. Brain Dev 30: 584-588

[13] Elefteriou F, Benson MD, Sowa H, Starbuck M, Liu X, Ron D, Parada LF, Karsenty G (2006) ATF4 mediation of NF1 functions in osteoblast reveals a nutritional basis for congenital skeletal dysplasiae. Cell Metab 4: 441-451

[14] Elefteriou F, Kolanczyk M, Schindeler A, Viskochil DH, Hock JM, Schorry EK, Crawford AH, Friedman JM, Little D, Peltonen J, Carey JC, Feldman D, Xijie Y, Armstrong L, Birch P, Kendler DL, Mundlos S, Yang FC, Agiostratidou G, Hunter-Schaedle K, Stevenson DA (2009) Skeletal abnormalities in neurofibromatosis type 1: approaches to therapeutic options. Am J Med Genet A 149A: 2327-2338

[15] El-Hoss J, Sullivan K, Cheng T, Yu NY, Bobyn JD, Peacock L, Mikulec K, Baldock P, Alexander IE, Schindeler A, Little DG (2012) A murine model of neurofibromatosis type 1 tibial pseudarthrosis featuring proliferative fibrous tissue and osteoclast-like cells. J Bone Miner Res. 27: 68-78

[16] Friedman JM, Birch PH (1997) Type 1 neurofibromatosis: a descriptive analysis of the disorder in 1728 patients. Am J Med Genet 70: 138-143

[17] Gutmann DH, Aylsworth A, Carey JC, Korf B, Marks J, Pyeritz RE, Rubenstein A, Viskochil D (1997) The diagnostic evaluation and multidisciplinary management of neurofibromatosis 1 and neurofibromatosis 2. JAMA 278: 51-57

[18] Heervä E, Alanne MH, Peltonen S, Kuorilehto T, Hentunen T, Väänänen K, Peltonen J (2010) Osteoclasts in neurofibromatosis type 1 display enhanced resorption capacity, aberrant morphology, and resistance to serum deprivation. Bone 47: 583-590

[19] Illes T, Halmai V, de Jonge T, Dubousset J (2001) Decreased bone mineral density in neurofibromatosis-1 patients with spinal deformities. Osteoporos Int 12: 823-827

[20] Ippolito E, Corsi A, Grill F, Wientroub S, Bianco P (2000) Pathology of bone lesions associated with congenital pseudarthrosis of the leg. J Pediatr Orthop B 9: 3-10

[21] Johnson B, MacWilliams B, Carey JC, Viskochil DH, D'Astous JL, Stevenson DA (2010) Examination of motor proficiency in children with neurofibromatosis type 1. Pediatr Phys Ther 22: 344-348

[22] Kolanczyk M, Kossler N, Kühnisch J, Lavitas L, Stricker S, Wilkening U, Manjubala I, Fratzl P, Spörle R, Herrmann BG, Parada LF, Kornak U, Mundlos S (2007) Multiple roles for neurofibromin in skeletal development and growth. Hum Mol Genet 16: 874-886

[23] Kolanczyk M, Kühnisch J, Kossler N, Osswald M, Stumpp S, Thurisch B, Kornak U, Mundlos S (2008) Modelling neurofibromatosis type 1 tibial dysplasia and its treatment with lovastatin. BMC Med 6: 21

[24] Kossler N, Stricker S, Rödelsperger C, Robinson PN, Kim J, Dietrich C, Osswald M, Kühnisch J, Stevenson DA, Braun T, Mundlos S, Kolanczyk M (2011) Neurofibromin (Nf1) is required for normal skeletal muscle development. Hum Mol Genet 20: 2697-2709

[25] Kuorilehto T, Nissinen M, Koivunen J, Benson MD, Peltonen J (2004) NF1 tumor suppressor protein and mRNA in skeletal tissues of developing and adult normal mouse and NF1-deficient embryos. J Bone Miner Res 19: 983-989

[26] Kuorilehto T, Pöyhönen M, Bloigu R, Heikkinen J, Väänänen K, Peltonen J (2005) Decreased bone mineral density and content in neurofibromatosis type 1: lowest local values are located in the load-carrying parts of the body. Osteoporos Int 16: 928-936

[27] Lakkis MM, Epstein JA (1998) Neurofibromin modulation of ras activity is required for normal endocardial-mesenchymal transformation in the developing heart. Development 125: 4359-4367

[28] Lammert M, Kappler M, Mautner VF, Lammert K, Störkel S, Friedman JM, Atkins D (2005) Decreased bone mineral

[28] density in patients with neurofibromatosis 1. Osteoporos Int 16: 1161-1166
[29] Mariaud-Schmidt RP, Rosales-Quintana S, Bitar E, Fajardo D, Chiapa-Robles G, Gonzalez-Mendoza A, Barros-Nunuz P (2005) Hamartoma involving the pseudarthrosis site in patients with neurofibromatosis type 1. Pediatr Dev Pathol 8: 190-196
[30] Ruggieri M, Pavone V, De Luca D, Franzo A, Tine A, Pavone L (1999) Congenital bone malformations in patients with neurofibromatosis type 1 (Nf1). J Pediatr Orthop 19: 301-305
[31] Sakamoto A, Yoshida T, Yamamoto H, Oda Y, Tsuneyoshi M, Iwamoto Y (2007) Congenital pseudarthrosis of the tibia: analysis of the histology and the NF1 gene. J Orthop Sci 12: 361-365
[32] Schindeler A, Morse A, Harry L, Godfrey C, Mikulec K, McDonald M, Gasser J, Little D (2008a) Models of tibial fracture healing in normal and Nf1-deficient mice. J Orthop Res 26: 1053-1060
[33] Schindeler A, Ramachandran M, Godfrey C, Morse A, McDonald M, Mikulec K, Little DG (2008b) Modeling bone morphogenetic protein and bisphosphonate combination therapy in wild-type and Nf1 haploinsufficient mice. J Orthop Res 26: 65-74
[34] Schindeler A, Birke O, Yu NY, Morse A, Ruys A, Baldock PA, Little DG (2011) Distal tibial fracture repair in a neurofibromatosis type 1-deficient mouse treated with recombinant bone morphogenetic protein and a bisphosphonate. J Bone Joint Surg Br 93: 1134-1139
[35] Seitz S, Schnabel C, Busse B, Schmidt HU, Beil FT, Friedrich RE, Schinke T, Mautner VF, Amling M (2010) High bone turnover and accumulation of osteoid in patients with neurofibromatosis 1. Osteoporos Int 21: 119-127
[36] Souza JF, Passos RL, Guedes AC, Rezende NA, Rodrigues LO (2009) Muscular force is reduced in neurofibromatosis type 1. J Musculoskelet Neuronal Interact 9: 15-17
[37] Stevenson DA, Yang FC (2011) The musculoskeletal phenotype of the RASopathies. Am J Med Genet C 157: 90-103
[38] Stevenson DA, Birch PH, Friedman JM, Viskochil DH, Balestrazzi P, Boni S, Buske A, Korf BR, Niimura M, Pivnick EK, Schorry EK, Short MP, Tenconi R, Tonsgard JH, Carey JC (1999) Descriptive analysis of tibial pseudarthrosis in patients with neurofibromatosis 1. Am J Med Genet 84: 413-419
[39] Stevenson DA, Moyer-Mileur LJ, Carey JC, Quick JL, Hoff CJ, Viskochil DH (2005) Case-control study of the muscular compartments and osseous strength in neurofibromatosis type 1 using peripheral quantitative computed tomography. J Musculoskelet Neuron Interact 5: 145-149
[40] Stevenson DA, Zhou H, Ashrafi S, Messiaen LM, Carey JC, D'Astous JL, Santora SD, Viskochil DH (2006) Double inactivation of NF1 in tibial pseudarthrosis. Am J Hum Genet 79: 143-148
[41] Stevenson DA, Moyer-Mileur LJ, Murray M, Slater H, Sheng X, Carey JC, Dube B, Viskochil DH (2007a) Bone mineral density in children and adolescents with neurofibromatosis type 1. J Pediatr 150: 83-88
[42] Stevenson DA, Viskochil DH, Schorry EK, Crawford AH, D'Astous J, Murray KA, Friedman JM, Armstrong L, Carey JC (2007b) The use of anterolateral bowing of the lower leg in the diagnostic criteria for neurofibromatosis type 1. Genet Med 9: 409-412
[43] Stevenson DA, Schwarz EL, Viskochil DH, Moyer-Mileur LJ, Murray M, Firth SD, D'Astous JL, Carey JC, Pasquali M (2008) Evidence of increased bone resorption in neurofibromatosis type 1 using urinary pyridinium crosslink analysis. Pediatr Res 63: 697-701
[44] Stevenson DA, Viskochil DH, Carey JC, Slater H, Murray M, Sheng X, D'Astous J, Hanson H, Schorry E, Moyer-Mileur LJ (2009) Tibial geometry in individuals with neurofibromatosis type 1 without anterolateral bowing of the lower leg using peripheral quantitative computed tomography. Bone 44: 585-589
[45] Stevenson DA, Schwarz EL, Carey JC, Viskochil DH, Hanson H, Bauer S, Weng HYC, Greene T, Reinker K, Swensen J, Chan RJ, Yang FC, Senbanjo L, Yang Z, Mao R, Pasquali M (2011a) Bone resorption in syndromes of the Ras/MAPK Pathway. Clin Genet 80: 566-573
[46] Stevenson DA, Yan J, He Y, Li H, Liu Y, Jing Y, Guo Z, Zhang Q, Zhang W, Yang D, Wu X, Hanson H, Li X, Staser K, Viskochil DH, Carey JC, Chen S, Miller L, Roberson K, Moyer-Mileur L, Yang FC (2011b) Increased multiple osteoclast functions in individuals with neurofibromatosis type 1. Am J Med Genet A 155: 1050-1059
[47] Tucker T, Schnabel C, Hartmann M, Friedrich RE, Frieling I, Kruse HP, Mautner VF, Friedman JM (2009) Bone health and fracture rate in individuals with neurofibromatosis 1 (NF1). J Med Genet 46: 259-265
[48] Vitale MG, Guha A, Skaggs DL (2002) Orthopaedic manifestations of neurofibromatosis in children: an update. Clin Orthop Relat Res 401: 107-118
[49] Wang W, Nyman JS, Moss HE, Gutierrez G, Mundy GR, Yang X, Elefteriou F (2010) Local lowdose lovastatin delivery improves the bone-healing defect caused by Nf1 loss of function in osteoblasts. J Bone Miner Res 25: 1658-1667
[50] Wang W, Nyman JS, Stevenson DA, Moss H, Yang X, Elefteriou F (2011) Mice lacking Nf1 in osteochondroprogenitor cells display skeletal dysplasia similar to patients with neurofibromatosis type 1. Hum Mol Genet 20: 3910-3924
[51] Wu X, Estwick SA, Chen S, Yu M, Ming W, Nebesio TD, Li Y, Yuan J, Kapur R, Ingram D, Yoder MC, Yang FC (2006) Neurofibromin plays a critical role in modulating osteoblast differentiation of mesenchymal stem/progenitor cells. Hum Mol Genet 15: 2837-2845
[52] Wu X, Chen S, He Y, Rhodes SD, Mohammad KS, Li X, Yang X, Jiang L, Nalepa G, Snider P, Robing AG, Clapp DW, Conway SJ, Guise TA, Yang FC (2011) The haploinsufficient hematopoietic microenvironment is critical to the pathological fracture repair in murine models of neurofibromatosis type 1. PLoS One 6: e24917
[53] Yan J, Chen S, Zhang Y, Li X, Li Y, Wu X, Yuan J, Robling AG, Kapur R, Chan RJ, Yang FC (2008) Rac1 mediates the osteoclast gains-in-function induced by haploinsufficiency of Nf1. Hum Mol Genet 17: 936-948
[54] Yang FC, Chen S, Robling AG, Yu X, Nebesio TD, Yan J, Morgan T, Li X, Yuan J, Hock J, Ingram DA, Clapp DW (2006) Hyperactivation of p21ras and PI3K cooperate to alter murine and human neurofibromatosis type 1-haploinsufficient osteoclast functions. J Clin Invest 116: 2880-2891
[55] Yilmaz K, Ozmen M, Bora Goksan S, Eskiyurt N (2007) Bone mineral density in children with neurofibromatosis 1.

Acta Paediatr 96: 1220-1222

[56] Young H, Hyman S, North K (2002) Neurofibromatosis 1: clinical review and exceptions to the rules. J Child Neurol 17: 613-621

[57] Yu X, Chen S, Potter OL, Murthy SM, Li J, Pulcini JM, Ohashi N, Winata T, Everett ET, Ingram D, Clapp WD, Hock JM (2005) Neurofibromin and its inactivation of Ras are prerequisites for osteoblast functioning. Bone 36: 793-802

[58] Zhang W, Rhodes SD, Zhao L, He Y, Zhang Y, Shen Y, Yang D, Wu X, Li X, Yang X, Park SJ, Chen S, Turner C, Yang FC (2011) Primary osteopathy of vertebrae in a neurofibromatosis type 1 murine model. Bone 48: 1378-1387

[59] Zhu Y, Romero MI, Ghosh P, Ye Z, Charnay P, Rushing EJ, Marth JD, Parada LF (2001) Ablation of NF1 function in neurons induces abnormal development of cerebral cortex and reactive gliosis in the brain. Genes Dev 15: 859-876

第22章 1型神经纤维瘤病相关视神经胶质瘤
NF1 – Associated Optic Glioma

Anne C. Solga and David H. Gutmann

22.1 引言

1型神经纤维瘤病（NF1）是一种常见的具有肿瘤易感性的、常染色体显性遗传的综合征，患者有罹患良性和恶性肿瘤的风险。

在中枢神经系统（central nervous system，CNS）中，累及视路的星形（胶质）细胞瘤（即视路胶质瘤，optic pathway gliomas，OPG）最为常见，可见于15%～20%的NF1患者（图22.1）。世界卫生组织（WHO）认定的Ⅰ级胶质瘤可位于从视神经到视交叉后视束视路的任何部位（Listernick et al. 1995）。大多数患者是7岁以下的儿童（Listernick et al. 2007）。与散发OPG病例相反，NF1相关的OPG大多数不会导致进行性的视力损害。在首诊时，近一半患NF1相关OPG的儿童会出现视力损害，但只有不到1/3的患儿会出现进一步的视力下降（Listernick et al. 1997）。大多数累及视交叉前和视交叉的OPG不会出现进展，但累及视束（视交叉后方）的OPG更容易出现病变进展（Balcer et al. 2001）并需要治疗。这些肿瘤的一线治疗都是卡铂/长春新碱化学治疗（Demaerel et al. 2002；Kato et al. 1998）。

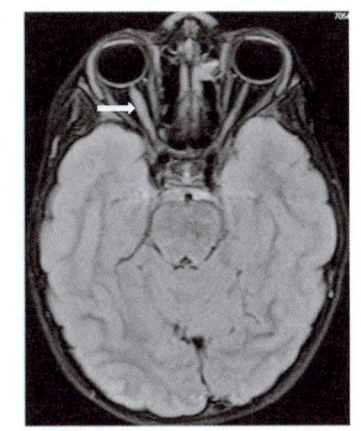

图22.1 NF1相关的OPG。磁共振成像显示右侧视神经胶质瘤。箭头所指为右侧视神经胶质瘤所致视神经增粗

22.2 神经胶质瘤发生的决定因素

NF1相关胶质瘤在幼儿视路中好发的这一特征性现象，支持胶质瘤的形成需要多种必要条件结合的理论，必要条件包括：对不同生长调节通路易感的细胞、特定的促生长的微环境和基因组修饰因子（图22.2）。

22.2.1 神经纤维瘤蛋白生长控制通路

*NF1*基因产物（神经纤维瘤蛋白，neurofibromin）最初被鉴定为一种大小为220 kDa的大细胞质蛋白，含有与Ras负性调节蛋白共有的结构域（Xu et al. 1990b）。与其他GTP酶激活蛋白（GTPase-activating protein，GAP）分子类似，神经纤维瘤蛋白通过将活性GTP结合型Ras转化为非活性GDP结合型，从而加速Ras的失活（Xu et al. 1990a）。在某些细胞中，神经纤维瘤蛋白的缺失

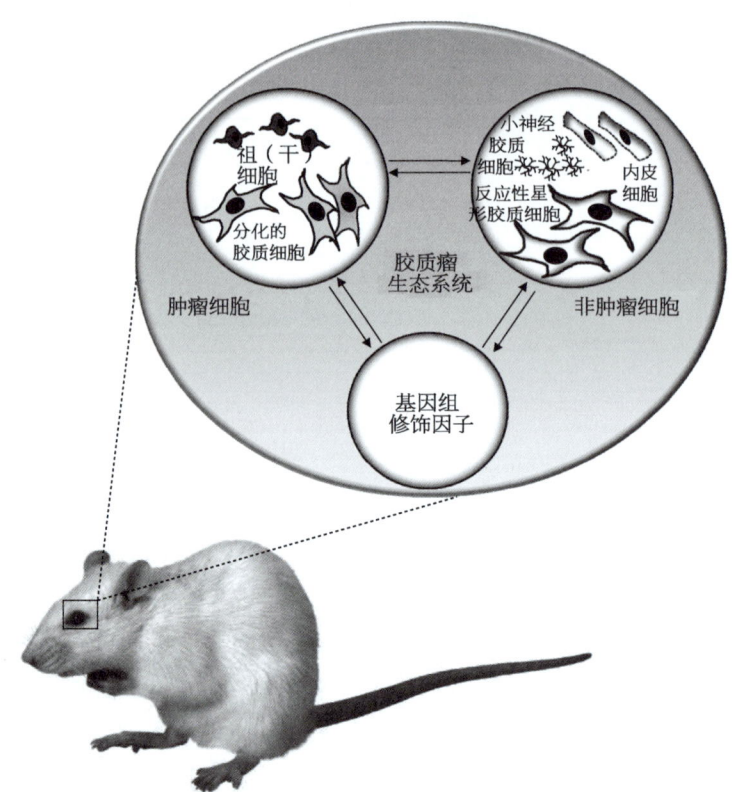

图 22.2 NF1 相关胶质瘤发生的必要条件。视路胶质瘤的发生是受基因组中的修饰基因、肿瘤微环境中的非肿瘤细胞以及癌前/肿瘤细胞协同影响的结果。在易感的癌前/肿瘤细胞中,肿瘤的发生伴随着 *Nf1* 抑癌基因表达的缺失。这些 *Nf1* 缺陷的神经胶质细胞会产生一些分子,来招募或激活小胶质细胞和其他基质细胞(内皮细胞和活性星形胶质细胞),从而创造一个有利于肿瘤发生的微环境。肿瘤微环境中的非肿瘤细胞反过来也会产生更多的分子("胶质诱导剂"),进一步促进肿瘤胶质细胞的生长、肿瘤转化和肿瘤进展。基因组修饰因子通过目前尚未明确的方式导致肿瘤易感性及促进肿瘤生长

会导致 Ras 活性升高、细胞生长失调和致癌性转化,故神经纤维瘤蛋白具有肿瘤抑制蛋白的作用。

虽然神经纤维瘤蛋白可以通过抑制 Ras 通路信号来对细胞生长进行负调节,但在不同类型细胞中,Ras 的下游效应蛋白却各不相同。例如,神经纤维瘤蛋白调控造血细胞生长依赖于 Ras/MEK 通路的激活(Bollag et al. 1996),而对星形胶质细胞的生长调控则依赖于 Akt 介导的哺乳动物雷帕霉素靶标(mammalian target of rapamycin, mTOR)通路的激活(Dasgupta et al. 2005)。此外,神经纤维瘤蛋白调节 Akt/mTOR 相关生长调节的机制在不同类型的细胞中也不尽相同。在已建立的细胞系和恶性周围神经鞘膜瘤(MPNST)细胞中,*NF1* 基因失活会导致结节性硬化症复合体(tuberous sclerosis complex, TSC)蛋白的 Akt 磷酸化,并增加脑中富集的 Ras 同源物(Ras homolog enriched in brain, Rheb)和 Rheb 介导的 mTOR 的激活(Johannessen et al. 2005)。相反,神经纤维瘤蛋白对于星形胶质细胞的生长调节无须 TSC/Rheb 信号通路(Banerjee et al. 2011)(图 22.3a)。

mTOR 是一种重要的丝氨酸/苏氨酸激酶,它与许多其他蛋白质组成复合物来共同调节细胞生长。当它与 raptor 蛋白结合时(Kim et al. 2002),mTOR 复合物 1(mTOR complex 1,mTORC1)会使核糖体 S6 激酶和 4EBP1 磷酸化,从而调节蛋白质翻译和核糖体的生物生成(Hara et al. 1997)。

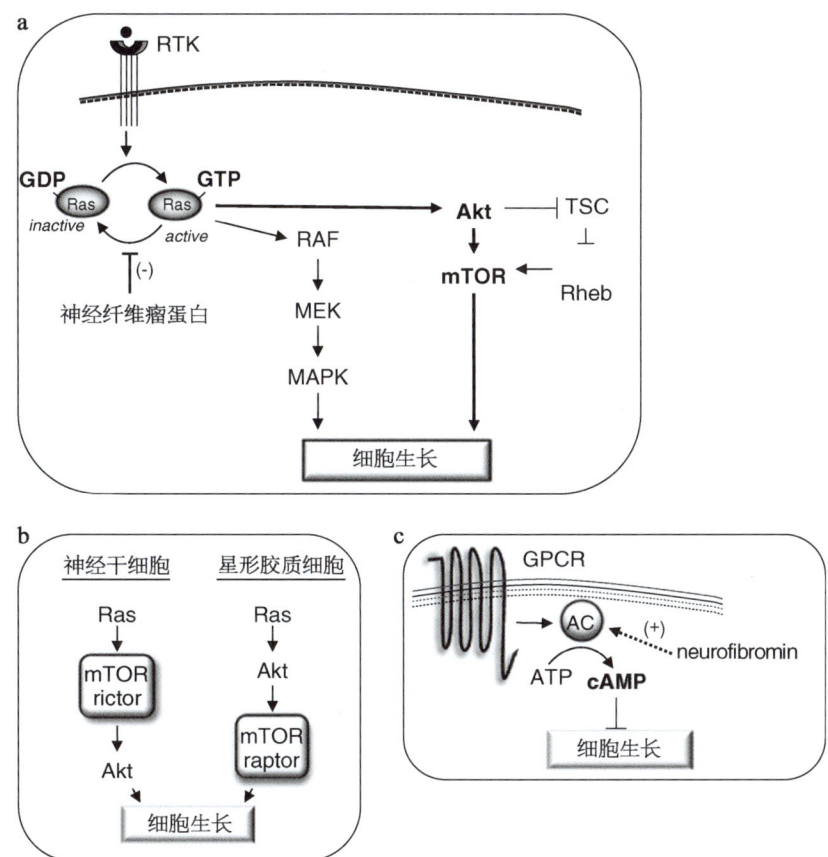

图 22.3 神经纤维瘤蛋白相关信号通路。神经纤维瘤蛋白可通过受体酪氨酸激酶(RTK)和 G 蛋白偶联受体(GPCR)来调控细胞内信号通路。a. NF1 基因产物,神经纤维瘤蛋白是 Ras 原癌基因的负调控因子,它可加速活性的 GTP 结合型 Ras 向非活性的 GDP 结合型 Ras 转化。活性 Ras 通过激活 RAF/MEK/MAPK 和 Akt/mTOR 通路启动下游信号转导。b. 在脑干的神经干细胞中,细胞生长受 rictor(TORC2)介导的 Akt 激活的调节,而在星形胶质细胞中,细胞生长则依赖于 Akt 介导的 TORC1 复合物(raptor)激活来调。c. 神经纤维瘤蛋白还能正向调节腺苷酸环化酶(AC)的活性,导致细胞内环状 AMP(cAMP)的水平升高。在星形胶质细胞中,cAMP 可促进细胞增殖和存活

当 mTOR 与 rictor 蛋白结合时(Sarbassov et al. 2004),mTOR 复合物 2(mTOR complex 2,mTORC2)通过 Rac1 调节 Akt 的活化以及肌动蛋白的细胞骨架功能(Sarbassov et al. 2005)。在星形胶质细胞中,神经纤维瘤蛋白通过 Rac1-(Sandsmark et al. 2007)和 STAT3 依赖的通路(Banerjee et al. 2010)调节细胞生长,而在神经干细胞(neural stem cell, NSC)中,神经纤维瘤蛋白通过 Akt 依赖的通路来调节细胞生长(Lee et al. 2010)(图 22.3b)。

由于 Ras-GAP 结构域只占整个神经纤维瘤蛋白多肽的 10%,因此该分子的其他区域也很可能对其功能起着重要作用。早期在黑腹果蝇中进行的研究表明,神经纤维瘤蛋白能调节环磷酸腺苷(cyclic AMP,cAMP)信号转导(The et al. 1997;Guo et al. 1997)。在小鼠神经元和星形胶质细胞中,神经纤维瘤蛋白也能正向调节细胞内 cAMP 的水平(Tong et al. 2002;Dasgupta et al. 2003)。在星形胶质细胞中,神经纤维瘤蛋白是 cAMP 生成的正向调节因子(Dasgupta et al. 2003),因此 Nf1 缺失会导致细胞内 cAMP 水平降低和细胞存活不良(图 22.3c)。同样,在神经元中,神经纤维瘤蛋白表达下降会导致 Rho-相关激酶(Rho-associated kinase,ROCK)的 cAMP/PKA 激活下降和肌球蛋白轻链(myosin light chain,MLC)磷酸化的减少,从而导

致神经元生长受限（Brown et al. 2010，2011）。尽管目前还不清楚神经纤维瘤蛋白是如何激活腺苷酸环化酶的，但可能与至少两种不同的机制相关。第一种与受体酪氨酸激酶激活相关，其作用独立于G蛋白偶联受体（G-protein-coupled receptor，GPCR），并可能与Ras通路相关。第二种机制涉及GPCR信号通路，且与Ras无关（Hannan et al. 2006）。

22.2.2 视路胶质瘤的细胞异质性

与其他实体瘤类似，OPG也是含有非肿瘤细胞和癌前/肿瘤细胞的混合物。非肿瘤（基质）部分由免疫系统细胞（小胶质细胞）、正常细胞（神经元）、反应性星形胶质细胞和肿瘤相关血管（内皮细胞）组成。肿瘤部分包含祖（干）细胞和分化的神经胶质细胞。这些不同类型的细胞都可能影响胶质瘤的形成和生长。

22.2.2.1 肿瘤细胞成分

研究表明，来自不同脑区的小鼠星形胶质细胞和神经干细胞（neural stem cell，NSC）对 $Nf1$ 基因失活的促增殖能力的反应各不相同，这也印证了NF1中癌前/肿瘤细胞的异质性有助于胶质瘤发生。小鼠视神经和脑干的星形胶质细胞中表达神经纤维瘤蛋白，而新大脑皮质星形胶质细胞（在儿童中，胶质瘤很少发生在此处）的 $Nf1$ 基因表达水平较低（Yeh et al. 2009）。与神经纤维瘤蛋白表达差异模式相一致的是，在 $Nf1$ 基因缺失后，脑干和视神经的星形胶质细胞在体外和体内都会出现增殖，而新大脑皮质的星形胶质细胞则不会出现增殖（Yeh et al. 2009）。

同样，来自 $Nf1$ 缺陷小鼠脑干的神经干细胞在体外的增殖能力增强，在体内分化不同胶质细胞的能力增强。相反，来自 $Nf1$ 缺陷小鼠大脑皮质的神经干细胞却没有这种特性。这种对 $Nf1$ 缺陷的不同反应是因为脑干神经干细胞中 rictor 表达增加，从而导致 TORC2 介导的 Akt 磷酸化以及神经干细胞生长和胶质分化的增加（Lee da et al. 2010）。

综上所述，虽然 $Nf1$ 失活是神经胶质瘤发生过程中的必经步骤，但它必须在一种能够对神经纤维瘤蛋白表达丧失做出增殖反应的细胞中发生才行。

22.2.2.2 非肿瘤细胞成分

除了有易感的癌前细胞外，胶质瘤的形成和生长还需要非肿瘤性的肿瘤微环境（基质）。基因工程小鼠（genetically-engineered mouse，GEM）实验首次揭示了这种基质依赖性：在胶质纤维酸性蛋白（glial fibrillary acidic protein，GFAP）阳性的胶质祖细胞中，$Nf1$ 基因表达缺失并不会导致视路胶质瘤的发生（Bajenaru et al. 2002）。在小鼠中，只有在神经胶质祖细胞 $Nf1$ 缺陷与 $Nf1$ 杂合性同时存在的情况下，才会导致胶质瘤，这与NF1患儿情况类似（Bajenaru et al. 2003）。非肿瘤细胞中 $Nf1$ 基因表达减少的必要性提示：胶质瘤的发生需要 $Nf1^{+/-}$ 的基质细胞与 $Nf1$ 缺陷的癌前/肿瘤细胞的协同作用。

这些基质细胞类型之一是小胶质细胞（单核细胞类似细胞）（Markovic et al. 2009），它们占人类低级别胶质瘤总细胞数的30%，也存在于Nf1小鼠视路神经胶质瘤中（Simmons et al. 2011）。多项实验证据表明，小胶质细胞在Nf1视路胶质瘤的生长中起关键作用。第一，$Nf1^{+/-}$，非野生型，小胶质细胞在体外能促进 $Nf1^{-/-}$ 星形胶质细胞的增殖。第二，使用四环素类似物米诺环素抑制小胶质细胞功能后能在体内抑制视神经胶质瘤的生长（Daginakatte and Gutmann 2007）。第三，药物阻断对 $Nf1^{+/-}$ 小胶质细胞功能至关重要的 c–Jun 氨基末端激酶（Jun N-terminal Kinase，JNK）信号通路能减少体内视神经胶质瘤的生长（Daginakatte et al. 2008）。第四，在体内，基因沉默小胶质细胞会抑制视神经胶质瘤的生长（Simmons et al. 2011）。

与胶质瘤相关的小胶质细胞能够产生大量生长因子和细胞因子，包括肿瘤坏死因子α（tumor necrosis factor α，TNF–α）、表皮生长因子（epidermal growth factor，EGF）和趋化因子（如 CXCL12），这些因子与神经胶质细胞上的受体结合以促进其生长和存活（Sawada et al. 1989）。CXCL12通过cAMP依赖的途径促进 $Nf1^{-/-}$ 星形胶质细胞的存活。最近，有研究发现通过药理学干预来恢复正常的cAMP水平后，可抑制小鼠视路胶质瘤的生长，这也强调了CXCL12和cAMP在NF1胶质瘤形成中的重要性。相反，在Nf1视路胶质瘤小鼠的皮质中,一种降解 cAMP 的酶(磷酸二酯酶-4 PDE4)的异常表达会导致胶质瘤的形成(Warrington et al. 2010)。

22.2.3 基因组对视路胶质瘤发生的贡献

多项研究均强调了遗传修饰因子的重要性。第一,Easton 及其同事发现,包括视路胶质瘤在内的 4 种 NF1 的临床特征具有显著的家族聚集性,这提示上位基因与 *NF1* 位点分离(Easton et al. 1993)。第二,GeneNetwork 数据库(Chesler et al. 2005)的微阵列数据显示,不同小鼠品系之间的 *Nf1* 表达水平存在差异。第三,Reilly 及其同事的研究显示,C57BL/6 基因工程小鼠中形成星形细胞瘤的概率较高,而在 129S4 基因工程小鼠中则对胶质瘤的形成相对耐受(Reilly et al. 2000)。尽管这些胶质瘤的修饰基因尚未被明确,但 *NF1* 基因表达的自然差异与潜在的基因位点被认为是影响 NF1 患儿胶质瘤形成的必要条件。

22.3 用于临床前药物研究的 *Nf1* 基因工程鼠

开始治疗的时机主要基于临床表现进展,最常见的是视力下降。对于 NF1 患儿的 OPG,通常采用化学治疗,而非手术或放射治疗。尽管卡铂/长春新碱是 OPG 的初始治疗方案,但对于临床上病情进展的儿童,往往需要额外的基因毒性治疗,这可能导致对学习和行为十分重要的增殖区(干细胞微环境)的继发性损害。

尽管针对有前景的抗肿瘤药物的初步评估通常基于异种移植物或细胞培养,但缺乏低级别胶质瘤的模型。因此,Nf1 视路胶质瘤的基因工程鼠应运而生。这些模型为我们在启动人体临床试验之前来评估新药的治疗方案提供了前所未有的机会。

22.3.1 靶向肿瘤细胞

由于神经纤维瘤蛋白是 Ras 的负调节因子,最初的治疗研究集中于 Ras 的抑制剂。Ras 必须通过翻译后异戊二烯化才能定位于细胞质膜,后向其下游效应器传递信号。因此,早期的 NF1 临床试验集中于法尼基转移酶抑制剂,但遗憾的是,这并没有减少肿瘤生长(Widemann et al. 2006)。

Ras 抑制剂在临床试验中的效果不佳,促使研究者进一步探索神经纤维瘤蛋白的调控靶点。通过蛋白质组学对 *Nf1* 缺陷的星形胶质细胞中差异表达蛋白的筛选分析,最终鉴定出 mTOR 是神经纤维瘤蛋白生长调控的下游效应物(Dasgupta et al. 2005)。结合其他人的相似工作(Johannessen et al. 2005),使用 mTOR 抑制剂雷帕霉素的临床前研究已开展。雷帕霉素治疗能减少 Nf1 视路胶质瘤小鼠的肿瘤细胞增殖以及缩小肿瘤体积,并呈现剂量依赖性(Hegedus et al. 2008)。这些令人振奋的结果推进了雷帕霉素类似物治疗 NF1 相关的丛状神经纤维瘤和低级别胶质瘤的临床试验。

对 mTOR 调控 *Nf1* 缺陷星形胶质细胞生长的进一步研究表明,mTOR 依赖的生长调控需要 Rac1 的激活(Sandsmark et al. 2007)。通过高通量化合物筛选分析,葫芦素-Ⅰ被认为是 *Nf1* 缺陷星形胶质细胞生长的抑制剂。葫芦素-Ⅰ抑制 STAT3 的激活,而 STAT3 是 mTOR 的下游效应物(Banerjee et al. 2010)。未来的临床前研究拟评估抑制 mTOR 的药物在 Nf1 视路胶质瘤小鼠中的功效。

22.3.2 瞄准肿瘤微环境

几十年来,化学治疗主要针对癌症中的肿瘤细胞。Judah Folkman 首次开创性地提出可以利用肿瘤与内皮细胞之间的相互作用,通过减少血管生成(Folkman, 1972),来破坏肿瘤内的干细胞微环境(Calabrese et al. 2007)。近来,对低级别胶质瘤的化学治疗方法采用了阿瓦斯汀(avastin)来抑制血管内皮生长因子(vascular endothelial growth factor, VEGF)及其受体(Packer et al. 2009)。除了靶向血管内皮细胞,小胶质细胞也可能是未来针对 NF1 相关视路胶质瘤基质靶向疗法的合理靶点(见 22.2.2)。

22.3.3 神经保护策略

虽然标准化学治疗能使 60%～80% 的 NF1 相关 OPG 儿童的肿瘤稳定,但仅少量(20%)患者的视力得到改善(Dalla Via et al. 2007)。在 Nf1 视路胶质瘤小鼠中，胶质瘤形成早期可以观察到视神经轴突的超微结构损伤和视网膜神经节细胞（retinal ganglion cell，RGC）的不可逆损失（凋亡）（Hegedus 等，2009）。这种 $Nf1^{+/-}$ RGC 神经细胞死亡是由于 cAMP 水平降低引起的，因此通过药理学方法提高 cAMP 水平可在体内减轻凋亡（Brown et al. 2010）。这些发现提出了一种令人振奋的可能疗法，即将神经保护疗法与靶向肿瘤细胞和非肿瘤细胞的新化学治疗方法相结合，可能改善儿童 NF1 相关 OPG 的疗效。

22.3.4 瞄准肿瘤生态系统

治疗儿童低级别胶质瘤充满挑战，这也提示我们需要考虑其他的替代疗法。鉴于繁多的细胞类型和基因组之间存在复杂的交互作用，治疗需要将胶质瘤视为一个生态系统。

生态系统是由相互作用的生物体和非生物的物理环境成分组成。不同成分之间的有机分工和合作是生态系统的关键特征之一。这在群居性昆虫世界中得到了很好的展现：巢穴由成百上千只具有专业分工的动物个体组成——包括生殖（王后）和非生殖阶层（Thorne et al. 2003；Amdam and Page 2010；Hartmann and Heinze 2003）。

同样地，胶质瘤也是具有高度异质性的组织，它由具有不同等级的细胞组织和特定功能的不同细胞类型（"阶层"）组成。一些细胞主要负责繁殖（肿瘤细胞），而其他细胞则负责维护（非肿瘤细胞）。所有这些不同类型细胞间的协同（相互）作用对于维持整个肿瘤的健康完整至关重要。

在这一概念框架下，未来 OPG 的治疗将需要更详细地了解每种细胞类型的独立作用和在肿瘤整体中发挥的团体作用。此外，由于肿瘤生态系统依赖关系网络运行，因此有必要开发能够破坏这些关系网络并重建肿瘤组织新稳态的治疗方法。

这种生态系统疗法可能会减少当前疗法对发育中大脑的毒性，从而降低胶质瘤治疗相关的长期认知后遗症的发生。

22.4 NF1 相关 OPG 治疗的未来

在过去的 10 年里，我们对视路胶质瘤形成的遗传基础，以及特定非肿瘤细胞和肿瘤细胞对胶质瘤发生和维持作用的认识有了极大的提高。科学水平的进步也让我们发现了几种有前景的治疗 NF1 相关肿瘤（包括 OPG）的药物，并进行了临床前和临床评估。随着快速筛选靶向药物的高通量技术的应用、有效的临床前药物测试模型、多中心 NF 临床试验联盟的建立，未来很有希望能将基础研究成果高效地转化到临床予以应用。尽管目前仍未明确，但前沿的个性化治疗正在路上，我们有望通过基因分析、先进的神经影像研究和预测性生物标志物，将患者分层为对特定靶向疗法具有高反应性的临床亚组。可靠的小动物模型、先进的多重高通量技术以及专业治疗中心的融合，将使研究人员和临床医师能够将最先进的方法应用于脑肿瘤的管理，不仅限于 NF1 儿童患者，还可能包括散发性儿童和成人脑肿瘤患者。

致谢：我们感谢古特曼实验室成员在本章编写过程中提出的有用意见。这项工作得到了美国国立癌症研究所（U01‑CA141549）和詹姆斯‑麦克唐纳基金会（James S. McDonnell Foundation）的部分资助。

（赵培泉，彭婕　译）

参考文献

[1] Amdam GV, Page RE (2010) The developmental genetics and physiology of honeybee societies. Anim Behav 79：973 - 980

[2] Bajenaru ML, Zhu Y, Hedrick NM, Donahoe J, Parada LF, Gutmann DH (2002) Astrocyte-specific inactivation of the neurofibromatosis 1 gene (NF1) is insufficient for astrocytoma formation. Mol Cell Biol 22：5100 - 5113

[3] Bajenaru ML, Hernandez MR, Perry A, Zhu Y, Parada LF, Garbow JR, Gutmann DH (2003) Optic nerve glioma in mice requires astrocyte Nf1 gene inactivation and Nf1 brain heterozygosity. Cancer Res 63：8573 - 8577

[4] Balcer LJ, Liu GT, Heller G, Bilaniuk L, Volpe NJ, Galetta SL, Molloy PT, Phillips PC, Janss AJ, Vaughn S, Maguire MG (2001) Visual loss in children with neurofibromatosis type 1 and optic pathway gliomas：relation to tumor location by magnetic resonance imaging. Am J Ophthalmol 131：442 - 445

[5] Banerjee S, Byrd JN, Gianino SM, Harpstrite SE, Rodriguez FJ, Tuskan RG, Reilly KM, Piwnica-Worms DR, Gutmann DH (2010) The neurofibromatosis type 1 tumor suppressor

controls cell growth by regulating signal transducer and activator of transcription-3 activity in vitro and in vivo. Cancer Res 70: 1356-1366
[6] Banerjee S, Crouse NR, Emnett RJ, Gianino SM, Gutmann DH (2011) Neurofibromatosis-1 regulates mTOR-mediated astrocyte growth and glioma formation in a TSC/Rheb-independent manner. Proc Natl Acad Sci USA 108: 15996-16001
[7] Bollag G, Clapp DW, Shih S, Adler F, Zhang YY, Thompson P, Lange BJ, Freedman MH, McCormick F, Jacks T, Shannon K (1996) Loss of NF1 results in activation of the Ras signaling pathway and leads to aberrant growth in haematopoietic cells. Nat Genet 12: 144-148
[8] Brown JA, Gianino SM, Gutmann DH (2010) Defective cAMP generation underlies the sensitivity of CNS neurons to neurofibromatosis-1 heterozygosity. J Neurosci 30: 5579-5589
[9] Brown JA, Diggs-Andrews KA, Gianino SM, Gutmann DH (2012) Neurofibromatosis-1 hetero-zygosity impairs CNS neuronal morphology in a cAMP/PKA/ROCK-dependent manner. Mol Cell Neurosci 49: 13-22
[10] Calabrese C, Poppleton H, Kocak M, Hogg TL, Fuller C, Hamner B, Oh EY, Gaber MW, Finklestein D, Allen M, Frank A, Bayazitov IT, Zakharenko SS, Gajjar A, Davidoff A, Gilbertson RJ (2007) A perivascular niche for brain tumor stem cells. Cancer Cell 11: 69-82
[11] Chesler EJ, Lu L, Shou S, Qu Y, Gu J, Wang J, Hsu HC, Mountz JD, Baldwin NE, Langston MA, Threadgill DW, Manly KF, Williams RW (2005) Complex trait analysis of gene expression uncovers polygenic and pleiotropic networks that modulate nervous system function. Nat Genet 37: 233-242
[12] Daginakatte GC, Gutmann DH (2007) Neurofibromatosis-1 (Nf1) heterozygous brain microglia elaborate paracrine factors that promote Nf1-deficient astrocyte and glioma growth. Hum Mol Genet 16: 1098-1112
[13] Daginakatte GC, Gianino SM, Zhao NW, Parsadanian AS, Gutmann DH (2008) Increased c-Jun-NH2-kinase signaling in neurofibromatosis-1 heterozygous microglia drives microglia activation and promotes optic glioma proliferation. Cancer Res 68: 10358-10366
[14] Dalla Via P, Opocher E, Pinello ML, Calderone M, Viscardi E, Clementi M, Battistella PA, Laverda AM, Da Dalt L, Perilongo G (2007) Visual outcome of a cohort of children with neurofibromatosis type 1 and optic pathway glioma followed by a pediatric neuro-oncology program. Neuro Oncol 9: 430-437
[15] Dasgupta B, Dugan LL, Gutmann DH (2003) The neurofibromatosis 1 gene product neurofibromin regulates pituitary adenylate cyclase-activating polypeptide-mediated signaling in astrocytes. J Neurosci 23: 8949-8954
[16] Dasgupta B, Yi Y, Chen DY, Weber JD, Gutmann DH (2005) Proteomic analysis reveals hyperactivation of the mammalian target of rapamycin pathway in neurofibromatosis 1-associated human and mouse brain tumors. Cancer Res 65: 2755-2760
[17] Demaerel P, de Ruyter N, Casteels I, Renard M, Uyttebroeck A, van Gool S (2002) Visual pathway glioma in children treated with chemotherapy. Eur J Paediatr Neurol 6: 207-212
[18] Easton DF, Ponder MA, Huson SM, Ponder BA (1993) An analysis of variation in expression of neurofibromatosis (NF) type 1 (NF1): evidence for modifying genes. Am J Hum Genet 53: 305-313
[19] Folkman J (1972) Anti-angiogenesis: new concept for therapy of solid tumors. Ann Surg 175: 409-416
[20] Guo HF, The I, Hannan F, Bernards A, Zhong Y (1997) Requirement of Drosophila NF1 for activation of adenylyl cyclase by PACAP38-like neuropeptides. Science 276: 795-798
[21] Hannan F, Ho I, Tong JJ, Zhu Y, Nurnberg P, Zhong Y (2006) Effect of neurofibromatosis type I mutations on a novel pathway for adenylyl cyclase activation requiring neurofibromin and Ras. Hum Mol Genet 15: 1087-1098
[22] Hara K, Yonezawa K, Kozlowski MT, Sugimoto T, Andrabi K, Weng QP, Kasuga M, Nishimoto I, Avruch J (1997) Regulation of eIF-4E BP1 phosphorylation by mTOR. J Biol Chem 272: 26457-26463
[23] Hartmann A, Heinze J (2003) Lay eggs, live longer: division of labor and life span in a clonal ant species. Evolution 57: 2424-2429
[24] Hegedus B, Banerjee D, Yeh TH, Rothermich S, Perry A, Rubin JB, Garbow JR, Gutmann DH (2008) Preclinical cancer therapy in a mouse model of neurofibromatosis-1 optic glioma. Cancer Res 68: 1520-1528
[25] Hegedus B, Hughes FW, Garbow JR, Gianino S, Banerjee D, Kim K, Ellisman MH, Brantley MA Jr, Gutmann DH (2009) Optic nerve dysfunction in a mouse model of neurofibromatosis-1 optic glioma. J Neuropathol Exp Neurol 68: 542-551
[26] Johannessen CM, Reczek EE, James MF, Brems H, Legius E, Cichowski K (2005) The NF1 tumor suppressor critically regulates TSC2 and mTOR. Proc Natl Acad Sci USA 102: 8573-8578
[27] Kato T, Sawamura Y, Tada M, Ikeda J, Ishii N, Abe H (1998) Cisplatin/vincristine chemotherapy for hypothalamic/visual pathway astrocytomas in young children. J Neurooncol 37: 263-270
[28] Kim DH, Sarbassov DD, Ali SM, King JE, Latek RR, Erdjument-Bromage H, Tempst P, Sabatini DM (2002) mTOR interacts with raptor to form a nutrient-sensitive complex that signals to the cell growth machinery. Cell 110: 163-175
[29] Lee DY, Yeh TH, Emnett RJ, White CR, Gutmann DH (2010) Neurofibromatosis-1 regulates neuroglial progenitor proliferation and glial differentiation in a brain region-specific manner. Genes Dev 24: 2317-2329
[30] Listernick R, Darling C, Greenwald M, Strauss L, Charrow J (1995) Optic pathway tumors in children: the effect of neurofibromatosis type 1 on clinical manifestations and natural history. J Pediatr 127: 718-722
[31] Listernick R, Louis DN, Packer RJ, Gutmann DH (1997) Optic pathway gliomas in children with neurofibromatosis 1: consensus statement from the NF1 Optic Pathway Glioma Task Force. Ann Neurol 41: 143-149
[32] Listernick R, Ferner RE, Liu GT, Gutmann DH (2007) Optic pathway gliomas in neurofibromatosis-1: controversies and recommendations. Ann Neurol 61: 189-198
[33] Markovic DS, Vinnakota K, Chirasani S, Synowitz M, Raguet H, Stock K, Sliwa M, Lehmann S, Kalin R, van Rooijen N, Holmbeck K, Heppner FL, Kiwit J, Matyash V, Lehnardt S, Kaminska B, Glass R, Kettenmann H (2009) Gliomas induce and exploit microglial MT1-MMP expression for tumor expansion. Proc Natl Acad Sci USA 106: 12530-12535
[34] Packer RJ, Jakacki R, Horn M, Rood B, Vezina G, MacDonald T, Fisher MJ, Cohen B (2009) Objective response of multiply recurrent low-grade gliomas to bevacizumab and irinotecan. Pediatr Blood Cancer 52: 791-795

[35] Reilly KM, Loisel DA, Bronson RT, McLaughlin ME, Jacks T (2000) Nf1;Trp53 mutant mice develop glioblastoma with evidence of strain-specific effects. Nat Genet 26: 109-113

[36] Sandsmark DK, Zhang H, Hegedus B, Pelletier CL, Weber JD, Gutmann DH (2007) Nucleophosmin mediates mammalian target of rapamycin-dependent actin cytoskeleton dynamics and proliferation in neurofibromin-deficient astrocytes. Cancer Res 67: 4790-4799

[37] Sarbassov DD, Ali SM, Kim DH, Guertin DA, Latek RR, Erdjument-Bromage H, Tempst P, Sabatini DM (2004) Rictor, a novel binding partner of mTOR, defines a rapamycin-insensitive and raptor-independent pathway that regulates the cytoskeleton. Curr Biol 14: 1296-1302

[38] Sarbassov DD, Guertin DA, Ali SM, Sabatini DM (2005) Phosphorylation and regulation of Akt/PKB by the rictor-mTOR complex. Science 307: 1098-1101

[39] Sawada M, Kondo N, Suzumura A, Marunouchi T (1989) Production of tumor necrosis factor-alpha by microglia and astrocytes in culture. Brain Res 491: 394-397

[40] Simmons GW, Pong WW, Emnett RJ, White CR, Gianino SM, Rodriguez FJ, Gutmann DH (2011) Neurofibromatosis-1 heterozygosity increases microglia in a spatially and temporally restricted pattern relevant to mouse optic glioma formation and growth. J Neuropathol Exp Neurol 70: 51-62

[41] The I, Hannigan GE, Cowley GS, Reginald S, Zhong Y, Gusella JF, Hariharan IK, Bernards A (1997) Rescue of a Drosophila NF1 mutant phenotype by protein kinase A. Science 276: 791-794

[42] Thorne BL, Breisch NL, Muscedere ML (2003) Evolution of eusociality and the soldier caste in termites: influence of intraspecific competition and accelerated inheritance. Proc Natl Acad Sci USA 100: 12808-12813

[43] Tong J, Hannan F, Zhu Y, Bernards A, Zhong Y (2002) Neurofibromin regulates G protein-stimulated adenylyl cyclase activity. Nat Neurosci 5: 95-96

[44] Warrington NM, Gianino SM, Jackson E, Goldhoff P, Garbow JR, Piwnica-Worms D, Gutmann DH, Rubin JB (2010) Cyclic AMP suppression is sufficient to induce gliomagenesis in a mouse model of neurofibromatosis-1. Cancer Res 70: 5717-5727

[45] Widemann BC, Salzer WL, Arceci RJ, Blaney SM, Fox E, End D, Gillespie A, Whitcomb P, Palumbo JS, Pitney A, Jayaprakash N, Zannikos P, Balis FM (2006) Phase I trial and pharmacokinetic study of the farnesyltransferase inhibitor tipifarnib in children with refractory solid tumors or neurofibromatosis type I and plexiform neurofibromas. J Clin Oncol 24: 507-516

[46] Xu GF, Lin B, Tanaka K, Dunn D, Wood D, Gesteland R, White R, Weiss R, Tamanoi F (1990a) The catalytic domain of the neurofibromatosis type 1 gene product stimulates ras GTPase and complements ira mutants of S. cerevisiae. Cell 63: 835-841

[47] Xu GF, O'Connell P, Viskochil D, Cawthon R, Robertson M, Culver M, Dunn D, Stevens J, Gesteland R, White R et al (1990b) The neurofibromatosis type 1 gene encodes a protein related to GAP. Cell 62: 599-608

[48] Yeh TH, da Lee Y, Gianino SM, Gutmann DH (2009) Microarray analyses reveal regional astrocyte heterogeneity with implications for neurofibromatosis type 1 (NF1)-regulated glial proliferation. Glia 57: 1239-1249

第23章 1型神经纤维瘤病患者心血管异常的分子基础
Molecular Basis of Cardiovascular Abnormalities in NF1

Brian K. Stansfield, David A. Ingram, Simon J. Conway, and Jan M. Friedman

大多数 NF1 患者的血管病变涉及多个动脉，呈斑点状分布。NF1 的血管病变通常是无症状的，尽管首次临床表现可能是危及生命或致命的事件。NF1 患者的血管病变可能出现在任何部位，但最常见于肾动脉，通常与高血压有关。脑血管疾病通常导致颈内动脉、大脑中动脉或大脑前动脉狭窄，并常伴有烟雾病。

目前没有针对 NF1 患者所有部位的血管病变进行系统筛查的队列研究，因此 NF1 患者中血管病变的整体发病率尚不清楚。在儿童、青少年或成年早期死亡的 NF1 患者中，血管病变是一个出乎意料的常见死因。

我们对神经纤维瘤蛋白在心血管系统发育中作用的理解大多来自对靶向小鼠突变体的研究。杂合子 $Nf1^{+/-}$ 小鼠并未发生自发性心血管疾病，而纯合 $Nf1^{-/-}$ 突变体在中期妊娠死于双出口右心室、膜性室间隔缺损和心内膜垫的比例增大。对谱系限制纯合子基因敲除小鼠的研究表明，内皮细胞在这些心脏畸形的发病机制中起着关键作用，pERK 激活导致心内膜垫过度增殖。

小鼠模型显示，杂合子 $Nf1^{+/-}$ 内皮细胞表型和功能正常，但这些细胞对环境变化和生长因子较为敏感。NF1 的成年人外周血中内皮集落形成细胞的数量正常，但这些细胞在血管生成生长因子的作用下表现出 ERK 活化增强、增殖和迁移增强。

血管壁中的每一种细胞类型，包括内皮细胞、血管平滑肌细胞（vascular smoothmuscle cell，VSMC）和周细胞，都已经证明具有增殖潜能。人类 NF1 血管病变的特征性病变是内膜增生和新内膜形成，内膜 VSMC 的类似增殖已经在小鼠模型中使用多种技术得到证实。对谱系限制性敲除小鼠的研究表明，在 VSMC 中 Ras-Mek-ERK 信号通路被放大，可能在新内膜形成中发挥重要作用。过继性骨髓移植实验证明，骨髓中 Nf1 的杂合灭活也是损伤后新生内膜形成所必需的。一个关键因素可能是骨髓来源的巨噬细胞产生的细胞因子刺激 VSMC 增殖。

尽管心血管异常作为 NF1 的一个特征已被认识超过 65 年（Reubi 1945；Feyrter 1949），但对于这些病变的频率和自然发展过程仍然了解不完全。然而，最近的研究为部分 NF1 患者发生的先天性心脏缺陷和血管病变的分子发病机制提供了重要见解。

23.1 先天性心脏缺陷

在已报道的 NF1 患者系列中，临床上明显的先天性心脏缺陷（congenital heart defects，CHD）的患病率为 0.4%～6.4%（Lin et al. 2000）。报道频率差异较大的原因可能是心脏缺陷的确定方法不同、患者年龄以及诊断标准差异。Tedesco 等（2002）对 48 例非选择性 NF1 儿童和青少年进行了二维超声心动图和彩色多普勒研究，发现 4 例（8%）心血管疾病：1 例肺动脉狭窄，1 例主动脉缩窄，2 例肥厚性心肌病，而在 30 名同龄儿童对照组中未发现异常。

事实上，NF1 与 CHD 相关的最有力证据是，这些患者中有相当高比例的先天性心脏病是肺动脉狭窄，通常是瓣膜型。在 NF1 患者中，肺动脉狭窄约占所有 CHD 的 1/4（Lin et al. 2000），是 NF1-Watson 综合征、NF1-Noonan 综合征和 NF1 基因大片段缺失个体三种临床亚型的公认特征。瓣膜型肺动脉狭窄也是 Noonan 综合征、LEOPARD 综合征或心脏-面部-皮肤综合征患者的共同特征，这些疾病与 NF1 一样，是导致 Ras/MAPK 通路失调的遗传性疾病（Zenker 2011）。

主动脉缩窄在 NF1 患者中已被反复报道（Lin et al. 2000），然而这些患者的狭窄通常为长梭状形。这在解剖学上不同于其他主动脉缩窄患者中最常见的突发性节段性缩窄。肥厚性心肌病在一些 NF1 患者中也有报道，但比较少见（Friedman et al. 2002）。

右心室双出口是一种圆锥动脉干畸形，发生在纯合子 Nf1 "敲除"小鼠胚胎中（Brannan et al. 1994；Jacks et al. 1994），但在 NF1 患者中似乎相当罕见。事实上，引人注意的是，任何类型的复杂 CHD 在 NF1 患者中均较为少见（Lin et al. 2000；Friedman et al. 2002）。

23.2 NF1 血管病变

NF1 血管病变可累及从小动脉到近端主动脉的各种大小动脉。体循环受累的发生率远高于肺动脉，尽管后者也可能受累。病变也可能累及心脏的流出道或静脉。大多数 NF1 患者血管病变累及多支血管（Friedman et al. 2002；Oderich et al. 2007）。

NF1 血管病变患者通常无症状，但其首发临床症状即有可能是致命的。据报道，NF1 型血管病变的年轻患者可因大动脉破裂、脑缺血或出血以及心肌梗死而猝死（Friedman et al. 2002）。NF1 血管病变的病理结果可能包括动脉狭窄、闭塞、动脉瘤、假性动脉瘤、血管破裂或瘘管形成。这种情况有时会进展，随着时间的推移，病变变得更加严重，或者在最初看似有效的治疗后复发（Criado et al. 2002；Rea et al. 2009；Ghosh et al. 2012）。

NF1 患者的血管病变最常见于肾动脉，约 1%～5% 的 NF1 患者患有肾动脉疾病（Friedman et al. 2002），NF1 患者高血压的发生可能是由于近端肾动脉狭窄、肾实质内动脉异常或两者兼而有之。肾血管性高血压通常出现在 NF1 患者的儿童期、青少年期或成年早期；在妊娠期，有时会被认为是子痫或恶性高血压（Dugoff and Sujansky 1996）。

NF1 患者的脑血管异常通常由颈内动脉、大脑中动脉或大脑前动脉狭窄或闭塞引起（Friedman et al. 2002）。狭窄区域周围可形成细小的毛细血管扩张，在脑血管造影上看起来像一团烟雾。NF1 患者似乎异常容易出现这种被称为"烟雾病"的表现，这是脑对缺氧（Wu et al. 2006）或放射损伤（Ullrich et al. 2007；Milewicz et al. 2010）的反应。

23.3 NF1 血管病变的患病率、发病率和死亡率

目前尚无针对 NF1 患者的人群队列进行系统性的血管病筛查，但有一些研究评估了临床系列中血管病变的不同特征。在一个病例系列中，在接受 MRI 检查的 398 例 NF1 患儿中，有 15 人（3.8%）出现颅内动脉狭窄或闭塞，或者有烟雾病（Ghosh et al. 2012）。Rosser 等（2005）检查了 316 例未经选择的 NF1 患儿的颅脑 MRI，发现 8 例（2.5%）有脑血管异常。在另一个病例系列，在 144 名接受颅脑

MRI 检查的 NF1 患者中，有 7 人(4.9%)出现了脑动脉发育不良(Cairns and North 2008)。大多数研究对象的动脉病变并没有引发症状。

在另外一项研究中，接受 MRI 检查的 266 名 NF1 患儿中，有 17 名(6.4%)出现了一条或多条颅内动脉狭窄、烟雾病或动脉瘤(Rea et al. 2009)。这些患者大多因中枢神经系统症状而进行影像学检查，17 名患者中有 15 名同时患有视神经胶质瘤，但是没有相关放射治疗的信息。

接受过颅内肿瘤放射治疗的患者患烟雾病的风险增加(Milewicz et al. 2010)，这在 NF1 患者中尤为常见(Ullrich et al. 2007)。这种关联的病理基础尚不清楚，可能原因包括放射损伤诱发 NF1 患者血管损伤增加、血管异常修复或新血管增殖增加。

Fossali 等(2000)筛选了 27 名非选择性 NF1 患儿，发现其中 3 人(11%)患有高血压，另外 2 人患有临界性高血压。其中 13 例患者接受了静脉数字减影血管造影检查，发现 7 例肾动脉狭窄和 1 例主动脉缩窄。对两组年轻 NF1 患者进行了 24 小时血压监测，分别包括 20 名和 73 名受试者(Fossali et al. 2000；Tedesco et al. 2005)。24 小时血压测量值异常在较小的系列中为 40%，在较大的系列中为 16%。部分 24 小时监测异常的患者基础血压测量值正常。

肺动脉高压也可能发生在 NF1 患者中，尽管其发生率远低于动脉高血压(Stewart et al. 2007；Montani et al. 2011)。与动脉性高压不同，肺动脉高压在 50 岁以下 NF1 患者中罕见，常合并肺实质疾病。

在儿童期、青少年期或成年早期死亡的 NF1 患者中，血管病变似乎是一个出乎意料的常见死亡原因(Rasmussen et al. 2001)。在 NF1 患者中，50 岁之前死亡的人数大幅度增加(Rasmussen et al. 2001)。这种超额死亡率大部分可归因于肿瘤，特别是恶性周围神经鞘膜瘤，但与血管疾病相关的死亡在 NF1 年轻成年人中也比预期更常见(Sørensen et al. 1986；Rasmussen et al. 2001；Evans et al. 2011)。

在一组未经筛选的尸检病例中，Salyer 和 Salyer(1974)发现 18 名 NF1 患者中有 8 名出现血管病变的组织学病变，这些患者死亡时的中位年龄为 24 岁(4~69 岁)。这些患者中只有 1 人死于血管疾病；其他 7 名受影响患者的血管病变没有症状。8 名 NF1 患者中有 6 名肾脏受累，在他们之中，多条动脉受到影响，包括心脏、胰腺、甲状腺、回肠、脾脏和脑膜等部位的动脉。

23.4 胚胎学

神经纤维瘤蛋白在胚胎发育和心血管发育中起着至关重要的作用。在动物模型中，心血管畸形是由于神经纤维瘤蛋白活性显著或完全丧失，以及胚胎中关键心血管谱系内异常增殖的组成性 Ras 刺激引起的(Viskochil, 2002)。然而，神经纤维瘤蛋白半失活对心脏发育和功能的作用尚不清楚。

我们对 NF1 在子宫内作用的大部分认识来自动物研究，主要是针对小鼠突变体和最近的斑马鱼结果(Brannan et al. 1994；Jacks et al. 1994；Gitler et al. 2003；Ismat et al. 2006；Xu et al. 2007；Padmanabhan et al. 2009)。有些令人惊讶的是，Nf1 杂合小鼠在出生后可存活，并且没有表现出任何子宫内心血管异常。小鼠和人类 NF1 杂合子心血管发育表型之间脱节的原因尚不清楚，可能是由于所使用的小鼠遗传背景的近交性质或缺乏复杂的实验工具来分析和绘制部分外显表型所致。

然而，系统性 Nf1 缺失突变体可表现出妊娠中期致死性和流出道分隔缺陷(右心室双出口/膜性室间隔缺损)，并伴有心内膜垫扩大(Brannan et al. 1994；Jacks et al. 1994)。虽然 Nf1 缺失妊娠中期死亡的确切原因尚不清楚，但胚胎的显著水肿表明心功能不良或反流异常、舒张功能障碍可能导致胚胎子宫内死亡(Conway et al. 2003；Phoon et al. 2004)。

考虑到神经嵴在 NF1 肿瘤形成和流出道分隔缺陷发病机制中的作用，以及周围神经系统中神经嵴来源的细胞具有最高的神经纤维瘤蛋白表达水平，这些心血管缺陷被推测起源于心脏神经嵴细胞(Kirby et al. 1983；Daston and Ratner 1992；Zhu et al. 2002；Hutson and Kirby 2003；Snider et al. 2007；Yang et al. 2008)。尽管神经嵴限制性失活导致周围神经组织过度生长，然而，最近的谱系限制性小鼠基因敲除方法令人意外地揭示，使用 Tie2-cre 介导的 Nf1 失活在内皮谱系内的组织特异性失活再现了子宫内 Nf1 缺失的心脏异常（Gitler et al. 2003；Ismat et al. 2006）。

此外，这些转基因小鼠显示，胚胎心内膜（心脏瓣膜的前体）中 Nf1 的缺失直接导致活化 GTP 结合的 Ras 增加。由此产生的 MAPK 信号通路刺激导致流出道隔膜异常扩大。内皮细胞中神经纤维瘤蛋白 GTP 酶激活蛋白（GTPaseactivating protein，GAP）相关结构域的恢复足以调节 Ras 活性并挽救 Nf1 基因缺失胚胎中观察到的 CHD（Ismat et al. 2006）。

尽管这些精细的转基因数据表明 NF1 在胚胎内皮中具有细胞自主作用，并且可能提供潜在的治疗靶点，但应该注意的是，这些研究中使用的 Tie2 启动子在胚胎和胚胎外内皮谱系中都有表达，并且已知在造血干细胞中也有活性（Forde et al. 2002）。因此，考虑到 NF1 的骨髓增殖特征以及单倍不足的造血微环境对 NF1 疾病进展的重要性，心血管内皮在 NF1 缺陷型 CHD 发病机制中的确切作用仍有待验证。同样，在心血管形态发生过程中，Nf1 缺陷的增殖性神经嵴谱系的潜在修饰作用和子宫内效应，以及它与邻近的心内膜和内皮谱系的相互作用也仍然未知（Gitler et al. 2002；Wang et al. 2005）。

神经纤维瘤蛋白作为 Ras 通路的调节因子的功能和 ERK 超活化的证明具有一致性，有人将其与 Noonan 综合征进行了类比（Mangues et al. 1998；Friedman et al. 2002；Araki et al. 2004；Lasater et al. 2008）。Noonan 综合征是一种常染色体显性遗传病，特征为身材矮小、面部畸形、心脏缺陷，并可能增加患白血病的风险（Araki et al. 2004）。约 50% 的 Noonan 综合征患者可发生 PTPN11 突变，并导致肺动脉瓣狭窄、肥厚型心肌病、房间隔缺损、法洛四联症、主动脉缩窄以及二尖瓣异常（Marino et al. 1999）。除了表现出类似的心血管表型范围外，NF1 和 Noonan 综合征的小鼠模型都具有增大的心内膜垫，ERK 表达增加，这与右心室双出口和流出道垫增厚一致（Araki et al. 2004）。此外，最近有一份报告提到 1 名早期死亡的婴儿患有严重的心血管缺陷，并被发现携带了 NF1 基因的一个错义突变和 PTPN11 基因的一个致病突变（Prada et al. 2011）。

因此，Nf1 缺失小鼠的子宫内心血管表现似乎是由一条调控 CHD 的通路引起的，在这个通路中，内皮驱动的内膜垫过度增殖与 pERK 激活相关。该机制与 NF1 基因单倍不足患者中 CHD 的发病机制之间的关系有待进一步研究，但在人类中，CHD 可能也涉及多种细胞谱系，这些细胞谱系以基因剂量依赖性和通路选择性的方式做出回应。

23.5　血管生成

血管的形成和增殖是实体瘤生长的重要组成部分，是肿瘤治疗的重要靶点。形成离散的、独立的血管网络的能力，被称为"血管生成开关"，是肿瘤传播所必需的，并已在各种 NF1 相关肿瘤中得到证实。施万细胞是神经纤维瘤的主要细胞类型，已在许多动物模型和人类肿瘤样本中显示发生了血管生成转换（Sheela et al. 1990；Kim et al. 1997；Mashour et al. 1999；Munchhof et al. 2006）。Sheela 等（1990）利用 NF1 患者的肿瘤样本首次证明了神经纤维瘤能够在不依赖其他生长因子的情况下刺激血管发育的能力。在发育中的鸡胚的绒毛膜尿囊膜（chorioallantoic membrane，CAM）上孵育单细胞集落表明，野生型（wild-type，WT）施万细胞、成纤维细胞和来自非 NF1 患者的肿瘤碎片未能诱导血管生成反应。然而，来自 NF1 患者的肿瘤碎片刺激了新生血管的强劲增殖，这样的增殖在 48 小时内就可以很容易看到，在 10 天内就已经非常普遍。添加成纤维细胞生长因子（fibroblast growth factor，bFGF），一种已知的血管生成生长因子，显著增强了这种反应。对来自神经纤维瘤的施万细胞和成纤维细胞的单细胞系的应用显示，富含施万细胞的培养物具有很高的血管生成能力，并经常侵入 CAM 的中胚层，而神经纤维瘤中的另一常见细胞群成纤维细胞未能诱导血管形成（Sheela et al. 1990）。

对 NF1$^{-/-}$ 施万细胞培养的条件培养基的检查表明，血管生成生长因子的平衡发生了改变，有利于增殖。与 WT 条件培养基相比，NF1$^{-/-}$ 施万细胞条件培养基中的血小板反应蛋白-1、血小板衍生生长因子β和中期因子 mRNA 表达升高（Mashour et al. 2001）。此外，内皮细胞（endothelial cell，EC）与 NF1$^{-/-}$ 施万细胞条件培养基孵育产生了高增殖的内皮细胞表型，类似于受血管内皮生长因子（vascular endothelial growth factor，VEGF）或成纤维细胞生长因子-2（fibroblast growth factor-2，FGF-2）刺激。这种反应是通过 Ras-Mek-ERK 信号的过度激活介导的，并且可以在体内使用 Mek-ERK 信号的特异性抑制剂来消除（Munchhof et al. 2006）。这是一个重要的观察结果，因为在一些肿瘤血管生成模型中已经观察到内皮细胞表型的改变。在神经纤维瘤的发展过程中，每一个或所有这些生长因子在促进血管生成中的作用，以及血管生成转换促进肿瘤生长的机制仍然是未来研究的领域。

尽管早期的实验集中在 Nf1 纯合缺失的突变细胞系上，但越来越多的证据表明，基质细胞的单倍体不足对 Nf1 肿瘤的增殖和血管生成具有重要意义。小鼠新生血管模型已经证明，杂合子内皮细胞、周细胞和异常的新生血管网络对缺氧的反应是过度增殖的，而同窝对照组在含氧环境中不存在这种现象（Wu et al. 2006；Ozerdem 2004）。此外，与对照组相比，Nf1$^{+/-}$ 小鼠在角膜植入含有 bFGF 或 VEGF 微球后，角膜新生血管形成、内皮细胞增殖和迁移显著增加（Munchhof et al. 2006；Wu et al. 2006）。

重要的是，与野生型对照相比，Nf1$^{-/-}$ 施万细胞条件培养基中含有浓度增加的几种促血管生成肽，通过放大 Ras-Mek-ERK 信号通路进一步放大了杂合子小鼠的血管生成（Mashour et al. 2001；Munchhof et al. 2006）。特别有趣的是，Wu 等（2006）注意到，与对照组相比，Nf1$^{+/-}$ 角膜的新生血管区域中的巨噬细胞数量增加近 5 倍，伴有显著的肥大细胞浸润。这是一个重要的观察结果，因为巨噬细胞和肥大细胞在肿瘤生长和新生血管生成中发挥关键作用。这些研究共同表明，杂合内皮细胞的表型和功能正常，但与野生型对照相比，对环境变化和生长因子的反应过度。

总体而言，有大量的小鼠和人类数据表明神经纤维瘤的血管生成潜力增加。此外，循环祖细胞在血管发育和血管生成中起着重要作用，是几种肿瘤类型的敏感生物标志物。具体而言，内皮祖细胞可以从成人外周血中分离出来，并含有具有增殖潜力和从头形成血管能力的新型内皮集落形成细胞（endothelial colony-forming cell，ECFC）群（Ingram 等，2004）。尽管 NF1 患者外周血中的 ECFC 数量正常，但与年龄和性别匹配的对照组相比，NF1 患者对血管生成因子 VEGF 和 bFGF 的反应显示出 ECFC 增殖和迁移增加。此外，从 NF1 患者中分离出的 ECFC 表现出 ERK 活化增加，但当与 Mek-ERK 信号转导的特异性抑制剂一起孵育时，它们的增殖潜力降低至非 NF1 水平。这与使用转导的人类细胞系的体外和体内研究类似，并为先前的模型系统提供了验证。

23.6 NF1 心血管疾病模型

NF1 的基因产物，神经纤维瘤蛋白，在构成血管壁的每一种细胞类型中都有表达，包括内皮细胞、血管平滑肌细胞（vascular smooth muscle cell，VSMC）和周细胞（Norton et al. 1995；Ozerdem 2004；Li et al. 2006；Munchhof et al. 2006）。这些细胞系的高增殖潜力，以及循环骨髓来源的细胞（它们提供维持血管壁稳态的生长因子和细胞因子），已经在体外实验中得到证实（Ozerdem 2004；Li et al. 2006；Munchhof et al. 2006；Xu et al. 2007）。然而，由于纯合突变小鼠的致死性，建立临床前 NF1 相关心血管疾病的小鼠模型很困难（Friedman et al. 2002）。此外，NF1 纯合性缺失是人类动脉疾病的不准确代表，因为患者的 NF1 纯合性缺失可能会导致显性（而非轻微）疾病。因此，重点放在利用杂合背景和谱系限制性 Nf1 失活的小鼠模型上，提供了更为可行和准确的研究代表。

Nf1 相关心血管疾病的特征性表型是由内膜增生（或新内膜形成）引起的动脉狭窄（Hamilton and Friedman 2000；Friedman et al. 2002）。在小鼠模型中，VSMC 在内膜层的增殖已经通过多种技术得到证实。两种损伤机制（使用串珠导丝的内皮剥脱和颈总动脉分叉近端结扎）在 NF1 新生内膜形成的研究中特别有用。此外，使用谱系限制的转基因小鼠提供了一个易于操作的平台，以细胞特异性方式测试神经纤维瘤蛋白杂合子和纯合子缺失对血管重塑的贡献。

为了建立新生内膜增生的初步模型，Xu 等（2007）通过将 α-平滑肌肌动蛋白 cre（SM22a-Cre）小鼠与 $Nf1^{fl/-}$ 小鼠（带有单个 floxed 等位基因的杂合子小鼠）进行杂交，产生了叠加在 $Nf1$ 单倍不足背景上的在 VSMC 中具有谱系限制的 $Nf1$ 纯合缺失的后代。这些小鼠以预期的孟德尔比率出生，出生时表型正常，并适当发育（Xu et al. 2007）。心血管系统的检查显示，大动脉呈现正常的表型，类似于野生型小鼠（Xu et al. 2007）。作为对颈动脉结扎后的反应，$Nf1^{fl/-}$；SM22a-Cre 小鼠的内膜增厚程度以及内膜/中膜比例较野生型小鼠增加了 2.5 倍，表明增殖仅限于内膜层，而中膜层并未同时增殖（Xu et al. 2007）。平滑肌细胞是新生内膜中最常见的细胞类型，与野生型对照相比，平滑肌细胞的数量和增殖指数显著增加（Xu et al. 2007）。然而，这个模型产生的表型只在单倍不足背景下才明显，这表明另一细胞谱系是 NF1 血管病变的主要效应细胞。

新生内膜层中 VSMC 的积聚表明 NF1 在 VSMC 的增殖、迁移和存活中起着至关重要的作用（Li et al. 2006；Xu et al. 2007）。几项研究表明，与野生型相比，小鼠和人类 VSMC 的增殖和迁移明显增加，并对生长因子有反应（Xu et al. 2007；Munchhof et al. 2006；Li et al. 2006；Lasater et al. 2010）。有趣的是，与野生型 VSMC 相比，用 PDGFBB 刺激 $Nf1$ 单倍体不足的小鼠 VSMC 会激活 Ras-ERK 和 PI-3 激酶 AKT 通路，导致增殖增加 2 倍，迁移增加 4 倍。这些表型变化可能是通过 Ras-ERK 信号通路介导的，因为使用特定的 Mek 抑制剂和恢复 $Nf1$ GAP 相关结构域会导致明显的 ERK 失活，并将 $Nf1$ 杂合子 VSMC 的增殖和迁移恢复到野生型对照组的水平。

对 $Nf1^{fl/-}$；SM22a-Cre 小鼠新生物内膜的检查显示，pERK 阳性细胞明显多于 WT 小鼠，表明 Ras-Mek-ERK 信号通路被放大，可能在新生内膜形成和血管修复中发挥重要作用（Xu et al. 2007）。此外，$Nf1$ GAP 相关结构域的修复将新生内膜形成降至与 WT 小鼠相同的水平（Xu et al. 2007）。这些观察引人关注，并为 NF1 血管病变的演变提供了见解，因为携带 PDGF-BB-Ras-ERK 轴信号转导增加的基因突变的小鼠会出现过度的新生内膜形成和动脉闭塞，类似于 NF1 血管病变患者的表现（Jin et al. 2000；Zhang et al. 2008）。

为了单独研究 $Nf1$ 杂合性的作用，Lasater 等（2008）在 $Nf1^{+/-}$ 和 WT 小鼠中使用导丝对颈总动脉进行了内皮剥脱。作为对损伤的反应，$Nf1^{+/-}$ 小鼠内膜面积和内膜-中膜比例显著增加，与其他模型和 NF1 血管病变患者类似（图 23.1）。与之前的报道一样，增殖的 VSMC 占新生内膜细胞的 75% 以上，并观察到显著的 pERK 染色（Lasater et al. 2008）。有趣的是，在损伤前使用 PDGF 信号抑制剂格列卫进行预处理，$Nf1^{+/-}$ 中新生内膜的形成显著减少。这意味着，新生内膜形成，或者更具体地说，VSMC 的增殖，可能是通过 Ras-Mek-ERK 信号通路介导的（Lasater et al. 2008）。这是一个重要的心血管疾病模型，表明在无已知风险因素的无症状 NF1 患者中可能存在异常血管重塑的表现。

为了进一步明确神经纤维瘤蛋白在血管壁稳态和重塑中的作用，Lasater 等（2010）建立了仅在内皮细胞和平滑肌细胞缺失单个 Nf1 等位基因的小鼠模型。作为对颈动脉结扎的反应，$Nf1^{fl/+}$；Tie2Cre（ECs）、$Nf1^{fl/+}$；SM22Cre（VSMCs）和 $Nf1^{fl/+}$；Tie2；SM22Cre（EC 和 VSMC）小鼠与 WT 小鼠有相似的新生内膜形成；与 $Nf1^{+/-}$ 小鼠相比，这些基因型中的内膜增殖明显减少，这表明新生内膜形成和 VSMC 增殖并非主要通过血管壁内 $Nf1$ 的杂合性缺失介导（Lasater et al. 2010）。然而，使用过继造血干细胞移植技术，与用 $Nf1^{+/-}$ 骨髓重构的 $Nf1^{+/-}$ 小鼠相比，用 WT 骨髓重构的 $Nf1^{+/-}$ 小鼠新生内膜面积减少了 10 倍，I/M 比例降低了 9 倍（Lasater et al. 2010）（图 23.2）。此外，与用 $Nf1^{+/-}$ 骨髓移植的 $Nf1^{+/-}$ 小鼠相比，用 $Nf1^{+/-}$ 骨髓移植的 WT 小鼠新生内膜形成增加（Lasater et al. 2010)(图23.2)。

这些使用过继骨髓移植的实验强烈表明,骨髓中 $Nf1$ 的杂合失活在损伤反应性新内膜形成中起着关键作用(Lasater et al. 2010)。正如先前关于血管重塑的研究中所指出的,巨噬细胞是新生内膜内最常见的骨髓来源造血细胞(Wu et al. 2006; Lasater et al. 2010)。这是一个重要的观察结果,因为新内膜内的巨噬细胞产生刺激 VSMC 增殖的细胞因子,并产生金属蛋白酶,而这些是新生内膜形成中细胞外基质重塑所必需的(Bendeck et al. 1994)。

小鼠模型为我们理解 NF1 心血管疾病的发病机制做出了重要贡献,但一些重要问题仍未得到解答。参与 VSMC 增殖和新生内膜形成的原代骨髓来源的造血细胞尚未正式确定。谱系限制的转基因小鼠将继续在鉴定主要细胞方面发挥核心作用,因为巨噬细胞、肥大细胞和淋巴细胞都被认为是血管重塑的重要因素(Strom et al. 2007;Swirski et al. 2007)。

我们对介导新生内膜内 VSMC 增殖的信号通路的性质仍然知之甚少。ERK 染色在新生内膜中显著增加,且细胞培养实验表明 Ras‑Mek‑ERK 信号通路在 VSMC 增殖和迁移中起到了重要作用,尽管通过分子治疗或使用转基因小鼠来使 ERK 信号通路失活尚未在体内得到证实。这些实验对于理解疾病发病机制、合理设计生物标志物以及为 NF1 血管病变患者开发潜在的治疗策略是必要的。

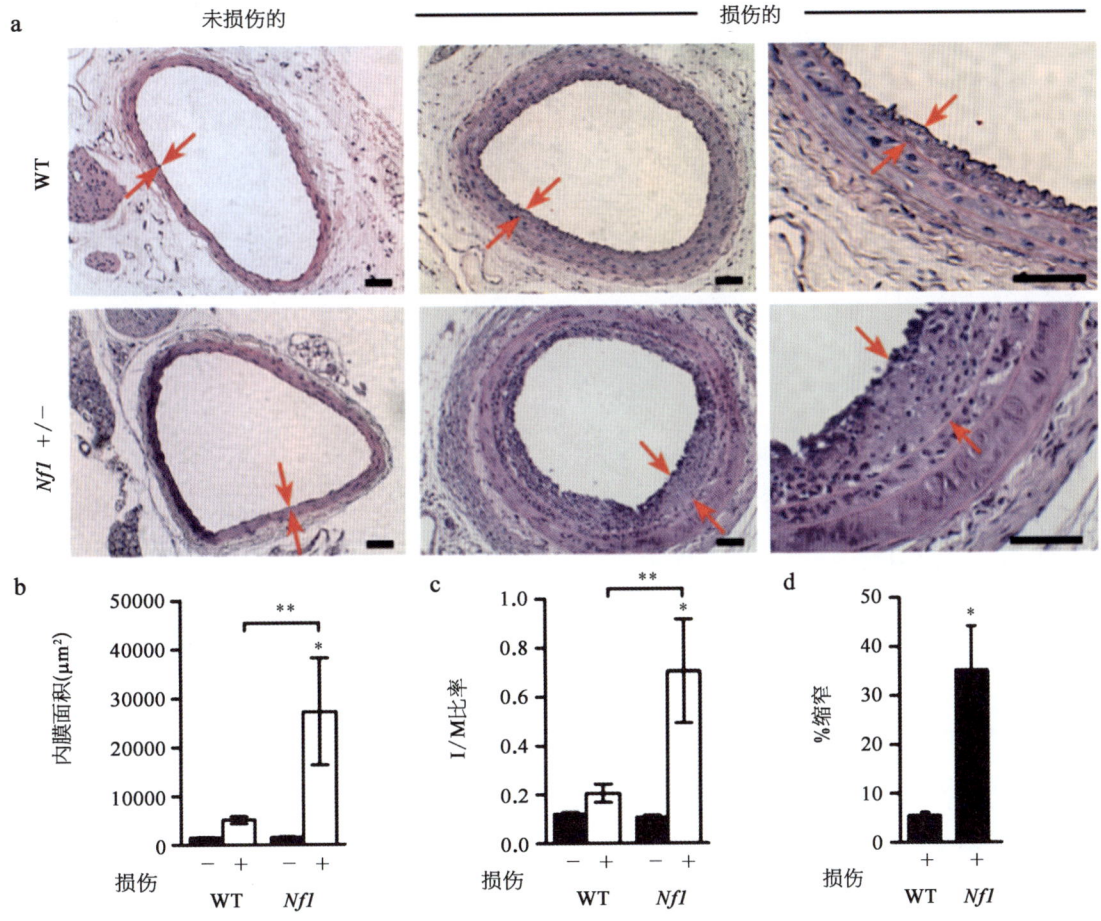

图23.1 WT 和 $Nf1^{+/-}$ 小鼠颈动脉损伤的组织学和形态计量学分析。a. 代表性的颈动脉显微照片,WT(上排)和 $Nf1^{+/-}$(下排)。红色箭头表示新生内膜的边界。b. WT 和 $Nf1^{+/-}$ 小鼠未损伤和损伤颈动脉横断面的内膜面积。c. WT 和 $Nf1^{+/-}$ 小鼠颈动脉未损伤和损伤横断面的 I/M 比值。d. WT 和 $Nf1^{+/-}$ 小鼠损伤后 21 天颈动脉狭窄百分比($*<0.05$;$**<0.005$)

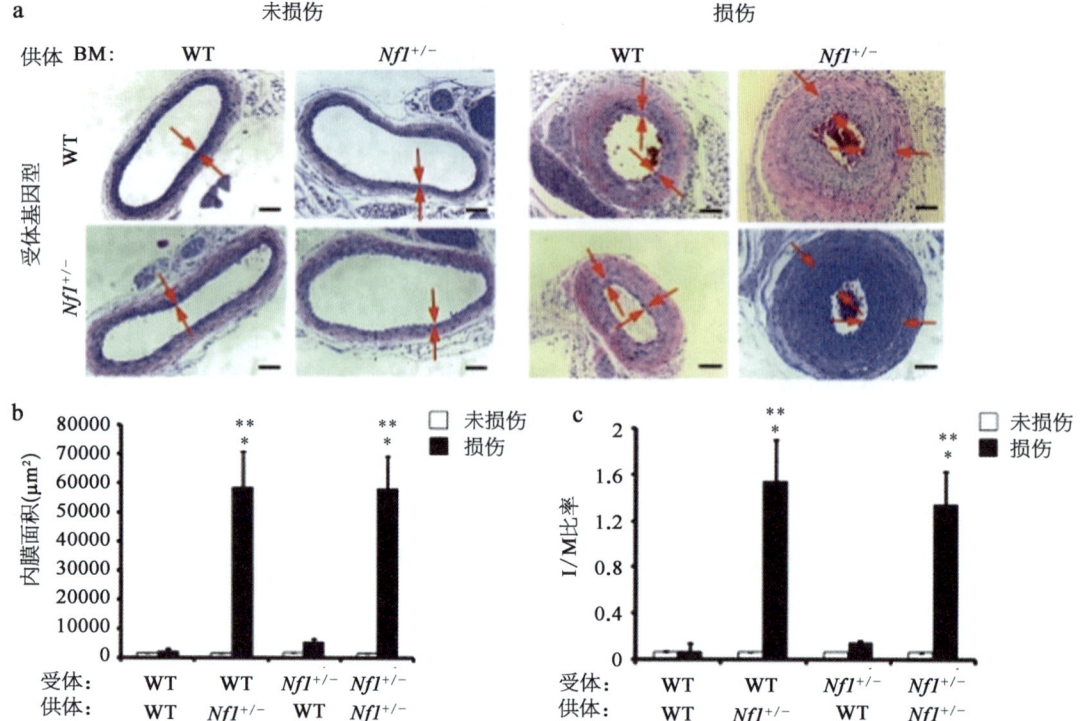

图 23.2 移植 WT 和 $Nf1^{+/-}$ 骨髓的 WT 和 $Nf1^{+/-}$ 小鼠的组织学和形态计量学分析。a. 移植 WT 或 $Nf1^{+/-}$ 骨髓的 WT 和 $Nf1^{+/-}$ 小鼠未损伤和损伤颈动脉的代表性苏木精-伊红染色横断面。红色箭头表示新生内膜的边界。比例尺：50 mm。b、c. 对接受 WT 或 $Nf1^{+/-}$ 骨髓移植的 WT 或 $Nf1^{+/-}$ 受体未损伤和损伤颈动脉新生内膜面积(b)和 I/M 比值(c)的量化(* <0.05；** <0.005)

（郑胜武，黄雄梅 译）

参考文献

[1] Araki T, Mohi MG, Ismat FA et al (2004) Mouse model of Noonan syndrome reveals cell type- and gene dosage-dependent effects of Ptpn11 mutation. Nat Med 10：849-857

[2] Bendeck MP, Zempo N, Clowes AW et al (1994) Smooth muscle cell migration and matrix metalloproteinase expression after arterial injury in the rat. Circ Res 75：539-545

[3] Brannan CI, Perkins AS, Vogel KS et al (1994) Targeted disruption of the neurofibromatosis type-1 gene leads to developmental abnormalities in heart and various neural crest-derived tissues. Genes Dev 8：1019-1029

[4] Cairns AG, North KN (2008) Cerebrovascular dysplasia in neurofibromatosis type 1. J Neurol Neurosurg Psychiatry 79：1165-1170

[5] Conway SJ, Kruzynska-Frejtag A, Kneer PL et al (2003) What cardiovascular defect does my prenatal mouse mutant have, and why? Genesis 35：1-21

[6] Criado E, Izquierdo L, Luján S, Puras E, del Mar Espino M (2002) Abdominal aortic coarctation, renovascular, hypertension, and neurofibromatosis. Ann Vasc Surg 16：363-367

[7] Daston MM, Ratner N (1992) Neurofibromin, a predominantly neuronal GTPase activating protein in the adult, is ubiquitously expressed during development. Dev Dyn 195：216-226

[8] Dugoff L, Sujansky E (1996) Neurofibromatosis type 1 and pregnancy. Am J Med Genet 66：7-10

[9] Evans DG, O'Hara C, Wilding A et al (2011) Mortality in neurofibromatosis 1：in North West England：an assessment of actuarial survival in a region of the UK since 1989. Eur J Hum Genet 19：1187-1191

[10] Feyrter F (1949) Über die vaskuläre Neurofibromatose, nach Untersuchungen am menschlichen Magen-Darmschlauch. Virchow Arch Pathol Anat 317：221-265

[11] Forde A, Constien R, Grone HJ, Hammerling G, Arnold B (2002) Temporal Cre-mediated recombination exclusively in endothelial cells using Tie2 regulatory elements. Genesis 33：191-197

[12] Fossali E, Signorini E, Intermite RC et al (2000) Renovascular disease and hypertension in children with neurofibromatosis. Pediatr Nephrol 14：806-810

[13] Friedman JM, Arbiser J, Epstein JA et al (2002) Cardiovascular disease in neurofibromatosis 1：report of the NF1 Cardiovascular Task Force. Genet Med 4：105-111

[14] Ghosh PS, Rothner AD, Emch TM, Freidman NR, Moodley M (2012) Cerebral vasculopathy in children with neurofibromatosis type 1. J Child Neurol (in press)

[15] Gitler AD, Brown CB, Kochilas L et al (2002) Neural crest migration and mouse models of congenital heart disease. Cold Spring Harb Symp Quant Biol 67：57-62

[16] Gitler AD, Zhu Y, Ismat FA et al (2003) Nf1 has an essential

role in endothelial cells. Nat Genet 33：75－79

[17] Hamilton SJ, Friedman JM (2000) Insights into the pathogenesis of neurofibromatosis 1 vasculopathy. Clin Genet 58：341－344

[18] Hutson MR, Kirby ML (2003) Neural crest and cardiovascular development：a 20-year perspec-tive. Birth Defects Res C Embryo Today 69：2－13

[19] Ingram DA, Mead LE, Tanaka H et al (2004) Identification of a novel hierarchy of endothelial progenitor cells using human peripheral and umbilical cord blood. Blood 104：2752－2760

[20] Ismat FA, Xu J, Lu MM, Epstein JA (2006) The neurofibromin GAP-related domain rescues endothelial but not neural crest development in Nf1 mice. J Clin Invest 116：2378－2384

[21] Jacks T, Shih TS, Schmitt EM et al (1994) Tumour predisposition in mice heterozygous for a targeted mutation in Nf1. Nat Genet 7：353－361

[22] Jin G, Chieh-Hsi Wu J et al (2000) Effects of active and negative mutants of Ras on rat arterial neointima formation. J Surg Res 94：124－132

[23] Kim HA, Ling B, Ratner N (1997) Nf1-deficient mouse Schwann cells are angiogenic and invasive and can be induced to hyperproliferate：reversion of some phenotypes by an inhibitor of farnesyl protein transferase. Mol Cell Biol 17：862－872

[24] Kirby ML, Gale TF, Stewart DE (1983) Neural crest cells contribute to normal aorticopulmonary septation. Science 220：1059－1061

[25] Lasater EA, Bessler WK, Mead LE et al (2008) Nf1$^{+/-}$ mice have increased neointima formation via hyperactivation of a Gleevec sensitive molecular pathway. Hum Mol Genet 17：2336－2344

[26] Lasater EA, Li F, Bessler WK et al (2010) Genetic and cellular evidence of vascular inflammation in neurofibromin-deficient mice and humans. J Clin Invest 120：859－870

[27] Li F, Munchhof AM, White HA et al (2006) Neurofibromin is a novel regulator of RAS-induced signals in primary vascular smooth muscle cells. Hum Mol Genet 15：1921－1930

[28] Lin AE, Birch PH, Korf BR et al (2000) Cardiovascular malformations and other cardiac abnormalities in neurofibromatosis 1 (NF1). Am J Med Genet 95：108－117

[29] Mangues R, Corral T, Lu S et al (1998) NF1 inactivation cooperates with N-ras in in vivo lymphogenesis activating ERK by a mechanism independent of its Ras-GTPase accelerating activity. Oncogene 17：1705－1716

[30] Marino B, Digilio MC, Toscano A et al (1999) Congenital heart diseases in children with Noonan syndrome：an expanded cardiac spectrum with high prevalence of atrioventricular canal. J Pediatr 135：703－706

[31] Mashour GA, Wang HL, Cabal-Manzano R et al (1999) Aberrant cutaneous expression of the angiogenic factor midkine is associated with neurofibromatosis type-1. J Invest Dermatol 113：398－402

[32] Mashour GA, Ratner N, Khan GA et al (2001) The angiogenic factor midkine is aberrantly expressed in NF1-deficient Schwann cells and is a mitogen for neurofibroma-derived cells. Oncogene 20：97－105

[33] Milewicz DM, Kwartler CS, Papke CL et al (2010) Genetic variants promoting smooth muscle cell proliferation can result in diffuse and diverse vascular diseases：evidence for a hyperplastic vasculomyopathy. Genet Med 12：196－203

[34] Montani D, Coulet F, Girerd B et al (2011) Pulmonary hypertension in patients with neurofibro-matosis type I. Medicine (Baltimore) 90：201－211

[35] Munchhof AM, Li F, White HA et al (2006) Neurofibroma-associated growth factors activate a distinct signaling network to alter the function of neurofibromin-deficient endothelial cells. Hum Mol Genet 15：1858－1869

[36] Norton KK, Xu J, Gutmann DH (1995) Expression of the neurofibromatosis I gene product, neurofibromin, in blood vessel endothelial cells and smooth muscle. Neurobiol Dis 2：13－21

[37] Oderich GS, Sullivan TM, Bower TC et al (2007) Vascular abnormalities in patients with neurofibro-matosis syndrome type I：clinical spectrum, management, and results. J Vasc Surg 46：475－484

[38] Ozerdem U (2004) Targeting neovascular pericytes in neurofibromatosis type 1. Angiogenesis 7：307－311

[39] Padmanabhan A, Lee JS, Ismat FA et al (2009) Cardiac and vascular functions of the zebrafish orthologues of the type I neurofibromatosis gene NFI. Proc Natl Acad Sci USA 106：22305－22310

[40] Phoon CK, Ji RP, Aristizabal O et al (2004) Embryonic heart failure in NFATc1$^{-/-}$ mice：novel mechanistic insights from in utero ultrasound biomicroscopy. Circ Res 95：92－99

[41] Prada CE, Zarate YA, Hagenbuch S et al (2011) Lethal presentation of neurofibromatosis and Noonan syndrome. Am J Med Genet A 155A：1360－1366

[42] Rasmussen SA, Yang Q, Friedman JM (2001) Mortality in neurofibromatosis 1：an analysis using U.S. death certificates. Am J Hum Genet 68：1110－1118

[43] Rea D, Brandsema JF, Armstrong D et al (2009) Cerebral arteriopathy in children with neurofi-bromatosis type 1. Pediatrics 124：e476－e483

[44] Reubi F (1945) Neurofibromatose et lésions vasculaires. Schweiz Med Wochenschr 75：463－465

[45] Rosser TL, Vezina G, Packer RJ (2005) Cerebrovascular abnormalities in a population of children with neurofibromatosis type 1. Neurology 64：553－555

[46] Salyer WR, Salyer DC (1974) The vascular lesions of neurofibromatosis. Angiology 25：510－519

[47] Sheela S, Riccardi VM, Ratner N (1990) Angiogenic and invasive properties of neurofibroma Schwann cells. J Cell Biol 111：645－653

[48] Snider P, Olaopa M, Firulli AB, Conway SJ (2007) Cardiovascular development and the colonizing cardiac neural crest lineage. ScientificWorldJournal 7：1090－1113

[49] Sørensen SA, Mulvihill JJ, Nielsen A (1986) Long-term follow-up of von Recklinghausen neurofibromatosis：survival and malignant neoplasms. N Engl J Med 314：1010－1015

[50] Stewart DR, Cogan JD, Kramer MR et al (2007) Is pulmonary arterial hypertension in neurofibro-matosis type 1 secondary to a plexogenic arteriopathy? Chest 132：798－808

[51] Strom A, Wigren M, Hultgardh-Nilsson A et al (2007) Involvement of the CD1d-natural killer T cell pathway in neointima formation after vascular injury. Circ Res 101：e83－e89

[52] Swirski FK, Libby P, Aikawa E et al (2007) Ly-6Chi monocytes dominate hypercholesterolemia-associated monocytosis and give rise to macrophages in atheromata. J Clin Invest 117：195－205

[53] Tedesco MA, Di Salvo G, Natale F et al (2002) The heart in neurofibromatosis type 1：an echocardiographic study. Am Heart J 143：883－888

[54] Tedesco MA, Di Salvo G, Natale F, Graziano L, Grassia C, Calabrò R, Lama G (2005) Early cardiac morphologic and functional changes in neurofibromatosis type 1 hypertensives：

an echocardiographic and tissue Doppler study. Int J Cardiol 101: 243-247
[55] Ullrich NJ, Robertson R, Kinnamon DD et al (2007) Moyamoya following cranial irradiation for primary brain tumors in children. Neurology 68: 932-938
[56] Viskochil D (2002) Genetics of neurofibromatosis 1 and the *NF1* gene. J Child Neurol 17: 562-570, discussion 71-72, 646-651
[57] Wang Y, Nicol GD, Clapp DW, Hingtgen CM (2005) Sensory neurons from *Nf1* haploinsufficient mice exhibit increased excitability. J Neurophysiol 94: 3670-3676
[58] Wu M, Wallace MR, Muir D (2006) Nf1 haploinsufficiency augments angiogenesis. Oncogene 25: 2297-2303
[59] Xu J, Ismat FA, Wang T et al (2007) NF1 regulates a Ras-dependent vascular smooth muscle proliferative injury response. Circulation 116: 2148-2156
[60] Yang FC, Ingram DA, Chen S et al (2008) Nf1-dependent tumors require a microenvironment containing $Nf1^{+/-}$ and c-kit-dependent bone marrow. Cell 135: 437-448
[61] Zenker M (2011) Clinical manifestations of mutations in RAS and related intracellular signal transduction factors. Curr Opin Pediatr 23: 443-451
[62] Zhang LN, Parkinson JF, Haskell C, Wang YX (2008) Mechanisms of intimal hyperplasia learned from a murine carotid artery ligation model. Curr Vasc Pharmacol 6: 37-43
[63] Zhu Y, Ghosh P, Charnay P et al (2002) Neurofibromas in NF1: Schwann cell origin and role of tumor environment. Science 296: 920-922

第24章 血管球瘤的分子基础
Molecular Basis of Glomus Tumours

Hilde Brems, Eric Legius, and Douglas R. Stewart

24.1 引言

1型神经纤维瘤病（NF1）是一种常染色体显性遗传病，出生发病率为1/3 000，并伴有肿瘤易感性增加（Huson et al. 1989）。NF1相关肿瘤是由抑癌基因 NF1 的体细胞突变引起的。NF1患者发生神经系统和非神经系统组织来源的良性和恶性肿瘤的风险增加（Brems et al. 2009a）。手指和足趾的血管球瘤是由于 NF1 双等位基因失活引起的，属于NF1肿瘤谱系的一部分（Brems et al. 2009b）。

血管球瘤是来源于球状体的小型良性肿瘤（<5 mm），最常见于四肢。球状体是存在于手指和足趾的体温调节分流器，是一种参与体温调节的动静脉吻合器，由血管结构、神经细胞和平滑肌细胞组成。平滑肌细胞来源于神经嵴，多能神经嵴干细胞可以分化为神经元、施万细胞和α-平滑肌肌动蛋白（alpha-smooth muscle actin, αSMA）阳性的平滑肌样成肌纤维细胞（Morrison et al. 1999）。平滑肌层因热刺激而收缩，导致分流器关闭，使毛细血管网络中的血流冷却下来。而当暴露于低温时，肌肉层松弛，血液从皮肤中分流，以防止热量流失。源自球状体的血管球瘤应与历史上也曾称作"血管球瘤"的肾上腺和肾上腺外副神经节瘤相区别（Strauchen 2002）。

血管球瘤通常表现为典型的三联症状：剧烈疼痛、局部压痛和冷敏感。唯一的治疗方法是手术切除，完全切除手指和足趾的血管球瘤是防止复发的必要手段（Lin et al. 2010）。血管球瘤的诊断往往会被延误。一项关于手指散发性血管球瘤的大样本量病例研究发现，平均每位患者在确诊前咨询了2.5位医师（范围：0～7位），包括精神科医师。诊断前的症状持续时间平均可长达10年（范围：1～40年）（Van Geertruyden et al. 1996）。

手指和足趾的散发性血管球瘤通常是单发的，并好发于中年女性（Rettig and Strickland 1977；Tsuneyoshi and Enjoji 1982；Van Geertruyden et al. 1996）。在两项大型回顾性研究中（86例）均未发现多发性血管球瘤的病例（Tsuneyoshi and Enjoji 1982；Van Geertruyden et al. 1996）。

Klaber首次报道了1例同时具有NF1特征和血管球瘤的13岁女孩，该女孩在右颈部、双下肢和左足跟处发现血管球瘤（Klaber 1938）。在本章中，我们提供了位于手指和足趾的NF1相关血管球瘤的最新信息。迄今为止,英文文献中已报道24例存在手指或足趾血管球瘤的NF1病例(表24.1)(Oughterson and Tennant 1939; Park et al. 1994; Sawada et al. 1995; Okada et al. 1999; Kim 2000; De Smet et al. 2002; Brems et al. 2009b; Stewart et al. 2010,2012; Leonard and Harrington 2010)。

24.2 诊断和临床表现

对于NF1的患者来说,血管球瘤可能与神经纤维瘤混淆。一般来说,血管球瘤的诊断基于局部压痛、冷敏感性和阵发性剧烈疼痛等症状。值得注意的是,患者可能已经忍受了很长时间的疼痛,因此需要特别询问他们有关这些症状的情况。血管球瘤合并的疼痛通常是持续的,患者可能会因为想要保护他们的手指而不愿握手。疼痛的发作可能由寒冷的温度(如伸手进冰箱)或轻微的振动(如转动门把手)诱发,持续时间较短,但会使患者感到虚弱和恐惧,需要数小时才能恢复。Love测试有助于血管球瘤的诊断。测试时,使用细小仪器(如铅笔尖或针)轻轻按压患处,诱发局部压痛,该操作不会引起按压点附近紧邻区域的疼痛(Love 1944)。若Love测试阳性,患者会在血管球瘤部位感到剧烈疼痛,并会立即缩回手(或脚)。根据Bhaskaranand和Navadgi(2002)的研究,Love测试的灵敏性为100%,准确性为78%。此外,Hildreth测试和冷敏感性测试也可用于帮助做出正确诊断。Hildreth测试是指将止血带绑在患指(趾)根部,重复Love测试,Love测试阳性患者的血管球瘤部位的疼痛感应消失。Hildreth测试的灵敏性为71%,特异性为100%(Bhaskaranand and Navadgi,2002)。冷敏感性测试是将患手(或脚)放入冷水中,使患有血管球瘤的手指(或足趾)受到冷刺激而产生剧烈疼痛。值得注意的是,冷敏感性测试的敏感性、特异性和准确性均为100%(Bhaskaranand and Navadgi 2002)。

表24.1总结了有手指或足趾血管球瘤的NF1患者的临床表现(Oughterson and Tennant 1939; Park et al. 1994; Sawada et al. 1995; Okada et al. 1999; Kim 2000; De Smet et al. 2002; Brems et al. 2009b; Stewart et al. 2010,2012; Leonard and Harrington 2010)。共报告了24例病例,女性患者较多(17/24,占71%),与散发性血管球瘤相关的研究结果相似(134/161,占83%)(Van Geertruyden et al. 1996; Lee et al. 2011)。NF1患者的平均诊断年龄为36岁,与散发性血管球瘤患者的平均诊断年龄(44岁和42岁)相似(Van Geertruyden et al. 1996; Lee et al. 2011)。值得注意的是,2例NF1的儿童(病例♯14和♯23)在11岁时被诊断出血管球瘤;病例♯13被诊断为节段型NF1,没有满足NIH的NF1诊断标准。Stewart等(2010)没有发现咖啡牛奶斑、神经纤维瘤严重程度与手指或足趾血管球瘤发展之间存在相关性。

与已被报道的散发性血管球瘤经验一致,大多数有血管球瘤的NF1患者满足血管球瘤三联征中的两个或更多(局部压痛、冷敏感和阵发性剧烈疼痛)(Stewart et al. 2010),并且在确诊前可能已经忍受了多年疼痛(从1年到40多年不等)(Van Geertruyden et al. 1996)(表24.1)。手指或足趾的外观通常正常,偶尔可以观察到指甲变蓝,但很少能触及肿瘤结节。由于血管球瘤未被充分认识,导致了许多病例被误诊为血管瘤,而使其发病率偏高,且使患者经历了不必要的手术(Sawada et al. 1995)。因此我们提倡建立筛查工作(Stewart et al. 2010),应在NF1的成人和儿童患者的常规护理中询问一个简单的问题:"您的指尖是否会感到疼痛,特别是受到寒冷刺激或碰撞时?"

24例NF1患者中发现有2例患者患有足趾血管球瘤(病例♯2和♯16,表24.1),有23例患者患有手指血管球瘤。同样,在非NF1患者中,血管球瘤更常见于手指(106/110)而非足趾(4/110)(Lee et al. 2011)。NF1合并血管球瘤的患者也符合肿瘤易感综合征的特点,42%(10/24)的NF1患者存在多个手指受累,但散发性血管球瘤患者中并未出现这种情况(Tsuneyoshi and Enjoji 1982; Van Geertruyden et al. 1996)。表24.1显示血管球瘤在左手和右手间的分布较为一致,第四和第五指较其他手指更容易受累。

过去曾采用X线、磁共振成像(magnetic resonance imaging,MRI)和超声等成像技术对血

表 24.1 已发表的 NF1 相关手指和足趾血管球瘤的总结

编号	参考文献	性别	年龄	NIH NF1 诊断标准	临床表现	症状持续年数	受累手指和足趾数量	受累手指或足趾	确诊的血管球瘤	切除术	疼痛/压痛缓解	复发	胚系 NF1 突变	体细胞 NF1 突变
1	Oughterson (1939) 病例 2	男	28	咖啡牛奶斑	压痛+进行性疼痛	16	1	LF1	LF1	LF1	是	否	未分析	未分析
2	Park (1994) 病例 2	女	17	咖啡牛奶斑，皮肤型神经纤维瘤，雀斑	压痛+疼痛	3	6	RF2, RF3, RF4, RF5, LF3,RT1	RF2, RF3, RF4, RF5, LF3,RT1	活检	未标明	未标明	未分析	未分析
3	Sawada (1995) 病例 1	男	45	咖啡牛奶斑，皮肤型神经纤维瘤	压痛+疼痛	20	5	RF2, RF4, RF5, LF1, LF4	RF2, RF4, RF5, LF1, LF4	RF2, RF4, RF5, LF1, LF4	是	未标明	未分析	未分析
4	Sawada (1995) 病例 2	女	28	咖啡牛奶斑，皮肤型神经纤维瘤	压痛	未标明	5	RF3, RF4, RF5, LF2, LF5	RF2, RF4, RF5, LF1, LF4	LF5	是，部分减轻压痛	未标明	未分析	未分析
5	Sawada (1995) 病例 3	女	39	NF1 家族史	剧烈疼痛+压痛	未标明	1	RF3	否	否	是，卡马西平+星状神经节阻滞治疗	未标明	未分析	未分析
6	Okada (1999) 病例 1	女	22	咖啡牛奶斑	疼痛	3	6	RF4, LF1, LF2, LF3, LF4,LF5	LF3	RF4, LF1, LF2, LF3, LF4,LF5	是	否	未分析	未分析
7	Kim (2000) 病例 1	女	34	咖啡牛奶斑，皮肤型神经纤维瘤	剧烈疼痛+压痛	未标明	1	RT2	RT2	活检	未标明	未标明	未分析	未分析
8	De Smet (2002) 病例 1 = Brems (2009b) NF1-G3 = Stewart (2010) Leu-3 = Stewart (2012)	女	53	>6 个咖啡牛奶斑，Lisch 结节，皮肤型神经纤维瘤，雀斑，1 度	进行性和局部疼痛（LF3, RF4）；分裂指甲和进行性局部疼痛（LF4）	1	2+1	2, LF3,RF4 2	LF3, RF4, LF4	是，2次；第一次，LF3，RF4，6 年后 2 个肿瘤在 LF4	是，需 2 次手术	否	c. 2546dupG	LF3 未分析；RF4 未分析；LF4 c. 5545C>A, c. 5539_5546dup8

续表

编号	参考文献	性别	年龄	NIH NF1诊断标准	临床表现	症状持续年数	受累手和足指趾数量	受累手指或足趾	确诊的血管球瘤	切除术	疼痛/压痛缓解	复发	胚系NF1突变	体细胞NF1突变
9	De Smet (2002)病例2 = Brems (2009b) NF1-G2 = Stewart (2010) Leu-2	男	35	>6个咖啡牛奶斑,Lisch结节,皮肤型神经纤维瘤,雀斑,1度	进行性+局部疼痛,剧烈疼痛	2~3	2	RF3,RF4	RF3,RF4	RF3,RF4	是	否	c. 7395_7404del10 c. 7395-2A>G	RF3 LOH intron 27-38;RF4未分析
10	Brems (2009b) NF1-G1 = Stewart (2010) Leu-1 = Stewart (2012)	女	42	+(包括神经纤维瘤)	进行性+局部疼痛	1~2	2	RF4,RF5	RF4,RF5	RF4,RF5	是	否	部分跳过外显子29 c. 2256A>G	RF4 c. 403 del; RF5未分析
11	Brems (2009b) NF1-G4=Stewart (2010) Leu-4	男	57	+(包括神经纤维瘤)	进行性+局部疼痛,受冷加重,指甲床变形,指甲弯曲度增加	>5	1	RF4	RF4	RF4	是	否	c. 2252-11 T>G c. 2256A>G	未检测
12	Brems (2009b) NF1-G5=Stewart (2010) Leu-5	女	41	+(包括神经纤维瘤)	远节指骨进行性+局部疼痛,受冷加重	4	1	LF3	LF3 2次	LF3 2次,间隔13个月,同一部位	是,需2次手术	是	c. 4515-2A>T	LF3 (1st) c. 3113+1 G>C; LF3 (2nd)未分析
13	Brems (2009b) NF1-G6=Maertens (2007) SNF1-1 = Stewart (2010) Leu-6	女	46	神经纤维瘤和仅3个咖啡牛奶斑,不符合诊断标准	远节指骨进行性+局部疼痛,冬季加重,伴少量皮肤型神经纤维瘤;节段型NF1	1~2	1	RF3	RF3	RF3	是	否	c. 2041C>T (<50%)镶嵌	未检测
14	Brems (2009b) NF1-G7=Stewart (2010) Leu-7	女	11	+	远节指骨剧烈疼痛+远节指骨肿胀,LF5轻度缩短	2~3	1	RF5	RF5	RF5	是	否	c. 2304dupT	未检测

续 表

编号	参考文献	性别	年龄	NIH NF1 诊断标准	临床表现	症状持续年数	受累手指和足趾数量	受累手指或足趾	确诊的血管球瘤	切除术	疼痛/压痛缓解	复发	胚系NF1突变	体细胞NF1突变
15	Brems (2009b) NF1-G8=Stewart (2010) Hamburg-1=Stewart (2012)	女	26	+（包括咖啡牛奶斑、神经纤维瘤）	不明原因疼痛，患者出现抑郁	5	1	LF4	LF4	LF4	是	否	c.311 T>G	c.7727C>A
16	Brems (2009b) NF1-G9=Stewart (2010) Hamburg-2	女	57	+（包括咖啡牛奶斑、神经纤维瘤）	疼痛	1	1	RT1	RT1	RT1	是	否	c.1541_1542delAG	未检测
17	Brems (2009b) NF1-G10=Stewart (2010) NIH-1=Soto (2012) NF1-G10	女	35	+（包括咖啡牛奶斑、神经纤维瘤）	双手剧烈、致残性疼痛，伴复杂区域疼痛综合征	5	6	LF3, LF4, LF5, RF3, RF4, RF5	LF4(2个同时出现), LF5, RF3	手术1: LF4, LF5, RF3;手术2: LF4, LF3, RF4, RF5; 手术3: LF4, LF3, LF5	是，需要3次手术，同时使用氯胺酮止痛	是	c.6789_6792delTTAC	RF3 未检测; LF5 c.204+1 G>A; LF4 c.7600_7621del22
18	Brems (2009b) NF1-G11=Stewart (2010) NIH-2	男	50	+（包括咖啡牛奶斑、神经纤维瘤）	左手和右拇指剧烈、进行性疼痛，左手和手臂复杂区域疼痛综合征	20(左手), 5(右拇指)	6	LF2, LF3, LF4, RF1, RF4, RF5	LF2, LF4, RF1, RF4	手术1: LF2, LF4, RF1;手术2: LF2, LF4, RF1, LF3;手术3: RF1, RF4, RF5	需要3次手术切除所有血管球瘤，但仍有持续性神经性疼痛。最后一次手术后不久因胶质母细胞瘤去世	是	c.7723_delG	LF2 未分析; LF4 未分析; RF1 未分析; RF4 未分析
19	Stewart (2010) NIH-3	女	28	+（包括咖啡牛奶斑、神经纤维瘤）	复杂区域疼痛综合征	4	3	LF3, LF4, RF4	LF3	LF3, LF4, RF4	是	否	未分析	未分析
20	Stewart (2010) NIH-4	女	49	+（包括咖啡牛奶斑、神经纤维瘤）	疼痛	>40	1	LF3	LF3	LF3	是，随访18个月无痛	否，但随访时间短	未分析	未分析

续 表

编号	参考文献	性别	年龄	NIH NF1 诊断标准	临床表现	症状持续年数	受累手指和足趾数量	受累手指或足趾	确诊的血管球瘤	切除术	疼痛/压痛缓解	复发	胚系 NF1 突变	体细胞 NF1 突变
21	Stewart (2010) NIH-5	女	35	+（包括咖啡牛奶斑）	疼痛	18	1	LF3	LF3	LF3	是，随访18个月无痛	否，但随访时间短	未分析	未分析
22	Stewart (2010) Leu-8=NF1-G12 Stewart (2012)	女	34	+（包括神经纤维瘤）	疼痛	4	1	LF4	LF4	LF4	是	否，但随访时间短	c.4368-1 G>C	有丝分裂重组 17q
23	Leonard (2010)病例1	男	11	>6个咖啡牛奶斑，Lisch结节，皮肤型神经纤维瘤，雀斑，1度	进行性疼痛+拇指敏感	1.5	1	LF1	LF1	LF1	是	未标明	未分析	未分析
24	Stewart (2012) NF1-G13	男	40	+	进行性剧烈疼痛	8	1	RF5	RF5	RF5	是，但随访时间短	否，但随访时间短	c.3113+1 G>A	有丝分裂重组 17q

注：L，左；R，右；F，手指；T，足趾；NIH NF1 诊断标准+，满足这些标准。

管球瘤进行可视化定位,不同成像技术的成功率各不相同,取决于病灶的大小。有典型症状且无并发症的血管球瘤,可能不需要影像学检查。然而,在更复杂的情况下(如症状复发、慢性疼痛),由于体格检查的预测力下降,所以可能更需要影像学检查(尤其是MRI)来辅助诊断(Stewart et al. 2010)。血管球瘤在MRI的T2加权像上呈结节状高信号(图24.1);T1序列增强后通常显示肿瘤轻到中度增强。偶尔在X线平片中可以观察到血管球瘤引起的骨侵蚀(5/24;表24.1)。总体而言,X线的灵敏度低于MRI,在4例患者的8个手指中仅检测到2个血管球瘤,而遗漏了6个病灶(Stewart et al. 2010)。

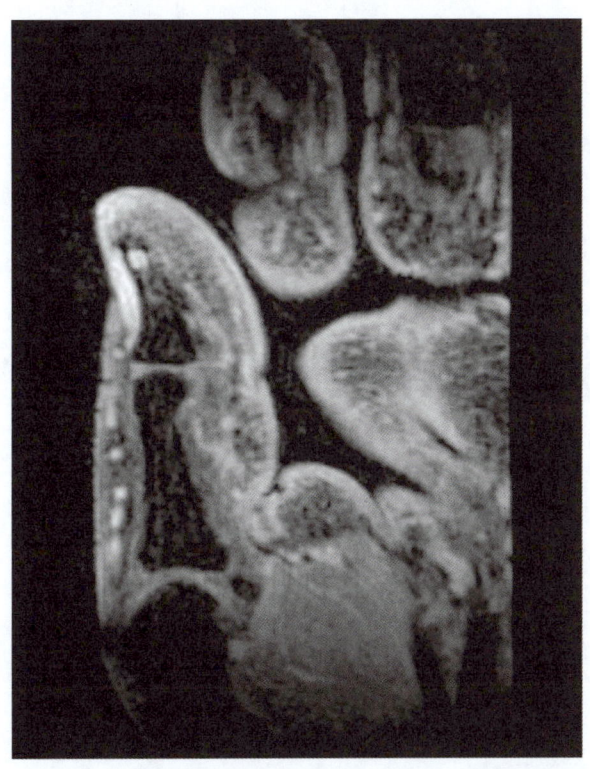

图24.1 病例♯17的磁共振成像(表24.1),1名50岁1型神经纤维瘤病的男性,其左手第二指和第四指的远节指骨有长达20年的阵发性剧烈疼痛史,右手拇指的远节指骨有长达5年的类似疼痛史(如图所示)。由于病痛,他的左手几乎无法使用,并因残疾提前退休;双手体格检查提示存在与复杂区域疼痛综合征一致的废用性萎缩和异常疼痛症状。右手拇指冠状位T1增强后MRI显示1个清晰可见的约5 mm皮质下骨内病变。在普通X线片上(未展示),在病变部位有1个3~4 mm边界清晰的透亮病灶,周围有硬化缘,可能是继发于骨侵蚀。随后进行的手术(图24.2)和病理检查结果与血管球瘤一致

24.3 治疗、并发症和预后

据已发表的文献报道,24例NF1患者中有21例患者的血管球瘤接受切除术治疗(表24.1),2例患者(病例♯2和♯7)行活检术,1例患者(病例♯5)未接受手术治疗,而接受口服卡马西平联合星状神经节阻滞治疗。21例患者在手术和(或)药物治疗后疼痛或压痛症状减轻(表24.1)。

根据我们的经验,手术切除是血管球瘤唯一的治疗方法(图24.2),大多数患者术后疼痛和压痛症状明显改善。根据血管球瘤的位置,需要采取不同的手术方法。直接经甲切除术适用于甲下血管球瘤;侧向骨膜下切口适用于甲下或指腹的血管球瘤,侧向切口可能减少指甲畸形的风险,但切除不完全的风险较高,因此复发的风险较高(Vasisht et al. 2004)。血管球瘤通常有一个假包膜,便于切除。当肿瘤靠近骨骼时,需要进行骨刮除术以减少复发的风险。

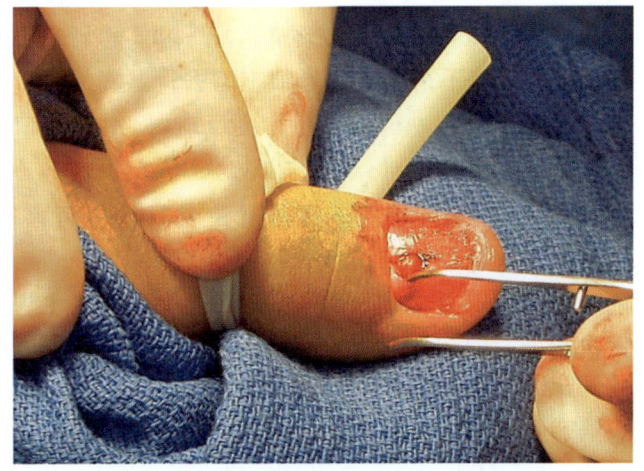

图24.2 图24.1中描述的50岁男性右手拇指的术中照片。已移除指甲床,右侧镊子尖端旁靠近中线处可见一约5 mm的肿瘤。病灶的病理检查结果与血管球瘤一致。血管球瘤通常具有假包膜,如本例所示,更易于切除。尽管进行了切除和骨刮除术,但患者的肿瘤复发,并在8个月后接受了第二次手术。照片已进行数字化处理以去除患者身份标识

大多数血管球瘤手术切除顺利且无复发。一项纳入75例散发性手指血管球瘤的回顾性研究显示,17%的患者出现了肿瘤复发(Lin et al. 2010)。根

据我们的经验,血管球瘤复发可能发生在早期(数周或数月,可能是由于切除不完全)或晚期(数年,可能是由于新肿瘤的形成)。表 24.1 显示,24 例 NF1 患者中有 6 例未出现肿瘤复发。在已知复发结局的 18 例患者中,少数患者(3/18,占 17%)报告了肿瘤复发,而大多数(15/18,占 83%)未报告复发。然而,未报告复发的 15 例患者中有 4 例仅进行了短期随访。

在 NF1 并伴有血管球瘤患者中,复杂区域疼痛综合征(complex regional pain syndrome,CRPS)是一种较为罕见但可能更具破坏性的并发症,尽管进行了充分的肿瘤切除,但患者仍出现复发性疼痛。CRPS 是一种病因不明、临床异质性较高的慢性疼痛综合征,影响一个或多个肢体。以前称为反射性交感神经营养不良(reflex sympathetic dystrophy,RSD)或灼痛症。CRPS 表现为痛觉过敏、感觉过度和(或)感觉异常,继发于急性或慢性疼痛的刺激。在总结的 24 例患者中,3 例 NF1 并伴有血管球瘤的患者(病例♯17、18 和 19)在血管球瘤切除术后发展为 CRPS(表 24.1)(Stewart et al. 2010)。其中 2 例 CRPS 患者进行了 3 次手术以切除所有血管球瘤,但仍有持续性的神经性疼痛。1 例 NF1 患者在最后一次手术后不久因胶质母细胞瘤去世。病例♯17 的慢性疼痛对多种药物治疗均无反应,但最终对口服氯胺酮有反应(Soto et al. 2012)。

CRPS 的最佳治疗方法是避免或消除疼痛源,但由于血管球瘤在临床上未被充分认识,患者确诊前可能已经忍受多年的痛苦,这种治疗方法往往具有挑战性。因此,我们主张对有症状的血管球瘤及时行手术切除。对于既往已行手术切除但仍有疼痛复发的血管球瘤患者,可使用 MRI 区分肿瘤复发和 CRPS。长期有症状的散发性血管球瘤患者可能会进展为 CRPS,也可能不会进展为 CRPS(Nebreda et al. 2000;Longdon et al. 2007;Cooke et al. 1995)。由于神经纤维瘤蛋白在痛觉感觉神经元的兴奋性调节中起关键作用,NF1 患者可能有更高的风险发展为慢性疼痛综合征,如 CRPS(Hingtgen 2008)。

24.4 病理学

表 24.1 列出了 43 例组织学确诊的血管球瘤。在病理学上,无法区分 NF1 相关的血管球瘤与散发性血管球瘤(Stewart et al. 2012)。血管球瘤的诊断通常可以通过苏木精-伊红染色完成(图 24.3a、b)。肿瘤由分支的血管通道组成,周围是成团或成片的血管球瘤细胞。血管球瘤细胞呈立方形,具有良性外观的圆形细胞核,胞质丰富呈嗜酸性,使用 αSMA 抗体进行免疫染色通常显示胞质呈阳性(图 24.4)。只有少数血管球瘤呈现非典型或恶性特征,通常不存在有丝分裂、非典型或坏死(Folpe et al. 2001)。

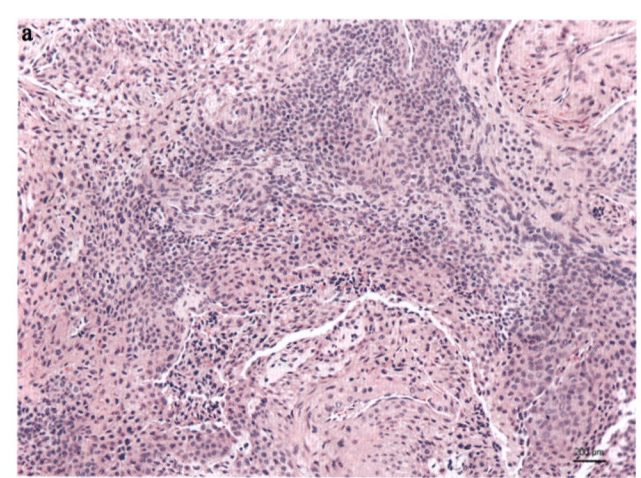

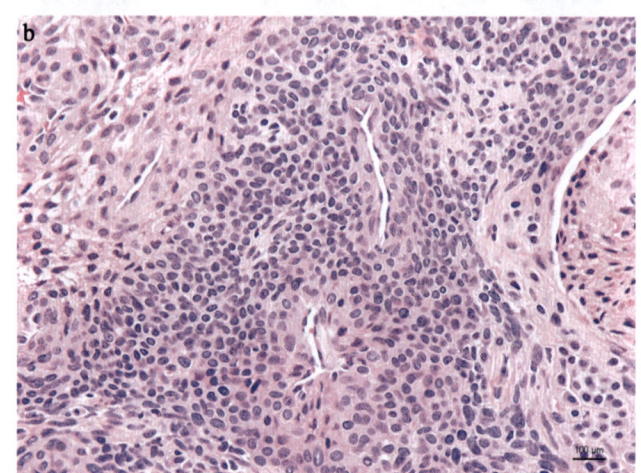

图 24.3 苏木精-伊红染色的血管球瘤显微照片。血管球瘤由中度至高度细胞密集的立方形细胞组成,这些细胞成片或成团排列,部分包绕血管。病灶组织的细胞显示圆形细胞核和不明显的核仁,胞质丰富呈嗜酸性。细胞学异型性很小;无坏死,也没有发现有丝分裂活性增加。病灶组织的细胞间也存在疏松基质组织。原始放大倍数为 20 倍(a)和 40 倍(b)。比例尺分别为 200 μm(a)和 100 μm(b)。显微照片由 C. Richard Lee,M. D.,Ph. D.(美国国家癌症研究所病理实验室)提供

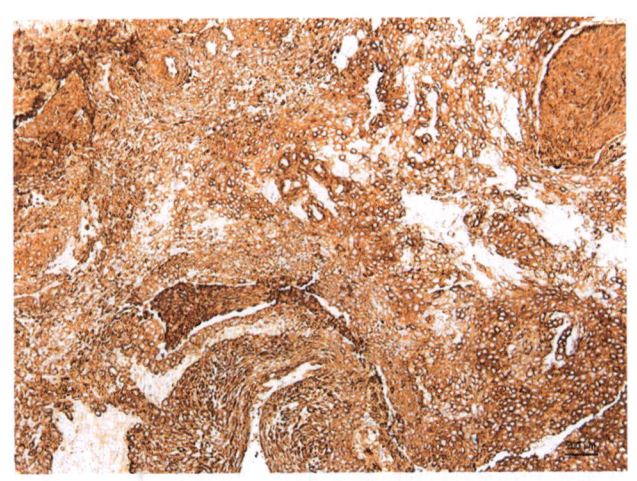

图 24.4 α-平滑肌肌动蛋白染色的血管球瘤显微照片。血管球瘤中的肿瘤细胞通常显示均一的 αSMA 胞质染色阳性。原始放大倍数为 20 倍。比例尺为 200 μm。显微照片由 C. Richard Lee, M. D., Ph. D. (美国国家癌症研究所病理实验室)提供

24.5 分子和功能特征

对 24 例 NF1 和血管球瘤患者中的 13 例进行了种系 NF1 突变分析(表 24.1)。13 例患者中,有 12 例患者的白细胞 DNA 发现了致病性胚系 NF1 突变。1 例节段性 NF1 的患者,在不到 50% 的白细胞中观察到致病性 NF1 突变(表 24.1,病例 13)。在同一患者的 2 个不同神经纤维瘤的施万细胞中培养鉴定出相同的 NF1 突变(Maertens et al. 2007)。在所有已鉴定的突变中,未发现 NF1 微缺失。突变分布于整个基因,通常是截断突变。这与随机选择的 NF1 患者群体的预期结果非常相似。尚无已知的基因型、表型相关性,尽管这可能由于报告的胚系突变数量较少。

由于血管球瘤通常是小病灶,往往很难获得足够的 DNA、RNA 或蛋白质进行体细胞 NF1 突变检测和功能分析。此外,尚未有 NF1 动物模型报道指出同时存在血管球瘤。在一项证明人类血管球瘤中 NF1 双等位基因失活的研究中,使用了两种不同策略收集肿瘤 DNA(Brems et al. 2009b)。首先,收集手术切除的新鲜血管球瘤组织,分离并培养血管球瘤细胞,后提取 DNA 或 RNA。血管球瘤细胞在免疫染色中呈 αSMA 阳性。其次,通过激光捕获显微镜(LCM)对石蜡包埋组织中的肿瘤细胞进行显微切割;如有需要,提取的 DNA 将进行全基因组扩增。

结合这两种技术,对 14 例经组织学确诊的血管球瘤进行了体细胞 NF1 突变分析(表 24.1)。这 14 例肿瘤中有 5 例未检测到 NF1 体细胞突变。这 9 例存在体细胞 NF1 突变或杂合性缺失,和致病性 NF1 突变的肿瘤中,有 6 例存在点突变或小插入或缺失事件(来自病例♯8、10、12、15、17 的肿瘤)[病例♯17 在两个手指的两个不同血管球瘤中鉴定出两种不同的体细胞 NF1 突变(Brems et al. 2009b)]。这些突变因产生过早终止密码子(4/14)或替代剪接位点(2/14),预计会导致 NF1 完全失活。有 1 例肿瘤(来自病例♯9)被发现存在跨越内含子 27 至 38 的杂合性缺失,预计导致 NF1 等位基因的丧失。有 2 例肿瘤(来自病例♯22 和 24)发生了染色体臂 17q 的有丝分裂重组,导致胚系突变 NF1 等位基因的复制,从而使 NF1 双等位基因失活。有丝分裂重组已在许多其他 NF1 相关肿瘤中报告,在本系列中,有 22% 的血管球瘤观察到该重组(Stewart et al. 2012)。在 2 例 NF1 相关的血管球瘤中,通过分离分析证明种系和体细胞 NF1 突变发生在 2 个不同的染色体上,确定了 NF1 的双等位基因失活(Brems et al. 2009b)。如果 NF1 相关的血管球瘤是由 NF1 双等位基因失活引起的,那么应该有单克隆扩展的证据,表明肿瘤来源于单个细胞。与这一预测一致,在 1 例女性(病例♯17)的 3 个手指的 3 个不同血管球瘤中,使用甲基化和未甲基化特异性引物对检测到单个等位基因(Brems et al. 2009b)。在 2 例散发性血管球瘤的血管球瘤细胞或成纤维细胞中未鉴定出体细胞 NF1 突变,表明其致病机制不同(Brems et al. 2009b)。

由于 NF1 完全失活会导致神经纤维瘤蛋白的丢失和 RAS-MAPK 通路的过度激活,因此研究了以下几种细胞的过度激活情况:NF1 相关的血管球瘤衍生的血管球瘤细胞($NF1^{-/-}$)、NF1 相关的血管球瘤衍生的成纤维细胞($NF1^{+/-}$)、散发性血管球瘤衍生的血管球瘤细胞($NF1^{+/+}$)和对照皮肤成纤维细胞($NF1^{+/+}$)(Brems et al. 2009b)。该研究监测了酸性成纤维细胞生长因子对培养细胞的影响。结果发现,$NF1^{-/-}$ 血管球瘤细胞中 MEK 和 ERK 的激活强度和持续时间比 $NF1^{+/-}$ 成纤维细

胞、$NF1^{+/+}$ 血管球瘤细胞和 $NF1^{+/+}$ 成纤维细胞更强、更长，这与 NF1 对 RAS-MAPK 通路调控的丧失一致。

一项研究对 5 例 NF1 相关血管球瘤（已证实 NF1 双等位基因失活）进行核型和拷贝数分析，发现其中 4 例肿瘤为二倍体，且几乎不存在细胞遗传学异常，这与其良性组织学和自然病史相符 (Stewart et al. 2012)。第 5 例肿瘤（来自病例 ♯22）所有染色体均为极端多倍体（近四倍体、近六倍体或近七倍体），但没有重排或形态异常。这一肿瘤的发生与染色体臂 17q 的有丝分裂重组有关；作者假设有丝分裂重组还"揭示"（即降低为纯合子）了位于染色体臂 17q 上的一个与染色体不稳定性相关的低表达胚系等位基因，导致了极端多倍体。

为了确定其他引起肿瘤发生的基因组事件，两项研究使用比较基因组杂交（SNP 阵列）来确定血管球瘤中的拷贝数 (Brems et al. 2009b；Stewart et al. 2012)。在两个 NF1 相关的血管球瘤（来自病例 ♯17）中，通过 LCM 获得的 DNA 中鉴定出 CRTAC1 的 3′端扩增和 WASF1 的 5′端缺失，并通过定量 PCR 进一步确认其结果 (Brems et al. 2009b)。WASF1 与其位于 5′端的 CDC40 形成双向基因对，WASF1 和 CDC40 的双向启动子位于两个血管球瘤中的假定缺失区内。尽管双向启动子在良性肿瘤发生中的作用尚不明确，但其与癌症相关基因有关。WASF1 在卵巢癌中下调，而 CDC40 的酵母同源基因是细胞周期停滞的调控者，这 2 个基因都是进一步研究血管球瘤的候选基因。第二项研究使用培养的血管球瘤细胞，通过 2 种不同的分析方法，在 6 个肿瘤中的至少 3 个鉴定出两个基因（WDR17 和 C16orf11）和 1 个 miRNA（MIR1267）的缺失 (Stewart et al. 2012)。

24.6 未解决的问题和未来方向

von Recklinghausen 描述 NF1 后 100 多年，血管球瘤才被确认为 NF1 肿瘤谱系的一部分。这提醒我们，即使面对熟悉的表型，敏锐的临床观察也发挥着重要作用。目前尚不清楚为什么如此小的病灶会引起如此剧烈的疼痛，以及为什么有些患者会发展为 CRPS，而其他患者不会进展为 CRPS。血管球瘤在 NF1 人群中女性较为多见的原因，以及其真实发病率和流行病学也尚不明确。尽管手术对许多患者具有治愈作用，但在确诊之前，血管球瘤会给患者带来严重的病痛和不必要的痛苦。如果能及时识别血管球瘤的体征和症状，就可以避免大部分这种情况的发生。我们期待未来对这些肿瘤的独特分子特征进行研究（例如肿瘤测序），并鼓励护理人员在对成人和儿童 NF1 患者的常规护理中关注患者手指和足趾疼痛的情况。

致谢：HB 是佛兰德斯研究基金会（FWO）在鲁汶大学的博士后研究员。

基金：本工作得到了佛兰德斯科学研究基金会（Fonds voor Wetenschappelijk Onderzoek, FWO）-Vlaanderen(G.0578.06)(EL)、癌症基金会"Stichting tegen Kanker"(C.0011-204-208)(EL) 和鲁汶大学协同行动计划 (GOA/11/010) 的资助。

本研究部分由美国国家癌症研究所校内研究计划（DRS）的癌症流行病学和遗传学部门（Division of Cancer Epidemiology and Genetics，DCEG）资助。本出版物的内容不一定反映美国卫生与公众服务部的观点或政策，提及商品名称、商业产品或组织也不代表美国政府的认可。

（吉毅，张梓欣 译）

参考文献

[1] Bhaskaranand K, Navadgi BC (2002) Glomus tumour of the hand. J Hand Surg 27：229–231

[2] Brems H, Beert E, de Ravel T, Legius E (2009a) Mechanisms in the pathogenesis of malignant tumours in neurofibromatosis type 1. Lancet Oncol 10：508–515

[3] Brems H, Park C, Maertens O, Pemov A, Messiaen L, Upadhyaya M, Claes K, Beert E, Peeters K, Mautner V, Sloan JL, Yao L, Lee CC, Sciot R, De Smet L, Legius E, Stewart DR (2009b) Glomus tumors in neurofibromatosis type 1：genetic, functional, and clinical evidence of a novel association. Cancer Res 69：7393–7401

[4] Cooke ED, Harris J, Fleming CE, Steinberg MD, Foster JM (1995) Correlation of pain with temperature and blood-flow changes in the lower limb following chemical lumbar sympathectomy in reflex sympathetic dystrophy. A case report. Int Angiol 14：226–228

[5] De Smet L, Sciot R, Legius E (2002) Multifocal glomus tumours of the fingers in two patients with neurofibromatosis type 1. J Med Genet 39: e45

[6] Folpe AL, Fanburg-Smith JC, Miettinen M, Weiss SW (2001) Atypical and malignant glomus tumors: analysis of 52 cases, with a proposal for the reclassification of glomus tumors. Am J Surg Pathol 25: 1-12

[7] Hingtgen CM (2008) Neurofibromatosis: the role of guanosine triphosphatase activating proteins in sensory neuron function. Sheng Li Xue Bao 60: 581-583

[8] Huson SM, Compston DA, Clark P, Harper PS (1989) A genetic study of von Recklinghausen neurofibromatosis in south east Wales. I. Prevalence, fitness, mutation rate, and effect of parental transmission on severity. J Med Genet 26: 704-711

[9] Kim YC (2000) An additional case of solitary subungual glomus tumor associated with neurofi-bromatosis 1. J Dermatol 27: 418-419

[10] Klaber R (1938) Morbus Recklinghausen with glomoid tumours. Proc R Soc Med 31: 347

[11] Lee DW, Yang JH, Chang S, Won CH, Lee MW, Choi JH, Moon KC (2011) Clinical and pathological characteristics of extradigital and digital glomus tumours: a retrospective comparative study. J Eur Acad Dermatol Venereol 25: 1392-1397

[12] Leonard M, Harrington P (2010) Painful glomus tumour of the thumb in an 11-year-old child with neurofibromatosis 1. J Hand Surg Eur Vol 35: 319-320

[13] Lin YC, Hsiao PF, Wu YH, Sun FJ, Scher RK (2010) Recurrent digital glomus tumor: analysis of 75 cases. Dermatol Surg 36: 1396-1400

[14] Longdon EJ, McCulloch TA, Perks AG, Ubhi CS, Morgan WE (2007) Multiple glomus tumors: an unusual presentation of chronic regional pain. Anesth Analg 105: 554-555

[15] Love JG (1944) Glomus tumors: diagnosis and treatment. Proc Staff Meet Mayo Clin 19: 113-116

[16] Maertens O, De Schepper S, Vandesompele J, Brems H, Heyns I, Janssens S, Speleman F, Legius E, Messiaen L (2007) Molecular dissection of isolated disease features in mosaic neurofibro-matosis type 1. Am J Hum Genet 81: 243-251

[17] Morrison SJ, White PM, Zock C, Anderson DJ (1999) Prospective identification, isolation by flow cytometry, and in vivo self-renewal of multipotent mammalian neural crest stem cells. Cell 96: 737-749

[18] Nebreda CL, Urban BJ, Taylor AE (2000) Upper extremity pain of 10 years duration caused by a glomus tumor. Reg Anesth Pain Med 25: 69-71

[19] Okada O, Demitsu T, Manabe M, Yoneda K (1999) A case of multiple subungual glomus tumors associated with neurofibromatosis type 1. J Dermatol 26: 535-537

[20] Oughterson AW, Tennant R (1939) Angiomatous tumors of the hands and feet. Surgery 5: 73-100

[21] Park YH, Choi SW, Cho BK, Houh W (1994) Solitary type of glomus tumor developed in multiple sites. Ann Dermatol 6: 225-229

[22] Rettig AC, Strickland JW (1977) Glomus tumor of the digits. J Hand Surg Am 2: 261-265

[23] Sawada S, Honda M, Kamide R, Niimura M (1995) Three cases of subungual glomus tumors with von Recklinghausen neurofibromatosis. J Am Acad Dermatol 32: 277-278

[24] Soto E, Stewart DR, Mannes AJ, Ruppert SL, Baker K, Zlott D, Handel D, Berger AM (2012) Oral ketamine in the palliative care setting: a review of the literature and case report of a patient with neurofibromatosis type 1 and glomus tumor-associated complex regional pain syndrome. Am J Hosp Palliat Care 29(4): 308-317

[25] Stewart DR, Sloan JL, Yao L, Mannes AJ, Moshyedi A, Lee CC, Sciot R, De Smet L, Mautner VF, Legius E (2010) Diagnosis, management, and complications of glomus tumours of the digits in neurofibromatosis type 1. J Med Genet 47: 525-532

[26] Stewart DR, Pemov A, Van Loo P, Beert E, Brems H, Sciot R, Claes K, Pak E, Dutra A, Lee CC, Legius E (2012) Mitotic recombination of chromosome 17q as a common cause of loss of heterozygosity of NF1 in neurofibromatosis type 1-associated glomus tumors. Genes Chromosomes Cancer 51: 429-437

[27] Strauchen JA (2002) Germ-line mutations in nonsyndromic pheochromocytoma. N Engl J Med 347: 854-855

[28] Tsuneyoshi M, Enjoji M (1982) Glomus tumor: a clinicopathologic and electron microscopic study. Cancer 50: 1601-1607

[29] Van Geertruyden J, Lorea P, Goldschmidt D, de Fontaine S, Schuind F, Kinnen L, Ledoux P, Moermans JP (1996) Glomus tumours of the hand. A retrospective study of 51 cases. J Hand Surg Br 21: 257-260

[30] Vasisht B, Watson HK, Joseph E, Lionelli GT (2004) Digital glomus tumors: a 29-year experience with a lateral subperiosteal approach. Plast Reconstr Surg 114: 1486-1489

第25章 嗜铬细胞瘤和1型神经纤维瘤病
Pheochromocytoma and NF1

Birke Bausch and Hartmut P. H. Neumann

25.1 引言

1型神经纤维瘤病（Neurofibromatosis type 1，NF1）又称雷克林豪森病（von Recklinghausen disease），是一种常见的常染色体显性遗传病。其发生与嗜铬细胞瘤相关，而嗜铬细胞瘤是一种罕见的神经内分泌肿瘤，可分泌儿茶酚胺类激素，既有散发性发病，也有家族遗传性发病。1型神经纤维瘤病是目前已知最早的遗传性嗜铬细胞瘤相关综合征，这类疾病还包括：多发性内分泌肿瘤2型（multiple endocrine neoplasia type 2，MEN2）、希佩尔-林道综合征（von Hippel-Lindau disease，VHL）、嗜铬细胞瘤（pheochromocytoma）/副神经节瘤综合征（paraganglioma syndromes，PGL1-4）和家族性嗜铬细胞瘤综合征（familial pheochromocytoma Syndromes）。它们具有典型的临床特征和分子遗传学基础。与这类综合征有关的嗜铬细胞瘤在发病年龄、肿瘤发生部位和恶性潜能方面存在差异。在嗜铬细胞瘤患者中，持续或间歇性的高血压是影响患者生存率的高危因素。而在NF1患者中，几乎一半的高血压病都由伴发的嗜铬细胞瘤所导致。尽管

我们发现只在少数NF1患者中伴发嗜铬细胞瘤，但其实两种疾病的历史同样悠久，而且存在一些显著的共同特征。

25.2 历史背景

NF1是历史上首个被报道的遗传性嗜铬细胞瘤相关综合征。它与嗜铬细胞瘤的第一次临床报道，不仅发表在同一个世纪，而且相距不超过10年。1882年，德国病理学家Friedrich Daniel von Recklinghausen（1833—1910）首次发表了一篇关于神经纤维瘤病的详细报道，并以他的名字命名了这种疾病（von Recklinghausen 1882）。4年后，Felix Fränkel发表了1篇关于1名有双侧肾上腺肉瘤和血管肉瘤病患者（Minna Roll，18岁）的临床报道（Fränkel 1886）。这篇文章通常被认为是对嗜铬细胞瘤的首次报道。但121年后，根据目前的认知和诊断方案，此患者应被诊断为MEN2（Neumann et al. 2007）。1910年，Suzuki首次报道了同时发生嗜铬细胞瘤与NF1患者的临床表现。他详细描述了该患者右侧肾上腺嗜铬细胞瘤和皮肤型神经纤维瘤病的临床症状和体征（Suzuki 1910）。自1911年

后，嗜铬细胞瘤被逐渐认为是 NF1 的一种罕见但具有特异性的临床特征。

25.3 流行病学和病因学

NF1 是常见的常染色体显性遗传病之一，其外显率为 100%（Lammert et al. 2005），发病率在 1/3 000 至 1/2 600 之间。NF1 和嗜铬细胞瘤发病的主要原因均为神经嵴细胞的恶性增殖。一般来说，嗜铬细胞瘤是指具有内分泌活性的、可分泌儿茶酚胺类激素的、肾上腺或肾上腺外的交感副神经节肿瘤；而副神经节瘤是指不具有内分泌活性的副交感副神经节肿瘤，其主要发生在头颈部（Neumann 2008）。嗜铬细胞瘤的发病率远低于 NF1，为（2~8）/100 万（Beard et al. 1983）。25%~30% 的嗜铬细胞瘤伴有遗传性嗜铬细胞瘤相关的综合征（NF1、MEN2、VHL、PGL1-4 和家族性嗜铬细胞瘤综合征）（Neumann et al. 2002；Karasek et al. 2010）。在 2%~4% 的嗜铬细胞瘤中，NF1 基因是该肿瘤发病的遗传学基础（Bausch et al. 2006a,b；Mannelli et al. 2009）。据估计，在 NF1 患者中伴发嗜铬细胞瘤的概率为 0.1%~5.7%（Walther et al. 1999）。

25.4 临床特点

NF1 和嗜铬细胞瘤都具有显著的临床症状和体征。NF1 最显著的特点就是其临床异质性：在两个不相关的患者之间，或具有血缘关系的不同患者之间，甚至在同一个患者的不同时间段，都具有不同的临床表现或体征。也正是因为这一特点，NF1 患者又被称为"假面具者"。在临床上，由于部分 NF1 患者体内大量分泌肾上腺素、去甲肾上腺素和多巴胺这些儿茶酚胺类激素，大约 24% 的患者都会出现心悸、头痛和出汗的典型三联征（Plouin et al. 1981；Mannelli et al. 1999）。分泌过量的儿茶酚胺类激素甚至会导致心律失常或心力衰竭，从而危及生命。此外，几乎所有的 NF1 患者都有持续性或间歇性高血压。

NF1 患者的典型临床特征还包括：皮肤色素异常（其可表现为咖啡牛奶斑、腋窝或腹股沟雀斑）、神经纤维瘤、丛状神经纤维瘤、视路胶质瘤和 Lisch 虹膜结节等临床症状及体征。大约有 50% 的 NF1 患者可伴有学习障碍，同时伴有发生骨骼异常或血管疾病的风险。相对于正常人群，NF1 患者发生高血压的概率要大得多（Lynch et al. 1972；Walther et al. 1999），而且在大多数情况下，只能用肾动脉狭窄或主动脉缩窄来解释，而没有明确的高血压致病原因。在所有 NF1 患者中，嗜铬细胞瘤的发生率为 0.1%~5.7%，这一概率要远小于高血压病 NF1 患者中嗜铬细胞瘤的发生率（20%~50%）（Lynch et al. 1972；Kalff et al. 1982；Walther et al. 1999）。

25.5 分子基础

NF1 及其相关的嗜铬细胞瘤，都是由位于染色体 17q11.2 上的肿瘤抑制基因 *NF1* 杂合性失活突变导致的。针对 *NF1* 基因的突变分析，目前比较耗时，因为该基因本身较大而嗜铬细胞瘤在 NF1 患者中发病率较低（0.1%~5.7%），所以该基因的突变分析存在一定的困难，因此较少进行。这类患者的基因突变谱与一般 NF1 患者的基因突变谱相似。超过 80% 的基因突变是无义突变，或者是移码突变（可能产生截断的无功能的神经纤维瘤蛋白）（图 25.1）。只有大约 10% 的基因突变表现为缺失或重复，其能够影响 1~>50 个外显子基因序列（Bausch et al. 2007）（图 25.1）。而尚未发现全基因缺失或大规模的基因重排，与嗜铬细胞瘤发生相关的特定基因突变也未明确。

在 2%~4% 的嗜铬细胞瘤患者中，NF1 被认为是发病的遗传学基础。就目前而言，针对散发性嗜铬细胞瘤患者的 *NF1* 基因突变分析并不罕见。有研究报道了 NF1 基因错义突变导致双侧良性嗜铬细胞瘤的病例。但对该患者重新进行临床评估时，发现了微弱但极具特征性的 NF1 临床表现。因此，我们不仅可以通过分子遗传学分析，还可以借助其典型的临床特征，对这类嗜铬细胞瘤进行鉴别诊断（图 25.2）（Bausch et al. 2006a,b）

作为已知最早的遗传性嗜铬细胞瘤相关综合征，NF1 必须与其他嗜铬细胞瘤相关的综合征结合

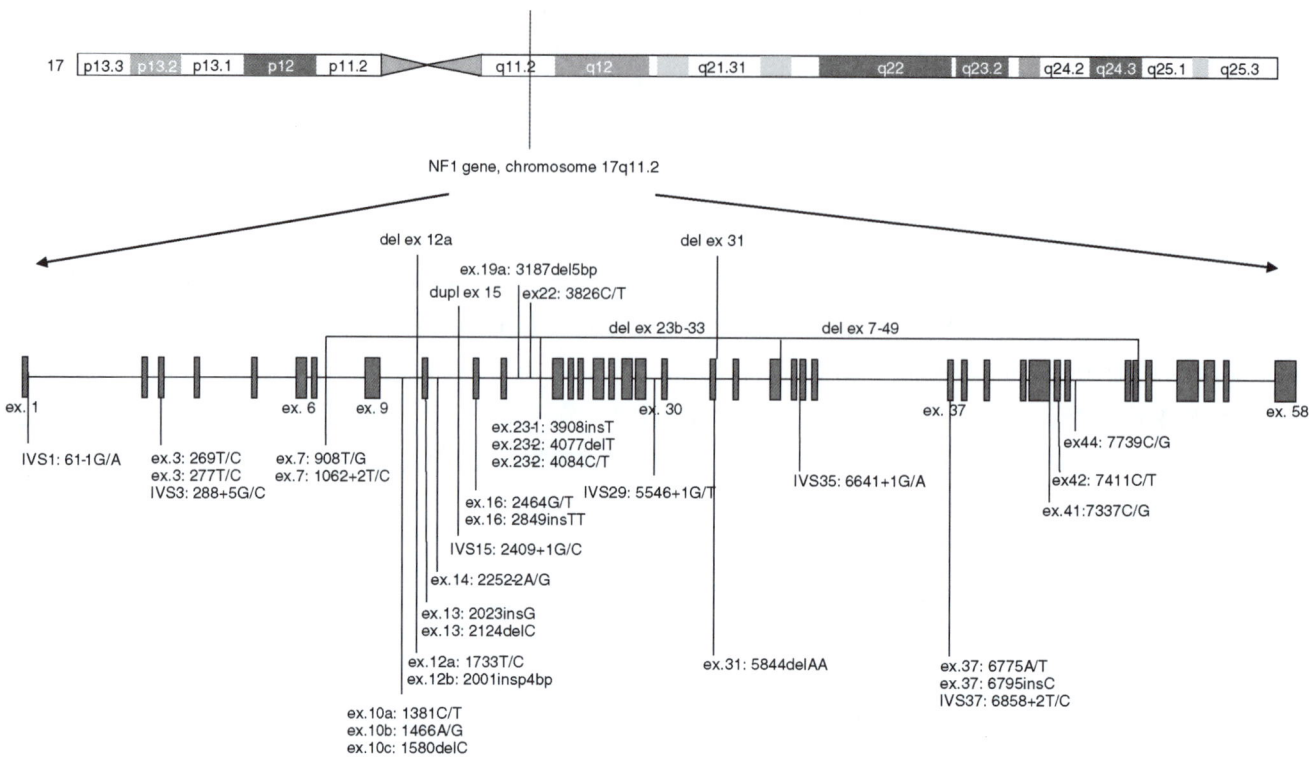

图 25.1　NF1 和嗜铬细胞瘤患者的基因突变图谱

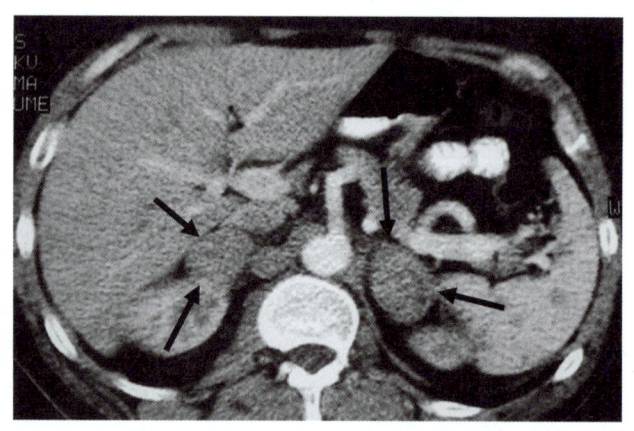

图 25.2　双侧嗜铬细胞瘤的 CT 扫描

起来综合分析。它们的特征在于不同的临床特征和分子遗传学基础。NF1 基因是与嗜铬细胞瘤发病相关的 10 个肿瘤易感基因之一（Neumann et al. 2004；Benn and Robinson 2006；Mannelli et al. 2007；Bayley et al. 2010；Burnichon et al. 2010；Qin et al. 2010；Comino-Mendez et al. 2011）（表 25.1）。其余基因包括：VHL、MAX、TMEM127 和 SDH（琥珀酸脱氢酶）复合物亚基（SDHA、SDHB、SDHC、SDHD 和 SDHAF2）基因的杂合性失活突变，可导致 VHL、PGL（1-4）型综合征以及家族性嗜铬细胞瘤综合征（表 25.1）。RET 原癌基因的突变，则可导致 RET 蛋白过度激活，从而导致 MEN 2A 或 MEN 2B 的发生（表 25.1）。在遗传模式上，除了 PGL 1 型或 PGL 2 型以及 MAX 基因相关的家族性嗜铬细胞瘤综合征，同时遵循常染色体显性遗传或染色体的亲缘效应（为母系印记）以外，其余综合征均只遵循常染色体显性遗传。只有从父亲处获得的基因突变，才会发生肿瘤（Hensen et al. 2004；Bayley et al. 2010；Comino-Mendez et al. 2011）。与 NF1 相比，其余综合征的致病基因比 NF1 基因相对更小，而且有更明确的基因型-表型相关性。因此在怀疑患者有 VHL、MEN2 或 PGL（1-4）综合征时，可以进行基因突变分析以明确诊断，并确定临床危险度分级。而由 TMEM127、MAX 和 SDHA 基因突变引起的家族性嗜铬细胞瘤综合征的主要表型，尚未明确定义，因此一般不进行基因筛查。在目前的临床和科研工作中，由于 NF1 基因较大和缺乏明确的基因型-表型相关性的缘故，我们很少采用分子遗传学分析，而是根据其临床特征和表现，对 NF1 患者进行诊断和鉴别诊断。

表 25.1 遗传性嗜铬细胞瘤综合征的分子遗传学基础

项目	NF1	VHL	MEN2	PGL1	PGL2	PGL3	PGL4	家族性嗜铬细胞瘤综合征		
遗传模式	常染色体显性遗传	常染色体显性遗传	常染色体显性遗传	常染色体显性遗传+母系遗传印记	常染色体显性遗传+母系遗传印记	常染色体显性遗传	常染色体显性遗传	常染色体显性遗传	常染色体显性遗传	常染色体显性遗传+母系遗传印记
基因类型	肿瘤抑制基因	肿瘤抑制基因	原癌基因	肿瘤抑制基因	肿瘤抑制基因	肿瘤抑制基因	肿瘤抑制基因		肿瘤抑制基因	
基因	NF1	VHL	RET	SDHD	SDHAF2	SDHC	SDHB	TMEM127	SDHA	MAX
染色体位置	17q11.2	3p25.5	10q11.2	11q23	11q13.1	1q21	1p35–p36	2q11.2	5p15.33	14q23
外显子	60	3	21	4	4	6	8	4	15	5
突变类型	功能丧失性突变	功能丧失性突变	功能获得性突变	功能缺失性突变	功能缺失性突变	功能缺失性突变	功能缺失性突变		功能缺失性突变	

25.6 发生机制

肿瘤抑制基因 *NF1* 的突变主要导致神经纤维瘤蛋白功能的缺失。在嗜铬细胞瘤中，由于体细胞的二次打击和剩余野生型等位基因的缺失（Knudson 1971；Bausch et al. 2007），可导致 *NF1* 基因杂合性的缺失，其遵循 Knudson 于 1971 年提出的"二次打击理论"。在肿瘤发生的机制上，由于神经纤维瘤蛋白是 GTPase 酶蛋白家族中的一种，这类蛋白质可下调原癌基因 p21-ras 的表达。P21-ras 基因可通过激活不同的信号通路，如：干细胞因子（stem cell factor，SCF）/c-kit 信号通路、mTOR 和 MAP 激酶通路等，对细胞的生长和调节具有重要的影响。神经纤维瘤蛋白功能的缺失可导致 p21-ras 基因过表达，从而导致细胞恶性增殖。此外，通过对全基因组表达的研究，我们对遗传性嗜铬细胞瘤相关综合征的发生机制有了新的认识。根据基因转录组分析结果，其主要可分为两个亚组（Burnichon et al. 2011）。一组为 *VHL* 或 *SDHx* 基因突变导致的肿瘤，可在低氧环境下进行转录增殖，主要特征包括氧化还原酶活性降低、缺氧以及血管生成增加；另一组为 *RET*、*NF1* 和 *TMEM127* 基因突变导致的肿瘤，其特征主要表现为 p21-ras 基因介导的 MAP 信号通路激活，从而导致细胞恶性增殖。

25.7 NF1 患者中嗜铬细胞瘤的临床特征

嗜铬细胞瘤一般为散发的，或者是遗传性肿瘤综合征的一部分。大多数散发性嗜铬细胞瘤患者的诊断年龄在 40～50 岁之间，其临床特征具有"10% 规律"，即：10% 为双侧肾上腺肿瘤；10% 为胸、腹、肾上腺外的交感副神经节肿瘤；10% 为恶性肿瘤。由于良性和恶性嗜铬细胞瘤都具有相同的组织学或生化特征，所以很难据此进行鉴别诊断。唯一可行的办法就是观察其是否存在淋巴结转移或远处转移（Tischler 2008）。

25%～30% 的嗜铬细胞瘤是家族性的，或者与遗传性嗜铬细胞瘤相关综合征有关，如：NF1、VHL、MEN2、副神经节瘤综合征或家族性嗜铬细胞瘤综合征等（表 25.2）。NF1 患者中伴发嗜铬细胞瘤的比例为 0.1%～5.7%，VHL 患者中的比例为 10%～20%，MEN2 患者中的比例约为 50%（Walther et al. 1999；Dluhy 2002）。与 NF1 一样，这类遗传性嗜铬细胞瘤相关综合征具有一些显著的特异性临床症状（表 25.2）。VHL 患者可出现视网膜或小脑血管母细胞瘤、肾透明细胞癌和胰岛细胞瘤。MEN 2A 患者则可出现甲状腺髓样癌（medullary thyroid carcinoma，MTC）以及甲状旁腺功能亢进的临床症状；MEN 2B 除了与 MTC 相关之外，还与多发性黏膜神经瘤和 Marfanoid 体质相关。PGL（1 至 4）型综合征典型的临床表现为头颈部的副交感神经节瘤。

副神经节瘤是一种主要发生在头颈部，不具有内分泌活性的副交感神经节肿瘤。它不仅与 PGL（1 至 4）型综合征相关，而且与嗜铬细胞瘤密切相关。这两类肿瘤都起源于神经嵴细胞，因此具有相同的组织病理学背景，通常被认为是嗜铬细胞瘤发生的遗传学基础。此外，它也有发生遗传性嗜铬细胞瘤相关综合征的显著临床特征，其患病率取决于潜在的家族性嗜铬细胞瘤综合征。绝大多数的头颈部副神经节瘤都是由 *SDHx* 基因突变导致的，因此也与 PGL（1 至 4）型综合征相关。副神经节瘤在 VHL 患者中的患病率约为 8/1 000。1987 年，DeAngelis 报道了一例 NF1 患者伴有肺副神经节瘤、颈静脉球瘤和嗜铬细胞瘤的临床病例。这也是 MEN 2 型患者或 NF1 患者中唯一伴发副神经节瘤的病例（DeAngelis et al. 1987；Boedeker et al. 2009）。

遗传性嗜铬细胞瘤相关综合征在诊断年龄、肿瘤发生部位和恶性程度上存在差异（Neumann et al. 2002；Bausch et al. Et al. 2006a,b）（表 25.2）。与散发性嗜铬细胞瘤相比，遗传性嗜铬细胞瘤患者的诊断年龄更低，发生在双侧及肾上腺外的更为常见，且恶性程度更高，其发病年龄比散发性嗜铬细胞瘤小 15 岁左右，最小年龄的患者为 1 名 VHL 病患者（16 岁）。在 *MAX* 基因突变相关的嗜铬细胞瘤中，至少有 67% 的患者有双侧嗜铬细胞瘤。家族性嗜铬细胞瘤发生在肾上腺外的概率超过 10%，其中

表 25.2 遗传性嗜铬细胞瘤相关综合征的临床特点

项目	散发性	NF1	VHL	MEN2	PGL1	PGL2	PGL3	PGL4	家族性嗜铬细胞瘤综合征	
									TMEM127	SDHA
基因	—	NF1	VHL	RET	SDHD	SDHAF2	SDHC	SDHB	TMEM127	SDHA
嗜铬细胞瘤患病率	100%	0.1%~5.7%	10%~20%	50%	34%	0	单病例	37%	100%	单病例
平均诊断年龄（岁）	40~50	43	16	34	26	23	41	34	43	—
单侧肾上腺	90%	84%~95%	92%	97%	86%	—	—	42%	100%	单病例
双侧肾上腺	10%	5%~15%	55%	65%	48%	—	—	12%	35%	—
肾上腺外定位	10%	6%	17%	3%	57%	—	单病例	58%	—	单病例
恶性嗜铬细胞瘤	10%	3%~12%	4%	3%	0%	—	0	24%	5%	单病例
头颈部副神经节瘤	—	单病例	很少	单病例	48%	100%	>90%	6%	单病例	单病例
其他临床特征	—	咖啡斑、腋窝或腹股沟雀斑、神经纤维瘤、丛状神经纤维瘤、视神经胶质瘤、Lisch结节	眼睛和中枢神经系统的血管母细胞瘤、肾透明细胞癌、胰岛细胞瘤、内淋巴囊肿瘤	甲状腺髓样癌、A型、甲状旁腺功能亢进、B型、多发性神经瘤、Marfanoid体质	胃肠道间质瘤		胃肠道间质瘤	肾细胞癌、胃肠道间质瘤		

伴发4型副神经节瘤综合征的概率可高达58%,而伴发 MEN 2型的概率仅为3%。遗传性嗜铬细胞瘤中出现恶性肿瘤的概率较大。而 MAX 基因突变或4型 PGL 相关的嗜铬细胞瘤,出现恶性肿瘤的概率分别为37%或24%。与之相反的是,NF1相关的嗜铬细胞瘤与散发性嗜铬细胞瘤存在很多的相似之处(Walther et al. 1999;Bausch et al. 2006a,b)。其平均诊断年龄约为43岁,相对较晚。84%~95%的肿瘤局限于肾上腺,仅有约6%的肿瘤发生于肾上腺外,5%~15%的患者表现为双侧嗜铬细胞瘤。在恶性肿瘤的发生率上,有3%~12%的NF1相关性嗜铬细胞瘤中出现恶性肿瘤(图25.3),虽然这已经是遗传性嗜铬细胞瘤中发病率高的综合征之一,但却与散发性嗜铬细胞瘤的发生率更加相似。

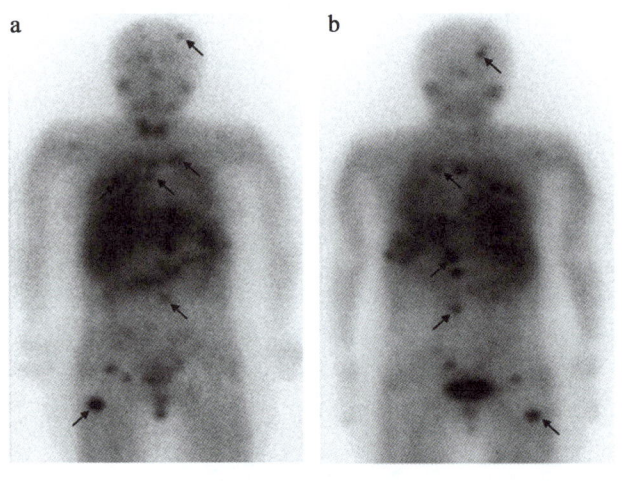

图25.3 恶性嗜铬细胞瘤的 MIBG 显像

25.8 诊断方法

NF1的诊断主要根据1987年 NIH 共识会议上制订的临床标准(1997年更新)(Anonymous 1988;Gutmann et al. 1997)。根据该标准,在没有其他临床诊断的前提下,至少满足以下两个特征才能被诊断为 NF1:① 6个或以上咖啡牛奶斑(CALM),在青春期前直径>5 mm 或在青春期后直径>15 mm;② 2个或以上任何类型的神经纤维瘤,或1个丛状神经纤维瘤(pNF);③ 腋窝或腹股沟区雀斑;④ 视路胶质瘤(optic pathway glioma,OPG),或2个或以上 Lisch 结节(虹膜错构瘤)。嗜铬细胞瘤的诊断主要依据生化检查和影像学检查。首先,根据嗜铬细胞瘤分泌去甲肾上腺素、肾上腺素和多巴胺这些儿茶酚胺类激素的特点,可以检测甲氧基肾上腺素和甲氧基去甲肾上腺素(肾上腺素和去甲肾上腺素的代谢产物)在体内的水平。24小时尿游离儿茶酚胺和总甲氧基肾上腺素测定的灵敏性约为90%;血浆游离甲氧基肾上腺素测定的灵敏性约为97%。这些检查通常用作诊断嗜铬细胞瘤的初步筛查。在生化检查以后,可以进行放射学评估。计算机断层扫描(computed tomography,CT 扫描)和磁共振成像(magnetic resonance imaging,MRI)都能有98%~100%的灵敏性和70%的特异性。而对可能发生在非典型部位的肿瘤、多发性嗜铬细胞瘤、恶性嗜铬细胞瘤,MRI 和 CT 扫描结果阴性但有明确的临床证据和生化指标异常结果时,通常采用 MIBG 显像检查或 ^{18}F-FDG PET 检查。

在20%~50%的高血压病 NF1患者中,嗜铬细胞瘤通常是高血压病的致病因素,严重时甚至会危及生命,但仍有治愈的可能。根据嗜铬细胞瘤在 NF1患者中的临床特点,我们可对年龄在43岁左右的高血压病 NF1患者进行嗜铬细胞瘤的筛查。具体流程可根据嗜铬细胞瘤的诊断方案,首先进行24小时尿游离儿茶酚胺和总甲氧基肾上腺素水平测定,或血浆游离甲氧基肾上腺素测定,之后再进行 CT 或 MRI 扫描。在大多数情况下,NF1患者发生的嗜铬细胞瘤局限于肾上腺,恶性肿瘤的概率约为12%。虽然我们可对 NF1 患者的基因突变进行分子遗传学分析,但由于 NF1 基因型与表型并不具有明确的相关性,且具有高度异质性(同一家族的患者都可能有不同的临床表现或病理),所以分子遗传学分析并不常用。

在临床病例中,仅有2%~4%的 NF1与嗜铬细胞瘤相关。因此在目前的临床及科研工作中,NF1主要的诊断依据仍然是其特殊的临床表现。值得注意的是,在诊断嗜铬细胞瘤患者时,应仔细筛查是否具有该病的特异性临床特征。

(顾松 译)

参考文献

[1] Anonymous (1988) Neurofibromatosis. Conference statement. National Institutes of Health Consensus Development Conference. Arch Neurol 45(5):575-578

[2] Bausch B, Borozdin W et al (2006a) Clinical and genetic characteristics of patients with neurofi-bromatosis type 1 and pheochromocytoma. N Engl J Med 354(25):2729-2731

[3] Bausch B, Koschker AC et al (2006b) Comprehensive mutation scanning of NF1 in apparently sporadic cases of pheochromocytoma. J Clin Endocrinol Metab 91(9):3478-3481

[4] Bausch B, Borozdin W et al (2007) Germline *NF1* mutational spectra and loss-of-heterozygosity analyses in patients with pheochromocytoma and neurofibromatosis type 1. J Clin Endocrinol Metab 92(7):2784-2792

[5] Bayley JP, Kunst HP et al (2010) *SDHAF2* mutations in familial and sporadic paraganglioma and phaeochromocytoma. Lancet Oncol 11:366-372

[6] Beard CM, Sheps SG et al (1983) Occurrence of pheochromocytoma in Rochester, Minnesota, 1950 through 1979. Mayo Clin Proc 58(12):802-804

[7] Benn DE, Robinson BG (2006) Genetic basis of phaeochromocytoma and paraganglioma. Best Pract Res Clin Endocrinol Metab 20(3):435-450

[8] Boedeker CC, Erlic Z et al (2009) Head and neck paragangliomas in von Hippel-Lindau disease and multiple endocrine neoplasia type 2. J Clin Endocrinol Metab 94(6):1938-1944

[9] Burnichon N, Briere JJ et al (2010) *SDHA* is a tumor suppressor gene causing paraganglioma. Hum Mol Genet 19:3011-3020

[10] Burnichon N, Vescovo L et al (2011) Integrative genomic analysis reveals somatic mutations in pheochromocytoma and paraganglioma. Hum Mol Genet 20(20):3974-3985

[11] Cichowski K, Shih TS et al (1999) Mouse models of tumor development in neurofibromatosis type 1. Science 286(5447):2172-2176

[12] Comino-Mendez I, Gracia-Aznarez FJ et al (2011) Exome sequencing identifies MAX mutations as a cause of hereditary pheochromocytoma. Nat Genet 43:663-667

[13] DeAngelis LM, Kelleher MB et al (1987) Multiple paragangliomas in neurofibromatosis: a new neuroendocrine neoplasia. Neurology 37(1):129-133

[14] Dluhy R (2002) Pheochromocytoma-death of an axiom. N Engl J Med 346:1486

[15] Fränkel F (1886) Ein Fall von doppelseitigem, völlig latent verlaufenen Nebennierentumor und gleichzeitiger Nephritis mit Veränderungen am Circulationsapparat und Retinitis. Arch Pathol Anat Physiol Klin Med 103:244-263

[16] Gutmann DH, Aylsworth A et al (1997) The diagnostic evaluation and multidisciplinary management of neurofibromatosis 1 and neurofibromatosis 2. JAMA 278(1):51-57

[17] Hensen EF, Jordanova ES et al (2004) Somatic loss of maternal chromosome 11 causes parent-of-origin-dependent inheritance in SDHD-linked paraganglioma and phaeochromocytoma families. Oncogene 23(23):4076-4083

[18] Kalff V, Shapiro B et al (1982) The spectrum of pheochromocytoma in hypertensive patients with neurofibromatosis. Arch Intern Med 142(12):2092-2098

[19] Karasek D, Frysak Z et al (2010) Genetic testing for pheochromocytoma. Curr Hypertens Rep 12:456-464

[20] Knudson AG Jr (1971) Mutation and cancer: statistical study of retinoblastoma. Proc Natl Acad Sci USA 68:820-823

[21] Lammert M, Friedman JM et al (2005) Prevalence of neurofibromatosis 1 in German children at elementary school enrollment. Arch Dermatol 141(1):71-74

[22] Lynch JD, Sheps SG et al (1972) Neurofibromatosis and hypertension due to pheochromocytoma or renal-artery stenosis. Minn Med 55(1):25-31

[23] Mannelli M, Ianni L et al (1999) Pheochromocytoma in Italy: a multicentric retrospective study. Eur J Endocrinol 141(6):619-624

[24] Mannelli M, Ercolino T et al (2007) Genetic screening for pheochromocytoma: should SDHC gene analysis be included? J Med Genet 44(9):586-587

[25] Mannelli M, Castellano M et al (2009) Clinically guided genetic screening in a large cohort of italian patients with pheochromocytomas and/or functional or nonfunctional paragangliomas. J Clin Endocrinol Metab 94(5):1541-1547

[26] Martin GA, Viskochil D et al (1990) The GAP-related domain of the neurofibromatosis type 1 gene product interacts with ras p21. Cell 63(4):843-849

[27] Neumann H (2008) Pheochromocytoma. In: Fauci A, Longo DL, Braunwald E (eds) Harrison's principles of internal medicine, 17th edn. McGraw-Hill, New York

[28] Neumann HP, Bausch B et al (2002) Germ-line mutations in nonsyndromic pheochromocytoma. N Engl J Med 346(19):1459-1466

[29] Neumann HP, Pawlu C et al (2004) Distinct clinical features of paraganglioma syndromes associated with *SDHB* and *SDHD* gene mutations. JAMA 292(8):943-951

[30] Neumann HP, Vortmeyer A et al (2007) Evidence of MEN-2 in the original description of classic pheochromocytoma. N Engl J Med 357(13):1311-1315

[31] Plouin PF, Degoulet P et al (1981) Screening for phaeochromocytoma: in which hypertensive patients? A semiological study of 2585 patients, including 11 with phaeochromocytoma (author's transl). Nouv Presse Med 10(11):869-872

[32] Qin Y, Yao L et al (2010) Germline mutations in *TMEM127* confer susceptibility to pheochromocytoma. Nat Genet 42:229-233

[33] Suzuki S (1910) Über zwei Tumoren aus Nebennierenmarkgewebe. Berlin Klein Wchnschr 47:1623

[34] Tischler AS (2008) Pheochromocytoma and extra-adrenal paraganglioma: updates. Arch Pathol Lab Med 132(8):1272-1284

[35] von Recklinghausen F (1882) Über die multiplen Fibrome der Haut und ihre Beziehung zu den multiplen Neuromen. 3-18 Berlin: Hirschwald

[36] Walther MM, Herring J et al (1999) von Recklinghausen's disease and pheochromocytomas. J Urol 162(5):1582-1586

[37] Weiss B, Bollag G et al (1999) Hyperactive Ras as a therapeutic target in neurofibromatosis type 1. Am J Med Genet 89(1):14-22

第26章 人皮肤型神经纤维瘤的分子和细胞基础及发生

Molecular and Cellular Basis of Human Cutaneous Neurofibromas and Their Development

Juha Peltonen, Eeva-Mari Jouhilahti, and Sirkku Peltonen

26.1 引言

多发性皮肤型神经纤维瘤是 1 型神经纤维瘤病的两个典型特征之一，也是该病命名的由来。尽管皮肤型神经纤维瘤不会对生命构成严重威胁，但已成为大多数成年 NF1 患者的主要疾病负担。与丛状神经纤维瘤可能发生恶变不同，皮肤型神经纤维瘤是良性肿瘤，从不发生恶性转化。皮肤型神经纤维瘤常在青春期开始出现，数量随年龄增长不断增加，可多达数千个（图 26.1）。神经纤维瘤最常见于躯干，也可以出现在所有皮肤区域。然而，皮肤型神经纤维瘤的生长潜力有限，直径很少超过 2~3 cm。肿瘤可以无蒂、有蒂或只位于皮内，呈紫色，按压时出现纽孔征。可有瘙痒或疼痛感，但大多数没有症状。

皮肤型神经纤维瘤是由施万细胞、成纤维细胞、神经束膜细胞、肥大细胞和轴突组成的混合细胞肿瘤。这些细胞嵌在丰富的胶原细胞外基质中，这使神经纤维瘤具有特征的橡胶弹性。从人神经纤维瘤中培养的施万细胞携带具有二次打击的 NF1 基因。传统观点认为，神经纤维瘤的发生是皮肤小神经分支被破坏和随后局部细胞增殖的过程。最近利用基因工程小鼠和从人神经纤维瘤中培养的细胞进行的研究显示多能前体细胞可能在肿瘤的起始和细胞表型数目惊人的神经纤维瘤的发生中起关键作用。

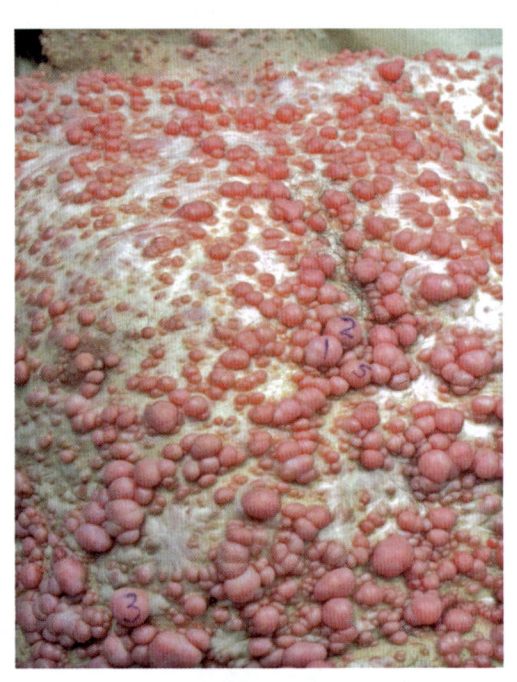

图 26.1 一例肿瘤负担相对较重的皮肤型神经纤维瘤

J. Peltonen (*) • E.-M. Jouhilahti
Department of Cell Biology and Anatomy, University of Turku, Turku, Finland
e-mail: juhpel@utu.fi

S. Peltonen
Department of Dermatology, University of Turku and Turku University Hospital, Turku, Finland

M. Upadhyaya and D. N. Cooper (eds.), *Neurofibromatosis Type 1*,
DOI 10.1007/978-3-642-32864-0_26, # Springer-Verlag Berlin Heidelberg 2012

26.2 神经纤维瘤的分子和细胞组成

对神经纤维瘤的分子水平研究可以解释这些肿瘤的物理特征,并根据其特定的基因表达谱来识别细胞表型。事实上,如果没有分子标记,识别神经纤维瘤组织中的单个细胞是很困难的。值得注意的是,NF1 基因的蛋白质产物神经纤维瘤蛋白作为生物标志物的价值很小,原因是它广泛表达,不具有细胞类型特异性。此外,体外研究表明,NF1 的表达受到严格的时间调控,阴性细胞可能在短时间内转化为阳性细胞;反之亦然(Cichowski et al. 2003;Kaufmann et al. 1999;Pummi et al. 2000)。

26.2.1 皮肤型神经纤维瘤的细胞外基质

神经纤维瘤含有丰富的细胞外基质,包括占无脂干重 30%~45% 的胶原蛋白(Peltonen et al. 1986)。这大约是皮肤对应值的一半,但却是人类神经内膜的 2 倍。经典的 Ⅰ 型和 Ⅲ 型胶原纤维在神经纤维瘤中最常见,且 Ⅲ 型胶原的相对含量高。这类似于结缔组织形成或愈合过程。

神经纤维瘤中的胶原原纤维形成松散排列的网络,不形成明显的胶原束。这与在光镜下组织学评估中观察到的瘤体上方有厚厚的胶原纤维束的皮肤形成鲜明对比。电子显微镜下示神经纤维瘤中胶原纤维的直径通常为 30~40 nm(Lassmann et al. 1976),小于人类皮肤(60 nm)或神经外膜(80~100 nm),但与神经内膜的胶原纤维相当。

在神经纤维瘤中也很容易检测到 Ⅵ 型胶原蛋白和 mRNA(Peltonen et al. 1990)。Ⅵ 型胶原呈细珠状,在神经纤维瘤中 Ⅵ 型胶原可以形成 Luse 小体,电镜下可以观察到典型的斑马样外观。成纤维细胞、施万细胞和神经束膜细胞都可以表达 Ⅰ 型、Ⅲ 型和 Ⅵ 型胶原(Jaakkola et al. 1989a,b)。成纤维细胞和神经束膜细胞可能是神经纤维瘤中纤维连接蛋白的来源。肿瘤的大多数细胞被基底膜覆盖,因此基底膜特异性 Ⅳ 型胶原在神经纤维瘤中很容易检测到。除了作为细胞外基质的组成部分,Ⅳ 型胶原蛋白似乎更像是一种细胞生物标志物。例如,施万细胞和神经束膜细胞被基底膜包裹,因此可以通过对 Ⅳ 型胶原、特定的层粘连蛋白和巢蛋白进行免疫标记来检测。

神经纤维瘤中的蛋白多糖/胶原蛋白比值是周围真皮组织的 4~10 倍(Peltonen et al. 1986)。这在一定程度上解释了神经纤维瘤的柔软特性,并可能为肿瘤生长提供有利环境。

神经纤维瘤的大部分体积是由细胞外基质组成的。因此下调相关基因可能达到控制肿瘤大小的目的。

26.2.2 皮肤型神经纤维瘤的细胞分化

神经纤维瘤由具有施万细胞、神经束膜细胞、成纤维细胞和肥大细胞表型特征的细胞组成的瘤体(图 26.2),类似于周围神经的结缔组织(Peltonen et al. 1988)。散在的巨噬细胞和淋巴细胞并不少见。此外,皮肤的附属器,如毛囊和腺体结构,也是典型表现。

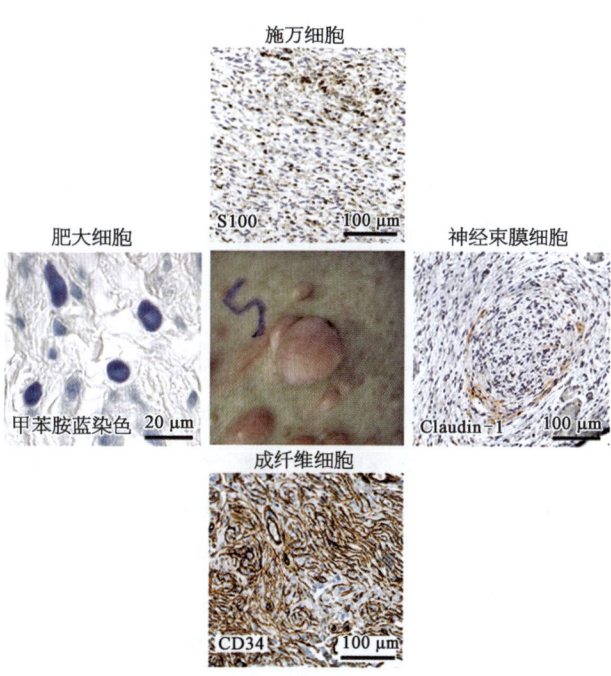

图 26.2 S100、Claudin-1、CD34 和甲苯胺蓝染色显示皮肤型神经纤维瘤中的施万细胞、神经束膜细胞、成纤维细胞和肥大细胞

26.2.2.1 施万细胞

光镜和电镜检查可见大量神经纤维瘤细胞的形态与施万细胞表型一致。在超微结构水平上,致瘤性施万细胞具有复杂的分枝状细胞质突起,这些突起被连续的基底膜覆盖(Hirose et al. 1986;

Lassmann et al. 1976)。肿瘤施万细胞表达 S100β，通过对 S100 蛋白的免疫标记估计施万细胞占神经纤维瘤细胞总数的 60%～80%（Peltonen et al. 1988）。然而，肿瘤内 S100 标记信号的强度存在显著差异，与神经相关的施万细胞相比，致瘤性施万细胞表达 S100 的水平较低（Peltonen et al. 1988）。施万细胞也有基底膜成分的阳性表达，如Ⅳ型胶原蛋白和层粘连蛋白链。值得注意的是，神经纤维瘤中Ⅳ型胶原阳性细胞的数量很容易超过 S100 阳性细胞的数量。这一发现说明神经束膜细胞可能是 S100 阴性、Ⅳ型胶原阳性细胞。与正常的施万细胞相反，神经纤维瘤施万细胞表达神经生长因子（nerve growth factor，NGF）受体（Ross et al. 1986）。

一项重要的体外研究发现，从皮肤型神经纤维瘤中培养的细胞亚群携带双重失活的 *NF1* 基因（Serra et al. 2000）。这些细胞 S100β 阳性，其形态与施万细胞一致。

26.2.2.2 神经束膜细胞

在正常的神经中，神经束膜细胞层围绕轴突-施万细胞单位形成一个紧密的鞘，从而勾画出神经束。在超微结构水平上，神经束膜细胞被连续的基底膜覆盖，有细长的细胞突起和大量的细胞内囊泡。神经纤维瘤中孤立的神经束膜细胞可能有不连续的基底膜，与正常的神经束膜细胞相比，胞饮泡数量可能更少（Erlandson and Woodruff 1982；Lassmann et al. 1976）。成纤维细胞不被基底膜覆盖，因此神经束膜细胞上的基底膜可以明确区分神经束膜细胞和成纤维细胞。由于缺乏特征性生物标志物，研究和鉴定神经纤维瘤中的神经束膜细胞一直很困难。一组分子标志物，如葡萄糖转运体 1（glucose transporter 1，Glut-1）、上皮膜抗原（epithelial membrane antigen，EMA）和Ⅳ型胶原，被用于鉴定神经纤维瘤中的神经束膜细胞（Hirose et al. 2003；Peltonen et al. 1988；Perentes et al. 1987）。一个有潜力的神经束膜细胞标志物是紧密连接蛋白 claudin-1（Pummi et al. 2006）。神经束膜细胞紧密连接蛋白的表达与之前的超微结构观察结果一致，相邻神经束膜细胞重叠的突起有时会通过紧密连接连接起来（Erlandson 1985）。

结合抗原标志物的研究表明，所有神经纤维瘤中都存在神经束膜细胞，但它们的数量在不同个体和肿瘤的不同区域之间有所不同（Peltonen et al. 1988；Pummi et al. 2006）。所有神经纤维瘤中都有向神经束膜细胞分化的区域。通过免疫标记 S100β 阴性同时 EMA 和 claudin-1 阳性的细胞来估计，大约 10% 的神经纤维瘤细胞为神经束膜细胞亚群（Peltonen et al. 1988；Pummi et al. 2006）。因为致瘤性施万细胞可以穿过神经纤维瘤的神经周围屏障并在被破坏的神经束外增生，神经束膜细胞被认为在神经纤维瘤发生中起到纵容作用。

26.2.2.3 成纤维细胞

神经纤维瘤成纤维细胞起源于神经内成纤维细胞。它们合成肿瘤中的纤维性胶原和纤维连接蛋白。成纤维细胞有丰富的细胞质和细胞器，但缺乏基底膜。免疫组化检测成纤维细胞表达 CD34（Hirose et al. 2003；Lassmann et al. 1976）。

26.2.2.4 肥大细胞

肥大细胞前体离开骨髓，迁移到组织中，并发育成熟。肥大细胞参与多种免疫、自身免疫和过敏机制。被激活的肥大细胞选择性地从颗粒中释放多种生物活性介质和细胞因子来参与这些过程。肥大细胞在正常皮肤中含量丰富，位于毛囊附近。它们与皮肤中的感觉神经有功能上的联系，也存在于神经干中。在神经纤维瘤和其他周围神经鞘膜瘤中肥大细胞数量丰富。肥大细胞可通过特定的 Kit 配体介导机制向神经纤维瘤迁移（Yang et al. 2003）。在光镜下，可通过其典型的胞质颗粒识别肥大细胞，并可以通过 pH1 的阿利新蓝染色、甲苯胺蓝染色或免疫标记Ⅷ因子相关抗原来观察（Peltonen et al. 1988）。后文分子机制会讨论 *NF1* 单倍体不足的肥大细胞如何促进神经纤维瘤的生长。

26.3 皮肤型神经纤维瘤的发生

目前，基于对条件敲除小鼠的研究和对培养的人神经纤维瘤细胞的遗传分析，我们认为施万细胞在神经纤维瘤的发展中起关键作用（Maertens et al. 2006；Serra et al. 2000；Zhu et al. 2002）。这些研究共同表明，*NF1* 基因的双等位基因失活是神经纤维瘤形成的先决条件，但肿瘤只发生于基因型为 $NF1^{+/-}$ 的背景下。

26.3.1 体外培养神经纤维瘤细胞是神经纤维瘤病因学研究的关键

几十年来，从 NF1 患者神经纤维瘤处及外观正常的组织提取 NF1 相关细胞进行培养的工作一直受到关注，但结果有限。使用添加 FCS 的 DMEM 标准培养流程可促进成纤维细胞的生长。研究结果表明，NF1 基因缺失可导致成纤维细胞产生过多的Ⅰ型和Ⅲ型纤维胶原（Peltonen et al. 1986）。早期传代细胞具有施万细胞、成纤维细胞和神经束膜细胞的特征（Jaakkola et al. 1989a）。尽管有大量证据表明肿瘤抑制模型（NF1 基因双等位失活）与神经纤维瘤的发生有关，但混合细胞组成阻碍了对 NF1 二次打击存在于特定细胞类型的解释。

通过富集两个不同神经纤维瘤施万细胞群的研究发现，具有施万细胞特征的神经纤维瘤细胞亚群会对 NF1 基因造成二次打击，导致出现 $NF1^{-/-}$ 基因型（Serra et al. 2000）。在肿瘤施万细胞亚群中检测到对 NF1 基因的二次打击，但在人神经纤维瘤培养的其他细胞亚群中没有检测到（Maertens et al. 2006；Serra et al. 2000）。进一步的研究结果显示，NF1 基因的二次打击在每个皮肤型神经纤维瘤中是独特的（Maertens et al. 2006）。还需要注意的是，在每个肿瘤中只发现了一种二次打击，这表明具有 NF1 二次打击的施万细胞群是克隆性的（Maertens et al. 2006）。

另外一项对神经纤维瘤来源细胞的研究表明，神经纤维瘤含有 $NF1^{+/-}$ 基因型的多能细胞-神经纤维瘤来源前体细胞（neurofibroma-derived precursor cell，NFP），NFP 具有强大的增生能力和分化为施万细胞、神经元、上皮细胞和脂肪的能力（Jouhilahti et al. 2011）。

基于对不同皮肤型神经纤维瘤来源的施万细胞培养的观察，发现携带 $NF1^{+/-}$ 和 $NF1^{-/-}$ 基因型的施万细胞在不同的神经纤维瘤中相对比例存在差异（Serra et al. 2000）。$NF1^{-/-}$ 基因型细胞具有生长优势，但目前尚不清楚在皮肤型神经纤维瘤中携带 $NF1^{-/-}$ 基因型的施万细胞比例，同时也不了解随着携带 $NF1^{+/-}$ 基因型细胞比例的增大会多大程度上影响肿瘤的生长。

26.3.2 靶向小鼠神经纤维瘤的发生

多个 Nf1 小鼠模型被用于对肿瘤发生的研究。Krox20 是一种周围神经髓鞘形成的相关基因，在 5%～10% 的施万细胞和施万细胞前体中表达。Krox20 启动子元件的下游插入 Cre 构建的 $NF1^{flox/flox}$ 小鼠出现了神经纤维瘤表现（Staser et al. 2012；Zhu et al. 2002）。在这个小鼠模型中，肿瘤仅发生在 Nf1 杂合突变的背景下。小鼠研究表明肿瘤微环境在神经纤维瘤的发生发展中起重要作用。更具体地说，该小鼠实验模型进一步表明，丛状神经纤维瘤的形成需要 NF1 单倍不足和 c-kit 功能正常的造血系统，包括肥大细胞（Yang et al. 2008）。然而，值得注意的是，大多数小鼠研究都集中在丛状神经纤维瘤上，其研究结果可能只部分适用于人 1 型神经纤维瘤病的共性和人皮肤型神经纤维瘤的特性。

26.3.3 神经纤维瘤发生的其他解释

既往研究表明，皮肤型神经纤维瘤起源于青春期和成年期的小周围神经，因为神经纤维瘤包含了以随意方式排列的正常周围神经具有的所有细胞类型。然而，成年施万细胞并不表现为持续分裂的细胞群，这使得它们不太可能出现二次打击。皮肤型神经纤维瘤在青春期开始生长的事实反映了 NF1 二次打击突变出现时间较晚。此外，皮肤型神经纤维瘤的生长有限可能与 $NF1^{-/-}$ 施万细胞的克隆性分裂潜能有限相关。

26.3.3.1 神经纤维瘤发生中的多能前体细胞

最近的研究表明，在人类和 NF1 小鼠模型中，多能前体细胞是皮肤型神经纤维瘤的一部分，也是这些肿瘤的潜在细胞来源（Jouhilahti et al. 2011；Le et al. 2009）。皮肤型神经纤维瘤的细胞来源问题已经通过使用具有 $Nf1^{+/-}$ 基因型，且使用他莫昔芬诱导真皮干细胞/祖细胞二次打击的小鼠模型来研究（Le et al. 2009）。在这些小鼠局部应用他莫昔芬导致 Nf1 基因双等位失活后发生皮肤型神经纤维瘤。

人皮肤型神经纤维瘤含有多能前体细胞 NFP，

NFP 具有分化为神经纤维瘤中多种细胞类型的潜力（Jouhilahti et al. 2011）。然而，NFP 具有 $NF1^{+/-}$ 基因型，进而推测人皮肤型神经纤维瘤中的 $NF1^{-/-}$ 施万细胞也可能来自多能祖细胞，这些祖细胞发生了 NF1 二次突变，进而分化为施万样细胞。因为在每个肿瘤中只发现了一种二次打击，故认为单个 $NF1^{-/-}$ 基因型细胞克隆性增生形成施万细胞群。然而，对于人体组织而言，恢复肿瘤形成的起始阶段并分离出具有 $NF1^{-/-}$ 基因型的单个多能细胞是有挑战的。

为了进一步明确神经纤维瘤来源前体细胞的潜在位置，我们研究了皮肤型神经纤维瘤的结构。组织学分析显示，毛囊结构嵌入皮肤型神经纤维瘤，甚至 NF1 患者在肿瘤发生早期外观正常皮肤的毛囊附近的皮肤也会出现微小的神经纤维瘤（Jouhilahti et al. 2011；Karvonen et al. 2000）。早期研究已经确定了皮肤来源的前体细胞（skin-derived precursor cell，SKP）特征，这种细胞可能存在于小鼠的毛根中，并有能力生成表达神经元、神经胶质细胞、平滑肌和脂肪细胞标记的细胞亚群（Fernandes et al. 2004，2008；Toma et al. 2005）。综上所述，这些结果提示毛囊中的多能细胞可能与皮肤型神经纤维瘤的发生有关。

26.3.4 炎症

在癌症生物学中，炎症细胞在肿瘤发生中的作用已得到认可（Hanahan and Weinberg 2011）。人类和小鼠研究均证明，神经纤维瘤的肿瘤间质中存在肥大细胞（Jouhilahti et al. 2011；Peltonen et al. 1988；Yang et al. 2008；Zhu et al. 2002）。据推测，肥大细胞通过分泌炎症介质、血管生成促进因子和血管内皮生长因子，在肿瘤的发生和维持中发挥积极作用（Yang et al. 2008）。此外，肥大细胞还会释放 PDGF-BB 和 TGF-β，这些因素共同促进了施万细胞、成纤维细胞和神经束膜细胞的增生和存活，并促进成纤维细胞合成胶原蛋白。

最近的研究结果揭示了另外一种在神经纤维瘤发生中具有潜在作用的炎症成分。神经纤维瘤来源的施万细胞的基因表达谱揭示具有 $NF1^{-/-}$ 基因型的施万细胞表达 HLA Ⅱ 类基因。此外，免疫组化分析显示，神经纤维瘤中散在分布 T 淋巴细胞。先前的研究表明，施万细胞有能力完成整个免疫反应过程，包括抗原提呈和识别，通过分泌可溶性因子调节免疫反应，以及通过 Fas 和 FasL 的相互作用终止免疫反应（Meyer zu Hörste et al. 2008）。我们认为有 $NF1^{-/-}$ 基因型的肿瘤施万细胞可能作为树突状或非专职抗原提呈细胞，参与由调节性 T 细胞介导的免疫耐受。

26.4 结论

综上所述，皮肤型神经纤维瘤是一种良性肿瘤，不会发生恶性转化。尽管它们不会对生命构成威胁，但由于它们数量众多，皮肤型神经纤维瘤是大多数成年 NF1 患者的主要疾病负担。目前认为，皮肤型神经纤维瘤的发生需要 $NF1^{+/-}$ 和 $NF1^{-/-}$ 基因型的多种类型施万细胞之间的相互作用。多能前体细胞是这些肿瘤的潜在细胞起源。此外，炎症成分在肿瘤发生中的作用增加了发病机制的复杂性。

（徐学刚，高兴华 译）

参考文献

[1] Cichowski K, Santiago S, Jardim M, Johnson B, Jacks T (2003) Dynamic regulation of the Ras pathway via proteolysis of the NF1 tumor suppressor. Genes Dev 17: 449-454

[2] Erlandson RA (1985) Peripheral nerve sheath tumors. Ultrastruct Pathol 9: 113-122

[3] Erlandson RA, Woodruff JM (1982) Peripheral nerve sheath tumors: an electron microscopic study of 43 cases. Cancer 49: 273-287

[4] Fernandes K, McKenzie I, Mill P, Smith K, Akhavan M, Barnabé-Heider F, Biernaskie J, Junek A, Kobayashi N, Toma J, Kaplan D, Labosky P, Rafuse V, Hui C, Miller F (2004) A dermal niche for multipotent adult skin-derived precursor cells. Nat Cell Biol 6: 1082-1093

[5] Fernandes K, Toma J, Miller F (2008) Multipotent skin-derived precursors: adult neural crest-related precursors with therapeutic potential. Philos Trans R Soc Lond B Biol Sci 363: 185-198

[6] Hanahan D, Weinberg RA (2011) Hallmarks of cancer: the next generation. Cell 144: 646-674

[7] Hirose T, Sano T, Hizawa K (1986) Ultrastructural localization of S-100 protein in neurofibroma. Acta Neuropathol 69: 103-110

[8] Hirose T, Tani T, Shimada T, Ishizawa K, Shimada S, Sano T (2003) Immunohistochemical demonstration of EMA/Glut1-positive perineurial cells and CD34-positive fibroblastic cells in peripheral nerve sheath tumors. Mod Pathol 16: 293-298

[9] Jaakkola S, Peltonen J, Riccardi V, Chu M, Uitto J (1989a) Type 1 neurofibromatosis: selective expression of extracellular matrix genes by Schwann cells, perineurial cells, and fibroblasts in mixed cultures. J Clin Invest 84: 253-261

[10] Jaakkola S, Peltonen J, Uitto JJ (1989b) Perineurial cells coexpress genes encoding interstitial collagens and basement membrane zone components. J Cell Biol 108: 1157-1163

[11] Jouhilahti EM, Peltonen S, Callens T, Jokinen E, Heape AM, Messiaen L, Peltonen J (2011) The development of cutaneous neurofibromas. Am J Pathol 178: 500-505

[12] Karvonen S, Kallioinen M, Ylä-Outinen H, Pöyhönen M, Oikarinen A, Peltonen J (2000) Occult neurofibroma and increased S100 protein in the skin of patients with neurofibromatosis type 1: new insight to the etiopathomechanism of neurofibromas. Arch Dermatol 136: 1207-1209

[13] Kaufmann D, Bartelt B, Hoffmeyer S, Müller R (1999) Posttranslational regulation of neurofibromin content in melanocytes of neurofibromatosis type 1 patients. Arch Dermatol Res 291: 312-317

[14] Lassmann H, Jurecka W, Gebhart W (1976) Some electron microscopic and autoradiographic results concerning cutaneous neurofibromas in von Recklinghausen's disease. Arch Dermatol Res 255: 69-81

[15] Le L, Shipman T, Burns D, Parada L (2009) Cell of origin and microenvironment contribution for NF1-associated dermal neurofibromas. Cell Stem Cell 4: 453-463

[16] Maertens O, Brems H, Vandesompele J, De Raedt T, Heyns I, Rosenbaum T, De Schepper S, De Paepe A, Mortier G, Janssens S, Speleman F, Legius E, Messiaen L (2006) Comprehensive NF1 screening on cultured Schwann cells from neurofibromas. Hum Mutat 27: 1030-1040

[17] Meyer zu Hörste G, Hu W, Hartung HP, Lehmann HC, Kieseier BC (2008) The immunocompetence of Schwann cells. Muscle Nerve 37: 3-13

[18] Peltonen J, Penttinen R, Larjava H, Aho H (1986) Collagens in neurofibromas and neurofibroma cell cultures. Ann NY Acad Sci 486: 260-270

[19] Peltonen J, Jaakkola S, Lebwohl M, Renvall S, Risteli L, Virtanen I, Uitto J (1988) Cellular differentiation and expression of matrix genes in type 1 neurofibromatosis. Lab Invest 59: 760-771

[20] Peltonen J, Jaakkola S, Hsiao LL, Timpl R, Chu ML, Uitto J (1990) Type VI collagen. In situ hybridizations and immunohistochemistry reveal abundant mRNA and protein levels in human neurofibroma, schwannoma and normal peripheral nerve tissues. Lab Invest 62: 487-492

[21] Perentes E, Nakagawa Y, Ross GW, Stanton C, Rubinstein LJ (1987) Expression of epithelial membrane antigen in perineurial cells and their derivatives. An immunohistochemical study with multiple markers. Acta Neuropathol 75: 160-165

[22] Pummi K, Ylä-Outinen H, Peltonen J (2000) Oscillation and rapid changes of NF1 mRNA steadystate levels in cultured human keratinocytes. Arch Dermatol Res 292: 422-424

[23] Pummi K, Aho H, Laato M, Peltonen J, Peltonen S (2006) Tight junction proteins and perineurial cells in neurofibromas. J Histochem Cytochem 54: 53-61

[24] Ross AH, Herlyn M, Maul GG, Koprowski H, Bothwell M, Chao M, Pleasure D, Sonnenfeld KH (1986) The nerve growth factor receptor in normal and transformed neural crest cells. Ann NY Acad Sci 486: 115-123

[25] Serra E, Rosenbaum T, Winner U, Aledo R, Ars E, Estivill X, Lenard H, Lázaro C (2000) Schwann cells harbor the somatic NF1 mutation in neurofibromas: evidence of two different Schwann cell subpopulations. Hum Mol Genet 9: 3055-3064

[26] Staser K, Yang FC, Clapp DW (2012) Pathogenesis of plexiform neurofibroma: tumor-stromal/hematopoietic interactions in tumor progression. Annu Rev Pathol 7: 469-495

[27] Toma J, McKenzie I, Bagli D, Miller F (2005) Isolation and characterization of multipotent skinderived precursors from human skin. Stem Cells 23: 727-737

[28] Yang F, Ingram D, Chen S, Hingtgen C, Ratner N, Monk K, Clegg T, White H, Mead L, Wenning M, Williams D, Kapur R, Atkinson S, Clapp D (2003) Neurofibromin-deficient Schwann cells secrete a potent migratory stimulus for $Nf1^{+/-}$ mast cells. J Clin Invest 112: 1851-1861

[29] Yang F, Ingram D, Chen S, Zhu Y, Yuan J, Li X, Yang X, Knowles S, Horn W, Li Y, Zhang S, Yang Y, Vakili S, Yu M, Burns D, Robertson K, Hutchins G, Parada L, Clapp D (2008) Nf1-dependent tumors require a microenvironment containing $Nf1^{+/-}$ and c-kit-dependent bone marrow. Cell 135: 437-448

[30] Zhu Y, Ghosh P, Charnay P, Burns D, Parada L (2002) Neurofibromas in NF1: Schwann cell origin and role of tumor environment. Science 296: 920-922

第27章 体细胞拷贝数改变：1型神经纤维瘤病相关的恶性周围神经鞘膜瘤中基因和蛋白质的表达

Somatic Copy Number Alterations: Gene and Protein Expression Correlates in NF1-Associated Malignant Peripheral Nerve Sheath Tumors

Meena Upadhyaya and David N. Cooper

27.1 引言

1型神经纤维瘤病（NF1）与良性和恶性肿瘤的生长有关（Upadhyaya and Cooper 1998；Bennett et al. 2009；reviewed by Upadhyaya 2010）。10%~15%的NF1患者会发展为恶性周围神经鞘膜瘤（MPNST）（Evans et al. 2002）。MPNST是一类软组织肉瘤（Barretina et al. 2010），大约一半的MPNST与NF1有关，患者预后较差。NF1-MPNST通常与先前存在的丛状神经纤维瘤（plexiform neurofibroma，PNF）或局部皮肤型神经纤维瘤有关。通过全身MRI扫描发现体内多个PNF的患者，其发展为MPNST的风险增加20倍（Tucker et al. 2005），这强调了对这些患者进行定期临床监测的必要性。不与NF1相关的散发性MPNST一开始就表现为恶性肿瘤（reviewed by Upadhyaya 2011）。许多MPNST直到晚期或原发肿瘤已经转移时才被诊断出，最常见的转移部位是肺、肝转移和脑转移较为少见。

目前对NF1-MPNST的诊断和临床管理状态并不理想，恶性转化的分子机制也尚未完全明确。为了识别NF1患者肿瘤形成过程中的关键基因，以及与MPNST发展相关的特定诊断和预后生物标志物，确定基因组中发生频繁改变的染色体区域是非常重要的。

直到最近，人们普遍认为每个基因的2个拷贝几乎在每个人类基因组中都存在。然而，最近的发现表明，大段的DNA片段，其大小范围从几千到几百万个碱基不等，可以在拷贝数量上有所不同。由于这种拷贝数变异（copy number variation，CNV）可以涵盖整个基因，这会导致个体间基因数量和基因表达的显著差异。曾被认为每个基因组中存在2个拷贝的基因现在发现可以存在于1个或3个或更多的拷贝中（Beroukhim et al. 2010）。

先天性拷贝数变异（CNV）可以代表良性多态性变体，或可能与疾病相关，包括癌症易感性。体系拷贝数改变（somatic copy number alteration，SCNA）不同于胚系拷贝数改变，因为它们仅存在于体细胞组织中。SCNA在癌症中极为常见［Kuo et

---

M. Upadhyaya • D. N. Cooper
Institute of Medical Genetics, School of Medicine, Cardiff University, Cardiff CF14 4XN, UK
e-mail: upadhyaya@cardiff.ac.uk

M. Upadhyaya and D. N. Cooper (eds.), *Neurofibromatosis Type 1*,
DOI 10.1007/978-3-642-32864-0_27, # Springer-Verlag Berlin Heidelberg 2012

al. 2009；Rothenberg and Settleman 2010；Kuiper et al. 2010；Shlien and Malkin 2009，2010；Baudis 2007；Henrichsen et al. 2009a，b；癌症染色体异常数据库（Database of Chromosome Aberrations in Cancer），2000（http：//cgap. nci. nih. gov/Chromosomes/Mitelman）]。与其他肿瘤相关的基因变化一样，这些SCNA（由于其所包含的基因）可以在细胞增殖、生存和克隆方面提供选择性优势。SCNA也在非癌症研究中有报道。Bruder等（2008）发现，在没有任何已知疾病的11对同卵双胞胎成员之间的多个位点存在拷贝数差异。随后，该小组检测到来自1个人在死后不同组织之间的拷贝数差异，但这些拷贝数差异被认为与疾病无关（Piotrowski et al. 2008）。根据这一发现，很明显，一些疾病可能确实是由拷贝数变化引起的，这些拷贝数改变存在于特定的组织但不存在于血液或口腔黏膜细胞，而血液或口腔黏膜组织常用于基因组分析（Dear 2009）。

肿瘤的基因组在遗传上是异质性的（Ding et al. 2008；Kan et al. 2010），其不同的重排（Campbell et al. 2008）和SCNA（Beroukhim et al. 2010）使其有所区分。SCNA分析可以识别不同肿瘤中反复出现的异常。在某些情况下，SCNA导致了新型致癌基因的发现，这反过来又提出了特定的治疗途径（Beroukhim et al. 2010；Valsesia et al. 2011）。

各种基于芯片的方法已被开发出来以检测CNV和SCNA。早期研究已经证实，由重叠的人类BAC克隆构建的比较基因组杂交阵列（array-CGH）是成功的。最近，结合高密度SNP和CNV基因分型芯片已被采用。这种高密度芯片，通常包含数百万个单独的标记，现在可以同时用于评估与特定肿瘤类型相关的可遗传拷贝数变异和体系SCNA相关的表达变化（Lebron et al. 2011）。用于CNV/SCNA分析的其他方法包括显微镜、荧光原位杂交（fluorescence in situ hybridisation，FISH）、DNA印迹法（Southern blotting）、基于PCR的方法（包括实时PCR、MLPA）、分子拷贝数计数（Daser et al. 2006）、高分辨率芯片技术和高通量测序（Campbell et al. 2008；Meyerson et al. 2010）。

本章讨论了体系拷贝数改变（SCNA）在良性神经纤维瘤转化为恶性周围神经鞘膜瘤中的潜在作用，并重点介绍了MPNST和相关癌症的基因表达以及基于蛋白质的研究。

27.2 体系拷贝数改变（SCNA）如何提高我们对MPNST分子基础的认识

尽管神经纤维瘤蛋白功能的丧失是NF1肿瘤发生的主要事件（reviewed by Upadhyaya 2011），但其他遗传病变也在影响细胞生长、分化和凋亡方面发挥了作用，这些过程是促进丛状和非典型神经纤维瘤恶性转化所必需的。基于芯片的技术使得在一次实验中同时分析来自MPNST和其他癌症的RNA或DNA中的多个基因和许多不同的基因组区域成为可能。这种基于芯片的分析使我们能够全面概览可能与肿瘤发生相关的所有基因表达和拷贝数变化。已经有几项研究分析了肿瘤DNA和RNA，以寻找能够区分MPNST和良性神经纤维瘤的潜在分子特征（表27.1）。

表27.1 NF1相关的MPNST中CNA和基因以及蛋白质表达分析

参考文献	肿瘤类型	分析方法	基因或染色体改变	
			扩增	缺失
Lothe等（1995，1996）	神经纤维瘤（15） MPNST（9）	17q LOH FISH		6个NF1相关的MPNST中有4个存在17q等位基因不平衡
Lothe等（1996）	MPNST（7）	染色体CGH	7个肿瘤中有5个17q24-ter拷贝数增加	10个MPNST中有6个存在13q14-q21区域缺失

续 表

参考文献	肿瘤类型	分析方法	基因或染色体改变	
			扩 增	缺 失
Mechtersheimer 等(1999)	MPNST(19) 神经纤维瘤(10)	染色体 CGH	17q24-q25,7p11-p13,5p15,8q22-q24,12q21-q24	9p21-24,13q14-q22,1p
Kourea 等(1999)	MPNST(11) 原发肿瘤(8) 复发肿瘤(3)	在 DNA 印迹法中使用 INK4A cDNA 探针		许多 MPNST 中存在 INK4A(*CDKN2A*)基因缺失
Nielsen 等(1999)	MPNST(6)	多重 PCR		3 个 MPNST 中存在 *CDKN2A* 基因纯合缺失
Plaat 等(1999)	MPNST(7)	计算机辅助细胞遗传学分析	7q1	1p3,9p1,11q1,12q2,17p1,18q1-q2,19p1,22q1,X,Y
Mertens 等(2000)	MPNST(20) 良性神经纤维瘤(46)	染色体带型分析	7 号染色体	22 号染色体
Schmidt 等(2000)	MPNST(14)	染色体 CGH	Chr 7;8q;15q;17q 扩增	
Koga 等(2002)	MPNST(9) 神经纤维瘤(27) 施万细胞瘤(14)	染色体 CGH	17q 和 X	
Mawrin 等(2002)	MPNST(12)	杂合型丧失		*TP53*,*RB1*
Frank 等(2003)	MPNST(3)	核型分析	7,8	1p,10q,9,15
Perrone 等(2003)	MPNST(20) 神经纤维瘤(14) 散发性 MPNST(12)	基于 PCR 的分子分析 FISH		*CDKN2A* 及其变异体(P15^{INK4b},p14^{ARF})
Skotheim 等(2003)	MPNST(14) MPNST(16) MPNST(44)	综合分析(1)染色体 17 特异性 cDNA 芯片(2)FISH 分析(3)组织芯片	大多数 MPNST 中 *TOP2A* 过表达	
Bridge 等(2004)	MPNST(21)	细胞遗传学和 FISH 分析	7/7q,8/8q,*EGFR*	1p36,3p21-pter,9p23-pter,10,11q23-qter,16/16q24,17,22/22q
Lévy 等(2004)	MPNST(9) PNF(16) CNF(10)	实时定量 PCR	*MK167*、*BIRC5*、*MMP13*、*SPP1*、*MMP9*、*TERT*、*TERC*、*TOP2A*、*SPP2*、*FOXM1*、*FOXA2/HNF3B*、*HMMR/RHAMM*、*CXCL5*、*OSF2*、*CCNE2*、*EPHA7* 和 *TP73* 仅在 MPNSTs 中上调	*ITGB4*、*CMA1*、*L1CAM*、*MPZ*、*DHH*、*S100B*、*ERBB3*、*RASSF2*、*PTCH2*、*TPSB*、*TIM4* 和 *SOX10* 仅在 MPNSTs 中下调
Watson 等(2004)	MPNST(25) 散发型 MPNST(25)	寡核苷酸芯片分析	*NCAM*,*MBP*,*L1CAM*,*PIP*	*IGF2*,*FGFR1*,*MDK*,*MKI67*

续表

参考文献	肿瘤类型	分析方法	基因或染色体改变	
			扩增	缺失
Adamowicz 等(2006)	软组织肉瘤(34) 包括 MPNST(10)	染色体 5p BAC 芯片	*TRIO*、*IRX2* 和 *NKD2* 均位于 5p15.3 并发生扩增	
Miller 等(2006)	原发 MPNST(44) MPNST 细胞系(8) 正常施万细胞系(7)	基因表达谱分析（Affymetrix 芯片）	*EDGRE*,*SOX9*,*TWIST1*	*SOX10*,*CNP*,*PMP2*
Storlazzi 等(2006)	MPNST(28) 原发肿瘤(25) 复发肿瘤(2) 转移肿瘤(1)	使用 BAC 探针对 17q 进行间断 FISH 分析	17q12-17q25 扩增,包含 *ERBB2*、*TOP2A*、*BIRC5*	
Lévy 等(2007)	CNF PNF MPNST	Agilent 22K	*TNXC*	*TNXB*
Kresse 等(2008)	高级别 MPNST(7)	比较基因组杂交	*LOXL2*,*TOP2A*,*ETV4* 和 *BIRC5*	
Tabone-Eglinger 等(2008)	MPNST(42)	FISH	*EGFR*	
Mantripragada 等(2008)	MPNST(35) PNF(16) CNF(8)	靶向基因阵列	*ITGB4*,*PDGFRA*,*MET*,*HGF* 和 *TP73*	*NF1*,*HMMR*,*MMP13*,*INK4A* 和 *CDKN2B*
Fang 等(2009)	MPNST 细胞系(3)	分子细胞遗传学	17q25,17p	9p,12q21-32,X
Perrone 等(2009)	散发型 MPNST(11) NF1 型 MPNST(16)	综合分析（1）FISH（2）基因激活（3）突变分析	*PDGFRA* 和 *PDGFRB*、*EGFR* 拷贝数	
Mantripragada 等(2009)	MPNST(24)	32K BAC 全基因组阵列	*NEDL1*,*AP3B1* 和 *CUL1*	*CDKN2A* 和 *CDKN2B*
Miller 等(2009)	MPNST 细胞系(13) 神经纤维瘤施万细胞系(22) 原发 MPNST(6)	基因表达谱分析（Affymetrix 芯片）	*SOX9*,*TWIST1*	
Brekke 等(2010)	神经纤维瘤(10) MPNST(48)	染色体和比较基因组杂交	8q,17q,7p,10,16,X	9p,11q,17p
Yang 等(2011)	MPNST(51)		*IGF1R*,*EGFR*,*BRAF*,*ETV1*,*MET*,*AKAP*	*CDKN2A*,*CDKN2B*
Yu 等(2011)	MPNST(125)	Affymetrix 全基因组 500K SNP 分析	*CDK4*,*FOXM1*,*SOX5*,*NOL1*,*MLF2*,*FKBP4*,*TSPAN31*	*ERBB2*,*MYC*,*TP53*

续 表

参考文献	肿瘤类型	分析方法	基因或染色体改变	
			扩 增	缺 失
Beert 等(2011)	MPNST(34) 良性神经纤维瘤(15)	Agilent 244K 微阵列	PDGFRA/KIT,TWIST1, EGFR, MET, MYC, CCND2 MDM2,14q,15q, 17q,20q 和 21q	CDKN2A、CDKN2B、TP53、PRDM2、CDKN2C、RNF11、EPS15、NFIA、PGM1、ROR1、UBE2U、CACHD1、RAVER2 和 JAK1。LSAMP(3q13.31)、EPHB1(3q22.2)和 STAG1(3q22.3)。SMARCD1(4q22.3)和 SPRY1(4q28.1)、RB1(13q14.2)、SPRY2(13q31.1)和 SUZ12 基因(17q11.2)在 12、14 和 17 个高等级 MPNSTs 中缺失,CHEK2(22q12.1)和 NF2(22q12.2)、PTEN、RB1
Upadhyaya 等(2012)	MPNST(15)	Affymetrix 全基因组 SNP 6.0 分析	RAC1, ROCK2, PTK2, LIMK1, PRKCA, ACTB, ACTG1, TRID	MMP12,TP53,CDKN2A, HMMR,RB1

注:PNF,丛状神经纤维瘤;CNF,皮肤型神经纤维瘤。

27.3 细胞遗传学和染色体比较基因组杂交研究

对 NF1 - MPNST 的细胞遗传学和 FISH 研究揭示了包括易位、重复以及数目增减在内的广泛染色体变异。大多数 MPNST 具有复杂的核型(Glover et al. 1991;Plaat et al. 1999;Mechtersheimer et al. 1999;Mertens et al. 2000),这使得确定哪些改变具有真正的生物学意义变得很难。在早期研究中,包含潜在相关原癌基因的候选扩增区域包括染色体带 17q24 - q25、7、7p11 - p13、8、5p15、8q22 - q24、12q21 - q24、8/8q 和 15q(Mertens et al. 2000; Frank et al. 2003;Bridge et al. 2004;Lothe et al. 1995,1996),而那些可能包含抑癌基因的缺失区域为 9p21 - p24、13q14 - q22、1p、10q、11q1、15、17p1、17q、18q1 - q2、19p1、22q1、X 和 Y(Mechtersheimer et al. 1999;Lothe et al. 1996;Plaat et al. 1999; Schmidt et al. 2000;Koga et al. 2002)(表 27.1)。与滑膜肉瘤和其他肉瘤中发现的特定染色体易位相比(Barretina et al. 2010),尚未发现与 MPNST 相关的致病染色体变异,尽管已有报道指出存在一些小的重复染色体改变(表 27.1)。最初使用细胞遗传学和 FISH 来识别 NF1 - MPNST 中的大型基因组改变(Mechtersheimer et al. 1999;Lothe et al. 1995;Plaat et al. 1999;Mertens et al. 2000; Skotheim et al. 2003;Frank et al. 2003;Perrone et al. 2003;Bridge et al. 2004;Tabone-Eglinger et al. 2008),后续的研究采用染色体比较基因组杂交(Schmidt et al. 2000;Koga et al. 2002;Lothe et al. 1996)和 BAC 芯片(Adamowicz et al. 2006; Storlazzi et al. 2006;Kresse et al. 2008; Mantripragada et al. 2009)(表 27.1)。然而,这些研究要么分辨率有限,要么仅评估了少数基因区域。最近,已经有研究采用了高分辨率寡核苷酸芯片分析来筛选 NF1 肿瘤中特定的 DNA 拷贝数变化

(Mantripragada et al. 2008；Yu et al. 2011；Beert et al. 2011；Upadhyaya et al. 2012)。

27.4 分子研究

从分子层面来说，MPNST 是复杂的肿瘤。约 95% 的 MPNST 在 NF1 位点存在体系大范围缺失（Upadhyaya et al. 2008）。已有研究报道 NF1 相关 MPNST 中存在不同范围的 NF1 位点重排（Pasmant et al. 2011a）。然而，在这项研究中，MPNST 相关的缺失点并未涉及大多数胚系 NF1 缺失中涉及的同源重复序列或 SUZ12 和 SUZ12P 序列。

20 多年前已经有研究指出肿瘤抑制基因 CDKN2A、TP53 和 RB1 的缺失与 MPNST 相关（reviewed by Upadhyaya 2011）。在几项 NF1 相关的 MPNST 研究中，使用低分辨率和高分辨率技术已发现 9p21 区域的频繁缺失与 CDKN2A（p16）基因的下调有关（Cairns et al. 1995；Kourea et al. 1999；Nielsen et al. 1999；Perrone et al. 2003；Frahm et al. 2004；Sabah et al. 2006；Mantripragada et al. 2008，2009；Beert et al. 2011；Yu et al. 2011）。

已发现许多 NF1 相关的 MPNST 中包含 TP53 基因的 17p13 区域的缺失（Legius et al. 1994；Upadhyaya et al. 2008；Mantripragada et al. 2008）。虽然 TP53 基因常因等位基因缺失或更微妙的病变而失活，但 NF1 相关的 MPNST 中很少发生双等位基因 TP53 失活。p53 的功能缺失导致总体基因组不稳定性增加，表现为基因扩增、非整倍体或其他染色体重排的增加。NF1 小鼠模型证实了 TP53 丧失与 NF1 失活在 MPNST 发展中的积极作用（Cichowski et al. 1999；Vogel et al. 1999），尽管尚不清楚是否存在其他明确的遗传修饰因子也可能导致 NF1-MPNST 的发展。

视网膜母细胞瘤（retinoblastoma，Rb）通路的破坏在 NF1 相关的 MPNST 中很常见。在一项基于 12 名 MPNST 患者的研究中，发现 RB1 基因的破坏在 NF1-MPNST 中很常见；在很多 NF1-MPNST 病例中报道了涉及 RB1 基因的杂合性缺失（Mawrin et al. 2002；Berner et al. 1999）。在一项比较基因组杂交研究中，35 个 MPNST 中有 8 个存在 RB1 基因缺失（Mantripragada et al. 2008）。

因此，MPNST 中 p16INK4A/CDKN2A、RB1 和 TP53 基因的缺失验证了 NF1、TP53 和（或）RB1 通路共失活模型对调控细胞生长和凋亡的影响。Holtkamp 等（2008）报道，可能涉及丛状神经纤维瘤恶性转化的候选基因包括 PDGFRA、PDGF 和 KIT。已有研究指出在 NF1 相关的 MPNST 中 BIRC5 和 TNC 上调，但在神经纤维瘤中未发现这种情况（Karube et al. 2006）。BIRC5 编码的蛋白 Survivin 抑制凋亡，BIRC5 上调在包括 NF1 相关的 MPNST 在内的许多癌症中是频发事件（Mantripragada et al. 2009；Storlazzi et al. 2006）。在我们自己的研究中，还发现了两个凋亡基因，BIRC5 和 TP73 的扩增（Mantripragada et al. 2008）。MPNST 中观察到的 TP73 基因扩增暗示编码的 DNp73 蛋白（一种凋亡抑制剂）可能在恶性施万细胞中上调（Mantripragada et al. 2008）。拓扑异构酶 II alpha（TOP2A）基因也由于 17q21-q22 区域的扩增在许多 NF1 相关的 MPNST 中上调（Latres et al. 1994；Skothei met al. 2003；Kresse et al. 2008）。在包括 NF1-MPNST 在内的软组织肉瘤中，也有研究报道了 TRIO（5p15.2）、NKD2（5p15.33）和 IRX2（5p15.33）的扩增（Adamowicz et al. 2006）。

我们最初在 57 个 MPNST DNA 样本中使用靶向基因阵列来筛选可能的基因改变，发现了肝细胞生长因子基因（hepatocyte growth factor gene，HGF）在 7q21.11 位置的共同扩增、c-MET 原癌基因/肝细胞生长因子受体（c-MET proto-oncogene/hepatocyte growth factor receptor，MET）在 7q31.2 位置的扩增以及血小板衍生生长因子受体 α 多肽基因（platelet-derived growth factor receptor alpha polypeptide gene，PDGFRA）在 4q12 位置的扩增（Mantripragada et al. 2008）。MET 是一种酪氨酸激酶受体，而 HGF 是 MET 的唯一已知配体。通常，只有干细胞表达 MET，使这些细胞能够在胚胎中生长并分化为新组织或进行组织再生。然而，癌症干细胞被认为获得了正常干胞表达 MET 的能力，从而导致肿瘤的进展和转移。通过 HGF 结合激活后，c-Met 自磷酸化，招募其他下游蛋白，激活多个信号通路（如 Ras-MAPK、PI3K、AKT 和 STAT3/5），从而调节细胞生长、运动以及形态改变。

在分析的约一半 MPNST 中还发现了位于 5q34 的透明质酸介导运动受体（hyaluronan-mediated motility receptor，HMMR）基因的半合子缺失（Mantripragada et al. 2008）。已发现几种癌症中 HMMR 过表达，包括 NF1 相关的 MPNST（Kalmyrzaev et al. 2008）。然而，HMMR 基因的半合子缺失不太可能导致该基因的过表达。MPNST 特异性 HMMR 缺失的识别使 HMMR 成为 NF1 患者恶性转化或发展的有力候选基因。随后使用 32K BAC 阵列分析了 25 个 MPNST 的 DNA，发现了在 9p21.3 区域存在约 540 kb 的缺失，该区域包含 CDKN2A、CDKN2B 和 MTAP 基因（Mantripragada et al. 2009）。在我们对 3 个肿瘤样本的研究中发现了这三个基因的双等位基因丧失，并在 8 个 MPNST 中发现了单拷贝缺失（Mantripragada et al. 2009）。

Yu 等（2011）最近的一项研究评估了 38 名 MPNST 患者，其中 23 名（60%）为 NF1 相关型，其余 15 名（40%）为散发病例。这些研究人员鉴定了一些已知对 NF1-MPNST 发展至关重要的位点，包括 17q11.2 上 NF1 的缺失和 9p21 上 CDKN2A 的缺失，以及 7p、8q、12 和 17q 的扩增。CDK4（12q14）的扩增和 FOXM1 蛋白表达的增加是 MPNST 患者预后不良的重要独立预测因子。

27.5 从非典型神经纤维瘤到 MPNST 的转变

非典型神经纤维瘤是有症状的、多细胞的周围神经鞘膜瘤，由染色质异常增多的细胞组成，但没有有丝分裂现象（Beert et al. 2011）。关于 NF1 患者中非典型神经纤维瘤的起源、性质和病理知之甚少。在有些研究中，Beert 等（2011）的研究显示非典型神经纤维瘤是恶性肿瘤的前体肿瘤，CDKN2A/B 的缺失是向 MPNST 进展的第一步。在这项研究中，在 15 个非典型神经纤维瘤中检测到了包含 CDKN2A 和 CDKN2B 的染色体 9p21.3 中的最小重复区域（MOR）缺失（Beert et al. 2011），但在良性神经纤维瘤中未检测到。在另一项研究中（Spurlock et al. 2010），揭示了从良性丛状神经纤维瘤通过非典型丛状神经纤维瘤转化为侵袭性恶性肿瘤的遗传过程，包括 TP53、RB1、CDKN2A 以及若干原癌基因和细胞周期基因的缺失（Spurlock et al. 2010）。

27.6 潜在的 MPNST 特异性通路

Yang 等（2011）对 51 个 NF1 相关的 MPNST 组织样本进行了基因组分析，发现了包含 2 599 个基因的频繁扩增区域以及包含 4 901 个基因的缺失区域。他们还确定了涉及胰岛素样生长因子 1 受体（insulin-like growth factor 1 receptor，IGF1R）通路的基因拷贝数显著增加，包括 IGF1R 基因本身的频繁扩增。为了验证 IGF1R 通路作为 MPNST 潜在靶点的可能性，Yang 等（2011）使用免疫组织化学方法确认了高 IGF1R 蛋白表达与患者更差的无瘤生存期相关。使用小干扰 RNA 或 IGF1R 抑制剂能够显著减少细胞增殖、侵袭和迁移，以及导致 PI3K/AKT、MAPK 通路的表达下降。

在最近对 NF1 肿瘤的研究中，Upadhyaya 等（2012）使用了比比较基因组杂交更密集的 SNP 阵列，并提供了同时检测染色体杂合性丧失（loss of heterozygosity，LOH）和单亲二倍体（uniparental Disomy，UPD）以及拷贝数变化的额外优势。使用人类全基因组 SNP-Array-6.0，对从 15 个 MPNST、5 个良性丛状神经纤维瘤（PNF）和患者匹配的淋巴细胞中分离的 DNA 进行单核苷酸多态性分型和拷贝数改变（SCNA）、杂合性丧失（LOH）和拷贝数中性 LOH（CNN-LOH）分析（Upadhyaya et al. 2012）。MPNST 表现出高水平、高频率的 LOH，这在 PNF 中没有出现。CNN-LOH 在 MPNST 中较为明显，但频率低于基因组缺失。涉及 ITGB8、PDGFA、RAC1（7p21-p22）、PDGFRL（8p22-p21.3）和 MMP12（11q22.3）基因的 SCNA 是 MPNST 特有的。通路分析显示了 MPNST 特异性的7个Rho-GTPase通路基因和若干细胞骨架重塑/细胞黏附基因的扩增。在使用短发夹RAC1、ROCK、PTK2和LIMK1 RNA转染对照和MPNST来源的细胞系的敲低实验中，MPNST细胞系中细胞黏附显著增加，而伤口愈合、细胞迁移和侵袭则减少，这与Rho-GTPase通路基因在MPNST发展和转移中的作用一致。这些结果表明了MPNST中新的治疗干预靶点(Upadhyaya et al. 2012)。

综合上述分子研究结果，似乎除了NF1之外，没有任何单一基因在所有NF1相关的MPNST中呈现出一致性的改变。

27.7 NF1-MPNST中的基因表达和蛋白质分析

证据表明，DNA拷贝数的变化可以直接影响这些基因组变化中涉及的基因的表达(Riddick and Fine 2011)，这促使人们将基于芯片的基因表达研究应用于许多不同类型的癌症。在NF1的背景下，一项定量RT-PCR研究测量了NF1-MPNST和丛状神经纤维瘤中489个基因的表达水平，发现与PNF相比，28个基因在MPNST中表现出显著不同的表达水平，其中16个基因上调，12个基因下调(Lévy et al. 2004)。这些不同表达水平的基因中，有2个涉及Ras信号通路(*RASSF2*和*HMMR*)，2个涉及Hedgehog-Gli信号通路(*DHH*和*PTCH2*)，其他基因则涉及细胞增殖(*MKI67*、*TOP2A*、*CCNE2*)、衰老(*TERT*、*TERC*)、凋亡(*BIRC5*、*TP73*)和细胞外基质重塑(*MMP13*、*MMP9*、*TIMP4*、*ITGB3*)。MPNST的活跃生长需要血管生成的增加，而已知活化的Ras上调*VEGF*(血管内皮生长因子)表达(Gesundheit et al. 2010)。在MPNST中，*VEGF*表达和肿瘤血管化显著增加(Angelov et al. 1999; Kranenburg et al. 2004)。

一项基因表达分析研究对散发型和与NF1相关MPNST的RNA"转录组"进行了类似的比较，尽管未能检测到任何差异，但成功地识别出了一个包含159个基因的分子特征，这有助于将MPNST细胞系与正常的施万细胞区分开来(Miller et al. 2006)。施万细胞分化标记(*SOX10*、*CNP*、*PMP22*和*NGFR*)在MPNST中下调，而神经嵴干细胞标记*SOX9*和*TWIST1*过表达。*TWIST1*基因在抑制凋亡、化学治疗耐药和转移中起作用(Maestro et al. 1999)。然而，使用小干扰RNA沉默MPNST细胞中的*TWIST1*表达，并未影响凋亡或化学治疗抵抗，尽管细胞趋化性受到抑制。

同一个研究团队进行的另一项相关基因表达谱研究分析了正常施万细胞(10个)、来自原发性良性(包括皮肤和丛状)神经纤维瘤的施万细胞(22个)、MPNST(6个)和从MPNST衍生的细胞系(13个)(Miller et al. 2009)。在良性皮肤型神经纤维瘤和丛状性神经纤维瘤之间没有发现差异。将*NF1*的基因表达谱与培养的正常原发性施万细胞进行比较，鉴定出了1 108个独特的基因特征，可以区分NF1肿瘤样本与正常施万细胞。发现*SOX9*基因在神经纤维瘤和MPNST组织中均有强表达；施万细胞瘤表达低水平的*SOX9*，而在组织学上与MPNST类似的滑膜肉瘤中，*SOX9*完全阴性。*SOX9*编码一种神经嵴转录因子，对干细胞的存活是必需的(Cheung et al. 2005)。在MPNST样本中，*SOX9*的平均表达值至少是神经纤维瘤样本的两倍。使用小发夹RNA(shRNA)在MPNST细胞系中减少*SOX9*表达，结果显示细胞迅速死亡。

Miller等(2010)最近的一项研究报告了MPNST中*DACH1*表达的减少和*PAX6*、*EYA1*、*EYA2*、*EYA4*和*SIX1-4*表达的增加。*EYA4*在肿瘤细胞系中的表达增加了20倍；在使用*EYA4*特异性小干扰RNA(siRNA)抑制其表达后，处理的细胞表现出黏附和迁移减少以及细胞死亡增加，但似乎并未影响细胞增殖或凋亡，这表明*EYA4*通路可能是一个潜在的治疗靶点。

在NF1相关肿瘤中，已有研究显示*NF1*微缺失区域内基因存在差异表达。因此，Pasmant等(2011b)通过实时定量反转录聚合酶链反应(reversetranscription polymerase chain reaction, RT-PCR)在大量人类皮肤和丛状神经纤维瘤及MPNST中研究了*NF1*、其他16个编码蛋白的基因和2个miRNA的表达。发现5个基因显著上调：丛状神经纤维瘤中的 OMG 和 SUZ12 以及 MPNST 中的 ATAD5、EVI2A 和 C17orf79。在从 MPNST 穿刺中衍生的肿瘤施万细胞和 MPNST 细胞系中，两个基因（RNF135 和 CENTA2）显著下调。然而，需要进一步的研究来确认这些发现。

所有基于芯片的肿瘤组织分析的一个主要问题是，在拷贝数和基因表达方面通常发现大量的基因和基因组区域发生改变。因此，这使得在大量其他"携带突变（passenger mutations）"的改变中识别出相对较少的致病"驱动"基因变得困难。这强调了需要对这些变化进行严格的功能分析以支持芯片数据。

一项基于肉瘤的研究，包括 NF1 相关的 MPNST，发现相较于 HIF1A 蛋白低表达，HIF1A 蛋白（通过免疫组织化学测定）中度至高表达的患者，其生存率显著降低（Shintani et al. 2006）。

据报道，与未恶性转化的施万细胞相比，人类和小鼠 MPNST 细胞系和肿瘤样本中 RalA 显著激活（Bodempudi et al. 2009）。RalA 是 Ras 样（Ras-like, Ral）蛋白家族的关键成员，在肿瘤发生中起着关键作用，其在 MPNST 细胞中的失活显著减弱了细胞增殖和肿瘤侵袭性。由于 Ral 鸟苷酸交换因子是 Ras 的直接效应物，Ral 信号通路可能被视为 Ras 的效应通路。Bodempudi 等（2009）的研究显示 RalA 在小鼠和人类 NF1－MPNST 中均过度激活，但这需要在更大规模的 NF1 患者研究中得到确认。

Cabibi 等的研究（2009）发现，CD10 在 NF1 相关的 MPNST 和非典型神经纤维瘤中表达，而在神经纤维瘤中没有。

总之，迄今为止，只有少数研究评估了不同蛋白质在 MPNST 发展中的作用。

27.8　微小 RNA 在 NF1－MPNST 形成中的作用

已知微小 RNA（miRNA）调节许多癌症基因的表达（Calin et al. 2002；Bottoni et al. 2005；Lamy et al. 2006；Zhang et al. 2006；Weiler et al. 2006；Wu and Mo 2009；Wu et al. 2009；Marcinkowska et al. 2011）。miRNA 可以调节许多蛋白质编码基因，沉默多个目标 mRNA（Lim et al. 2005）。据估计，约 1/3 的蛋白质编码基因的表达是由大约 1 000 个 miRNA 调节的（Lewis et al. 2005）。在人类基因组中已知约有 2 000 个 miRNA 基因（Kozomara and Griffiths-Jones 2011）。很多 miRNA 基因会经历拷贝数扩增或缺失，导致上调或下调。

癌症基因组中反复扩增或缺失的 miRNA 基因可以代表原癌基因或抑癌基因，其扩增或缺失将促进细胞增殖（Bottoni et al. 2005；He et al. 2005）。Dong 等（2010）整合了 miRNA、体系突变、SCNA 和基因表达数据，以重建与胶质瘤肿瘤起始和进展相关的网络。

由于 miRNA 在癌症发展中起重要作用，所以评估神经纤维瘤和 MPNST 中的 miRNA 表达谱可以提供有用的诊断标志物，并有助于识别额外的治疗靶点。已知几种不同的肉瘤组织学亚型表现出不同的 miRNA 表达谱（Subramanian et al. 2008），最近的研究表明 miRNA－34a 在 NF1－MPNST 中下调，但在 NF1 相关的神经纤维瘤中不下调（Subramanian et al. 2010），而 miRNA－10b 在原发性 MPNST 组织及其衍生的细胞系中上调，以及在神经纤维瘤衍生的施万细胞中上调（Chai et al. 2010）。进一步的研究应重点关注参与 MPNST 发展调节的 miRNA，以识别潜在的治疗靶点。

27.9　整合肿瘤发生中的拷贝数变异和基因表达数据

许多研究表明，CNV/SCNA 可以以拷贝数依赖的方式影响蛋白质编码基因的表达（Pollack et al. 2002；Zheng et al. 2004；Perry et al. 2007；Gonzalez et al. 2005；Bergamaschi et al. 2006；Stranger et al. 2007；Lee et al. 2008；Barretina et al. 2010；Beroukhim et al. 2010；Huang et al. 2011）。国家癌症研究所的癌症基因组图谱项目（http://cancergenome.nih.gov/）正在为各种不同的癌症生成多种数据类型（包括基因表达和拷贝数数据）。对于一些癌症，已证实基因拷贝数和表达水平相关（Santarius et al. 2010；Schlattl et al. 2011）。据估计，大约 60% 的基因在表达差异上与

其拷贝数状态一致（Huang et al. 2012），具体取决于所采用的癌症类型和分析方法。尽管拷贝数对基因表达的影响正在探索中（Goh et al. 2011），但目前仍然缺乏足够的信息来评估 LOH 和 UPD 对基因表达的影响。使用以上策略，可以识别特定的良性、癌前和恶性状态的基因缺失和扩增模式（Nigro et al. 2005；Yi et al. 2005；Lu et al. 2011；Chu et al. 2011）。

SCNA 和基因表达数据的结合可能提供区分驱动突变和携带突变（passenger mutations）的有用信息。实际上，我们推测 SCNA 和基因表达的一致性减少假阳性的数量（Riddick and Howard 2011）。在 NF1 中，MPNST 芯片中鉴定的几个基因的拷贝数变化与以前研究中的表达数据之间似乎存在一些一致性。例如，*BIRC5*、*CCNE2*、*FOXA2*、*MMP9*、*SOX10*、*SPP1*、*TERT* 和 *TP73* 基因的扩增与基因表达研究中这些基因的上调相一致（Mantripragada et al. 2008，2009；Lévy et al. 2004）。同样，*L1CAM2*、*PTCH2*、*RB1* 和 *TIMP4* 的缺失与以前的报告中显示这些基因在 MPNST 中下调的结果一致（Mantripragada et al. 2008；Mawrin et al. 2002）。然而，无论是比较基因组杂交（Mantripragada et al. 2008，2009）还是表达研究（Miller et al. 2009）都未能在皮肤和丛状神经纤维瘤之间鉴定出任何 SCNA 和基因表达方面的差异。

人们希望快速下降的二代测序成本将进一步促进基因表达/SCNA 研究。基于 RNA 的二代测序还将提供关于可变剪接和 mRNA 表达的信息。

27.10 线粒体 DNA 的体系拷贝数变化

在一系列原发性人类癌症中，越来越多的研究报告了线粒体 DNA（mitochondrial DNA，mtDNA）拷贝数的增加或减少，这表明 mtDNA 数量的变化可能是癌症发病和进展中的一个关键因素（Carew and Huang 2002；Yu 2011）。然而，mtDNA 拷贝数变化在驱动肿瘤形成过程中的确切作用仍然未知。虽然 mtDNA 拷贝数改变可能在 MPNST 发展的致病机制中起作用，但迄今为止，这一问题尚未得到证实。研究者已经在良性 NF1 相关肿瘤中寻找体系 mtDNA 突变（Kurtz et al. 2004）。在这项研究中，NF1 患者的皮肤和丛状神经纤维瘤中均发现了线粒体突变。Detjen 等（2007）研究了 4 对不一致的 NF1 单卵双胞胎及其中 1 对双胞胎的皮肤型神经纤维瘤的有核血细胞。他们未能检测到同一对双胞胎个体之间的 mtDNA 序列差异或异质性差异。为了评估线粒体 DNA 在 MPNST 发展中的作用，基于 NF1-MPNST 和良性神经纤维瘤之间的线粒体拷贝数变化的比较研究正在进行中（Upadhyaya et al. unpublished data）。

27.11 未来的发展与挑战

我们仍然不知道有多少驱动突变参与了 NF1 肿瘤发生（Stratton et al. 2009）。许多常见的人类癌症中的局部缺失表明它们具有携带突变（passenger mutations）的特征。因此，这些改变通常是半合子的，且似乎针对缺乏肿瘤抑制功能的基因（Beroukhim et al. 2010；Bignell et al. 2010）。虽然许多癌症中报告了若干原癌基因的扩增（Santarius et al. 2010），但扩增的 SCNA 包含许多功能未得到充分定义的其他基因。在之前的一项 NF1 相关 MPNST 研究中，报道了 1q25、3p26、3q13、5p12、5q11.2-q14、5q21-23、5q31-33、6p23-p21、6p12、6q15、6q23-q24、7p22、7p14-p13、7q21、7q36、8q22-q24、14q22 和 17q21-q25 的拷贝数扩增（Mantripragada et al. 2009）。若干原癌基因定位于这些区域，包括 *NEDL1*（7p14）、*AP3B1*（5q14.1）和 *CUL1*（7q36.1），涉及这些基因的拷贝数扩增已在超过 63% 的 MPNST 中得到鉴定。然而，尚不清楚这些区域的基因中有多少比例代表驱动突变。

2008 年，国际癌症研究基因组（International Cancer Research Genome，ICGC）成立，旨在标准化识别人类癌症基因组改变的方法（http://www.icgc.org），包括胰腺、卵巢、胃、肝脏、乳腺及口腔的癌症和慢性淋巴细胞白血病。需要注意的是，NF1 相关肿瘤没有得到类似的关注，因为根据定义，它们相对较为罕见，限于 NF1 患者。因此，迫切需要 NF1 研究人员组成一个联盟，仔细评估这些肿瘤的基因组图谱。

MPNST 像许多其他肿瘤一样，表现出比其相应的淋巴细胞 DNA（用于胚系基因组分析）更大的细胞异质性（Thomas et al. 2012；Gerlinger et al. 2012）。事实上，一个给定的 MPNST 样本总是包含恶性和非恶性细胞的混合物（Thomas et al. 2012）。这对于在 MPNST 中检测 SCNA/基因表达分析具有重要意义。

因此，人们逐渐认识到 MPNSTs 中的体细胞改变既包括小规模的变化，也包括大规模的变化（Upadhyaya et al. 2008；Bottillo et al. 2009）。将二代测序应用于整个基因组、外显子组和转录组已提高了与肿瘤发生相关的不同病变的分辨率和检测能力（Campbell et al. 2008）。因此，NF1 相关肿瘤也需要类似的方法。二代测序的另一个优势是其数字特性使我们能够估计基因组位点的肿瘤-正常拷贝数比率。DNA 拷贝数数据与基因表达、蛋白质表达和甲基化数据的整合分析，对 NF1 相关肿瘤是必要的，正如在胶质母细胞瘤、白血病、肺癌、卵巢癌和神经母细胞瘤中的研究所揭示的那样（Parsons et al. 2008；Ding et al. 2008；Sangha et al. 2008；Haferlach et al. 2010；Wang et al. 2011）。显然，跨学科合作努力对于完全了解 NF1-MPNST 发展的复杂分子基础至关重要。这不仅有助于识别与 NF1 肿瘤发生相关的驱动基因，还可能识别出新的肿瘤特异性信号通路和治疗靶点。

（杨吉龙，刘昊天　译）

参考文献

[1] Adamowicz M, Radlwimmer B, Rieker RJ, Mertens D, Schwarzbach M, Schraml P, Benner A, Lichter P, Mechtersheimer G, Joos S (2006) Frequent amplifications and abundant expression of TRIO, NKD2, and IRX2 in soft tissue sarcomas. Genes Chromosomes Cancer 45: 829–838

[2] Angelov L, Salhia B, Roncari L, McMahon G, Guha A (1999) Inhibition of angiogenesis by blocking activation of the vascular endothelial growth factor receptor 2 leads to decreased growth of neurogenic sarcomas. Cancer Res 59: 5536–5541

[3] Barretina J, Taylor BS, Banerji S, Ramos AH, Lagos-Quintana M, Decarolis PL, Shah K, Socci ND, Weir BA, Ho A, Chiang DY, Reva B, Mermel CH, Getz G, Antipin Y, Beroukhim R, Major JE, Hatton C, Nicoletti R, Hanna M, Sharpe T, Fennell TJ, Cibulskis K, Onofrio RC, Saito T, Shukla N, Lau C, Nelander S, Silver SJ, Sougnez C, Viale A, Winckler W, Maki RG, Garraway LA, Lash A, Greulich H, Root DE, Sellers WR, Schwartz GK, Antonescu CR, Lander ES, Varmus HE, Ladanyi M, Sander C, Meyerson M, Singer S (2010) Subtype-specific genomic alterations define new targets for soft-tissue sarcoma therapy. Nat Genet 42: 715–721

[4] Baudis M (2007) Genomic imbalances in 5918 malignant epithelial tumors: an explorative metaanalysis of chromosomal CGH data. BMC Cancer 7: 226

[5] Beert E, Brems H, Daniëls B, De Wever I, Van Calenbergh F, Schoenaers J, Debiec-Rychter M, Gevaert O, De Raedt T, Van Den Bruel A, de Ravel T, Cichowski K, Kluwe L, Mautner V, Sciot R, Legius E (2011) Atypical neurofibromas in neurofibromatosis type 1 are premalignant tumors. Genes Chromosomes Cancer 50: 1021–1032

[6] Bennett E, Thomas NS, Upadhyaya M (2009) Neurofibromatosis type 1: its association with the Ras/MAPK pathway syndromes. J Pediatr Neurol 7: 105–115

[7] Bergamaschi A, Kim YH, Wang P, Sørlie T, Hernandez-Boussard T, Lonning PE, Tibshirani R, Børresen-Dale AL, Pollack JR (2006) Distinct patterns of DNA copy number alteration are associated with different clinicopathological features and gene-expression subtypes of breast cancer. Genes Chromosomes Cancer 45: 1033–1040

[8] Berner JM, Sorlie T, Mertens F, Henriksen J, Sater G, Mandahl N, Brogger A, Myklebost O, Lothe RA (1999) Chromosome band 9p21 is frequently altered in malignant peripheral nerve sheath tumors: studies of CDKN2A and other genes of the pRB pathway. Genes Chromosomes Cancer 26: 151–160

[9] Beroukhim R, Mermel CH, Porter D, Wei G, Raychaudhuri S, Donovan J, Barretina J, Boehm JS, Dobson J, Urashima M, Mc Henry KT, Pinchback RM, Ligon AH, Cho YJ, Haery L, Greulich H, Reich M, Winckler W, Lawrence MS, Weir BA, Tanaka KE, Chiang DY, Bass AJ, Loo A, Hoffman C, Prensner J, Liefeld T, Gao Q, Yecies D, Signoretti S, Maher E, Kaye FJ, Sasaki H, Tepper JE, Fletcher JA, Tabernero J, Baselga J, Tsao MS, Demichelis F, Rubin MA, Janne PA, Daly MJ, Nucera C, Levine RL, Ebert BL, Gabriel S, Rustgi AK, Antonescu CR, Ladanyi M, Letai A, Garraway LA, Loda M, Beer DG, True LD, Okamoto A, Pomeroy SL, Singer S, Golub TR, Lander ES, Getz G, Sellers WR, Meyerson M (2010) The landscape of somatic copy-number alteration across human cancers. Nature 463: 899–905

[10] Bignell GR, Greenman CD, Davies H, Butler AP, Edkins S, Andrews JM, Buck G, Chen L, Beare D, Latimer C, Widaa S, Hinton J, Fahey C, Fu B, Swamy S, Dalgliesh GL, Teh BT, Deloukas P, Yang F, Campbell PJ, Futreal PA, Stratton MR (2010) Signatures of mutation and selection in the cancer genome. Nature 463: 893–898

[11] Bodempudi F, Yamoutpoor W, Pan A, Dudek T, Esfandyari M, Piedra D, Babovick-Vuksanovic R, Woo V, Mautner L, Kluwe D, Clapp GD, Vries S, Thomas A, Kurtz LP, Farassati F (2009) Ral overactivation in malignant peripheral nerve sheath tumors. Mol Cell Biol 29: 3964–3974

[12] Bottillo I, Ahlquist T, Brekke H, Danielsen SA, van den Berg E, Mertens F, Lothe RA, Dallapiccola B (2009) Germline and somatic NF1 mutations in sporadic and NF1-associated malignant peripheral nerve sheath tumours. J Pathol 217: 693–701

[13] Bottoni A, Piccin D, Tagliati F, Luchin A, Zatelli MC, Degli Uberti EC (2005) miR-15a and miR-16-1 down-regulation in pituitary adenomas. J Cell Physiol 204: 280-285

[14] Brekke HR, Ribeiro FR, Kolberg M, Agesen TH, Lind GE, Eknaes M, Hall KS, Bjerkehagen B, van den Berg E, Teixeira MR, Mandahl N, Smeland S, Mertens F, Skotheim RI, Lothe RA (2010) Genomic changes in chromosomes 10, 16, and X in malignant peripheral nerve sheath. Tumors identify a high-risk patient group. JCO 20: 1573-1582

[15] Bridge RS Jr, Bridge JA, Neff JR, Naumann S, Althof P, Bruch LA (2004) Recurrent chromosomal imbalances and structurally abnormal breakpoints within complex karyotypes of malignant peripheral nerve sheath tumor and malignant triton tumor: a cytogenetic and molecular cytogenetic study. J Clin Pathol 57: 1172-1178

[16] Bruder CE, Piotrowski A, Gijsbers AA, Andersson R, Erickson S, Diaz de Ståhl T, Menzel U, Sandgren J, von Tell D, Poplawski A, Crowley M, Crasto C, Partridge EC, Tiwari H, Allison DB, Komorowski J, van Ommen GJ, Boomsma DI, Pedersen NL, den Dunnen JT, Wirdefeldt K, Dumanski JP (2008) Phenotypically concordant and disconcordant monozygotic twins display different DNA copy-number variation profiles. Am J Hum Genet 82: 763-771

[17] Cabibi D, Zerilli M, Caradonna G, Schillaci L, Belmonte B, Rodolico V (2009) Diagnostic and prognostic value of CD10 in peripheral nerve sheath tumors. Anticancer Res 29: 3149-3155

[18] Cairns P, Polascik TJ, Eby Y, Tokino K, Califano J, Merlo A, Mao L, Herath J, Jenkins R, Westra W (1995) Frequency of homozygous deletion at p16/CDKN2 in primary human tumors. Nat Genet 11: 210-212

[19] Calin GA, Dumitru CD, Shimizu M, Bichi R, Zupo S, Noch E, Aldler H, Rattan S, Keating M, Rai K, Rassenti L, Kipps T, Negrini M, Bullrich F, Croce CM (2002) Frequent deletions and down-regulation of micro-RNA genes miR15 and miR16 at 13q14 in chronic lymphocytic leukemia. Proc Natl Acad Sci USA 99: 15524-15529

[20] Campbell PJ, Stephens PJ, Pleasance ED, O'Meara S, Li H, Santarius T, Stebbings LA, Leroy C, Edkins S, Hardy C, Teague JW, Menzies A, Goodhead I, Turner DJ, Clee CM, Quail MA, Cox A, Brown C, Durbin R, Hurles ME, Edwards PA, Bignell GR, Stratton MR, Futreal PA (2008) Identification of somatically acquired rearrangements in cancer using genome-wide massively parallel paired-end sequencing. Nat Genet 40: 722-729

[21] Carew JS, Huang P (2002) Mitochondrial defects in cancer. Mol Cancer 1: 9

[22] Chai G, Liu N, Ma J, Li H, Oblinger JL, Prahalad AK, Gong M, Chang LS, Wallace M, Muir D, Guha A, Phipps RJ, Hock JM, Yu X (2010) MicroRNA-10b regulates tumorigenesis in neurofibromatosis type 1. Cancer Sci 101: 1997-2004

[23] Cheung M, Chaboissier MC, Mynett A, Hirst E, Schedl A, Briscoe J (2005) The transcriptional control of trunk neural crest induction, survival, and delamination. Dev Cell. 8: 179-192

[24] Chu F, Feng Q, Qian Y, Zhang C, Fang Z, Shen G (2011) ERBB2 gene amplification in oral squamous cell malignancies: a correlation with tumor progression and gene expression. Oral Surg Oral Med Oral Pathol Oral Radiol Endod 112: 90-95

[25] Cichowski K, Shih T, Schmitt E, Santiago S, Reilly K, McLaughlin ME, Bronson RT, Jacks T (1999) Mouse models of tumor development in neurofibromatosis type 1. Science 286: 2172-2176

[26] Daser A, Thangavelu M, Pannell R, Forster A, Sparrow L, Chung G, Dear PH, Rabbitts TH (2006) Interogation of genomes by molecular copy number counting (MCC). Nat Methods 3: 447-453

[27] Dear PH (2009) Copy-number variation: the end of the human genome? Trends Biotechnol 27: 448-454

[28] Detjen AK, Tinschert S, Kaufmann D, Algermissen B, Nürnberg P, Schuelke M (2007) Analysis of mitochondrial DNA in discordant monozygotic twins with neurofibromatosis type 1. Twin Res Hum Genet 10: 486-495

[29] Ding L, Getz G, Wheeler DA, Mardis ER, McLellan MD, Cibulskis K, Sougnez C, Greulich H, Muzny DM, Morgan MB, Fulton L, Fulton RS, Zhang Q, Wendl MC, Lawrence MS, Larson DE, Chen K, Dooling DJ, Sabo A, Hawes AC, Shen H, Jhangiani SN, Lewis LR, Hall O, Zhu Y, Mathew T, Ren Y, Yao J, Scherer SE, Clerc K, Metcalf GA, Ng B, Milosavljevic A, Gonzalez-Garay ML, Osborne JR, Meyer R, Shi X, Tang Y, Koboldt DC, Lin L, Abbott R, Miner TL, Pohl C, Fewell G, Haipek C, Schmidt H, Dunford-Shore BH, Kraja A, Crosby SD, Sawyer CS, Vickery T, Sander S, Robinson J, Winckler W, Baldwin J, Chirieac LR, Dutt A, Fennell T, Hanna M, Johnson BE, Onofrio RC, Thomas RK, Tonon G, Weir BA, Zhao X, Ziaugra L, Zody MC, Giordano T, Orringer MB, Roth JA, Spitz MR, Wistuba II, Ozenberger B, Good PJ, Chang AC, Beer DG, Watson MA, Ladanyi M, Broderick S, Yoshizawa A, Travis WD, Pao W, Province MA, Weinstock GM, Varmus HE, Gabriel SB, Lander ES, Gibbs RA, Meyerson M, Wilson RK (2008) Somatic mutations affect key pathways in lung adenocarcinoma. Nature 455: 1069-1075

[30] Dong H, Luo L, Hong S, Siu H, Xiao Y, Jin L, Chen R, Xiong M (2010) Integrated analysis of mutations, miRNA and mRNA expression in glioblastoma. BMC Syst Biol 4: 163

[31] Evans DG, Baser ME, McGaughran J, Sharif S, Howard E, Moran A (2002) Malignant peripheral nerve sheath tumors in neurofibromatosis 1. J Med Genet 39: 311-314

[32] Fang Y, Elahi A, Denley RC, Rao PH, Brennan MF, Jhanwar SC (2009) Molecular characterization of permanent cell lines from primary, metastatic and recurrent malignant peripheral nerve sheath tumors (MPNST) with underlying neurofibromatosis-1. Anticancer Res 29: 1255-1262

[33] Frahm S, Mautner V, Brems H, Legius E, Debiec-Rychter M, Friedrich R, Knöfel W, Peiper M, Kluwe L (2004) Genetic and phenotypic characterization of tumor cells derived from malignant peripheral nerve sheath tumors of neurofibromatosis type-1 patients. Neurobiol Dis 16: 85-91

[34] Frank D, Gunawan B, Holtrup M, Füzesi L (2003) Cytogenetic characterization of three malignant peripheral nerve sheath tumors. Cancer Genet Cytogenet 144: 18-22

[35] Gerlinger M, Rowan AJ, Horswell S, Math M, Larkin J, Endesfelder D, Gronroos E, Martinez P, Matthews N, Stewart A, Tarpey P, Varela I, Phillimore B, Begum S, McDonald NQ, Butler A, Jones D, Raine K, Latimer C, Santos CR, Nohadani M, Eklund AC, Spencer-Dene B, Clark G, Pickering L, Stamp G, Gore M, Szallasi Z, Downward J, Futreal PA, Swanton C (2012) Intratumour heterogeneity and branched evolution revealed by multiregion sequencing. N Engl J Med 366: 883-892

[36] Gesundheit B, Parkin P, Greenberg M, Baruchel S, Senger C, Kapelushnik J, Smith C, Klement GL (2010) The role of angiogenesis in the transformation of plexiform neurofibroma into-malignant peripheral nerve sheath tumors in children with

neurofibromatosis type 1. J Pediatr Hematol Oncol 32: 548-553

[37] Glover TW, Stein CK, Legius E, Andersen LB, Brereton A, Johnson S (1991) Molecular and cytogenetic analysis of tumors in von Recklinghausen neurofibromatosis. Genes Chromosomes Cancer 3: 62-70

[38] Goh XY, Rees JR, Paterson AL, Chin SF, Marioni JC, Save V, O'Donovan M, Eijk PP, Alderson D, Ylstra B, Caldas C, Fitzgerald RC (2011) Integrative analysis of array-comparative genomic hybridisation and matched gene expression profiling data reveals novel genes with prognostic significance in oesophageal adenocarcinoma. Gut 60: 1317-1326

[39] Gonzalez E, Kulkarni H, Bolivar H, Mangano A, Sanchez R, Catano G, Nibbs RJ, Freedman BI, Quinones MP, Bamshad MJ, Murthy KK, Rovin BH, Bradley W, Clark RA, Anderson SA, O'connell RJ, Agan BK, Ahuja SS, Bologna R, Sen L, Dolan MJ, Ahuja SK (2005) The influence of *CCL3L1* gene-containing segmental duplications on HIV-1/AIDS susceptibility. Science 307: 1434-1440

[40] Haferlach C, Dicker F, Kohlmann A, Schindela S, Weiss T, Kern W, Schnittger S, Haferlach T (2010) AML with *CBFB-MYH11* rearrangement demonstrate RAS pathway alterations in 92% of all cases including a high frequency of *NF1* deletions. Leukemia 24: 1065-1069

[41] He L, Thomson JM, Hemann MT, Hernando-Monge E, Mu D, Goodson S, Powers S, Cordon-Cardo C, Lowe SW, Hannon GJ, Hammond SM (2005) A microRNA polycistron as a potential human oncogene. Nature 435: 828-833

[42] Henrichsen CN, Chaignat E, Reymond A (2009a) Copy number variants, diseases and gene expression. Hum Mol Genet 18: R1-R8

[43] Henrichsen CN, Vinckenbosch N, Zöllner S, Chaignat E, Pradervand S, Schütz F, Ruedi M, Kaessmann H, Reymond A (2009b) Segmental copy number variation shapes tissue transcriptomes. Nat Genet 41: 424-429

[44] Holtkamp N, Malzer E, Zietsch J, Okuducu AF, Mucha J, Mawrin C, Mautner VF, Schildhaus HU, von Deimling A (2008) EGFR and erbB2 in malignant peripheral nerve sheath tumors and implications for targeted therapy. Neuro Oncol 10: 946-957

[45] Huang YT, Lin X, Chirieac LR, McGovern R, Wain JC, Heist RS, Skaug V, Zienolddiny S, Haugen A, Su L, Christiani DC (2011) Impact on disease development, genomic location and biological function of copy number alterations in non-small cell lung cancer. PLoS One 6: e22961

[46] Huang N, Shah PK, Li C (2012) Lessons from a decade of integrating cancer copy number alterations with gene expression profiles. Brief Bioinform, 13: 305-316

[47] Kalmyrzaev B, Pharoah PD, Easton DF, Ponder BA, Dunning AM, SEARCH Team (2008) Hyaluronan-mediated motility receptor gene single nucleotide polymorphisms and risk of breast cancer. Cancer Epidemiol Biomarkers Prev 17: 3618-3620

[48] Kan Z, Jaiswal BS, Stinson J, Janakiraman V, Bhatt D, Stern HM, Yue P, Haverty PM, Bourgon R, Zheng J, Moorhead M, Chaudhuri S, Tomsho LP, Peters BA, Pujara K, Cordes S, Davis DP, Carlton VE, Yuan W, Li L, Wang W, Eigenbrot C, Kaminker JS, Eberhard DA, Waring P, Schuster SC, Modrusan Z, Zhang Z, Stokoe D, de Sauvage FJ, Faham M, Seshagiri S (2010) Diverse somatic mutation patterns and pathway alterations in human cancers. Nature 466: 869-873

[49] Karube K, Nabeshima K, Ishiguro M, Harada M, Iwasaki H (2006) cDNA microarray analysis of cancer associated gene expression profiles in malignant peripheral nerve sheath tumours. J Clin Pathol 59: 160-165

[50] Koga T, Iwasaki H, Ishiguro M, Matsuzaki A, Kikuchi M (2002) Frequent genomic imbalances in chromosomes 17, 19, and 22q in peripheral nerve sheath tumors detected by comparative genomic hybridization analysis. J Pathol 197: 98-107

[51] Kourea HP, Orlow I, Scheithauer BW, Cordon-Cardo C, Woodruff JM (1999) Deletions of the INK4A gene occur in malignant peripheral nerve sheath tumors but not neurofibromas. Am J Pathol 155: 1855-1860

[52] Kozomara A, Griffiths-Jones S (2011) miRBase: integrating microRNA annotation and deep-sequencing data. Nucleic Acids Res 39: D152-D157

[53] Kranenburg O, Gebbink MF, Voest EE (2004) Stimulation of angiogenesis by Ras proteins. Biochim Biophys Acta 1654: 23-37

[54] Kresse SH, Skårn M, Ohnstad HO, Namløs HM, Bjerkehagen B, Myklebost O, Meza-Zepeda LA (2008) DNA copy number changes in high-grade malignant peripheral nerve sheath tumors by array CGH. Mol Cancer 7: 48

[55] Kuiper RP, Ligtenberg MJ, Hoogerbrugge N, Geurts van Kessel A (2010) Germline copy number variation and cancer risk. Curr Opin Genet Dev 20: 282-289

[56] Kuo KT, Guan B, Feng Y, Mao TL, Chen X, Jinawath N, Wang Y, Kurman RJ, IeM S, Wang TL (2009) Analysis of DNA copy number alterations in ovarian serous tumors identifies new molecular genetic changes in low-grade and high-grade carcinomas. Cancer Res 69: 4036-4042

[57] Kurtz A, Lueth M, Kluwe L, Zhang T, Foster R, Mautner VF, Hartmann M, Tan DJ, Martuza RL, Friedrich RE, Driever PH, Wong LJ (2004) Somatic mitochondrial DNA mutations in neurofi-bromatosis type 1-associated tumors. Mol Cancer Res 2: 433-441

[58] Lamy P, Andersen CL, Dyrskjøt L, Tørring N, Ørntoft T, Wiuf C (2006) Are microRNAs located in genomic regions associated with cancer? Br J Cancer 95: 1415-1418

[59] Latres E, Drobnjak M, Pollack D, Oliva MR, Ramos M, Karpeh M, Woodruff JM, Cordon-Cardo C (1994) Chromosome 17 abnormalities and *TP53* mutations in adult soft tissue sarcomas. Am J Pathol 145: 345-355

[60] LeBron C, Pal P, Brait M, Dasgupta S, Guerrero-Preston R, Looijenga LH, Kowalski J, Netto G, Hoque MO (2011) Genome-wide analysis of genetic alterations in testicular primary seminoma using high resolution single nucleotide polymorphism arrays. Genomics 97: 341-349

[61] Lee H, Kong SW, Park PJ (2008) Integrative analysis reveals the direct and indirect interactions between DNA copy number aberrations and gene expression changes. Bioinformatics 24: 889-896

[62] Legius E, Dierick H, Wu R, Hall B, Marynen P, Cassiman J, Glover T (1994) *TP53* mutations are frequent in malignant NF1 tumors. Genes Chromosomes Cancer 10: 250-255

[63] Lévy P, Vidaud D, Leroy K, Laurendeau I, Wechsler J, Bolasco G, Parfait B, Wolkenstein P, Vidaud M, Bièche I (2004) Molecular profiling of malignant peripheral nerve sheath tumors associated with neurofibromatosis type 1, based on large-scale real-time RT-PCR. Mol Cancer 3: 20

[64] Lévy P, Ripoche H, Laurendeau I, Lazar V, Ortonne N, Parfait B, Leroy K, Wechsler J, Salmon I, Wolkenstein P, Dessen P, Vidaud M, Vidaud D, Bièche I (2007) Microarray-based identification of tenascin C and tenascin XB, genes

possibly involved in tumorigenesis associated with neurofibromatosis type 1. Clin Cancer Res 13: 398-407

[65] Lewis BP, Burge CB, Bartel DP (2005) Conserved seed pairing often flanked by adenosine, indicates that thousands of human genes are microRNA targets. Cell 120: 15-20

[66] Lim L, Lau N, Garrett-Engele P, Grimson A, Schelter J, Castle J, Bartel D, Linsley P, Johnson J (2005) Microarray analysis shows that some microRNA down-regulate large numbers of target mRNAs. Nature 433: 769-773

[67] Lothe RA, Slettan A, Saeter G, Brøgger A, Børresen AL, Nesland JM (1995) Alterations at chromosome 17 loci in peripheral nerve sheath tumors. J Neuropathol Exp Neurol 54: 65-73

[68] Lothe RA, Karhu R, Mandahl N, Mertens F, Saeter G, Heim S, Borresen-Dale AL, Kallioniemi OP (1996) Gain of 17q24-qter detected by comparative genomic hybridization in malignant tumors from patients with von Recklinghausen's neurofibromatosis. Cancer Res 56: 4778-4781

[69] Lu TP, Lai LC, Tsai MH, Chen PC, Hsu CP, Lee JM, Hsiao CK, Chuang EY (2011) Integrated analyses of copy number variations and gene expression in lung adenocarcinoma. PLoS One 6: e24829

[70] Maestro R, Dei Tos AP, Hamamori Y, Krasnokutsky S, Sartorelli V, Kedes L, Doglioni C, Beach DH, Hannon GJ (1999) *Twist* is a potential oncogene that inhibits apoptosis. Genes Dev 13: 2207-2217

[71] Mantripragada KK, Spurlock G, Kluwe L, Chuzhanova N, Ferner RE, Frayling IM, Dumanski JP, Guha A, Mautner V, Upadhyaya M (2008) High-resolution DNA copy number profiling of malignant peripheral nerve sheath tumors using targeted microarray-based comparative genomic hybridization. Clin Cancer Res 14: 1015-1024

[72] Mantripragada KK, de Ståhl TD, Patridge C, Menzel U, Andersson R, Chuzhanova N, Kluwe L, Guha A, Mautner V, Dumanski JP, Upadhyaya M (2009) Genome-wide high-resolution analysis of DNA copy number alterations in NF1-associated malignant peripheral nerve sheath tumors using the 32K BAC array. Genes Chromosomes Cancer 48: 897-907

[73] Marcinkowska M, Szymanski M, Krzyzosiak WJ, Kozlowski P (2011) Copy number variation of microRNA genes in the human genome. BMC Genomics 12: 183

[74] Mawrin C, Kirches E, Boltze C, Dietzmann K, Roessner A, Schneider-Stock R (2002) Immuno-histochemical and molecular analysis of p53, RB, and PTEN in malignant peripheral nerve sheath tumors. Virchows Arch 440: 610-615

[75] Mechtersheimer G, Otaño-Joos M, Ohl S, Benner A, Lehnert T, Willeke F, Möller P, Otto HF, Lichter P, Joos S (1999) Analysis of chromosomal imbalances in sporadic and NF1-associated peripheral nerve sheath tumors by comparative genomic hybridization. Genes Chromosomes Cancer 25: 362-369

[76] Mertens F, Dal Cin P, De Wever I, Fletcher CD, Mandahl N, Mitelman F, Rosai J, Rydholm A, Sciot R, Tallini G, van Den Berghe H, Vanni R, Willén H (2000) Cytogenetic characterization of peripheral nerve sheath tumours: a report of the CHAMP study group. J Pathol 190: 31-38

[77] Meyerson M, Gabriel S, Getz G (2010) Advances in understanding cancer genomes through second generation sequencing. Nat Rev Genet 11: 685-696

[78] Miller SJ, Rangwala F, Williams J, Ackerman P, Kong S, Jegga AG, Kaiser S, Aronow BJ, Frahm S, Kluwe L, Mautner V, Upadhyaya M, Muir D, Wallace M, Hagen J, Quelle DE, Watson MA, Perry A, Gutmann DH, Ratner N (2006) Large-scale molecular comparison of human Schwann cells to malignant peripheral nerve sheath tumor cell lines and tissues. Cancer Res 66: 2584-2591

[79] Miller S, Walter JJ, Mehta T, Hardiman A, Sites E, Kaiser S, Jegga A, Li H, Upadhyaya M, Giovannini M, Muir D, Wallace M, Lopez E, Serra E, Lazaro C, Stemmer-Rachamimov PG, Aronow BJ, Ratner N (2009) Integrative genomic analyses show altered Schwann cell development in neurofibromatosis tumors and implicate *SOX9* as an addicting oncogene. EMBO Mol Med 1: 236-248

[80] Miller S, Lan Z, Hardiman A, Wu J, Kordich J, Patmore D, Hegde R, Cripe T, Cancelas J, Collins M, Ratner N (2010) Inhibition of Eyes Absent Homolog 4 expression induces malignant peripheral nerve sheath tumor necrosis. Oncogene 29: 368-379

[81] Nielsen GP, Stemmer-Rachamimov AO, Ino Y, Moller MB, Rosenberg AE, Louis DN (1999) Malignant transformation of neurofibromas in neurofibromatosis 1 is associated with *CDKN2A*/p16 inactivation. Am J Pathol 155: 1879-1884

[82] Nigro JM, Misra A, Zhang L, Smirnov I, Colman H, Griffin C, Ozburn N, Chen M, Pan E, Koul D, Yung WK, Feuerstein BG, Aldape KD (2005) Integrated array-comparative genomic hybridization and expression array profiles identify clinically relevant molecular subtypes of glioblastoma. Cancer Res 65: 1678-1686

[83] Parsons D, Jones S, Zhang X, Lin J, Leary R, Angenendt P, Mankoo P, Carter H, Siu I, Gallia G, Olivi A, McLendon R, Rasheed B, Keir S, Nikolskaya T, Nikolsky Y, Busam D, Tekleab H, Diaz LJ, Hartigan J, Smith D, Strausberg R, Marie S, Shinjo S, Yan H, Riggins G, Bigner D, Karchin R, Papadopoulos N, Parmigiani G, Vogelstein B, Velculescu V, Kinzler K (2008) An integrated genomic analysis of human glioblastoma multiforme. Science 321: 1807-1812

[84] Pasmant E, Vidaud D, Harrison M, Upadhyaya M (2011a) Different sized somatic NF1 locus rearrangements in neurofibromatosis1-associated malignant peripheral nerve sheath tumours. J Neurooncol 102: 341-346

[85] Pasmant E, Masliah-Planchon J, Lévy P, Laurendeau I, Ortonne N, Parfait B, Valeyrie-Allanore L, Leroy K, Wolkenstein P, Vidaud M, Vidaud D, Bièche I (2011b) Identification of genes potentially involved in the increased risk of malignancy in NF1-microdeleted patients. Mol Med 17: 79-87

[86] Perrone F, Tabano S, Colombo F, Dagrada G, Birindelli S, Gronchi A, Colecchia M, Pierotti M, Pilotti S (2003) p15INK4b, p14ARF, and p16INK4a inactivation in sporadic and neurofibromatosis type-1-related malignant peripheral nerve sheath tumors. Clin Cancer Res 9: 4132-4138

[87] Perrone F, Da Riva L, Orsenigo M, Losa M, Jocollè G, Millefanti C, Pastore E, Gronchi A, Pierotti MA, Pilotti S (2009) *PDGFRA*, *PDGFRB*, *EGFR*, and downstream signalling activation in malignant peripheral nerve sheath tumor. Neuro Oncol 11: 725-736

[88] Perry GH, Dominy NJ, Claw KG, Lee AS, Fiegler H, Redon R, Werner J, Villanea FA, Mountain JL, Misra R, Carter NP, Lee C, Stone AC (2007) Diet and the evolution of human amylase gene copy number variation. Nat Genet 39: 1256-1260

[89] Piotrowski A, Bruder CE, Andersson R, Diaz de Ståhl T, Menzel U, Sandgren J, Poplawski A, von Tell D, Crasto C, Bogdan A, Bartoszewski R, Bebok Z, Krzyzanowski M, Jankowski Z, Partridge EC, Komorowski J, Dumanski JP

[90] Plaat BE, Molenaar WM, Mastik MF, Hoekstra HJ, te Meerman GJ, van den Berg E (1999) Computer-assisted cytogenetic analysis of 51 malignant peripheral-nerve-sheath tumors: sporadic vs. neurofibromatosis-type-1-associated malignant schwannomas. Int J Cancer 83: 171-178

[91] Pollack JR, Sorlie T, Perou CM, Rees CA, Jeffrey SS, Lonning PE, Tibshirani R, Botstein D, Borresen-Dale AL, Brown PO (2002) Microarray analysis reveals a major direct role of DNA copy number alteration in the transcriptional program of human breast tumors. Proc Natl Acad Sci USA 99: 12963-12968

[92] Riddick G, Fine HA (2011) Integration and analysis of genome-scale data from gliomas. Nat Rev Neurol 7: 439-450

[93] Rothenberg SM, Settleman J (2010) Discovering tumor suppressor genes through genome-wide copy number analysis. Curr Genomics 11: 297-310

[94] Sabah M, Cummins R, Leader M, Kay E (2006) Loss of p16 (INK4A) expression is associated with allelic imbalance/loss of heterozygosity of chromosome 9p21 in microdissected malignant peripheral nerve sheath tumors. Appl Immunohistochem Mol Morphol 14: 97-102

[95] Sangha N, Wu R, Kuick R, Powers S, Mu D, Fiander D, Yuen K, Katabuchi H, Tashiro H, Fearon E, Cho K (2008) Neurofibromin 1 (NF1) defects are common in human ovarian serous carcinomas and co-occur with TP53 mutations. Neoplasia 10: 1362-1372

[96] Santarius T, Shipley J, Brewer D, Stratton MR, Cooper CS (2010) A census of amplified and overexpressed human cancer genes. Nat Rev Cancer 10: 59-64

[97] Schlattl A, Anders S, Waszak SM, Huber W, Korbel JO (2011) Relating CNVs to transcriptome data at fine resolution: assessment of the effect of variant size, type and overlap with functional regions. Genome Res 21: 2004-2013

[98] Schmidt H, Taubert H, Meye A, Würl P, Bache M, Bartel F, Holzhausen HJ, Hinze R (2000) Gains in chromosomes 7, 8q, 15q and 17q are characteristic changes in malignant but not in benign peripheral nerve sheath tumors from patients with Recklinghausen's disease. Cancer Lett 155: 181-190

[99] Shintani K, Matsumine A, Kusuzaki K, Matsubara T, Satonaka H, Wakabayashi T, Hoki Y, Uchida A (2006) Expression of hypoxia-inducible factor (HIF)-1alpha as a biomarker of outcome in soft-tissue sarcomas. Virchows Arch 449: 673-681

[100] Shlien A, Malkin D (2009) Copy number variations and cancer. Genome Med 1: 62

[101] Shlien A, Malkin D (2010) Copy number variations and cancer susceptibility. Curr Opin Oncol 22: 55-63

[102] Skotheim R, Kallioniemi A, Bjerkhagen B, Mertens F, Brekke H, Monni O, Mousses S, Mandahl N, Soeter G, Nesland J, Smeland S, Kallioniemi O, Lothe R (2003) Topoisomerase-II alpha is upregulated in malignant peripheral nerve sheath tumors and associated with clinical outcome. J Clin Oncol 21: 4586-4591

[103] Spurlock G, Knight SJ, Thomas N, Kiehl TR, Guha A, Upadhyaya M (2010) Molecular evolution of a neurofibroma to malignant peripheral nerve sheath tumor (MPNST) in an NF1 patient: correlation between histopathological, clinical and molecular findings. J Cancer Res Clin Oncol 136: 1869-1880

[104] Storlazzi CT, Brekke HR, Mandahl N, Brosjö O, Smeland S, Lothe RA, Mertens F (2006) Identification of a novel amplicon at distal 17q containing the BIRC5/SURVIVIN gene in malignant peripheral nerve sheath tumors. J Pathol 209: 492-500

[105] Stranger BE, Forrest MS, Dunning M, Ingle CE, Beazley C, Thorne N, Redon R, Bird CP, de Grassi A, Lee C, Tyler-Smith C, Carter N, Scherer SW, Tavaré S, Deloukas P, Hurles ME, Dermitzakis ET (2007) Relative impact of nucleotide and copy number variation on gene expression phenotypes. Science 315: 848-853

[106] Stratton MR, Campbell PJ, Futreal PA (2009) The cancer genome. Nature 458: 719-724

[107] Subramanian S, Lui W, Lee C, Espinosa I, Nielsen TO, Heinrich MC, Corless CL, Fire AZ, van de Rijn M (2008) MicroRNA expression signature of human sarcomas. Oncogene 27: 2015-2026

[108] Subramanian S, Thayanithy V, West RB, Lee CH, Beck AH, Zhu S, Downs-Kelly E, Montgomery K, Goldblum JR, Hogendoorn PC, Corless CL, Oliveira AM, Dry SM, Nielsen TO, Rubin BP, Fletcher JA, Fletcher CD, van de Rijn M (2010) Genome-wide transcriptome analyses reveal p53 inactivation mediated loss of miR-34a expression in malignant peripheral nerve sheath tumors. J Pathol 220: 58-70

[109] Tabone-Eglinger S, Bahleda R, Côté JF, Terrier P, Vidaud D, Cayre A, Beauchet A, Théou-Anton N, Terrier-Lacombe MJ, Lemoine A, Penault-Llorca F, Le Cesne A, Emile JF (2008) Frequent EGFR positivity and overexpression in high-grade areas of human MPNSTs. Sarcoma 2008: 849156

[110] Thomas L, Mautner VF, Cooper DN, Upadhyaya M (2012) Molecular heterogeneity in malignant peripheral nerve sheath tumors (MPNSTs) associated with neurofibromatosis type 1 (NF1). Hum Genomics 6: 18

[111] Tucker T, Wolkenstein P, Revuz J, Zeller J, Friedman J (2005) Association between benign and malignant peripheral nerve sheath tumors in NF1. Neurology 65: 205-211

[112] Upadhyaya M, Cooper DN (1998) Neurofibromatosis type 1: from genotype to phenotype. In: Upadhyaya M, Cooper DN (eds) BIOS Scientific Publishers, Oxford

[113] Upadhyaya M (2010) Neurofibromatosis type 1: diagnosis and recent advances. Expert Opin Med Diagn 4: 307-322

[114] Upadhyaya M (2011) Genetic basis of tumorigenesis in NF1 malignant peripheral nerve sheath tumors. Front Biosci 16: 937-951

[115] Upadhyaya M, Kluwe L, Spurlock G, Monem B, Majounie E, Mantripragada K, Ruggieri M, Chuzhanova N, Evans DG, Ferner R, Thomas N, Guha A, Mautner V (2008) Germline and somatic NF1 gene mutation spectrum in NF1-associated malignant peripheral nerve sheath tumors (MPNSTs). Hum Mutat 29: 74-82

[116] Upadhyaya M, Spurlock G, Thomas L, Thomas N, Richards M, Mautner VF, Cooper DN, Guha A, Yan J (2012) Microarray-based copy number analysis of neurofibromatosis type-1 (NF1)-associated malignant peripheral nerve sheath tumours (MPNSTs) reveals a role for Rho-GTPase pathway genes in NF1 tumorigenesis. Hum Mutat 33: 763-776

[117] Valsesia A, Rimoldi D, Martinet D, Ibberson M, Benaglio P, Quadroni M, Waridel P, Gaillard M, Pidoux M, Rapin B, Rivolta C, Xenarios I, Simpson AJ, Antonarakis SE, Beckmann JS, Jongeneel CV, Iseli C, Stevenson BJ (2011) Network-guided analysis of genes with altered somatic copy number and gene expression reveals pathways ommonly perturbed in metastatic melanoma. PLoS One 6: e18369

[118] Vogel K, Klesse L, Velasco-Miguel S, Meyers K, Rushing EJ, Parada LF (1999) Mouse tumor model for

neurofibromatosis type 1. Science 286: 2176-2179

[119] Wang K, Diskin SJ, Zhang H, Attiyeh EF, Winter C, Hou C, Schnepp RW, Diamond M, Bosse K, Mayes PA, Glessner J, Kim C, Frackelton E, Garris M, Wang Q, Glaberson W, Chiavacci R, Nguyen L, Jagannathan J, Saeki N, Sasaki H, Grant SF, Iolascon A, Mosse YP, Cole KA, Li H, Devoto M, McGrady PW, London WB, Capasso M, Rahman N, Hakonarson H, Maris JM (2011) Integrative genomics identifies *LMO1* as a neuroblastoma oncogene. Nature 469: 216-220

[120] Watson A, Perry A, Tihan T, Prayson R, Guha A, Bridge J, Ferner R, Gutmann D (2004) Gene expression profiling reveals unique molecular subtypes of neurofibromatosis type I-associated and sporadic malignant peripheral nerve sheath tumors. Brain Pathol 14: 297-303

[121] Weiler J, Hunziker J, Hall J (2006) Anti-miRNA oligonucleotides (AMOs): ammunition to target miRNAs implicated in human disease? Gene Ther 13: 496-502

[122] Wu H, Mo YY (2009) Targeting miR-205 in breast cancer. Expert Opin Ther Targets 13: 1439-1448

[123] Wu X, Wu S, Tong L, Luan T, Lin L, Lu S, Zhao W, Ma Q, Liu H, Zhong Z (2009) miR-122 affects the viability and apoptosis of hepatocellular carcinoma cells. Scand J Gastroenterol 44: 1332-1339

[124] Yang J, Ylipää A, Sun Y, Zheng H, Chen K, Nykter M, Trent J, Ratner N, Lev DC, Zhang W (2011) Genomic and molecular characterization of malignant peripheral nerve sheath tumor identifies the IGF1R pathway as a primary target for treatment. Clin Cancer Res 17: 7563-7573

[125] Yi Y, Mirosevich J, Shyr Y, Matusik R, George AL Jr (2005) Coupled analysis of gene expression and chromosomal location. Genomics 85: 401-412

[126] Yu M (2011) Generation, function and diagnostic value of mitochondrial DNA copy number alterations in human cancers. Life Sci 89: 65-71

[127] Yu J, Deshmukh H, Payton JE, Dunham C, Scheithauer BW, Tihan T, Prayson RA, Guha A, Bridge JA, Ferner RE, Lindberg GM, Gutmann RJ, Emnett RJ, Salavaggione L, Gutmann DH, Nagarajan R, Watson MA, Perry A (2011) Array-based comparative genomic hybridization identifies *CDK4* and *FOXM1* alterations as independent predictors of survival in malignant peripheral nerve sheath tumor. Clin Cancer Res 17: 1924-1934

[128] Zhang L, Huang J, Yang N, Greshock J, Megraw MS, Giannakakis A, Liang S, Naylor TL, Barchetti A, Ward MR, Yao G, Medina A, O'brien-Jenkins A, Katsaros D, Hatzigeorgiou A, Gimotty PA, Weber BL, Coukos G (2006) microRNAs exhibit high frequency genomic alterations in human cancer. Proc Natl Acad Sci USA 103: 9136-9141

[129] Zheng M, Simon R, Mirlacher M, Maurer R, Gasser T, Forster T, Diener PA, Mihatsch MJ, Sauter G, Schraml P (2004) *TRIO* amplification and abundant mRNA expression is associated with invasive tumor growth and rapid tumor cell proliferation in urinary bladder cancer. Am J Pathol 165: 63-66

第28章 1型神经纤维瘤病相关周围神经鞘膜瘤的病理学和分子诊断特征

Pathologic and Molecular Diagnostic Features of Peripheral Nerve Sheath Tumors in NF1

Anat Stemmer-Rachamimov and G. Petur Nielse

28.1 神经纤维瘤的病理学

神经纤维瘤（neurofibroma）是常见的良性肿瘤，可表现为与遗传综合征无关的孤立性病变，也可表现为与1型神经纤维瘤病（neurofibromatosis type I，NF1）相关的多发性病变。神经纤维瘤是 NF1 的特征性表现。

28.1.1 神经纤维瘤的大体和临床特征

神经纤维瘤根据临床表现、影像学检查和（或）组织学形态有多种分类（Riccardi 1992；Scheithauer et al. 1999a，b；Barbarot et al. 2007；Weiss and Goldblum 2008）。不同学科的亚专科（皮肤病学、神经病学、神经病理学、影像学和基础研究）各自采用或提出了自己的诊断术语，妨碍不同学科亚专科之间以及临床医师和基础研究者之间的交流（特别是在试图整合人类和小鼠模型病变的数据时）。

神经纤维瘤有三种生长方式：局限性（结节状、散在性）（localized）、弥漫性（diffuse）和丛状（plexiform）。

28.1.1.1 局限性（结节状、散在性）神经纤维瘤

局限性神经纤维瘤（localized neurofibroma）是非 NF1 患者（散发性）中最常见的神经纤维瘤。局限性神经纤维瘤表现为边界清楚的结节，但无包膜（图 28.1）。局限性神经纤维瘤多发生于皮肤真皮或皮下组织的小神经，可发生于躯体任何部位，但最常见于躯干。肿瘤的数量随年龄增长而增加，30 岁以上患者可超过 100 个（Huson et al. 1988）。

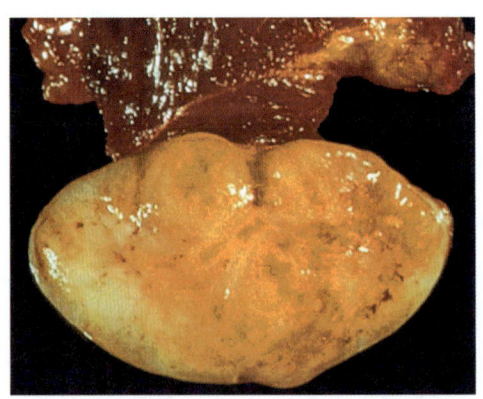

图 28.1 局限性（结节状）神经纤维瘤肉眼观。肿瘤边界清楚，与邻近软组织分界清晰。切面呈均质淡黄色，有光泽

发生于深部较大神经的局限性神经内神经纤维瘤(intraneural, localized neurofibroma)肉眼上呈梭形，在病变的近端和远端可见神经穿入和穿出。因局限性神经纤维瘤位于神经内，肿瘤被神经外膜所包裹。

在NF1患者中，皮肤和皮下神经纤维瘤最为常见。当肿瘤数量非常多时，可导致毁容和精神心理障碍，有时与局部持续性瘙痒相关(Riccardi 1981)。皮肤和皮下神经纤维瘤多在青春期较为明显，数量和大小随年龄增长而增加和增大。妊娠期间可快速生长(Huson et al. 1988)。

28.1.1.2 弥漫性神经纤维瘤

弥漫性神经纤维瘤(diffuse neurofibroma)可发生于非NF1的年轻患者中，但在NF1患者中更常见。弥漫性神经纤维瘤表现为边界不清的质硬斑块，受累区域呈弥漫性增大(图28.2)。弥漫性神经纤维瘤可发生于皮肤、软组织或内脏。胃肠道是最好发的内脏器官(Hochberg et al. 1974)。

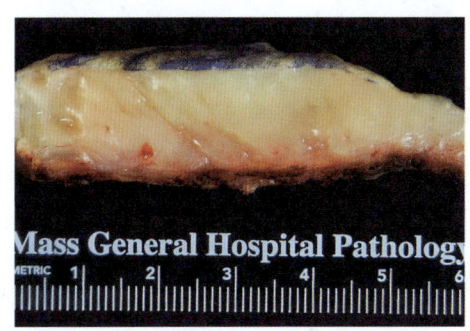

图28.2 皮肤弥漫性神经纤维瘤。肿瘤弥漫累及真皮层，使之增厚变硬

28.1.1.3 丛状神经纤维瘤（内在性，深部神经纤维瘤）

丛状神经纤维瘤(plexiform neurofibroma)几乎总与NF1相关。因丛状神经纤维瘤多在儿童早期发生，而被认为是先天性的。肿瘤沿大神经生长，使后者变粗大和扭曲，类似麻绳(丛状)，累及多个神经束时可形成"一袋蠕虫"("a bag of worms")样外观(图28.3)。体积较大的丛状神经纤维瘤可发生于脊髓神经、脑神经或周围神经。当肿瘤累及整个神经丛时，大的神经丛(臂、腰椎)可被弥漫性累及。当肿瘤位于浅表时，被覆表皮增厚，并有色素沉着。在NF1相关的"脊髓神经纤维瘤病"中，肿瘤可累及双侧多个脊神经根。

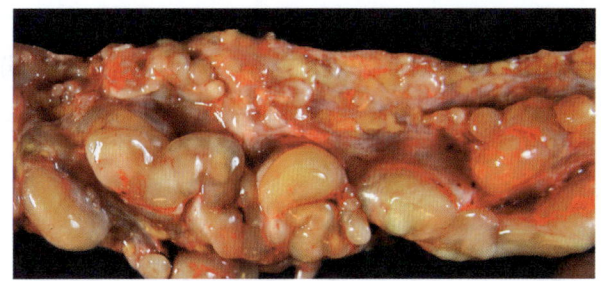

图28.3 丛状神经纤维瘤肉眼观。肿瘤累及多个神经，使之膨大呈多结节状，缠绕在一起，类似"一袋蠕虫"

临床上，丛状神经纤维瘤在NF1患者中的发生率为30%(Huson et al. 1988)，但并非所有丛状神经纤维瘤都有临床症状。如通过影像学检查，丛状神经纤维瘤在NF1患者中的发生率可达到40%。

肿瘤体积较大时可引起疼痛、神经功能缺损或压迫邻近结构。少数情况下，肿瘤引起周围软组织和骨骼过度增生，导致肢体不成比例生长(软组织巨神经纤维瘤，神经瘤性象皮病)。软组织巨神经纤维瘤仅见于NF1患者。

丛状神经纤维瘤是神经纤维瘤中发生恶性转化的一种高危类型。NF1患者发生恶性周围神经鞘膜瘤(malignant peripheral never sheath tumor, MPNST)的累积终生风险为4%～5%(Ducatman et al. 1986)，但新近研究显示风险可达8%～12%(Evans et al. 2002)。

28.1.2 神经纤维瘤组织学

孤立性神经纤维瘤和丛状神经纤维瘤在组织学上相同，由两种成分组成：间质和细胞。间质含有比例不等的细胞外黏液样基质和胶原纤维。肿瘤内的细胞成分呈异质性，由不同类型细胞构成，包括肿瘤性施万细胞和多种非肿瘤细胞(非单一性)。神经纤维瘤中的细胞主要为施万细胞和成纤维细胞，其他细胞包括神经束膜细胞、内皮细胞、平滑肌细胞、周皮细胞、肥大细胞、淋巴细胞和神经轴突。肿瘤的组织学表现可能因基质的类型和数量以及基质与细胞成分的比例而有所不同。经典的形态表现为大量黏液样基质、胡萝卜丝样胶原纤维、散在的瘤细胞(图28.4)。其中的细胞成分包括波浪状和核细长的瘤细胞，核呈短小逗号样的瘤细胞，以及散在的肥大细胞。部分肿瘤内的黏液样基质稀少，主要由致密的胶原纤维组成。间质成分较少而以瘤细胞成分为主时称为富细胞性神经纤维瘤。孤立性（散发性）神经纤维瘤和 NF1 相关神经纤维瘤在组织学上相似。NF1 相关的神经纤维瘤并无特有的组织学特征。

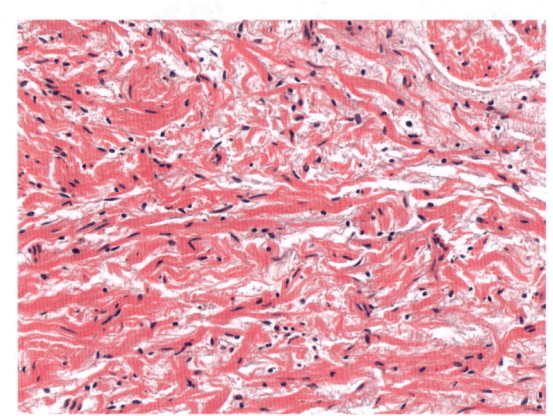

图 28.4　经典的神经纤维瘤组织学形态。镜下瘤细胞密度低，间质呈黏液样，可见胶原纤维，瘤细胞核小，呈特征的逗号样

弥漫性神经纤维瘤弥漫浸润软组织，围绕（但不破坏）毛囊和腺体，并在脂肪细胞或肌肉组织之间浸润性生长（图 28.5）。

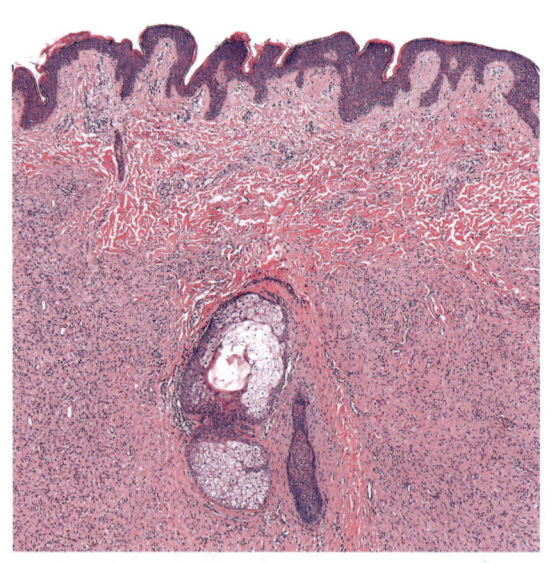

图 28.5　弥漫性神经纤维瘤的镜下形态。肿瘤浸润皮肤，并围绕在皮肤附件（毛囊）周围，但并不破坏后者

丛状神经纤维瘤的组织学形态与弥漫性和局限性神经纤维瘤有所不同。丛状神经纤维瘤位于受累的神经束内，使神经膨大并扭曲。在早期阶段，增多的基质使神经内膜受到扩张，轴突之间的间距明显加大。

丛状神经纤维瘤可位于神经内（神经束内），也可累及至神经外膜外，弥漫浸润邻近软组织（弥漫性，神经束外）（图 28.6）。浸润至神经束外的肿瘤成分在组织学上与弥漫性神经纤维瘤难以区分。因此在诊断丛状神经纤维瘤时需有位于神经内的丛状结构。

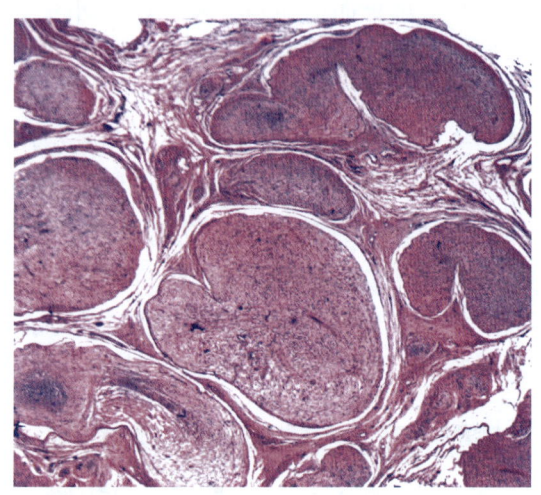

图 28.6　丛状神经纤维瘤的镜下形态。神经因被肿瘤替代而膨大。肿瘤越过神经外膜累及至神经周围的软组织内，并围绕神经束

28.1.3　神经纤维瘤和恶性周围神经鞘膜瘤的分子病理

尽管不同亚型的神经纤维瘤在组织学形态和细胞组成上相似，但临床观察和实验小鼠数据提示在生物学行为上有所不同。这些差异反映在肿瘤的恶性转化率和对激素的反应上，并可能是对各自不同的始祖细胞或微环境潜在差异的一种反映。

28.1.3.1　恶性转化

皮肤型神经纤维瘤不发生恶性转化。极少情况下，恶性转化可发生于神经内局限性神经纤维瘤和皮下神经纤维瘤（Scheithauer et al. 1999a, b）。恶性转化风险最高的是丛状神经纤维瘤（8%～13%）（Evans et al. 2002）。尚不清楚为何神经纤维瘤的某些亚型会发展成恶性周围神经鞘膜瘤（MPNST）。从神经纤维瘤发展成 MPNST 被认为涉及抑癌基因的突变以及生长因子或其受体信号通路发生异常。其中的一些分子变化可通过相应的免疫组织化学标记应用于病理诊断中。MPNST 中 *TP53* 的分子改变很常见,约见于 75% 病例(Birindelli et al. 2001；Menon et al. 1990；Holtkamp et al. 2007；Upadhyaya et al. 2008)。*TP53* 的改变也可以通过肿瘤细胞中 p53 的表达来识别,p53 在 68% 的 MPNST 中(通过免疫化学)表达(Hlling et al. 1996)。另一可通过免疫组织化学显示的分子改变是 p16^{INK4A}(*CDKN2A*),50% 的 MPNST p16 蛋白失表达(Nielsen et al. 1999；Kourea et al. 1999),提示基因失活。

p53 和 p16 标记有助于周围神经鞘膜瘤的病理诊断,包括富细胞性或非典型神经纤维瘤与低级别 MPNST 的鉴别诊断。对疑似肿瘤,p53 表达和(或)p16 表达缺失支持早期恶性转化的诊断。

28.1.3.2　激素对生长的影响

临床观察发现皮肤型神经纤维瘤在青春期起病且在妊娠期间数量增加,提示激素驱动性生长(Ferner 2007；Lakkis and Tennekoon 2000)。其他支持激素对皮肤型神经纤维瘤生长影响的证据包括瘤细胞高比例表达孕酮受体,体外被孕酮作用促使施万细胞增殖率升高(McLaughlin and Jacks 2003)。最近,激素对真皮神经纤维瘤的生长促进作用在动物实验中也得到了验证,相比非妊娠的 NF1 小鼠模型,妊娠小鼠中的皮肤型神经纤维瘤数量增加(Zhu et al. 2002)。

相比之下,丛状神经纤维瘤在青春期或孕期间的生长并没有增加,意味着对激素水平不敏感。

28.1.3.3　神经纤维瘤的起源细胞(小鼠模型)

基因工程小鼠(genetically engineered mouse models, GEMS)发生的 NF1 相关丛状神经纤维瘤和 MPNST 在组织学上与发生于人类的丛状神经纤维瘤和 MPNST 相似(Stemmer-Rachamimov et al. 2004)。

关于丛状神经纤维瘤的起源细胞存有争议,但多数小鼠研究均指向未成熟的施万细胞(Wu et al. 2008)或非髓鞘施万细胞(Zheng et al. 2008)。尽管 NF1 小鼠模型可发生丛状神经纤维瘤和 MPNST,但大多数小鼠模型并不发生皮肤型神经纤维瘤。Le 和其同事们推测不同的始祖细胞引发真皮神经纤维瘤和丛状神经纤维瘤,真皮中的一组干细胞(皮肤源性前驱细胞)在 *NF1* 丢失后形成皮肤型神经纤维瘤(Le et al. 2009)。然而,微环境(神经内或神经外)也可能对神经纤维瘤的生物学、生长模式和亚型起决定性影响(Le et al. 2009)。

28.1.4　神经纤维瘤的诊断挑战

28.1.4.1　神经鞘瘤——神经纤维瘤——杂合瘤?

经典的神经鞘瘤和神经纤维瘤在组织学上不相同,并且有不同的潜在遗传学改变。神经纤维瘤与 1 型神经纤维瘤病(NF1)相关,具有 *NF1* 基因的双等位基因改变,神经鞘瘤与 2 型神经纤维瘤病(NF2)和神经鞘瘤病相关,由 *NF2* 基因的双等位基因丢失所致。区分这两种形式的肿瘤在多发性神经鞘膜肿瘤(综合征性)的患者中至关重要,病理诊断可能可以决定 NF1 或 NF2(或神经鞘瘤病)的临床诊断。这在其他临床体征/症状出现模棱两可的情况下尤为重要,这些患者往往难以根据临床表现进行归类(例如,疾病特征在年轻患者中尚未完全表现出来,或表现为嵌合型/马赛克型)。

神经鞘瘤和神经纤维瘤在组织学上可通过以下形态进行鉴别：间质类型、肿瘤构成以及肿瘤与其起源神经的关系。与神经纤维瘤中大量的细胞外黏液样基质不同,神经鞘瘤极少含有细胞外基质,瘤细胞多形成实性肿块。神经鞘瘤中的组成比较单一,只有施万细胞。但在神经纤维瘤中,细胞组成复杂多样。这种形态特征可通过 S100 标记肿瘤内的施万细胞显现出来。此外,神经纤维瘤在神经内和神经轴突之间生长,使它们在肿瘤内分开,而神经鞘瘤则呈膨胀性生长,将轴突推至肿瘤外围。NF 标记可显示位于肿瘤内或周边的轴突。

某些类型的神经鞘瘤类似神经纤维瘤；反之亦然。如常与神经鞘瘤病相关的黏液样神经鞘瘤即与神经纤维瘤难以区分。同样,在一些被指定为"富施万细胞"的神经纤维瘤中,增生的施万细胞形成致密结节(图 28.7),与神经鞘瘤也难以区分。

混杂性神经纤维瘤/神经鞘瘤(hybrid neurofibroma/schwannoma)是一种良性周围神经肿瘤,由两部分组成：一部分具有神经纤维瘤的组

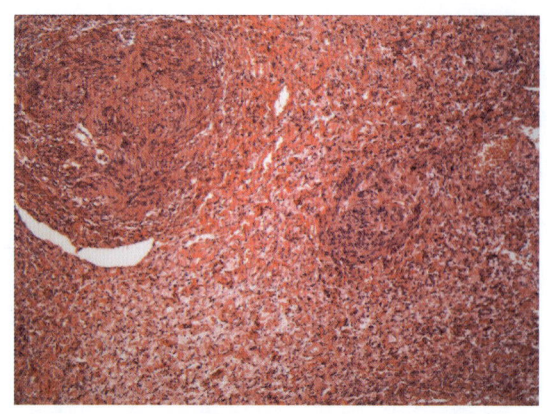

图28.7 神经纤维瘤与施万细胞结节的显微镜下表现。和神经鞘瘤不同，神经纤维瘤中施万细胞结节表现突出。如果肿瘤同时具有神经鞘瘤和神经纤维瘤的特征，则称为"杂合瘤"

织学特征，一部分具有神经鞘瘤的组织学特征。该名称由Feany等提出（1998）。目前尚不清楚混杂性肿瘤是否代表真正的第三种类型，或为神经鞘瘤和神经纤维瘤的特殊亚型。新近一项有关混杂性肿瘤的研究发现，肿瘤多发生于NF2和神经鞘瘤病背景中。然而，少数混杂性肿瘤也与NF1相关（Harder et al. 2012）。

28.2 恶性周围神经鞘膜瘤病理学

MPNST是一种起自神经，或起自良性神经鞘膜肿瘤（通常为神经纤维瘤），或在组织学、免疫组化和超微结构上显示施万细胞分化的恶性肿瘤。文献上其他的曾用名包括恶性神经鞘瘤、神经源性肉瘤和神经纤维肉瘤。

28.2.1 MPNST的大体和临床特征

散发性MPNST（sporadic MPNST，non-NF1 MPNST）很少见，仅占所有软组织肉瘤的5%（Ducatman et al. 1984）。半数MPNST与NF1有关（NF1-associated MPNST），起自既有的神经纤维瘤，10%病例为放射诱导MPNST（radiation induced MPNST），其余病例为特发性（idiopathic MPNST）（Ducatman et al. 1986）。NF1患者发生MPNST的终生风险为8%～13%（Evans et al. 2002）。MPNST多发生于成人（20～50岁），但也可发生于青少年（Ducatman et al. 1984）。神经纤维瘤发生恶变最重要的临床症状表现为出现疼痛（Korf 1999）。其他提示性体征包括神经功能缺损或近期内丛状神经纤维瘤快速生长。

MPNST多发生于四肢大神经（臂丛、坐骨神经）。脑神经很少受累。

大体上，肿瘤呈梭形，与其他类型的软组织肉瘤相似。体积较大，切面呈不均质性，棕褐色或灰白色，质硬，可伴有坏死和出血（图28.8）。

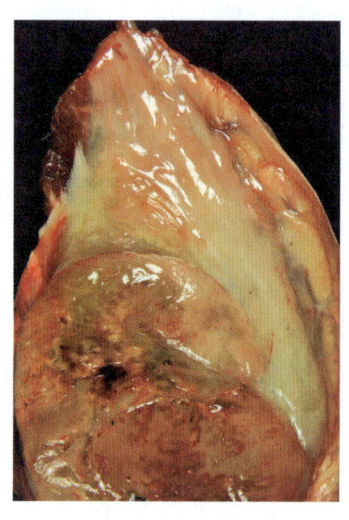

图28.8 MPNST肉眼观。起自丛状神经纤维瘤的MPNST。与质地均匀的神经纤维瘤区域（右上）不同，MPNST区域（左下）可见出血和坏死

28.2.2 MPNST组织学

镜下，瘤细胞较为丰富，由梭形细胞和多形性细胞组成，常伴有地图状坏死和出血。细胞丰富区域和细胞稀疏区常呈交替性分布。部分MPNST由条束状或鱼骨样梭形细胞组成，形态上类似纤维肉瘤。少数MPNST中的瘤细胞显示明显的多形性，形态上类似多形性未分化肉瘤。

与神经纤维瘤不同，半数以上的MPNST不表达S100。S100在MPNST中的阳性表达多为局灶性。大多数MPNST病例p53阳性，p16阴性。

MPNST中可见异向分化，导致镜下形态呈异质性。15%的MPNST显示异源性间叶性分化，如骨骼肌、骨骼和软骨。

28.2.2.1 恶性蝾螈瘤

恶性蝾螈瘤(malignant triton tumor)指的是伴有横纹肌分化的 MPNST。该型非常罕见，常发生于 NF1 患者(Ducatman and Scheithauer 1984)。最常见部位为头颈部和躯干。镜下，在 MPNST 的背景中可见胞质嗜伊红色的横纹肌母细胞。偶见横纹（图 28.9）。结蛋白(desmin)、MyoD1 和肌生成素(mygogenin)可清晰显示肿瘤内的横纹肌母细胞成分（图 28.10）。恶性蝾螈瘤侵袭性高，预后差。

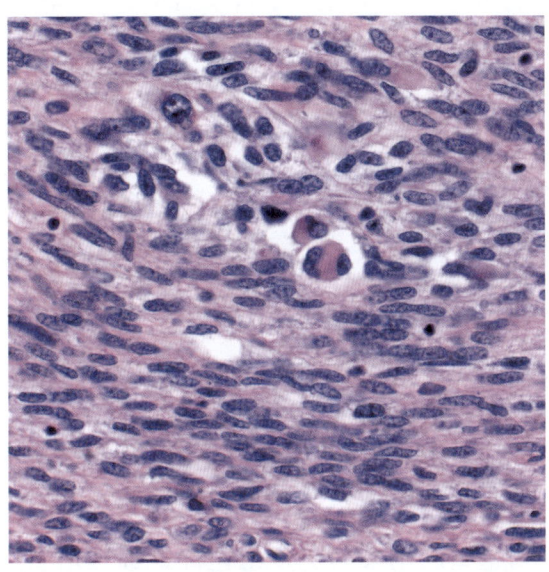

图 28.9 恶性蝾螈瘤镜下形态。伴有异源性（横纹肌）分化的 MPNST。镜下可见散在分布的胞质嗜伊红色横纹肌母细胞

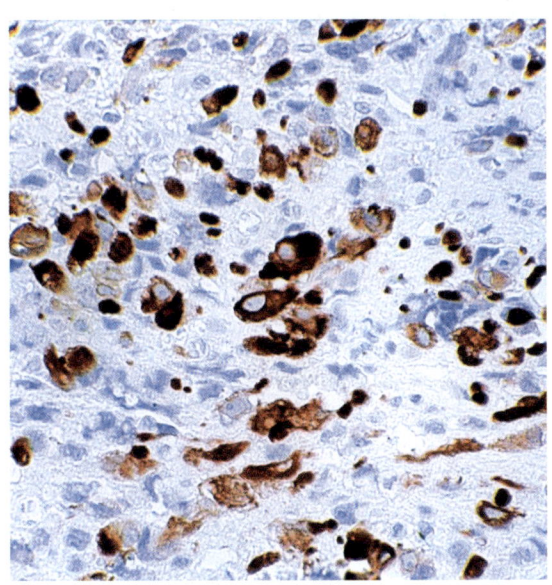

图 28.10 恶性蝾螈瘤镜下形态。Desmin 标记显示肿瘤内的横纹肌母细胞

28.2.2.2 腺样 MPNST

腺样 MPNST(glandular MPNST)指的是在 MPNST 的梭形细胞背景中可见散在分布的高分化腺体。腺体内衬立方上皮，腔内可含有黏蛋白。该亚型极为罕见，几乎均发生于 NF1 患者(Woodruff and Christensen 1993)（图 28.11）。细胞角蛋白和 CEA 可显示肿瘤内的腺体成分。

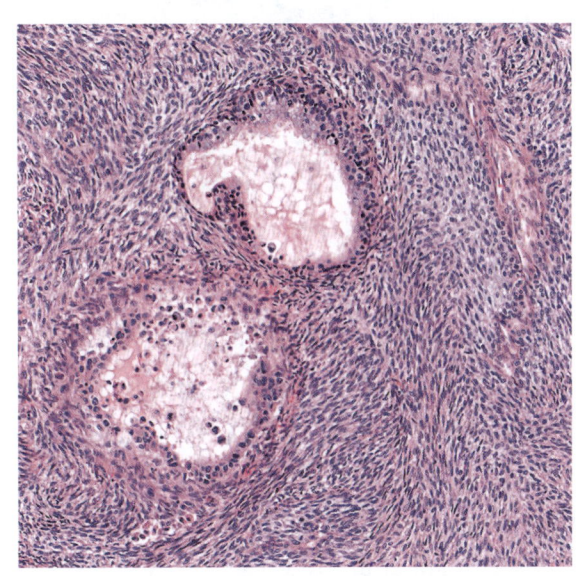

图 28.11 腺样 MPNST 镜下形态。肿瘤内含有高分化腺体。本亚型少见，多见于 NF1 患者

28.2.2.3 上皮样 MPNST

上皮样 MPNST(epithelioid MPNST)是 MPNST 的一种少见亚型(<5%)，由胞质嗜伊红色的上皮样细胞组成。上皮样 MPNST 与 NF1 无相关性。瘤细胞弥漫表达 S100 和 SOX10，常失表达 SMARCB1(INI1)。

28.2.2.4 伴有血管肉瘤的 MPNST

伴有血管肉瘤的 MPNST(MPNST with angiosarcoma)非常罕见，肿瘤内可见 MPNST 和血管肉瘤两种区域。多与 NF1 相关，并发生于青年人（图 28.12）。

28.2.2.5 MPNST 的分级

MPSNT 采用的分级系统与其他类型的软组织肉瘤相同，主要基于几个形态标准。软组织肉瘤按 3 级系统分级，1 级为低级别，3 级为高级别（差分化）。最常用的两个分级系统分别为美国国家癌症研究所(National Cancer Institute, NCI)分级系统和法国癌症中心肉瘤组织联合会(French Federation of

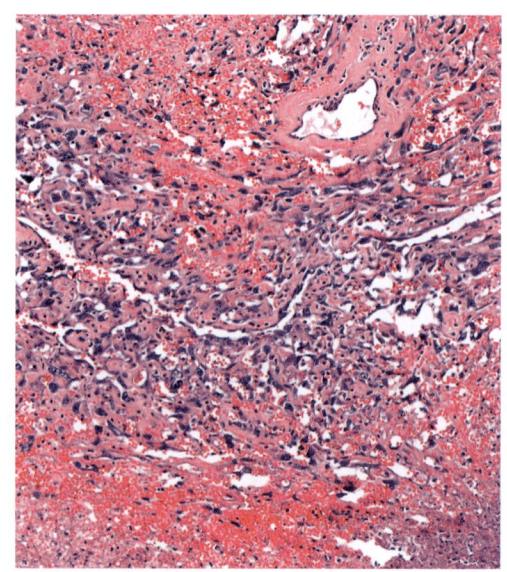

图 28.12 伴有血管肉瘤的 MPSNT 镜下形态

Cancer Centers Sarcoma Group，FNCLCC）分级系统。分级系统参考了组织学诊断、瘤细胞密度、细胞多形性和核分裂象。这些分级系统在预测肿瘤转移率和总生存期上具有预后价值。分级应包含在 MPNST 的诊断中（Trojani et al. 1984；Guillou et al. 1997；Costa et al. 1984）。

28.2.3 MPNST 的诊断挑战性

28.2.3.1 神经纤维瘤——非典型性神经纤维瘤——MPNST?

组织学上，丛状神经纤维瘤发生恶性转化常形成一个瘤谱，较难在良性和恶性之间有明确的界限。与恶性转化相关的非典型性形态包括：细胞密度增加，可见核分裂象，瘤细胞显示异型性。

仅有 1 个非典型性形态尚不足以诊断 MPNST。细胞密度增加可见于富细胞神经纤维瘤，核异型性也可为退行性改变。诊断 MPNST 需要同时具有细胞密度增加、可见核分裂象、瘤细胞显示异型性这 3 个非典型性形态。但如仅有 2 个非典型性形态时在诊断上就有困难，对诊断为伴有非典型性的神经纤维瘤还是 MPNST 就会有争议（Scheithauer et al. 1999a，b；Weiss and Goldblum 2008）（图 28.13）。

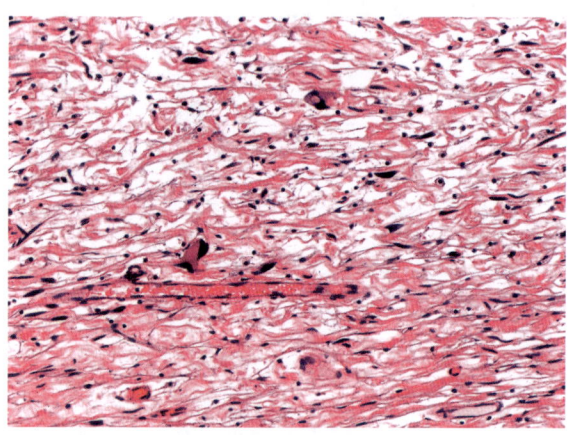

图 28.13 神经纤维瘤内可见核大深染的细胞，但无核分裂象，细胞密度不高，也无坏死，提示为退行性改变，非恶性转化

对这些病例采用免疫组化标记细胞增殖指数（Ki67 或 MIB1）可能会有帮助，在评估瘤细胞的增殖率上比计数核分裂象更为敏感。其他支持恶性转化的形态证据包括瘤细胞失表达 S100（提示发生去分化）。如前所述，免疫组化标记 p53 和（或）p16 也可用于 MPNST 的辅助诊断（Nielsen et al. 1999）。

（王坚，朱培培　译）

参考文献

[1] Barbarot S, Nicol C et al (2007) Cutaneous lesions in neurofibromatosis 1: confused terminology. Br J Dermatol 157(1): 183-184

[2] Birindelli S, Perrone F et al (2001) Rb and TP53 pathway alterations in sporadic and NF1-related malignant peripheral nerve sheath tumors. Lab Invest 81(6): 833-844

[3] Costa J, Wesley RA et al (1984) The grading of soft tissue sarcomas. Results of a clinicohisto-pathologic correlation in a series of 163 cases. Cancer 53(3): 530-541

[4] Ducatman BS, Scheithauer BW (1984) Malignant peripheral nerve sheath tumor with divergent differentiation. Cancer 54: 1049

[5] Ducatman BS, Scheithauer BW et al (1984) Malignant peripheral nerve sheath tumors in child-hood. J Neurooncol 2: 241-248

[6] Ducatman BS, Scheithauer BW et al (1986) Malignant peripheral nerve sheath tumors. A clinico-pathologic study of 120 cases. Cancer Cell 57: 2006-2021

[7] Evans DG, Baser ME et al (2002) Malignant peripheral nerve sheath tumours in neurofibromatosis 1. J Med Genet 39(5): 311-314

[8] Feany MB, Anthony DC et al (1998) Nerve sheath tumours with hybrid features of neurofibroma and schwannoma: a conceptual challenge. Histopathology 32(5): 405-410

[9] Ferner RE (2007) Neurofibromatosis 1 and neurofibromatosis 2: a twenty first century perspective. Lancet Neurol 6(4):

[10] Guillou L, Coindre JM et al (1997) Comparative study of the National Cancer Institute and French Federation of Cancer Centers Sarcoma Group grading systems in a population of 410 adult patients with soft tissue sarcoma. J Clin Oncol 15(1): 350-362

[11] Harder A, Wesemann M et al (2012) Hybrid Neurofibroma/Schwannoma is overrepresented among schwannomatosis and neurofibromatosis patients. Am J Surg Pathol 36(5): 702-709

[12] Hlling KC, Scheithauer BW et al (1996) p53 Expression in neurofibroma and malignant peripheral nerve sheath tumor. An immunohistochemical study of sporadic and NF1-associated tumors. Am J Clin Pathol 106(3): 271-272

[13] Hochberg FH, Dasilva AB et al (1974) Gastrointestinal involvement in von Recklinghausen's neurofibromatosis. Neurology 24(12): 1144-1151

[14] Holtkamp N, Atallah I et al (2007) MMP-13 and p53 in the progression of malignant peripheral nerve sheath tumors. Neoplasia 9(8): 671-677

[15] Huson SM, Harper PS et al (1988) Von Recklinghausen neurofibromatosis. A clinical and population study in southeast Wales. Brain 111(Pt 6): 1355-1381

[16] Korf B (1999) Neurofibromas and malignant tumors of the peripheral nerve sheath. In: Friedman JM, Gutmann DH, MacCollin M, Riccardi VM (eds) Neurofibromatosis: phenotype, natural history and pathogenesis. The John Hopkins University Press, Baltimore, pp 142-161

[17] Kourea HP, Orlow I et al (1999) Deletions of the INK4A gene occur in malignant peripheral nerve sheath tumors but not in neurofibromas. Am J Pathol 155(6): 1855-1860

[18] Lakkis MM, Tennekoon GI (2000) Neurofibromatosis type 1. I. General overview. J Neurosci Res 62(6): 755-763

[19] Le LQ, Shipman T et al (2009) Cell of origin and microenvironment contribution for NF1-associated dermal neurofibromas. Cell Stem Cell 4(5): 453-463

[20] McLaughlin ME, Jacks T (2003) Progesterone receptor expression in neurofibromas. Cancer Res 63(4): 752-755

[21] Menon AG, Gusella JF et al (1990) Progress toward the isolation and characterization of the genes causing neurofibromatosis. Brain Pathol 1(1): 33-40

[22] Nielsen GP, Stemmer-Rachamimov AO et al (1999) Malignant transformation of neurofibromas in neurofibromatosis 1 is associated with CDKN2A/p16 inactivation. Am J Pathol 155(6): 1879-1884

[23] Riccardi VM (1981) Cutaneous manifestation of neurofibromatosis: cellular interaction, pigmentation, and mast cells. Birth Defects Orig Artic Ser 17(2): 129-145

[24] Riccardi VM (1992) The prenatal diagnosis of NF-1 and NF-2. J Dermatol 19(11): 885-891

[25] Scheithauer BW, Woodruff JM et al (1999a) Neurofibroma. In: Scheithauer BW, Woodruff JM, Erlandosn RA (eds) Tumors of the peripheral nervous system. Armed Forces Institute of Pathology, Washington, DC, pp 156-157

[26] Scheithauer BW, Woodruff JM et al (1999b) Tumors of the peripheral nervous system. Atlas of tumor pathology. Armed Forces Institute of Pathology, Bethesda, MD

[27] Stemmer-Rachamimov AO, Louis DN et al (2004) Comparative pathology of nerve sheath tumors in mouse models and humans. Cancer Res 64(10): 3718-3724

[28] Trojani M, Contesso G et al (1984) Soft-tissue sarcomas of adults: study of pathological prognostic variables and definition of a histopathological grading system. Int J Cancer 33(1): 37-42

[29] Upadhyaya M, Kluwe L et al (2008) Germline and somatic NF1 gene mutation spectrum in NF1-associated malignant peripheral nerve sheath tumors (MPNSTs). Hum Mutat 29(1): 74-82

[30] Weiss SW, Goldblum JR (2008) Benign tumors of peripheral nerves. In: Weiss SW, Goldblum JR (eds) Enzinger and Weiss's soft tissue tumors. Mosby Elsevier, North Point, Hong Kong, pp 825-903

[31] Woodruff JM, Christensen WN (1993) Glandular peripheral nerve sheath tumors. Cancer 72: 3618-3628

[32] Wu J, Williams JP et al (2008) Plexiform and dermal neurofibromas and pigmentation are caused by Nf1 loss in desert hedgehog-expressing cells. Cancer Cell 13(2): 105-116

[33] Zheng H, Chang LS et al (2008) Induction of abnormal proliferation by nonmyelinating Schwann cells triggers neurofibroma formation. Cancer Cell 13: 117-128

[34] Zhu Y, Ghosh P et al (2002) Neurofibromas in NF1: Schwann cell origin and role of tumor environment. Science 296(5569): 920-922

第29章 恶性周围神经鞘膜瘤：预后和诊断标志物以及治疗靶点

Malignant Peripheral Nerve Sheath Tumors: Prognostic and Diagnostic Markers and Therapeutic Targets

Holly Meany, Brigitte C. Widemann, and Nancy Ratner

29.1 引言

恶性周围神经鞘膜瘤（MPNST）是最常见的NF1相关恶性肿瘤。目前，彻底的手术切除是MPNST唯一有效的治疗方法，无法切除、复发或转移性MPNST预后仍然很差。MPNST患者中近一半发生于NF1个体中，尤其是从丛状神经纤维瘤到非典型神经纤维瘤之间。由于NF1相关MPNST的预后似乎比散发性肿瘤更差，所以许多MPNST研究都使用了NF1模型，并将散发性MPNST和NF1相关MPNST进行对比。最近的分子分析已经开始帮助识别MPNST中的基因组异常。重要的是，临床前测试已开始发现靶向这类侵袭性肿瘤的有希望的治疗方法。整合基因组的发现、临床前测试、确定的MPNST流行病学、临床表现、诊断和预后因素，有望更早发现MPNST并更成功地治疗。

29.2 NF1相关MPNST和散发性MPNST的流行病学和临床表现

MPNST占所有软组织肉瘤的5%～10%，是常见的非横纹肌肉瘤软组织肉瘤之一（Ferrari et al. 2011）。在所有软组织肉瘤组织学中，MPNST具有最大的肉瘤特异性死亡风险（Kattan et al. 2002）。大约50%的MPNST是在NF1的患者中诊断出来的；NF1患者终身罹患MPNST的风险为8%～13%，而一般人群的风险为0.001%（Ducatman et al. 1986; Evans et al. 2002）。MPNST是NF1患者死亡的主要原因：死亡率分析表明，NF1患者的死亡证明上列出恶性结缔组织或其他软组织肿瘤的可能性是非NF1患者的34倍（Rasmussen et al. 2001）。散发性MPNST通常在成年晚期诊断出来，而NF1患者的MPNST诊断高峰年龄更年轻，一般在成年早期（20～50岁），10%～20%的病例报告年龄甚至

H. Meany
Pediatric Oncology Branch, National Cancer Institute, Bethesda, MD, USA

Children's National Medical Center, Washington, DC, USA

B. C. Widemann
Pediatric Oncology Branch, National Cancer Institute, Bethesda, MD, USA

N. Ratner
Division of Experimental Hematology and Cancer Biology, Cincinnati Children's Research Foundation, Cincinnati Children's Hospital Medical Center, University of Cincinnati College of Medicine, Cincinnati, OH 45229, USA
e-mail: Nancy.Ratner@cchmc.org3

M. Upadhyaya and D. N. Cooper (eds.), *Neurofibromatosis Type 1*,
DOI 10.1007/978-3-642-32864-0_29, # Springer-Verlag Berlin Heidelberg 2012

更小(1～19岁)。在诊断时,NF1相关的MPNST往往体积大(>5 cm)、具有侵袭性且无法切除(Carli et al. 2005)。散发性MPNST通常位于躯干(34%～55%)、四肢(30%～45%)和头/颈部(14%～19%),相比散发性MPNST,NF1-MPNST在躯干中更常见(55%)(Stucky et al. 2012;Zou et al. 2009a)。这一点很重要并可能影响结果,因为与四肢病变相比,中轴部位病变可能更不易于手术治疗(Ducatman et al. 1986;Sordillo et al. 1981)。

MPNST的局部复发风险(43%)和远处转移风险(40%)较高(Wong et al. 1998)。NF1-MPNST预后比散发性MPNST差的另外一个可能原因是NF1-MPNST可能具有更大的转移倾向。在62例NF1-MPNST患者中,39%出现转移性疾病;而在58例散发性MPNST患者中,只有16%出现转移(Ducatman et al. 1986)。成人MPNST转移至肺,其次为软组织、骨、肝、腹腔、肾上腺、横膈膜、纵隔、脑、卵巢、肾和腹膜后(Ducatman et al. 1986)。儿童MPNST可出现同样部位的转移(包括淋巴结、肝脏、骨、软组织和脑)(Meis et al. 1992)。

NF1-MPNST预后可能比散发性MPNST更差的第3个原因是,大多数(65%～88%)NF1-MPNST发生于先前已存在的丛状神经纤维瘤中(Ducatman et al. 1986;Hruban et al. 1990;Meis et al. 1992;King et al. 2003)。MPNST的相关症状可能与良性丛状神经纤维瘤症状重叠,而且难以区分。因为这两种情况均表现为肿块增大、神经根性疼痛、感觉异常、运动无力或其他神经系统症状。NF1中与肿块相关的疼痛被描述为MPNST的最大风险因素(King et al. 2003)。

29.3 MPNST的诊断和进展风险

大多数MPNST发生在NF1和丛状神经纤维瘤的个体中。对丛状神经纤维瘤患者进行MRI纵向评估表明,成人中丛状神经纤维瘤的生长并不常见,应怀疑其有恶变可能(Tucker et al. 2009)。对NF1患者正在进行的前瞻性研究中,对NF1的患者进行全身MRI纵向评估,可能确定其应用于早期发现丛状神经纤维瘤恶变(例如生长)中的作用。内部丛状神经纤维瘤的存在也与MPNST的发展密切相关(Tucker et al. 2005)。NF1患者的高总肿瘤负荷也可能是MPNST的风险因素。NF1发生MPNST的其他重要危险因素包括 *NF1* 基因片段的微缺失(De Raedt et al. 2003;Leppig et al. 1997)和之前接受过放射治疗(Ducatman and Scheithauer 1983;Foley et al. 1980;Meadows et al. 1985)。

29.3.1 MPNST的早期诊断

早期诊断MPNST至关重要,因为只有彻底手术切除才能治愈。NF1相关MPNST的活检部位必须认真选择,因为当MPNST出现在组织学良性的丛状神经纤维瘤中时,NF1中的MPNST诊断可能难以确定和(或)延迟,并且恶性肿瘤的临床指标也可能是先前存在的良性丛状神经纤维瘤的特征。NF1且伴有较大肿瘤负荷的患者,在开始治疗之前进行FDG-PET扫描可能很有价值(见下文)。虽然影像学检查可用于辅助诊断MPNST和选择最合适的肿瘤区域进行活检,但MPNST的诊断需要组织病理学确认。活检方式必须经过肿瘤外科医师批准,以免影响后续手术治疗。

常用的组织病理学分级系统(Costa et al. 1984;Parham et al. 1995;Trojani et al. 1984)包括评估肿瘤的组织学类型或亚型、坏死量、细胞数、有丝分裂数和核多形性。最近对周围神经肿瘤的病理学进行了详细的回顾(Rodriguez et al. 2012)。大多数MPNST是高级别肿瘤,其特征是细胞丰富、核分裂和坏死率高。MPNST最常用的分期是美国癌症联合委员会(American Joint Committee on Cancer,AJCC)软组织肉瘤分期系统(Scaife and Pisters 2003),结合了肿瘤大小(≤5 cm *vs.* >5 cm)、深度(浅表对比深层)、级别(1至4级)以及有无转移等临床、病理特征,分为4期(Ⅰ至Ⅳ)。施万细胞标志物S100β的表达或肿瘤与神经束的关联可有助于诊断。诊断评估除对原发灶进行详细的影像学检查外,应包括胸部CT扫描,以评估是否出现肺转移。

磁共振成像(MRI)是评估良性丛状神经纤维瘤和MPNST的常用影像学检查。不均匀病变(由于坏死和出血)和斑块状强化灶被描述为 MPNST 的特征(Friedrich et al. 2005)。然而,MPNST 在 MRI 上的成像特征并不一致。恶性病变可具有不规则的肿瘤形状、浸润性边缘、周边强化模式、病变周围水肿样区域、肿瘤内囊变或分叶、T1 加权图像上存在不均匀的高信号强度区域、T2 加权图像上缺乏靶征或对比后有不均匀强化(Bhargava et al. 1997;Chhabra et al. 2011;Li et al. 2008;Matsumine et al. 2009;Wasa et al. 2010)。最近的多变量分析得出结论,肿瘤内分叶和 T1 加权图像上存在高信号强化区域可诊断 MPNST(Matsumine et al. 2009)。

良性神经纤维瘤是周围神经或脑神经的一部分,因此具有明确的边缘、分裂脂肪征和中央点征(神经中心区域信号强度降低)(Korf 1999;Li et al. 2008)。MRI 上存在边界清晰的(结节性)病变≥3 cm,但缺乏中央点征也需要注意。对结节性快速生长病变(超过其起源的丛状神经纤维瘤的生长速度)的活检组织学分析显示,存在良性神经纤维瘤区域,但也存在非典型神经纤维瘤和(或)MPNST(Meany et al. 2012)。这些广泛的研究表明,MRI 通常无法可靠地将 MPNST 与丛状神经纤维瘤区分开来。因此,丛状神经纤维瘤的生长速度增加,特别是在成人中,应该怀疑是恶变(Dombi et al. 2007;Tucker et al. 2009)。

用于检测 NF1 患者中伴发 MPNST 的另外一种有价值但尚不完善的方法是 ^{18}F-脱氧葡萄糖正电子发射断层扫描(FDG-PET)。该方法对 MPNST 诊断的灵敏性为 89%~100%,特异性为 72%~95%,阴性预测值为 95%~100%,阳性预测值为 50%~71%(Bensaid et al. 2007;Bredella et al. 2007;Ferner et al. 2008)。多项研究一致认为,SUV_{max} 升高可预测恶性肿瘤;恶性病变的平均值为 5.4~7.0 g/mL,良性肿瘤的平均值为 1.5~2.0 g/mL(Benz et al. 2010)。然而,在 SUV_{max} 为 2.5~3.5 g/mL 的范围内,良性和恶性病变均可发现(Ferner et al. 2000, 2008;Karabatsou et al. 2009;Warbey et al. 2009)。例如,在 105 例 NF1 和症状性丛状神经纤维瘤的患者中,利用 FDG-PET 确定了 34 个 FDG 亲和部位,报道 28 个为恶性病灶(26 个 MPNST 和 2 个其他恶性肿瘤)(Ferner et al. 2008),并且所有恶性病变的 SUV_{max} 均≥2.5 g/mL。然而,在其余 6 个病变中,活检显示 4 个为良性丛状神经纤维瘤,2 个 SUV_{max}>3.5 g/mL 的非典型神经纤维瘤。非典型神经纤维瘤中 FDG 的高摄取与最近的描述一致,即这些病变是癌前病变,并且转化为 MPNST 的风险很高(Beert et al. 2011)。最近的一项研究证实,与活检诊断为良性神经纤维瘤的患者相比,NF1 患者中伴有生长或疼痛的结节性丛状神经纤维瘤的非典型神经纤维瘤和 MPNST,在 FDG-PET 上的平均 SUV_{max} 更高(Meany et al. 2012)。

29.4　MPNST 血清生物标志物

由于目前的成像方式很难对 MPNST 做出确诊,加之生存率低,所以人们试图寻找可能预示丛状神经纤维瘤内 MPNST 生长的生物标志物。这方面的分析尚处于起步阶段。肾上腺髓质素是一种由 52 个氨基酸组成的分泌肽,属于降钙素超家族,在 NF1 患者血清中存在差异表达,在少数 MPNST 患者中显著升高(Hummel et al. 2010),但这尚未在大样本患者队列中得到证实。在另外一项研究中,与正常对照组相比,生长因子中期因子(midkine)在 NF1 患者中升高,且在少数视神经胶质瘤和 MPNST 的 NF1 患者中进一步升高(Mashour et al. 2004)。

29.5　预后因素

MPNST 患者与疾病特异性生存相关的不良预后因素包括:伴有 NF1、诊断时肿瘤直径>10 cm、原发于躯干部位、手术切缘阳性、高级别肿瘤、肿瘤 S100β 染色阴性和 p53 阳性。对于 NF1 相关的 MPNST,p53 免疫反应性和不良预后之间的关系尤其密切(Brekke et al. 2009)。在大多数系列研究中,MPNST 患者的 5 年总体生存率为 21%~52%,NF1-MPNST 患者的生存率更差(Carli et al. 2005;deCou et al. 1995;Ducatman et al. 1986;Moretti et al. 2011;Widemann 2009;Wong et al.

1998；Zou et al. 2009a）。然而，其他研究未能确定散发性 MPNST 和 NF1 相关 MPNST 的预后差异（Cashen et al. 2004；Hruban et al. 1990）。肿瘤分期也是预后因素，起病时伴有转移的患者，其 2 年、5 年和 10 年疾病特异性生存率分别为 28%、23% 和 8%，而局限性患者则为 54%、39% 和 26%（$P = 0.0025$）（Zou et al. 2009a）。在分子水平上，基于 38 例 MPNST 的阵列比较基因组杂交数据，位于染色体 12q14.1 上的 *CDK4* 基因获得/扩增和染色体 12p13.3 上 *FOXMI* 基因的上调是 87 例 MPNST 患者不良生存的显著独立预测因素（Yu et al. 2011）。10q 和 Xq 染色体的丢失以及 16p 的增加也与 MPNST 患者生存率降低有关（Brekke et al. 2010）。

虽然尚未发现女性和男性间罹患 NF1-MPNST 的风险存在显著差异，但最近的一项研究发现，在诊断后的 5 年和 10 年，女性患者的存活率（分别为 46% 和 41.5%）高于男性 MPNST 患者（分别为 22% 和 8.2%）（$P = 0.05$）（Ingham et al. 2011）。X 染色体位点的丢失主要发生在女性身上，这可能是造成这种差异的原因（Brekke et al. 2010）。最后，两项大型研究（Carli et al. 2005；Ferrari et al. 2011）显示，NF1 相关 MPNST 对化学治疗的反应明显比散发性 MPNST 更差。在计算了其他预后因素后，尚不清楚 NF1 相关 MPNST 的结果是否比散发性 MPNST 更差。

29.6　MPNST 的治疗

彻底手术切除是散发性和 NF1 相关 MPNST 的唯一治愈方法（Carli et al. 2005；Ferner and Gutmann 2002；Longhi et al. 2010）。手术目的是在安全外科边界下切除 MPNST。如果不能实现肿瘤完整手术切除，术后放射治疗有助于提高局部控制率（Wong et al. 1998）。临床试验表明，除保肢手术外，外照射或近距离放射治疗可提高软组织肉瘤患者的局部控制率（Pisters et al. 1996；Yang et al. 1998）。因此，建议对边缘切除、肿瘤>5 cm 的中度至高度恶性病变进行辅助放射治疗以改善局部控制率（Pisters et al. 1996；Wong et al. 1998；Yang et al. 1998；Ferner and Gutmann 2002）。有临床研究报告显示，应用治疗儿童和成人软组织肉瘤的标准化学治疗药物来治疗 MPNST 是有效的（Carli et al. 2005；Edmonson et al. 1989；Ferrari et al. 2011；Raney et al. 1987；Valdes and Maurer 1970），但化学治疗反应率尚未在 MPNST 特异性试验获得前瞻性评价。因此，一项正在进行的针对高级别不可切除 MPNST 化学治疗的临床试验中，将患者分为散发性和 NF1 相关 MPNST，因为回顾性研究表明 NF1 相关 MPNST 对化学治疗的反应明显低于散发性 MPNST（Ferrari et al. 2011；Carli et al. 2005）。

基于非典型神经纤维瘤是 MPNST 癌前病变的证据（Beert et al. 2011；见下文），如果可行且没有过多的并发症，应考虑手术切除这些病变。即使密切监测也可能不足以及时发现非典型神经纤维瘤恶变而进行彻底手术切除。以 1 例伴有 NF1 且长期无症状骶前非典型神经纤维瘤的患者为例（图 29.1），非典型神经纤维瘤突然生长后，手术切除显示阳性切缘。

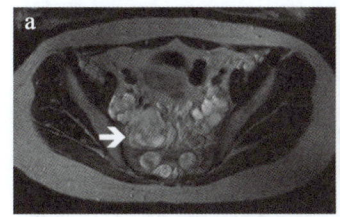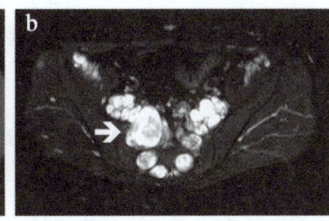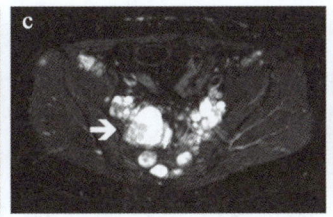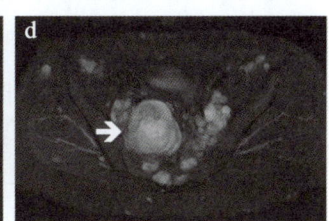

图 29.1　非典型神经纤维瘤进展为 MPNST。1 名 23 岁男性，患有 NF1 和广泛的丛状神经纤维瘤，对其骨盆进行连续纵向 MRI 检查。右侧骶前活检证实的非典型神经纤维瘤（箭头）保持稳定，并且在 8 年的体积 MRI 分析中显示出相似的成像特征（a），2003 年，47 mL；活检证实的非典型神经纤维瘤（箭头）(b) 2009 年，50 mL；活检再次证实非典型神经纤维瘤（箭头）(c)，2011 年，47 mL；(d) 6 个月后的 2012 年，患者抱怨左小腿疼痛，肿瘤大小增加一倍至 98 mL，活检证实为高级别 MPNST。患者接受手术切除，切缘阳性。重要的是，在 8 年的时间段内，FDG-PET 对 FDG 的摄取

29.7 NF1 突变导致 MPNST 发病

由于 MPNST 对 NF1 患者生存的毁灭性影响，为发现导致 MPNST 发生和发展的分子异常提供了强大的动力。起始突变中主要是 NF1 基因本身的突变，因为至少 95% 的 NF1 患者携带位于 17 号染色体长臂（17q11.2）上的肿瘤抑制基因 NF1 的结构性突变以及该基因的功能拷贝数变异（Messiaen et al. 2000），并且至少 40%~90% 的 NF1 MPNST 中发现了第二等位基因的突变或功能性缺失（Upadhyaya et al. 2008、Bottillo et al. 2009）。尽管 NF1 患者的结构性突变发生在整个 NF1 基因位点中（Messiaen et al. 2000），但在 5% 结构性突变涉及全部基因缺失的 NF1 患者中，发生 MPNST 则更为普遍（Wimmer et al. 2006，De Raedt et al. 2003）。关于 NF1 相邻基因的共同缺失增加恶性转化风险的可能性，相关研究正在进行中；与正常施万细胞相比，RNF125 和 CENTA2 两个基因在常见区域的缺失导致其在 MPNST 细胞中的表达降低（Pasmant et al. 2011a）。

重要的是，最近在散发性 MPNST 中也发现了 NF1 突变，至少在一定程度上解释了为什么 NF1 和散发性肿瘤中的基因表达和基因组变化会出现重叠（Brekke et al. 2010；Miller et al. 2006；Watson et al. 2004）。在迄今为止最大规模的研究中，Bottillo 等（2009）发现 9/22（41%）的散发性 MPNST 存在 NF1 突变。NF1 和散发性 MPNST 中的 NF1 体细胞突变通常是 NF1 中的大基因组拷贝数变化，可能包括相邻基因的共缺失（Upadhyaya et al. 2008；Pasmant et al. 2011c）。

29.8 形成 MPNST 的其他途径

在一些缺乏 NF1 突变的散发性 MPNST 中，Ras 突变或 Ras 通路基因可能导致 MPNST 肿瘤的发生。在大型 MPNST 病例系列中，尚未报道散发性 MPNST 中的 Ras 突变量，但在少数散发性病例中，发现了 Ras 激活突变[N-Ras(1/11)或 K-Ras(1/11)]（Perrone et al. 2009）或 B-Raf 突变（1/13MPNST）（Bottillo et al. 2009）。miRNA miR-10b 可以靶向 NF1 mRNA（Chai et al. 2010）；原则上，靶向 NF1 的 miR 也可能导致 NF1 肿瘤发生。

29.9 神经纤维瘤和 MPNST 中间状态：非典型神经纤维瘤

除 NF1 基因位点外，神经纤维瘤中尚未发现其他基因组异常，但在 MPNST 中却很多。因此，神经纤维瘤发展为 MPNST 必定涉及一系列基因组改变。重要的是，在 16 例非典型神经纤维瘤中，有 15 例检测到 9p21.3 染色体上 CDKN2A 基因的复发性纯合缺失（Beert et al. 2011）。相比之下，相邻的 CDKN2B 基因座并未复发性缺失。CDKN2A 基因编码 p16^{INK4A}，这是一种细胞周期抑制剂，可抑制细胞周期蛋白依赖性激酶 4（CDK4）和 6（CDK6）的作用。CDKN2A 基因还编码 p14^{ARF}，它与 MDM2 泛素连接酶结合并抑制该酶，从而稳定 p53。有报道称，在一些神经纤维瘤病例中，长非编码 RNA（LncRNA）在 CDKN2A/B 基因位点的丢失可能表明一些手术切除的丛状神经纤维瘤包含非典型神经纤维瘤区域，这再次强调了神经纤维瘤组织病理学分析的关键重要性（Pasmant et al. 2011b）。在没有其他基因组变化（除 NF1 基因本身外）的情况下，CDKN2A 基因的早期缺失强烈支持非典型神经纤维瘤是良性神经纤维瘤和 MPNST 之间的中间过渡的观点，并表明 CDKN2A 丢失是神经纤维瘤向 MPNST 发展的关键早期步骤。毫不奇怪，大约 50% 的 MPNST 存在 CDKN2A 基因缺失（Kourea et al. 1999；Nielsen et al. 1999）。小鼠模型支持该基因在 MPNST 中的重要性，因为 $Nf1^{+/-}$；$Ink4a/Arf-1^{-/-}$ 小鼠发生了 MPNST，而不是神经纤维瘤（Joseph et al. 2008）。

29.10 MPNST 的全基因组分析

与大多数肉瘤一样，MPNST 中的染色体增加、丢失和重排具有高度可变性（Wallace et al. 2000）。不同肿瘤中，染色体的增加和丢失具有高度可变性，这表明有一系列以上的突变导致 MPNST。MPNST 通常具有亚二倍体或近三倍体的核型，染色体 7、8q 和 15q 上经常出现增加,而染色体的丢失会影响许多染色体区域(1p、9p、11、12p、14q、17q、18、22q、X 和 Y)(Forus et al. 1995；Lothe et al. 1996；Mechtersheimer et al. 1999；Mertens et al. 1995；2000；Plaat et al. 1999；Schmidt et al. 1999，2000，2001)。目前,正在致力于对 MPNST 细胞系和原发性肿瘤进行全基因组分析,以便更全面地描述与 MPNST 发病机制相关的癌基因和抑癌基因。我们预计将发表几项使用阵列 CGH、大规模 SNP 分析和全基因组测序的研究,以帮助识别 MPNST 中的驱动突变。GEO 上已经有多个数据系列。这包括人类 mRNA 基因表达分析、DNA 阵列比较基因组杂交、BAC 阵列和 MPNST 甲基化数据集,以及来自大鼠和斑马鱼 MPNST 样肿瘤的数据(表 29.1)。

表 29.1 已发表的 MPNST 数据集

数据类型	数据系列	种 属	样本量	实 验 小 结	引 自
甲基化组	GSE21714	人属	3	对比分析良性和恶性周围神经鞘膜瘤的甲基组	Feber 等(2011)
基因表达	GSE36144	褐家鼠	19	从大鼠三叉神经经 ENU 诱导的 MPNST 和正常组织	N/A
基因表达	GSE14038	人属	86	86 个微阵列,由 77 个样品和 9 批参考样品组成：10 个 NHSC,11 个 dNFSC,11 个 pNFSC,13 个 MPNST 细胞系,13 个 dNF,13 个 pNF,6 个 MPNST	Miller 等(2009)
基因表达	GSE11493	斑马鱼	11	对比由 rp 突变引起的 6 个斑马鱼 MPNST 的 mRNA(3 个来自 rpL35,1 个来自 rpL14,1 个来源 rpS5,1 个源自 rpS11)和由 p53 M214K/M214K 突变引起的 3 个 MPNSTs 的 mRNA	MacInnes 等(2008)
基因表达	GSE6481	人属	105	使用 Affymetrix HG-U133A 阵列检测 105 例肉瘤,包括 3 例 MPNST,16 例滑膜肉瘤,19 例黏液脂肪肉瘤,3 例脂肪瘤,3 例高分化脂肪瘤,15 例去分化脂肪肉瘤,15 例黏液纤维肉瘤,6 例平滑肌肉瘤,4 例纤维肉瘤,21 例恶性纤维组织	Nakayama 等(2007)
拷贝数变异	GSE33881	人属	51	对 MPNST 的组织样本进行基于微阵列比较基因组杂交分析	Yang 等(2011)
拷贝数变异	GSE16041	人属	27	比较 24 个 MPNST 样本与 NF1 患者的 3 个良性神经纤维瘤的拷贝数变化,与人类 32K BAC 平铺路径阵列杂交	Mantripragada 等(2009)

值得注意的是,对神经纤维瘤和 MPNST 进行的基因组体细胞拷贝数改变(CNA)和杂合性缺失(LDH)联合性分析证实,神经纤维瘤中不存在复发性或重叠的 CNA,而 MPNST 显示了 232 个 CNA(涵盖超过 2 900 个基因,并且超过 500 个基因表现出一致的 LOH(Upadhyaya et al. 2012)。

29.11 MPNST 中细胞周期基因的常见基因组变化

人们普遍认为,在大多数 MPNST 中存在 TP53 基因功能缺失。重要的是,在 18/20 MPNST 样本中发现了"p53 失活相关增殖"基因表达特征,且 p53 失活导致 miR-34a 下调,从而阻止组织培养中的 MPNST 细胞凋亡(Subramanian et al. 2010)。TP53 基因的双等位基因失活在 MPNST 中很少见(Lothe et al. 2001),因此提示半合子 TP53 突变可能导致进展至 MPNST(Upadhyaya et al. 2008)。然而,在小鼠模型中,只有 Tp53 的完全缺失才与 MPNST 形成相关(此外没有 Nf1；Cichowski et al. 1999；Vogel et al. 1999)。

在染色体水平上,TP53 失活似乎由多种机制引起，包括缺失和突变导致 17p13.1 染色体上的 TP53 抑癌基因功能丧失。这些在神经纤维瘤或非典型神经纤维瘤中未发现，但在 MPNST 中很常见 (Birindelli et al. 2001; Legius et al. 1994; Menon et al. 1990)。对 MPNST 伴有具 TP53 基因组改变的预测变异度很大，一些预测报告中 MPNST 的 TP53 突变高达 75%（Holtkamp et al. 2007; Upadhyaya et al. 2008），而其他的估计值要低得多 (24%, Verdijk et al. 2010)。这些差异可能是由于每项研究中通常分析的肿瘤数量较少，以及使用不同的抗体来检测 p53 表达作为基于 DNA 方法的替代，和（或）肿瘤内的区域差异(Brekke et al. 2009; Riddle et al. 2010; Verdijk et al. 2010; Zhou et al. 2003)。p53 的稳定性可由 MDM2 通过 $p14^{ARF}$ 调节。由于 $p14^{ARF}$ 保留在某些 MPNST 中，这种机制可能部分解释在没有稳定的 TP53 突变的情况下 p53 的高表达。

视网膜母细胞瘤(Rb)蛋白是一种阻碍细胞周期进程的分子，在 25% 的 MPNST 中表达缺失 (Mantripragada et al. 2008; Mawrin et al. 2002)。PTEN 基因作为 PI3K 信号转导的关闭信号，是人类癌症中第二最常突变的肿瘤抑制因子。在 MPNST 中发现了 PTEN 位点的频繁单体性 (Holtkamp et al. 2008; Perrone et al. 2009)，小鼠中 Nf1 和 Pten 的共同缺失导致了神经纤维瘤和 MPNST 的形成 (Keng et al. 2012)；K-RasG12D 的激活与 Pten 的缺失相结合也导致了 GEM-PNST(Gregorian et al. 2009)。目前还不清楚 PI3K 通路如何以及在人类 MPNST 肿瘤形成的哪个阶段失调(Perrone et al. 2009); Perrone 等人的研究未发现 MPNST 中 PI3KCA 或 PTEN 突变。

29.12 MPNST 的细胞起源和标记

MPNST 的确切细胞起源仍不清楚。施万细胞标志物 S100β 表达于一半以上的 MPNST 中。神经嵴细胞、施万细胞前体、未成熟施万细胞或成熟施万细胞去分化等都可能是其细胞起源。对源自鼠类 NPCis(GEM-PNST)肿瘤的永久细胞系进行检查表明，肿瘤细胞表达神经嵴细胞、施万细胞和成肌细胞的特征性标志物(Vogel et al. 1999)。对人类 MPNST 肿瘤和 MPNST 细胞系进行基因分析后显示，神经嵴细胞标志物的表达是一个突出的特征 (Miller et al. 2006, 2009)。多项基因表达研究已证实，神经嵴标志物 SOX9 和 TWIST1 在 MPNST 中显著上调（Carbonnelle-Puscian et al. 2011; Miller et al. 2006, 2009; Pytel et al. 2010)。在 MPNST 中，细胞似乎依赖于这些神经嵴基因的表达，因为 SOX9 的下调会导致细胞死亡，TWIST1 的下调会降低细胞迁移能力 (Miller et al. 2006, 2009)。一项包含 34 例 MPNST 的病例系列描述，与神经纤维瘤相比，MPNST 中谱系标志物 FOXD3、PAX7、SOX5 和 AP-2α 的免疫反应表达增高(Pytel et al. 2010)。基板标志物 EYA/SIX 在 MPNST 细胞和肿瘤中也上调（Miller et al. 2010)。使用 shRNA 来减少 EYA4 表达可防止肿瘤形成并导致坏死。这很有趣，因为 EYA 是一种磷酸酶，原则上可以作为治疗的靶点。

除了谱系标记之外，MPNST 的其他标记也已被描述。通过二维凝胶和对 1 500 个蛋白质点的检查，MPNST 最类似于滑膜肉瘤和透明细胞癌(Kawai et al. 2008)。Wilms 肿瘤 1 (WT1)在所有神经施万细胞、神经纤维瘤和 MPNST 细胞中均有表达(Schittenhelm et al. 2010)。使用抗体染色，TLE 表达于 30% 的 MPNST(Kosemehmetoglu et al. 2009)。6/6 MPNST 表达 Tenascin-C（一种细胞外基质糖蛋白）和 NNAT（神经胶原蛋白），而这些标志物并未在神经纤维瘤中表达(Dugu et al. 2010)。组织蛋白酶 K 是降解胶原蛋白和弹性蛋白的半胱氨酸蛋白酶，同样在 6/6 MPNST 中表达，但在神经纤维瘤中没有表达(Yan et al. 2010)。在单个病例中，MPNST 而非相邻的神经纤维瘤显示了血管生成开关的标志物：SMA、vWF、VEGF 以及 VEGF 受体 Flt1 和 Flk1 的表达均上调(Gesundheit et al. 2010)。许多生长中或非典型神经纤维瘤和 MPNST CD10 抗体染色阳性(Cabibi et al. 2009)。一些神经纤维瘤和 MPNST 表达 hTERT(Patel and Folpe 2009)。最后，c-Fos 在小鼠 PNST 中表达，并且是 GEM-PNST 形成所必需的，并在 1 例人类 MPNST 中高度表达(Silvestre et al. 2010)。由于

AP-1转录因子(包括c-fos),作用于Ras信号的下游,这一发现与神经纤维瘤蛋白作为Ras-GAP的主要作用一致。我们的目标仍然是确定将MPNST与滑膜肉瘤和透明细胞肉瘤区分开来的标志物,并明确将其与周围的神经纤维瘤区分开来。

29.13 MPNST中的生长因子受体扩增

大量证据表明,生长因子和生长因子受体激活的异常信号转导是MPNST的发病机制。EGFR基因扩增很常见(Perry et al. 2002; Holtkamp et al. 2008),一项研究(Keizman et al. 2009)表明EGFR过表达与预后较差有关,但在另一项研究中并非如此(Tabone-Eglinger et al. 2008)。Perrone等(2009)研究了27例MPNST,在所有散发性MPNST和一半NF1 MPNST中发现EGFR扩增。重要的是,在许多独立研究中,未检测到EGFR的激活突变,这表明受体扩增加上EGFR配体(包括TGFa和HBEGF)的自分泌和旁分泌表达可能促进肿瘤生长。激活EGFR的配体表达于90%的MPNST中,这表明MPNST细胞中存在自分泌环(Holtkamp et al. 2008)。相反,相关的神经调节蛋白-1辅助受体erbB2的扩增却很少见(Storlazzi et al. 2006; Holtkamp et al. 2008)。

4q12染色体上的扩增子编码三个相邻的酪氨酸激酶受体基因:*PDGFRA*、*KIT*和*VEGFR-2/KDR*。在MPNST小系列样本中,15%存在扩增子(Zietsch et al. 2010)。在这3个基因中,*PDGFRA*扩增最频繁(Badache and De Vries 1998; Holtkamp et al. 2006; Mantripragada et al. 2008)且很少发生突变(Holtkamp et al. 2006)。*PDGFRA*和*PDGFRB*在6/24MPNST中共扩增;2/24仅有*DGFRA*扩增(Holtkamp et al. 2008)。虽然c-Kit扩增可能发生,但这是一种罕见事件(Holtkamp et al. 2006)。

在MPNST中肝细胞生长因子表达且其c-Met受体(Mantripragada et al. 2008)扩增。Torres等(2011)最近的一项研究表明,尽管仅在肿瘤显著生长之前给药,靶向MET的短发夹RNA和XL184(一种靶向MET和VEGFR2的化合物)均可降低移植瘤中MPNST细胞的生长。

使用MPNST细胞系进行的体外研究支持这些扩增基因编码的分子具有功能性作用的结论。在有限量血清存在下生长的MPNST细胞的增殖依赖于外源性EGF;在较高的血清浓度下,这些细胞不需要外源性EGF,但它们的增殖仍然受到针对EGFR的小分子抑制剂和中和抗体的抑制(DeClue et al. 2000; Johansson et al. 2008; Dilworth et al. 2008)。靶向神经调节蛋白-1受体(Stonecypher et al. 2005)、c-Kit(Badache and De Vries 1998)和PDGF受体(Holtkamp et al. 2006)的抑制剂同样抑制MPNST有丝分裂。PDGF(Aoki et al. 2007)和c-Met(Su et al. 2004)也与MPNST细胞侵袭有关。目前,尚不清楚所有这些生长因子和生长因子受体是否都是MPNST发病所必需的,或者是否存在不同的MPNST亚群,其肿瘤的发生仅依赖于其中的一些分子。此外,针对PDGFR、C-KIT和EGFR的多项组织特异性试验已完成,所有单药均未获得反应或有意义的疾病稳定(Albritton et al. 2006; Chugh et al. 2009; Maki et al. 2009; Schuetze et al. 2010)。

29.14 MPNST的临床前治疗:细胞内通路

人们已经探索了活化受体的下游信号通路,包括Ras、PI3K、ERK、mTOR、Akt和Ral。这一点尤其重要,因为Nf1的缺失预计会激活Ras-GTP的下游信号通路。一篇出色的综述(Katz et al. 2009)总结了这几年的研究结果;在任何情况下,任何单一药物都不能超过暂时性地阻止GEM或异种移植模型中的MPNST生长(Zou et al. 2009b)。更新的研究发现更有希望的结果,PI3K/mTOR抑制剂PI-103可诱导MPNST细胞中的G1细胞周期停滞和自噬。使用透明质酸寡聚体可抑制药物转运蛋白活性并抑制MPNST异体移植瘤的生长,寡聚体和阿霉素之间有协同作用(Slomiany et al. 2009)。在为期18天的测定中,将MPNST细胞暴露于4-OH-他莫昔芬或钙调蛋白抑制剂氟拉嗪和W-7可模拟这种对小鼠坐骨神经移植瘤中MPNST增殖和凋亡的影响(Byer et al. 2011)。使用MLN2036

抑制极光激酶导致异种移植模型中 9/10 小鼠的 MPNST 生长停滞时间延长，从而导致细胞停滞在细胞周期的 G2/M 期（Patel et al. 2012）。组蛋白去乙酰化酶抑制剂 PC-24791（可促进自噬）与自噬阻断剂氯喹的联合，可消除 MPNST 异种移植物的生长并促进细胞凋亡；但是，由于试验时间很短，因此反应的持久性尚不清楚（Lopez et al. 2011）。使用雷帕霉素或其类似物 RAD001，只能暂时阻断 GEM-PNST 的 NPCis 模型、异种移植瘤模型和皮下成瘤模型中的 MPNST 生长（Johannessen et al. 2008; Johansson et al. 2008; Bhola et al. 2010）。在一个令人兴奋的新进展中，雷帕霉素的细胞抑制作用通过与促进蛋白毒性/内质网（ER）应激的药物结合转化为细胞毒性作用，这是一种癌细胞由于 ER 中未折叠蛋白的积累而表现出的应激类型（De Raedt et al. 2011）。使用 HSP90 抑制剂进一步增强 ER 应激，再加上雷帕霉素，导致该模型中的肿瘤急剧消退，这与 ER 和线粒体的严重损伤以及细胞死亡相关。抗氧化剂治疗阻止了这种情况，表明其依赖于活性氧物质。基于这些重要数据，正在考虑进行组合临床试验。

29.15　结论

MPNST 仍然与不良预后相关，对 NF1 的个体则更为显著。为了更早期诊断 MPNST，例如① 识别生物标志物，以便将丛状神经纤维瘤与 MPNST 区分开来，② 使用纵向 MRI 监测 NF1 丛状神经纤维瘤的个体，以发现提示恶变的变化，以及③ 使用 FDG-PET 评估神经纤维瘤负担和代谢，并提高对肿块不断增大或疼痛的患者发生恶变可能的认识，可能使手术治疗更加成功。在纳入 MPNST 的特异性试验中，对患者临床表现的详细描述，包括 NF1 表现的细节，例如体内肿瘤负担、性别、针对 NF1 和散发性肿瘤的不同治疗反应，将有助于进一步了解散发性和 NF1 相关肿瘤。MPNST 中基因组水平改变的信息正在不断被完善，有助于了解 MPNST 的分子发病机制。在有意义的临床前模型中对靶向药物进行的临床前评估，支持了联合疗法对参与 MPNST 临床试验患者的潜在效用。

致谢：作者感谢 Kwangmin Choi 博士编制表 29.1，以及 Eva Dombi 博士编制图 29.1。Ratner 博士关于神经纤维瘤和 MPSNT 的工作得到了美国国立卫生研究院（R01 NS28840 和 P50 NS057531 至 N. R.）、国防部神经纤维瘤病计划（W81XWH-11-1-0057 和 W81XWH08-1-0052）以及儿童肿瘤基金会的支持。Ratner 博士还要感谢部分支持她工作的癌症生物学 Beatrice Lampkin 主席。Widemann 博士的研究得到了 NCI 癌症研究中心内部研究项目的支持。

（周宇红　译）

参考文献

[1] Albritton K, Rankin C, Coffin C, Ratner N, Budd T, Schuetze S, Randall R, DeClue J, Borden E (2006) Phase II trial of erlotinib in metastatic or unresectable malignant peripheral nerve sheath tumor (MPNST). ASCO, Alexandria, VA

[2] Aoki M, Nabeshima K, Koga K, Hamasaki M, Suzumiya J, Tamura K, Iwasaki H (2007) Imatinib mesylate inhibits cell invasion of malignant peripheral nerve sheath tumor induced by platelet-derived growth factor-BB. Lab Invest 87(8): 767-779

[3] Badache A, De Vries GH (1998) Neurofibrosarcoma-derived Schwann cells overexpress platelet-derived growth factor (PDGF) receptors and are induced to proliferate by PDGF BB. J Cell Physiol 177(2): 334-342

[4] Beert E, Brems H, Daniels B, De Wever I, Van Calenbergh F, Schoenaers J, Debiec-Rychter M, Gevaert O, De Raedt T, Van Den Bruel A, de Ravel T, Cichowski K, Kluwe L, Mautner V, Sciot R, Legius E (2011) Atypical neurofibromas in neurofibromatosis type 1 are premalignant tumors. Genes Chromosomes Cancer 50(12): 1021-1032

[5] Bensaid B, Giammarile F, Mognetti T, Galoisy-Guibal L, Pinson S, Drouet A, Combemale P (2007) Utility of 18 FDG positon emission tomography in detection of sarcomatous transfor-mation in neurofibromatosis type 1. Ann Dermatol Venereol 134(10 Pt 1): 735-741

[6] Benz MR, Czernin J, Dry SM, Tap WD, Allen-Auerbach MS, Elashoff D, Phelps ME, Weber WA, Eilber FC (2010) Quantitative F18-fluorodeoxyglucose positron emission tomography accurately characterizes peripheral nerve sheath tumors as malignant or benign. Cancer 116(2): 451-458

[7] Bhargava R, Parham DM, Lasater OE, Chari RS, Chen G, Fletcher BD (1997) MR imaging differentiation of benign and malignant peripheral nerve sheath tumors: use of the target sign. Pediatr Radiol 27(2): 124-129

[8] Bhola P, Banerjee S, Mukherjee J, Balasubramanium A, Arun V, Karim Z, Burrell K, Croul S, Gutmann DH, Guha A (2010) Preclinical in vivo evaluation of rapamycin in human malignant peripheral nerve sheath explant xenograft. Int J Cancer 126(2): 563-571

[9] Birindelli S, Perrone F, Oggionni M, Lavarino C, Pasini B, Vergani B, Ranzani GN, Pierotti MA, Pilotti S (2001) Rb and TP53 pathway alterations in sporadic and NF1-related malignant peripheral nerve sheath tumors. Lab Invest 81(6): 833-844

[10] Bottillo I, Ahlquist T, Brekke H, Danielsen SA, van den Berg E, Mertens F, Lothe RA, Dallapiccola B (2009) Germline and somatic NF1 mutations in sporadic and NF1-associated malignant peripheral nerve sheath tumours. J Pathol 217(5): 693-701

[11] Bredella MA, Torriani M, Hornicek F, Ouellette HA, Plamer WE, Williams Z, Fischman AJ, Plotkin SR (2007) Value of PET in the assessment of patients with neurofibromatosis type 1. Am J Roentgenol 189(4): 928-935

[12] Brekke HR, Kolberg M, Skotheim RI, Hall KS, Bjerkehagen B, Risberg B, Domanski HA, Mandahl N, Liestol K, Smeland S, Danielsen HE, Mertens F, Lothe RA (2009) Identification of p53 as a strong predictor of survival for patients with malignant peripheral nerve sheath tumors. Neuro Oncol 11(5): 514-528

[13] Brekke HR, Ribeiro FR, Kolberg M, Agesen TH, Lind GE, Eknaes M, Hall KS, Bjerkehagen B, van den Berg E, Teixeira MR, Mandahl N, Smeland S, Mertens F, Skotheim RI, Lothe RA (2010) Genomic changes in chromosomes 10, 16, and X in malignant peripheral nerve sheath tumors identify a high-risk patient group. J Clin Oncol 28(9): 1573-1582

[14] Byer SJ, Eckert JM, Brossier NM, Clodfelder-Miller BJ, Turk AN, Carroll AJ, Kappes JC, Zinn KR, Prasain JK, Carroll SL (2011) Tamoxifen inhibits malignant peripheral nerve sheath tumor growth in an estrogen receptor-independent manner. Neuro Oncol 13(1): 28-41

[15] Cabibi D, Zerilli M, Caradonna G, Schillaci L, Belmonte B, Rodolico V (2009) Diagnostic and prognostic value of CD10 in peripheral nerve sheath tumors. Anticancer Res 29(8): 3149-3155. doi: 29/8/3149 [pii]

[16] Carbonnelle-Puscian A, Vidal V, Laurendeau I, Valeyrie-Allanore L, Vidaud D, Bieche I, Leroy K, Lantieri L, Wolkenstein P, Schedl A, Ortonne N (2011) SOX9 expression increases with malignant potential in tumors from patients with neurofibromatosis 1 and is not correlated to desert hedgehog. Hum Pathol 42(3): 434-443

[17] Carli M, Ferrari A, Mattke A, Zanetti I, Casanova M, Bisogno G, Cecchetto G, Alaggio R, De Sio L, Koscielniak E, Sotti G, Treuner J (2005) Pediatric malignant peripheral nerve sheath tumor: the Italian and German soft tissue sarcoma cooperative group. J Clin Oncol 23(33): 8422-8430

[18] Cashen DV, Parisien RC, Raskin K, Hornicek FJ, Gebhardt MC, Mankin HJ (2004) Survival data for patients with malignant schwannoma. Clin Orthop Relat Res 426: 69-73

[19] Chai G, Liu N, Ma J, Li H, Oblinger JL, Prahalad AK, Gong M, Chang LS, Wallace M, Muir D, Guha A, Phipps RJ, Hock JM, Yu X (2010) MicroRNA-10b regulates tumorigenesis in neurofi-bromatosis type 1. Cancer Sci 101(9): 1997-2004

[20] Chhabra A, Soldatos T, Durand DJ, Carrino JA, McCarthy EF, Belzberg AJ (2011) The role of magnetic resonance imaging in the diagnostic evaluation of malignant peripheral nerve sheath tumors. Indian J Cancer 48(3): 328-334

[21] Chugh R, Wathen JK, Maki RG, Benjamin RS, Patel SR, Meyers PA, Priebat DA, Reinke DK, Thomas DG, Keohan ML, Samuels BL, Baker LH (2009) Phase II multicenter trial of imatinib in 10 histologic subtypes of sarcoma using a bayesian hierarchical statistical model. J Clin Oncol 27(19): 3148-3153

[22] Cichowski K, Shih TS, Schmitt E, Santiago S, Reilly K, McLaughlin ME, Bronson RT, Jacks T (1999) Mouse models of tumor development in neurofibromatosis type 1. Science 286(5447): 2172-2176

[23] Costa J, Wesley RA, Glatstein E, Rosenberg SA (1984) The grading of soft tissue sarcomas. Results of a clinicohistopathologic correlation in a series of 163 cases. Cancer 53(3): 530-541

[24] De Raedt T, Brems H, Wolkenstein P, Vidaud D, Pilotti S, Perrone F, Mautner V, Frahm S, Sciot R, Legius E (2003) Elevated risk for MPNST in NF1 microdeletion patients. Am J Hum Genet 72(5): 1288-1292

[25] De Raedt T, Walton Z, Yecies JL, Li D, Chen Y, Malone CF, Maertens O, Jeong SM, Bronson RT, Lebleu V, Kalluri R, Normant E, Haigis MC, Manning BD, Wong KK, Macleod KF, Cichowski K (2011) Exploiting cancer cell vulnerabilities to develop a combination therapy for ras-driven tumors. Cancer Cell 20(3): 400-413

[26] DeClue JE, Heffelfinger S, Benvenuto G, Ling B, Li S, Rui W, Vass WC, Viskochil D, Ratner N (2000) Epidermal growth factor receptor expression in neurofibromatosis type 1-related tumors and NF1 animal models. J Clin Invest 105(9): 1233-1241

[27] deCou JM, Rao BN, Parham DM, Lobe TE, Bowman L, Pappo AS, Fontanesi J (1995) Malignant peripheral nerve sheath tumors: the St. Jude Children's Research Hospital experience. Ann Surg Oncol 2(6): 524-529

[28] Dilworth JT, Wojtkowiak JW, Mathieu P, Tainsky MA, Reiners JJ Jr, Mattingly RR, Hancock CN (2008) Suppression of proliferation of two independent NF1 malignant peripheral nerve sheath tumor cell lines by the pan-ErbB inhibitor CI-1033. Cancer Biol Ther 7(12): 1938-1946

[29] Dombi E, Solomon J, Gillespie AJ, Fox E, Balis FM, Patronas N, Korf BR, Babovic-Vuksanovic D, Packer RJ, Belasco J, Goldman S, Jakacki R, Kieran M, Steinberg SM, Widemann BC (2007) NF1 plexiform neurofibroma growth rate by volumetric MRI: relationship to age and body weight. Neurology 68(9): 643-647

[30] Ducatman BS, Scheithauer BW (1983) Postirradiation neurofibrosarcoma. Cancer 51(6): 1028-1033

[31] Ducatman BS, Scheithauer BW, Piepgras DG, Reiman HM, Ilstrup DM (1986) Malignant peripheral nerve sheath tumors. A clinicopathologic study of 120 cases. Cancer 57(10): 2006-2021

[32] Dugu L, Hayashida S, Nakahara T, Xie L, Iwashita Y, Liu X, Uchi H, Tateuchi S, Takahara M, Oda Y, Moroi Y, Furue M (2010) Aberrant expression of tenascin-c and neuronatin in malignant peripheral nerve sheath tumors. Eur J Dermatol 20(5): 580-584

[33] Edmonson JH, Buckner JC, Long HJ, Loprinzi CL, Schaid DJ (1989) Phase II study of ifosfamide-etoposide-mesna in adults with advanced nonosseous sarcomas. J Natl Cancer Inst 81(11): 863-866

[34] Evans DG, Baser ME, McGaughran J, Sharif S, Howard E, Moran A (2002) Malignant peripheral nerve sheath tumours in neurofibromatosis 1. J Med Genet 39(5): 311-314

[35] Feber A, Wilson GA, Zhang L, Presneau N, Idowu B, Down

TA, Rakyan VK, Noon LA, Lloyd AC, Stupka E, Schiza V, Teschendorff AE, Schroth GP, Flanagan A, Beck S (2011) Comparative methylome analysis of benign and malignant peripheral nerve sheath tumors. Genome Res 21(4): 515-524

[36] Ferner RE, Gutmann DH (2002) International consensus statement on malignant peripheral nerve sheath tumors in neurofibromatosis. Cancer Res 62(5): 1573-1577

[37] Ferner RE, Lucas JD, O'Doherty MJ, Hughes RA, Smith MA, Cronin BF, Bingham J (2000) Evaluation of (18) fluorodeoxyglucose positron emission tomography ((18)FDG PET) in the detection of malignant peripheral nerve sheath tumours arising from within plexiform neurofibromas in neurofibromatosis 1. J Neurol Neurosurg Psychiatry 68(3): 353-357

[38] Ferner RE, Golding JF, Smith M, Calonje E, Jan W, Sanjayanathan V, O'Doherty M (2008) [18F] 2-fluoro-2-deoxy-D-glucose positron emission tomography (FDG PET) as a diagnostic tool for neurofibromatosis 1 (NF1) associated malignant peripheral nerve sheath tumours (MPNSTs): a long-term clinical study. Ann Oncol 19(2): 390-394

[39] Ferrari A, Miceli R, Rey A, Oberlin O, Orbach D, Brennan B, Mariani L, Carli M, Bisogno G, Cecchetto G, De Salvo GL, Casanova M, Vannoesel MM, Kelsey A, Stevens MC, Devidas M, Pappo AS, Spunt SL (2011) Non-metastatic unresected paediatric non-rhabdomyosarcoma soft tissue sarcomas: results of a pooled analysis from United States and European groups. Eur J Cancer 47(5): 724-731

[40] Foley KM, Woodruff JM, Ellis FT, Posner JB (1980) Radiation-induced malignant and atypical peripheral nerve sheath tumors. Ann Neurol 7(4): 311-318

[41] Forus A, Weghuis DO, Smeets D, Fodstad O, Myklebost O, van Kessel AG (1995) Comparative genomic hybridization analysis of human sarcomas: I. Occurrence of genomic imbalances and identification of a novel major amplicon at 1q21-q22 in soft tissue sarcomas. Genes Chromosomes Cancer 14(1): 8-14

[42] Friedrich RE, Kluwe L, Funsterer C, Mautner VF (2005) Malignant peripheral nerve sheath tumors (MPNST) in neurofibromatosis type 1 (NF1): diagnostic findings on magnetic resonance images and mutation analysis of the NF1 gene. Anticancer Res 25(3A): 1699-1702

[43] Gesundheit B, Parkin P, Greenberg M, Baruchel S, Senger C, Kapelushnik J, Smith C, Klement GL (2010) The role of angiogenesis in the transformation of plexiform neurofibroma into malignant peripheral nerve sheath tumors in children with neurofibromatosis type 1. J Pediatr Hematol Oncol 32(7): 548-553

[44] Gregorian C, Nakashima J, Dry SM, Nghiemphu PL, Smith KB, Ao Y, Dang J, Lawson G, Mellinghoff IK, Mischel PS, Phelps M, Parada LF, Liu X, Sofroniew MV, Eilber FC, Wu H (2009) PTEN dosage is essential for neurofibroma development and malignant transformation. Proc Natl Acad Sci USA 106(46): 19479-19484

[45] Holtkamp N, Okuducu AF, Mucha J, Afanasieva A, Hartmann C, Atallah I, Estevez-Schwarz L, Mawrin C, Friedrich RE, Mautner VF, von Deimling A (2006) Mutation and expression of PDGFRA and KIT in malignant peripheral nerve sheath tumors, and its implications for imatinib sensitivity. Carcinogenesis 27: 664-671

[46] Holtkamp N, Atallah I, Okuducu AF, Mucha J, Hartmann C, Mautner VF, Friedrich RE, Mawrin C, von Deimling A (2007) MMP-13 and p53 in the progression of malignant peripheral nerve sheath tumors. Neoplasia 9(8): 671-677

[47] Holtkamp N, Malzer E, Zietsch J, Okuducu AF, Mucha J, Mawrin C, Mautner VF, Schildhaus HU, von Deimling A (2008) EGFR and erbB2 in malignant peripheral nerve sheath tumors and implications for targeted therapy. Neuro Oncol 10(6): 946-957

[48] Hruban RH, Shiu MH, Senie RT, Woodruff JM (1990) Malignant peripheral nerve sheath tumors of the buttock and lower extremity. A study of 43 cases. Cancer 66(6): 1253-1265

[49] Hummel TR, Jessen WJ, Miller SJ, Kluwe L, Mautner VF, Wallace MR, Lazaro C, Page GP, Worley PF, Aronow BJ, Schorry EK, Ratner N (2010) Gene expression analysis identifies potential biomarkers of neurofibromatosis type 1 including adrenomedullin. Clin Cancer Res 16(20): 5048-5057

[50] Ingham S, Huson SM, Moran A, Wylie J, Leahy M, Evans DGR (2011) Malignant peripheral nerve sheath tumours in NF1: improved survival in women and in recent years. Eur J Cancer 47(18): 2723-2728

[51] Johannessen CM, Johnson BW, Williams SM, Chan AW, Reczek EE, Lynch RC, Rioth MJ, McClatchey A, Ryeom S, Cichowski K (2008) TORC1 is essential for NF1-associated malignancies. Curr Biol 18(1): 56-62

[52] Johansson G, Mahller YY, Collins MH, Kim MO, Nobukuni T, Perentesis J, Cripe TP, Lane HA, Kozma SC, Thomas G, Ratner N (2008) Effective in vivo targeting of the mammalian target of rapamycin pathway in malignant peripheral nerve sheath tumors. Mol Cancer Ther 7(5): 1237-1245

[53] Joseph NM, Mosher JT, Buchstaller J, Snider P, McKeever PE, Lim M, Conway SJ, Parada LF, Zhu Y, Morrison SJ (2008) The loss of Nf1 transiently promotes self-renewal but not tumorigenesis by neural crest stem cells. Cancer Cell 13(2): 129-140

[54] Karabatsou K, Kiehl TR, Wilson DM, Hendler A, Guha A (2009) Potential role of 18fluorodeoxyglucose-positron emission tomography/computed tomography in differentiating benign neurofibroma from malignant peripheral nerve sheath tumor associated with neurofi-bromatosis 1. Neurosurgery 65(4 Suppl): A160-A170

[55] Kattan MW, Leung DH, Brennan MF (2002) Postoperative nomogram for 12-year sarcoma-specific death. J Clin Oncol 20(3): 791-796

[56] Katz D, Lazar A, Lev D (2009) Malignant peripheral nerve sheath tumour (MPNST): the clinical implications of cellular signalling pathways. Expert Rev Mol Med 11: e30

[57] Kawai A, Kondo T, Suehara Y, Kikuta K, Hirohashi S (2008) Global protein-expression analysis of bone and soft tissue sarcomas. Clin Orthop Relat Res 466(9): 2099-2106

[58] Keizman D, Issakov J, Meller I, Maimon N, Ish-Shalom M, Sher O, Merimsky O (2009) Expression and significance of EGFR in malignant peripheral nerve sheath tumor. J Neurooncol 94(3): 383-388

[59] Keng VW, Rahrmann EP, Watson AL, Tschidal BR, Moerte CL, Jessen WJ, Rizvi TA, Collins MH, Ratner N, Largaespada D (2012) PTEN and NF1 inactivation in Schwann cells produces a severe phenotype in the peripheral nervous system that promotes the development and malignant progression of peripheral nerve sheath tumors. Cancer Res 72(13): 3405-3413 (Epub 2012 June 14)

[60] King A, Listernick R, Charrow J, Piersall L, Gutmann DH (2003) Optic pathway gliomas in neurofibromatosis type 1: the effect of presenting symptoms on outcome. Am J Med Genet A 122(2): 95-99

[61] Korf BR (1999) Plexiform neurofibromas. Am J Med Genet 89(1): 31-37

[62] Kosemehmetoglu K, Vrana JA, Folpe AL (2009) TLE1 expression is not specific for synovial sarcoma: a whole section study of 163 soft tissue and bone neoplasms. Mod Pathol 22 (7): 872-878

[63] Kourea HP, Orlow I, Scheithauer BW, Cordon-Cardo C, Woodruff JM (1999) Deletions of the INK4A gene occur in malignant peripheral nerve sheath tumors but not in neurofibromas. Am J Pathol 155(6): 1855-1860

[64] Legius E, Dierick H, Wu R, Hall BK, Marynen P, Cassiman JJ, Glover TW (1994) TP53 mutations are frequent in malignant NF1 tumors. Genes Chromosomes Cancer 10(4): 250-255

[65] Leppig KA, Kaplan P, Viskochil D, Weaver M, Ortenberg J, Stephens K (1997) Familial neurofibromatosis 1 microdeletions: cosegregation with distinct facial phenotype and early onset of cutaneous neurofibromata. Am J Med Genet 73(2): 197-204

[66] Li CS, Huang GS, Wu HD, Chen WT, Shih LS, Lii JM, Duh SJ, Chen RC, Tu HY, Chan WP (2008) Differentiation of soft tissue benign and malignant peripheral nerve sheath tumors with magnetic resonance imaging. Clin Imaging 32(2): 121-127

[67] Longhi A, Errani C, Magagnoli G, Alberghini M, Gambarotti M, Mercuri M, Ferrari S (2010) High grade malignant peripheral nerve sheath tumors: outcome of 62 patients with localized disease and review of the literature. J Chemother 22 (6): 413-418

[68] Lopez G, Torres K, Liu J, Hernandez B, Young E, Belousov R, Bolshakov S, Lazar AJ, Slopis JM, McCutcheon IE, McConkey D, Lev D (2011) Autophagic survival in resistance to histone deacetylase inhibitors: novel strategies to treat malignant peripheral nerve sheath tumors. Cancer Res 71(1): 185-196

[69] Lothe RA, Karhu R, Mandahl N, Mertens F, Saeter G, Heim S, Borresen-Dale AL, Kallioniemi OP (1996) Gain of 17q24-qter detected by comparative genomic hybridization in malignant tumors from patients with von Recklinghausen's neurofibromatosis. Cancer Res 56(20): 4778-4781

[70] Lothe RA, Smith-Sorensen B, Hektoen M, Stenwig AE, Mandahl N, Saeter G, Mertens F (2001) Biallelic inactivation of TP53 rarely contributes to the development of malignant peripheral nerve sheath tumors. Genes Chromosomes Cancer 30(2): 202-206

[71] MacInnes AW, Amsterdam A, Whittaker CA, Hopkins N, Lees JA (2008) Loss of p53 synthesis in zebrafish tumors with ribosomal protein gene mutations. Proc Natl Acad Sci USA 105(30): 10408-10413

[72] Maki RG, D'Adamo DR, Keohan ML, Saulle M, Schuetze SM, Undevia SD, Livingston MB, Cooney MM, Hensley ML, Mita MM, Takimoto CH, Kraft AS, Elias AD, Brockstein B, Blachere NE, Edgar MA, Schwartz LH, Qin LX, Antonescu CR, Schwartz GK (2009) Phase II study of sorafenib in patients with metastatic or recurrent sarcomas. J Clin Oncol 27(19): 3133-3140

[73] Mantripragada KK, Spurlock G, Kluwe L, Chuzhanova N, Ferner RE, Frayling IM, Dumanski JP, Guha A, Mautner V, Upadhyaya M (2008) High-resolution DNA copy number profiling of malignant peripheral nerve sheath tumors using targeted microarray-based comparative genomic hybridization. Clin Cancer Res 14(4): 1015-1024

[74] Mantripragada KK, Diaz de Stahl T, Patridge C, Menzel U, Andersson R, Chuzhanova N, Kluwe L, Guha A, Mautner V, Dumanski JP, Upadhyaya M (2009) Genome-wide high-resolution analysis of DNA copy number alterations in NF1-associated malignant peripheral nerve sheath tumors using 32K BAC array. Genes Chromosomes Cancer 48(10): 897-907

[75] Mashour GA, Driever PH, Hartmann M, Drissel SN, Zhang T, Scharf B, Felderhoff-Muser U, Sakuma S, Friedrich RE, Martuza RL, Mautner VF, Kurtz A (2004) Circulating growth factor levels are associated with tumorigenesis in neurofibromatosis type 1. Clin Cancer Res 10(17): 5677-5683

[76] Matsumine A, Kusuzaki K, Nakamura T, Nakazora S, Niimi R, Matsubara T, Uchida K, Murata T, Kudawara I, Ueda T, Naka N, Araki N, Maeda M, Uchida A (2009) Differentiation between neurofibromas and malignant peripheral nerve sheath tumors in neurofibromatosis 1 evaluated by MRI. J Cancer Res Clin Oncol 135(7): 891-900

[77] Mawrin C, Kirches E, Boltze C, Dietzmann K, Roessner A, Schneider-Stock R (2002) Immuno-histochemical and molecular analysis of p53, RB, and PTEN in malignant peripheral nerve sheath tumors. Virchows Arch 440(6): 610-615

[78] Meadows AT, Baum E, Fossati-Bellani F, Green D, Jenkin RD, Marsden B, Nesbit M, Newton W, Oberlin O, Sallan SG et al (1985) Second malignant neoplasms in children: an update from the Late Effects Study Group. J Clin Oncol 3(4): 532-538

[79] Meany H, Dombi E, Reynolds J, Whatley M, Kurwa A, Tsokos M, Salzer W, Gillespie A, Baldwin A, Derdak J, Widemann B (2013) 18-Fluorodeoxyglucose-positron emission tomography (FDG-PET) Evaluation of nodular lesions in patients with neurofibromatosis type 1 and plexiform neurofibromas (PN) or malignant peripheral nerve sheath tumors (MPNST). Pediatr Blood Cancer 60: 59-64

[80] Mechtersheimer G, Otano-Joos M, Ohl S, Benner A, Lehnert T, Willeke F, Moller P, Otto HF, Lichter P, Joos S (1999) Analysis of chromosomal imbalances in sporadic and NF1-associated peripheral nerve sheath tumors by comparative genomic hybridization. Genes Chromosomes Cancer 25(4): 362-369

[81] Meis JM, Enzinger FM, Martz KL, Neal JA (1992) Malignant peripheral nerve sheath tumors (malignant schwannomas) in children. Am J Surg Pathol 16(7): 694-707

[82] Menon AG, Anderson KM, Riccardi VM, Chung RY, Whaley JM, Yandell DW, Farmer GE, Freiman RN, Lee JK, Li FP et al (1990) Chromosome 17p deletions and p53 gene mutations associated with the formation of malignant neurofibrosarcomas in von Recklinghausen neuro-fibromatosis. Proc Natl Acad Sci USA 87(14): 5435-5439

[83] Mertens F, Rydholm A, Bauer HF, Limon J, Nedoszytko B, Szadowska A, Willen H, Heim S, Mitelman F, Mandahl N (1995) Cytogenetic findings in malignant peripheral nerve sheath tumors. Int J Cancer 61(6): 793-798

[84] Mertens F, Dal Cin P, De Wever I, Fletcher CD, Mandahl N, Mitelman F, Rosai J, Rydholm A, Sciot R, Tallini G, van Den Berghe H, Vanni R, Willen H (2000) Cytogenetic characterization of peripheral nerve sheath tumours: a report of the CHAMP study group. J Pathol 190(1): 31-38

[85] Messiaen LM, Callens T, Mortier G, Beysen D, Vandenbroucke I, Van Roy N, Speleman F, Paepe AD (2000) Exhaustive mutation analysis of the NF1 gene allows identification of 95% of mutations and reveals a high frequency

of unusual splicing defects. Hum Mutat 15(6): 541-555

[86] Miller SJ, Rangwala F, Williams J, Ackerman P, Kong S, Jegga AG, Kaiser S, Aronow BJ, Frahm S, Kluwe L, Mautner V, Upadhyaya M, Muir D, Wallace M, Hagen J, Quelle DE, Watson MA, Perry A, Gutmann DH, Ratner N (2006) Large-scale molecular comparison of human schwann cells to malignant peripheral nerve sheath tumor cell lines and tissues. Cancer Res 66(5): 2584-2591

[87] Miller SJ, Jessen WJ, Mehta T, Hardiman A, Sites E, Kaiser S, Jegga AG, Li H, Upadhyaya M, Giovannini M, Muir D, Wallace MR, Lopez E, Serra E, Nielsen GP, Lazaro C, Stemmer-Rachamimov A, Page G, Aronow BJ, Ratner N (2009) Integrative genomic analyses of neurofibromatosis tumours identify SOX9 as a biomarker and survival gene. EMBO Mol Med 1(4): 236-248

[88] Miller SJ, Lan ZD, Hardiman A, Wu J, Kordich JJ, Patmore DM, Hegde RS, Cripe TP, Cancelas JA, Collins MH, Ratner N (2010) Inhibition of Eyes Absent Homolog 4 expression induces malignant peripheral nerve sheath tumor necrosis. Oncogene 29(3): 368-379

[89] Moretti VM, Crawford EA, Staddon AP, Lackman RD, Ogilvie CM (2011) Early outcomes for malignant peripheral nerve sheath tumor treated with chemotherapy. Am J Clin Oncol 34(4): 417-421

[90] Nakayama R, Nemoto T, Takahashi H, Ohta T, Kawai A, Seki K, Yoshida T, Toyama Y, Ichikawa H, Hasegawa T (2007) Gene expression analysis of soft tissue sarcomas: characterization and reclassification of malignant fibrous histiocytoma. Mod Pathol 20(7): 749-759

[91] Nielsen GP, Stemmer-Rachamimov AO, Ino Y, Moller MB, Rosenberg AE, Louis DN (1999) Malignant transformation of neurofibromas in neurofibromatosis 1 is associated with CDKN2A/p16 inactivation. Am J Pathol 155(6): 1879-1884

[92] Parham DM, Webber BL, Jenkins JJ 3rd, Cantor AB, Maurer HM (1995) Nonrhabdomyosar-comatous soft tissue sarcomas of childhood: formulation of a simplified system for grading. Mod Pathol 8(7): 705-710

[93] Pasmant E, Masliah-Planchon J, Levy P, Laurendeau I, Ortonne N, Parfait B, Valeyrie-Allanore L, Leroy K, Wolkenstein P, Vidaud M, Vidaud D, Bieche I (2011a) Identification of genes potentially involved in the increased risk of malignancy in NF1-microdeleted patients. Mol Med 17(1-2): 79-87

[94] Pasmant E, Sabbagh A, Masliah-Planchon J, Ortonne N, Laurendeau I, Melin L, Ferkal S, Hernandez L, Leroy K, Valeyrie-Allanore L, Parfait B, Vidaud D, Bieche I, Lantieri L, Wolkenstein P, Vidaud M (2011b) Role of noncoding RNA ANRIL in genesis of plexiform neurofibromas in neurofibromatosis type 1. J Natl Cancer Inst 103(22): 1713-1722

[95] Pasmant E, Vidaud D, Harrison M, Upadhyaya M (2011c) Different sized somatic NF1 locus rearrangements in neurofibromatosis 1-associated malignant peripheral nerve sheath tumors. J Neurooncol 102(3): 341-346

[96] Patel RM, Folpe AL (2009) Immunohistochemistry for human telomerase reverse transcriptase catalytic subunit (hTERT): a study of 143 benign and malignant soft tissue and bone tumours. Pathology 41(6): 527-532

[97] Patel AV, Eaves D, Jessen WJ, Rizvi TA, Ecsedy JA, Qian MG, Aronow BJ, Perentesis JP, Serra E, Cripe TP, Miller SJ, Ratner N (2012) Ras-driven transcriptome analysis identifies aurora kinase A as a potential malignant peripheral nerve sheath tumor therapeutic target. Clin Cancer Res 18(18): 5020-5030

[98] Perrone F, Da Riva L, Orsenigo M, Losa M, Jocolle G, Millefanti C, Pastore E, Gronchi A, Pierotti MA, Pilotti S (2009) PDGFRA, PDGFRB, EGFR, and downstream signaling activation in malignant peripheral nerve sheath tumor. Neuro Oncol 11(6): 725-736

[99] Perry A, Kunz SN, Fuller CE, Banerjee R, Marley EF, Liapis H, Watson MA, Gutmann DH (2002) Differential NF1, p16, and EGFR patterns by interphase cytogenetics (FISH) in malignant peripheral nerve sheath tumor (MPNST) and morphologically similar spindle cell neoplasms. J Neuropathol Exp Neurol 61(8): 702-709

[100] Pisters PW, Leung DH, Woodruff J, Shi W, Brennan MF (1996) Analysis of prognostic factors in 1,041 patients with localized soft tissue sarcomas of the extremities. J Clin Oncol 14(5): 1679-1689

[101] Plaat BE, Molenaar WM, Mastik MF, Hoekstra HJ, te Meerman GJ, van den Berg E (1999) Computer-assisted cytogenetic analysis of 51 malignant peripheral-nerve-sheath tumors: sporadic vs neurofibromatosis-type-1-associated malignant schwannomas. Int J Cancer 83(2): 171-178

[102] Pytel P, Karrison T, Can G, Tonsgard JH, Krausz T, Montag AG (2010) Neoplasms with schwannian differentiation express transcription factors known to regulate normal schwann cell development. Int J Surg Pathol 18(6): 449-457. doi: 1066896909351698 [pii]

[103] Raney B, Schnaufer L, Ziegler M, Chatten J, Littman P, Jarrett P (1987) Treatment of children with neurogenic sarcoma. Experience at the Children's Hospital of Philadelphia, 1958-1984. Cancer 59(1): 1-5

[104] Rasmussen SA, Yang Q, Friedman JM (2001) Mortality in neurofibromatosis 1: an analysis using U.S. death certificates. Am J Hum Genet 68(5): 1110-1118

[105] Riddle ND, Gorden L, Rojiani MV, Hakam A, Rojiani AM (2010) CD44 and p53 immunoexpression patterns in NF1 neoplasms-indicators of malignancy and infiltration. Int J Clin Exp Pathol 3(5): 515-521

[106] Rodriguez FJ, Folpe AL, Giannini C, Perry A (2012) Pathology of peripheral nerve sheath tumors: diagnostic overview and update on selected diagnostic problems. Acta Neuropathol 123(3): 295-319

[107] Scaife CL, Pisters PW (2003) Combined-modality treatment of localized soft tissue sarcomas of the extremities. Surg Oncol Clin N Am 12(2): 355-368

[108] Schittenhelm J, Thiericke J, Nagel C, Meyermann R, Beschorner R (2010) WT1 expression in normal and neoplastic cranial and peripheral nerves is independent of grade of malignancy. Cancer Biomark 7(2): 73-77

[109] Schmidt H, Wurl P, Taubert H, Meye A, Bache M, Holzhausen HJ, Hinze R (1999) Genomic imbalances of 7p and 17q in malignant peripheral nerve sheath tumors are clinically relevant. Genes Chromosomes Cancer 25(3): 205-211

[110] Schmidt H, Taubert H, Meye A, Wurl P, Bache M, Bartel F, Holzhausen HJ, Hinze R (2000) Gains in chromosomes 7, 8q, 15q and 17q are characteristic changes in malignant but not in benign peripheral nerve sheath tumors from patients with Recklinghausen's disease. Cancer Lett 155(2): 181-190

[111] Schmidt H, Taubert H, Wurl P, Bache M, Bartel F, Holzhausen HJ, Hinze R (2001) Cytogenetic characterization of six malignant peripheral nerve sheath tumors: comparison of karyotyping and comparative genomic hybridization.

Cancer Genet Cytogenet 128(1): 14–23
[112] Schuetze S, Wathen S, Choy E, Samuels B, Ganjoo K, Staddon A, von Mehren M, Chow W, Trent J, Baker L (2010) Results of a Sarcoma Alliance for Research through Collaboration (SARC) phase II trial of dasatinib in previously treated, high-grade, advanced sarcoma. ASCO J Clin Oncol 28: 15s (suppl; abstr 10009)
[113] Silvestre DC, Gil GA, Tomasini N, Bussolino DF, Caputto BL (2010) Growth of peripheral and central nervous system tumors is supported by cytoplasmic c-Fos in humans and mice. PLoS One 5(3): e9544
[114] Slomiany MG, Dai L, Bomar PA, Knackstedt TJ, Kranc DA, Tolliver L, Maria BL, Toole BP (2009) Abrogating drug resistance in malignant peripheral nerve sheath tumors by disrupting hyaluronan-CD44 interactions with small hyaluronan oligosaccharides. Cancer Res 69(12): 4992–4998
[115] Sordillo PP, Helson L, Hajdu SI, Magill GB, Kosloff C, Golbey RB, Beattie EJ (1981) Malignant schwannoma-clinical characteristics, survival, and response to therapy. Cancer 47(10): 2503–2509
[116] Stonecypher MS, Byer SJ, Grizzle WE, Carroll SL (2005) Activation of the neuregulin-1/ErbB signaling pathway promotes the proliferation of neoplastic Schwann cells in human malignant peripheral nerve sheath tumors. Oncogene 24(36): 5589–5605
[117] Storlazzi CT, Brekke HR, Mandahl N, Brosjo O, Smeland S, Lothe RA, Mertens F (2006) Identification of a novel amplicon at distal 17q containing the BIRC5/SURVIVIN gene in malignant peripheral nerve sheath tumours. J Pathol 209(4): 492–500
[118] Stucky CC, Johnson KN, Gray RJ, Pockaj BA, Ocal IT, Rose PS, Wasif N (2012) Malignant peripheral nerve sheath tumors (MPNST): the Mayo Clinic experience. Ann Surg Oncol 19(3): 878–885
[119] Su W, Gutmann DH, Perry A, Abounader R, Laterra J, Sherman LS (2004) CD44-independent hepatocyte growth factor/c-Met autocrine loop promotes malignant peripheral nerve sheath tumor cell invasion in vitro. Glia 45(3): 297–306
[120] Subramanian S, Thayanithy V, West RB, Lee CH, Beck AH, Zhu S, Downs-Kelly E, Montgomery K, Goldblum JR, Hogendoorn PC, Corless CL, Oliveira AM, Dry SM, Nielsen TO, Rubin BP, Fletcher JA, Fletcher CD, van de Rijn M (2010) Genome-wide transcriptome analyses reveal p53 inactivation mediated loss of miR-34a expression in malignant peripheral nerve sheath tumours. J Pathol 220(1): 58–70
[121] Tabone-Eglinger S, Bahleda R, Cote JF, Terrier P, Vidaud D, Cayre A, Beauchet A, Theou-Anton N, Terrier-Lacombe MJ, Lemoine A, Penault-Llorca F, Le Cesne A, Emile JF (2008) Frequent EGFR Positivity and Overexpression in High-Grade Areas of Human MPNSTs. Sarcoma 2008: 849156
[122] Torres KE, Zhu QS, Bill K, Lopez G, Ghadimi MP, Xie X, Young ED, Liu J, Nguyen T, Bolshakov S, Belousov R, Wang S, Lahat G, Hernandez B, Lazar AJ, Lev D (2011) Activated MET is a molecular prognosticator and potential therapeutic target for malignant peripheral nerve sheath tumors. Clin Cancer Res 17(12): 3943–3955
[123] Trojani M, Contesso G, Coindre JM, Rouesse J, Bui NB, de Mascarel A, Goussot JF, David M, Bonichon F, Lagarde C (1984) Soft-tissue sarcomas of adults; study of pathological prognostic variables and definition of a histopathological grading system. Int J Cancer 33(1): 37–42
[124] Tucker T, Wolkenstein P, Revuz J, Zeller J, Friedman JM (2005) Association between benign and malignant peripheral nerve sheath tumors in NF1. Neurology 65(2): 205–211
[125] Tucker T, Friedman JM, Friedrich RE, Wenzel R, Funsterer C, Mautner VF (2009) Longitudinal study of neurofibromatosis 1 associated plexiform neurofibromas. J Med Genet 46(2): 81–85
[126] Upadhyaya M, Kluwe L, Spurlock G, Monem B, Majounie E, Mantripragada K, Ruggieri M, Chuzhanova N, Evans DG, Ferner R, Thomas N, Guha A, Mautner V (2008) Germline and somatic NF1 gene mutation spectrum in NF1-associated malignant peripheral nerve sheath tumors (MPNSTs). Hum Mutat 29(1): 74–82
[127] Upadhyaya M, Spurlock G, Thomas L, Thomas NS, Richards M, Mautner VF, Cooper DN, Guha A, Yan J (2012) Microarray-based copy number analysis of neurofibromatosis type-1 (NF1)-associated malignant peripheral nerve sheath tumors reveals a role for Rho-GTPase pathway genes in NF1 tumorigenesis. Hum Mutat 33(4): 763–776
[128] Valdes OS, Maurer HM (1970) Combination therapy with vincristine sulfate (NSC-67574) and cyclophosphamide (NSC-26271) for generalized malignant schwannoma-a case report. Cancer Chemother Rep 54(1): 65–68
[129] Verdijk RM, den Bakker MA, Dubbink HJ, Hop WC, Dinjens WN, Kros JM (2010) TP53 mutation analysis of malignant peripheral nerve sheath tumors. J Neuropathol Exp Neurol 69(1): 16–26
[130] Vogel KS, Klesse LJ, Velasco-Miguel S, Meyers K, Rushing EJ, Parada LF (1999) Mouse tumor model for neurofibromatosis type 1. Science 286(5447): 2176–2179
[131] Wallace MR, Rasmussen SA, Lim IT, Gray BA, Zori RT, Muir D (2000) Culture of cytogeneti-cally abnormal schwann cells from benign and malignant NF1 tumors. Genes Chromosomes Cancer 27(2): 117–123
[132] Warbey VS, Ferner RE, Dunn JT, Calonje E, O'Doherty MJ (2009) [18F]FDG PET/CT in the diagnosis of malignant peripheral nerve sheath tumours in neurofibromatosis type-1. Eur J Nucl Med Mol Imaging 36(5): 751–757
[133] Wasa J, Nishida Y, Tsukushi S, Shido Y, Sugiura H, Nakashima H, Ishiguro N (2010) MRI features in the differentiation of malignant peripheral nerve sheath tumors and neurofibromas. Am J Roentgenol 194(6): 1568–1574
[134] Watson MA, Perry A, Tihan T, Prayson RA, Guha A, Bridge J, Ferner R, Gutmann DH (2004) Gene expression profiling reveals unique molecular subtypes of Neurofibromatosis Type I-associated and sporadic malignant peripheral nerve sheath tumors. Brain Pathol 14(3): 297–303
[135] Widemann BC (2009) Current status of sporadic and neurofibromatosis type 1-associated malignant peripheral nerve sheath tumors. Curr Oncol Rep 11(4): 322–328
[136] Wimmer K, Yao S, Claes K, Kehrer-Sawatzki H, Tinschert S, De Raedt T, Legius E, Callens T, Beiglbock H, Maertens O, Messiaen L (2006) Spectrum of single- and multiexon NF1 copy number changes in a cohort of 1,100 unselected NF1 patients. Genes Chromosomes Cancer 45(3): 265–276
[137] Wong WW, Hirose T, Scheithauer BW, Schild SE, Gunderson LL (1998) Malignant peripheral nerve sheath tumor: analysis of treatment outcome. Int J Radiat Oncol Biol Phys 42(2): 351–360
[138] Yan X, Takahara M, Dugu L, Xie L, Gondo C, Endo M, Oda Y, Nakahara T, Uchi H, Takeuchi S, Tu Y, Moroi Y, Furue M

(2010) Expression of cathepsin K in neurofibromatosis 1-associated cutaneous malignant peripheral nerve sheath tumors and neurofibromas. J Dermatol Sci 58(3): 227-229

[139] Yang JC, Chang AE, Baker AR, Sindelar WF, Danforth DN, Topalian SL, DeLaney T, Glatstein E, Steinberg SM, Merino MJ, Rosenberg SA (1998) Randomized prospective study of the benefit of adjuvant radiation therapy in the treatment of soft tissue sarcomas of the extremity. J Clin Oncol 16(1): 197-203

[140] Yang J, Ylipaa A, Sun Y, Zheng H, Chen K, Nykter M, Trent J, Ratner N, Lev DC, Zhang W (2011) Genomic and molecular characterization of malignant peripheral nerve sheath tumor identifies the IGF1R pathway as a primary target for treatment. Clin Cancer Res 17(24): 7563-7573

[141] Yu J, Deshmukh H, Payton JE, Dunham C, Scheithauer BW, Tihan T, Prayson RA, Guha A, Bridge JA, Ferner RE, Lindberg GM, Gutmann RJ, Emnett RJ, Salavaggione L, Gutmann DH, Nagarajan R, Watson MA, Perry A (2011) Array-based comparative genomic hybridization-identifies CDK4 and FOXM1 alterations as independent predictors of survival in malignant peripheral nerve sheath tumor. Clin Cancer Res 17(7): 1924-1934

[142] Zhou H, Coffin CM, Perkins SL, Tripp SR, Liew M, Viskochil DH (2003) Malignant peripheral nerve sheath tumor: a comparison of grade, immunophenotype, and cell cycle/growth activation marker expression in sporadic and neurofibromatosis 1-related lesions. Am J Surg Pathol 27(10): 1337-1345

[143] Zietsch J, Ziegenhagen N, Heppner FL, Reuss D, von Deimling A, Holtkamp N (2010) The 4q12 amplicon in malignant peripheral nerve sheath tumors: consequences on gene expression and implications for sunitinib treatment. PLoS One 5(7): e11858

[144] Zou C, Smith KD, Liu J, Lahat G, Myers S, Wang WL, Zhang W, McCutcheon IE, Slopis JM, Lazar AJ, Pollock RE, Lev D (2009a) Clinical, pathological, and molecular variables predictive of malignant peripheral nerve sheath tumor outcome. Ann Surg 249(6): 1014-1022

[145] Zou CY, Smith KD, Zhu QS, Liu J, McCutcheon IE, Slopis JM, Meric-Bernstam F, Peng Z, Bornmann WG, Mills GB, Lazar AJ, Pollock RE, Lev D (2009b) Dual targeting of AKT and mammalian target of rapamycin: a potential therapeutic approach for malignant peripheral nerve sheath tumor. Mol Cancer Ther 8(5): 1157-1168

第30章 血液恶性肿瘤中的 NF1 突变
NF1 Mutations in Hematologic Cancers

Tiffany Chang and Kevin Shannon

30.1 引言

1958年，一篇描述1名有咖啡牛奶斑和罕见骨髓增生性肿瘤（myeloproliferative neoplasm，MPN）幼儿的文章提出了1型神经纤维瘤病（NF1）与血液肿瘤之间可能存在潜在的相互作用（Royer et al. 1958）。而后来的临床和流行病学研究证实，这种侵袭性MPN即现在的幼年型粒-单核细胞白血病（juvenile myelomonocytic leukemia，JMML），在NF1儿童中的发病率增加了200～500倍（Bader and Miller 1978; Stiller et al. 1994），所以NF1具有显性遗传的癌症易感性。此外，人们还发现，NF1基因胚系突变失活的患者和NF1基因遗传的患者都有可能患上癌症（Marchuk et al. 1991; Viskochil et al. 1990; Wallace et al. 1990）。NF1基因产物神经纤维瘤蛋白为Ras编码的一种GTPase激活蛋白（GTPase-activating protein，GAP）（Basu et al. 1992; DeClue et al. 1991; Xu et al. 1990a, b），这表明NF1是一种肿瘤抑制基因（tumor suppressor gene，TSG）。事实上，对JMML骨髓的遗传分析表明，在多个NF1患儿中，NF1基因座上都出现了常染色体杂合缺失（loss of constitutional heterozygosity，LOH），在家族病例中，这无一例外地涉及正常亲代等位基因的缺失（Miles et al. 1996; Shannon et al. 1994）。随后的一项研究表明，JMML细胞中NF1基因的双等位基因失活，从遗传学角度证明了NF1基因是一种"典型的"隐性TSG，在癌细胞中会发生体细胞功能缺失（Side et al. 1997）。重要的是，对NF1患儿的白血病细胞进行的生化分析表明，神经纤维瘤蛋白特异性GAP活性降低，Ras-GTP水平升高，Raf/MEK/ERK激酶效应器途径异常激活（Bollag et al. 1996）。总之，这些数据确定了NF1是造血细胞中的TSG，并表明Raf/MEK/ERK信号转导异常可导致白血病的发生。如下所述，最近在JMML小鼠模型中进行的临床前研究有力地支持了这一假设，并为在这种侵袭性癌症中实施MEK抑制剂的临床试验提供了依据。

将异常Ras信号转导定义为NF1与JMML的分子机制，也为白血病的发生提供了新的见解。特别是，目前已明确，JMML从本质上是一种Ras过度激活的疾病，在超过90%的病例中发现了NRAS、KRAS、PTPN11和CBL基因的胚系或体细胞突变（Lauchle et al. 2006; Loh 2011）。所有患

T. Chang
Department of Pediatrics, University of California, San Francisco, CA 94158, USA

K. Shannon (*)
Department of Pediatrics, University of California, San Francisco, CA 94158, USA

Comprehensive Cancer Center, University of California, San Francisco, CA 94158, USA
e-mail: shannonk@peds.ucsf.edu

者几乎仅出现一种基因突变,这与 JMML 中突变基因所编码的蛋白成分是一种保守的生化网络的观点相一致,该网络调节造血干细胞(hematopoietic stem cells,HSC)及其子代细胞的增殖、分化和存活。

NF1 与 JMML 的关联也为发育与癌症之间的联系提供了清晰的证据之一。如第 32 章所述,NF1 是引发一系列具有表型重叠特征和胚系突变的遗传性疾病的关键基因,胚系突变会导致 Ras/Raf/MEK/ERK 信号转导失调。其他已知的 JMML 相关基因也可能引发努南综合征谱系中的发育性疾病 (Cirstea et al. 2010;Niemeyer et al. 2010;Schubbert et al. 2006;Tartaglia et al. 2001)。然而,有趣的是,这些胚系 PTPN11、NRAS 和 KRAS 基因突变编码的蛋白质的生化功能增强通常比在 JMML 中发现的相应体细胞突变要弱 (Cirstea et al. 2010;Keilhack et al. 2005;Kratz et al. 2005;Schubbert et al. 2006)。事实上,只有 NF1 的幼儿的血液肿瘤风险显著增加,这一观察尤为引人注目,因为造血是一个高度动态的过程,每天需要大量未成熟细胞不断增殖和成熟,以替代数十亿的白细胞、红细胞和血小板。这揭示了一个有趣的"种子与土壤"相互作用现象,体细胞 NF1 失活仅在特定发育环境或特殊条件下才可能引发白血病。

体细胞突变是人类细胞恶性转化的关键事件。NF1 患者遗传一个等位基因的胚系突变后,常会发生"二次打击",这通常通过 LOH 或体细胞突变使剩余正常等位基因失活,从而赋予细胞生长优势,导致肿瘤的发生。由于 NF1 基因体积庞大且在许多组织中的表达水平较低,鉴定 NF1 患者肿瘤中的体细胞"二次打击"突变一直是一项挑战。然而,体细胞突变的分类对于理解肿瘤发生的复杂分子机制至关重要。近年来的癌症基因组测序研究显示,NF1 也与无神经纤维瘤病患者所发生的散发性恶性肿瘤的发病机制相关,这与神经纤维瘤蛋白在细胞功能中的核心作用相一致(Cancer Genome Atlas Network 2008)。

最近,一些综述文章探讨了遗传易感性与 Ras 信号异常及白血病之间的相互关系,以及 JMML 的生物学特征和治疗策略(Lauchle et al. 2006;Loh 2011;Schubbert et al. 2007)。在本文中,我们将重点讨论 NF1 基因突变在血液恶性肿瘤中的作用,强调该领域的最新进展、治疗潜力、亟待解决的问题及未来研究方向。

30.2　NF1 中的血液恶性肿瘤

JMML 是一种侵袭性的髓系恶性肿瘤,主要发生在幼儿中,年发病率为 1.2/100 万,诊断时的中位年龄为 2 岁(Lauchle et al. 2006;Loh 2011)。因其骨髓中原始细胞比例较低、血液中存在未成熟单核细胞,以及由于白血病细胞浸润引起的显著脾肿大,早期报道将 JMML 称为"幼年型慢性粒细胞白血病"(juvenile chronic myeloid leukemia,JCML)。随着时间的推移,当慢性髓系白血病在所有年龄组被重新定义为由 BCR-ABL 融合基因驱动的独特分子和临床实体时,这一名称也随之被重新考虑(Sawyers 1999)。在成人血液肿瘤中,JMML 与慢性粒细胞白血病(chronic myelomonocytic leukemia,CMML)的增殖亚型最为相似,因此这两种疾病现在被世界卫生组织归类为"重叠综合征",因其同时展现了 MPN 和骨髓增生异常综合征(myelodysplastic syndrome,MDS)的临床和病理特征。研究表明,JMML 和 CMML 中的 NRAS 和 CBL 基因的频繁突变,突显了这两种疾病之间的共同分子基础(Dunbar et al. 2008;Kalra et al. 1994;Loh et al. 2009;Miyauchi et al. 1994;Onida et al. 2002;Sanada et al. 2009)。

1991 年,Emanuel 及其同事报道,在含有低浓度生长因子粒细胞-巨噬细胞集落刺激因子(granulocyte-macrophage colony-stimulating factor,GM-CSF)的甲基纤维素培养基中,JMML 细胞能够选择性地形成异常数量的集落和单位粒细胞-巨噬细胞(colony-forming-unit granulocyte-macrophage,CFU-GM)。CFU-GM 的高敏感性使其依然是用于建立 JMML 诊断时使用的一种方法,然而,由于这一现象可能与慢性感染、遗传性或获得性免疫缺陷综合征以及其他血液系统恶性肿瘤重叠,导致诊断上存在挑战。分子检测在 JMML 的诊断中同样至关重要，检测到 NF1、NRAS、KRAS、PTPN11 或 CBL 基因的突变可以有力地支持临床上已有提示性结果的患者诊断为 JMML（Loh 2011）。Kotecha 等（2008）的研究显示，JMML、CMML 和急性髓系白血病（acute myeloid leukemia，AML）M4 或 M5 亚型患者的骨髓细胞中，$CD33^+$ $CD14^+$ $CD38^{lo}$ 细胞亚群对 GM-CSF 的反应呈现独特的 STAT5 过度磷酸化模式。这种生化特征在包括 NF1 在内的多种基因突变导致的 JMML 患者中也得到了确认。

虽然 NF1 家族史有助于确诊 JMML，但许多病例是由新突变引起的，且 NF1 的主要表型特征在幼儿中可能并不明显或缺失。此外，努南综合征谱系中的发育障碍可能表现出一些 NF1 的特征（Schubbert et al. 2007）。展示胚系突变（包括特定的氨基酸替代）对于临床管理具有重要意义，因为在 PTPN11 基因突变的患者中，MPN 很可能会自发消退，而 KRAS 和 CBL 基因突变患者也观察到了类似现象（Loh 2011；Niemeyer et al. 2010；Schubbert et al. 2006）。这些患者在出生后几周内通常会出现类似 JMML 的髓系疾病，但仅接受积极的支持性治疗，而不进行细胞毒性化学治疗或造血干细胞移植（hematopoietic stem cell transplantation，HSCT）。相比之下，被诊断为 JMML 的 NF1 儿童往往年龄较大，目前尚未发现任何正常 NF1 等位基因缺失的病例能够不经治疗而自行痊愈。

简单的数学计算显示，NF1 和 JMML 之间的相互作用相当复杂，因为 JMML 的年发病率（约为 1/100 万）远低于 NF1 的发病率（1/3 000）。此外，NF1 基因突变只占 JMML 病例的 10%～15%。基于这些数据，JMML 在 NF1 患者中的个体风险非常低，约为 1/2 500。这与 RB1 或 WT1 等 TSG 有很大不同，在这些胚系突变的患者中，视网膜母细胞瘤或 Wilms 肿瘤的发病率高达 80% 或更高，并提出了有哪些其他因素可能导致 JMML 易感性的问题。约 75% 的 JMML 患者为男孩（Loh 2011）。在 NF1 患者中，男性比例始终较高（Shannon et al. 1992），这在其他发育障碍中也有所观察到。例如，Niemeyer 等（2010）最近报告了一个引人注目的、具有 CBL 胚系突变的多代家系，只有男性成员罹患 JMML。除了男性性别外，目前尚无证据支持存在与 NF1 共同参与白血病发生的修饰突变，尤其没有关于 NF1 谱系中有多个儿童患上 JMML 的报道。其他可能解释 NF1 中 JMML 风险相对较低的模型包括：① 在正常 NF1 等位基因发生体细胞缺失后，和（或）只有极少数发育受限的易感靶细胞可以启动 JMML。② 除 NF1 失活外，完全白血病转化可能还需要联合突变。约 30% 的 JMML 病例存在体细胞 7 号染色体缺失（7 号单体），这与第二种可能性相符（Loh 2011）。最近，全基因组和外显子组测序技术的广泛应用，使研究人员在未来几年内可以更深入地探讨这一问题。

如前所述，对 NF1 患者的 JMML 标本进行分子分析时，常常发现 LOH。在家族病例中，这种缺失总是涉及从未受影响的父母遗传的 NF1 等位基因（Miles et al. 1996；Shannon et al. 1994；Side et al. 1997）。早期研究并未发现某些病例存在 NF1 双等位基因失活现象（Miles et al. 1996；Shannon et al. 1994；Side et al. 1997）。然而，最近 Steinemann 等（2010）对 10 例患者进行的研究中，采用先进的测序和定位小缺失技术，发现 NF1 突变中有 5 例正常等位基因缺失、3 例复合杂合突变和 2 例间隙杂合缺失。这些数据表明，NF1 双等位基因失活是 NF1 患者 JMML 的一个显著特征，同时也提出了一种可能性，即偶尔出现的无 NF1 改变的病例可能因其他发育障碍而被误诊为 NF1。值得注意的是，影响 NF1 位点及其位于 17q 染色体上一大段侧翼序列的单亲二体（uniparental disomy，UPD）被认为是导致 JMML 中正常 NF1 等位基因体细胞缺失的原因（Flotho et al. 2007；Stephens et al. 2006）。有趣的是，CBL 突变的 CMML 和 JMML 患者也表现出类似的遗传机制（Dunbar et al. 2008；Loh et al. 2009；Sanada et al. 2009）。

目前，JMML 的治疗效果并不理想。针对 AML 的细胞毒性化学治疗方案大多效果欠佳，而造血干细胞移植（hematopoietic stem cell transplantation，HSCT）被认为是标准治疗方案（Loh 2011）。尽管 HSCT 可治愈约 50% 的患者，但对年幼儿童来说，后期不良反应的风险仍然较高。那些在造血干细胞移植后病情未缓解或复发的患者预后较差,绝大多数最终死于加速型 JMML 或演变为 AML,且在转变为 AML 的病例中常可检测到单体 7(Kaneko et al. 1989)。鉴于我们目前对 JMML 发病机制的了解,利用小分子抑制剂靶向 Ras 激活的激酶效应途径成为一种颇具吸引力的治疗选择。

临床观察显示,NF1 的儿童和成人在接受不同原发性癌症的基因毒性治疗后,罹患 MDS 和 AML 的风险增加。Maris 及其同事(Maris et al. 1997)报道了 5 名儿童患者,他们在接受原发性实体瘤的多模式积极治疗后,转化为 MDS 或 AML。有趣的是,这些患者的骨髓均显示为单体 7 型,同时保留了正常的 NF1 等位基因。此外,2 名 NF1 的成人在接受 AML 治疗后,也迅速发展为 MDS(Papageorgio et al. 1999)。尽管尚无定论,但这些在 NF1 患者中观察到的令人振奋的结果与本章后面提到的小鼠研究结果相一致,这些研究结果表明,Nf1 杂合性缺失与辐射密切相关,从而诱发 MDS 及其他常见的治疗相关的人类癌症。

30.3 血液肿瘤中的 NF1 体细胞突变

最近的研究报告指出,肺腺癌、乳腺癌、卵巢浆液性癌(ovarian serous carcinoma, OSC)、神经母细胞瘤以及白血病中均发现了体细胞 NF1 突变(Ding et al. 2008; Haferlach et al. 2010; Holzel et al. 2010; Laycock-van Spyk et al. 2011; Parsons et al. 2008; Sangha et al. 2008)。这些肿瘤中 NF1 突变的发生相对频繁,可能会具有重要的预后和诊断意义。例如,癌症基因组图谱网络(Cancer Genome Atlas Network)发现新生多形性胶质母细胞瘤(glioblastoma multiforme, GBM)中 NF1 基因突变的发生率较高,在分析的 206 例患者样本中,至少有 23%(47/206)携带体细胞 NF1 基因突变或缺失(Cancer Genome Atlas Network 2008; Parsons et al. 2008)。同样,在 22% 的原发性 OSC(9/41)中检测到体细胞 NF1 突变,其中包括 6 例显示出双等位基因失活特征的癌症(Sangha et al. 2008)。值得注意的是所有 9 个 OSC 样本均含有 TP53 突变,这与对 NF1 患者中恶性周围神经鞘膜瘤的研究结果一致(Menon et al. 1990)。

大多数 NF1 突变为基因内突变,分布于整个基因,通常导致剪接突变,从而导致神经纤维瘤蛋白的编码发生截断和失活。另外一种遗传异常是影响整个 NF1 位点的微缺失,这可能导致更为复杂的发育表型,并增加了罹患 JMML 和进一步发展为 AML 的风险。这些机制包括点突变、缺失以及体细胞重组导致 UPD 发生(Ding et al. 2008; Haferlach et al. 2010; Holzel et al. 2010; Laycock-van Spyk et al. 2011; Parsons et al. 2008; Sangha et al. 2008; Side et al. 1998)。先前的一项研究显示,缺乏 NF1 临床证据的 JMML 患者中会出现 NF1 双等位基因失活,尽管这些患者的发病年龄较早,但并不能排除胚系突变的可能性(Side et al. 1998)。

或许关于血液恶性肿瘤中 NF1 体细胞突变的最佳数据来源于 Parkin 等(2010)的一项研究。该研究发现,在成年 AML 患者中存在一个亚群,其 NF1 功能失活,导致 Ras 信号转导增强,并对 mTOR 抑制剂表现出敏感性。研究人员通过高密度 SNP 微阵列分析了 95 名成年 AML 患者的纯化幼稚细胞及配对的口腔 DNA 样本,发现在 17q 染色体上存在复发性、体细胞获得性的微缺失,其中约 0.9 Mb 的缺失区域包括 NF1 位点。在该队列的 95 例白血病样本中,有 11 例(12%)显示 NF1 的体细胞拷贝数改变,其中 10 例为杂合缺失,1 例为拷贝数扩增。研究者发现,在 10 名杂合缺失患者中,有 3 名 AML 患者的幼稚细胞中 NF1 表达水平降低,而在 3 个 NF1 拷贝数正常的样本中也观察到了 NF1 表达的缺失。这表明,在 NF1 表达缺失的 AML 病例中,Ras-GTP 的水平显著增加。此外,NF1 缺失的 AML $CD34^+/CD38^-$ 细胞对雷帕霉素治疗表现出高度敏感,提示 mTOR 可能是该亚组成年 AML 患者的潜在治疗靶点,同时也可能揭示 NF1 在成人 AML 中的致病作用。与 NF1 体细胞突变在成人髓系恶性肿瘤中的作用相一致,Kolquist 等(2011)通过比较基因组杂交微阵列分析了 35 例成人 MDS 患者骨髓,发现其中 3 例患者存在涉及 17q11.2 带上 NF1 位点的复发性隐性变化或缺失。

对儿童患者的研究进一步揭示了 NF1 体细胞突变在血液恶性肿瘤中的作用。最近的一项报告描述了与白血病相关的 NF1 失活现象，涉及 T 细胞急性淋巴细胞白血病（T-cell acute lymphoblastic leukemia，T-ALL）及 MLL 重排 AML（Balgobind et al. 2008）。对 103 例儿童 T-ALL 患者和 71 例 MLL 重排 AML 患者进行的高分辨率基因组筛查发现，3 例 T-ALL 患者和 2 例 MLL 重排 AML 患者中存在复发性隐性缺失，即 del(17)(q11.2)。与保留两个 NF1 等位基因的白血病患者相比，del(17)(q11.2)阳性的 T-ALL 和 MLL 重排 AML 患者的 NF1 表达显著降低。NF1 体细胞突变的 T-ALL 样本还伴随有 NOTCH1 及其他基因的联合突变。突变分析显示，在 4 例 del(17)(q11.2)阳性患者中，有 3 例发生了破坏 NF1 编码区的小框移突变，导致 NF1 双等位基因失活，而在这些患者中未发现 NF1 体细胞纯合突变，表明双等位基因失活的频率很低。不过，研究者指出，包括 UPD 在内的其他 NF1 失活机制可能被忽略了（Balgobind et al. 2008）。有趣的是，最近对没有潜在 NF1 突变的儿童 ALL 和 JMML 患者进行的 SNP 分析显示，NF1 区域并未涉及 UPD。此外，约 20% 的成人 AMLs 患者存在大片的 UPD 区域，但均不涉及 NF1 位点（Mullighan et al. 2007）。这些研究表明，NF1 位点的 UPD 在体细胞突变来源的白血病中可能很罕见。

30.4 动物模型的启示

1994 年，两个研究小组通过破坏 Nf1 基因的第 31 号外显子，建立了 NF1 的"第一代"小鼠模型（Brannan et al. 1994；Jacks et al. 1994）。纯合子 Nf1 突变体（$Nf1^{-/-}$）胚胎会在子宫内因心脏缺陷而死亡。在 C57Bl/6×129Sv 株背景下，约 10% 的 Nf1 杂合突变小鼠（$Nf1^{+/-}$）在出生后第二年自发发展为 JMML 样 MPN，这与野生型等位基因的体细胞丢失相关（Jacks et al. 1994）。重要的是，$Nf1^{-/-}$ 胎儿的造血细胞在 GM-CSF 的刺激下表现出与 JMML 骨髓细胞相似的 CFU-GM 集落生长模式（Bollag et al. 1996；Largaespada et al. 1996），此外，将 Nf1 缺陷胚胎的胎儿肝细胞移植到接受了辐射的受体中，不仅恢复了造血功能，还有效诱导了 JMML 样 MPN（Largaespada et al. 1996；Zhang et al. 1998）。研究表明，Nf1 失活导致该小鼠模型多个造血区生长紊乱，并在竞争性再增殖试验中赋予造血细胞持久的增殖优势（Zhang et al. 1998，2001）。通过交叉和过继性转移实验进一步证明，GM-CSF 信号通路在体内驱动 Nf1 突变体造血细胞的异常生长中起着核心作用（Birnbaum et al. 2000；Kim et al. 2007）。总之，这些研究提供了有力证据，表明神经纤维瘤蛋白通过负调控 Ras 信号通路来抑制髓系细胞的生长，而 Nf1 的失活足以在体内外重现 JMML 的主要特征。

$Nf1^{+/-}$ 小鼠模型被用于验证临床观察的生物学意义，相关研究显示，NF1 患者使用基因毒性治疗后，易患髓系恶性肿瘤及其他继发性癌症（Maris et al. 1997；Papageorgio et al. 1999）。Mahgoub 等（1999a）的一项初步研究表明，烷化剂（如环磷酰胺）或拓扑异构酶 II 抑制剂（如依托泊苷）在白血病发生过程中与 Nf1 杂合缺失之间存在协同作用。这些化学治疗相关的白血病大多表现出野生型 Nf1 等位基因的缺失，荧光原位杂交（fluorescence in situ hybridization，FISH）显示获得性 UPD 是其潜在的遗传机制（Mahgoub et al. 1999a）。在该模型中，环磷酰胺的作用更为显著，无论有无 NF1 突变的患者，烷化剂与单体 7 都密切相关（Le Beau et al. 1996；Smith et al. 2003）。基于这些数据，Chao 等（2005）将 $Nf1^{+/-}$ 小鼠及其野生型小鼠随机分成四组，分别接受环磷酰胺、低剂量全身照射、低剂量全身照射＋环磷酰胺或不接受任何治疗。研究发现，Nf1 杂合缺失与辐射及辐射联合使用环磷酰胺的作用显著协同，导致了多种继发性癌症谱，模拟出人类治疗相关性的癌症。在这些小鼠模型中，MDS 和 MPN 较为常见（Chao et al. 2005）。最近，Nakamura 及其团队（2011）开发了一种新技术，把 300 cGy 的辐射剂量分次对小鼠进行局部照射。这一方案精准模拟了当前人类癌症放射治疗的实际操作。与以往研究结果一致，$Nf1^{+/-}$ 小鼠易罹患多种辐射诱导的癌症，包括鳞状细胞癌、肉瘤和 MDS。有趣的是，该研究确定了辐射剂量与血液肿瘤发生之间存在密切关系,接受1 500 cGy总剂量的小鼠其血液系统肿瘤的发病率较高,而3 000 cGy总剂量的小鼠则主要发生实体肿瘤。Chao等和Nakamura等的研究表明,大多数实体瘤样本表现出正常$Nf1$等位基因的体细胞缺失,然而在血液肿瘤中却未发现LOH现象。目前尚不清楚$Nf1$单倍体缺失在白血病发生过程中是否与其他基因毒性诱导的突变起到协同作用,或正常$Nf1$等位基因是否因点突变或其他遗传机制而失活。然而,值得注意的是,迄今为止,在人类治疗相关的髓系恶性肿瘤研究中并未发现$NF1$基因位点上的LOH。总之,这些研究确立了$Nf1^{+/-}$小鼠作为一个可操作的体内模型,可用以探究治疗相关的人类癌症机制并评估预防策略。

为了解决纯合子$Nf1$基因失活所导致的胚胎致死表型,Zhu及其同事(Zhu et al. 2001)在$Nf1$基因座中引入了LoxP位点,从而开发出一个条件性突变体的$Nf1$等位基因。在这种"第二代"小鼠模型中,$Nf1^{flox}$等位基因在基础状态下保持了野生型功能。通过在特定细胞类型中表达Cre重组酶,实现了组织特异性的$Nf1$体细胞失活(Zhu et al. 2001,2002)。利用干扰素诱导的Mx1-Cre小鼠(Kuhn et al. 1995),在造血细胞中敲除$Nf1$,可导致MPN的发生,其特征包括白细胞增多、脾脏肿大、增殖过度、凋亡受损,以及骨髓CFU-GM祖细胞对细胞因子的超敏反应(Le et al. 2004)。

Lauchle等(2009)使用MOL4070LTR反转录病毒对$Nf1$突变小鼠进行插入突变,模拟了从JMML到AML的进展。在因Mx1-Cre表达导致$Nf1$失活的细胞中,选择反转录病毒插入以实现协同突变。结果表明,注射MOL4070LTR的$Mx1$-Cre、$Nf1^{flox/flox}$小鼠显示出更高的AML发病率和更短的潜伏期。MPN仅能移植到经过致死性辐射处理的宿主中(Le et al. 2004),而在接受亚致死剂量辐射(450 cGy)的受体小鼠中注射AML细胞后,3~6周内会发展为白血病。使用能够检测MOL4070LTR序列的探针进行的DNA印迹分析显示,移植受体中的克隆整合模式是稳定的。此外,通过反转录病毒插入导致破坏或激活的克隆基因,发现了可能在白血病发生过程中与$Nf1$失活起协同作用的候选基因。这进一步证明,MOL4070LTR诱导的AML模型模拟了晚期人类癌症中的遗传多样性。

30.5　临床前试验和治疗意义

对$NF1$基因突变引起的人类血液肿瘤进行的遗传学、细胞生物学和生物化学研究,以及小鼠模型提供的大量数据,均表明Ras信号通路过度激活是这些癌症异常生长的主要"驱动因素"。尽管理论上通过基因治疗或其他手段恢复神经纤维瘤蛋白的功能具有潜在的价值,但目前缺乏实际可行性。因此,研究者们积极开发抑制Ras及其下游效应分子的治疗策略。

首次对基因工程$Nf1$突变小鼠进行的临床前试验中,研究者将$Nf1$缺陷胎儿肝细胞移植到接受辐射的小鼠体内,以建立JMML模型(Largaespada et al. 1996),并评估了法尼基转移酶抑制剂L-744832的疗效(Mahgoub et al. 1999b)。法尼基转移酶是$NF1$突变肿瘤药物设计的重要靶点,因为它催化Ras的翻译后修饰,直接影响其膜定位和生物活性(Gibbs et al. 1994)。尽管L-744832能够以剂量依赖的方式抑制CFU-GM集落的生长,但对$Nf1$突变祖细胞集落并未表现出选择性。在最大耐受剂量(maximally tolerated dose,MTD)下的体内治疗可以抑制小鼠体内的H-Ras异戊烯化,但$Nras$和$Kras$的活性保持正常。在两项对照的临床前研究中,22名接受胎儿肝细胞移植的受体每日接受40 mg/kg或80 mg/kg的L-744832治疗后,在白细胞计数或脾肿大方面未见改善。观察到的治疗效果不明显可能是由于存在一种替代酶(香叶基转移酶),该酶能在法尼基转移酶被阻断时有效进行N-Ras和K-Ras的异戊烯化(Downward 2003;James et al. 1996)。这些临床前数据初步表明,法尼基转移酶抑制剂在体内并未有效降低Ras信号转导,这可能对治疗NF1患者的癌症和肿瘤带来挑战(Mahgoub et al. 1999b)。这一预测后来在临床试验中得到了验证(Downward 2003)。使用移植的胎儿肝细胞进行试验时所面临的挑战,也突显了开发更好JMML临床前模型的必要性,而这一目标通过使用$Mx1\text{-}Cre$、$Nf1^{flox/flox}$菌株使得后续研究得以实现(Le et al. 2004)。

Lauchle等(2009)从辉瑞公司获得了MEK抑制剂CI-1040,发现25~50 mM的CI-1040在GM-CSF作用下,可抑制$Mx1\text{-}Cre$、$Nf1^{flox/flox}$骨髓中CFU-GM集落的形成。然而,与法尼基转移酶试验类似,CI-1040在体外也未表现出有益的治疗指数,因为在相似浓度下,野生型骨髓中的CFU-GM生长亦受到抑制。在一项随机临床前试验中,MPN的$Mx1\text{-}Cre$、$Nf1^{flox/flox}$小鼠接受CI-1040治疗(最大剂量为100 mg/kg,每天2次),结果显示白细胞计数或脾巨细胞计数未见改善。药效学分析表明,CI-1040能够短暂抑制小鼠骨髓细胞中的MEK激酶活性,这种抑制可通过测量GM-CSF提高磷酸化ERK(phosphorylated ERK, pERK)水平的变化来评估(Lauchle et al. 2009)。

使用$Mx1\text{-}Cre$激活内源性致癌$Kras^{G12D}$的表达会导致小鼠出现类似JMML的MPN,病情发展迅速,通常在4个月大时死亡(Braun et al. 2004; Chan et al. 2004)。与CI-1040在$Mx1\text{-}Cre$、$Nf1^{flox/flox}$ MPN小鼠模型中治疗失败的结果(Lauchle et al. 2009)不同,在JMML的$Mx1\text{-}Cre$、$Kras^{G12D}$模型中,901的治疗意外地诱导了血液学改善并提高了生存率(Lyubynska et al. 2011)。有趣的是,这种有益的治疗效果与$Kras^{G12D}$造血细胞的持续存在相关,表明MEK抑制改变了突变细胞的生长,但并未消除这些细胞。所以为了探讨CI-1040和901的不同疗效是否源于潜在的基因型($Nf1$与$Kras$),还是由于接受901治疗的小鼠抑制时间更长,Chang等(2011)最近在$Mx1\text{-}Cre$、$Nf1^{flox/flox}$ MPN小鼠模型中测试了901。结果显示,901可使小鼠的血液学状况显著改善,表明持续的MEK抑制对于该模型的治疗反应至关重要。与接受901治疗的$Kras$突变小鼠一样,这些动物的骨髓中仍然持续存在$Nf1$突变细胞(Chang et al. 2011)。

除了在MPN的$Mx1\text{-}Cre$、$Nf1^{flox/flox}$小鼠中评估CI-1040外,Lauchle和同事(2009)还评估了MEK抑制剂对$Mx1\text{-}Cre$、$Nf1^{flox/flox}$小鼠注射MOL4070LTR反转录病毒后对AML的影响。出乎意料的是,与野生型或MPN骨髓相比,体外幼稚细胞集落在更低药物浓度(0.25~5 mM)下就完全被抑制,这表明$Mx1\text{-}Cre$、$Nf1^{flox/flox}$ AML更依赖于Raf/MEK/ERK信号转导。为了在体内验证这一假设,研究者将25只接受了四种独立白血病移植的受体小鼠随机分为两组,一组接受MTD的CI-1040,另一组接受对照药物。结果显示,CI-1040对AML的生长产生了显著影响,接受治疗的小鼠血液细胞计数明显减少,存活时间显著延长(24天 vs. 7天)。这些数据表明,针对分子靶向抑制剂的生物学反应受到疾病始动突变所处遗传背景的强烈调控。具体而言,尽管$Nf1$失活诱导的MPN对CI-1040并不敏感,但发展为AML后却增强了对该药物的敏感性。

尽管接受CI-1040治疗的AML小鼠始终对治疗有反应,但所有小鼠最终仍会复发并死于该疾病。有趣的是,这些复发的白血病在体外对CI-1040的敏感性显著降低,并且对后续治疗也无反应。随后进行的遗传分析显示,在对CI-1040耐药的白血病中,存在反转录病毒整合,而对药物敏感的亲本AML未见这种整合,提示在治疗过程中存在克隆选择的过程。研究人员进一步鉴定并验证了$RasGRP$家族成员和$Mapk14$(编码p38)对CI-1040耐药的潜在作用。值得一提的是,与MPN的$Mx1\text{-}Cre$、$Nf1^{flox/flox}$小鼠相比,PD0325901在控制$Nf1$突变AML生长方面并不优于CI-1040(Lauchle et al. 2009)。

30.6 总结与未来方向

NF1与JMML的关联对于阐明Ras过度激活在MPN乃至广义的髓系白血病发病中的分子机制所发挥的核心作用至关重要(Sawyers and Denny 1994; Van Etten and Shannon 2004)。令人意外的是,NF1患者罹患白血病的风险较低,而其局限于狭窄发育窗口期的原因尚不清楚。通过阐述胎儿和成人造血干细胞生长控制机制的不同,可能有助于理解丛状神经纤维瘤及NF1在生命早期引发的其他并发症的成因。

直到最近,$NF1$基因片段过大以及其在许多组织中的低表达水平成为研究体细胞突变在散发性人类癌症中作用的重大障碍。而随着高灵敏度 SNP 阵列和高效癌症基因组测序技术的出现，这一领域的研究发生了重大变化，NF1 已成为包括白血病在内多种人类癌症中失活突变的常见靶点。随着越来越多样本的测序，NF1 体细胞突变在血液系统恶性肿瘤中的发生率预计将在未来几年显著上升。随着这项工作的深入，一个重要的问题是确定体细胞突变是否会导致两个等位基因失活，或者 NF1 是否通过单倍体缺失引发恶性生长。根据其他肿瘤抑制基因的研究，这个问题的答案很可能是"两者兼有"。尽管 NF1 失活在 NF1 患者中启动了肿瘤发生，但在白血病和其他散发性癌症中，它更可能是一种作为后期事件获得的协同突变。这反过来又会显著影响 NF1 缺失对肿瘤生物学和药物反应的影响。

从治疗的角度来看，现有的遗传、生化和临床前数据表明，异常的 Raf/MEK/ERK 信号通路在驱动 Nf1 缺失型造血细胞的异常生长中起着关键作用。特别是，Kras 和 Nf1 突变小鼠在 MPN 治疗中对 PD0325901 表现出的显著反应，以及早期数据，都强烈支持在 NF1 和非 NF1 的 JMML 患者中开展 MEK 抑制剂的临床试验。此外，尽管 901 治疗在 Nf1 突变的 AML 中诱导了短暂的缓解，但这些白血病总是不可避免地复发。这些数据与其他情况下信号转导抑制剂的临床前和临床试验结果基本一致，表明开发以胚系或体细胞 NF1 突变为特征的晚期癌症的有效治疗将需要联合用药。最后，虽然神经纤维瘤蛋白在调控 Ras GTP 酶开关中发挥着重要作用，但 NF1 失活的生化后果与致癌的 NRAS 和 KRAS 突变存在显著差异。尤其是，致癌的 Ras 蛋白由于内在水解缺陷和对 GAP 的抗性而"锁定"在 GTP 构象中。相比之下，NF1 缺失细胞中的 Ras 蛋白在本质上是正常的，鸟嘌呤核苷酸交换因子（guanine nucleotide exchange factor, GNEF）在循环中起应答作用，并能受到其他细胞 GAP 的调节。这些细微差别可能会影响治疗反应，甚至可能影响有效药物的类型。例如，美国基因泰克公司的研究人员最近报告了一类通过干扰 SOS GNEF 抑制 Ras 信号转导的小分子药物（Maurer et al. 2012）。与 NRAS 或 KRAS 突变引起的恶性肿瘤相比，NF1 突变的癌症中 Ras 信号转导过度激活更依赖于生长因子介导的核苷酸交换，这种类型的化合物对 NF1 突变的癌症应更有效。因此，NF1 失活的独特后果以及与致癌 Ras 信号网络的相似性可能会影响血液肿瘤和其他恶性肿瘤对靶向抗癌药物的反应。

致谢：本章所介绍的我们实验室的工作部分由美国陆军神经纤维瘤病研究计划（项目 DAMD17-02-1-0638）、美国国立卫生研究院（NIH）资助的 CA72614 和 U0184221 以及儿童肿瘤基金会资助。T. C. 是圣鲍德里克基金会（St. Baldrick's Foundation）的奖学金获得者，K. S. 是美国癌症协会（American Cancer Society）的研究教授。

（袁晓军，张鑫 译）

参考文献

[1] Bader JL, Miller RW (1978) Neurofibromatosis and childhood leukemia. J Pediatr 92: 925-929

[2] Balgobind BV, Van Vlierberghe P, van den Ouweland AM, Beverloo HB, Terlouw-Kromosoeto JN, van Wering ER, Reinhardt D, Horstmann M, Kaspers GJ, Pieters R, Zwaan CM, Van den Heuvel-Eibrink MM, Meijerink JP (2008) Leukemia-associated NF1 inactivation in patients with pediatric T-ALL and AML lacking evidence for neurofibromatosis. Blood 111: 4322-4328

[3] Basu TN, Gutmann DH, Fletcher JA, Glover TW, Collins FS, Downward J (1992) Aberrant regulation of ras proteins in malignant tumour cells from type 1 neurofibromatosis patients. Nature 356: 713-715

[4] Birnbaum RA, O'Marcaigh A, Wardak Z, Zhang YY, Dranoff G, Jacks T, Clapp DW, Shannon KM (2000) Nf1 and Gmcsf interact in myeloid leukemogenesis. Mol Cell 5: 189-195

[5] Bollag G, Clapp DW, Shih S, Adler F, Zhang Y, Thompson P, Lange BJ, Freedman MH, McCormick F, Jacks T, Shannon K (1996) Loss of NF1 results in activation of the Ras signaling pathway and leads to aberrant growth in murine and human hematopoietic cells. Nat Genet 12: 144-148

[6] Brannan CI, Perkins AS, Vogel KS, Ratner N, Nordlund ML, Reid SW, Buchberg AM, Jenkins N, Parada L, Copeland N (1994) Targeted disruption of the neurofibromatosis type 1 gene leads to developmental abnormalities in heart and various neural crest-derived tissues. Genes Dev 8: 1019-1029

[7] Braun BS, Tuveson DA, Kong N, Le DT, Kogan SC, Rozmus J, Le Beau MM, Jacks TE, Shannon KM (2004) Somatic activation of oncogenic Kras in hematopoietic cells initiates a rapidly fatal myeloproliferative disorder. Proc Natl Acad Sci

USA 101: 597-602
[8] Cancer Genome Atlas Network (2008) Comprehensive genomic characterization defines human glioblastoma genes and core pathways. Nature 455: 1061-1068
[9] Chan IT, Kutok JL, Williams IR, Cohen S, Kelly L, Shigematsu H, Johnson L, Akashi K, Tuveson DA, Jacks T, Gilliland DG (2004) Conditional expression of oncogenic K-ras from its endogenous promoter induces a myeloproliferative disease. J Clin Invest 113: 528-538
[10] Chang T, Krisman K, Braun BS, Shannon K (2011) MEK inhibition modulates the growth of $Nf1$ mutant hematopoietic cells and induces clinical improvement in a murine model of JMML (abstract). Blood 118: 797
[11] Chao RC, Pyzel U, Fridlyand J, Kuo YM, Teel L, Haaga J, Borowsky A, Horvai A, Kogan SC, Bonifas J, Huey B, Jacks TE, Albertson DG, Shannon KM (2005) Therapy-induced malignant neoplasms in Nf1 mutant mice. Cancer Cell 8: 337-348
[12] Cirstea IC, Kutsche K, Dvorsky R, Gremer L, Carta C, Horn D, Roberts AE, Lepri F, Merbitz-Zahradnik T, Konig R, Kratz CP, Pantaleoni F, Dentici ML, Joshi VA, Kucherlapati RS, Mazzanti L, Mundlos S, Patton MA, Silengo MC, Rossi C, Zampino G, Digilio C, Stuppia L, Seemanova E, Pennacchio LA, Gelb BD, Dallapiccola B, Wittinghofer A, Ahmadian MR, Tartaglia M, Zenker M (2010) A restricted spectrum of NRAS mutations causes Noonan syndrome. Nat Genet 42: 27-29
[13] DeClue JE, Cohen BD, Lowy DR (1991) Identification and characterization of the neurofibromatosis type 1 protein product. Proc Natl Acad Sci USA 88: 9914-9918
[14] Ding L, Getz G, Wheeler DA, Mardis ER, McLellan MD, Cibulskis K, Sougnez C, Greulich H, Muzny DM, Morgan MB, Fulton L, Fulton RS, Zhang Q, Wendl MC, Lawrence MS, Larson DE, Chen K, Dooling DJ, Sabo A, Hawes AC, Shen H, Jhangiani SN, Lewis LR, Hall O, Zhu Y, Mathew T, Ren Y, Yao J, Scherer SE, Clerc K, Metcalf GA, Ng B, Milosavljevic A, Gonzalez-Garay ML, Osborne JR, Meyer R, Shi X, Tang Y, Koboldt DC, Lin L, Abbott R, Miner TL, Pohl C, Fewell G, Haipek C, Schmidt H, Dunford-Shore BH, Kraja A, Crosby SD, Sawyer CS, Vickery T, Sander S, Robinson J, Winckler W, Baldwin J, Chirieac LR, Dutt A, Fennell T, Hanna M, Johnson BE, Onofrio RC, Thomas RK, Tonon G, Weir BA, Zhao X, Ziaugra L, Zody MC, Giordano T, Orringer MB, Roth JA, Spitz MR, Wistuba B II, Ozenberger PJ, Good AC, Chang DG, Beer MA, Watson M, Ladanyi S, Broderick A, Yoshizawa WD, Travis W, Pao MA, Province GM, Weinstock HE, Varmus SB, Gabriel ES, Lander RA, Gibbs MM, Wilson RK (2008) Somatic mutations affect key pathways in lung adenocarcinoma. Nature 455: 1069-1075
[15] Downward J (2003) Targeting RAS signalling pathways in cancer therapy. Nat Rev Cancer 3: 11-22
[16] Dunbar AJ, Gondek LP, O'Keefe CL, Makishima H, Rataul MS, Szpurka H, Sekeres MA, Wang XF, McDevitt MA, Maciejewski JP (2008) 250K single nucleotide polymorphism array karyotyping identifies acquired uniparental disomy and homozygous mutations, including novel missense substitutions of c-Cbl, in myeloid malignancies. Cancer Res 68: 10349-10357
[17] Emanuel PD, Bates LJ, Castleberry RP, Gualtieri RJ, Zuckerman KS (1991) Selective hypersensitivity to granulocyte-macrophage colony stimulating factor by juvenile chronic myeloid leukemia hematopoietic progenitors. Blood 77: 925-929
[18] Flotho C, Steinemann D, Mullighan CG, Neale G, Mayer K, Kratz CP, Schlegelberger B, Downing JR, Niemeyer CM (2007) Genome-wide single-nucleotide polymorphism analysis in juvenile myelomonocytic leukemia identifies uniparental disomy surrounding the NF1 locus in cases associated with neurofibromatosis but not in cases with mutant RAS or PTPN11. Oncogene 26: 5816-5821
[19] Gibbs JB, Oliff A, Kohl NE (1994) Farnesyltransferase inhibitors: Ras research yields a potential cancer therapeutic. Cell 77: 175-178
[20] Haferlach C, Dicker F, Kohlmann A, Schindela S, Weiss T, Kern W, Schnittger S, Haferlach T (2010) AML with CBFB-MYH11 rearrangement demonstrate RAS pathway alterations in 92% of all cases including a high frequency of NF1 deletions. Leukemia 24: 1065-1069
[21] Holzel M, Huang S, Koster J, Ora I, Lakeman A, Caron H, Nijkamp W, Xie J, Callens T, Asgharzadeh S, Seeger RC, Messiaen L, Versteeg R, Bernards R (2010) NF1 is a tumor suppressor in neuroblastoma that determines retinoic acid response and disease outcome. Cell 142: 218-229
[22] Jacks T, Shih S, Schmitt EM, Bronson RT, Bernards A, Weinberg RA (1994) Tumorigenic and developmental consequences of a targeted $Nf1$ mutation in the mouse. Nat Genet 7: 353-361
[23] James G, Goldstein JL, Brown MS (1996) Resistance of K-RasBv12 proteins to farnesyl-transferase inhibitors in Rat1 cells. Proc Natl Acad Sci USA 93: 4454-4458
[24] Kalra R, Paderanga D, Olson K, Shannon KM (1994) Genetic analysis is consistent with the hypothesis that NF1 limits myeloid cell growth through p21^{ras}. Blood 84: 3435-3439
[25] Kaneko Y, Maseki N, Sakuri M, Shibuya A, Shinohara T, Fujimoto T, Kanno H, Nishikawa A (1989) Chromosome patterns in juvenile chronic myelogenous leukemia, myelodysplastic syndrome, and acute leukemia associated with neurofibromatosis. Leukemia 3: 36-41
[26] Keilhack H, David FS, McGregor M, Cantley LC, Neel BG (2005) Diverse biochemical properties of Shp2 mutants: implications for disease phenotypes. J Biol Chem 280: 30984-30993
[27] Kim A, Morgan K, Hasz DE, Wiesner SM, Lauchle JO, Geurts JL, Diers MD, Le DT, Kogan SC, Parada LF, Shannon K, Largaespada DA (2007) Beta common receptor inactivation attenuates myeloproliferative disease in Nf1 mutant mice. Blood 109: 1687-1691
[28] Kolquist KA, Schultz RA, Furrow A, Brown TC, Han JY, Campbell LJ, Wall M, Slovak ML, Shaffer LG, Ballif BC (2011) Microarray-based comparative genomic hybridization of cancer targets reveals novel, recurrent genetic aberrations in the myelodysplastic syndromes. Cancer Genet 204: 603-628
[29] Kotecha N, Flores NJ, Irish JM, Simonds EF, Sakai DS, Archambeault S, Diaz-Flores E, Coram M, Shannon KM, Nolan GP, Loh ML (2008) Single-cell profiling identifies aberrant STAT5 activation in myeloid malignancies with specific clinical and biologic correlates. Cancer Cell 14: 335-343
[30] Kratz CP, Niemeyer CM, Castleberry RP, Cetin M, Bergstrasser E, Emanuel PD, Hasle H, Kardos G, Klein C, Kojima S, Stary J, Trebo M, Zecca M, Gelb BD, Tartaglia M, Loh ML (2005) The mutational spectrum of PTPN11 in juvenile myelomonocytic leukemia and Noonan syndrome/myeloproliferative disease. Blood 106: 2183-2185
[31] Kuhn R, Schwenk F, Aguet M, Rajewsky K (1995) Inducible

gene targeting in mice. Science 269: 1427-1429

[32] Largaespada DA, Brannan CI, Jenkins NA, Copeland NG (1996) Nf1 deficiency causes Ras-mediated granulocyte-macrophage colony stimulating factor hypersensitivity and chronic myeloid leukemia. Nat Genet 12: 137-143

[33] Lauchle JO, Braun BS, Loh ML, Shannon K (2006) Inherited predispositions and hyperactive Ras in myeloid leukemogenesis. Pediatr Blood Cancer 46: 579-585

[34] Lauchle JO, Kim D, Le DT, Akagi K, Crone M, Krisman K, Warner K, Bonifas JM, Li Q, Coakley KM, Diaz-Flores E, Gorman M, Przybranowski S, Tran M, Kogan SC, Roose JP, Copeland NG, Jenkins NA, Parada L, Wolff L, Sebolt-Leopold J, Shannon K (2009) Response and resistance to MEK inhibition in leukaemias initiated by hyperactive Ras. Nature 461: 411-414

[35] Laycock-van Spyk S, Thomas N, Cooper DN, Upadhyaya M (2011) Neurofibromatosis type 1-associated tumours: their somatic mutational spectrum and pathogenesis. Hum Genomics 5: 623-690

[36] Le Beau MM, Espinosa R 3rd, Davis EM, Eisenbart JD, Larson RA, Green ED (1996) Cytogenetic and molecular delineation of a region of chromosome 7 commonly deleted in malignant myeloid diseases. Blood 88: 1930-1935

[37] Le DT, Kong N, Zhu Y, Lauchle JO, Aiyigari A, Braun BS, Wang E, Kogan SC, Le Beau MM, Parada L, Shannon KM (2004) Somatic inactivation of Nf1 in hematopoietic cells results in a progressive myeloproliferative disorder. Blood 103: 4243-4250

[38] Loh ML (2011) Recent advances in the pathogenesis and treatment of juvenile myelomonocytic leukaemia. Br J Haematol 152: 677-687

[39] Loh ML, Sakai DS, Flotho C, Kang M, Fliegauf M, Archambeault S, Mullighan CG, Chen L, Bergstraesser E, Bueso-Ramos CE, Emanuel PD, Hasle H, Issa JP, van den Heuvel-Eibrink MM, Locatelli F, Stary J, Trebo M, Wlodarski M, Zecca M, Shannon KM, Niemeyer CM (2009) Mutations in CBL occur frequently in juvenile myelomonocytic leukemia. Blood 114: 1859-1863

[40] Lyubynska N, Gorman MF, Lauchle JO, Hong WX, Akutagawa JK, Shannon K, Braun BS (2011) A MEK inhibitor abrogates myeloproliferative disease in Kras mutant mice. Sci Transl Med 3: 76ra27

[41] Mahgoub N, Taylor B, Le Beau M, Gratiot M, Carlson K, Jacks T, Shannon KM (1999a) Myeloid malignancies induced by alkylating agents in Nf1 mice. Blood 93: 3617-3623

[42] Mahgoub N, Taylor BR, Gratiot M, Kohl NE, Gibbs JB, Jacks T, Shannon KM (1999b) In vitro and in vivo effects of a farnesyltransferase inhibitor on Nf1-deficient hematopoietic cells. Blood 94: 2469-2476

[43] Marchuk DA, Saulino AM, Tavakkol R, Swaroop M, Wallace MR, Andersen LB, Mitchell AL, Gutmann DH, Boguski M, Collins FS (1991) cDNA cloning of the type 1 neurofibromatosis gene: complete sequence of the NF1 gene product. Genomics 11: 931-940

[44] Maris JM, Wiersma SR, Mahgoub N, Thompson P, Geyer RJ, Lange BJ, Shannon KM (1997) Monosomy 7 myelodysplastic syndrome and other second malignant neoplasms in children with neurofibromatosis type 1. Cancer 79: 1438-1446

[45] Maurer T, Garrenton LS, Oh A, Pitts K, Anderson DJ, Skelton NJ, Fauber BP, Pan B, Malek S, Stokoe D, Ludlam MJ, Bowman KK, Wu J, Giannetti AM, Starovasnik MA, Mellman I, Jackson PK, Rudolph J, Wang W, Fang G (2012) Small-molecule ligands bind to a distinct pocket in Ras and inhibit SOS-mediated nucleotide exchange activity. Proc Natl Acad Sci USA 109: 5299-5304

[46] Menon AG, Anderson KM, Riccardi VM, Chung RY, Whaley JM, Yandell DW, Farmer GE, Freiman RN, Lee JK, Li FP et al (1990) Chromosome 17p deletions and p53 gene mutations associated with the formation of malignant neurofibrosarcomas in von Recklinghausen neuro-fibromatosis. Proc Natl Acad Sci USA 87: 5435-5439

[47] Miles DK, Freedman MH, Stephens K, Pallavicini M, Sievers E, Weaver M, Grunberger T, Thompson P, Shannon KM (1996) Patterns of hematopoietic lineage involvement in children with neurofibromatosis, type 1, and malignant myeloid disorders. Blood 88: 4314-4320

[48] Miyauchi J, Asada M, Sasaki M, Tsunematsu Y, Kojima S, Mizutani S (1994) Mutations of the N-ras gene in juvenile chronic myelogenous leukemia. Blood 83: 2248-2254

[49] Mullighan CG, Goorha S, Radtke I, Miller CB, Coustan-Smith E, Dalton JD, Girtman K, Mathew S, Ma J, Pounds SB, Su X, Pui CH, Relling MV, Evans WE, Shurtleff SA, Downing JR (2007) Genome-wide analysis of genetic alterations in acute lymphoblastic leukaemia. Nature 446: 758-764

[50] Nakamura JL, Phong C, Pinarbasi E, Kogan SC, Vandenberg S, Horvai AE, Faddegon BA, Fiedler D, Shokat K, Houseman BT, Chao R, Pieper RO, Shannon K (2011) Dose-dependent effects of focal fractionated irradiation on secondary malignant neoplasms in Nf1 mutant mice. Cancer Res 71: 106-115

[51] Niemeyer CM, Kang MW, Shin DH, Furlan I, Erlacher M, Bunin NJ, Bunda S, Finklestein JZ, Sakamoto KM, Gorr TA, Mehta P, Schmid I, Kropshofer G, Corbacioglu S, Lang PJ, Klein C, Schlegel PG, Heinzmann A, Schneider M, Stary J, van den Heuvel-Eibrink MM, Hasle H, Locatelli F, Sakai D, Archambeault S, Chen L, Russell RC, Sybingco SS, Ohh M, Braun BS, Flotho C, Loh ML (2010) Germline CBL mutations cause developmental abnormalities and predispose to juvenile myelomonocytic leukemia. Nat Genet 42: 794-800

[52] Onida F, Kantarjian HM, Smith TL, Ball G, Keating MJ, Estey EH, Glassman AB, Albitar M, Kwari MI, Beran M (2002) Prognostic factors and scoring systems in chronic myelomonocytic leukemia: a retrospective analysis of 213 patients. Blood 99: 840-849

[53] Papageorgio C, Seiter K, Feldman EJ (1999) Therapy-related myelodysplastic syndrome in adults with neurofibromatosis. Leuk Lymphoma 32: 605-608

[54] Parkin B, Ouillette P, Wang Y, Liu Y, Wright W, Roulston D, Purkayastha A, Dressel A, Karp J, Bockenstedt P, Al-Zoubi A, Talpaz M, Kujawski L, Shedden K, Shakhan S, Li C, Erba H, Malek SN (2010) NF1 inactivation in adult acute myelogenous leukemia. Clin Cancer Res 16: 4135-4147

[55] Parsons DW, Jones S, Zhang X, Lin JC, Leary RJ, Angenendt P, Mankoo P, Carter H, Siu IM, Gallia GL, Olivi A, McLendon R, Rasheed BA, Keir S, Nikolskaya T, Nikolsky Y, Busam DA, Tekleab H, Diaz LA Jr, Hartigan J, Smith DR, Strausberg RL, Marie SK, Shinjo SM, Yan H, Riggins GJ, Bigner DD, Karchin R, Papadopoulos N, Parmigiani G, Vogelstein B, Velculescu VE, Kinzler KW (2008) An integrated genomic analysis of human glioblastoma multiforme. Science 321: 1807-1812

[56] Royer P, Blondet C, Guihard J (1958) Xantholeucemie du nourrisson et neurofibromatose de Recklinghausen. Ann Pediatr 24: 1504-1513

[57] Sanada M, Suzuki T, Shih LY, Otsu M, Kato M, Yamazaki S, Tamura A, Honda H, Sakata-Yanagimoto M, Kumano K, Oda H, Yamagata T, Takita J, Gotoh N, Nakazaki K, Kawamata N, Onodera M, Nobuyoshi M, Hayashi Y, Harada H, Kurokawa M, Chiba S, Mori H, Ozawa K, Omine M, Hirai H, Nakauchi H, Koeffler HP, Ogawa S (2009) Gain-of-function of mutated C-CBL tumour suppressor in myeloid neoplasms. Nature 460: 904-908

[58] Sangha N, Wu R, Kuick R, Powers S, Mu D, Fiander D, Yuen K, Katabuchi H, Tashiro H, Fearon ER, Cho KR (2008) Neurofibromin 1 (NF1) defects are common in human ovarian serous carcinomas and co-occur with TP53 mutations. Neoplasia 10: 1362-1372

[59] Sawyers CL (1999) Chronic myeloid leukemia. N Engl J Med 340: 1330-1340

[60] Sawyers CL, Denny CT (1994) Chronic myelomonocytic leukemia: tel-a-kinase what ets all about. Cell 77: 171-173

[61] Schubbert S, Zenker M, Rowe SL, Boll S, Klein C, Bollag G, van der Burgt I, Musante L, Kalscheuer V, Wehner LE, Nguyen H, West B, Zhang KY, Sistermans E, Rauch A, Niemeyer CM, Shannon K, Kratz CP (2006) Germline *KRAS* mutations cause Noonan syndrome. Nat Genet 38: 331-336

[62] Schubbert S, Shannon K, Bollag G (2007) Hyperactive Ras in developmental disorders and cancer. Nat Rev Cancer 7: 295-308

[63] Shannon KM, Watterson J, Johnson P, O'Connell P, Lange B, Shah N, Kan YW, Priest JR (1992) Monosomy 7 myeloproliferative disease in children with neurofibromatosis, type 1: epidemiology and molecular analysis. Blood 79: 1311-1318

[64] Shannon KM, O'Connell P, Martin GA, Paderanga D, Olson K, Dinndorf P, McCormick F (1994) Loss of the normal *NF1* allele from the bone marrow of children with type 1 neurofibromatosis and malignant myeloid disorders. N Engl J Med 330: 597-601

[65] Side L, Taylor B, Cayouette M, Conner E, Thompson P, Luce M, Shannon K (1997) Homozygous inactivation of the *NF1* gene in bone marrow cells from children with neurofibromatosis type 1 and malignant myeloid disorders. N Engl J Med 336: 1713-1720

[66] Side LE, Emanuel PD, Taylor B, Franklin J, Thompson P, Castleberry RP, Shannon KM (1998) Mutations of the NF1 gene in children with juvenile myelomonocytic leukemia without clinical evidence of neurofibromatosis, type 1. Blood 92: 267-272

[67] Smith SM, Le Beau MM, Huo D, Karrison T, Sobecks RM, Anastasi J, Vardiman JW, Rowley JD, Larson RA (2003) Clinical-cytogenetic associations in 306 patients with therapy-related myelodysplasia and myeloid leukemia: the University of Chicago series. Blood 102: 43-52

[68] Steinemann D, Arning L, Praulich I, Stuhrmann M, Hasle H, Stary J, Schlegelberger B, Niemeyer CM, Flotho C (2010) Mitotic recombination and compound-heterozygous mutations are predominant *NF1*-inactivating mechanisms in children with juvenile myelomonocytic leukemia and neurofibromatosis type 1. Haematologica 95: 320-323

[69] Stephens K, Weaver M, Leppig KA, Maruyama K, Emanuel PD, Le Beau MM, Shannon KM (2006) Interstitial uniparental isodisomy at clustered breakpoint intervals is a frequent mechanism of *NF1* inactivation in myeloid malignancies. Blood 108: 1684-1689

[70] Stiller CA, Chessells JM, Fitchett M (1994) Neurofibromatosis and childhood leukemia/lymphoma: a population-based UKCCSG study. Br J Cancer 70: 969-972

[71] Tartaglia M, Mehler EL, Goldberg R, Zampino G, Brunner HG, Kremer H, van der Burgt I, Crosby AH, Ion A, Jeffery S, Kalidas K, Patton MA, Kucherlapati RS, Gelb BD (2001) Mutations in *PTPN11*, encoding the protein tyrosine phosphatase SHP-2, cause Noonan syndrome. Nat Genet 29: 465-468

[72] Van Etten RA, Shannon KM (2004) Focus on myeloproliferative diseases and myelodysplastic syndromes. Cancer Cell 6: 547-552

[73] Viskochil D, Buchberg AM, Xu G, Cawthon RM, Stevens J, Wolff RK, Culver M, Carey JC, Copeland NG, Jenkins NA, White R, O'Connell P (1990) Deletions and a translocation interrupt a cloned gene at the neurofibromatosis type 1 locus. Cell 62: 187-192

[74] Wallace MR, Marchuk DA, Andersen LB, Letcher R, Odeh HM, Saulino AM, Fountain JW, Brereton A, Nicholson J, Mitchell AL, Brownstein BH, Collins FS (1990) Type 1 neurofibro-matosis gene: identification of a large transcript disrupted in three NF1 patients. Science 249: 181-186

[75] Xu G, Lin B, Tanaka K, Dunn D, Wood D, Gesteland R, White R, Weiss R, Tamanoi F (1990a) The catalytic domain of the neurofibromatosis type 1 gene product stimulates *ras* GTPase and complements *ira* mutants of *S. cerevisiae*. Cell 63: 835-841

[76] Xu G, O'Connell P, Viskochil D, Cawthon R, Robertson M, Culver M, Dunn D, Stevens J, Gesteland R, White R, Weiss R (1990b) The neurofibromatosis type 1 gene encodes a protein related to GAP. Cell 62: 599-608

[77] Zhang Y, Vik TA, Ryder JW, Srour EF, Jacks T, Shannon K, Clapp DW (1998) Nf1 regulates hematopoietic progenitor cell growth and Ras signaling in response to multiple cytokines. J Exp Med 187: 1893-1902

[78] Zhang Y, Taylor BR, Shannon K, Clapp DW (2001) Quantitative effects of Nf1 inactivation on in vivo hematopoiesis. J Clin Invest 108: 709-715

[79] Zhu Y, Romero MI, Ghosh P, Ye Z, Charnay P, Rushing EJ, Marth JD, Parada LF (2001) Ablation of NF1 function in neurons induces abnormal development of cerebral cortex and reactive gliosis in the brain. Genes Dev 15: 859-876

[80] Zhu Y, Ghosh P, Charnay P, Burns DK, Parada LF (2002) Neurofibromas in NF1: Schwann cell origin and role of tumor environment. Science 296: 920-922

第31章 Legius 综合征：诊断与病理
Legius Syndrome: Diagnosis and Pathology

Hilde Brems, Ludwine Messiaen, and Eric Legius

31.1 引言

1型神经纤维瘤病（NF1）（MIM♯162200）是一种常见的遗传性疾病，在新生儿中的发病率为1/3 000（Huson et al. 1989）。典型的临床表现为多发性咖啡牛奶斑（CALM）、腋窝或腹股沟斑点、虹膜Lisch结节（虹膜错构瘤）、神经纤维瘤和视神经胶质瘤。其他与NF1相关的临床表现包括大头畸形、身材矮小、脊柱侧弯、学习障碍和独特的骨病变。此外，NF1患者罹患特定恶性肿瘤的风险也会增加（Brems et al. 2009）。美国国立卫生研究院（National Institutes of Health，NIH）规定了NF1的诊断标准（No Authors 1988）。NF1属于RASopathies综合征的一种，RASopathies综合征是一类因编码RAS/MAPK通路的基因突变而引起的遗传综合征（Zenker，2011）。除此之外，RASopathies综合征还包括努南综合征、心-面-皮肤综合征（cardio-facio-cutaneous，CFC）、LEOPARD综合征、科斯特罗综合征（Costello）、毛细血管畸形-动静脉畸形综合征（capillary malformation-arteriovenous malformation，CM-AVM）、CBL基因突变相关综合征和遗传性牙龈纤维瘤病。这些综合征的临床表现有重叠之处。2007年，研究人员发现了一种新的与SPRED1种系失活突变有关的RASopathies综合征。最初，该综合征被命名为1型神经纤维瘤样综合征（MIM ♯611431），但后来又被重新命名为Legius综合征（Upadhyaya 2008；Stevenson and Viskochil 2009）。Legius综合征也是RASopathies综合征的一种。

31.2 临床表现

1型神经纤维瘤样综合征（Legius综合征）最早是在5个家族（37人）和6名无亲属关系的人身上发现的（Brems et al. 2007）。由于其临床表现与NF1有极大的相似之处，因此无法仅根据临床特征来诊断该综合征。Legius综合征患者表现为多发性咖啡牛奶斑，伴有或不伴有腋窝或腹股沟斑块（图31.1）。在最初的报告中，31名患者中13名出现大头畸形，5名患者出现努南样特征，6名患儿存在学习问题和（或）注意力缺陷，1名患儿出现发育迟缓，14名患儿出现脂肪瘤，3名患儿表现出轻度鸡胸，各有1名患者患儿童肾癌、肺癌和结肠腺瘤。而其他

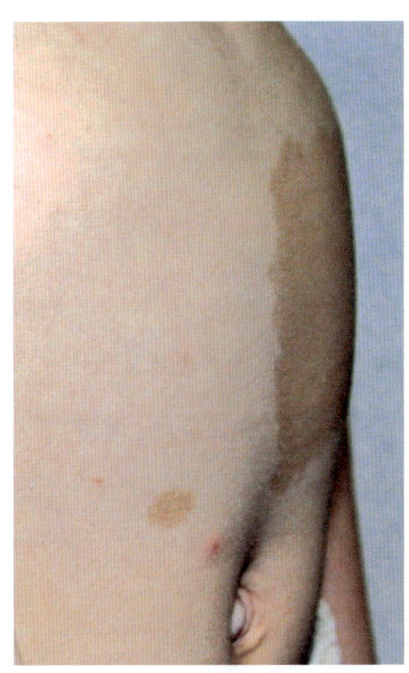

图 31.1　Legius 综合征患儿腹部的典型咖啡牛奶斑

典型的 NF1 相关特征均不存在，如 Lisch 结节、神经纤维瘤、特殊骨病变、视神经胶质瘤和恶性周围神经鞘膜瘤。

随后发表的 7 篇论文则证实了第一份报告的结论。文章中报道了以下临床表现：多发性咖啡牛奶斑（108/119）伴（53/115）或不伴腋窝或腹股沟斑块，以及大头畸形（15/93）和努南样特征（14/89）（Pasmant et al. 2009a，b；Spurlock et al. 2009；Messiaen et al. 2009；Muram-Zborovski et al. 2010；Denayer et al. 2011a；Laycock-Van Spyk et al. 2011；Spencer et al. 2011）。此外，学习障碍（24/115）、发育迟缓（20/85）和注意力缺陷（15/87）也常见报道（Pasmant et al. 2009a，b；Messiaen et al. 2009；Muram-Zborovski et al. 2010；Denayer et al. 2011a；Laycock-Van Spyk et al. 2011；Spencer et al. 2011）。15 名 Legius 综合征患者出现了认知障碍（Denayer et al. 2011b）。与未受影响的家庭成员相比，Legius 综合征患儿的平均智商较低。与 NF1 相比，Legius 综合征的认知障碍表现较轻。

文章中提到的其他临床表现包括：漏斗胸或鸡胸 12/87（Messiaen et al. 2009；Denayer et al. 2011a；Laycock-Van Spyk et al. 2011；Spencer et al. 2011）和单侧多指畸形（3/159）（Messiaen et al. 2009；Denayer et al. 2011b）。在一些 Legius 综合征患者中诊断出脂肪瘤（Pasmant et al. 2009a；Messiaen et al. 2009；Denayer et al. 2011a，b；Spencer et al. 2011）。

目前尚不清楚恶性肿瘤是否与 Legius 综合征有关。个别案例仅报道过 1 次：单倍体急性白血病（Pasmant et al. 2009a，b；同一人）、巨细胞瘤、卵巢皮样瘤、乳腺癌（Messiaen et al. 2009）、前庭分裂瘤和类脂膜瘤（Denayer et al. 2011a）。在单核细胞性急性白血病（Pasmant et al. 2009a，b；同一人）中没有发现 SPRED1 的其他基因突变位点，在一小部分幼年骨髓细胞白血病病例中也未发现 SPRED1 突变（Batz et al. 2010）。

目前没有证据表明以上临床表现由 Legius 综合征引起。由于报道的病例总数相对较少（159 例：各年龄段），而且大部分确诊病例为儿童，成人的罕见并发症可能会被遗漏。如要发现发病率为 1% 的罕见并发症，至少需要调查 250 名 Legius 综合征成人患者（Messiaen et al. 2009）。因此，继续收集新诊断出的 Legius 综合征患者的详细临床信息非常重要。

31.3　SPRED1 的分子遗传学

31.3.1　SPRED1 的基因组组织和分子检测

SPRED1 位于 15q13.2 染色体带，基因组序列跨度为 104.4 kb，包含 7 个外显子。转录本长度为 7 255 bp，开放阅读框编码 444 个氨基酸。外周血白细胞中提取的 DNA 或 RNA 可以进行分子基因检测（Brems et al. 2007；Messiaen et al. 2009）。通过多重连接依赖性探针扩增（multiplex ligationdependent probe amplification，MLPA）、阵列比较基因组杂交（array comparative genomic hybridisation，arrayCGH）或其他技术可以检测拷贝数变化（copy number changes，CNC），如多外显子缺失和整个 SPRED1 基因缺失（Spencer et al. 2011）。

与 NF1 基因突变相比，SPRED1 基因突变非常罕见。在 43% 的伴咖啡牛奶斑、伴或不伴斑块且无其他 NF1 诊断标准的散发性病例中发现了致病性 NF1 突变。而在具有以上临床表现的病例中，仅有 1.3% 的病例检测出了致病性 SPRED1 突变。在具有相同表现的家族性病例中，73% 的病例发现了致病性 NF1 突变，19% 的病例发现了致病性 SPRED1 突变（Messiaen et al. 2009）。在有 Lisch 结节、神经纤维瘤或视神经胶质瘤的患者中，没有发现致病性 SPRED1 突变的报道。

31.3.2 基因突变谱和多态性

尽管家族性和散发性 Legius 综合征病例均有报道，其中最大的一项研究描述了在 SPRED1 突变阳性组中有 39%（13/33）的散发性病例（Messiaen et al. 2009），但这项研究对散发性病例有所偏倚。Leiden 开放变异数据库（Leiden Open Variation Database, LOVD）汇总了所有已知的 SPRED1 突变和多态性，并将定期更新。该数据库（http://www.lovd.nl/SPRED1）可在线访问，于 2012 年 4 月建立之初录入了在 146 名无关个体中发现的 89 种不同突变（Brems et al. 2012）。其突变遵循 HGVS 命名法，并根据 SPRED1 cDNA 参考序列（NM_152594.2）进行编号，A 为起始密码子+1。

该数据库包含大量突变（Brems et al. 2012），包括 29 个错义突变（33%）、28 个框移码突变（31%）、19 个无义突变（21%）、8 个 CNC 突变（9%）、2 个剪接突变（2%）、1 个沉默突变（<1%）、1 个框内缺失突变（<1%）和 1 个影响起始密码子的突变（<1%）。突变遍布整个基因。大多数突变为截断突变或可能会导致 SPRED1 蛋白合成缺失的突变（28 个移帧突变、19 个无义突变、8 个 CNC 突变、2 个剪接突变、1 个影响起始密码子的突变）。在 29 个错义突变中，8 个可能是良性罕见变异，3 个明显致病，1 个可能致病（基于氨基酸保守性和在一个大家族中的分离情况）。有 17 个错义突变仍未分类，需要进一步研究。只有少数错义突变被归类为致病性突变。

公共数据集 dbSNP135 中描述了多态性，其中包括 3 个经过验证的中性错义变体（p. Asp274Gly、p. Val309Ala 和 p. Pro315Leu）。p. Asp274Gly 和 p. Pro315Leu 很可能是良性的罕见变异，因为在怀疑 Legius 综合征的患者中没有检测到它们（L. M.，个人通信），对 p. Val309Ala 的错义变异进行的功能分析证实了它的中性作用（H. B.，个人通信）。

迄今为止，仅 Brems 等（2007）的论文中报道了 1 例体细胞突变。

黑色素细胞是从 1 名 Legius 综合征患者的咖啡牛奶斑组织中培养出来的。除了胚系 SPRED1 突变（p. Arg24*）外，还发现了一个体细胞框架移位 SPRED1 突变（c. 304dupA；p. Thr102Asnfs*7）。

31.3.3 基因型与表型的相关性

目前尚未有报道证实 SPRED1 突变的基因型与表型的具体相关性。Spencer 等（2011）报道了 7 例多外显子或全 SPRED1 缺失，这些个体的表型与 SPRED1 点突变个体的表型没有差异。

31.4 生物学基础

31.4.1 蛋白质结构和功能

SPRED1 是 Sprouty/SPRED 蛋白家族中的 1 个 55 kDa 亚型。SPRED 家族有 3 个亚型（SPRED1-3），Sprouty 家族有 4 个亚型（SPRY1-4）。人类 SPRED1 包含 444 个氨基酸。已确定 3 个功能域，即 N 端 EVH-1 域、中央 c-KIT 结合域（KBD）和 C 端 SPRY 相关域（SPR）（reviewed by Bundschu et al. 2007）。

大多数报道都集中于小鼠 Spred1 蛋白，关于人类 SPRED1 的数据非常有限。小鼠 Spred1 主要在大脑和一些胎儿组织中表达。在神经发生过程中，它富集于中枢神经系统的生殖区（Kato et al. 2003; Engelhardt et al. 2004; Phoenix and Temple 2010）。Spred1 可抑制大脑皮质祖细胞的自我更新和增殖，并维持脑室区的结构（Phoenix and Temple 2010）。Spred1 在白细胞介素-3 依赖性小鼠造血细胞系和骨髓肥大细胞中高度表达（Nonami et al. 2004）。

Spred1 是 Ras-MAPK 信号通路的负调控分子（Wakioka et al. 2001）。生长因子介导的 Spred1 表达可抑制生长因子刺激后 Raf 的磷酸化和活化，从而抑制 MAPK 的活化（图 31.2）。KBD 对 ERK

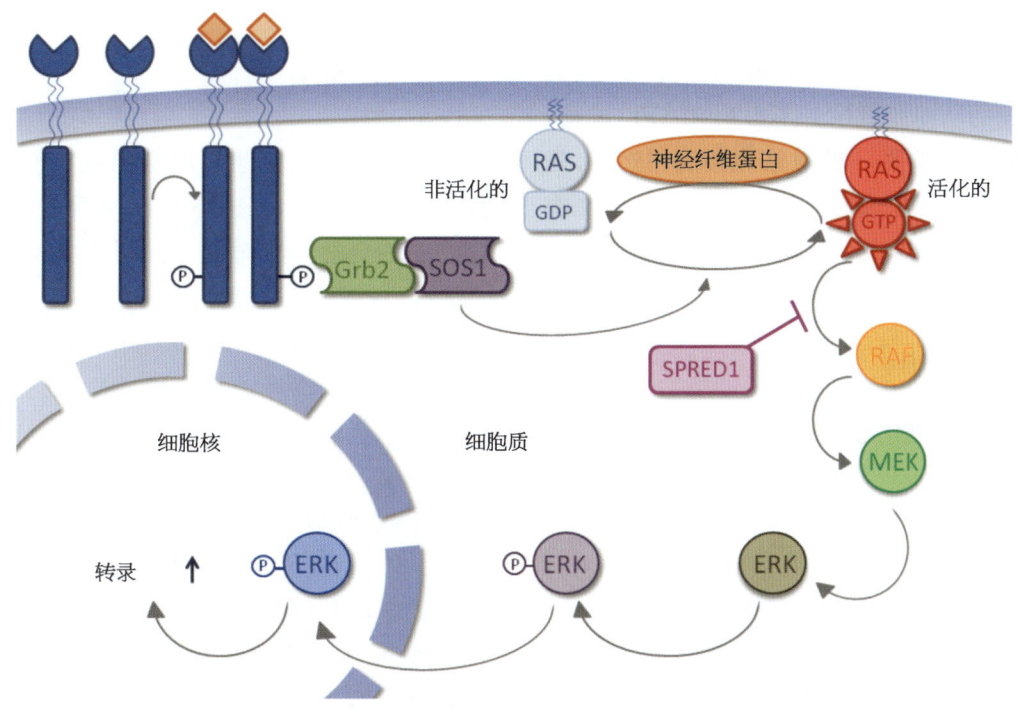

图 31.2 生长因子结合导致受体酪氨酸激酶生长因子受体二聚化。这导致受体磷酸化并激活适配蛋白(GRB2、SOS1)。活化的 RAS 与 GTP 结合,而非活化 RAS 则与 GDP 结合。神经纤维瘤蛋白刺激 RAS 固有的 GTP 酶活性,并激活 RAS 转换为与 GDP 结合的非活性形式。SPRED1 通过激活 GTP 结合的 RAS 从而抑制 RAF 的激活

的抑制并不是必不可少的,但对其有贡献(Wakioka et al. 2001;Nonami et al. 2004),其对 Akt 或 Rac 的激活没有影响。Spred1 定位于脂筏/洞穴小体,与洞穴素共同抑制 Erk 的活化(Nonami et al. 2005)。EVH-1 和 KBD 对肌动蛋白细胞骨架有影响,EVH-1 和 SPR 结构域会影响应力纤维的形成(Miyoshi et al. 2004)。

目前已发现多个 Spred1 的相互作用分子:如微管相关蛋白/微管亲和性调节激酶激活激酶(microtubule affinity-regulating kinase-activating kinase,MARKK)、睾丸特异性蛋白激酶(TESK1)(Johne et al. 2008)、成纤维细胞生长因子受体样-1(fibroblast growth factor receptor like-1,FGFRL1)(Zhuang et al. 2011)、DYRK1A(Li et al. 2010)和 SHP2(Quintanar-Audelo et al. 2011)。

有两种不同的微小 RNA 与 Spred1 有关,即 miR-126 和 miR-212。MiRNA-126 通过抑制 Spred1 的表达促进血管生成(Wang et al. 2008)。Spred1 负向调节肥大细胞活化,而肥大细胞活化受 miR126 调节(Ishizaki et al. 2011)。在长期摄入可卡因的大鼠背侧纹状体中检测到 miRNA-212 上调(Hollander et al. 2010)。MiRNA-212 通过抑制 Spred1 从而激活 Raf1 并放大 CREB-TORC 级联反应。

人类野生型 SPRED1 可抑制生长因子诱导的 RAS-MAPK 激活。EVH-1 和 SPR 结构域似乎都是这种抑制作用所必需的(Brems et al. 2007)。SPRED1 表达于人类黑色素细胞(Brems et al. 2007)。我们比较了对照组皮肤($SPRED1^{+/+}$)、正常皮肤($SPRED1^{+/-}$)和来自同一 Legius 综合征患者的咖啡牛奶斑($SPRED1^{-/-}$)的黑色素细胞培养物(Brems et al. 2007)。用干细胞因子刺激后,$SPRED1^{-/-}$ 黑色素细胞中活化的 MEK 和 ERK 水平最高。$SPRED1^{+/+}$ 黑色素细胞的 MEK 和 ERK 活化水平最低,$SPRED1^{+/-}$ 黑色素细胞则处于中等水平。

31.4.2 错义突变的功能分析

只有一小部分检测到的错义突变可被归类为致病性突变。我们建议结合家族分离数据、氨基酸进化保守性和两种不同的 MAPK 通路功能测试来对

SPRED1 错义突变进行分类(分类方法见在线数据库 http://www.lovd.nl/SPRED1)。有些错义突变在两种不同的功能测试中并不影响 MAPK 通路,但仍有可能通过影响另一种通路而致病。然而,目前所有与表型分离的已知家族性 *SPRED1* 错义突变和所有新发的错义突变都在至少两种 MAPK 途径功能测试中显示出功能缺陷。

31.4.3 小鼠模型

Spred1 蛋白在进化过程中高度保守,人与小鼠的蛋白质相似度为 93.5%。小鼠 *Spred1* mRNA 在胎儿脑、心、肺、肝和骨中表达(Engelhardt et al. 2004)。在成体组织中,*Spred1* 主要在大脑中表达(Kato et al. 2003;Engelhardt et al. 2004)。*Spred1* 基因敲除小鼠有生育能力,但体重较轻,脸部较短(Inoue et al. 2005,Brems et al. 2007)。

对 Spred1 小鼠模型进行了多项学习任务的海马依赖性学习和记忆研究(Denayer et al. 2008)。在隐藏版的莫里斯水迷宫中,$Spred1^{-/-}$ 小鼠的学习和记忆能力都有所下降。在视觉辨别任务(T 型迷宫)中,$Spred1^{-/-}$ 小鼠在视觉辨别训练的几乎所有阶段的表现都明显较差。在最后的混合试验演示中,$Spred1^{-/-}$ 小鼠没有表现出任何学习能力。$Spred1^{+/-}$ 小鼠的表现介于 $Spred1^{-/-}$ 和 $Spred1^{+/+}$ 小鼠之间。

对 *Spred1* 基因敲除小鼠海马脑切片的电生理记录发现了短期和长期突触可塑性缺陷(Denayer et al. 2008),包括 CA1 区 Schaffer 副线的长期电位(long-term potentiation,LTP)和长期抑制(long-term depression,LTD)缺陷。

这些发现与 $Nf1^{+/-}$ 小鼠的学习和突触可塑性缺陷相当(Cui et al. 2008),证实了 RAS-MAPK 通路在学习和记忆中的重要性。成年 $Nf1^{+/-}$ 小鼠的学习和突触可塑性缺陷可以通过洛伐他汀治疗得到有效缓解(Cui et al. 2008)。类似的实验在 *Spred1* 小鼠中尚未见报道。

31.5 管理和随访

Legius 综合征患者不会出现 NF1 中常见的肿瘤并发症。因此,采用不同的、强度较低的医疗随访似乎更为合适。然而,在撰写本章时,只获得了 159 名 Legius 综合征患者的临床数据。因此,有必要收集更多患者的信息,并对 Legius 综合征患者进行临床监测。由于临床数据有限,罕见的并发症可能会被遗漏。正确的诊断对预后、咨询和产前诊断具有重要意义。Legius 综合征的诊断可减轻家庭的心理负担,否则他们将面临更严重的 NF1 相关肿瘤并发症。不过,我们建议特别关注 Legius 综合征患儿潜在的学习和行为问题。我们希望临床试验能显示出针对 NF1 儿童认知和行为问题的特定治疗方法的益处。希望 NF1 和 Legius 综合征患儿都能获得此类特殊治疗。

在致病性 *NF1* 和 *SPRED1* 基因突变阴性的群体中,仍有一小部分未分类的家族性多发性咖啡牛奶斑患者。在散发性病例中,可能存在 *NF1* 基因突变的嵌合体,这一现象能够解释为何在白细胞中检测不到 *NF1* 基因突变的情况下患者仍表现出 NF1 症状(Maertens et al. 2007)。一些有多发性咖啡牛奶斑但没有 *NF1* 或 *SPRED1* 基因突变的患者可能存在与 RAS-MAPK 通路相关的基因突变,最近 *CBL* 突变相关综合征的病例证明了这一观点(Niemeyer et al. 2010;Pérez et al. 2010)。

致谢:HB 是 Flanders 研究基金会(FWO)在 KULeuven 大学的博士后研究员。本研究得到了 Flanders 研究基金会(Fonds voor Wetenschappelijk Onderzoek,FWO)-Vlaanderen(G.0578.06)(EL)、癌症基金会"Stichting tegen Kanker"(C.0011-204-208)(EL)和 KULeuven 的联合行动资助(GOA/11/010)的支持。

(孙家明,孙谛 译)

参考文献

[1] Batz C, Hasle H, Bergsträsser E, van den Heuvel-Eibrink MM, Zecca M, Niemeyer CM, Flotho C (2010) European Working Group of Myelodysplastic Syndromes in Childhood (EWOG-MDS) Does SPRED1 contribute to leukemogenesis in juvenile myelomonocytic leukemia (JMML)? Blood 115:2557-2558

[2] Brems H, Chmara M, Sahbatou M, Denayer E, Taniguchi K, Kato R, Somers R, Messiaen L, De Schepper S, Fryns JP, Cools J, Marynen P, Thomas G, Yoshimura A, Legius E (2007) Germline loss-of-function mutations in SPRED1 cause a neurofibromatosis 1-like phenotype. Nat Genet 33: 1538-1546

[3] Brems H, Beert E, de Ravel T, Legius E (2009) Mechanisms in the pathogenesis of malignant tumours in neurofibromatosis type 1. Lancet Oncol 10: 508-515

[4] Brems H, Legius E, Messiaen L (2012) Review and update of SPRED1 mutations causing Legius syndrome. Hum Mutat 33: 1538-1546

[5] Bundschu K, Walter U, Schuh K (2007) Getting a first clue about SPRED functions. Bioessays 29: 897-907

[6] Cui Y, Costa RM, Murphy GG, Elgersma Y, Zhu Y, Gutmann DH, Parada LF, Mody I, Silva AJ (2008). Neurofibromin regulation of ERK signaling modulates GABA release and learning. Cell 135: 549-60

[7] Denayer E, Ahmed T, Brems H, Van Woerden G, Borgesius NZ, Callaerts-Vegh Z, Yoshimura A, Hartmann D, Elgersma Y, D'Hooge R, Legius E, Balschun D (2008) Spred1 is required for synaptic plasticity and hippocampus-dependent learning. J Neurosci 28: 14443-14449

[8] Denayer E, Chmara M, Brems H, Kievit AM, van Bever Y, Van den Ouweland AM, Van Minkelen R, de Goede-Bolder A, Oostenbrink R, Lakeman P, Beert E, Ishizaki T, Mori T, Keymolen K, Van den Ende J, Mangold E, Peltonen S, Brice G, Rankin J, Van Spaendonck-Zwarts KY, Yoshimura A, Legius E (2011a) Legius syndrome in fourteen families. Hum Mutat 32: E1985-E1998

[9] Denayer E, Descheemaeker MJ, Stewart DR, Keymolen K, Plasschaert E, Ruppert SL, Snow J, Thurm AE, Joseph LA, Fryns JP, Legius E (2011b) Observations on intelligence and behavior in 15 patients with Legius syndrome. Am J Med Genet C Semin Med Genet 157: 123-128

[10] Engelhardt CM, Bundschu K, Messerschmitt M, Renné T, Walter U, Reinhard M, Schuh K (2004) Expression and subcellular localization of Spred proteins in mouse and human tissues. Histochem Cell Biol 122: 527-538

[11] Hollander JA, Im HI, Amelio AL, Kocerha J, Bali P, Lu Q, Willoughby D, Wahlestedt C, Conkright MD, Kenny PJ (2010) Striatal microRNA controls cocaine intake through CREB signalling. Nature 466: 197-202

[12] Huson SM, Compston DA, Clark P, Harper PS (1989) A genetic study of von Recklinghausen neurofibromatosis in south east Wales. I. Prevalence, fitness, mutation rate, and effect of parental transmission on severity. J Med Genet 26: 704-711

[13] Inoue H, Kato R, Fukuyama S, Nonami A, Taniguchi K, Matsumoto K, Nakano T, Tsuda M, Matsumura M, Kubo M, Ishikawa F, Moon BG, Takatsu K, Nakanishi Y, Yoshimura A (2005) Spred-1 negatively regulates allergen-induced airway eosinophilia and hyperresponsiveness. J Exp Med 201: 73-82

[14] Ishizaki T, Tamiya T, Taniguchi K, Morita R, Kato R, Okamoto F, Saeki K, Nomura M, Nojima Y, Yoshimura A (2011) miR126 positively regulates mast cell proliferation and cytokine production through suppressing Spred1. Genes Cells 16: 803-814

[15] Johne C, Matenia D, Li XY, Timm T, Balusamy K, Mandelkow EM (2008) Spred1 and TESK1-two new interaction partners of the kinase MARKK/TAO1 that link the microtubule and actin cytoskeleton. Mol Biol Cell 19: 1391-1403

[16] Kato R, Nonami A, Taketomi T, Wakioka T, Kuroiwa A, Matsuda Y, Yoshimura A (2003) Molecular cloning of mammalian Spred-3 which suppresses tyrosine kinase-mediated Erk activation. Biochem Biophys Res Commun 302: 767-772

[17] Laycock-van Spyk S, Jim HP, Thomas L, Spurlock G, Fares L, Palmer-Smith S, Kini U, Saggar A, Patton M, Mautner V, Pilz DT, Upadhyaya M (2011) Identification of five novel SPRED1 germline mutations in Legius syndrome. Clin Genet 80: 93-96

[18] Li D, Jackson RA, Yusoff P, Guy GR (2010) Direct association of Sprouty-related protein with an EVH1 domain (SPRED) 1 or SPRED2 with DYRK1A modifies substrate/kinase interactions. J Biol Chem 285: 35374-35385

[19] Maertens O, De Schepper S, Vandesompele J, Brems H, Heyns I, Janssens S, Speleman F, Legius E, Messiaen L (2007) Molecular dissection of isolated disease features in mosaic neurofibro-matosis type 1. Am J Hum Genet 81: 243-251

[20] Messiaen L, Yao S, Brems H, Callens T, Sathienkijkanchai A, Denayer E, Spencer E, Arn P, Babovic-Vuksanovic D, Bay C, Bobele G, Cohen BH, Escobar L, Eunpu D, Grebe T, Greenstein R, Hachen R, Irons M, Kronn D, Lemire E, Leppig K, Lim C, McDonald M, Narayanan V, Pearn A, Pedersen R, Powell B, Shapiro LR, Skidmore D, Tegay D, Thiese H, Zackai EH, Vijzelaar R, Taniguchi K, Ayada T, Okamoto F, Yoshimura A, Parret A, Korf B, Legius E (2009) Clinical and mutational spectrum of neurofibromatosis type 1-like syndrome. JAMA 302: 2111-2118

[21] Miyoshi K, Wakioka T, Nishinakamura H, Kamio M, Yang L, Inoue M, Hasegawa M, Yonemitsu Y, Komiya S, Yoshimura A (2004) The Sprouty-related protein, Spred, inhibits cell motility, metastasis, and Rho-mediated actin reorganization. Oncogene 23: 5567-55676

[22] Muram-Zborovski TM, Stevenson DA, Viskochil DH, Dries DC, Wilson AR, Mao R (2010) SPRED1 mutations in a neurofibromatosis clinic. J Child Neurol 25: 1203-1209

[23] Niemeyer CM, Kang MW, Shin DH, Furlan I, Erlacher M, Bunin NJ, Bunda S, Finklestein JZ, Sakamoto KM, Gorr TA, Mehta P, Schmid I, Kropshofer G, Corbacioglu S, Lang PJ, Klein C, Schlegel PG, Heinzmann A, Schneider M, Starý J, van den Heuvel-Eibrink MM, Hasle H, Locatelli F, Sakai D, Archambeault S, Chen L, Russell RC, Sybingco SS, Ohh M, Braun BS, Flotho C, Loh ML (2010) Germline CBL mutations cause developmental abnormalities and predispose to juvenile myelomonocytic leukemia. Nat Genet 42: 794-800

[24] No Authors (1988) National Institutes of Health Consensus Development Conference Statement. Bethesda, MD, USA, July 13-15, 1987. Neurofibromatosis 1: 172-178

[25] Nonami A, Kato R, Taniguchi K, Yoshiga D, Taketomi T, Fukuyama S, Harada M, Sasaki A, Yoshimura A (2004) Spred-1 negatively regulates interleukin-3-mediated ERK/mitogen-activated protein (MAP) kinase activation in hematopoietic cells. J Biol Chem 279: 52543-52551

[26] Nonami A, Taketomi T, Kimura A, Saeki K, Takaki H, Sanada T, Taniguchi K, Harada M, Kato R, Yoshimura A (2005) The Sprouty-related protein, Spred-1, localizes in a lipid raft/caveola and inhibits ERK activation in collaboration with caveolin-1. Genes Cells 10: 887-895

[27] Pasmant E, Sabbagh A, Hanna N, Masliah-Planchon J, Jolly E, Goussard P, Ballerini P, Cartault F, Barbarot S, Landman-Parker J, Soufir N, Parfait B, Vidaud M, Wolkenstein P, Vidaud D, France RN (2009a) SPRED1

germline mutations caused a neurofibromatosis type 1 overlapping phenotype. J Med Genet 46: 425-430

[28] Pasmant E, Ballerini P, Lapillonne H, Perot C, Vidaud D, Leverger G, Landman-Parker J (2009b) SPRED1 disorder and predisposition to leukemia in children. Blood 114: 1131

[29] Pérez B, Mechinaud F, Galambrun C, Ben Romdhane N, Isidor B, Philip N, Derain-Court J, Cassinat B, Lachenaud J, Kaltenbach S, Salmon A, Désirée C, Pereira S, Menot ML, Royer N, Fenneteau O, Baruchel A, Chomienne C, Verloes A, Cavé H (2010) Germline mutations of the *CBL* gene define a new genetic syndrome with predisposition to juvenile myelomonocytic leukaemia. J Med Genet 47: 686-691

[30] Phoenix TN, Temple S (2010) Spred1, a negative regulator of Ras-MAPK-ERK, is enriched in CNS germinal zones, dampens NSC proliferation, and maintains ventricular zone structure. Genes Dev 24: 45-56

[31] Quintanar-Audelo M, Yusoff P, Sinniah S, Chandramouli S, Guy GR (2011) Sprouty-related Ena/vasodilator-stimulated phosphoprotein homology 1-domain-containing protein (SPRED1), a tyrosine-protein phosphatase non-receptor type 11 (SHP2) substrate in the Ras/extracellular signal-regulated kinase (ERK) pathway. J Biol Chem 286: 23102-23112

[32] Spencer E, Davis J, Mikhail F, Fu C, Vijzelaar R, Zackai EH, Feret H, Meyn MS, Shugar A, Bellus G, Kocsis K, Kivirikko S, Pöyhönen M, Messiaen L (2011) Identification of *SPRED1* deletions using RT-PCR, multiplex ligation-dependent probe amplification and quantitative PCR. Am J Med Genet A 155A: 1352-1359

[33] Spurlock G, Bennett E, Chuzhanova N, Thomas N, Jim HP, Side L, Davies S, Haan E, Kerr B, Huson SM, Upadhyaya M (2009) *SPRED1* mutations (Legius syndrome): another clinically useful genotype for dissecting the neurofibromatosis type 1 phenotype. J Med Genet 46: 431-437

[34] Stevenson D, Viskochil D (2009) Pigmentary findings in neurofibromatosis type 1-like syndrome (Legius syndrome): potential diagnostic dilemmas. JAMA 302: 2150-2151

[35] Upadhyaya M (2008) 13th Annual European Neurofibromatosis Meeting, Killarney, Ireland Wakioka T, Sasaki A, Kato R, Shouda T, Matsumoto A, Miyoshi K, Tsuneoka M, Komiya S, Baron R, Yoshimura A (2001) Spred is a Sprouty-related suppressor of Ras signalling. Nature 412: 647-651

[36] Wang S, Aurora AB, Johnson BA, Qi X, McAnally J, Hill JA, Richardson JA, Bassel-Duby R, Olson EN (2008) The endothelial-specific microRNA miR-126 governs vascular integrity and angiogenesis. Dev Cell 15: 261-271

[37] Zenker M (2011) Clinical manifestations of mutations in RAS and related intracellular signal transduction factors. Curr Opin Pediatr 23: 443-451

[38] Zhuang L, Villiger P, Trueb B (2011) Interaction of the receptor FGFRL1 with the negative regulator Spred1. Cell Signal 23: 1496-1504

第32章 RAS 病:Ras/MAPK 通路失调的综合征
The RASopathies: Syndromes of Ras/MAPK Pathway Dysregulation

William E. Tidyman and Katherine A. Rauen

32.1 RAS 病

RAS 病是一类由编码 Ras/丝裂原活化蛋白激酶(mitogenactivated protein kinase,MAPK)通路成分的基因发生胚系突变引起的发育性疾病。Ras/MAPK 通路是研究得最透彻的信号转导途径之一,在细胞周期调控、分化、增殖和细胞衰老中起关键作用,这些过程对于正常哺乳动物的发育至关重要(图 32.1)。因此,不难理解其调节失常可能对发育产生深远影响。这些 RAS 病可表现各异。然而,由于 Ras 途径调节失常的机制相同,它们具有许多重叠特征,包括颅面畸形,心脏畸形,皮肤、骨骼和眼部异常,神经认知障碍,低肌张力以及罹患癌症的风险增加。总体而言,RAS 病是已知的大的畸形综合征群之一,1 000 个人中就可能有 1 个人罹患 RAS 病。1 型神经纤维瘤病(NF1)是第一个被确定为由 Ras/MAPK 途径中基因种系突变引起的综合征(Cawthon et al. 1990;Viskochil et al. 1990;Wallace et al. 1990),此后又识别出许多其他综合

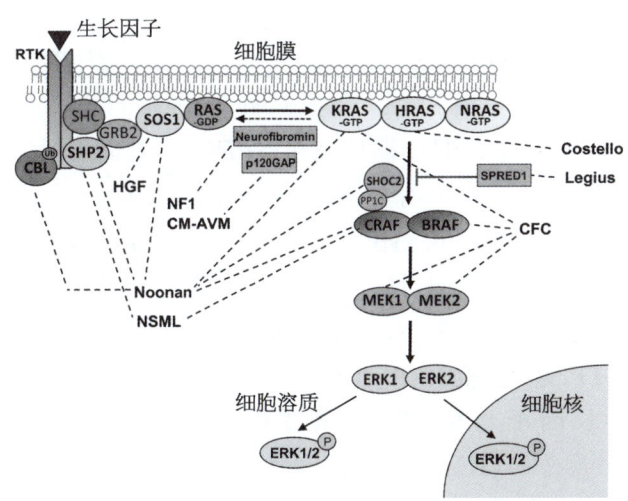

图 32.1 Ras/丝裂原活化蛋白激酶(MAPK)信号转导通路。MAPK 信号通路的蛋白激酶对细胞增殖、分化、运动、细胞凋亡和衰老至关重要。RAS 病是由 Ras/MAPK 通路中的各种基因突变所致(用虚线表示)。这些综合征包括:努南综合征、多发性雀斑样痣努南综合征(NSML)、1 型遗传性牙龈纤维瘤病(HGF)、1 型神经纤维瘤病(NF1)、毛细血管畸形-小静脉畸形(CM-AVM)、Costello 综合征、心-面-皮综合征(CFC)和 Legius 综合征

W. E. Tidyman
Department of Orofacial Science, University of California, San Francisco, CA, USA

K. A. Rauen
Department of Pediatrics, Division of Medical Genetics, University of California, San Francisco, CA, USA

UCSF Helen Diller Family Comprehensive Cancer Center, 2340 Sutter Street, Room S429, Box 0706, San Francisco, CA 94115, USA
e-mail: rauenk@peds.ucsf.edu

M. Upadhyaya and D. N. Cooper (eds.), *Neurofibromatosis Type 1*,
DOI 10.1007/978-3-642-32864-0_32, # Springer-Verlag Berlin Heidelberg 2012

征,这些综合征包括① 由 PTPN11 (Tartaglia et al. 2001)、SOS1 (Roberts et al. 2007; Tartaglia et al. 2007)、RAF1 (Pandit et al. 2007; Razzaque et al. 2007)、KRAS (Schubbert et al. 2006)、NRAS (Cirstea et al. 2010)、SHOC2 (Cordeddu et al. 2009)和 CBL (Martinelli et al. 2010; Niemeyer et al. 2010)的激活突变引起的努南综合征(Noonan syndrome, NS);② 由 PTPN11 (Digilio et al. 2002)和 RAF1 (Pandit et al. 2007)突变引起的多发性雀斑样痣努南综合征;③ 由 RASA1 基因单倍体不足引起的毛细血管畸形-动静脉畸形(Eerola et al. 2003);④ 由 HRAS 激活突变引起的 Costello 综合征(Aoki et al. 2005);⑤ BRAF (Niihori et al. 2006; Rodriguez-Viciana et al. 2006b)和 MEK1/MEK2 (Rodriguez-Viciana et al. 2006b)激活突变引起的心-面-皮综合征(cardio-facio-cutaneous syndrome, CFC);⑥ 以及由 SPRED1 基因失活突变引起的 Legius 综合征(Brems et al. 2007)。

Ras/MAPK 途径由细胞外生长因子激活,在发育中起关键作用(图 32.1)。Ras 基因是多基因家族,包括 HRAS、NRAS 和 KRAS。Ras 蛋白是小 GTP 酶,是细胞内的重要信号枢纽。Ras 蛋白通过生长因子与酪氨酸激酶受体(receptor tyrosine kinase, RTK)、G 蛋白偶联受体、细胞因子受体和细胞外基质受体结合而被激活。Ras 蛋白存在两种状态,与 GTP 结合时处于活跃状态,和 GDP 结合时则呈失活状态。RAS 蛋白的激活通过 RTK 与生长因子结合引起的 RTK 自磷酸化,以及与接头蛋白 GRB2 相互作用。GRB2 与 SOS 结合,随后被募集到质膜。SOS 蛋白是鸟嘌呤核苷酸交换因子(guanosine nucleotide exchange factor, GEF),可促进 Ras 将 GDP 转化为 GTP,导致活性 GTP 结合形式的 Ras 增加。MAPK 途径是 Ras 的关键下游信号级联中的一个。活跃的 Ras 导致途径中的第一个 MAPK 激酶激酶激活,即 Raf[ARAF、BRAF 和(或)CRAF]。Raf 磷酸化并激活 MEK1 和(或)MEK2(MAPK 激酶),后者进一步磷酸化并激活 ERK1 和(或)ERK2。ERK1 和 ERK2 是最终的效应物,对大量下游分子(包括细胞核和细胞质中的分子)发挥作用。ERK1/2 底物包括核成分、转录因

子、膜蛋白和蛋白激酶,这些底物控制关键的细胞功能,包括细胞周期进程、分化和细胞生长(Yoon and Seger 2006)。Ras/MAPK 途径在肿瘤发生中的研究非常广泛,因此其调节失常是癌症的主要原因之一。在 20% 的恶性肿瘤中可发现 RAS 体细胞突变,因此,RAS 病作为一个整体被认为是癌症综合征,大多数与 RAS 病相关的突变可导致信号通路激活增强或失调(Bos 1989)。然而,生物化学研究表明,该途径中新发现的胚系突变的大部分并不像肿瘤发生相关突变那样具有强烈的激活作用。这可能是因为当发生胚系突变时,常出现胚胎致死。

32.2　1 型神经纤维瘤病:第一个 RAS 病

1 型神经纤维瘤病(NF1)是一种常染色体显性疾病,新生儿罹患率大约为 1/3 000,其中约一半的 NF1 突变源自父母[见综述 Williams et al. (2009)]。NF1 的临床诊断基于临床表现——存在咖啡牛奶斑、皱褶部位雀斑、神经纤维瘤和丛状神经纤维瘤、虹膜 Lisch 结节、骨骼发育异常、视神经通路胶质瘤和(或)一级亲属患有 NF1(图 32.2),这些

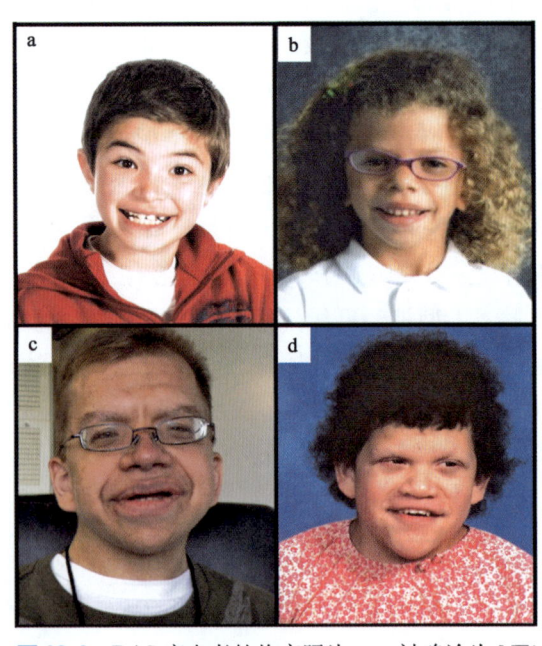

图 32.2　RAS 病患者的临床照片。a. 被确诊为 NF1 的 7 岁男孩。b. 7 岁女孩,努南综合征,携带 PTPN11 基因突变。c. Costello 综合征的 27 岁男性,携带常见的 p.G12S HRAS 突变。d. 心-面-皮综合征的 14 岁女孩,携带 1 个新发 BRAF 突变

是 NF1 最常见的相关症状和体征。NF1 患者可能还有其他表现，包括心脏畸形、心血管疾病、血管病、高血压、维生素 D 缺乏、脑发育异常和癫痫。此外，患者可能具有类似努南综合征的颅面畸形、轻度神经认知障碍以及发展为某些恶性肿瘤的倾向（Huffmeier et al. 2006；Stevenson et al. 2006）。节段性 NF1 和镶嵌型 NF1 并不罕见，生殖细胞嵌合现象也有所报道。

NF1 是第一个与 Ras/MAPK 途径种系突变相关的多发性先天异常综合征。NF1 由 *NF1* 基因突变引起，约一半的突变为新发突变（Cawthon et al. 1990；Viskochil et al. 1990；Wallace et al. 1990）。*NF1* 编码神经纤维瘤蛋白，一种 RasGAP，即 Ras 的 GTP 酶激活蛋白，是 Ras 的负调控因子（图 32.1；表 32.1）。*NF1* 的错义突变导致神经纤维瘤蛋白的功能丧失，造成细胞内单倍体剂量不足，即降低了 RasGTP 酶活性，从而导致与 GTP 结合的活跃状态 Ras 总体增加。

表 32.1 RAS/MAPK 通路相关遗传综合征

综合征	RAS 通路基因	染色体位置	蛋白质	蛋白质功能	参考文献
1 型神经纤维瘤病	*NF1*	17q11.2	神经纤维瘤蛋白	RasGAP	Cawthon 等（1990），Viskochil 等（1990），Wallace 等（1990）
努南综合征	*PTPN11*	12q24.1	SHP2	磷酸酯酶	Tartaglia 等（2001）
	SOS1	2p22.1	SOS1	RasGEF	Roberts 等（2007）
	RAF1	3p25.1	CRAF	激酶	Tartaglia 等（2007）
	KRAS	12p12.1	KRAS	GTPase	Pandit 等（2007）
	NRAS	1p13.2	NRAS	GTPase	Cirstea 等（2010）
	SHOC2	10q25.2	SHOC2	支架蛋白	Cordeddu 等（2009）
	CBL	11q23.3	CBL	E3 泛素连接酶	Martinelli 等（2010），Niemeyer 等（2010）
多发性痣样努南综合征	*PTPN11*	12q24.1	SHP2	磷酸酯酶	Digilio 等（2002）
	RAF1	3p25.1	RAF1/CRAF	激酶	Pandit 等（2007）
1 型遗传性牙龈纤维瘤病	*SOS1*	2p22.1	SOS1	RasGEF	Hart 等（2002）
毛细血管畸形-房室畸形	*RASA1*	5q14.3	p120Gap	RasGAP	Eerola 等（2003）
Costello 综合征	*HRAS*	11p15.5	HRAS	GTPase	Aoki 等（2005）
心-面-皮综合征	*BRAF*	7q34	BRAF	激酶	Niihori 等（2006），Rodriguez-Viciana 等（2006b）
	MAP2K1	15q22.31	MEK1	激酶	Rodriguez-Viciana 等（2006b）
	MAP2K2	19p13.3	MEK2	激酶	Rodriguez-Viciana 等（2006b）
	KRAS	12p12.1	KRAS	GTPase	Niihori 等（2006）
Legius 综合征	*SPRED1*	15q14	SPRED1	Sprouty 相关	Brems 等（2007）

NF1 是一种遗传性癌症综合征[见综述 Brems et al. (2009)]。NF1 患者相比普通人群更容易罹患恶性肿瘤。在儿童中，恶性肿瘤包括视神经通路胶质瘤、横纹肌肉瘤（rhabdomyosarcoma, RMS）、神经母细胞瘤和青少年性骨髓单核细胞白血病（juvenile myelomonocytic leukemia, JMML）；而在成人中，恶性肿瘤包括恶性周围神经鞘膜瘤、胃肠道间质瘤、生长抑素瘤、嗜铬细胞瘤和乳腺癌。

32.3 Legius 综合征

Legius 综合征（Legius Syndrome，正式名称为 NF1 样综合征）是一种新发现的常染色体显性遗传疾病。它与 NF1 以及其他 RAS 病共享许多相似的表型特征。患者可能有咖啡牛奶斑、皮肤皱褶处雀斑、轻度神经认知障碍和巨头症，以及部分患者具有类似努南综合征的颅面畸形。然而，NF1 常见的肿瘤特征如神经纤维瘤、丛状神经纤维瘤、虹膜 Lisch 结节和中枢神经系统肿瘤似乎与该综合征无关。Legius 综合征是由 *SPRED1* 基因的杂合失活突变引起（Brems et al. 2007）（图 32.1；表 32.1）。*SPRED1* 编码 SPRED1 蛋白，该蛋白质具有一个与 SPROUTY 相关的 N 端 EVH1 结构域，作为 Ras 的负调节因子，通过抑制 Raf 的磷酸化来发挥功能（Wakioka et al. 2001）。大多数与 Legius 综合征相关的 *SPRED1* 突变会产生截短蛋白，导致 SPRED1 功能丧失并引起 Ras/MAPK 通路的信号失调。尽管已有若干患者系列的研究报告，但仍不清楚携带 *SPRED1* 胚系突变的个体是否更容易罹患癌症（Denayer et al. 2011）。

32.4 努南综合征

努南综合征（Noonan syndrome，NS）是一种常染色体显性遗传病，患病率为 1/2 000~1/1 000。NS 的临床表现具有广泛的变异性，但通常具有一些显著的颅面部特征，包括宽额、眼距增宽、眼裂向下倾斜以及耳朵低位后旋（图 32.2）。其他重要的表型特征包括先天性心脏缺陷、身材矮小、出血性疾病和不同程度的神经认知发育迟缓[见综述 Romano et al. (2010)]。此外，NS 患者罹患癌症概率增加。目前已知有 7 个基因与 NS 相关：*PTPN11*（Tartaglia et al. 2001）、*KRAS*（Schubbert et al. 2006）、*NRAS*（Cirstea et al. 2010）、*SOS1*（Roberts et al. 2007；Tartaglia et al. 2007）、*RAF1*（Pandit et al. 2007；Razzaque et al. 2007）、*SHOC2*（Cordeddu et al. 2009）和 *CBL*（Martinelli et al. 2010；Niemeyer et al. 2010）。这些基因均存在杂合性种系突变，并编码 Ras/MAPK 信号通路的各种组成部分或相关蛋白质（图 32.1，表 32.1）。

PTPN11 是 NS 中最常见的突变基因，约占所有 NS 病例的 50%（Tartaglia et al. 2001）。*PTPN11* 编码的 SHP2 蛋白是一个非受体蛋白酪氨酸磷酸酶，包含 N 端和 C 端的 SH2 结构域以及催化蛋白酪氨酸磷酸酶（PTP）结构域。大多数导致 NS 的 *PTPN11* 错义突变集中在 N-SH2 和 PTP 结构域之间的相互作用区域。该区域的突变破坏了催化活性形式的稳定性，导致蛋白质从活性构象转向非活性构象的能力受损（Keilhack et al. 2005；Tartaglia et al. 2006），导致 Ras/MAPK 信号通路的过度激活。

SOS1 错义突变是导致 NS 的第二常见原因，约占 NS 病例的 15%（Roberts et al. 2007；Tartaglia et al. 2007）。*SOS1* 编码 RasGEF（鸟嘌呤核苷酸交换因子）蛋白 SOS1，该蛋白质负责促进 Ras 从非活性 GDP 结合态转变为活性 GTP 结合态。大多数 SOS1 基因的错义突变发生在特定氨基酸残基的密码子中，这些密码子编码能够稳定蛋白质处于抑制状态的蛋白质，这些突变破坏了 SOS1 RasGEF 活性的自我抑制，导致 SOS1 功能增强以及 Ras/MAPK 信号通路的过度激活。

KRAS 突变是 NS 的一个罕见原因（Schubbert et al. 2006）。*KRAS* 有两个剪接变体，其中 *KRASA* 在组织特异性表达和发育阶段限制性表达，*KRASB* 则在所有组织中广泛表达。导致 NS 的 *KRAS* 突变通过两种不同机制增强了 Ras/MAPK 信号通路的信号传递：一种是通过降低 GTP 酶活性（Schubbert et al. 2006, 2007），另一种是干扰 KRAS 与鸟嘌呤核苷酸的结合。这些突变引起的 Ras/MAPK 通路激活程度不及致癌 *KRAS* 的激活突变（Schubbert et al. 2006)。

NRAS 突变也在少数 NS 病例中被发现(Cirstea et al. 2010)。这些突变位于或靠近 NRAS 的开关Ⅱ区域,可能影响 GTP 酶功能,并已被证明可导致 MEK 和 ERK 的磷酸化增强。

RAF1 突变也是 NS 的一个致病原因(Pandit et al. 2007；Razzaque et al. 2007)。RAF1 编码的 RAF1(又称 CRAF)是一种丝氨酸/苏氨酸激酶,是 Ras 的直接下游效应器之一。大多数与 NS 相关的 RAF1 突变集中在两个区域：一个是位于 S259 附近的保守区域 2,另一个是围绕激活段的保守区域 3。这些突变导致 CRAF 功能的增强,因为 S259 和 S621 残基的磷酸化负责 CRAF 的调控。

最近发现一种罕见的努南综合征(NS)亚型,其具有一种独特的表型特征——松弛性附着发。这种表型是由 SHOC2 基因中的一个单点突变引起的,该突变导致 p.S2G 的氨基酸替换(Cordeddu et al. 2009)。SHOC2 即秀丽隐杆线虫(C. elegans)中的 SOC-2 同源基因,编码一种几乎完全由富含亮氨酸的重复序列组成的蛋白质。SHOC2 作为一种支架蛋白,将 RAS 与其下游效应蛋白 RAF1 连接(Rodriguez-Viciana et al. 2006a)。SHOC2 广泛表达,作为蛋白磷酸酶 1(PP1C)的调节亚单位,并介导 PP1C 转位至细胞膜,促进 PP1C 对 RAF1 的 Ser259 位点进行去磷酸化,这一过程对于 RAF1 的膜转位和催化活性是必需的。独特的 p.S2G 突变导致一个 14 碳饱和脂肪酸链——肉豆蔻酸,异常地附加到 SHOC2 的 N 端甘氨酸上。这种突变引起 SHOC2 异常地转位到细胞膜上,从而导致 PP1C 对 RAF1 的去磷酸化延长,导致 MAPK 信号通路的持续激活(Cordeddu et al. 2009)。

另外一种罕见的努南综合征(NS)发生原因是 CBL 突变,全称为肿瘤抑制基因 casitas B-lineage lymphoma (CBL)(Martinelli et al. 2010；Niemeyer et al. 2010)。这些患者还可能出现幼年期骨髓增生性疾病(JMML)在内的骨髓增生性疾病,这种情况也可以在 NF1 以及 NS 中观察到。CBL 基因编码一种 E3 泛素连接酶,它在受体酪氨酸激酶(RTK)激活后的信号转导中起到负调控作用,促使泛素与激活的 RTK 结合,这对受体的内化和降解至关重要(Dikic and Schmidt 2007)。CBL 基因突变导致活化的 RTK 的降解速率降低,因此这些突变总体上增加了 ERK 的活化水平。

32.5 多发性雀斑样痣努南综合征(豹斑综合征)

努南综合征合并多发性雀斑(Noonan syndrome with multiple lentigines，NSML),以前也被称为"LEOPARD"综合征,是一种罕见的常染色体显性遗传病。患者表现出努南综合征的颅面特征以及多发性雀斑、心电图异常、眼距宽、肺动脉瓣狭窄、生殖器异常、发育迟缓和耳聋。NSML 和努南综合征是等位基因疾病,由相同基因 PTPN11(Digilio et al. 2002；Legius et al. 2002)和 RAF1(Pandit et al. 2007)的不同杂合错义突变引起(图 32.1,表 32.1)。最常见的 NSML 相关的 PTPN11 突变影响催化型 PTP 结构域中的氨基酸,导致体外 SHP2 催化活性降低,从而引起功能缺失(Digilio et al. 2002；Kontaridis et al. 2006)。然而,果蝇模型的研究表明,NSML 突变型 SHP2 蛋白的残余催化活性足以在发育过程中产生功能获得性表型,这是由于该突变引起了 MAPK 信号通路的持续激活(Oishi et al. 2009)。

32.6 毛细血管畸形-动静脉畸形综合征

毛细血管畸形-动静脉畸形综合征(capillary malformation-arteriovenous malformation syndrome, CM-AVM)也是一种 RAS 病,是一种常染色体显性遗传性疾病。其特征是多发性的毛细血管畸形,并且可能伴有动静脉畸形和瘘管形成[见综述 Boon et al. (2005)]。CM-AVM 综合征由 RASA1 基因(Eerola et al. 2003)的杂合失活突变引起,该基因像 NF1 基因一样,编码一个 RasGAP 蛋白,具体来说是 p120-RasGTP 酶激活蛋白(p120-RasGAP)(图 32.1,表 32.1)。p120-RasGAP 蛋白的 N 末端包含 Src 同源区域,C 末端则含有 Pleckstrin 同源域和 RasGTP 酶激活域。RASA1 蛋白类似于神经纤维瘤蛋白(neurofibromin, NF1 的产物),能够将活跃的GTP结合型Ras转换为不活跃的GDP结合型Ras。RASA1是Ras/MAPK信号转导通路的负调节因子,这一通路对细胞的生长、分化和增殖至关重要。该综合征的主要特征是多发性畸形,即动静脉畸形可以发生在皮肤、肌肉、骨骼等多种组织中,以及心脏、大脑等各种内脏器官中。此外,RASA1突变还与Parkes-Weber综合征和Galen静脉畸形的发生有关(Revencu et al. 2008)。p120-RasGAP的单倍体不足会导致Ras-GTP的降解减少,因此增加了Ras/MAPK信号通路的活性。CM-AVM是一种常染色体显性遗传疾病,大多数患者有一个患病的父亲或母亲。但是,还有大约30%的病例是由新发突变引起。突变的类型多种多样,以无义突变、框移突变或剪接突变为主。除了动静脉畸形,患者还可能出现法洛四联症、房间隔缺损、心脏瓣膜异常等心血管畸形。具体机制尚不明确,CM-AVM患者与NF1和NF2患者类似,面临罹患肿瘤风险增加的可能性。

32.7　Costello综合征

Costello综合征(Costello syndrome,CS)比NF1更为罕见,但它也是一种多发性先天性异常综合征,与NF1有许多重叠的特征。尽管如此,CS的诊断标准与NF1完全不同,因此两者不易混淆。CS患者具有明显的发育异常性颅面特征,特别是在新生儿期出现生长发育迟缓、心脏、肌肉骨骼、外胚层和眼部异常、肌肉张力低下以及神经认知发育迟缓(图32.2)[见综述Rauen(2007)]。这些表型特征通常在围产期即显现,孕妇可能会出现羊水过多,许多胎儿会早产,并且出生体重大于正常水平。面部特征粗糙,通常包括前额突出的巨头畸形、眼角内侧的内眦赘皮、眼裂下斜、短鼻、鼻梁塌陷且鼻基部宽、耳朵位置较低、耳轮增厚且耳垂后旋。面颊可能显得丰满,嘴巴较大,嘴唇丰厚。与NF1类似,患者的皮肤表现有助于CS的临床诊断,表现为手背和足背皮肤松弛、多皱纹以及掌底和足底纹路深(Siegel et al. 2012)。大多数CS患者存在心脏异常,包括肥厚型心肌病(hypertrophic cardiomyopathy,HCM)、瓣膜异常、室间隔缺损以及心律失常(Lin et al. 2011)。

在早期婴儿期,可出现典型表现,即生长发育迟缓、胃肠功能障碍如胃食管反流、口腔回避和便秘。因此,大多数患者需要通过胃造口管进行喂养。

HRAS基因中的杂合激活性生殖系突变导致Costello综合征(CS)(Aoki et al. 2005)(图32.1,表32.1)。突变的分布图显示,超过80%的CS患者存在p.G12S的氨基酸替换,其次是最常见的p.G12A替换[见综述Tidyman and Rauen (2008)]。这些氨基酸替换破坏了鸟嘌呤核苷酸的结合,导致内源性GTP酶以及GAP诱导的GTP酶活性降低,从而使Ras保持在活跃状态(Gibbs et al. 1984)。此外,HRAS中也可能出现一些较少见的突变,包括p.K117R(Kerr et al. 2006)和p.A146T(Pandit et al. 2007),这些突变可能引发非典型表型。值得注意的是,在CS中最常见的氨基酸突变位置——第12位和第13位,也是致癌Ras中最常见的突变位置。Ras基因在第12、13或61位的突变约占所有肿瘤的20%(Bos 1989)。与NF1类似,CS患者面临着更高的肿瘤发生风险,包括良性和恶性肿瘤。CS中常见的良性肿瘤是皮肤乳头状瘤(Siegel et al. 2012)。大约72%的CS患者会出现皮肤乳头状瘤,其发病年龄范围从婴儿期到22岁。皮肤乳头状瘤最常见的位置是鼻部,也可以发生在身体的任何部位。重要的是,这些肿瘤在其他RAS病中并不常见。令人担忧的是,15%~20%的CS患者会发展为恶性肿瘤,其中最常见的肿瘤包括横纹肌肉瘤(RMS)、移行细胞癌(transitional cell carcinoma,TCC)和神经母细胞瘤(Gripp 2005)。有趣的是,RMS和神经母细胞瘤是儿童常见的恶性肿瘤,而TCC则不常见。CS中最常见的恶性肿瘤是胚胎性RMS,并且报告了HRAS野生型等位基因丧失的现象(Estep et al. 2006)。

Costello综合征的生殖系突变呈现出父源偏倚(Sol-Church et al. 2006;Zampino et al. 2007)。与NF1类似,Costello综合征中也发现了体细胞嵌合体,但是极为罕见(Gripp et al. 2006)。此外,还有一例报道报告了常染色体显性遗传的情况(Sol-Church et al. 2009),以及生殖细胞嵌合体的现象(Gripp et al. 2011)。

32.8 心-面-皮综合征

心-面-皮综合征（cardio-facio-cutaneous Syndrome，CFC）是一种罕见的疾病，类似于 Costello 综合征(CS)，与努南综合征(NS)、Costello 综合征(CS)以及 1 型神经纤维瘤病(NF1)出现重叠的表型特征。CFC 患者通常表现出类似努南综合征的面部特征，包括巨头、宽额、双侧颞部变窄、眼眶上缘发育不良、下斜眼裂伴眼睑下垂、短鼻伴有塌陷的鼻梁和前突的鼻孔、高拱的上颚、低位、向后旋转的耳朵及突出的耳轮（图 32.2）。外胚层表现通常包括稀疏的卷发、稀疏的眉毛和睫毛、角化过度、毛囊角化病、血管瘤、鱼鳞病以及逐渐形成的色素痣（Siegel et al. 2011）。心脏异常的发生概率与努南综合征、Costello 综合征相似，其中最常见的心脏异常包括肺动脉狭窄、室间隔缺损和肥厚型心肌病（HCM）。肌肉骨骼异常也很常见。此外，眼异常包括斜视、眼球震颤、近视、远视和散光。婴儿期通常表现为生长迟缓和胃肠功能障碍，如胃食管反流、呕吐、口腔回避和便秘。神经系统异常也普遍存在，表现为肌张力低下、运动发育迟缓、癫痫、语言发育迟缓、学习障碍（Yoon et al. 2007）。

CFC 综合征与 4 个编码 Ras/MAPK 通路下游蛋白的基因相关联：*BRAF*（Niihori et al. 2006；Rodriguez-Viciana et al. 2006b）、*MAP2K1* 和 *MAP2K2*（Rodriguez-Viciana et al. 2006b），以及 *KRAS*（Niihori et al. 2006）（表 32.1）。*KRAS* 在 CFC 中的作用仍不明确，因为临床诊断为 NS 的个体中也发现了 *KRAS* 突变（Schubbert et al. 2006）。在具有阳性突变的 CFC 患者中，大约 75％是 *BRAF* 杂合突变[见综述 Tidyman and Rauen (2009)]。*BRAF* 是一种丝氨酸/苏氨酸蛋白激酶，是 Ras 的直接下游效应器之一。BRAF 是已知的致癌蛋白，在多种癌症中均报道有 *BRAF* 体细胞突变，包括甲状腺癌、肺癌、卵巢癌和结肠直肠癌；然而，大多数与 CFC 相关的 *BRAF* 突变是新发现的。与癌症相关突变不同，大多数 CFC 中的 *BRAF* 突变聚集在第 6 号外显子的半胱氨酸富集结构域和蛋白激酶结构域。CFC 中最常见的 *BRAF* 突变是 p. Q257R。*BRAF* 突变蛋白的体外功能分析表明，大多数突变蛋白激酶活性增强；然而，少数突变蛋白激酶活性受损（Niihori et al. 2006；Rodriguez-Viciana et al. 2006b）。目前已证实，BRAF 激酶活性受损也会通过 CRAF 促进 MAPK 通路的信号转导（Heidorn et al. 2010）。CFC 突变的进一步体内研究表明，无论是激酶活性增强还是激酶活性受损的突变，在斑马鱼模型中均导致类似的 MAPK 信号转导异常表型（Anastasaki et al. 2009）。在已诊断的 CFC（心-面-皮综合征）患者中，大约 25％的个体存在 *MAP2K1*（*MEK1*）和 *MAP2K2*（*MEK2*）中的杂合错义突变[见综述 Tidyman and Rauen (2009)]。MEK1 和 MEK2 是苏氨酸/酪氨酸激酶，两个亚型均能磷酸化和激活 ERK1 和 ERK2。MEK 功能研究表明，在所有已确定的 CFC 突变中，所有这些突变蛋白均具有激活性（Rodriguez-Viciana et al. 2006b；Anastasaki et al. 2009）。

CFC 综合征以常染色体显性方式遗传（Rauen et al. 2010）。然而，在大多数情况下，CFC 综合征是由于新发的显性突变导致的，因为 CFC 综合征患者很少会生育后代。绝大多数 CFC 综合征患者都是由于新发突变引起而致病。尽管引起 CFC 的突变位于一个众所周知的致癌途径中，但目前仍不清楚 CFC 患者是否具有恶性肿瘤发生增加的风险。但 CFC 综合征显然不具有 NS、CS 和 NF1 那样的恶性肿瘤风险（Rauen et al. 2010；Kratz et al. 2011）。

32.9 遗传性牙龈纤维瘤病

遗传性牙龈纤维瘤病（hereditary gingival fibromatosis，HGF）与上述综合征表现不同，但考虑 RAS 病的完整性，也被归类为 RAS 病（Hart et al. 1998）。HGF 是一种罕见的、缓慢进展的良性角化牙龈纤维过度生长性疾病。由于其遗传异质性，HGF 的遗传方式既有常染色体显性，也有隐性。存在一种非常罕见的常染色体显性类型，即 1 型 HGF，是由 *SOS1* 基因的插入突变引起（Hart et al. 2002）（图 32.1，表 32.1）。这种罕见的 SOS1 插入突变导致了移码，即产生了 22 个新的氨基酸残基。然而，在产生一个提前终止密码子之前，该突变会使

C-末端的四个富含脯氨酸的 SH3 结合结构域被废除,这些结构域对 GRB2 结合至关重要(Hart et al. 2002)。突变 SOS1 蛋白体外表达显示,截短蛋白定位于细胞质膜上,但无生长因子结合。这导致了 Ras 激活和 Ras/MAPK 信号通路的持续信号转导(Jang et al. 2007)。迄今为止,与 HGF1 相关的新发 SOS1 突变尚未报道任何发育影响,这与 NS 相关的激活 SOS1 突变不同。然而,有趣的是,我们观察到许多 RAS 病患者也出现了非药物诱导的牙龈增生。

32.10 结论

RAS 病是由编码 Ras/MAPK 通路成分的种系突变引起,突显了该信号转导途径在胚胎发育和出生后生长中的关键作用。这些突变导致 Ras/MAPK 信号转导途径的失调,通常表现为信号通路活性增强。因此,许多这些综合征临床表现出现重叠,并且都有一定程度上罹患某些恶性肿瘤的倾向。这些综合征临床表现各异,这种差异与受影响基因的数量以及单个基因内突变的多样性密切相关。尽管一些激活性突变类似于癌症中的体细胞突变,但它们通常表现出较轻的活化水平,可能是由于在生殖细胞发育或早期发育阶段,严重的致癌突变被一定程度抑制。

对于 RAS 病患者,初步诊断主要基于临床表现。目前,分子遗传学检测也用于确诊。临床诊断与分子诊断之间的关联通常取决于所使用的临床诊断标准。此外,并非所有 RAS 病的致病基因都被确认。随着基因型与表型相关性的不断加强,分子诊断的重要性将进一步提升,并有助于克服临床诊断的局限性。这不仅有助于患者的治疗管理,而且有助于设计临床试验,以开发针对这些综合征的潜在治疗方法。

致谢:作者感谢 RAS 病的患者及其家属对遗传医学研究的支持。由于篇幅限制,未能引用所有相关文献,谨此致歉。

(林志淼,刘周亮 译)

参考文献

[1] Anastasaki C, Estep AL et al (2009) Kinase-activating and kinase-impaired cardio-facio-cutaneous syndrome alleles have activity during zebrafish development and are sensitive to small molecule inhibitors. Hum Mol Genet 18(14):2543-2554

[2] Aoki Y, Niihori T et al (2005) Germline mutations in HRAS proto-oncogene cause Costello syndrome. Nat Genet 37(10):1038-1040

[3] Boon LM, Mulliken JB et al (2005) RASA1:variable phenotype with capillary and arteriovenous malformations. Curr Opin Genet Dev 15(3):265-269

[4] Bos JL (1989) Ras oncogenes in human cancer:a review. Cancer Res 49(17):4682-4689

[5] Brems H, Chmara M et al (2007) Germline loss-of-function mutations in SPRED1 cause a neurofibromatosis 1-like phenotype. Nat Genet 39(9):1120-1126

[6] Brems H, Beert E et al (2009) Mechanisms in the pathogenesis of malignant tumours in neurofi-bromatosis type 1. Lancet Oncol 10(5):508-515

[7] Cawthon RM, Weiss R et al (1990) A major segment of the neurofibromatosis type 1 gene:cDNA sequence, genomic structure, and point mutations. Cell 62(1):193-201

[8] Cirstea IC, Kutsche K et al (2010) A restricted spectrum of NRAS mutations causes Noonan syndrome. Nat Genet 42(1):27-29

[9] Cordeddu V, Di Schiavi E et al (2009) Mutation of SHOC2 promotes aberrant protein N-myristoylation and causes Noonan-like syndrome with loose anagen hair. Nat Genet 41(9):1022-1026

[10] Denayer E, Chmara M et al (2011) Legius syndrome in fourteen families. Hum Mutat 32(1):E1985-E1998

[11] Digilio MC, Conti E et al (2002) Grouping of multiple-lentigines/LEOPARD and Noonan syndromes on the PTPN11 gene. Am J Hum Genet 71(2):389-394

[12] Dikic I, Schmidt MH (2007) Malfunctions within the Cbl interactome uncouple receptor tyrosine kinases from destructive transport. Eur J Cell Biol 86(9):505-512

[13] Eerola I, Boon LM et al (2003) Capillary malformation-arteriovenous malformation, a new clinical and genetic disorder caused by RASA1 mutations. Am J Hum Genet 73(6):1240-1249

[14] Estep AL, Tidyman WE et al (2006) HRAS mutations in Costello syndrome:detection of constitutional activating mutations in codon 12 and 13 and loss of wild-type allele in malig-nancy. Am J Med Genet A 140(1):8-16

[15] Gibbs JB, Sigal IS et al (1984) Intrinsic GTPase activity distinguishes normal and oncogenic ras p21 molecules. Proc Natl Acad Sci USA 81(18):5704-5708

[16] Gripp KW (2005) Tumor predisposition in Costello syndrome. Am J Med Genet C Semin Med Genet 137(1):72-77

[17] Gripp KW, Stabley DL et al (2006) Somatic mosaicism for an HRAS mutation causes Costello syndrome. Am J Med Genet A 140(20):2163-2169

[18] Gripp KW, Stabley DL et al (2011) Molecular confirmation of HRAS p. G12S in siblings with Costello syndrome. Am J Med Genet A 155A(9):2263-2268

[19] Hart TC, Pallos D et al (1998) Genetic linkage of hereditary

gingival fibromatosis to chromosome 2p21. Am J Hum Genet 62(4): 876-883

[20] Hart TC, Zhang Y et al (2002) A mutation in the SOS1 gene causes hereditary gingival fibromatosis type 1. Am J Hum Genet 70(4): 943-954

[21] Heidorn SJ, Milagre C et al (2010) Kinase-dead BRAF and oncogenic RAS cooperate to drive tumor progression through CRAF. Cell 140(2): 209-221

[22] Huffmeier U, Zenker M et al (2006) A variable combination of features of Noonan syndrome and neurofibromatosis type I are caused by mutations in the NF1 gene. Am J Med Genet A 140A(24): 2749-2756

[23] Jang SI, Lee EJ et al (2007) Germ line gain of function with SOS1 mutation in hereditary gingival fibromatosis. J Biol Chem 282(28): 20245-20255

[24] Keilhack H, David FS et al (2005) Diverse biochemical properties of Shp2 mutants. Implications for disease phenotypes. J Biol Chem 280(35): 30984-30993

[25] Kerr B, Delrue MA et al (2006) Genotype-phenotype correlation in Costello syndrome: HRAS mutation analysis in 43 cases. J Med Genet 43(5): 401-405

[26] Kontaridis MI, Swanson KD et al (2006) PTPN11 (Shp2) mutations in LEOPARD syndrome have dominant negative, not activating, effects. J Biol Chem 281(10): 6785-6792

[27] Kratz CP, Rapisuwon S et al (2011) Cancer in Noonan, Costello, cardiofaciocutaneous and LEOPARD syndromes. Am J Med Genet C Semin Med Genet 157(2): 83-89

[28] Legius E, Schrander-Stumpel C et al (2002) PTPN11 mutations in LEOPARD syndrome. J Med Genet 39(8): 571-574

[29] Lin AE, Alexander ME et al (2011) Clinical, pathological, and molecular analyses of cardiovas-cular abnormalities in Costello syndrome: a Ras/MAPK pathway syndrome. Am J Med Genet A 155A(3): 486-507

[30] Martinelli S, De Luca A et al (2010) Heterozygous germline mutations in the CBL tumorsuppressor gene cause a Noonan syndrome-like phenotype. Am J Hum Genet 87(2): 250-257

[31] Niemeyer CM, Kang MW et al (2010) Germline CBL mutations cause developmental abnormalities and predispose to juvenile myelomonocytic leukemia. Nat Genet 42(9): 794-800

[32] Niihori T, Aoki Y et al (2006) Germline KRAS and BRAF mutations in cardio-facio-cutaneous syndrome. Nat Genet 38(3): 294-296

[33] Oishi K, Zhang H et al (2009) Phosphatase-defective LEOPARD syndrome mutations in PTPN11 gene have gain-of-function effects during Drosophila development. Hum Mol Genet 18(1): 193-201

[34] Pandit B, Sarkozy A et al (2007) Gain-of-function RAF1 mutations cause Noonan and LEOPARD syndromes with hypertrophic cardiomyopathy. Nat Genet 39(8): 1007-1012

[35] Rauen KA (2007) HRAS and the Costello syndrome. Clin Genet 71(2): 101-108

[36] Rauen KA, Tidyman WE et al (2010) Molecular and functional analysis of a novel MEK2 mutation in cardio-facio-cutaneous syndrome: transmission through four generations. Am J Med Genet A 152A(4): 807-814

[37] Razzaque MA, Nishizawa T et al (2007) Germline gain-of-function mutations in RAF1 cause Noonan syndrome. Nat Genet 39(8): 1013-1017

[38] Revencu N, Boon LM et al (2008) Parkes Weber syndrome, vein of Galen aneurysmal malformation, and other fast-flow vascular anomalies are caused by RASA1 mutations. Hum Mutat 29(7): 959-965

[39] Roberts AE, Araki T et al (2007) Germline gain-of-function mutations in SOS1 cause Noonan syndrome. Nat Genet 39(1): 70-74

[40] Rodriguez-Viciana P, Oses-Prieto J et al (2006a) A phosphatase holoenzyme comprised of Shoc2/Sur8 and the catalytic subunit of PP1 functions as an M-Ras effector to modulate Raf activity. Mol Cell 22(2): 217-230

[41] Rodriguez-Viciana P, Tetsu O et al (2006b) Germline mutations in genes within the MAPK pathway cause cardio-facio-cutaneous syndrome. Science 311(5765): 1287-1290

[42] Romano AA, Allanson JE et al (2010) Noonan syndrome: clinical features, diagnosis, and management guidelines. Pediatrics 126(4): 746-759

[43] Schubbert S, Zenker M et al (2006) Germline KRAS mutations cause Noonan syndrome. Nat Genet 38(3): 331-336

[44] Schubbert S, Bollag G et al (2007) Biochemical and functional characterization of germ line KRAS mutations. Mol Cell Biol 27(22): 7765-7770

[45] Siegel DH, McKenzie J et al (2011) Dermatological findings in 61 mutation-positive individuals with cardiofaciocutaneous syndrome. Br J Dermatol 164(3): 521-529

[46] Siegel DH, Mann JA et al (2012) Dermatological phenotype in Costello syndrome: consequences of Ras dysregulation in development. Br J Dermatol 166(3): 601-607

[47] Sol-Church K, Stabley DL et al (2006) Paternal bias in parental origin of HRAS mutations in Costello syndrome. Hum Mutat 27(8): 736-741

[48] Sol-Church K, Stabley DL et al (2009) Male-to-male transmission of Costello syndrome: G12S HRAS germline mutation inherited from a father with somatic mosaicism. Am J Med Genet A 149A(3): 315-321

[49] Stevenson DA, Viskochil DH et al (2006) Clinical and molecular aspects of an informative family with neurofibromatosis type 1 and Noonan phenotype. Clin Genet 69(3): 246-253

[50] Tartaglia M, Mehler EL et al (2001) Mutations in PTPN11, encoding the protein tyrosine phosphatase SHP-2, cause Noonan syndrome. Nat Genet 29(4): 465-468

[51] Tartaglia M, Martinelli S et al (2006) Diversity and functional consequences of germline and somatic PTPN11 mutations in human disease. Am J Hum Genet 78(2): 279-290

[52] Tartaglia M, Pennacchio LA et al (2007) Gain-of-function SOS1 mutations cause a distinctive form of Noonan syndrome. Nat Genet 39(1): 75-79

[53] Tidyman WE, Rauen KA (2008) Noonan, Costello and cardio-facio-cutaneous syndromes: dysregulation of the Ras-MAPK pathway. Expert Rev Mol Med 10: e37

[54] Tidyman WE, Rauen KA (2009) Molecular cause of cardio-facio-cutaneous syndrome. In: Zenker M (ed) Monographs in human genetics: Noonan syndrome and related disorders—a matter of deregulated Ras signaling, vol 17. Bassel, Karger, Switzerland, pp 73-82

[55] Viskochil D, Buchberg AM et al (1990) Deletions and a translocation interrupt a cloned gene at the neurofibromatosis type 1 locus. Cell 62(1): 187-192

[56] Wakioka T, Sasaki A et al (2001) Spred is a Sprouty-related suppressor of Ras signalling. Nature 412(6847): 647-651

[57] Wallace MR, Marchuk DA et al (1990) Type 1 neurofibromatosis gene: identification of a large transcript disrupted in three NF1 patients. Science 249(4965): 181-186

[58] Williams VC, Lucas J et al (2009) Neurofibromatosis type 1 revisited. Pediatrics 123(1): 124-133

[59] Yoon S, Seger R (2006) The extracellular signal-regulated kinase: multiple substrates regulate diverse cellular functions. Growth Factors 24(1): 21-44

[60] Yoon G, Rosenberg J et al (2007) Neurological complications of cardio-facio-cutaneous syndrome. Dev Med Child Neurol 49(12): 894-899

[61] Zampino G, Pantaleoni F et al (2007) Diversity, parental germline origin, and phenotypic spectrum of *de novo* HRAS missense changes in Costello syndrome. Hum Mutat 28(3): 265-272

第33章 1型神经纤维瘤病动物模型的进展和经验教训
Advances in NF1 Animal Models and Lessons Learned

Ophelia Maertens and Karen Cichowski

33.1 NF1 的早期小鼠模型

最初在小鼠中模拟 NF1 时,尝试采用经典的基因敲除技术。有趣的是,这种方法揭示了 NF1 在早期胚胎发育中的作用,因为纯合突变胚胎在妊娠中期死于心脏畸形(Brannan et al. 1994)。然而,观察到 Nf1 杂合小鼠发生了几种恶性肿瘤,并且野生型 Nf1 等位基因在这些肿瘤中丢失,这提供了重要证据,证明 Nf1 是一种经典的肿瘤抑制基因(Jacks et al. 1994)。后来,通过将 $Nf1^{-/-}$ 胚胎干细胞注射到 $Nf1^{+/+}$ 胚泡中产生的嵌合小鼠进行的研究证实,野生型 Nf1 等位基因的缺失也是神经纤维瘤发育的限速步骤,这在当时是一个尚未解决的问题(Cichowski et al. 1999)。为了测试额外的突变是否会增强肿瘤易变性,学者们构建了在同一染色体上携带 Nf1 和 p53 肿瘤抑制基因的复合突变的小鼠(缩写为 NP 顺式小鼠)(Cichowski et al. 1999; Vogel et al. 1999)。这些小鼠出现了侵袭性恶性周围神经鞘膜瘤(MPNSTs),在组织学和遗传学上与人类同类肿瘤无法区分(Stemmer-Rachamimov et al. 2004)。除了证明 p53 突变在 MPNST 形成的因果关系外,该模型的成功还强调了与 NF1 相关的不同肿瘤类型的可处理小鼠模型的可行性。如下文讨论,NP 顺式小鼠已被广泛用于研究 MPNST 的发病机制和临床前研究。

33.2 从第二代神经纤维瘤模型中吸取的 2 个教训

为了开发 NF1 相关神经纤维瘤更易于处理和精确的模型,携带条件性 Nf1 等位基因的小鼠出现了,该等位基因可以通过 Cre 介导的重组在特定的细胞类型和特定的时间点呈现神经纤维瘤蛋白缺乏(Zhu et al. 2001)。广泛的条件性 NF1 小鼠神经纤维瘤模型的开发(表 33.1)提高了鉴定这些肿瘤的病理生理学起源细胞、环境线索和分子通路的可行性。其中许多模型的细节将在其他章节中讨论。然而,这些模型的汇总以及它们如何共同促进我们对神经纤维瘤发病机制的理解将在本章阐述。

尽管 Nf1 杂合子小鼠在成年后期死于各种恶性肿瘤,但他们没有发展出神经纤维瘤,这是 NF1 的特征(Jacks et al. 1994)。为了测试这种缺乏神经纤维瘤的现象是否可以通过小鼠获得第二次突变的能力有限来解释,研究人员生成了部分由 $Nf1^{-/-}$ 细胞组成的嵌合小鼠(Cichowski et al. 1999)。观察

表 33.1 丛状神经纤维瘤发育的条件性 NF1 小鼠模型

参考信息	基因类型	Cre 驱动程序	施万细胞阶段发展[a]	丛状神经纤维瘤	其他表现
Joseph 等(2008)	$Nf1^{flox/-}$	Wnt1-Cre	NCSC	没有	
Zheng 等(2008)	$Nf1^{flox/-}$	POA-Cre	SC 前体(早期)	是,贯穿周围神经系统	
Wu 等(2008)	$Nf1^{flox/flox}$	Dhh-Cre	SC 前体(晚期)	是,靠近 DRG[b],脊柱旁	皮肤型神经纤维瘤色素沉着
Zhu 等(2002)	$Nf1^{flox/flox}$ $Nf1^{flox/-}$	Krox20-Cre	SC 前体+未成熟 SC 系统	没有 是,靠近 DGR,脊柱旁	
Le 等(2011)	$Nf1^{flox/-}$	PLP-Cre/ERT[c]	SC 前体 不成熟 SC 成熟 SC	是,靠近 DGR,脊柱旁 是,靠近 DGR,脊柱旁 是,很少见	
Mayes 等(2011)	$Nf1^{flox/flox}$	PLP-Cre/ERT[c]	不成熟 SC 成熟 SC	是,贯穿神经轴 是,贯穿神经轴较大肿瘤	造血扩张,脾肿大

注:[a] 施万细胞发育的不同阶段:迁移性神经及干细胞(NCSC)在小鼠胚胎 E9 至 11 天神经形成之前穿过未成熟的结缔组织,然后在 E12 和 13 之间分化为施万细胞(SC)前体这些 SC 前体然后变成未成熟的施万细胞,从 E14 到早期新生儿阶段产生。未成熟施万细胞最终在出生后分化为成熟施万细胞(Carroll and Ratner 2008;Jessen and Mirsky 2005)。[b] DRG,背根神经节。[c] 他莫昔芬诱导型 PLP-Cre 驱动线。

到这些小鼠发生了许多神经纤维瘤,这表明野生型 $Nf1$ 等位基因的丢失确实是神经纤维瘤发展的限速步骤。然而,使用嵌合小鼠模型很难确定哪种细胞类型参与神经纤维瘤的发育,因为在这些小鼠中,几种细胞类型是 $Nf1$ 的纯合突变体。

神经纤维瘤由多种细胞类型组成,包括施万细胞、肥大细胞、神经周细胞、成纤维细胞和内皮细胞(Cichowski and Jacks 2001)。施万细胞是该复合体中最常见的细胞类型,并已被提出是致瘤细胞(Rutkowski et al. 2000;Serra et al. 2000)。一个突破性进展来自有条件地切除施万细胞谱系中的 Nf1,使用在前体/未成熟施万细胞中,特异性启动子 Krox20 控制下的 Cre 转基因的作用(Zhu et al. 2002)。Zhu 等发现丛状神经纤维瘤可以通过在施万细胞前体细胞群中敲除 $Nf1$ 来驱动。有趣的是,这些研究人员还发现,在该模型中周围细胞类型需要 $Nf1$ 单倍不足,因为神经纤维瘤仅在 $Nf1^{flox/-}$;Krox-20-cre 小鼠中出现,其中所有相邻细胞都是 Nf1 杂合子,而在 $Nf1^{flox/fox}$;Krox-20-cre 小鼠中,其相邻细胞为 Nf1 的野生型(Zhu et al. 2002)。周围细胞单倍不足的要求将在下文简要讨论,并在另一章中详细讨论。

NF1 患者的丛状神经纤维瘤被认为是先天性的(Riccatdi 1992)。在施万细胞前体群体中,在 $Nf1$ 在胚胎发育期间被消融的条件下,在小鼠中出现神经纤维瘤的观察结果与该假说一致(Zhu et al. 2002)。然而,在 NF1 患者中,可能在发育的任何阶段发生第二次 NF1 突变(例如从神经嵴细胞到成熟的施万细胞,见表 33.1)。不同的细胞来源可能会导致肿瘤发生机制的差异。为了确定可能作为神经纤维瘤起源细胞的细胞类型范围,研究人员现在已经生成了具有受控 Cre 驱动转基因的小鼠模型,这些基因在不同发展时间点消除了施万细胞谱系中的 $Nf1$ 功能(表 33.1)。使用 Wnt-1 启动子使胎儿神经嵴细胞(NCSC)中条件性缺失 $Nf1$,导致 NCSC 的频率和自我更新的短暂增加,但没有致瘤性,表明神经纤维瘤不能从这种不稳定的细胞中发出分化的细胞群(Joseph et al. 2008)。然而,除了 Krox20-Cre 模型外,其中在施万细胞发育的各个阶段(如 PO、Dhh 和诱导性 Plp)表达的启动子驱动 Cre 重组酶表达的小鼠也促进了丛状神经纤维的形成(Zhu et al. 2002;Wu et al. 2008;Zheng et al. 2008;Le et al. 2001;Mayes et al. 2011)。这些结果表明神经纤维瘤可以从施万细胞谱系中的一系列细胞类型发展而来。因此,这些模型中的每一个都可能代表在 NF1 患者中发展的神经纤维瘤的不同子集。重要的是,这些模型之间似乎在肿瘤治病方面存在一些差异。例如,由 Dhh-Cre 驱动的神经纤维瘤相对较大,并且似乎不需要周围细胞类型的单倍不足(Wu et al. 2008),而 Krox20-Cre 驱动的肿瘤确实需要这种单倍不足(Zhu et al. 2002)。因此,在设计和解释旨在确定潜在疗法的临床前研究时,应考虑这些差异。尽管如此,该领域将从研究几种不同的神经纤维瘤模型中受益,这些模型可以共同概括人类肿瘤的广谱。值得注意的是,真皮神经纤维瘤在这些模型中的任何一个都没有有效的发展,这表明这些肿瘤的起源细胞不同于引起丛状神经纤维瘤的群体。Parada 实验室的工作现在提供了强有力的证据,表面皮肤衍生的前体(SKP),一种位于真皮中的神经嵴样神经干细胞,可能是这种独特肿瘤类型的起源细胞(Le et al. 2009)。

33.3 识别合作遗传活动的小鼠模型的使用

NF1 的个体易发生恶性肿瘤,如 MPNST、视路神经胶质瘤、恶性星形细胞瘤、嗜铬细胞瘤和 JMML(Ferner 2007)。癌症是一个复杂的过程,需要一系列连续的遗传和表现遗传事件在一个允许的微环境中获得一组基本的功能(Hanahan and Weinberg 2011)。与这个多步骤癌症范例一致,在 NF1 缺陷的 MPNST 中经常发现 p53 和(或)INK4alARF 肿瘤抑制基因中的其他突变(Kourea et al. 1999; Legius et al. 1994; Menon et al. 1990; Nielsen et al 1999)。为了如实地再现人类肿瘤中的这些突变,产生了携带 Nf1 和 p53 或 Ink4alArf 复合突变的小鼠模型(Cichowski et al. 1999; Vogel et al. 1999; Josph et al. 2008)。重要的是,小鼠肿瘤显示了在这些肿瘤的人类对应物中描述的信号通路的改变(Miller et al. 2009),并且在组织学上与后者难以区分(Semmer-Rachamimov et al. 2004),说明了这些小鼠模型如何准确地模拟人类条件,并确定这些基因在肿瘤进展中的因果作用。

随着我们对人类 MPNST 的生物学和遗传学更多的了解,我们可以使用这些模型来评估其他基因在此过程中的贡献。例如,通过将 NP cis 小鼠与携带 EGFR 突变的小鼠杂交,研究人员表明 EGFR 有助于 MPNST 的发展(Ling et al. 2005),最终可能被用于开发未来的治疗方法。此外,NF1 的一个标志是极端的临床异质性,即使在携带相同体质 NF1 突变的相关个体中也是如此。流行病学研究表明,这种表性变异背后的分子基础在很大程度上是修饰位点的基因型决定的(Easton et al. 1993)。NP 损失模型中遗传研究已经证明了小鼠遗传背景菌株对肿瘤表型的修饰作用(Reilly et al. 2000, 2004)。这些小鼠现在被用来识别遗传修饰因子,这可能最终证明介导 NF1 患者疾病表达的遗传修饰物(Reilly et al. 2006)。因此,这些模型可用于遗传和治疗研究,这将在下面进一步讨论。

需要注意的是,有一部分 NF1 患者可能提供了一些遗传提示,这些提示涉及神经纤维瘤和 MPNST 的发展微缺失患者是携带 NF1 和 12 个周围基因缺失的 NF1 患者的一个子集(De Raedt et al. 2004)。值得注意的是,这些患者会发展成数百个神经纤维瘤,并且发展 MPNST 的可能性增加了两倍以上(De Raedt et al. 2003),表明在该区域存在另外的肿瘤抑制因子。因此,可用神经纤维瘤和 MPNST 小鼠模型去观察这些周围基因的参与能力。

33.4 使用小鼠模型进行治疗开发

忠实地再现 NF1 相关肿瘤发生的小鼠模型有可能提供对肿瘤起始和进展过程中改变的信号通路的见解。同时,这些小鼠模型可以作为临床前工具,开始评估最有希望的 NF1 靶向治疗。值得注意的是,在过去 5 年中,这些模型的临床前研究已经开始直接影响 NF1 患者临床试验的发展。

基于发现神经纤维瘤蛋白关键调节 mTOR 通路,并且 mTOR 在 Nf1 缺陷的肿瘤中过度激活(Dasgupta et al. 2005; Johannessen et al. 2005),在 Nf1/p53 突变 MPNST 模型中评估了雷帕霉素(一种有效的 mTOR 抑制剂)的治疗潜力(Johannessen et al. 2008)和 $Nf1^{flox-}$；$GFAR-Cre$ 神经胶质瘤模型（Hegedus et al. 2008）。值得注意的是，雷帕霉素在两种模型中迅速而有效地抑制了肿瘤生长（Johannessen et al. 2008；Hegedus et al. 2008）。这些研究激发了在 NF1 患者中使用 mTOR 抑制剂的四项临床试验的发展（Clinicaltrys.gov）。尽管这些实验仍在进行中，但这些努力强调了如何使用小鼠模型来指导靶向药物的临床试验开发。由于目前对大多数 NF1 相关症状的治疗效果有限，动物模型是识别和开发适当临床试验的重要工具。

临床试验也可以通过研究小鼠模型中对特定药物的治疗反应来改进/精炼。Johannessen 等发现，除了促进小鼠 MPNST 中有效的细胞抑制反应外，长时间暴露于雷帕霉素导致 $Nf1/p53$ MPNST 模型中肿瘤微血管的完全破坏（Johannessen et al. 2008）。此外，对雷帕霉素具有耐药性的肿瘤绕过了这些抗血管生成阻断并重新建立了它们的微血管系统（CMJ，KC 未发表的观察结果）。因此，有理由认为，防止这种血运重建的治疗策略可能会延迟或防止耐药肿瘤的出现。为了评估这种可能性，抗血管生成药物舒尼替尼与雷帕霉素在 NP 顺势模型中联合使用。虽然单独使用舒尼替尼对这些动物没有影响，但与雷帕霉素单药治疗相比，雷帕霉素和舒尼替尼有效地抑制了肿瘤生长并显著延长了生存期（Cichowski Laboratory，未发表数据）。值得注意的是，基于这些有希望的临床前数据，评估口服 mTOR 抑制剂依维莫司与抗血管生成药物贝伐珠单抗联合治疗的二期临床试验已在不可切除和转移性 MPNST 患者中开展。基于 NP 顺式模型的观察，预计这种组合虽然可能无法治愈，但将延迟进展并延长生存期。

现在出现了第二个令人兴奋的例子，说明如何使用小鼠模型来开发现在有希望的疗法。为了将雷帕霉素的细胞抑制作用转化为细胞毒性反应，在 NP 顺式小鼠中进一步评估了基于 mTOR 抑制剂的联合治疗。由于 Ras 的高度非整倍体和组成性激活，$Nf1$ 缺陷的 MPNST 表现出高水平的蛋白质毒性应激（De Raedt et al. 2001）。因此，这种癌细胞特异性脆弱性可以在治疗开发的背景下加以利用。事实上，阻断这些适应性途径的药物，无论是单独使用还是与抗肿瘤药物（例如雷帕霉素）联合使用，都可以在 MPNST 中触发细胞毒性反应。

为了研究这种治疗策略在侵袭性 MPNST 中的潜力，在体内评估了几种增强蛋白毒性应激的药物，这些 MPNST 通常对常规治疗无效（De Raedt et al. 2011）。重要的是，Hsp90 抑制剂 IPI-504 在 $Nf1/p53$ MPNST 小鼠模型中显著地诱导肿瘤消退，但仅在与雷帕霉素联合使用时。这种协同效应依赖于活性氧（reactive oxygen species，ROS）的积累，因为雷帕霉素消除了细胞中和 IPI-504 诱导的 ROS 的能力，导致细胞内 ROS 造成肿瘤中的内质网和线粒体灾难性损伤（De Raed et al. 2011）。这种联合治疗的疗效也可以扩展到 Kras 驱动的非小细胞肺癌（non-small cell lung cancer，NSCLC）小鼠模型（De Raedt et al. 2011）。在这些侵袭性肿瘤模型中，没有发现靶向治疗可促进肿瘤消退，这强调了这些发现的重要性以及对治疗开发的潜在影响。一项一期临床试验已经启动，以评估 IPI-504 和 mTOR 抑制剂依维莫司对 KRAS 突变 NSCLC 的活性，如果成功，将演变为 NCSCL 和 MPNST 的二期研究。

最后，正如将在另一章中详细介绍的那样，小鼠模型也可用于开发神经纤维瘤的潜在疗法。如前所述，Zhu 等发现周围微环境的单倍不足在 $Krox20-Cre$ 驱动模型中神经纤维瘤的发展中起着关键作用（Zhu et al. 2002）。通过一系列遗传研究，研究人员发现肥大细胞在神经纤维瘤的发展中起着关键作用（Yang et al. 2008）。因此，研究人员推断，靶向肿瘤微环境可能是治疗 NF1 相关神经纤维瘤的有效方法。因为肥大细胞受到 c-kit 受体的严格调节，在该小鼠神经纤维瘤模型中评估了 c-kit 抑制的治疗潜力（Yang et al. 2008）。$Nf1^{flox-}$；$Krox-20-cre$ 小鼠用甲磺酸伊马替尼治疗，伊马替尼是包括 c-kit 在内的几种酪氨酸激酶的强效抑制剂，并通过 FDG-PET 成像评估对神经纤维瘤负荷的影响（Yang et al. 2008）。总体而言，甲磺酸伊马替尼治疗的小鼠在治疗后 FDG-PET 摄取平均减少 50%（Yang et al. 2008）。引人注目的是，与小鼠模型的临床前研究一致，显示 3 年后肿瘤体积减小约 70%（Yang et al. 2008）。

为了进一步促进和加速对 NF1 的有效性新疗法

的开发，儿童肿瘤基金会开发了神经纤维瘤病临床前联盟（Neurofibromatosis Preclinical Consortium，NFPC）。这个多中心合作小组制作了一组 NF1 相关的小鼠模型，代表一组不同的 NF1 疾病症状，目前尚无治疗方法。到目前为止，NFPC 已经成功完成了与四家制药公司合作的许多临床前试验。其中一些临床前研究已经在 NF1 患者中进行了临床试验。基于所使用的动物模型的数量和该联盟目前的规模，这些努力可能会对 NF1 患者的临床策略产生重大影响。

33.5 结论和未来方向

很明显，复杂的 NF1 小鼠模型的发展，已经允许解剖广泛的 NF1 疾病表现发展的分子机制。它为 NF1 复杂病理生理学中涉及的遗传缺陷和细胞自主性以及非细胞自主性因素提供了具体见解。此外，这些真实再现人类条件特征的小鼠模型设计使研究人员能够开始使用这些作为准确的临床前工具，用于测试 NF1 最有希望的靶向治疗。

未来一个最令人兴奋的应用，是使用这些基因工程 NF1 小鼠模型进行转化研究。所描述的模型代表了一个强大的实验工具，因为它允许在基因明确定义的系统中评估候选药物，这些系统在适当的环境中和在存在完整免疫系统的情况下出现症状。此外，可以利用快速评估给定药剂的生物学效应的能力来确定针对最有希望的治疗靶点的最佳临床候选药物。最终，正如 MPNST 模型所示，获得的益处将超越对靶向单一疗法的反应，并可用于快速评估各种联合疗法的疗效，识别敏感性生物标志物，并开发克服对特定治疗的耐药性的疗法。因此，这些模型有可能成为成功预测临床试验中药物反应的优秀平台。

同时，扩大 NF1 小鼠模型的复杂性，无疑将有助于更深入地了解该疾病的基本机制。因此，可以预期，相关 NF1 小鼠模型的开发和研究将继续转化为基础和临床研究的重大进展。

（杨志国　译）

参考文献

[1] Brannan CI et al (1994) Targeted disruption of the neurofibromatosis type-1 gene leads to develop-mental abnormalities in heart and various neural crest-derived tissues. Genes Dev 8：1019

[2] Carroll SL, Ratner N (2008) How does the Schwann cell lineage form tumors in NF1? Glia 56：1590

[3] Cichowski K, Jacks T (2001) NF1 tumor suppressor gene function：narrowing the GAP. Cell 104：593

[4] Cichowski K et al (1999) Mouse models of tumor development in neurofibromatosis type 1. Science 286：2172

[5] Dasgupta B, Yi Y, Chen DY, Weber JD, Gutmann DH (2005) Proteomic analysis reveals hyperactivation of the mammalian target of rapamycin pathway in neurofibromatosis 1-associated human and mouse brain tumors. Cancer Res 65：2755

[6] De Raedt T et al (2003) Elevated risk for MPNST in NF1 microdeletion patients. Am J Hum Genet 72：1288

[7] De Raedt T et al (2004) Genomic organization and evolution of the NF1 microdeletion region. Genomics 84：346

[8] De Raedt T et al (2011) Exploiting cancer cell vulnerabilities to develop a combination therapy for ras-driven tumors. Cancer Cell 20：400

[9] Easton DF, Ponder MA, Huson SM, Ponder BA (1993) An analysis of variation in expression of neurofibromatosis (NF) type 1 (NF1)：evidence for modifying genes. Am J Hum Genet 53：305

[10] Ferner RE (2007) Neurofibromatosis 1. Eur J Hum Genet 15：131

[11] Hanahan D, Weinberg RA (2011) Hallmarks of cancer：the next generation. Cell 144：646

[12] Hegedus B et al (2008) Preclinical cancer therapy in a mouse model of neurofibromatosis-1 optic glioma. Cancer Res 68：1520

[13] Jacks T et al (1994) Tumour predisposition in mice heterozygous for a targeted mutation in Nf1. Nat Genet 7：353

[14] Jessen KR, Mirsky R (2005) The origin and development of glial cells in peripheral nerves. Nat Rev Neurosci 6：671

[15] Johannessen CM et al (2005) The NF1 tumor suppressor critically regulates TSC2 and mTOR. Proc Natl Acad Sci USA 102：8573

[16] Johannessen CM et al (2008) TORC1 is essential for NF1-associated malignancies. Curr Biol 18：56

[17] Joseph NM et al (2008) The loss of Nf1 transiently promotes self-renewal but not tumorigenesis by neural crest stem cells. Cancer Cell 13：129

[18] Kim I, Xu W, Reed JC (2008) Cell death and endoplasmic reticulum stress：disease relevance and therapeutic opportunities. Nat Rev Drug Discov 7：1013

[19] Kourea HP, Orlow I, Scheithauer BW, Cordon-Cardo C, Woodruff JM (1999) Deletions of the INK4A gene occur in malignant peripheral nerve sheath tumors but not in neurofibromas. Am J Pathol 155：1855

[20] Le LQ, Shipman T, Burns DK, Parada LF (2009) Cell of origin and microenvironment contribution for NF1-associated dermal neurofibromas. Cell Stem Cell 4：453

[21] Le LQ et al (2011) Susceptible stages in Schwann cells for

NF1-associated plexiform neurofi-broma development. Cancer Res 71: 4686
[22] Legius E et al (1994) TP53 mutations are frequent in malignant NF1 tumors. Genes Chromosomes Cancer 10: 250
[23] Ling BC et al (2005) Role for the epidermal growth factor receptor in neurofibromatosis-related peripheral nerve tumorigenesis. Cancer Cell 7: 65
[24] Mayes DA et al (2011) Perinatal or adult Nf1 inactivation using tamoxifen-inducible PlpCre each cause neurofibroma formation. Cancer Res 71: 4675
[25] Menon AG et al (1990) Chromosome 17p deletions and p53 gene mutations associated with the formation of malignant neurofibrosarcomas in von Recklinghausen neurofibromatosis. Proc Natl Acad Sci USA 87: 5435
[26] Miller SJ et al (2009) Integrative genomic analyses of neurofibromatosis tumours identify SOX9 as a biomarker and survival gene. EMBO Mol Med 1: 236
[27] Nielsen GP et al (1999) Malignant transformation of neurofibromas in neurofibromatosis 1 is associated with CDKN2A/p16 inactivation. Am J Pathol 155: 1879
[28] Reilly KM, Loisel DA, Bronson RT, McLaughlin ME, Jacks T (2000) Nf1; Trp53 mutant mice develop glioblastoma with evidence of strain-specific effects. Nat Genet 26: 109
[29] Reilly KM et al (2004) Susceptibility to astrocytoma in mice mutant for Nf1 and Trp53 is linked to chromosome 11 and subject to epigenetic effects. Proc Natl Acad Sci USA 101: 13008
[30] Reilly KM et al (2006) An imprinted locus epistatically influences Nstr1 and Nstr2 to control resistance to nerve sheath tumors in a neurofibromatosis type 1 mouse model. Cancer Res 66: 62
[31] Riccardi VM (1992) Neurofibromatosis: phenotype, natural history, and pathogenesis. Johns Hopkins Press, Baltimore
[32] Rutkowski JL, Wu K, Gutmann DH, Boyer PJ, Legius E (2000) Genetic and cellular defects contributing to benign tumor formation in neurofibromatosis type 1. Hum Mol Genet 9: 1059
[33] Serra E et al (2000) Schwann cells harbor the somatic NF1 mutation in neurofibromas: evidence of two different Schwann cell subpopulations. Hum Mol Genet 9: 3055
[34] Stemmer-Rachamimov AO et al (2004) Comparative pathology of nerve sheath tumors in mouse models and humans. Cancer Res 64: 3718
[35] Vogel KS et al (1999) Mouse tumor model for neurofibromatosis type 1. Science 286: 2176
[36] Wu J et al (2008) Plexiform and dermal neurofibromas and pigmentation are caused by Nf1 loss in desert hedgehog-expressing cells. Cancer Cell 13: 105
[37] Yang FC et al (2008) Nf1-dependent tumors require a microenvironment containing $Nf1^{+/-}$ and c-kit-dependent bone marrow. Cell 135: 437
[38] Zheng H et al (2008) Induction of abnormal proliferation by nonmyelinating schwann cells triggers neurofibroma formation. Cancer Cell 13: 117
[39] Zhu Y et al (2001) Ablation of NF1 function in neurons induces abnormal development of cerebral cortex and reactive gliosis in the brain. Genes Dev 15: 859
[40] Zhu Y, Ghosh P, Charnay P, Burns DK, Parada LF (2002) Neurofibromas in NF1: Schwann cell origin and role of tumor environment. Science 296: 920

第34章 果蝇：1型神经纤维瘤病的无脊椎动物模型
Drosophila: An Invertebrate Model of NF1

James A. Walker, Jean Y. Gouzi, and André Bernards

34.1 引言

如前所述，1型神经纤维瘤病（NF1）是一种与多种症状相关的多系统慢性遗传病。NF1的另外一个常见特征是其变异性和不可预测性。因此，患者通常只会表现出部分症状，并且个体症状的严重程度在不同患者之间也可能存在显著差异。单基因遗传疾病如NF1的可变表达可能由多个因素导致，包括不完全的基因外显率、致病基因缺陷、患者是否为体细胞嵌合体，以及患者是否携带遗传修饰因子或暴露于不同的环境。在NF1的病例中，所有上述因素都被认为起到了作用。因此，尽管携带 NF1 突变的个体会以完全外显率表现出部分症状，但随机的遗传或表观遗传事件可能导致某些症状的部分外显。例如，丛状神经纤维瘤，多数被认为是先天性发育的，只有约1/3的患者会发展出这些肿瘤，这可能反映了在有限的发育时期内，肿瘤前体细胞中野生型 NF1 等位基因丧失的概率有限。另外，虽然在NF1中基因型和表型的关联较少，但也存在一些显著的例外。首先，5%～10%的患者携带重复发生的1.2～1.4 Mb的微缺失，这些微缺失包括 NF1 基因及其周围的多个编码蛋白和微小RNA基因。

这些患者通常表现出特别严重的症状，包括智力障碍、畸形、儿童期过度生长以及大量早发性神经纤维瘤（Kayes et al. 1994；Pasmant et al. 2010）。支持相邻基因缺失可能导致或修饰这些缺陷的观点是，只去除 NF1 基因的患者并不会表现出这种更严重的表型。另外一个例子是发现21名不相关的NF1患者携带相同的单个氨基酸缺失，却没有明显的神经纤维瘤（Upadhyaya et al. 2007）。除了 NF1 基因本身的影响外，变异表达也可能反映在那些在合子后获得NF1突变的散发患者中的体细胞嵌合现象（Bernards and Gusella 1994）。早期的一项重要研究支持症状特异性遗传修饰因子在决定疾病结局中发挥重要作用的假设，该研究分析了175名来自48个 NF1 家族的患者，包括6对单卵双胞胎（monozygotic，MZ），5个二进制症状的有无，以及3个定量症状的严重程度。研究发现，4个二进制特征和2个定量特征（神经纤维瘤和咖啡牛奶斑的负担）在MZ双胞胎中的相关系数较高，而在一级亲属中的得分较低，在更远的家族成员中的值更低（Easton et al. 1993）。后续研究进一步支持了未链接修饰基因控制特定NF1症状的假设（Rieley et al. 2011；Szudek et al. 2002）。环境因素是导致变异表达的另外一个潜在原因。在NF1的情况下，观

J. A. Walker • J. Y. Gouzi • A. Bernards (✱)
Massachusetts General Hospital Center for Cancer Research and Harvard Medical School, Building 149, 13th Street, Charlestown, MA 02129, USA
e-mail: abernards@helix.mgh.harvard.edu

M. Upadhyaya and D. N. Cooper (eds.), *Neurofibromatosis Type 1*,
DOI 10.1007/978-3-642-32864-0_34, # Springer-Verlag Berlin Heidelberg 2012

察到神经纤维瘤在妊娠期间的大小和（或）数量增加是最清晰的非遗传因素影响疾病进展的例子（Roth et al. 2008）。

修饰基因的身份可能为疾病症状的机制提供线索，并且由于修饰基因执行限速功能，人类修饰基因代表了预先验证的治疗靶点。然而，当 NF1 基因在 1990 年被鉴定时，人类基因组序列和其他工具还无法有效调查不同受影响患者群体中的潜在修饰基因。因此，我们识别 NF1 修饰基因的策略涉及识别高度保守的果蝇 NF1（Drosophila NF1, dNF1）直系同源基因，生成突变体，分析表型，进行结构功能研究和遗传筛选。本章的剩余部分总结了迄今为止的研究成果，这些研究对那些对 NF1 感兴趣的人而言是有意义的。

34.2 果蝇 dNF1 的识别与结构

人类 NF1 基因序列表明其编码蛋白的功能是作为 Ras 的 GTP 酶激活蛋白（GTPase-activating protein, GAP）（Xu et al. 1990）。同样显而易见的是，尽管神经纤维瘤蛋白在约 360 个氨基酸的催化功能域上与几种物种的 RasGAP 具有相似性，但它在几乎一半的长度上与出芽酵母的 Ras 活性抑制蛋白 1 和 2（Inhibitor of Ras Activity-1 and -2, IRA1/2）表现出更广泛的相似性（Ballester et al. 1990）。这些发现促使我们研究在适合遗传分析的无脊椎动物物种中是否存在 NF1 直系同源物。在线虫（秀丽隐杆线虫）中没有发现 NF1 同源物。然而，在果蝇（黑腹果蝇）的 dNF1 基因中发现一种与人类神经纤维瘤蛋白在整个 2 802 个氨基酸长度上 55%相同和 69%相似的蛋白质（The et al. 1997）。如图 34.1 所示，果蝇神经纤维瘤蛋白的 IRA 相关中央片段与人类蛋白质最为相似，但在上下游也存在保守区域。反映出果蝇基因组的较小规模，dNF1 基因比人类对应基因更紧凑。因此，尽管人类 NF1 由分布在约 283 kb DNA 上的 60 个外显子组成，并在其内含子中拥有三个其他基因，但 dNF1 由 18 个外显子组成（图 34.1 中的交替白色/灰色框），且仅跨越 13 kb。在 2 个位置，dNF1 mRNA 是可变剪接的。可变剪接的 dNF1 外显子 14 的位置与人类外显子 43 的可变剪接位置非常接近（Thomson and Wallace 2002）。然而，尽管人类外显子 43 被认为提供了核定位信号（Vandenbroucke et al. 2004），dNF1 外显子 14 预测的 30 个氨基酸是否具有功能性后果仍有待确定。在可变剪接的人类外显子 48a 的确切位置，倒数第二个 dNF1 编码外显子 17 剪接到 3 个不同的终末外显子，生成预测具有 3 种不同 C-端的 mRNA。同样，这些 C-端异构体是否在功能上不同尚不清楚。在人类 NF1 中，在 GAP 相关域（GAP-related domain，GRD）中包含可变剪接的外显子 23a 会降低编码蛋白的催化活性（Andersen et al. 1993）。然而，外显子 23a 的位置在 dNF1 中并不对应任何剪接位点。最后，我们注意到，与疾病相关的错义突变不成比例地影响了果蝇 NF1 中保守的残基。例如，GRD 上游的大约 1 200 个氨基酸片段在人类和果蝇之间具有 46%的整体序列相似性，但该区域中的 47 个错义突变中有 35 个（74%）影响了果蝇中保守的残基。

34.3 dNF1 突变体与表型

由于不存在经典的 dNF1 突变体，我们使用 flanking P 转录子生成了两个破坏性的新整合 dNF1 突变体。$dNF1^{P1}$ 和 $dNF1^{P2}$ 等位基因在分子和遗传上表现出相似性。鉴于致癌 Ras 在果蝇眼睛中的表达会导致严重缺陷（Bishop and Corces 1988），但令人困惑的是 dNF1 的纯合子缺失并未导致任何异常情况。然而，这两种突变体在整个后胚胎发育的所有阶段线性尺寸都减少了 15%~20%，成年果蝇在释放后倾向于飞走（The et al. 1997）。由于这些和其他的 dNF1 表型可能受遗传背景的影响，并且 $dNF1^{P1}$ 等位基因还删除了 E(spl) 复合基因，我们通过同系果蝇的化学诱变产生了额外的等位基因。在 3 个新等位基因中，$dNF1^{E1}$ 是一个 C1045Y 错义突变，$dNF1^{E1}$ 和 $dNF1^{E2}$ 是 Q370* 和 Q1062* 无义突变（Walker et al. 2006）。

除了调用 Ras 独立功能之外，至少还有 2 个因素可能解释为什么 dNF1 的缺失和表达持续活性的 Ras 不会导致类似的缺陷。首先，果蝇基因组包含 5 个 RasGAP 基因（Gap1、Vap、dNF1、CG1657、

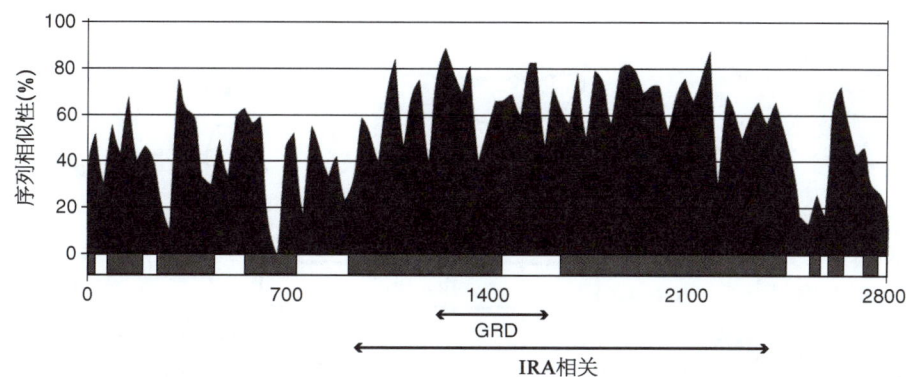

图 34.1 图表显示了果蝇和人类神经纤维瘤蛋白之间氨基酸序列的相似度。图表下方的交替灰色/白色框表示 18 个 dNF1 外显子的大小和位置。GRD 表示 GAP 相关域。图中还标示了与酿酒酵母 IRA1 和 IRA2 蛋白相关的蛋白质片段的范围

CG42684)和 2 个与质膜相关的潜在 RasGAP。相关基因的潜在功能也可能反映出 NF1 表现在神经系统中的限制(Walker et al. 2006)。虽然 dNF1 的缺失并未明显影响存活率、繁殖力或模式,但已识别出几种宏观、细胞和生化表型(图 34.2)。有趣的是,已经确定的 dNF1 缺陷对影响 Ras 信号强度的基因操作并不敏感。相反,这些缺陷可以通过增加 cAMP 依赖的蛋白激酶 A(protein kinase A, PKA)通路的信号来修复,并且通过减少该通路的信号来增强或模拟(Guo et al. 1997;The et al. 1997)。dNF1 与腺苷酸环化酶(adenylyl cyclase,AC)/PKA 信号通路之间的关联促使了大量后续研究。尽管 dNF1 的缺失毫无疑问会以某种方式影响 AC/PKA 信号,但我们和其他研究人员对 dNF1 是直接还是间接影响该通路存在矛盾的结论。在讨论这种差异的原因之前,以下部分首先简要描述了图 34.2 中所示的 dNF1 表型。

34.3.1 胚胎后期生长缺陷

dNF1 胚胎大小正常,但在随后的幼虫、蛹和成虫阶段,突变体都比对照组小 15%～20%。通过测量成翅细胞密度,这种缺陷被证明反映了细胞大小的减少,而不是细胞数量的减少。然而,较小的突变体眼睛由较少的正常大小的膜细胞组成,这表明不同的组织对 dNF1 的缺失有不同的反应。镶嵌分析首次表明,翅膀生长的减少涉及一种非细胞自主机制(The et al. 1997)。有证据表明,dNF1 的表达主要局限于神经系统(Walker et al. 2006),而且蝇或人 NF1 的神经元再表达足以恢复 dNF1 的生长(Tong et al. 2002;Walker et al. 2006)。dNF1 的生长缺陷不会因 Ras1 或 Ras 交换因子 Son-of-sevenless 的杂合性缺失而被抑制,也不会在携带功能增益 Raf 等位基因的突变体中增强。相反,低形态 PKA 催化亚基突变表征了 dNF1 的大小缺陷,在整个发育过程中表达组成型活性 PKA 转基因可部分恢复 dNF1 的生长(The et al. 1997)。

生物体的大小是生长速度和持续时间的函数。昆虫的生长主要发生在幼虫发育过程中,前者受胰岛素样肽控制,后者受激素级联控制,最终导致蜕皮激素的定时释放。目前还没有发现 dNF1 与这两种途径有关的确凿证据(Walker et al. 2006)。在各种 dNF1 表型中,生长缺陷是唯一一种容易进行遗传分析的表型。关注这一缺陷的另一个原因是,生长减慢是人类 NF1 和相关 RAS 疾病的常见症状(Szudek et al. 2000)。

34.3.2 行为缺陷

dNF1 突变体表现出微妙的行为缺陷。当飞虫被释放时,即使反复催促,仍有约 15% 的飞虫不会飞走(The et al. 1997)。当成虫被拍打到瓶中时,突变体需要更长的时间才能爬上来(Tong et al. 2007)。这些缺陷的解剖学基础尚未确定;突变体对视觉或嗅觉线索反应正常(The et al. 1997),并显示出正常的运动活动(Williams et al. 2001)。与生长减弱的表型一样,异常的攀爬反应也被归因于 AC/PKA 信号转导缺陷(Tong et al. 2007)。

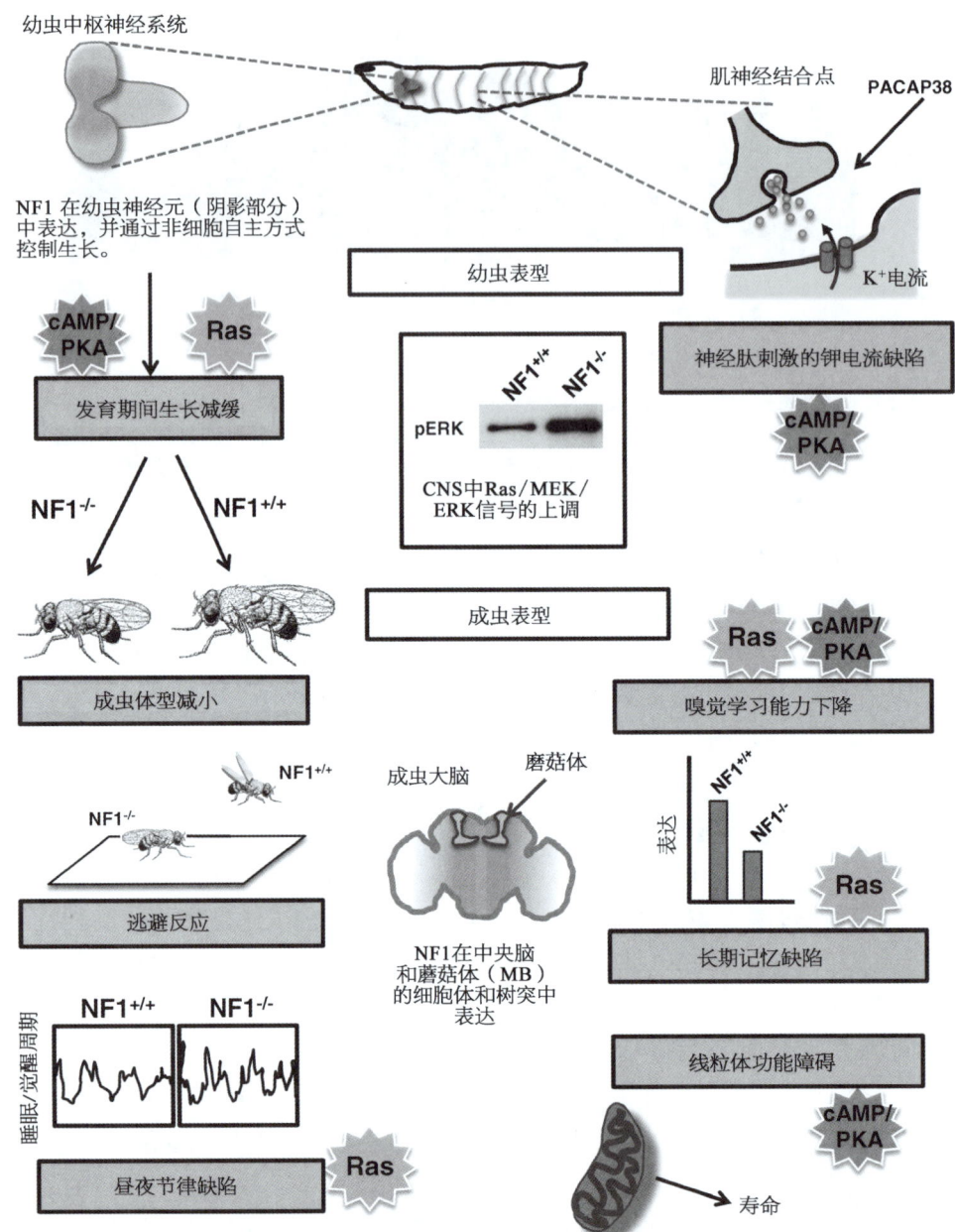

图 34.2 幼虫和成虫的纯合子缺失 dNF1 表型。dNF1 幼虫在体壁神经肌肉接点缺乏神经肽诱导的整流钾电流。幼虫、蛹和成虫的体型比同系野生型对照小 15%~20%，并且幼虫和成虫的 dNF1 脑部磷酸化 ERK 水平约为对照的 3 倍。成年 dNF1 果蝇缺乏正常的昼夜节律性运动行为，表现出较低的嗅觉联想学习/短期记忆能力，以及中期和长期记忆的缺陷。图示的成虫脑显示了蘑菇体（MB）的位置，MBs 在昆虫中的定位等同于脊椎动物的海马体。MB 在嗅觉学习中发挥重要作用，并优先表达多个 AC/PKA 通路蛋白。尽管 dNF1 在 MBs 中表达，但其与学习/记忆相关的功能是否涉及 MB 内部或外部的细胞仍存在争议（Buchanan and Davis 2010；Gouzi et al. 2011）。

34.3.3　神经肽刺激的 K^+-电流缺陷

dNF1 的缺失并不影响控制胚胎中光感受器细胞发育或躯干/Ras 信号转导的 sevenless 介导的 Ras 信号（The et al. 1997）。因此，为了分析 dNF1 是否会影响其他 Ras 通路，我们与 Yi Zhong 博士合作，他曾报告说，哺乳动物神经肽 PACAP38 在果蝇幼虫体壁神经肌肉接头制备物中引起的整流 K^+ 电流需要完整的 Ras 和 rutabagaAC 通路（Zhong 1995）。电生理分析表明，dNF1 突变体缺乏由

PACAP38 引发的电流，而通过操作 AC 而不是 Ras 信号转导，这种电流可以恢复（Guo et al. 1997）。在没有明显的果蝇 PACAP 受体同源物的情况下，哺乳动物的 PACAP38 是如何刺激反应的？

34.3.4 昼夜节律缺陷

昼夜节律钟控制着各种节律行为，包括运动活动的每日变化。在恒定黑暗条件下进行分析时，dNF1 突变体显示出周期和定时钟基因的正常循环，但完全（$NF1^{P1}$）或几乎完全（$NF1^{P2}$）心律失常。elav - GAL4 驱动的 UAS - dNF1 泛神经元表达可以恢复正常的节律行为，但昼夜节律钟的部位——大脑中枢侧神经元的限制性表达则不能恢复正常的节律行为。抗体染色显示，在含有色素分散因子（一种时钟细胞的分泌物）的神经末梢附近，磷酸化 ERK 存在昼夜节律振荡。因此，dNF1 缺失神经元中过量的 Ras/ERK 信号会影响昼夜节律时钟输出途径和昼夜节律运动活动（Williams et al. 2001）。

34.3.5 联想嗅觉学习和中短期记忆缺陷

果蝇被广泛用于研究学习和记忆的分子和细胞回路（Davis 2005）。由于对神经肌肉信号缺陷的分析表明，dNF1 与涉及芦柑 AC（一种著名的学习突变体）的通路有关，而且 NF1 与人和小鼠的学习缺陷有关（Hyman et al. 2005；Silva et al. 1997），因此 Zhong 研究小组在巴甫洛夫联想学习试验中对 dNF1 突变体进行了分析。在这项试验中，$NF1^{P1}$ 和 $NF1^{P2}$ 突变体的学习/短时记忆能力都明显下降。成人表达 hsp70 - dNF1 转基因抑制了这种学习缺陷，从而证明发育缺陷并不能解释这种缺陷。进一步的研究表明，在缺乏 dNF1 的小鼠中，除了短期（3 分钟）记忆外，3 小时和 8 小时的中期记忆保持也受到影响。这也与 AC/PKA 信号转导异常有关，学习和记忆缺陷都被 PKA 表达的增加所抑制（Guo et al. 2000）。

34.3.6 长期记忆缺陷

过多的 Ras/ERK 信号是 $Nf1^{+/-}$ 小鼠在评估空间学习能力的莫里斯水迷宫中表现下降的原因（Costa et al. 2002；Cui et al. 2008）。相比之下，AC 信号的缺陷似乎是 dNF1 嗅觉学习能力下降的原因（Guo et al. 2000）。与短期嗅觉学习试验不同，水迷宫中的表现需要依赖蛋白质合成的长期记忆（longterm memory，LTM）。dNF1 空缺突变体具有 LTM 缺陷，与短期学习和记忆缺陷不同，这种缺陷似乎依赖于 Ras（Ho et al. 2007）。其他人最近的研究进一步证实了 dNF1 在短期（3 分钟）、中期（3 小时）和 24 小时 LTM 中的作用，特别是在记忆获得而非衰减中的作用（Buchanan and Davis 2010）。

34.3.7 线粒体功能障碍

dNF1 突变体寿命缩短，更容易受到热或氧化应激的影响，同时线粒体呼吸减少，活性氧（reactive oxygen species，ROS）产生增加。相比之下，过表达 dNF1 能延长寿命，提高生殖能力，增强对热和氧化应激的抵抗力，同时线粒体呼吸作用增强，ROS 产生量减少 60%。与其他 dNF1 缺陷一样，这些表型也可以通过增加 cAMP/PKA 信号的药物或遗传操作来恢复。用催化抗氧化剂抵消 ROS 也能使同基因 dNF1 空缺突变体恢复正常寿命（Tong et al. 2007）。

34.4　dNF1 是直接还是间接影响 AC/PKA 信号

如上所述，遗传学证据有力地证明了 dNF1 与 AC/PKA 信号转导之间的联系。生化证据进一步支持了这种功能性联系，包括观察到在 $dNF1^{P1}$ 和 $dNF1^{P2}$ 脑膜制备物中，GTPgS 刺激的 AC 活性降低，但基础 AC 活性并不降低（Guo et al. 2000）。此外，在 E12.5 天的 $Nf1^{-/-}$ 鼠脑提取物中，也发现 GTPgS 刺激的 AC 活性和 cAMP 水平降低（Tong et al. 2002）。因此，尽管 AC 信号转导缺陷似乎是一种进化上保守的 NF1 表型（尽管是隐性的），但这些结果并未揭示神经溴素是如何影响 AC 活性的。与可能涉及非细胞自主机制的观点一致的是，GTPgS 刺激的 AC 活性不仅在果蝇大脑中降低，而且在腹部组织中也降低了（Guo et al. 2000），而在腹部组织中 dNF1 可能没有表达（Walker et al.

2006)。dNF1/PKA 介导的对线粒体呼吸的影响也与非细胞自主机制相吻合，该影响是在从全基因突变体中分离的线粒体实验中检测到的（Tong et al. 2007；Walker and Bernards 2007）。

在旨在确定 dNF1 如何影响 AC/PKA 信号转导的实验中，我们和其他人得出了相互矛盾的结论。因此，Zhong 小组的研究工作使他们推测，除了典型的 Gαs 依赖性途径外，还存在两种 dNF1 依赖性 AC 途径。第一种依赖 NF1 的途径受血清素和组胺的刺激，依赖于 Gαs，而另一种新型 AC 途径涉及 EGF 受体、NF1 和 Ras，但不依赖 Gαs。作者利用表达人类 NF1 缺失和点突变体的转基因小鼠报告说，NF1 介导的 Ras 调节对新型 EGF 受体刺激的 AC 通路至关重要，但对 NF1/Gαs 依赖的神经递质刺激的 AC 活性并不重要。此外，最清楚地证明 NF1 可能具有不依赖于 Ras 的功能的证据是，不包括 GRD 的人类神经纤维瘤蛋白 C 端片段能够挽救依赖 AC 的生物体生长（Hannan et al. 2006）和学习缺陷（Ho et al. 2007）。

我们得出的结论是，神经元 Ras/ERK 活性过剩是导致 dNF1 生长和学习表型的直接原因，这一结论是基于两项研究的结果。第一项研究侧重于 dNF1 的生长缺陷。在与人类 NF1 转基因类似的结构/功能研究中（Hannan et al. 2006），我们发现除 GRD 之外的大的 dNF1 片段对于生长调节是不可或缺的，几种 GAP 缺失的 dNF1 点突变体不能恢复生长，而仅代表 dNF1 GRD 的截短蛋白的表达足以抑制生长缺陷。此外，神经元表达果蝇 p120RasGAP 同源物也能抑制生长检测。为了研究为什么在早期研究中，Ras1 或其他典型 Ras 通路成分的缺失不能改变 dNF1 的生长缺陷，我们测试了一组全面的 Ras 通路单突变体和双突变体恢复 dNF1 生长的能力。作为分子关联，我们还分析了这些突变体恢复幼虫和成虫大脑磷酸-ERK 水平升高的能力。没有一个单突变体能改变这两种表型，这表明被测试的 Ras 通路成分要么没有参与，要么在导致 dNF1 大脑中 ERK 激活的通路中没有速率限制。支持后一种结论的是，一些确实恢复了正常 ERK 活性的双突变体也至少部分地挽救了生长缺陷（Walker et al. 2006）。因此，非细胞自主性 dNF1 机体生长缺陷的近因是神经元 Ras/ERK 信号过度传递（Walker et al. 2006）。

34.4.1 果蝇的 Alk/Ras 信号可能是 dNF1 生长和学习缺陷的原因

有进一步的证据表明，Ras/ERK 信号异常是导致 dNF1 缺陷的主要原因，这项工作始于观察到过量表达果蝇 Alk（Drosophila Alk，dAlk）受体酪氨酸激酶或其激活配体果冻腹（jelly belly，jeb）会使 dNF1 的生长和嗅觉学习表型发生改变。这一结果并不出人意料，因为之前的研究已经确定 dAlk 是体内 Ras/ERK 信号的激活剂（Loren et al. 2001）。然而，通过使用 dAlk 突变等位基因、dAlk shRNA 构建物、表达显性阴性的 dAlk 转基因或通过药物抑制来减弱 dAlk 的表达或活性，可以挽救 dNF1 的生长、嗅觉学习和脑 ERK 过度激活表型。dNF1 和 dAlk 的表达在幼虫和成虫大脑中广泛重叠，这支持了 dAlk 是 dNF1 调控的 Ras/ERK 信号的限速激活剂这一假说。此外，dAlk-GAL4 驱动的神经元 UAS-dNF1 表达足以恢复所有测试过的缺陷（Gouzi et al. 2011）。最后，尽管 dAlk 作为学习的负调控因子似乎并不寻常，但最近的研究表明，鼠类 Alk 可能也有类似的作用（Weiss et al. 2012）。

过量的 Alk/NF1/Ras 信号转导是否会导致人类 NF1 缺陷，这显然是下一个问题。耐人寻味的是，NF1 表达缺失在神经母细胞瘤中很常见，并与预后恶化有关（Holzel et al. 2010），其中很大一部分出现了 ALK 扩增或 ALK 功能增益突变 [reviewed by Azarova et al. (2011)]。ALK 过表达和 NF1 缺失同样与胶质母细胞瘤有关（Powers et al. 2002；Verhaak et al. 2010）。最后，哺乳动物的 ALK 可直接（Stoica et al. 2001，2002）或间接（Perez-Pinera et al. 2007）在人类 NF1 中过表达，并已被证明可作为 NF1 肿瘤细胞的氨原（Mashour et al. 2001，2004），这表明不适当的 ALK 信号转导可能有助于 NF1 肿瘤的发生。

34.5 结论

我们的研究得出结论，神经元过量的 Ras/ERK

信号是大多数（如果不是全部）dNF1 缺陷的根本原因。然而，几个重要的问题依然存在。最棘手的未决问题或许是 dNF1 如何影响 AC/PKA 信号转导。一种可能的机制是，dNF1 的缺失会导致一种或多种神经内分泌或神经递质信号缺陷。由于激素和神经递质通常通过 AC 耦合受体发出信号，这种缺陷可能通过增加 AC/PKA 信号转导而得到恢复。我们注意到，在该模型中，AC/PKA 信号缺陷并不一定涉及需要 NF1 的神经元。然而，尽管迄今为止没有任何结果正式排除了 dNF1 自主影响 AC/PKA 信号转导细胞的可能性，但我们的工作假设仍然是，不同神经元群之间的交叉对话可能参与产生了各种 Ras/ERK 和 AC/PKA 依赖性 dNF1 表型。除 dAlk 和 jeb 外，我们还在对 dNF1 表型的显性遗传修饰物进行遗传筛选，进行实验以确定修饰物的作用部位，并进行研究以确定增加 AC/PKA 信号可恢复 dNF1 缺陷的细胞，这些研究最终可能会揭示 dNF1 发挥其各种功能的神经元回路，并为导致人类 NF1 症状的分子和细胞途径提供更多线索。

（王智　译）

参考文献

[1] Andersen LB, Ballester R, Marchuk DA, Chang E, Gutmann DH, Saulino AM, Camonis J, Wigler M, Collins FS (1993) A conserved alternative splice in the von Recklinghausen neurofibromatosis (NF1) gene produces two neurofibromin isoforms, both of which have GTPase-activating protein activity. Mol Cell Biol 13: 487-495

[2] Azarova AM, Gautam G, George RE (2011) Emerging importance of ALK in neuroblastoma. Semin Cancer Biol 21: 267-275

[3] Ballester R, Marchuk D, Boguski M, Saulino A, Letcher R, Wigler M, Collins F (1990) The NF1 locus encodes a protein functionally related to mammalian GAP and yeast IRA proteins. Cell 63: 851-859

[4] Bernards A, Gusella JF (1994) The importance of genetic mosaicism in human disease. N Engl J Med 331: 1447-1449

[5] Bishop JG 3rd, Corces VG (1988) Expression of an activated ras gene causes developmental abnormalities in transgenic Drosophila melanogaster. Genes Dev 2: 567-577

[6] Buchanan ME, Davis RL (2010) A distinct set of Drosophila brain neurons required for neurofi-bromatosis type 1-dependent learning and memory. J Neurosci 30: 10135-10143

[7] Costa RM, Federov NB, Kogan JH, Murphy GG, Stern J, Ohno M, Kucherlapati R, Jacks T, Silva AJ (2002) Mechanism for the learning deficits in a mouse model of neurofibromatosis type 1. Nature 415: 526-530

[8] Cui Y, Costa RM, Murphy GG, Elgersma Y, Zhu Y, Gutmann DH, Parada LF, Mody I, Silva AJ (2008) Neurofibromin regulation of ERK signaling modulates GABA release and learning. Cell 135: 549-560

[9] Davis RL (2005) Olfactory memory formation in Drosophila: from molecular to systems neuro-science. Annu Rev Neurosci 28: 275-302

[10] Easton DF, Ponder MA, Huson SM, Ponder BA (1993) An analysis of variation in expression of neurofibromatosis (NF) type 1 (NF1): evidence for modifying genes. Am J Hum Genet 53: 305-313

[11] Gouzi JY, Moressis A, Walker JA, Apostolopoulou AA, Palmer RH, Bernards A, Skoulakis EM (2011) The receptor tyrosine kinase Alk controls neurofibromin functions in Drosophila growth and learning. PLoS Genet 7: e1002281

[12] Guo HF, The I, Hannan F, Bernards A, Zhong Y (1997) Requirement of Drosophila NF1 for activation of adenylyl cyclase by PACAP38-like neuropeptides. Science 276: 795-798

[13] Guo HF, Tong J, Hannan F, Luo L, Zhong Y (2000) A neurofibromatosis-1-regulated pathway is required for learning in Drosophila. Nature 403: 895-898

[14] Hannan F, Ho I, Tong JJ, Zhu Y, Nurnberg P, Zhong Y (2006) Effect of neurofibromatosis type I mutations on a novel pathway for adenylyl cyclase activation requiring neurofibromin and Ras. Hum Mol Genet 15: 1087-1098

[15] Ho IS, Hannan F, Guo HF, Hakker I, Zhong Y (2007) Distinct functional domains of neurofibro-matosis type 1 regulate immediate versus long-term memory formation. J Neurosci 27: 6852-6857

[16] Holzel M, Huang S, Koster J, Ora I, Lakeman A, Caron H, Nijkamp W, Xie J, Callens T, Asgharzadeh S et al (2010) NF1 is a tumor suppressor in neuroblastoma that determines retinoic acid response and disease outcome. Cell 142: 218-229

[17] Hyman SL, Shores A, North KN (2005) The nature and frequency of cognitive deficits in children with neurofibromatosis type 1. Neurology 65: 1037-1044

[18] Kayes LM, Burke W, Riccardi VM, Bennett R, Ehrlich P, Rubenstein A, Stephens K (1994) Deletions spanning the neurofibromatosis 1 gene: identification and phenotype of five patients. Am J Hum Genet 54: 424-436

[19] Loren CE, Scully A, Grabbe C, Edeen PT, Thomas J, McKeown M, Hunter T, Palmer RH (2001) Identification and characterization of DAlk: a novel Drosophila melanogaster RTK which drives ERK activation in vivo. Genes Cells 6: 531-544

[20] Mashour GA, Driever PH, Hartmann M, Drissel SN, Zhang T, Scharf B, Felderhoff-Muser U, Sakuma S, Friedrich RE, Martuza RL et al (2004) Circulating growth factor levels are associated with tumorigenesis in neurofibromatosis type 1. Clin Cancer Res 10: 5677-5683

[21] Mashour GA, Ratner N, Khan GA, Wang HL, Martuza RL, Kurtz A (2001) The angiogenic factor midkine is aberrantly expressed in NF1-deficient Schwann cells and is a mitogen for neurofibroma-derived cells. Oncogene 20: 97-105

[22] Pasmant E, Sabbagh A, Spurlock G, Laurendeau I, Grillo E, Hamel MJ, Martin L, Barbarot S, Leheup B, Rodriguez D et al (2010) NF1 microdeletions in neurofibromatosis type 1: from genotype to phenotype. Hum Mutat 31: E1506-E1518

[23] Perez-Pinera P, Zhang W, Chang Y, Vega JA, Deuel TF (2007) Anaplastic lymphoma kinase is activated through the

pleiotrophin/receptor protein-tyrosine phosphatase beta/zeta signaling pathway: an alternative mechanism of receptor tyrosine kinase activation. J Biol Chem 282: 28683-28690

[24] Powers C, Aigner A, Stoica GE, McDonnell K, Wellstein A (2002) Pleiotrophin signaling through anaplastic lymphoma kinase is rate-limiting for glioblastoma growth. J Biol Chem 277: 14153-14158

[25] Rieley MB, Stevenson DA, Viskochil DH, Tinkle BT, Martin LJ, Schorry EK (2011) Variable expression of neurofibromatosis 1 in monozygotic twins. Am J Med Genet A 155A: 478-485

[26] Roth TM, Petty EM, Barald KF (2008) The role of steroid hormones in the NF1 phenotype: focus on pregnancy. Am J Med Genet A 146A: 1624-1633

[27] Silva AJ, Frankland PW, Marowitz Z, Friedman E, Laszlo GS, Cioffi D, Jacks T, Bourtchuladze R (1997) A mouse model for the learning and memory deficits associated with neurofibromatosis type I. Nat Genet 15: 281-284

[28] Stoica GE, Kuo A, Aigner A, Sunitha I, Souttou B, Malerczyk C, Caughey DJ, Wen D, Karavanov A, Riegel AT et al (2001) Identification of anaplastic lymphoma kinase as a receptor for the growth factor pleiotrophin. J Biol Chem 276: 16772-16779

[29] Stoica GE, Kuo A, Powers C, Bowden ET, Sale EB, Riegel AT, Wellstein A (2002) Midkine binds to anaplastic lymphoma kinase (ALK) and acts as a growth factor for different cell types. J Biol Chem 277: 35990-35998

[30] Szudek J, Birch P, Friedman JM (2000) Growth in North American white children with neurofi-bromatosis 1 (NF1). J Med Genet 37: 933-938

[31] Szudek J, Joe H, Friedman JM (2002) Analysis of intrafamilial phenotypic variation in neurofi-bromatosis 1 (NF1). Genet Epidemiol 23: 150-164

[32] The I, Hannigan GE, Cowley GS, Reginald S, Zhong Y, Gusella JF, Hariharan IK, Bernards A (1997) Rescue of a Drosophila NF1 mutant phenotype by protein kinase A. Science 276: 791-794

[33] Thomson SA, Wallace MR (2002) RT-PCR splicing analysis of the NF1 open reading frame. Hum Genet 110: 495-502

[34] Tong J, Hannan F, Zhu Y, Bernards A, Zhong Y (2002) Neurofibromin regulates G protein-stimulated adenylyl cyclase activity. Nat Neurosci 5: 95-96

[35] Tong JJ, Schriner SE, McCleary D, Day BJ, Wallace DC (2007) Life extension through neurofibromin mitochondrial regulation and antioxidant therapy for neurofibromatosis-1 in Drosophila melanogaster. Nat Genet 39: 476-485

[36] Upadhyaya M, Huson SM, Davies M, Thomas N, Chuzhanova N, Giovannini S, Evans DG, Howard E, Kerr B, Griffiths S et al (2007) An absence of cutaneous neurofibromas associated with a 3-bp inframe deletion in exon 17 of the NF1 gene (c. 2970-2972 delAAT): evidence of a clinically significant NF1 genotype-phenotype correlation. Am J Hum Genet 80: 140-151

[37] Vandenbroucke I, Van Oostveldt P, Coene E, De Paepe A, Messiaen L (2004) Neurofibromin is actively transported to the nucleus. FEBS Lett 560: 98-102

[38] Verhaak RG, Hoadley KA, Purdom E, Wang V, Qi Y, Wilkerson MD, Miller CR, Ding L, Golub T, Mesirov JP et al (2010) Integrated genomic analysis identifies clinically relevant subtypes of glioblastoma characterized by abnormalities in PDGFRA, IDH1, EGFR, and NF1. Cancer Cell 17: 98-110

[39] Walker JA, Bernards A (2007) Drosophila melanogaster neurofibromatosis-1: ROS, not Ras? Nat Genet 39: 443-445

[40] Walker JA, Tchoudakova AV, McKenney PT, Brill S, Wu D, Cowley GS, Hariharan IK, Bernards A (2006) Reduced growth of Drosophila neurofibromatosis 1 mutants reflects a non-cell-autonomous requirement for GTPase-activating protein activity in larval neurons. Genes Dev 20: 3311-3323

[41] Weiss JB, Xue C, Benice T, Xue L, Morris SW, Raber J (2012) Anaplastic lymphoma kinase and leukocyte tyrosine kinase: functions and genetic interactions in learning, memory and adult neurogenesis. Pharmacol Biochem Behav 100: 566-574

[42] Williams JA, Su HS, Bernards A, Field J, Sehgal A (2001) A circadian output in Drosophila mediated by neurofibromatosis-1 and Ras/MAPK. Science 293: 2251-2256

[43] Xu GF, O'Connell P, Viskochil D, Cawthon R, Robertson M, Culver M, Dunn D, Stevens J, Gesteland R, White R et al (1990) The neurofibromatosis type 1 gene encodes a protein related to GAP. Cell 62: 599-608

[44] Zhong Y (1995) Mediation of PACAP-like neuropeptide transmission by coactivation of Ras/Raf and cAMP signal transduction pathways in Drosophila. Nature 375: 588-592

第35章 1型神经纤维瘤病的斑马鱼模型
Zebrafish Model for NF1

Arun Padmanabhan and Jonathan A. Epstein

35.1 引言

斑马鱼（Danio rerio）模型具有一些独特的生物学和遗传学特征，使其在与哺乳动物和无脊椎动物模型的比较中具有优势。这些鱼可以高密度养殖，生长周期短，产卵量大，再加上体外受精和快速发育的特点，使得脊椎动物斑马鱼成为在脊椎动物模型中基因筛查的有用工具（Driever et al. 1996；Haffter et al. 1996；Stainier et al. 1996）。胚胎和幼鱼的透明可视化以及通过转基因技术对特定细胞群体进行遗传标记的能力，使得可以在体内连续观察到诸如原始生殖细胞迁移或早期血管发育等复杂过程（Köprunner et al. 2001；Lawson and Weinstein 2002）。此外，斑马鱼已经成为一种有效的全机体脊椎动物模型，用于筛选大量已知的小分子化合物，并且已被证实具有识别抑制疾病表型或病理机制的化合物的能力（Peterson et al. 2004；Stern et al. 2005；Hong et al. 2006）。随着研究技术的快速发展，斑马鱼模型在基因靶向和基因转换等领域更加精准（Meng et al. 2008；Doyon et al. 2008；Foley et al. 2009；Zhu et al. 2011）。利用斑马鱼的这些优势来研究NF1，我们通过识别和鉴定人类NF1基因的斑马鱼同源物，分析其暂时缺失后出现的表型，以及培育基因突变导致功能缺失的斑马鱼品系，建立了斑马鱼NF1疾病模型（Zhu et al. 2011；Padmanabhan et al. 2009；Lee et al. 2010）。

35.2 斑马鱼基因组与人类 *NF1* 有两个同源基因

生物信息学分析发现斑马鱼基因组中存在两个与人类 *NF1* 基因高度同源的基因，在氨基酸水平上的相似度分别为90.4%和90.7%。这些基因分别命名为 *nf1a* 和 *nf1b*，它们之间具有很高的亲缘关系，相似度为87.4%，相似性为93.7%，并且具有相似的基因结构，每个基因都含有57个外显子（图35.1a、b）。*nf1a* 位于第15号染色体上（图35.1a），预测含有311 kDa的蛋白质，由2 755个氨基酸

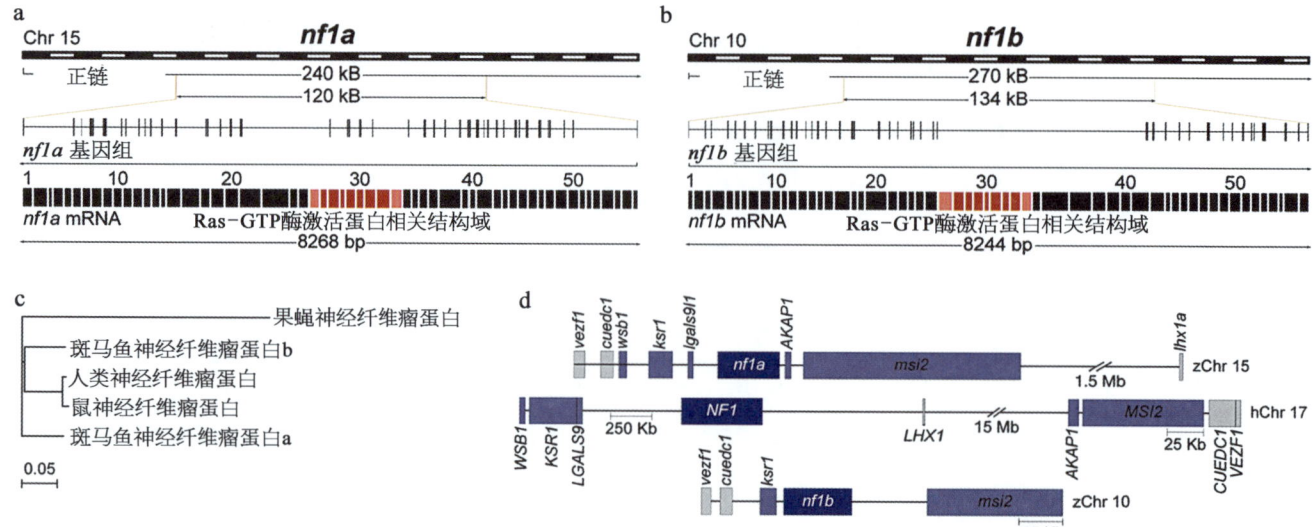

图 35.1 斑马鱼有两个与人类 NF1 基因相对应的同源基因。a、b. 斑马鱼 NF1 基因的基因组和 mRNA 结构。c. 比较斑马鱼、人类、小鼠和果蝇神经纤维瘤蛋白的进化树。d. 人类染色体 17（NF1）与斑马鱼染色体 15（nf1a）和 10（nf1b）的同源关系分析，相对基因组位置按比例绘制

组成，而 nf1b 位于第 10 号染色体上（图 35.1b），预测含有 310 kDa 的蛋白质，由 2 747 个氨基酸组成。一个进化树（图 35.1c）显示斑马鱼神经纤维瘤蛋白与其他哺乳动物神经纤维瘤蛋白的基因组有高度相关性，并且都来源于果蝇神经纤维瘤蛋白的同源物。对人类/斑马鱼同源图分析表明，nf1a 和 nf1b 很可能是通过基因复制产生的（图 35.1d），这与已知的早期硬骨鱼类染色体倍增现象相符（Amores et al. 1998）。NF1 基因位于第 17 号染色体上，其上游编码含 WD 重复 SOCS 框蛋白 1（WD repeat and SOCS box-containing 1，WSB1）、Ras 1 激酶抑制因子（Kinase suppressor of ras 1，KSR1）以及甘露糖结合蛋白 9（Galectin-9，LGALS9），而 NF1 下游则编码 A 激酶锚定蛋白 1（A kinase anchor protein 1，AKAP1）和 RNA 结合蛋白 Musashi 同源物 2（Musashi homolog 2，MSI2）。nf1a 两侧有与其相似的基因，而 nf1b 只有单侧有 KSR1 和 MSI2 的同源基因。这些基因在母体中表达（图 35.2a、b），并在早期发育过程中广泛表达，但随后其表达仅限于头部和前脑中枢神经系统的特定区域（图 35.2c~f）。

35.3 NF1a 和 NF1b 功能缺陷的表型与小鼠和人类 NF1 模型中相似性

反义磷酰二胺吗啉代寡聚核苷酸（morpholino phosphorodiamidate antisense oligonucleotides，MO）是一种常用的工具，可通过敲除特异性序列（Nasevicius and Ekker 2000）来研究斑马鱼的基因功能。经过对 nf1a 和 nf1b 多个 MO 的开发和验证，我们能够评估早期斑马鱼发育过程中缺失这些基因所导致的表型结果（Padmanabhan et al. 2009；Lee et al. 2010）。

35.3.1 NF1a 和 NF1b 的敲除导致了心血管缺陷

Nf1a 和 Nf1b 基因敲除的斑马鱼胚胎在受精

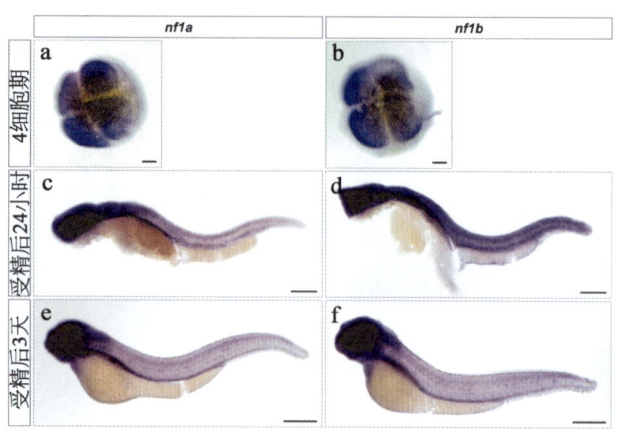

图 35.2 斑马鱼的 nf1a 和 nf1b 在胚胎发育期间表达。a~f. 经过斑马鱼胚胎的全胚原位杂交实验，我们可以观察到 nf1a 和 nf1b 基因在不同发育阶段（包括 4 细胞期、24 小时和 3 天）的时间和空间上的表达模式。标尺：25 μm

后 48 小时内呈现心血管发育异常,包括房室瓣缺损、大静脉淤血以及背侧主动脉和后主静脉血流减少。根据大体形态学分析显示,与对照组相比,在 48 小时后 nf1a 和 nf1b 敲除的斑马鱼心脏功能出现异常,同时心包积液的发生率增加(图 35.3a~c)。此外,在对受精后 3.5 天(dpf)对 nf1a 和 nf1b 基因敲除的斑马鱼进行组织学分析,观察到心室肌层变薄,并伴有明显的心包积液(图 35.3d、e)。这些发现与 NF1 小鼠模型的结果一致。而 NF1 模型小鼠在胚胎中期因严重心脏衰竭而死亡,并出现明显的心血管缺陷,包括心肌萎缩、异常的心脏瓣膜形态和心包积液。这些情况已被证明是由 Nf1 在内皮细胞中的细胞自主作用所导致的(Brannan et al. 1994;Jacks et al. 1994;Gitler et al. 2003)。尽管有心脏缺陷,但在前 3 天内胚胎的整体发育仍然呈现相对正常的状态。

在敲除 nf1a 和 nf1b 基因的斑马鱼胚胎中,将绿色荧光蛋白(green fluorescent protein,GFP)基因转入内皮细胞的细胞质,在胚胎发育的 48 和 72 小时,与对照组相比畸变体的间叶血管呈现明显异常的形态(图 35.3f~i)。在 NF1a MO 组的胚胎中,新生血管的尖端在 48 小时后呈现爪状突起(图 35.3g),无法正常形成背侧纵向吻合血管(dorsal longitudinal anastomotic vessel,DLAV)结构的完整形态,或只能形成最初略的结构在 72 小时后(图 35.3i)。这些异常在胚胎中很明显,尽管胚胎的整体大小和成熟度看起来正常,但在联合施用 nf1a 和 nf1b MO 或单独施用 nf1b MO 后,会出现相似的缺陷,尽管程度较轻。在没有心包积液或瓣膜功能不全的情况下,经常可以观察到血管异常的胚胎,这表明这些血管结构缺陷与心脏缺陷之间几乎没有或根本没有明显的相关性。虽然在胚胎中发现了孤立性的血管异常,但是其背侧主动脉和后侧主静脉内的仍然保持正常血流。在胚胎发育的 24 小时内,通过对表达核定位绿色荧光蛋白(GFP)的斑马鱼胚胎内皮细胞进行分析,发现突变体呈现出完全缺失的血管内皮细胞(图 35.3k),与对照组相比,可观察到胸主动脉发出的间叶血管部分呈现缺失(图 35.3j)。在单独的 NF1a MO 组与 NF1b MO 组中,这种表型呈现出的比例为 29% 和 33%(在注射的胚胎中),但是同时敲除这两种基因组产生了相加效应,比例达到了 51%(在注射胚胎中),表明两种基因在部分功能上有重叠。通过对具有血管损伤遗传背景的研究,进一步验证了 nf1a 和 nf1b 在血管发育调控中的作用。flt4 是斑马鱼 VEGF 受体-3 的同源物,之前的研究曾利用针对 flt4 的 MO(即突变体),以探讨斑马鱼动脉发育过程中的遗传相互作用(Covassin et al. 2006)。在斑马鱼胚

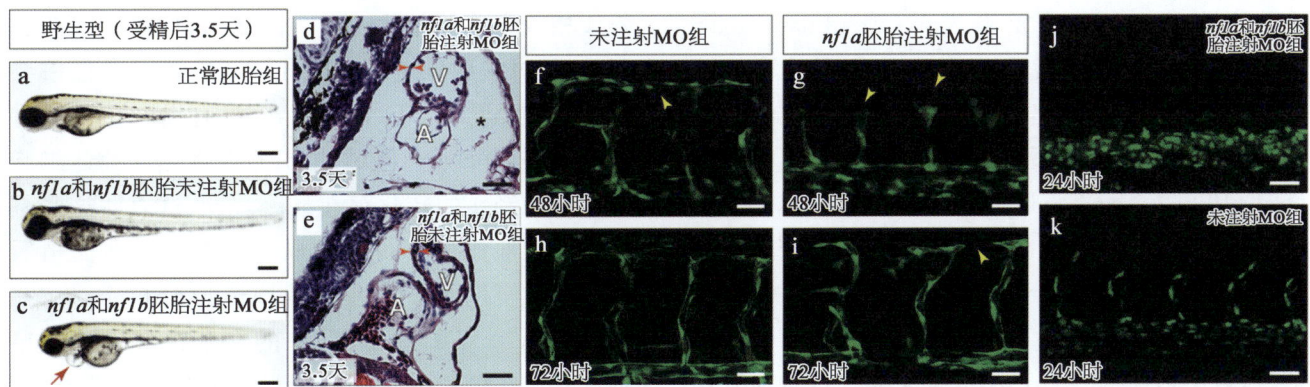

图 35.3 临时敲除 nf1a 和 nf1b 导致的心血管发育缺陷。a~c. (a) 正常胚胎组;(b) nf1a 和 nf1b 胚胎未注射 MO 组;(c) nf1a 和 nf1b 胚胎注射 MO 组,三组间在大体形态上未见明显缺陷,但 nf1a 和 nf1b 胚胎注射 MO 组出现心包腔扩张。d,e. 受精后 3.5 天,与对照组相比,nf1a/nf1b 复合突变胚胎的横切面显示室间隔心肌出现稀薄,并伴有心包积液(星号标注在左心房和右心室处)。f~i. 与对照样本(f)相比,受精后 48 小时,在发育过程中,经 nf1a 基因敲除后斑马鱼胚胎特异性表达 GFP 的间充质血管前端出现异常的爪状突起(g)。与对照组胚胎相比较(h),受精后 72 小时,Nf1a 基因敲除的胚胎仅呈现出一些原始的 DLAV 和躯干血管组织发育异常(i)。j,k. 与对照组相比(k),受精后 24 小时,nf1a/nf1b 基因突变的斑马鱼胚胎特异性内皮细胞 GFP 显示出间充质血管发育异常(j)。标尺:0.25 mm(a~c);25 μm(d~k)

胎中，单独注射 *Flt4* MO 或联合 *Nf1a* MO、*Nf1b* MO 注射或者 *NF1a* 和 *NF1b* MO 同时注射，将导致血管分流表型的出现，而对照组则不会有该表现。这些分流现象发生在背主动脉与背侧纵向吻合血管之间，通过节段动脉逆行回流至背主动脉或经节段静脉回流入后侧主静脉。在某些情况下，观察到背主动脉有中断现象。最重要的是，在 *Nf1* 缺陷的小鼠胚胎中尚未观察到血管发育缺陷的现象。由于观察到 *nf1a/nf1b* 敲除的斑马鱼胚胎中出现了周围血管发育缺陷的现象，之后在 *nf1* 敲除的小鼠中再次评估，发现在出现明显的心脏衰竭前其存在血管异常，包括整体血管数量的增加以及体节区域和头部原始血管丛的失效，导致无法进行适当的重构（Padmanabhan et al. 2009）。

这些结果的发现突出了研发斑马鱼 NF1 模型的优势。利用这些优势，可以区分原发性血管发育缺陷与由心脏衰竭引起的继发性表现，因为早期斑马鱼的血管发育只需要通过被动扩散提供足够的氧气即可，并不需要完整的血液循环来促进血管的发育（Vogel and Weinstein，2000）。但是，在小鼠模型中并非如此，在同时存在心功能异常和血管发育缺陷的疾病模型中，很难将原发性血管发育缺陷与继发于心脏功能障碍引起的血管异常区分开来。另外，在患病的个体中，血管发育缺陷也是 NF1 的众多临床表现中的一个重要表现（Friedman et al. 2002）。NF1 患者通常会出现一种典型的血管病变，称为"烟雾病"，其名称来源于在头部 CT 检查中血管的异常排列形态看起来像一团"烟雾"（Norton et al. 1995；Cairns and North 2008）。另外，也有其他血管异常的记录，如高血压和肾动脉狭窄。神经纤维瘤蛋白（neurofibromin）通过其 GAP 相关域（GAP-related domain，GRD）调节 ras 原癌基因的活性，有多项证据表明 Ras 信号通路在正常血管结构形成和发育中扮演着重要角色（Henkemeyer et al. 1995；Eerola et al. 2003；Liu et al. 2008；Revencu et al. 2008）。从以上结果表明，对 Ras 信号通路的严格调控对于正常的血管发育至关重要。在 *nf1a/nf1b* 敲除模型中观察到的各种血管发育缺陷可能反映了神经纤维瘤蛋白在血管系统中的不同功能，也可能是由共同的潜在机制引起的。与此同时，在不能排除其他解释的情况下，*Flt4* 与 *nf1a/nf1b* 之间的遗传相互作用表明这些分子可能参与共同的信号转导途径，并且可能与通过 Ras 激酶介导的 VEGF 受体信号通路相关联。

35.3.2 *nf1a* 和 *nf1b* 敲除导致少突胶质祖细胞缺陷

少突胶质细胞起源于脊髓腹侧的运动神经元祖细胞（pMN）区域，在这里首次观察到少突胶质细胞特异性关键转录因子 *olig2* 的表达（Lu et al. 2002；Rowitch 2004）。转基因的斑马鱼表达了由 *olig2* 调节序列驱动的 GFP，在脊髓背侧存在两类被标记的少突胶质祖细胞（oligodendrocyte progenitor cell，OPC），其中一类向背侧迁移并分化为少突胶质细胞，另一类则在原位与 GFP 阳性的运动神经元和中间神经元混合（Shin et al. 2003；Park et al. 2004）。在这一阶段，位于腹侧的 OPC 表达 Sox10，而运动神经元或中间神经元则不会表达。受精后 3 天，在 *olig2*：GFP 转基因的斑马鱼中，*nf1a*、*nf1b* 或两者同时被敲除会导致 OPC 数量增加，这可以通过体内观察背向迁移的 GFP 阳性细胞（图 35.4a、b）或通过脊髓横切的免疫组织化学分析对 Sox10/GFP 双阳性细胞进行定量评估（图 35.4c～h）。同样，同时敲除 *nf1a/nf1b* 复合突变胚胎中所产生的效应相较于单独敲除一个基因更为显著，在发育过程中对 OPC 数量进行负调控时存在部分功能重叠现象。在 NF1a/NF1b 敲除后，没有发现位于脊髓前角神经节（pMN）区域的 GFP 阳性共同前体细胞向运动神经元的转化存在显著差异，这表明这些基因特异性地作用于少突胶质细胞谱系。在受精后 80 小时，使用 BrdU 进行脉冲标记分析 BrdU 在 GFP/Sox10 双阳性 OPC 中的整合情况。结果显示，与对照组相比，*nf1a/nf1b* 复合突变胚胎的 OPC 增殖能力显著增强，从而解释了观察到的 OPC 数量增加的原因。这些数据与小鼠体外和体内研究一致，表明在 *Nf1* 杂合或纯合缺失后星形胶质细胞和少突胶质细胞过度增殖（Gutmann et al. 1999；Bennett et al. 2003；Zhu et al. 2005；Hegedus et al. 2007）。此外，NF1 患者容易发展为神经胶质肿

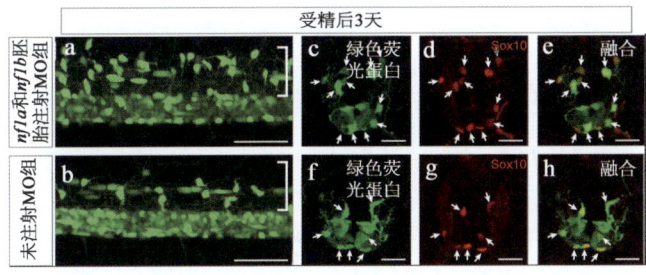

图 35.4 敲除 *nf1a* 和 *nf1b* 会导致 OPC 数量增加。a、b. 在携带 *p53* 基因突变以避免 MO 毒性的转基因胚胎中注射 *nf1a*＋*nf1b* MO olig2：GFP，观察受精 3 天后活体脊髓侧面观的共聚焦图像，与同时期的对照组比较（b），位于脊髓背侧位置的 OPC 数量增加（a）。c～h. *p53* 突变的斑马鱼胚胎中，使用 *olig2*：GFP 标记同时注射 *nf1a*＋*nf1b* MO，观察受精 3 天后脊髓横切面的免疫组化染色图片。（c～e）显示 GFP（绿色）/Sox10（红色）的增加，与同期对照组比较，双阳性细胞数量呈现显著增加（f～h）。标尺：50 μm（a、b）；20 μm（c～h）

瘤，包括视神经胶质瘤和星形细胞肿瘤（Gutmann et al. 2003；Listernick et al. 2007）。

这些表型评估依赖于神经纤维瘤蛋白对 Ras 信号的负向调节作用，通过 GAP 相关结构域（GRD）来调控（Ballester et al. 1990；Xu et al. 1990；Ismat et al. 2006）。在斑马鱼体模型中很容易实施，具体来说，通过编码分离的人类 NF1 GRD 的 RNA 同时注射到 *nf1a/nf1b* 复合突变胚胎中，然后评估脊髓背部的 OPC 数量。事实上，注射了人类 NF1 GRD RNA 的 *nf1a/nf1b* 复合突变胚胎显示出背侧脊髓 OPC 的减少（每个胚胎 67.7 对 48.5），与注射了 MO 组或 RNA 组的胚胎结果相似（图 35.5a～e）。这些数据表明，神经纤维瘤蛋白（neurofibromin）唯一的 GAP 活性能够充分促进由 *nf1a/nf1b* 基因敲除引起的 OPC 数量增加，提示 *nf1a* 和 *nf1b* 的 GAP 活性调节 OPC 的增殖。这一发现是值得注意的，因为已经观察到小鼠 *Nf1* 在发育中具有组织特异性作用，在某些情况下可能独立于 GRD 活性（Ismat et al. 2006）。

斑马鱼模型系统有独特的能力，允许对 *nf1a/nf1b* 敲除后 OPC 数量的增加进行更深入的分析，即通过直接可视化转基因胚胎中荧光标记细胞群的行为来评估体内复杂发育过程。对 *nf1a/nf1b* 复合突变 *Olig2*：GFP 胚胎进行 12 小时的延时成像，

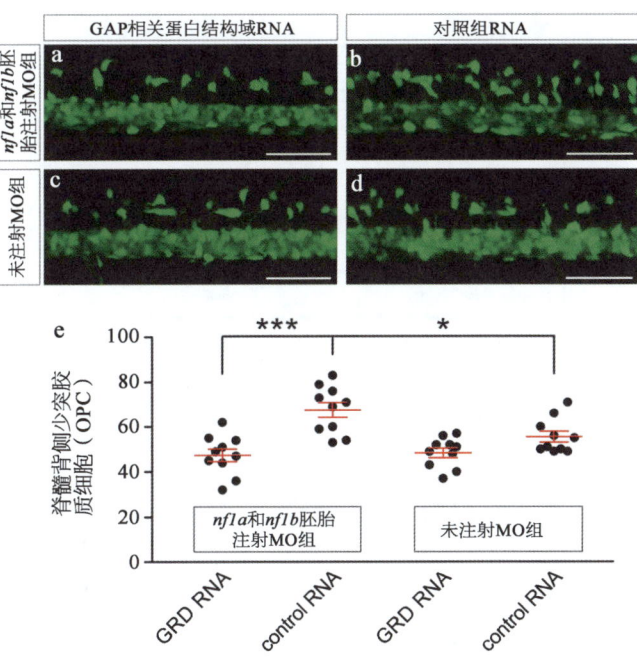

图 35.5 特异性的人 NF1 GRD 能够充分促进由 *nf1a/nf1b* 基因敲除引起的 OPC 数量增加。a～d. *p53* 突变的斑马鱼胚胎中，使用 *olig2*：GFP 转基因标记，观察受精 3 天后脊髓侧面观的共聚焦图像。人 NF1 GRD 的表达情况在注射 NF1a 和 NF1b MO 的胚胎中（a）OPC 数量降低与注射 MO 样本的对照组水平一致（c、d），与对照 RNA 相比注射 *nf1a/nf1b* MO 组的 OPC 数量增加（b）。e. 在受精 3 天后，各实验组胚胎脊髓背部 OPC 数量的定量评估（$^*P<0.05$；$^{***}P<0.001$）。标尺：50 μm

从受精后 60 小时进行定量分析。研究结果表明，与对照组相比，突变体 OPC 向背侧脊髓迁移的数量增加，且突变体 OPC 的迁移距离更长，停顿时间更短（图 35.6）。可以对单个 OPC 的迁移进行全面分析，从而构建迁移细胞轨迹（图 35.6a、b），以及测量总行进距离（图 35.6c）、主动迁移或停顿的时间（图 35.6d）和迁移速度（图 35.6e）。OPC 迁移的特点是频繁且有周期性间歇性的迁移活动。与对照组相比，敲除 *nf1a/nf1b* 以后，细胞暂停移动的频率和迁移速度无显著差异。这些数据与体外研究结果一致，NF1 基因的单倍体不足或者纯合子缺失，会增强星形胶质细胞的迁移能力（Gutmann et al. 2001）和施万细胞的侵袭性（Kim et al. 1997）。然而，这些细胞在体内如何运动尚未明确。通过敲除 *nf1a/nf1b* 以增强 OPC 的迁移能力代表了一种新的表型，可以通过在斑马鱼中建立 NF1 模型来论证。

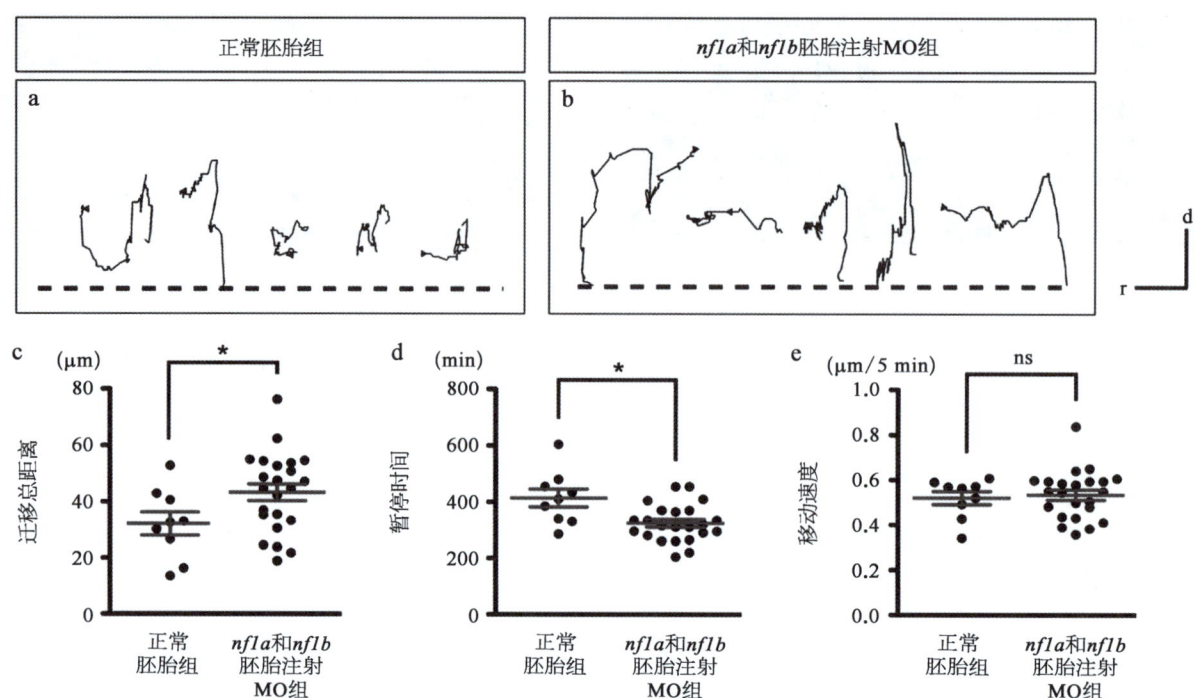

图 35.6 nf1a/nf1b 缺失影响 OPC 迁移。a、b. 5 个个体 OPC 在观察期间的细胞动态迁移大体的路径展示图例,其中(a)为未注射组的 olig2:GFP,p53 突变斑马鱼胚胎,(b)为 nf1a+nf1b MO 注射组的 olig2:GFP,p53 突变斑马鱼胚胎。箭头表示细胞迁移的终点,虚线表示在脊髓腹侧(上部、背部;左侧、头侧)GFP 标记区域的最大背侧部分。c. 对单个胚胎总的 OPC 迁移距离进行定量分析,结果显示,与未注射对照组比较,nf1a+nf1b MO 注射组的 OPC 增加了 35%($^*P<0.05$)。d. 对单个胚胎 OPC 暂停时间进行定量分析,结果显示,与未注射对照组比较,nf1a+nf1b MO 注射组的 OPC 总暂停时间减少了 22%($^*P<0.05$)。e. 与未注射对照组相比,nf1a+nf1b MO 注射组的胚胎中,未观察到单个 OPC 的速度有显著差异(ns 不具有统计学意义)。标尺:10 μm(c,d;x 轴);5 μm(c,d;y 轴)

35.4 培育稳定的 nf1a 和 nf1b 基因功能缺失的斑马鱼品种

上述研究表明利用斑马鱼胚胎临时敲除 nf1a 和 nf1b 的实验是可行的,并且可以利用这个实验模型来进行深入的机制研究和表型观察。然而,要充分利用斑马鱼系统的潜力,就需要培育 nf1a 和 nf1b 基因功能缺失的斑马鱼品种。利用最先进的转基因方法,已成功实现靶向 nf1a 和 nf1b 基因功能缺失的斑马鱼模型传代(Zhu et al. 2011)。尽管在斑马鱼中同源重组胚胎干细胞这种经典的基因靶向方法不能实施,但最近报道了利用锌指核酸酶进行靶向突变的替代方法。我们采用了这种方法来产生多个独立的 nf1a 和 nf1b 突变位点等位基因。此外,可使用化学诱变剂或插入性诱变引起的随机突变,然后进行基因测序,分离出具有特定基因突变的斑马鱼品种。例如,已有插入突变的 nf2 斑马鱼的描述(Amsterdam et al. 2004)。通过使用 TILLING 方法(Wienholds et al. 2002;Wienholds et al. 2003),我们在 nf1a 和 nf1b 中发现了几个错义基因突变,但是需要进一步特征描述。通过利用各种 nf1a 和 nf1b 稳定突变的等位基因进行初步研究,证实了 nf1a/nf1b MO 介导的基因敲除所产生的结果,这些结果与 NF1 基因中相关表型结果一致,提示 nf1a/nf1b 部分功能重叠。此外,对 nf1a/nf1b 胚胎的突变体 MO 分析一段时间,终于发现了色素细胞谱系中的新缺陷,从而建立了第一个能够再现 NF1 患者特征性咖啡牛奶斑的动物模型。

35.5 运用 NF1 斑马鱼模型的领域

在斑马鱼中模拟 NF1 可能有助于解决 NF1 领域中那些目前工具难以解决的问题。其中一个迫切需要解决的问题是，神经纤维瘤蛋白在调控 Ras 活性方面的功能在疾病中起到了多大的作用。多项证据表明，除了神经纤维瘤蛋白（NF1）功能域之外的区域也参与介导调控神经纤维瘤蛋白生物学活性（Ismat et al. 2006；Upadhyaya et al. 1997；Fahsold et al. 2000；Mattocks et al. 2004；Hannan et al. 2006；Ho et al. 2007）。具有 nf1a/nf1b 稳定突变的斑马鱼品种，是一种容易获取的用来识别和描述其他功能域的模型。由于在斑马鱼胚胎中蛋白质或蛋白质片段很容易进行过度表达，利用这个特点，可采用斑马鱼或人类 NF1 cDNA 构建体编码各种潜在的功能域，并进行功能补救实验。事实上，人类 NF1 cDNA 已被证明能够拯救突变果蝇的表型，这表明它在进化过程中具有足够的保守性，从而允许进行功能性替代（The et al. 1997）。

稳定的斑马鱼品种也有望作为一个高通量的发现平台，用于正向遗传方法和小分子筛选。在 nf1a/nf1b 缺失的背景下，正向遗传筛选将提供一种无偏倚的方法，用于发现能够增强或抑制 NF1 相关表型的新遗传位点。在同一 NF1 病变家族中，其临床表型呈现出显著的差异性，这提示存在不同的修饰位点来调控疾病特征的表达（Sabbagh et al. 2009）。识别这些修饰位点具有重要的诊断和预后价值，并可能发展成为新的治疗靶点。以斑马鱼为代表进行全动物筛选的方法具有启发性，因为它们融合了生物利用度的内在要求，可用于检测毒性和非靶向效应。在 nf1a/nf1b 缺失的背景下进行化学筛选有助于发现可能具有治疗效果的新型先进化合物，并有助于识别可能增强或改善 NF1 表型的分子途径。

（张家平，张璠 译）

参考文献

[1] Amores A, Force A, Yan YL, Joly L, Amemiya C, Fritz A, Ho RK, Langeland J, Prince V, Wang YL, Westerfield M, Ekker M, Postlethwait JH (1998) Zebrafish hox clusters and vertebrate genome evolution. Science 282：1711－1714

[2] Amsterdam A, Nissen RM, Sun Z, Swindell EC, Farrington S, Hopkins N (2004) Identification of 315 genes essential for early zebrafish development. Proc Natl Acad Sci USA 101：12792－12797

[3] Ballester R, Marchuk D, Boguski M, Saulino A, Letcher R, Wigler M, Collins F (1990) The NF1 locus encodes a protein functionally related to mammalian GAP and yeast IRA proteins. Cell 63：851－859

[4] Bennett MR, Rizvi TA, Karyala S, McKinnon RD, Ratner N (2003) Aberrant growth and differentiation of oligodendrocyte progenitors in neurofibromatosis type 1 mutants. J Neurosci 23：7207－7217

[5] Brannan CI, Perkins AS, Vogel KS, Ratner N, Nordlund ML, Reid SW, Buchberg AM, Jenkins NA, Parada L, Copeland NG (1994) Targeted disruption of the neurofibromatosis type-1 gene leads to developmental abnormalities in heart and various neural crest-derived tissues. Genes Dev 8：1019－1029

[6] Cairns AG, North KN (2008) Cerebrovascular dysplasia in neurofibromatosis type 1. J Neurol Neurosurg Psychiatr 79：1165－1170

[7] Covassin LD, Villefranc JA, Kacergis MC, Weinstein BM, Lawson ND (2006) Distinct genetic interactions between multiple Vegf receptors are required for development of different blood vessel types in zebrafish. Proc Natl Acad Sci USA 103：6554－6559

[8] Doyon Y, McCammon JM, Miller JC, Faraji F, Ngo C, Katibah GE, Amora R, Hocking TD, Zhang L, Rebar EJ, Gregory PD, Urnov FD, Amacher SL (2008) Heritable targeted gene disruption in zebrafish using designed zinc-finger nucleases. Nat Biotechnol 26：702－708

[9] Driever W, Solnica-Krezel L, Schier AF, Neuhauss SC, Malicki J, Stemple DL, Stainier DY, Zwartkruis F, Abdelilah S, Rangini Z, Belak J, Boggs C (1996) A genetic screen for mutations affecting embryogenesis in zebrafish. Development 123：37－46

[10] Eerola I, Boon LM, Mulliken JB, Burrows PE, Dompmartin A, Watanabe S, Vanwijck R, Vikkula M (2003) Capillary malformation—arteriovenous malformation, a new clinical and genetic -disorder caused by RASA1 mutations. Am J Hum Genet 73：1240

[11] Fahsold R, Hoffmeyer S, Mischung C, Gille C, Ehlers C, Kücükceylan N, Abdel-Nour M, Gewies A, Peters H, Kaufmann D, Buske A, Tinschert S, Nürnberg P (2000) Minor lesion mutational spectrum of the entire NF1 gene does not explain its high mutability but points to a functional domain upstream of the GAP-related domain. Am J Hum Genet 66：790－818

[12] Foley JE, Yeh J-RJ, Maeder ML, Reyon D, Sander JD, Peterson RT, Joung JK (2009) Rapid mutation of endogenous zebrafish genes using zinc finger nucleases made by Oligomerized Pool ENgineering (OPEN). PLoS One 4：e4348

[13] Friedman JM, Arbiser J, Epstein JA, Gutmann DH, Huot SJ, Lin AE, McManus B, Korf BR (2002) Cardiovascular disease in neurofibromatosis 1：report of the NF1 Cardiovascular Task Force. Genet Med 4：105－111

[14] Gitler AD, Zhu Y, Ismat FA, Lu MM, Yamauchi Y, Parada LF, Epstein JA (2003) Nf1 has an essential role in endothelial cells. Nat Genet 33：75－79

[15] Gutmann DH, Loehr A, Zhang Y, Kim J, Henkemeyer M, Cashen A (1999) Haploinsufficiency for the neurofibromatosis 1 (NF1) tumor suppressor results in increased astrocyte

proliferation. Oncogene 18: 4450-4459

[16] Gutmann DH, Wu YL, Hedrick NM, Zhu Y, Guha A, Parada LF (2001) Heterozygosity for the neurofibromatosis 1 (NF1) tumor suppressor results in abnormalities in cell attachment, spreading and motility in astrocytes. Hum Mol Genet 10: 3009-3016

[17] Gutmann DH, James CD, Poyhonen M, Louis DN, Ferner R, Guha A, Hariharan S, Viskochil D, Perry A (2003) Molecular analysis of astrocytomas presenting after age 10 in individuals with NF1. Neurology 61: 1397-1400

[18] Haffter P, Granato M, Brand M, Mullins MC, Hammerschmidt M, Kane DA, Odenthal J, van Eeden FJ, Jiang YJ, Heisenberg CP, Kelsh RN, Furutani-Seiki M, Vogelsang E, Beuchle D, Schach U, Fabian C, Nüsslein-Volhard C (1996) The identification of genes with unique and essential functions in the development of the zebrafish, Danio rerio. Development 123: 1-36

[19] Hannan F, Ho I, Tong JJ, Zhu Y, Nurnberg P, Zhong Y (2006) Effect of neurofibromatosis type I mutations on a novel pathway for adenylyl cyclase activation requiring neurofibromin and Ras. Hum Mol Genet 15: 1087-1098

[20] Hegedus B, Dasgupta B, Shin JE, Emnett RJ, Hart-Mahon EK, Elghazi L, Bernal-Mizrachi E, Gutmann DH (2007) Neurofibromatosis-1 regulates neuronal and glial cell differentiation from neuroglial progenitors in vivo by both cAMP- and Ras-dependent mechanisms. Cell Stem Cell 1: 443-457

[21] Henkemeyer M, Rossi DJ, Holmyard DP, Puri MC, Mbamalu G, Harpal K, Shih TS, Jacks T, Pawson T (1995) Vascular system defects and neuronal apoptosis in mice lacking ras GTPase-activating protein. Nature 377: 695-701

[22] Ho IS, Hannan F, Guo H-F, Hakker I, Zhong Y (2007) Distinct functional domains of neurofibro-matosis type 1 regulate immediate versus long-term memory formation. J Neurosci 27: 6852-6857

[23] Hong CC, Peterson QP, Hong J-Y, Peterson RT (2006) Artery/vein specification is governed by opposing phosphatidylinositol-3 kinase and MAP kinase/ERK signaling. Curr Biol 16: 1366-1372

[24] Ismat FA, Xu J, Lu MM, Epstein JA (2006) The neurofibromin GAP-related domain rescues endothelial but not neural crest development in Nf1 mice. J Clin Invest 116: 2378-2384

[25] Jacks T, Shih TS, Schmitt EM, Bronson RT, Bernards A, Weinberg RA (1994) Tumour predisposition in mice heterozygous for a targeted mutation in Nf1. Nat Genet 7: 353-361

[26] Kim HA, Ling B, Ratner N (1997) Nf1-deficient mouse Schwann cells are angiogenic and invasive and can be induced to hyperproliferate: reversion of some phenotypes by an inhibitor of farnesyl protein transferase. Mol Cell Biol 17: 862-872

[27] Köprunner M, Thisse C, Thisse B, Raz E (2001) A zebrafish nanos-related gene is essential for the development of primordial germ cells. Genes Dev 15: 2877-2885

[28] Lawson ND, Weinstein BM (2002) In vivo imaging of embryonic vascular development using transgenic zebrafish. Dev Biol 248: 307-318

[29] Lee J-S, Padmanabhan A, Shin J, Zhu S, Guo F, Kanki JP, Epstein JA, Look AT (2010) Oligodendrocyte progenitor cell numbers and migration are regulated by the zebrafish orthologs of the NF1 tumor suppressor gene. Hum Mol Genet 19: 4643-4653

[30] Listernick R, Ferner RE, Liu GT, Gutmann DH (2007) Optic pathway gliomas in neurofibromatosis-1: controversies and recommendations. Ann Neurol 61: 189-198

[31] Liu L, Zhu S, Gong Z, Low BC (2008) K-ras/PI3K-Akt signaling is essential for zebrafish hematopoiesis and angiogenesis. PLoS One 3: e2850

[32] Lu QR, Sun T, Zhu Z, Ma N, Garcia M, Stiles CD, Rowitch DH (2002) Common developmental requirement for Olig function indicates a motor neuron/oligodendrocyte connection. Cell 109: 75-86

[33] Mattocks C, Baralle D, Tarpey P, Ffrench-Constant C, Bobrow M, Whittaker J (2004) Automated comparative sequence analysis identifies mutations in 89% of NF1 patients and confirms a mutation cluster in exons 11-17 distinct from the GAP related domain. J Med Genet 41: e48

[34] Meng X, Noyes MB, Zhu LJ, Lawson ND, Wolfe SA (2008) Targeted gene inactivation in zebrafish using engineered zinc-finger nucleases. Nat Biotechnol 26: 695-701

[35] Nasevicius A, Ekker SC (2000) Effective targeted gene 'knockdown' in zebrafish. Nat Genet 26: 216-220

[36] Norton KK, Xu J, Gutmann DH (1995) Expression of the neurofibromatosis I gene product, neurofibromin, in blood vessel endothelial cells and smooth muscle. Neurobiol Dis 2: 13-21

[37] Padmanabhan A, Lee J, Ismat F, Lu M, Lawson N, Kanki J, Look A, Epstein J (2009) Cardiac and vascular functions of the zebrafish orthologues of the type I neurofibromatosis gene NFI. Proc Natl Acad Sci USA 106: 22305-22310

[38] Park HC, Shin J, Appel B (2004) Spatial and temporal regulation of ventral spinal cord precursor specification by Hedgehog signaling. Development 131: 5959-5969

[39] Peterson RT, Shaw SY, Peterson TA, Milan DJ, Zhong TP, Schreiber SL, Macrae CA, Fishman MC (2004) Chemical suppression of a genetic mutation in a zebrafish model of aortic coarctation. Nat Biotechnol 22: 595-599

[40] Revencu N, Boon LM, Mulliken JB, Enjolras O, Cordisco MR, Burrows PE, Clapuyt P, Hammer F, Dubois J, Baselga E, Brancati F, Carder R, Quintal JM, Dallapiccola B, Fischer G, Frieden IJ, Garzon M, Harper J, Johnson-Patel J, Labrèze C, Martorell L, Paltiel HJ, Pohl A, Prendiville J, Quere I, Siegel DH, Valente EM, Van Hagen A, Van Hest L, Vaux KK, Vicente A, Weibel L, Chitayat D, Vikkula M (2008) Parkes Weber syndrome, vein of Galen aneurysmal malformation, and other fast-flow vascular anomalies are caused by RASA1 mutations. Hum Mutat 29: 959-965

[41] Rowitch DH (2004) Glial specification in the vertebrate neural tube. Nat Rev Neurosci 5: 409-419

[42] Sabbagh A, Pasmant E, Laurendeau I, Parfait B, Barbarot S, Guillot B, Combemale P, Ferkal S, Vidaud M, Aubourg P, Vidaud D, Wolkenstein P (2009) Unravelling the genetic basis of variable clinical expression in neurofibromatosis 1. Hum Mol Genet 18: 2768-2778

[43] Shin J, Park HC, Topczewska JM, Mawdsley DJ, Appel B (2003) Neural cell fate analysis in zebrafish using olig2 BAC transgenics. Methods Cell Sci 25: 7-14

[44] Stainier DY, Fouquet B, Chen JN, Warren KS, Weinstein BM, Meiler SE, Mohideen MA, Neuhauss SC, Solnica-Krezel L, Schier AF, Zwartkruis F, Stemple DL, Malicki J, Driever W, Fishman MC (1996) Mutations affecting the formation and function of the cardiovascular system in the zebrafish embryo. Development 123: 285-292

[45] Stern HM, Murphey RD, Shepard JL, Amatruda JF, Straub CT, Pfaff KL, Weber G, Tallarico JA, King RW, Zon LI (2005) Small molecules that delay S phase suppress a zebrafish

bmyb mutant. Nat Chem Biol 1: 366 – 370
[46] The I, Hannigan GE, Cowley GS, Reginald S, Zhong Y, Gusella JF, Hariharan IK, Bernards A (1997) Rescue of a Drosophila NF1 mutant phenotype by protein kinase A. Science 276: 791 – 794
[47] Upadhyaya M, Osborn MJ, Maynard J, Kim MR, Tamanoi F, Cooper DN (1997) Mutational and functional analysis of the neurofibromatosis type 1 (NF1) gene. Hum Genet 99: 88 – 92
[48] Vogel AM, Weinstein BM (2000) Studying vascular development in the zebrafish. Trends Cardiovasc Med 10: 352 – 360
[49] Wienholds E, Schulte-Merker S, Walderich B, Plasterk RHA (2002) Target-selected inactivation of the zebrafish rag1 gene. Science 297: 99 – 102
[50] Wienholds E, van Eeden F, Kosters M, Mudde J, Plasterk RHA, Cuppen E (2003) Efficient target-selected mutagenesis in zebrafish. Genome Res 13: 2700 – 2707
[51] Xu GF, Lin B, Tanaka K, Dunn D, Wood D, Gesteland R, White R, Weiss R, Tamanoi F (1990) The catalytic domain of the neurofibromatosis type 1 gene product stimulates ras GTPase and complements ira mutants of S. cerevisiae. Cell 63: 835 – 841
[52] Zhu Y, Harada T, Liu L, Lush ME, Guignard F, Harada C, Burns DK, Bajenaru ML, Gutmann DH, Parada LF (2005) Inactivation of NF1 in CNS causes increased glial progenitor proliferation and optic glioma formation. Development 132: 5577 – 5588
[53] Zhu C, Smith T, McNulty J, Rayla AL, Lakshmanan A, Siekmann AF, Buffardi M, Meng X, Shin J, Padmanabhan A, Cifuentes D, Giraldez AJ, Look AT, Epstein JA, Lawson ND, Wolfe SA (2011) Evaluation and application of modularly assembled zinc-finger nucleases in zebrafish. Development 138: 4555 – 4564

第36章 起源细胞及微环境因素在1型神经纤维瘤病肿瘤发生中的作用及治疗意义

Cell of Origin and the Contribution of Microenvironment in NF1 Tumorigenesis and Therapeutic Implications

Johanna Buchstaller, D. Wade Clapp, Luis F. Parada, and Yuan Zhu

36.1 引言

1型神经纤维瘤病(neurofibromatosis type 1, NF1)是最常见的遗传性疾病之一,全球每3 500名新生儿中约有1名患有NF1(Riccardi 1992)。*NF1*基因的生殖系突变通常表现为失活或"功能丧失"突变,因此该基因被归类为肿瘤抑制基因。许多NF1相关的良性和恶性肿瘤都显示了杂合性缺失(loss of heterozygosity,LOH),即失去一个遗传型野生型等位基因或者*NF1*基因的第二个等位基因存在突变(Legius et al. 1993; Side et al. 1997; Xu et al. 1992)。NF1的一个显著临床特征是出现多发性良性周围神经鞘膜瘤,亦称为神经纤维瘤(Cichowski and Jacks 2001; Riccardi 1992; Zhu and Parada 2001)。其中,丛状神经纤维瘤(PNF)可能会经历额外的基因突变,进而发展为恶性周围神经鞘膜瘤(MPNST)(Woodruff 1999)。

36.2 皮肤型神经纤维瘤和丛状神经纤维瘤

神经纤维瘤有两个主要特征:首先,它们起源于周围神经或其分支;其次,它们是异质性肿块,包含了正常周围神经中的多种细胞组分,如施万细胞、神经元、成纤维细胞和肥大细胞等(Krone et al. 1983; Peltonen et al. 1988)。与NF1相关的神经纤维瘤主要有两个亚型,即皮肤型神经纤维瘤和丛状神经纤维瘤(Korf 1999)。皮肤型神经纤维瘤是最常见的类型,它们发生在皮肤真皮层或表皮中的小型周围神经枝。几乎所有的 NF1 患者在一生中的某个时期都会发展出多发性皮肤型神经纤维瘤。尽管可能导致外观畸形,但皮肤型神经纤维瘤很少对生命构成威胁。由于神经纤维瘤由多种细胞类型组成,并非所有细胞都缺乏 NF1 基因(Muir et al. 2001),因此只有少数皮肤型神经纤维瘤中检测到 LOH,比例在 13%~36%(Colman et al. 1995; Rasmussen et al. 2000; Serra et al. 1997; Thomas et al. 2012)。在对小鼠的遗传分析中发现,$Nf1$ 杂合缺失($Nf1^{+/-}$)小鼠或由 $Nf1^{-/-}$ 和 $Nf1^{+/+}$ 细胞组成的嵌合小鼠($Nf1^{-/-}$ $Nf1^{+/+}$)均未发展出皮肤型神经纤维瘤(Brannan et al. 1994; Cichowski et al. 1999; Jacks et al. 1994b)。小鼠模型研究表明,其他遗传因素、非遗传因素以及人类与小鼠皮肤之间的潜在物种差异可能有助于人类皮肤型神经纤维瘤的发展。临床研究表明,激素变化可能在皮肤型神经纤维瘤的形成中起到作用,因为 NF1 患者通常在青春期发展出皮肤型神经纤维瘤,而妊娠常常增加肿瘤的大小和数量(Ferner 2007,2010)。

30%~50% 的 NF1 患者发展为丛状神经纤维瘤,这些肿瘤沿着周围神经生长,可能涉及多个神经束或大神经的多个分支(Korf 1999)。尽管丛状神经纤维瘤与皮肤型神经纤维瘤具有相同的细胞组成,但它们的生长特性和对恶性进展的倾向是不同的。皮肤型神经纤维瘤通常是小型、局部的,并且不会进展为恶性肿瘤。相比之下,丛状神经纤维瘤通常更大且以扩散和浸润的方式生长,导致神经干和其分支的扩张。由于它们体积更大且位于体内较深的位置,这些肿瘤通常会影响正常的神经功能。此外,5%~10% 的丛状神经纤维瘤最终会发生恶性转化发展为 MPNST,这是与 NF1 相关的最常见的恶性肿瘤(Woodruff 1999)。更重要的是,MPNST 是 40 岁以下 NF1 患者最主要的死亡原因。目前,丛状神经纤维瘤的主要治疗方法是手术切除。然而,由于丛状神经纤维瘤常常发生在功能关键的神经中并且以扩散和浸润的方式生长,手术往往难以实现病变部位的完全切除,因此复发率较高。

目前为止,遗传分析尚未明确揭示丛状神经纤维瘤和皮肤型神经纤维瘤之间的显著差异。在三项独立研究中,发现 40%~50% 的丛状神经纤维瘤中存在 $NF1$ 位点的 LOH,这与皮肤病变中 LOH 的频率相当(Daschner et al. 1997; Kluwe et al. 1999; Rasmussen et al. 2000. Laycock-van Spyk et al. 2011)。值得注意的是,随着技术的改进,几乎所有人类神经纤维瘤中都发现了体细胞"第二次打击"$NF1$ 突变(Maertens et al. 2006,2007)。这些结果表明,双 NF1 等位基因失活驱动了人类皮肤型神经纤维瘤和丛状神经纤维瘤的形成。尽管与皮肤型神经纤维瘤相比,丛状神经纤维瘤细胞中更频繁地发现细胞遗传学异常,但丛状神经纤维瘤中并未发现特定的异常核型区域(Wallace et al. 2000)。此外,对嵌合 $Nf1^{-/-}$ $Nf1^{+/+}$ 小鼠的研究表明,$Nf1$ 的双等位基因失活足以诱导丛状神经纤维瘤的发展(Cichowski et al. 1999)。这些观察结果支持了 $NF1/Nf1$ 失活之外的其他因素对这两种神经纤维瘤发展的根本差异起到贡献的观点。临床上已经明确的一种差异是皮肤型神经纤维瘤和丛状神经纤维瘤的肿瘤发生时间(Korf 1999; Riccardi 1992)。

一个值得深入讨论的关键问题是,哪些细胞类型是神经纤维瘤形成和进一步发展为 MPNST 的起源细胞。由于施万细胞是神经纤维瘤的主要细胞群(40%~80%),且这些细胞表现出异常的侵袭性和血管生成性质,因此早期认为施万细胞是神经纤维瘤最可能的起源细胞(Sheela et al. 1990)。随后,从人类神经纤维瘤中分离出的细胞类型进行的遗传学研究为揭示起源细胞的性质提供了重要的见解(Rutkowski et al. 2000; Serra et al. 2000; Sherman et al. 2000)。此外,最近开发的在施万细胞谱系中不同发育阶段失活 $Nf1$ 的小鼠模型,允许对皮肤型神经纤维瘤、丛状神经纤维瘤以及 MPNST 起源细胞的性质进行进一步深入研究(Joseph et al. 2008; Le et al. 2009,2011; Mayes et al. 2011; Wu et al. 2008; Zheng et al. 2008; Zhu et al. 2002)。

36.3 皮肤型神经纤维瘤的起源细胞

通过对皮肤型神经纤维瘤中的施万细胞和成纤

维细胞进行培养，多个研究小组已经证明，从神经纤维瘤中分离的施万细胞通常缺乏 NF1 表达（Rutkowski et al. 2000），具有更高水平的 Ras-GTP 活性（Sherman et al. 2000），并往往携带双 NF1 等位基因突变（Serra et al. 2000）。临床研究表明，激素变化可能在肿瘤形成中起作用，因为 NF1 患者通常在青春期时发展出皮肤型神经纤维瘤，而妊娠通常会增加肿瘤的大小和数量（Ferner 2007，2010；Lakkis and Tennekoon 2000）。观察到皮肤型神经纤维瘤在生活的后期，即青春期时期出现，这引发了一种假设，即皮肤型神经纤维瘤可能起源于成年器官中的多能干细胞。在人类和小鼠皮肤中，已经发现了多能性神经嵴样干细胞和前体细胞，称为皮肤源前体细胞（skin-derived precursor cell，SKP），可以在悬浮培养中扩增（Fernandes et al. 2004；Sieber-Blum et al. 2004；Wong et al. 2006）。在皮肤中条件性失活 Nf1 的小鼠中可以观察到皮肤型神经纤维瘤的形成，而在培养的 SKP 中失活 Nf1 后，在周围神经移植实验中可观察到神经纤维瘤的形成（Le et al. 2009）。这些数据表明，皮肤型神经纤维瘤可能起源于 SKP 或其衍生的细胞。

36.4 丛状神经纤维瘤的起源细胞

与皮肤型神经纤维瘤通常在青春期和成年期发展不同，丛状神经纤维瘤通常在儿童早期即可被诊断。在一项基于临床的研究中（Waggoner et al. 2000），44%（32/72 名患者）的丛状神经纤维瘤在 5 岁之前被发现。最近的研究利用全身体积磁共振成像（MRI）显示，成年 NF1 患者中丛状神经纤维瘤的数量随时间变化不明显（Cai et al. 2009；Mautner et al. 2008）。这些观察结果支持了一个假设，即丛状神经纤维瘤可能是发育过程中从施万细胞谱系中形成的先天性病变（Riccardi 1992）。

36.4.1 施万细胞发育

施万细胞的发育是一个复杂的过程，包括从神经嵴干细胞、施万细胞前体、已分化的施万细胞，到两种成熟的细胞类型——有髓鞘形成的和无髓鞘形成的施万细胞（Jessen and Mirsky 2005）（图 36.1）。最近的研究着重于确定在施万细胞谱系中，NF1 基因失活发生的关键发育阶段，以有效地引发丛状神经纤维瘤的发生。

36.4.1.1 神经嵴干细胞

施万细胞的起源是神经嵴干细胞（图 36.1）。在脊椎动物的胚胎中，神经嵴细胞在神经管闭合后从背侧神经褶的末端分离出来，并沿着特定路径迁移到正在发育的胚胎中的特定位置，它们根据来自神经管的前后位置生成多种细胞类型（Dupin et al. 2006；Dupin and Sommer 2012；Morales et al. 2005）。躯干部位的神经嵴细胞经过分化成为皮肤的黑色素细胞、肾上腺和甲状腺的神经分泌细胞，以及感觉、自主和肠神经节中的周围神经元和神经胶质细胞。早期实验中，通过标记并追踪鸟类和小鼠胚胎中的单个预迁移和迁移细胞到它们的目标器官，表明迁移中的神经嵴细胞是多功能干细胞和已经定向于特定命运的细胞的混合（Bronner-Fraser and Fraser 1988，1989，1991；Serbedzija et al. 1994）。然而，最近的体内谱系追踪研究表明，神经嵴细胞的命运可能在脱层之前就已确定，并且取决于脱层的时间（Krispin et al. 2010）。尽管在体内，神经嵴细胞的命运可能受到限制，但至少其中一部分细胞在体外受到适当生长因子的刺激或者在体内移植到不同区域后，仍保留自我更新和分化为各种细胞谱系的潜力（Dupin et al. 1990；Shah et al. 1994；Sieber-Blum and Cohen 1980；Trentin et al. 2004）。在移植到前-后轴的不同区域后，迁移的神经嵴细胞可以倾向于它们所移植区域的命运（Le Douarin and Kalcheim 1999），晚期迁移的细胞也可在移植实验中取代早期迁移的细胞（Baker et al. 1997）。总之，这些数据表明在迁移过程中，不同环境信号的综合作用可能促使神经嵴细胞成熟为各种谱系（Jessen and Mirsky 2005）。

36.4.1.2 在胚胎和成体靶器官中持续存在的多能细胞

目前已经从各种胚胎和成体神经嵴靶器官中分离出具有自我更新和多种神经嵴谱系分化能力的干细胞，这些干细胞在体外培养和体内移植实验后展现了这种潜力。例如，这些干细胞来自背根神经节（dorsal root ganglia，DRG）（Hagedorn et al. 1999；

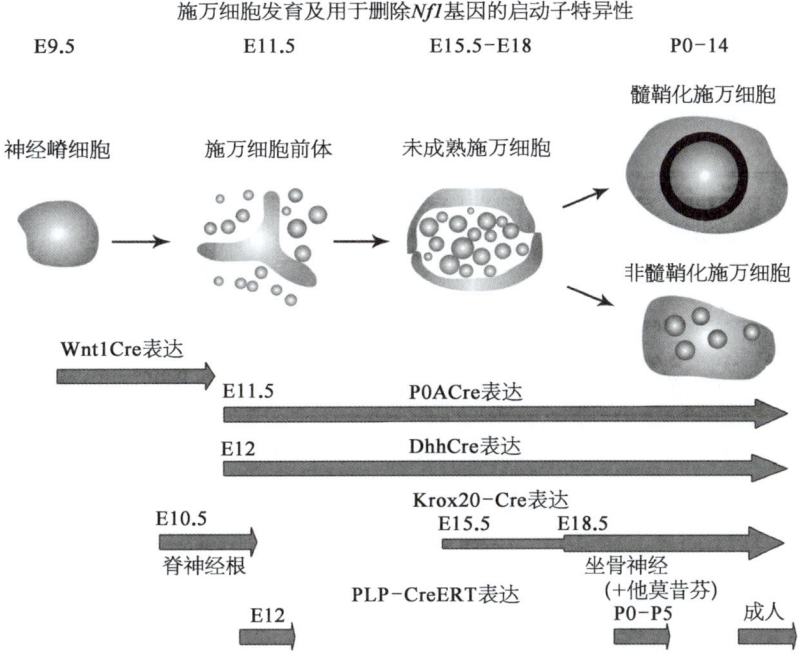

图 36.1　施万细胞的发育以及用于在施万细胞谱系中删除 $Nf1$ 的启动子[adapted from Jessen and Mirsky (2005)]。施万细胞来源于神经嵴干细胞,这些细胞在小鼠胚胎发育第 9 天(E9)从神经管背侧迁移出来。它们经过体节并在 E11.5 天与生长中的感觉和运动神经相关联,成为施万细胞前体细胞,尽管有些细胞仍然保持多能性(Morrison et al. 1999)。施万细胞前体细胞沿着轴突束迁移,在轴突信号的影响下增殖并在其谱系中进展,最终形成未成熟的施万细胞,这些细胞侵入轴突束,停止增殖,并根据轴突的直径进行排序(Jessen and Mirsky 2005)。在出生前后(出生后第 0 天),施万细胞与大直径轴突形成一对一的关系,这种相互作用在生命的前两周(P0 至 P14)内触发髓鞘的形成。多个小直径轴突被一个施万细胞包裹,这些施万细胞将保持非髓鞘化状态。使用在不同发育阶段表达 Cre 重组酶的小鼠,研究人员在施万细胞谱系中删除了 $Nf1$ 基因。通过使用 Wnt1‑cre,可以在迁移中的神经嵴细胞中删除 $Nf1$ 基因(Joseph et al. 2008),而 P0‑cre 和 Dhh‑cre 的表达则在周围神经中施万细胞发育的最早阶段删除了 $Nf1$ 基因(Joseph et al. 2008;Wu et al. 2008;Zheng et al. 2008)。Krox‑cre 在发育过程中在周围神经根中的多能边界帽细胞中表达,在 E15.5 至 E18 期间在未成熟施万细胞中低水平表达,最后在 E18 时在促髓鞘化施万细胞中高水平表达(Zhu et al. 2002)。Le 等(2011)和 Mayes 等(2011)使用了在更狭窄的时间窗口内通过给予他莫昔芬条件性灭活 $Nf1$ 基因的小鼠。除了 Wnt1‑cre;$Nf1^{flox/flox}$ 小鼠在出生时死亡而无法进一步分析外,所有其他 $Nf1$ 突变株都在 6 至 12 个月的潜伏期内发展出丛状神经纤维瘤

Nagoshi et al. 2008)、gut (Bixby et al. 2002;Kruger et al. 2002;Lo and Anderson 1995)、皮肤(Fernandes et al. 2004;Wong et al. 2006),以及胚胎坐骨神经(Bixby et al. 2002;Morrison et al. 1999)。尽管来自周围神经的神经嵴细胞在体内的分化命运受到一定限制,但仍然能够产生多种细胞类型。早期胚胎周围神经的神经嵴衍生细胞能够产生胶质细胞、内神经鞘成纤维细胞(Joseph et al. 2004),以及皮肤中的黑色素细胞(Adameyko et al. 2009),但在体内不形成神经元。在成体肠道中发现的神经嵴衍生细胞主要产生胶质细胞,即使在受伤或细菌感染后的再生过程中,成体肠道中的神经元再生现象也很少见(Joseph et al. 2011)。然而,迄今为止,尚未从成体坐骨神经中分离出自我更新和多系分化潜力的细胞(Kruger et al. 2002)。这可能是因为这种神经嵴靶器官缺乏类似成体干细胞的细胞,也可能是因为合适的生长和解离条件尚未完全确立。

36.4.1.3 施万细胞谱系的限制

神经胶质细胞的形成过程以及它们与多能神经嵴干细胞的分离时间点目前仍不明确(Jessen and Mirsky 2005)。当躯干神经嵴细胞到达体节后,它们会聚集形成背根神经节(DRG)。神经嵴衍生细

胞与从脊髓和脑神经发出的感觉神经相关联,并分化为施万细胞前体细胞,这些细胞沿着轴突束移动,紧随生长锥的尖端(Wanner et al. 2006)。虽然,神经的生长和到达目标区域并不一定需要施万细胞前体细胞(Grim et al. 1992;Riethmacher et al. 1997;Woldeyesus et al. 1999),施万细胞前体细胞却为感觉神经元和运动神经元的生存提供了营养支持,并对神经束的形成至关重要(Garratt et al. 2000)。在轴突信号的影响下,施万细胞前体细胞会增殖并逐步分化形成不成熟的施万细胞,这些细胞侵入轴突束并根据轴突的直径进行分类。与大直径轴突相关联的施万细胞会形成1∶1的施万细胞-轴突关系进行髓鞘化。直径较小的单个至超过50个轴突则被一种保持非髓鞘化状态的施万细胞包围,形成Remak束结构(Jessen and Mirsky 2005)(图36.1)。

36.4.1.4 施万细胞受损后可塑性

当施万细胞与轴突分离时,例如在损伤情况下,它们可能经历脱分化过程,表现出与未髓鞘化前的不成熟施万细胞相似但不完全相同的分子和形态表型(Jessen and Mirsky 2008)。这些施万细胞会开始增殖,并与浸润的巨噬细胞一同清除轴突和髓鞘残骸,形成管道,有助于轴突从损伤部位向上游再生(Jessen and Mirsky 2008;Mirsky et al. 2008;Zochodne 2012)。虽然受伤后的施万细胞具有重新进入细胞周期的能力,但在成熟神经中,施万细胞通常不会再有丝分裂了。这种特性,加上周围神经中尚未发现成体干细胞群体的事实,可能解释了在一般人群中罕见发生丛状神经纤维瘤的现象(Korf 1999)。因此,一个关键问题是,生殖细胞系 NF1 杂合突变如何使周围神经这一相对耐受肿瘤的器官变得高度易感于良性和恶性肿瘤的形成。进一步深入研究以确定 PNF 和 MPNST 的起源细胞可能会为解决这一基本问题提供有效指导。

36.4.2 丛状神经纤维瘤的细胞起源

癌症生物学中一个关键问题是确定哪种细胞类型是癌症发展的起源(Visvader 2011)。许多成体组织含有干细胞,它们具备自我更新和多向分化的能力以维持组织生命,尽管它们的数量随时间逐渐减少。相比之下,限制性祖细胞和分化细胞的寿命通常较短。由于癌症通常需要多次突变才能发生(Knudson 1993),有假设认为癌症的发展需要在具有强大自我更新能力的干细胞中积累突变(Clevers 2011)。系谱追踪实验在肠道中的隐窝干细胞中证实了这一假设(Barker et al. 2009)。然而,也有证据表明,某些癌症可能起源于限制性祖细胞或分化细胞,这些细胞通过突变获得了自我更新的能力(Cozzio et al. 2003;Huntly et al. 2004;Jamieson et al. 2004;Krivtsov et al. 2006;Magee et al. 2012;Visvader 2011;Yang et al. 2008b)。另一种可能性是,癌症作为一个多步骤过程,突变可能在干细胞中开始积累,但最终是祖细胞开始异常增殖(Pardal et al. 2003;Reya et al. 2001;Yang et al. 2008b)。起源细胞的性质影响了实验性小鼠模型中哪些类型的突变可以引起癌症(Heuser et al. 2009;Somervaille et al. 2009)。然而,这些数据是基于小鼠模型得出的,目前尚不清楚小鼠中起源细胞之间的生物学差异是否反映了人类癌症中细胞起源的差异(reviewed in Magee et al. 2012)。此外,有证据表明起源细胞的差异可能导致癌症生物学特性的差异(Magee et al. 2012;Visvader 2011)。

尽管已明确神经纤维瘤和MPNST中 NF1/Nf1 功能缺失发生在人类和小鼠的施万细胞谱系中,但在施万细胞发育过程中具体的肿瘤形成的具体时间点仍然不明确(Cichowski et al. 1999;Serra et al. 2000)。通过开发能够在不同细胞系和特定时间点条件性失活基因的小鼠模型,研究者们得以深入探究这一问题(图36.1)。因此,有研究者设计了一种多形性神经纤维瘤的小鼠模型,利用Krox20-cre转基因小鼠(Zhu et al. 2002),使 Nf1 突变靶向于施万细胞系。Krox20-cre 在早期胚胎发育期间开始表达,在胚胎第10.5天(E10.5)出现于脑神经和脊神经的神经根中,这里存在多能神经嵴干细胞(即界线帽细胞)(Maro et al. 2004)。在后期(E15.5-E18.5)表达水平较低的未成熟施万细胞中表达,并在髓鞘化开始时表达水平在前髓鞘化施万细胞中上升(Ghislain et al. 2002)。Krox20-cre驱动的 Nf1 条件性基因敲除小鼠(Krox20-cre+; $Nf1^{flox/-}$)在脑神经和脊神经的神经根中沿发育,以

100%的穿透率发展出丛状神经纤维瘤，然而在坐骨神经中尽管存在经历 $Nf1$ 缺失的细胞，但未检测到神经纤维瘤（Zhu et al. 2002）。这个模型中观察到的丛状神经纤维瘤在分子、组织学和超微结构特征上与人类对应物相似。这些数据提示神经纤维瘤不是起源于完全髓鞘化的施万细胞，而可能起源于 NCSC/SC 系谱中另一种细胞类型，这与丛状神经纤维瘤在人类中是先天性病变的假设相符（Korf 1999；Riccardi 1992）。

为了进一步研究神经纤维瘤的起源细胞，研究人员在发育中的神经嵴干细胞和施万细胞前体细胞中敲除了 $Nf1$（Joseph et al. 2008；Le et al. 2011；Mayes et al. 2011；Wu et al. 2008；Zheng et al. 2008）。在神经嵴干细胞中失活 $Nf1$ 导致了周围神经中神经嵴干细胞在胚胎阶段暂时扩张和自我更新能力增强。然而，出生后早期阶段未观察到肿瘤形成，并且将 $Nf1$ 缺失的神经嵴干细胞移植到野生型或 $Nf1$ 杂合小鼠的周围神经中也未导致肿瘤形成（Joseph et al. 2008）。出生后早期的死亡使本研究无法对这些动物进行后期的分析（Joseph et al. 2008）。通过使用具有更局部表达的不同 Cre 驱动转基因动物模型，研究者避免了胚胎早期 $Nf1$ 敲除的致死性，证明在发育中的神经嵴干细胞/施万细胞前体细胞失活 $Nf1$ 会导致神经纤维瘤形成，穿透率达到 100%，潜伏期为 4~12 个月（Wu et al. 2008）或 12~24 个月（Zheng et al. 2008）。一项研究分析了这些动物在完成髓鞘化后的神经中，在出生后第 22 天发现突变神经中的施万细胞数量与对照组和正常髓鞘化相比没有差异（Zheng et al. 2008）。然而，观察到一个微小的表型变化：一些突变的 Remak 束中施万细胞表现出髓鞘缺陷，这些区域包含了大量未分离的轴突，这一现象在正常神经中很少见（图 36.2a~c）。在 3 个月大时，突变神经中异常分化的 Remak 束退化，导致施万细胞分离和轴突丧失（图 36.2d~g）。神经纤维瘤形成过程中，非髓鞘化的施万细胞数量逐渐增加（Zheng et al. 2008）。这些数据表明，非髓鞘化的施万细胞可能是小鼠神经纤维瘤的起源细胞。因此，在胚胎期施万细胞系中失活 $Nf1$ 可能导致轴突的发育缺陷和轴突与非髓鞘化的施万细胞的异常相互作用，从而导致 Remak 束的退化和在增殖的非髓鞘化的施万细胞中肿瘤的形成。尽管如此，这些数据并不排除在成年施万细胞中失活 $Nf1$ 也可能导致肿瘤形成的可能性，尤其是在不同的条件下，例如受损伤时。近期，研究者使用时间和空间受控的 Cre 驱动转基因技术，在不同发育阶段的施万细胞中失活 $Nf1$（图 36.1）。在髓鞘化开始之前失活施万细胞前体细胞或未成熟施万细胞导致肿瘤发生率为 80%~100%（Le et al. 2011；Mayes et al. 2011）。当在成年施万细胞中敲除 $Nf1$ 时，也观察到肿瘤形成；然而，在一项研究中，只有 2% 的小鼠发展出肿瘤（Le et al. 2011），而在另一项研究中，100% 的小鼠发展出肿瘤（Mayes et al. 2011）。这些数据表明，在发育过程中的胚胎和出生后早期中施万细胞中失活 $Nf1$ 时对神经纤维瘤形成的易感性最大，但成年阶段细胞中发生突变也可能产生影响。未来的研究仍需确定在成年神经中失活 $Nf1$ 时受影响的细胞类型，可能是完全分化的成熟施万细胞（非髓鞘化或髓鞘化），也可能是去分化的施万细胞，或是在成年神经中持续存在的罕见的、更未成熟的细胞类型。在神经损伤的响应中，施万细胞可以去分化为类似于未成熟施万细胞的状态。已有研究表明，在体内和体外激活 Raf/MEK/ERK 信号通路足以诱导髓鞘化施万细胞去分化（Harrisingh et al. 2004；Napoli et al. 2012）。Lloyd 等的研究结果表明，未受伤的神经中短时间激活 Raf 激酶已足以推动髓鞘化施万细胞去分化为周围成年神经中的祖细胞样状态，且在受伤相关的情况下，神经纤维瘤可由髓鞘化施万细胞形成（Kalamarides et al. 2012）。综上所述，这些数据表明在施万细胞系中对 $Nf1$ 进行双等位失活会导致神经纤维瘤形成。在小鼠模型中，当在胚胎施万细胞中敲除 $Nf1$ 时，丛状神经纤维瘤穿透率最高，但在成年施万细胞中敲除 $Nf1$ 也可能导致肿瘤形成。这表明在不同发育阶段的细胞类型都具有形成肿瘤的潜力，尽管可能通过不同的机制实现，如异常的轴突分选、Remak 束缺陷、去分化和受伤后的异常增殖。

36.4.3 MPNST 的细胞起源

MPNST 在一般人群中发病率极低，仅为

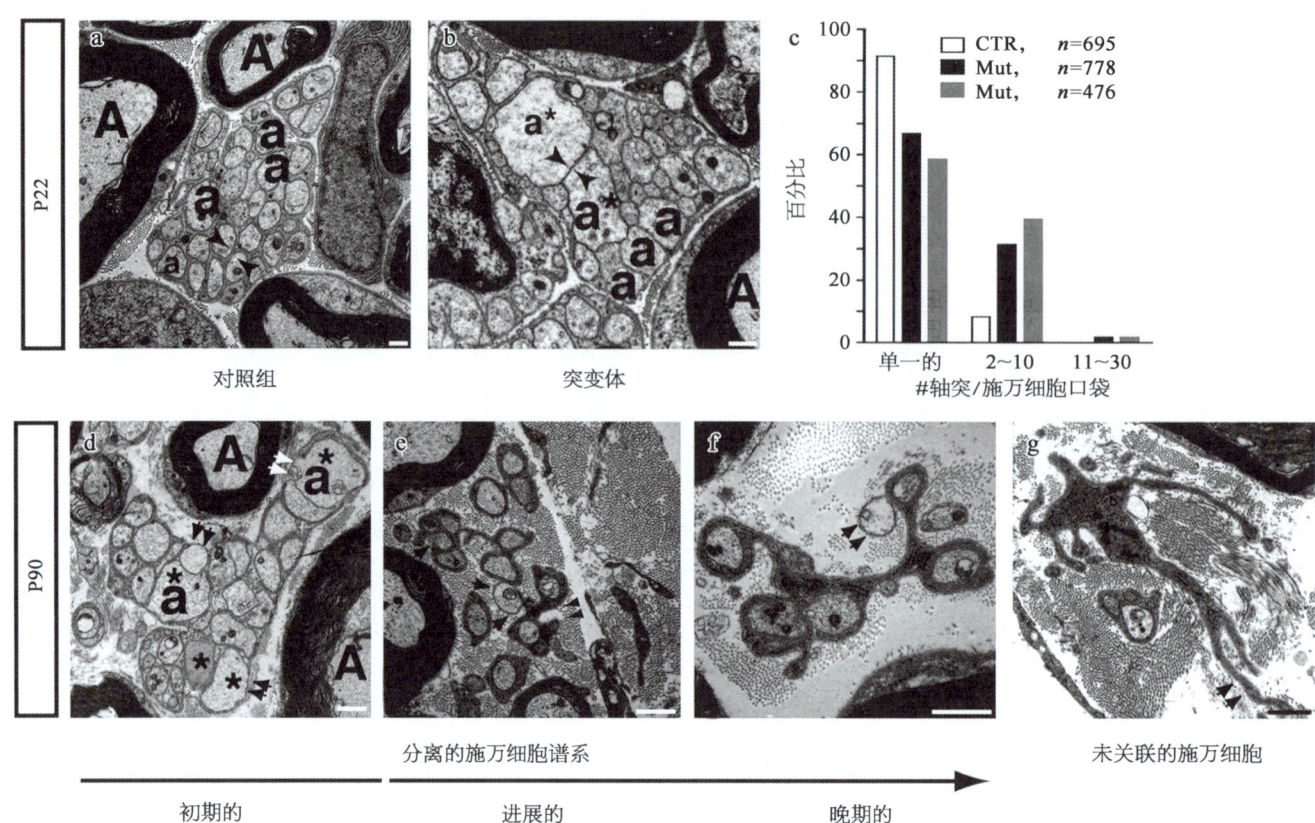

图 36.2 $Nf1$ 突变坐骨神经中异常的 Remak 束形成和退化[from Zheng et al. (2008)]。在出生后第 22 天(P22),通过透射电子显微镜分析 Remak 束在坐骨神经中的形成情况,发现 $Nf1$ 缺失小鼠(b)相比于对照组(a)存在异常分隔。比例尺在 a 和 b 中均为 1 mm。突变的施万细胞束中包含彼此直接相对的轴突(b 中的箭头),而在对照小鼠中,这些轴突被施万细胞质分隔开(a 中的箭头)。还观察到了异常扩张的轴突(a^*)。c. 显示了对照组和突变神经中每个施万细胞胞质通道内轴突的比例分布。与对照组相比,突变体 Remak 束中正确分隔的轴突数量显著减少,而含有 2 个以上未分隔轴突的束显著增加(卡方检验中 $P<0.000\,1$)。d~g. 电子显微照片显示了在 P90 时 $Nf1$ 缺失坐骨神经横截面上不同阶段的轴突束退化情况。d 中的箭头指向正在相互分离的未分隔轴突(星号)以及 e 和 f 中的裸露轴突,这些轴突缺乏施万细胞质。轴突退化可能导致在退化的晚期阶段出现游离或分隔的施万细胞(g),这些游离的施万细胞增殖并导致神经纤维瘤的形成。所有图板的比例尺均为 1 mm

0.001%,其发病高峰出现在 60~70 岁(Evans et al. 2002)。然而,对于 NF1 的个体而言,患上 MPNST 的终生风险则估计为 7%~13%,通常发生在较年轻的 20~40 岁的患者中(Evans et al. 2002)。尽管这种临床表型的机制尚不完全清楚,但在 NF1 患者的周围神经中存在 MPNST 的良性前体病变——丛状神经纤维瘤,而在正常个体中很少见,这为 NF1 相关的周围神经肿瘤易感性提供了基础。临床研究表明,大多数 MPNST 起源于 NF1 患者已存在的丛状神经纤维瘤(Woodruff 1999)。在 NF1 患者中,有丛状神经纤维瘤的患者比没有这种病变的患者发生 MPNST 的风险高出 20 倍(Szudek et al. 2003;Tucker et al. 2005)。这些观察结果支持这样一种观点:丛状神经纤维瘤的易感性是导致 NF1 个体周围神经高度易感于 MPNST 的主要潜在原因。此外,这些临床结果还表明,丛状神经纤维瘤是 MPNST 的一个来源。最近的研究使用基于阵列的比较基因组杂交(array-based comparative genomic hybridization,aCGH)揭示了自体丛状神经纤维瘤和 MPNST 中观察到的相同基因组微缺失,从而提供了确凿证据表明丛状神经纤维瘤和 MPNST 可能共享一个共同的肿瘤祖细胞(Beert et al. 2011)。未来利用下一代测序技术的研究应该能够提供更全面的基因组学资料,以更确切地确定丛状神经纤维瘤和 MPNST 之间的谱系关系。根据丛状神经纤维瘤起源于完全分化的非髓鞘化施万细胞的观点,最近的小鼠模型研究也表明 MPNST 源自分化的施万细胞,而不是神经嵴干细胞(Joseph et al. 2008)。

$NF1/Nf1$ 的双等位失活已被确定为导致人类和小鼠中丛状神经纤维瘤形成的原因(Cichowski et al. 1999; Zhu et al. 2002)。然而,导致 MPNST 恶性转化的分子机制目前尚不清楚。目前只有少数遗传变异被确定为 MPNST 发展中恶性转化的重要驱动因素。$p53$ 基因的突变仅在 MPNST 中发现,而在良性神经纤维瘤中未见,这表明 $p53$ 介导的途径可能涉及周围神经鞘膜瘤(peripheral nerve sheath tumor, PNST)的恶性转化(Legius et al. 1994; Menon et al. 1990)。与 $p53$ 在 PNST 发展后期阶段的作用相一致,无论是纯合子 $p53^{-/-}$ 突变还是杂合子 $p53^{+/-}$ 突变的小鼠都不会发展出神经纤维瘤或 MPNST(Donehower et al. 1992; Jacks et al. 1994a)。相反,在同一染色体上携带 $Nf1$ 和 $p53$ 突变的小鼠(所谓的"$Nf1/p53$ cis"小鼠)发展出 MPNST 的频率很高(Cichowski et al. 1999; Vogel et al. 1999)。因此,无论是人类遗传研究还是小鼠模型都支持了 PNST 发展的阶梯遗传模型:① $NF1$ 的丧失导致神经纤维瘤的形成。② PNST 的恶性转化需要额外的遗传突变,如 $p53$ 介导的途径。在 MPNST 中频繁检测到的 $CDKN2A/p16^{INK4a}$ 基因位点的遗传变异在神经纤维瘤中却罕见(Kourea et al. 1999b; Nielsen et al. 1999),表明该位点的缺陷也可能导致神经纤维瘤的恶性转化。$CDKN2A/p16^{INK4a}$ 基因位点编码两个独立的肿瘤抑制基因,$p14^{ARF}$ 和 $p16^{INK4a}$。$p14^{ARF}$ 基因产物(小鼠中的 $p19^{Arf}$)通过拮抗 Mdm2 介导的 p53 蛋白降解而正向调节 p53 功能(Sherr 2001)。因此,MPNST 中 $p14^{ARF}$ 功能的丧失与 p53 介导的肿瘤抑制途径在 PNST 的恶性转化中起着关键作用的假设一致。然而,在 MPNST 中发现了 50%~60% 的纯合子缺失(同时影响 $p14^{ARF}$ 和 $p16^{INK4a}$)(Kourea et al. 1999b; Nielsen et al. 1999),表明 $p16^{INK4a}$ 的丧失也可能导致 PNST 的恶性转化。与此一致的是,在人类肿瘤中,$p16^{INK4a}$ 的丧失仅在 MPNST 中发现,而在神经纤维瘤中则没有。此外,在缺乏 $p16^{INK4a}$ 突变的 MPNST 中检测到 RB 的遗传变异和 $CDK4$ 的扩增(Berner et al. 1999),表明 Rb 介导的 G1/S 检查点途径也可能在 PNST 的恶性转化中起到关键作用。此外,在大多数 MPNST 中(91%)发现了另一个 Rb 途径成分 $p27^{KIP1}$ 的丧失表达,而在神经纤维瘤中仅有 6%(Kourea et al. 1999a)。在小鼠中,$Nf1$ 杂合子背景中的 $p16^{Ink4a}$ 丧失或 $p19^{Arf}$ 丧失都不会诱导神经纤维瘤或 MPNST 的形成(Joseph et al. 2008; King et al. 2002)。然而,在 $Nf1$ 杂合子背景中,约 26% 的 $Ink4a/Arf^{-/-}$ 双突变小鼠发展出 MPNST(Joseph et al. 2008)。因此,这些研究表明,在小鼠中需要同时丧失 $p16^{Ink4a}$ 和 $p19^{Arf}$ 功能才能引发 $Nf1$ 介导的 MPNST 的形成,这进一步强调了 p53 介导的途径在 MPNST 发展中的重要性。最近对人类肿瘤的 aCGH 研究表明,虽然丛状神经纤维瘤几乎没有染色体异常,但 MPNST 的基因组具有复杂的染色体丢失或增加(Mantripragada et al. 2008, 2009)。一些频繁出现的染色体改变表明,潜在的癌基因和肿瘤抑制基因可能位于这些染色体区域,负责将丛状神经纤维瘤转化为 MPNST。最后,考虑到有相当数量的 MPNST 在没有丛状神经纤维瘤的证据下发生,由此可见,施万细胞系的细胞有能力直接经历恶性转化,而不必经过良性肿瘤阶段(Woodruff 1999)。神经嵴干细胞、施万细胞前体和成熟的非髓鞘化或髓鞘化施万细胞是否可以作为 MPNST 的起源细胞目前尚未确定。要解答这个问题,需要开发具有不同施万细胞发育阶段的有针对性突变的新型、高渗透性 MPNST 模型。

36.4.4 肿瘤微环境及治疗意义

NF1 相关肿瘤起源细胞的探索不仅将揭示 $NF1$ 在正常施万细胞发育和肿瘤形成中的基本机制,还将对治疗产生重大影响。正如前文所述,NF1 相关的 MPNST 可能是唯一具有确定发展基础和关键良性前体病变的软组织肉瘤(soft tissue sarcoma, STS)亚型。因此,设计早期化学预防策略以针对丛状神经纤维瘤和 MPNST 是切实可行的目标。由于丛状神经纤维瘤在早期出生后阶段是由非髓鞘化的施万细胞与轴突之间的异常相互作用引发的(Zheng et al. 2008),一种可能的策略是稳定轴突与施万细胞的互动,以此作为抑制神经纤维瘤发生的一种治疗方法。此外,相较于 MPNST,丛状神经纤维瘤基因相对稳定，基因改变较少（Mantripragada et al. 2008，2009）。这些特点表明丛状神经纤维瘤的发展可能高度依赖于其肿瘤微环境。事实上，使用小鼠模型的研究表明，丛状神经纤维瘤是在神经环境中形成的，其中包括神经退行和肥大细胞浸润，而且更重要的是，丛状神经纤维瘤的发展高度依赖于肿瘤微环境中的 $Nf1$ 杂合缺失细胞（Zheng et al. 2008；Zhu et al. 2002）。这些观察结果得到了体外和体内研究的支持，包括肿瘤微环境中的细胞类型（如纤维细胞、内皮细胞和肥大细胞）对于 $Nf1$ 缺失施万细胞的增殖和致瘤能力有更有效的促进作用（Ingram et al. 2000，2001；Staser et al. 2012；Yang et al. 2003，2006）（see review in Staser et al. 2012）。一项最新的研究利用相互骨髓移植和复合 $Nf1/c$-Kit 受体突变小鼠，将骨髓来源的表达 c-Kit 的 $Nf1$ 杂合子肥大细胞确定为丛状神经纤维瘤形成的关键因素（Yang et al. 2008a）。更重要的是，伊马替尼（格列卫）在一位无法手术的丛状神经纤维瘤 NF1 患者中显示出了治疗益处。考虑到 c-kit/kit-L 在预防丛状神经纤维瘤形成中的关键作用，一个可能的假设是伊马替尼通过破坏 SCF/c-kit 介导的肥大细胞形成和炎症，从而中断了致瘤施万细胞及其微环境所需的生长因子之间的关键联系。然而，可能还存在其他协同作用机制（Staser et al. 2012）。例如，伊马替尼在非受体酪氨酸激酶 c-abl 上的抑制作用可能还会干扰肿瘤基层中生化调节失衡的纤维细胞中的 TGF-b 介导的信号转导。此外，伊马替尼还可能抑制施万细胞高浓度表达的 PDGF 受体的信号转导（Demestre et al. 2010）。同样，在肿瘤微环境中普遍存在的血管细胞可能也依赖于 PDGF 受体信号转导，正如促进新血管生成的血管生成巨噬细胞（Li et al. 2006；Munchhof et al. 2006）。因此，伊马替尼可能通过作用于几种对肿瘤生长重要的细胞-受体系统来发挥作用，尽管基于移植和其他研究的数据强有力地表明破坏 SCF/c-kit 信号转导轴可能是最为重要的（Staser et al. 2012）。

综上所述，对 NF1 相关肿瘤起源细胞的研究将为预防和治疗这些不可治愈的人类肿瘤设计治疗方案提供重要的见解。

致 谢：感谢 Renee McKay 博士和 Meena Upadhyaya 对手稿的批阅。本研究得到了国防部（W81XWH-06-1-0293）、美国国立卫生研究院（1R01 NS073762）和美国癌症协会（RSG DDC-110857）的资助。J. Buchstaller 得到了儿童肿瘤基金会"青年研究员奖"的资助。

（黄薇，葛玲玲　译）

参考文献

[1] Adameyko I, Lallemend F, Aquino JB, Pereira JA, Topilko P, Muller T, Fritz N, Beljajeva A, Mochii M, Liste I et al (2009) Schwann cell precursors from nerve innervation are a cellular origin of melanocytes in skin. Cell 139：366-379

[2] Baker CV, Bronner-Fraser M, Le Douarin NM, Teillet MA (1997) Early- and late-migrating cranial neural crest cell populations have equivalent developmental potential in vivo. Development 124：3077-3087

[3] Barker N, Ridgway RA, van Es JH, van de Wetering M, Begthel H, van den Born M, Danenberg E, Clarke AR, Sansom OJ, Clevers H (2009) Crypt stem cells as the cells-of-origin of intestinal cancer. Nature 457(7229)：608-611

[4] Beert E, Brems H, Daniels B, De Wever I, Van Calenbergh F, Schoenaers J, Debiec-Rychter M, Gevaert O, De Raedt T, Van Den Bruel A et al (2011) Atypical neurofibromas in neurofibro-matosis type 1 are premalignant tumors. Genes Chromosomes Cancer 50：1021-1032

[5] Berner JM, Sorlie T, Mertens F, Henriksen J, Saeter G, Mandahl N, Brogger A, Myklebost O, Lothe RA (1999) Chromosome band 9p21 is frequently altered in malignant peripheral nerve sheath tumors：studies of CDKN2A and other genes of the pRB pathway. Genes Chromosomes Cancer 26：151-160

[6] Bixby S, Kruger GM, Mosher JT, Joseph NM, Morrison SJ (2002) Cell-intrinsic differences between stem cells from different regions of the peripheral nervous system regulate the generation of neural diversity. Neuron 35：643-656

[7] Brannan CI, Perkins AS, Vogel KS, Ratner N, Nordlund ML, Reid SW, Buchberg AM, Jenkins NA, Parada LF, Copeland NG (1994) Targeted disruption of the neurofibromatosis type-1 gene leads to developmental abnormalities in heart and various neural crest-derived tissues. Genes Dev 8：1019-1029 [published erratum appears in Genes Dev 1994；8(22)：2792]

[8] Bronner-Fraser M, Fraser SE (1988) Cell lineage analysis reveals multipotency of some avian neural crest cells. Nature 335：161-164

[9] Bronner-Fraser M, Fraser S (1989) Developmental potential of avian trunk neural crest cells in situ. Neuron 3：755-766

[10] Bronner-Fraser M, Fraser SE (1991) Cell lineage analysis of the avian neural crest. Development 2：17-22

[11] Cai W, Kassarjian A, Bredella MA, Harris GJ, Yoshida H, Mautner VF, Wenzel R, Plotkin SR (2009) Tumor burden in patients with neurofibromatosis types 1 and 2 and

schwannomatosis: determination on whole-body MR images. Radiology 250: 665-673

[12] Cichowski K, Jacks T (2001) NF1 tumor suppressor gene function: narrowing the GAP. Cell 104: 593-604

[13] Cichowski K, Shih TS, Schmitt E, Santiago S, Reilly K, McLaughlin ME, Bronson RT, Jacks T (1999) Mouse models of tumor development in neurofibromatosis type 1. Science 286: 2172-2176

[14] Clevers H (2011) The cancer stem cell: premises, promises and challenges. Nat Med 17: 313-319

[15] Colman SD, Williams CA, Wallace MR (1995) Benign neurofibromas in type 1 neurofibromatosis (NF1) show somatic deletions of the NF1 gene. Nat Genet 11: 90-92

[16] Cozzio A, Passegue E, Ayton PM, Karsunky H, Cleary ML, Weissman IL (2003) Similar MLL-associated leukemias arising from self-renewing stem cells and short-lived myeloid progenitors. Genes Dev 17: 3029-3035

[17] Daschner K, Assum G, Eisenbarth I, Krone W, Hoffmeyer S, Wortmann S, Heymer B, Kehrer-Sawatzki H (1997) Clonal origin of tumor cells in a plexiform neurofibroma with LOH in NF1 intron 38 and in dermal neurofibromas without LOH of the NF1 gene. Biochem Biophys Res Commun 234: 346-350

[18] Demestre M, Herzberg J, Holtkamp N, Hagel C, Reuss D, Friedrich RE, Kluwe L, Von Deimling A, Mautner VF, Kurtz A (2010) Imatinib mesylate (Glivec) inhibits Schwann cell viability and reduces the size of human plexiform neurofibroma in a xenograft model. J Neurooncol 98: 11-19

[19] Donehower LA, Harvey M, Slagle BL, McArthur MJ, Montgomery CA Jr, Butel JS, Bradley A (1992) Mice deficient for p53 are developmentally normal but susceptible to spontaneous tumours. Nature 356: 215-221

[20] Dupin E, Sommer L (2012) Neural crest progenitors and stem cells: from early development to adulthood. Dev Biol 366(1): 83-95

[21] Dupin E, Baroffio A, Dulac C, Cameron-Curry P, Le Douarin NM (1990) Schwann-cell differentiation in clonal cultures of the neural crest, as evidenced by the anti-Schwann cell myelin protein monoclonal antibody. Proc Natl Acad Sci USA 87: 1119-1123

[22] Dupin E, Creuzet S, Le Douarin NM (2006) The contribution of the neural crest to the vertebrate body. Adv Exp Med Biol 589: 96-119

[23] Evans DG, Baser ME, McGaughran J, Sharif S, Howard E, Moran A (2002) Malignant peripheral nerve sheath tumours in neurofibromatosis 1. J Med Genet 39: 311-314

[24] Fernandes KJ, McKenzie IA, Mill P, Smith KM, Akhavan M, Barnabe-Heider F, Biernaskie J, Junek A, Kobayashi NR, Toma JG et al (2004) A dermal niche for multipotent adult skinderived precursor cells. Nat Cell Biol 6: 1082-1093

[25] Ferner RE (2007) Neurofibromatosis 1 and neurofibromatosis 2: a twenty first century perspective. Lancet Neurol 6: 340-351

[26] Ferner RE (2010) The neurofibromatoses. Pract Neurol 10: 82-93

[27] Garratt AN, Voiculescu O, Topilko P, Charnay P, Birchmeier C (2000) A dual role of erbB2 in myelination and in expansion of the schwann cell precursor pool. J Cell Biol 148: 1035-1046

[28] Ghislain J, Desmarquet-Trin-Dinh C, Jaegle M, Meijer D, Charnay P, Frain M (2002) Characterisation of cis-acting sequences reveals a biphasic, axon-dependent regulation of Krox20 during Schwann cell development. Development 129: 155-166

[29] Grim M, Halata Z, Franz T (1992) Schwann cells are not required for guidance of motor nerves in the hindlimb in Splotch mutant mouse embryos. Anat Embryol (Berl) 186: 311-318

[30] Hagedorn L, Suter U, Sommer L (1999) P0 and PMP22 mark a multipotent neural crest-derived cell type that displays community effects in response to TGF-beta family factors. Development 126: 3781-3794

[31] Harrisingh MC, Perez-Nadales E, Parkinson DB, Malcolm DS, Mudge AW, Lloyd AC (2004) The Ras/Raf/ERK signalling pathway drives Schwann cell dedifferentiation. EMBO J 23: 3061-3071

[32] Heuser M, Sly LM, Argiropoulos B, Kuchenbauer F, Lai C, Weng A, Leung M, Lin G, Brookes C, Fung S et al (2009) Modeling the functional heterogeneity of leukemia stem cells: role of STAT5 in leukemia stem cell self-renewal. Blood 114: 3983-3993

[33] Huntly BJ, Shigematsu H, Deguchi K, Lee BH, Mizuno S, Duclos N, Rowan R, Amaral S, Curley D, Williams IR et al (2004) MOZ-TIF2, but not BCR-ABL, confers properties of leukemic stem cells to committed murine hematopoietic progenitors. Cancer Cell 6: 587-596

[34] Ingram DA, Yang FC, Travers JB, Wenning MJ, Hiatt K, New S, Hood A, Shannon K, Williams DA, Clapp DW (2000) Genetic and biochemical evidence that haploinsufficiency of the Nf1 tumor suppressor gene modulates melanocyte and mast cell fates in vivo. J Exp Med 191: 181-188

[35] Ingram DA, Hiatt K, King AJ, Fisher L, Shivakumar R, Derstine C, Wenning MJ, Diaz B, Travers JB, Hood A et al (2001) Hyperactivation of p21(ras) and the hematopoietic-specific Rho GTPase, Rac2, cooperate to alter the proliferation of neurofibromin-deficient mast cells in vivo and in vitro. J Exp Med 194: 57-69

[36] Jacks T, Remington L, Williams BO, Schmitt EM, Halachmi S, Bronson RT, Weinberg RA (1994a) Tumor spectrum analysis in p53-mutant mice. Curr Biol 4: 1-7

[37] Jacks T, Shih TS, Schmitt EM, Bronson RT, Bernards A, Weinberg RA (1994b) Tumour predisposition in mice heterozygous for a targeted mutation in Nf1. Nat Genet 7: 353-361

[38] Jamieson CH, Ailles LE, Dylla SJ, Muijtjens M, Jones C, Zehnder JL, Gotlib J, Li K, Manz MG, Keating A et al (2004) Granulocyte-macrophage progenitors as candidate leukemic stem cells in blast-crisis CML. N Engl J Med 351: 657-667

[39] Jessen KR, Mirsky R (2005) The origin and development of glial cells in peripheral nerves. Nat Rev Neurosci 6: 671-682

[40] Jessen KR, Mirsky R (2008) Negative regulation of myelination: relevance for development, injury, and demyelinating disease. Glia 56: 1552-1565

[41] Joseph NM, Mukouyama YS, Mosher JT, Jaegle M, Crone SA, Dormand EL, Lee KF, Meijer D, Anderson DJ, Morrison SJ (2004) Neural crest stem cells undergo multilineage differentiation in developing peripheral nerves to generate endoneurial fibroblasts in addition to Schwann cells. Development 131: 5599-5612

[42] Joseph NM, Mosher JT, Buchstaller J, Snider P, McKeever PE, Lim M, Conway SJ, Parada LF, Zhu Y, Morrison SJ (2008) The loss of Nf1 transiently promotes self-renewal but not tumorigenesis by neural crest stem cells. Cancer Cell 13: 129-140

[43] Joseph NM, He S, Quintana E, Kim YG, Nunez G, Morrison SJ (2011) Enteric glia are multipotent in culture but primarily form glia in the adult rodent gut. J Clin Invest 121: 3398-3411

[44] Kalamarides M, Acosta MT, Babovic-Vuksanovic D, Carpen O, Cichowski K, Evans DG, Giancotti F, Hanemann CO, Ingram D, Lloyd AC et al (2012) Neurofibromatosis 2011: a report of the Children's Tumor Foundation annual meeting. Acta Neuropathol 123: 369-380

[45] King D, Yang G, Thompson MA, Hiebert SW (2002) Loss of neurofibromatosis-1 and p19 (ARF) cooperate to induce a multiple tumor phenotype. Oncogene 21: 4978-4982

[46] Kluwe L, Friedrich RE, Mautner VF (1999) Allelic loss of the NF1 gene in NF1-associated plexiform neurofibromas. Cancer Genet Cytogenet 113: 65-69

[47] Knudson AG (1993) Antioncogenes and human cancer. Proc Natl Acad Sci USA 90: 10914-10921

[48] Korf BR (1999) Plexiform neurofibromas. Am J Med Genet 89: 31-37

[49] Kourea HP, Cordon-Cardo C, Dudas M, Leung D, Woodruff JM (1999a) Expression of p27 (kip) and other cell cycle regulators in malignant peripheral nerve sheath tumors and neurofibromas: the emerging role of p27 (kip) in malignant transformation of neurofibromas. Am J Pathol 155: 1885-1891

[50] Kourea HP, Orlow I, Scheithauer BW, Cordon-Cardo C, Woodruff JM (1999b) Deletions of the INK4A gene occur in malignant peripheral nerve sheath tumors but not in neurofibromas. Am J Pathol 155: 1855-1860

[51] Krispin S, Nitzan E, Kassem Y, Kalcheim C (2010) Evidence for a dynamic spatiotemporal fate map and early fate restrictions of premigratory avian neural crest. Development 137: 585-595

[52] Krivtsov AV, Twomey D, Feng Z, Stubbs MC, Wang Y, Faber J, Levine JE, Wang J, Hahn WC, Gilliland DG et al (2006) Transformation from committed progenitor to leukaemia stem cell initiated by MLL-AF9. Nature 442: 818-822

[53] Krone W, Jirikowski G, Muhleck O, Kling H, Gall H (1983) Cell culture studies on neurofibro-matosis (von Recklinghausen). II. Occurrence of glial cells in primary cultures of peripheral neurofibromas. Hum Genet 63: 247-251

[54] Kruger GM, Mosher JT, Bixby S, Joseph N, Iwashita T, Morrison SJ (2002) Neural crest stem cells persist in the adult gut but undergo changes in self-renewal, neuronal subtype potential, and factor responsiveness. Neuron 35: 657-669

[55] Lakkis MM, Tennekoon GI (2000) Neurofibromatosis type 1. I. General overview. J Neurosci Res 62: 755-763

[56] Laycock-van Spyk S, Thomas N, Cooper DN, Upadhyaya M (2011) Neurofibromatosis type 1-associated tumours: their somatic mutational spectrum and pathogenesis. Hum Genomics 5(6): 623-690

[57] Le Douarin NM, Kalcheim C (1999) The neural crest. Cambridge University Press, New York

[58] Le LQ, Shipman T, Burns DK, Parada LF (2009) Cell of origin and microenvironment contribution for NF1-associated dermal neurofibromas. Cell Stem Cell 4: 453-463

[59] Le LQ, Liu C, Shipman T, Chen Z, Suter U, Parada LF (2011) Susceptible stages in Schwann cells for NF1-associated plexiform neurofibroma development. Cancer Res 71: 4686-4695

[60] Legius E, Marchuk DA, Collins FS, Glover TW (1993) Somatic deletion of the neurofibromatosis type 1 gene in a neurofibrosarcoma supports a tumour suppressor gene hypothesis. Nat Genet 3: 122-126

[61] Legius E, Dierick H, Wu R, Hall BK, Marynen P, Cassiman JJ, Glover TW (1994) TP53 mutations are frequent in malignant NF1 tumors. Genes Chromosomes Cancer 10: 250-255

[62] Li F, Munchhof AM, White HA, Mead LE, Krier TR, Fenoglio A, Chen S, Wu X, Cai S, Yang FC et al (2006) Neurofibromin is a novel regulator of RAS-induced signals in primary vascular smooth muscle cells. Hum Mol Genet 15: 1921-1930

[63] Lo L, Anderson DJ (1995) Postmigratory neural crest cells expressing c-RET display restricted developmental and proliferative capacities. Neuron 15: 527-539

[64] Maertens O, Brems H, Vandesompele J, De Raedt T, Heyns I, Rosenbaum T, De Schepper S, De Paepe A, Mortier G, Janssens S et al (2006) Comprehensive NF1 screening on cultured Schwann cells from neurofibromas. Hum Mutat 27: 1030-1040

[65] Maertens O, De Schepper S, Vandesompele J, Brems H, Heyns I, Janssens S, Speleman F, Legius E, Messiaen L (2007) Molecular dissection of isolated disease features in mosaic neurofibromatosis type 1. Am J Hum Genet 81: 243-251

[66] Magee JA, Piskounova E, Morrison SJ (2012) Cancer stem cells: impact, heterogeneity, and uncertainty. Cancer Cell 21: 283-296

[67] Mantripragada KK, Spurlock G, Kluwe L, Chuzhanova N, Ferner RE, Frayling IM, Dumanski JP, Guha A, Mautner V, Upadhyaya M (2008) High-resolution DNA copy number profiling of malignant peripheral nerve sheath tumors using targeted microarray-based comparative genomic hybridization. Clin Cancer Res 14: 1015-1024

[68] Mantripragada KK, de Stahl TD, Patridge C, Menzel U, Andersson R, Chuzhanova N, Kluwe L, Guha A, Mautner V, Dumanski JP et al (2009) Genome-wide high-resolution analysis of DNA copy number alterations in NF1-associated malignant peripheral nerve sheath tumors using 32K BAC array. Genes Chromosomes Cancer 48: 897-907

[69] Maro GS, Vermeren M, Voiculescu O, Melton L, Cohen J, Charnay P, Topilko P (2004) Neural crest boundary cap cells constitute a source of neuronal and glial cells of the PNS. Nat Neurosci 7: 930-938

[70] Mautner VF, Asuagbor FA, Dombi E, Funsterer C, Kluwe L, Wenzel R, Widemann BC, Friedman JM (2008) Assessment of benign tumor burden by whole-body MRI in patients with neurofi-bromatosis 1. Neuro-oncology 10: 593-598

[71] Mayes DA, Rizvi TA, Cancelas JA, Kolasinski NT, Ciraolo GM, Stemmer-Rachamimov AO, Ratner N (2011) Perinatal or adult Nf1 inactivation using tamoxifen-inducible PlpCre each cause neurofibroma formation. Cancer Res 71: 4675-4685

[72] Menon AG, Anderson KM, Riccardi VM, Chung RY, Whaley JM, Yandell DW, Farmer GE, Freiman RN, Lee JK, Li FP et al (1990) Chromosome 17p deletions and p53 gene mutations associated with the formation of malignant neurofibrosarcomas in von Recklinghausen neuro-fibromatosis. Proc Natl Acad Sci USA 87: 5435-5439

[73] Mirsky R, Woodhoo A, Parkinson DB, Arthur-Farraj P, Bhaskaran A, Jessen KR (2008) Novel signals controlling embryonic Schwann cell development, myelination and dedifferentiation. J Peripher Nerv Syst 13: 122-135

[74] Morales AV, Barbas JA, Nieto MA (2005) How to become neural crest: from segregation to delamination. Semin Cell Dev Biol 16: 655-662

[75] Morrison SJ, White PM, Zock C, Anderson DJ (1999) Prospective identification, isolation by flow cytometry, and in vivo self-renewal of multipotent mammalian neural crest stem cells. Cell 96: 737-749

[76] Muir D, Neubauer D, Lim IT, Yachnis AT, Wallace MR (2001) Tumorigenic properties of neurofibromin-deficient neurofibroma Schwann cells. Am J Pathol 158: 501-513

[77] Munchhof AM, Li F, White HA, Mead LE, Krier TR, Fenoglio A, Li X, Yuan J, Yang FC, Ingram DA (2006) Neurofibroma-associated growth factors activate a distinct signaling network to alter the function of neurofibromin-deficient endothelial cells. Hum Mol Genet 15: 1858-1869

[78] Nagoshi N, Shibata S, Kubota Y, Nakamura M, Nagai Y, Satoh E, Morikawa S, Okada Y, Mabuchi Y, Katoh H et al (2008) Ontogeny and multipotency of neural crest-derived stem cells in mouse bone marrow, dorsal root ganglia, and whisker pad. Cell Stem Cell 2: 392-403

[79] Napoli I, Noon LA, Ribeiro S, Kerai AP, Parrinello S, Rosenberg LH, Collins MJ, Harrisingh MC, White IJ, Woodhoo A et al (2012) A central role for the ERK-signaling pathway in controlling Schwann cell plasticity and peripheral nerve regeneration in vivo. Neuron 73: 729-742

[80] Nielsen GP, Stemmer-Rachamimov AO, Ino Y, Moller MB, Rosenberg AE, Louis DN (1999) Malignant transformation of neurofibromas in neurofibromatosis 1 is associated with CDKN2A/p16 inactivation. Am J Pathol 155: 1879-1884

[81] Pardal R, Clarke MF, Morrison SJ (2003) Applying the principles of stem-cell biology to cancer. Nat Rev Cancer 3: 895-902

[82] Peltonen J, Jaakkola S, Lebwohl M, Renvall S, Risteli L, Virtanen I, Uitto J (1988) Cellular differentiation and expression of matrix genes in type 1 neurofibromatosis. Lab Invest 59: 760-771

[83] Rasmussen SA, Overman J, Thomson SA, Colman SD, Abernathy CR, Trimpert RE, Moose R, Virdi G, Roux K, Bauer M et al (2000) Chromosome 17 loss-of-heterozygosity studies in benign and malignant tumors in neurofibromatosis type 1. Genes Chromosomes Cancer 28: 425-431

[84] Reya T, Morrison SJ, Clarke MF, Weissman IL (2001) Stem cells, cancer, and cancer stem cells. Nature 414: 105-111

[85] Riccardi VM (1992) Neurofibromatosis: phenotype, natural history, and pathogenesis, 2nd edn. Johns Hopkins University Press, Baltimore

[86] Riethmacher D, Sonnenberg-Riethmacher E, Brinkmann V, Yamaai T, Lewin GR, Birchmeier C (1997) Severe neuropathies in mice with targeted mutations in the ErbB3 receptor. Nature 389: 725-730

[87] Rutkowski JL, Wu K, Gutmann DH, Boyer PJ, Legius E (2000) Genetic and cellular defects contributing to benign tumor formation in neurofibromatosis type 1. Hum Mol Genet 9: 1059-1066

[88] Serbedzija GN, Bronner-Fraser M, Fraser SE (1994) Developmental potential of trunk neural crest cells in the mouse. Development 120: 1709-1718

[89] Serra E, Puig S, Otero D, Gaona A, Kruyer H, Ars E, Estivill X, Lazaro C (1997) Confirmation of a double-hit model for the NF1 gene in benign neurofibromas. Am J Hum Genet 61: 512-519

[90] Serra E, Rosenbaum T, Winner U, Aledo R, Ars E, Estivill X, Lenard HG, Lazaro C (2000) Schwann cells harbor the somatic NF1 mutation in neurofibromas: evidence of two different Schwann cell subpopulations. Hum Mol Genet 9: 3055-3064

[91] Shah NM, Marchionni MA, Isaacs I, Stroobant P, Anderson DJ (1994) Glial growth factor restricts mammalian neural crest stem cells to a glial fate. Cell 77: 349-360

[92] Sheela S, Riccardi VM, Ratner N (1990) Angiogenic and invasive properties of neurofibroma Schwann cells. J Cell Biol 111: 645-653

[93] Sherman LS, Atit R, Rosenbaum T, Cox AD, Ratner N (2000) Single cell ras-GTP analysis reveals altered ras activity in a subpopulation of neurofibroma schwann cells but not fibroblasts [In Process Citation]. J Biol Chem 275: 30740-30745

[94] Sherr CJ (2001) The INK4a/ARF network in tumour suppression. Nat Rev Mol Cell Biol 2: 731-737

[95] Side L, Taylor B, Cayouette M, Conner E, Thompson P, Luce M, Shannon K (1997) Homozygous inactivation of the NF1 gene in bone marrow cells from children with neurofibromatosis type 1 and malignant myeloid disorders. N Engl J Med 336: 1713-1720

[96] Sieber-Blum M, Cohen AM (1980) Clonal analysis of quail neural crest cells: they are pluripotent and differentiate in vitro in the absence of noncrest cells. Dev Biol 80: 96-106

[97] Sieber-Blum M, Grim M, Hu YF, Szeder V (2004) Pluripotent neural crest stem cells in the adult hair follicle. Dev Dyn 231: 258-269

[98] Somervaille TC, Matheny CJ, Spencer GJ, Iwasaki M, Rinn JL, Witten DM, Chang HY, Shurtleff SA, Downing JR, Cleary ML (2009) Hierarchical maintenance of MLL myeloid leukemia stem cells employs a transcriptional program shared with embryonic rather than adult stem cells. Cell Stem Cell 4: 129-140

[99] Staser K, Yang FC, Clapp DW (2012) Pathogenesis of plexiform neurofibroma: tumor-stromal/hematopoietic interactions in tumor progression. Annu Rev Pathol 7: 469-495

[100] Szudek J, Evans DG, Friedman JM (2003) Patterns of associations of clinical features in neurofi-bromatosis 1 (NF1). Hum Genet 112: 289-297

[101] Thomas L, Spurlock G, Eudall C, Thomas NS, Mort M, Hamby SE, Chuzhanova N, Brems H, Legius E, Cooper DN, Upadhyaya M (2012) Exploring the somatic NF1 mutational spectrum associated with NF1 cutaneous neurofibromas. Eur J Hum Genet 20(4): 411-419

[102] Trentin A, Glavieux-Pardanaud C, Le Douarin NM, Dupin E (2004) Self-renewal capacity is a widespread property of various types of neural crest precursor cells. Proc Natl Acad Sci USA 101: 4495-4500

[103] Tucker T, Wolkenstein P, Revuz J, Zeller J, Friedman JM (2005) Association between benign and malignant peripheral nerve sheath tumors in NF1. Neurology 65: 205-211

[104] Visvader JE (2011) Cells of origin in cancer. Nature 469: 314-322

[105] Vogel KS, Klesse LJ, Velasco-Miguel S, Meyers K, Rushing EJ, Parada LF (1999) Mouse tumor model for neurofibromatosis type 1. Science 286: 2176-2179

[106] Waggoner DJ, Towbin J, Gottesman G, Gutmann DH (2000) Clinic-based study of plexiform neurofibromas in neurofibromatosis 1. Am J Med Genet 92: 132-135

[107] Wallace MR, Rasmussen SA, Lim IT, Gray BA, Zori RT, Muir D (2000) Culture of cytogenetically abnormal schwann cells from benign and malignant NF1 tumors. Genes Chromosomes Cancer 27: 117-123

[108] Wanner IB, Mahoney J, Jessen KR, Wood PM, Bates M, Bunge MB (2006) Invariant mantling of growth cones by Schwann cell precursors characterize growing peripheral nerve fronts. Glia 54: 424-438

[109] Woldeyesus MT, Britsch S, Riethmacher D, Xu L, Sonnenberg-Riethmacher E, Abou-Rebyeh F, Harvey R, Caroni P, Birchmeier C (1999) Peripheral nervous system defects in erbB2 mutants following genetic rescue of heart development. Genes Dev 13: 2538-2548

[110] Wong CE, Paratore C, Dours-Zimmermann MT, Rochat A, Pietri T, Suter U, Zimmermann DR, Dufour S, Thiery JP, Meijer D et al (2006) Neural crest-derived cells with stem cell features can be traced back to multiple lineages in the adult skin. J Cell Biol 175: 1005-1015

[111] Woodruff JM (1999) Pathology of tumors of the peripheral nerve sheath in type 1 neurofibromatosis. Am J Med Genet 89: 23-30

[112] Wu J, Williams JP, Rizvi TA, Kordich JJ, Witte D, Meijer D, Stemmer-Rachamimov AO, Cancelas JA, Ratner N (2008) Plexiform and dermal neurofibromas and pigmentation are caused by Nf1 loss in desert hedgehog-expressing cells. Cancer Cell 13: 105-116

[113] Xu W, Mulligan LM, Ponder MA, Liu L, Smith BA, Mathew CG, Ponder BA (1992) Loss of NF1 alleles in phaeochromocytomas from patients with type I neurofibromatosis. Genes Chromosomes Cancer 4: 337-342

[114] Yang FC, Ingram DA, Chen S, Hingtgen CM, Ratner N, Monk KR, Clegg T, White H, Mead L, Wenning MJ et al (2003) Neurofibromin-deficient Schwann cells secrete a potent migratory stimulus for $Nf1^{+/-}$ mast cells. J Clin Invest 112: 1851-1861

[115] Yang FC, Chen S, Clegg T, Li X, Morgan T, Estwick SA, Yuan J, Khalaf W, Burgin S, Travers J et al (2006) $Nf1^{+/-}$ mast cells induce neurofibroma like phenotypes through secreted TGF-beta signaling. Hum Mol Genet 15: 2421-2437

[116] Yang FC, Ingram DA, Chen S, Zhu Y, Yuan J, Li X, Yang X, Knowles S, Horn W, Li Y et al (2008a) Nf1-dependent tumors require a microenvironment containing $Nf1^{+/-}$ and c-kit-dependent bone marrow. Cell 135: 437-448

[117] Yang ZJ, Ellis T, Markant SL, Read TA, Kessler JD, Bourboulas M, Schuller U, Machold R, Fishell G, Rowitch DH et al (2008b) Medulloblastoma can be initiated by deletion of patched in lineage-restricted progenitors or stem cells. Cancer Cell 14: 135-145

[118] Zheng H, Chang L, Patel N, Yang J, Lowe L, Burns DK, Zhu Y (2008) Induction of abnormal proliferation by nonmyelinating schwann cells triggers neurofibroma formation. Cancer Cell 13: 117-128

[119] Zhu Y, Parada LF (2001) Neurofibromin, a tumor suppressor in the nervous system. Exp Cell Res 264: 19-28

[120] Zhu Y, Ghosh P, Charnay P, Burns DK, Parada LF (2002) Neurofibromas in NF1: Schwann cell origin and role of tumor environment. Science 296: 920-922

[121] Zochodne DW (2012) The challenges and beauty of peripheral nerve regrowth. J Peripher Nerv Syst 17: 1-18

第37章 与1型神经纤维瘤病和其他Ras信号通路相关疾病相关认知障碍的分子学和细胞学研究方法

Molecular and Cellular Approaches to Cognitive Impairments Associated with NF1 and Other Rasopathies

Yong-Seok Lee and Alcino J. Silva

37.1 引言

1型神经纤维瘤病(NF1)是一种常见的遗传性疾病,会影响包括神经系统、眼睛、骨骼、内分泌系统、血管和皮肤在内的多个系统(Ratner and North 2003)。咖啡牛奶斑等色素沉着异常是其特征之一。NF1患者会表现出多种神经心理症状,如学习障碍。

NF1是一种常染色体显性遗传病,由17号染色体上的 NF1 基因发生功能丧失型突变引起。该基因编码的神经纤维瘤蛋白参与多种信号通路,包括Ras-MAPK和腺苷酸环化酶-cAMP级联反应。人们对其Ras-GAP(GTP酶活化蛋白)功能进行了深入研究,并发现其可能在脑中起关键作用。NF1 Ras-GAP通过将激活状态的Ras-GTP转化成失活状态的Ras-GDP来负向调控Ras-MAPK信号转导(Weiss et al. 1999)。因此,NF1功能丧失会导致包括脑组织在内的许多组织中Ras信号异常增加。

还有一些发育性疾病表现出与NF1相同的症状,如先天性心脏病、发育迟缓和认知缺陷。这些疾病包括努南综合征(Noonan syndrome,NS)、Costello综合征、LEOPARD综合征、CFC综合征和Legius综合征。遗传学研究发现,这些疾病是由Ras-MAPK信号转导通路中各种组分的突变引起的。因此,这些疾病被称为RAS信号通路相关疾病(Zenker 2011)。分子层面上相似的发病机制使这些疾病表现出相似的临床症状。临床遗传学的进步不仅使我们能够对这一组患者进行更精确的诊断,还为我们提供了研究这些疾病的分子学和细胞学机制的绝佳机会。我们希望这些研究最终能为此类疾病带来更有效的治疗方法。

在过去10年中,不断涌现的分子学和细胞学研究成果使我们比以往任何时候都更深刻地理解与NF1和其他RAS信号通路相关疾病相关的认知障碍。动物模型,尤其是小鼠模型,在产生这些新发现的过程中发挥了重要作用。在本章中,我们将回顾对NF1及其他RAS信号通路相关疾病小鼠模型进行的分子、细胞和行为研究。这些研究极大改变了我们对此类疾病的机制和治疗方法的理解。此外,我们将讨论如何将小鼠模型的研究成果应用于人类。

37.2 与 NF1 和其他 RAS 信号通路相关疾病相关的认知症状

NF1 和其他 RAS 信号通路相关疾病都会影响多个器官,大脑是其中之一。但每种疾病会表现出不同类型的认知障碍。例如,在 NF1 中整体认知障碍(如智力障碍)相对少见,而在 CFC 综合征中则更为常见(Wieczorek et al. 1997)。即使是同一种疾病,其表型也有很大差异。下文中我们将以 NF1 和 NS 为重点,总结与 RAS 信号通路相关疾病的认知症状。

37.2.1 NF1

执行功能与目标导向行为相关,需要注意力、计划能力、组织能力和抑制控制力。虽然全面认知障碍(global intellectual impairment)在 NF1 中并不常见,但特定的执行功能异常往往与之相关。此外,一些研究发现,NF1 患者的言语智商和操作智商之间有差异(Eliason 1986),这表明他们在视间认知领域(visual-spatial domain)存在功能障碍。实际上,已有报告称 NF1 患者存在视空间障碍(Kelly 2004)。表现出视空间障碍的 NF1 患儿通常也表现出记忆缺陷(Eliason 1988)。

在 NF1 患者中,注意力缺陷较为突出,大约 40% 的患儿存在注意力问题。有研究发现 NF1 患者有持续性注意力、选择性注意力和分散性注意力方面的问题(Hyman et al. 2005;Mautner et al. 2002)。对有注意力问题的 NF1 患儿使用兴奋剂治疗后取得了一些积极效果(Aron et al. 1990;Mautner et al. 2002)。然而,需要进行更多的纵向随访研究,以准确评估兴奋剂对这一人群的获益和不良影响。

学习障碍在 NF1 患儿中非常常见。研究表明,与 NF1 相关的学习障碍发生率为 40%~60%(Ratner and North 2003)。学习障碍可大致分为言语型(基于语言)和非言语型。言语型障碍包括读、写问题,非言语型障碍包括视空间缺陷、空间学习困难和社交问题。值得注意的是,NF1 患者可同时出现言语和非言语学习障碍,这表明该类人群的学习障碍并不能归类于传统的诊断中。这与传统观点不同,即不同的学习障碍反映了特定的病理原因。在 NF1 中,单一基因的突变可导致多种类型的学习障碍(Shilyansky et al. 2010b)。

除了高级认知功能缺陷外,NF1 患者的运动协调能力也存在异常。例如,NF1 患儿会表现出平衡和步态问题(Hofman et al. 1994;North et al. 1994),这可能与非言语任务的学习困难有关。

37.2.2 努南综合征

努南综合征(NS)是 RAS 信号通路相关疾病中最常见的类型(1/2 500 活产儿)。临床特征包括面部畸形、身材矮小、运动迟缓、心脏缺陷和认知障碍(Noonan 1994;Romano et al. 2010;Tartaglia and Gelb 2005)。约 50% 的 NS 病例是由 *PTPN11* 基因突变引起的,该基因编码非受体蛋白酪氨酸磷酸酶 SHP-2。此外,有报道 *SOS1*、*KRAS*、*RAF1*、*BRAF*、*SHOC2*、*MEK1* 和 *CBL* 基因的胚系突变也会导致 NS。这些突变会影响 Ras-MAPK 级联反应的正调控因子。与 NF1 类似,这将导致 Ras-MAPK 信号转导增加。

对 NS 患者进行的 IQ 研究发现,患者智商异质性大,从低分的精神发育迟滞到正常范围不等。NS 患者的平均智商分数低于正常人群。虽然智力障碍在 NS 患者中较为常见(约 30% 的患者受影响),但通常程度较轻(Lee et al. 2005;van der Burgt et al. 1999)。最近的研究表明,这种认知能力的异质性可部分归因于特定的突变和受影响的基因(Cesarini et al. 2009;Pierpont et al. 2009)。

既往研究也观察到了 NS 患者的言语智商和非言语智商之间的差异现象(van der Burgt et al. 1999;Pierpont et al. 2009;but see Lee et al. 2005)。NS 患者还存在空间功能、注意力和其他执行功能(如计划能力)方面的问题。然而,多数研究结果来自小样本研究,需要通过更大规模的研究加以验证。

学习障碍在 NS 患者中较为常见。有 30%~50% 的患者需要接受特殊教育(Wingbermuehle et al. 2009;Zenker et al. 2004)。NS 患者存在语言发育障碍(Pierpont et al. 2010),也有较大比例的患

者存在运动延迟,如笨拙和协调能力差(Romano et al. 2010)。这些缺陷均会影响言语型和非言语型学习过程。

Alfieri 等对 NS 和 LEOPARD 综合征患者的长期记忆进行了评估(Alfieri et al. 2011)。他们通过延迟口头自由回忆任务来评估,结果发现大多数患者的海马体依赖性长时记忆受损。然而,识别性记忆却基本不受影响,这表明 NS 患者表现出一种特定模式的记忆缺陷。

此外,有研究表明 NS 患者在社会认知方面存在问题,如述情障碍(无法用言语表达情感),这可能导致他们出现社会适应延迟(Verhoeven et al. 2008; Wingbermuhle et al. 2011)。

37.2.3 其他 RAS 信号通路相关疾病中的认知问题

Costello 综合征是一种由 *HRAS* 基因发生胚系突变引起的罕见疾病。与 NF1 和 NS 一样,Costello 综合征也与心脏缺陷、生长迟缓和认知障碍有关。Costello 综合征患者会出现轻度至边缘性智力障碍(Axelrad et al. 2011)。患者还表现出言语和非言语认知方面的问题。也有报告称患者在语言、视空间学习测试中出现记忆障碍(Dileone et al. 2010)。然而,其他研究表明其学习和记忆能力处于轻度残疾到边缘范围(Axelrad et al. 2011)。也有报道称 Costello 综合征患者存在视觉运动技能、适应行为和焦虑方面的问题(Axelrad et al. 2011)。

最近被命名的 Legius 综合征(类似于 NF1 的综合征)是由 *SPRED1* 基因发生功能丧失性突变引起的,*SPRED1* 是 Ras-MAPK 信号转导过程中的另一个负调控因子(Brems et al. 2007)。与 NF1 一样,*SPRED1* 基因突变也导致 MEK/MAPK 信号的过度激活。Legius 综合征患者临床表现和 NF1 类似,但不会出现神经纤维瘤或中枢神经系统肿瘤(Brems et al. 2007)。患儿可表现出注意力缺陷和学习障碍(Brems et al. 2007; Pasmant et al. 2009)。

心-面-皮肤综合征(cardio-facio-cutaneous syndrome,CFC 综合征)是另一种由 *BRAF*、*MEK1* 或 *MEK2* 基因突变引起的罕见的 RAS 信号通路相关疾病。大多数患者有轻度至重度智力障碍(Papadopoulou et al. 2011)。

37.3 小鼠模型的认知测试

在发现了 RAS 信号通路相关疾病的相关基因后,小鼠动物模型开始被投入研究,希望更好地了解疾病的机制,从而开发更有针对性的治疗方法。突变型小鼠是研究认知障碍的有效工具,原因有以下几点。首先,可以设计行为任务来模拟人类的认知缺陷。重要的是,可以设计特定的行为测试来检测特定脑区的功能,包括海马体和前额叶皮质。其次,某些行为(如学习和记忆)相关的分子学和细胞学机制可被用于研究特定突变 RAS 信号通路相关疾病的致病机制。这可帮助我们发现行为表型与分子和细胞机制之间的联系。尽管小鼠和人类存在明显的差异,但两者之间仍有很大程度的进化保守性。这一点非常重要,因为有些关键研究可以在小鼠身上进行伦理上无法在人体上进行的试验。不过也有必要提醒一下:小鼠和人类之间存在巨大差距,这也就解释了为什么并非所有在小鼠模型中开发的疗法都对患者有效。

37.3.1 海马依赖性学习和记忆

海马在人类的空间学习中发挥着重要作用(Squire 1992)。可以通过隐蔽平台版本的 Morris 水迷宫任务来测试海马依赖性表型,如空间学习障碍(Morris et al. 1982)。在这个任务中,训练小鼠在圆形水池中找到并记住一个平台的位置。由于平台隐藏在不透明的水面下,小鼠必须利用放置在水池周围的空间线索来了解平台的位置。训练后,可以通过探索试验评估小鼠的记忆力:将平台从水池中移出,让小鼠在一小段时间内(通常为 60 秒)寻找平台。一般认为,更准确、更持久地寻找平台表明小鼠有更好的学习和记忆能力。这项任务的另一个版本是用可看到的标志标记出逃生平台的位置,用于作为空间学习所需的其他大脑功能的对照,如视觉、运动功能和动机。这些其他功能的缺陷会影响以上两种水迷宫任务表现。

情境恐惧条件反射是另一种广泛使用的用于评

估海马依赖性的学习和记忆的任务的测试(Phillips and LeDoux 1992)。在这项测试中,小鼠被放置在一个条件反射箱中进行训练。几分钟后,箱子的地板会施加轻微的电击,因此,小鼠会害怕这个箱子。当再次被放回训练箱时,小鼠会表现出冻结反应(恐惧的表现)。事实证明,这些测试对海马损伤显示出较高敏感性。

海马依赖性学习和记忆的机制研究(包括水迷宫和情境条件反射的研究)发现,长时程增强(long-term potentiation,LTP)是细胞水平的一个关键机制。海马LTP的缺陷通常会导致海马依赖性学习和记忆障碍,而大多数在海马学习和记忆方面强化的突变小鼠都被证明也有LTP的增强。此外,海马学习通常伴随着海马突触功能的增加,这与LTP的特性类似。值得注意的是,在许多认知障碍小鼠模型中都发现了LTP的损害(Matynia et al. 2002)。

37.3.2 注意力

注意力缺陷在NF1患者中较为常见(Ferner et al. 1996)。侧化反应时间人物可被用于测试啮齿动物的注意力缺陷(Jentsch et al. 2009a)。前额叶缺陷会影响啮齿动物和人类在这项任务中的表现。在这个任务中,将小鼠放置在操作箱中,训练它们将鼻子固定在中间的端口上,同时也注意两侧的其他两个端口。在短暂(但不固定)的时间间隔内,其中一个侧面的端口会亮光提示,小鼠需将鼻子放到刚刚亮起的端口上才能获得奖励。注意力缺陷会导致动物选择错误的端口或更常见的是对灯光无反应。注意力有问题的动物在灯光长时间亮起的状态下(如10秒)能够完成这项任务,但与正常动物相比,当亮灯时间很短(如1秒)时,它们会表现出明显的缺陷。

37.3.3 工作记忆

工作记忆系统可短暂地保存、更新信息。皮质-纹状体网络被认为在工作记忆中起重要的作用。可以使用延迟性胜利-变化辐射状8臂迷宫任务来测试啮齿动物的这种记忆形式。在这项任务的训练阶段,迷宫的8个臂中只有4个是开放的,实验小鼠需记住这些,以便在训练阶段和随后所有臂都开放的测试阶段中只进入未去过的臂。在每轮训练和测试阶段后,臂的开放和关闭模式就会发生变化,从而迫使实验对象使用工作记忆系统。在测试过程中,实验对象可能会犯两种错误:① 同阶段错误,在同一测试阶段中重新进入已经去过的臂(受皮质-纹状体损伤影响);② 跨阶段错误,重新进入在前期训练阶段去过的臂(受海马损伤影响)。

延迟非匹配位置测试也常用于测试啮齿动物的工作记忆(Jentsch et al. 2009b)。每次试验由样本阶段和选择阶段构成,中间有短暂的间隔(3～6秒)。在采样阶段,实验对象被放置在一个内含多个鼻触孔的操作箱中,其中一个孔被照亮。实验对象需要将鼻子探入该孔,然后在操作箱的另一侧获得奖励。在选择阶段,除了样本阶段被照亮的孔外,另一个孔(非匹配位置)也会被照亮。对非匹配孔做出反应(即将鼻子探入)会得到奖励(因此得名"非匹配样本")。有工作记忆问题的实验对象会做出更多错误选择,有更多遗漏(无反应)。

37.4 NF1的小鼠模型

大多数NF1突变是功能丧失性突变,产生截短的、无功能的神经纤维瘤蛋白(Shen et al. 1996; Thomson et al. 2002)。在人类和小鼠中,NF1基因的序列、转录调控和下游靶点高度保守(Bernards et al. 1993; Hajra et al. 1994)。为了研究NF1,通过在Nf1基因的第31号外显子中插入1个neo基因,产生了具有Nf1基因杂合无义突变的小鼠($Nf1^{+/-}$),这会产生一种不稳定且快速降解的转录本(Jacks et al. 1994)。这种突变小鼠表现出与人类NF1类似的认知缺陷,因此被广泛用于研究这些缺陷的细胞学和分子学机制(见下文)。

在小鼠Nf1基因的60个外显子中,外显子23a对于高效Ras-GAP的活性是必需的。Nf1 23a的同源异构体主要在神经元中表达。为了研究这种神经元特异性Nf1同源异构体的作用,Costa等培养了一种Nf1基因第23号外显子纯合缺失的突变小鼠(Costa等,2001)。这种突变小鼠表现出学习缺陷,但没有Nf1其他突变的后果,如肿瘤易感性增加(Costa et al. 2001),这表明NF1的学习缺陷是由NF1信号转导改变引起的,而非由肿瘤本身引起。

为了具体研究 Nf1 基因缺失对特定细胞类型的影响，Zhu 等使用 Cre-loxP 系统制作了条件性基因敲除突变体。他们培育出一种在 Nf1 基因第 31—32 号外显子之间夹有 loxP 位点（$Nf1^{flox/+}$）的突变小鼠（Zhu et al. 2001）。与在特定启动子下表达 Cre 重组酶的品系杂交，可以实现 Nf1 的时间特异性和细胞类型特异性缺失。这一系统已被广泛用于探究认知缺陷的细胞机制（见下文）。例如，Brown 等最近利用这种 Cre 系统研究出一种 $Nf1^{+/-}$ 突变体小鼠模型，这种模型在表达 GFAP 的胶质细胞中合并 Nf1 基因完全缺失（Nf1 OPG 小鼠）（Brown et al. 2010）。与 $Nf1^{+/-}$ 小鼠不同，Nf1 OPG 小鼠出现了视神经胶质瘤。重要的是，这种突变似乎还会导致纹状体多巴胺减少和注意力缺陷。

37.4.1 $Nf1^{+/-}$ 及其他 NF1 小鼠模型的行为表型

$Nf1^{+/-}$ 小鼠表现出多种与人类 NF1 认知症状类似的行为缺陷。首先，$Nf1^{+/-}$ 小鼠在隐蔽平台版本的 Morris 水迷宫（一个海马依赖性空间学习任务）中表现出缺陷（Costa et al. 2002；Cui et al. 2008；Li et al. 2005；Silva et al. 1997）（见 37.3.1）。在探索试验阶段，杂合突变体在训练阶段时平台所在的目标象限中花费的时间明显更少。重要的是，通过额外训练试验可以克服这种记忆缺陷。额外训练同样也能改善 NF1 的学习缺陷（Silva et al. 1997）。除了水迷宫外，当施加轻度训练条件时，$Nf1^{+/-}$ 小鼠表现出情境恐惧条件反射缺陷（Cui et al. 2008）。Park 等使用了与 Cui 等设计的（C57Bl/6×129T2/SvEmsJ F1 杂交）不同遗传背景（C57Bl/6）的 $Nf1^{+/-}$ 小鼠，并在训练后 7 天发现 $Nf1^{+/-}$ 小鼠的情境恐惧条件反射受损（Park et al. 2009）。有趣的是，$Nf1^{+/-}$ 小鼠的学习缺陷仅限于特定领域。比如，$Nf1^{+/-}$ 小鼠在可视平台版本的水迷宫或听觉恐惧条件反射中均没有表现出缺陷。与情境条件反射和空间版本的水迷宫不同，这两项任务并不依赖于海马功能。在 NF1 患者身上也发现了相同的特定领域的认知缺陷模式。此外，在 $Nf1^{23a-/-}$ 小鼠中也发现了类似的海马学习缺陷模式（Costa et al. 2001）。

NF1 的表达具有高度异质性（即不完全外显率）。这个情况也在小鼠模型中得到了确认。在 NMDA 受体亚基 NR1 基因发生杂合无义突变（$NR1^{+/-}$）没有表现出缺陷的条件下，同时具有 $Nf1^{+/-}$ 和 $NR1^{+/-}$ 基因的小鼠却表现出严重的空间学习和情境辨别缺陷（Frankland et al. 1998；Silva et al. 1997）。这些结果表明，遗传修饰因子（如 $NR1^{+/-}$）在 NF1 学习表型的外显率中发挥重要作用。可以推测，NF1 患者的突变可能无法直接导致学习能力缺陷（如 $NR1^{+/-}$ 突变），但这些突变会加重患者的学习和记忆表现。

多项任务测试被用于 $Nf1^{+/-}$ 小鼠的注意力评估（Brown et al. 2010），包括侧化反应时间任务（Li et al. 2005）。当亮灯提示时间<0.5 秒时，$Nf1^{+/-}$ 小鼠犯错误和遗漏的次数明显多于同窝野生型小鼠，这意味着 $Nf1^{+/-}$ 小鼠具有与 NF1 患者类似的注意力缺陷（Li et al. 2005）。如上所述，Nf1 突变影响小鼠注意力系统的研究发现与 Brown 等（2010）的最新结论一致。

Shilyansky 等测试了 $Nf1^{+/-}$ 小鼠的工作记忆（一种执行功能）（Shilyansky et al. 2010a）。在延迟性胜利-转移放射状臂迷宫任务的测试阶段，$Nf1^{+/-}$ 小鼠犯了更多同阶段错误，这表明 $Nf1^{+/-}$ 小鼠具有皮质依赖性工作记忆缺陷。为了确认这种缺陷，还对 $Nf1^{+/-}$ 小鼠进行了延迟非匹配位置测试。在采样阶段，$Nf1^{+/-}$ 小鼠的表现与同窝的野生型小鼠相当。然而，在选择阶段，$Nf1^{+/-}$ 小鼠犯的错误明显更多。这印证了 $Nf1^{+/-}$ 小鼠存在工作记忆缺陷的观点（Shilyansky et al. 2010a）。

Nf1 OPG 小鼠表现出与 $Nf1^{+/-}$ 小鼠类似的表型。Nf1 OPG 小鼠在海马依赖性行为任务中如隐藏平台版本的 Morris 水迷宫任务和物体位置测试表现出缺陷（Brown et al. 2010）。此外，这种小鼠模型在面对新环境和新位置的物体时表现出明显减少的直立频率，表明 Nf1 OPG 小鼠在非选择性和选择性注意力上都存在缺陷（Brown et al. 2010）。

需要注意的是，上述不同类型 Nf1 小鼠模型为我们理解与疾病相关的中枢神经系统表型做出了不同方面但同样重要的贡献。这些研究表明，单个小鼠模型不必显示出与某种疾病相关的所有表型，才能对该疾病的研究有用。在某些方面，一些小鼠模型仅表现出患者复杂表型中的一部分可能更好，因为这种简化有助于阐明与该疾病相关的复杂缺陷集合背后的多种因果关系。例如，上述各种 $Nf1$ 小鼠突变体并不像许多 NF1 患者那样有明显的肿瘤负荷，这说明肿瘤本身不能完全解释 NF1 中的学习和其他认知缺陷。与此观点一致，基于 NF1 患者的研究也未能发现肿瘤负荷与认知缺陷之间存在明确相关性。

37.4.2 $Nf1^{+/-}$ 行为缺陷的细胞学和分子学机制

37.4.2.1 Ras 功能增加和可塑性受损

由于 NF1 是由神经纤维瘤蛋白（Ras 信号转导的负向调控因子）的功能丧失性突变引起的，所以 Ras 信号转导增强是 $Nf1$ 小鼠认知障碍的关键机制。相应地，在 $Nf1^{+/-}$ 小鼠的海马和皮质中确实观察到了 Ras 活性及其下游信号成分（MEK/ERK）的增强（Li et al. 2005）。Ras 信号的增加是 $Nf1^{+/-}$ 小鼠认知缺陷的基础，这一观点也通过遗传学和药理学方法得到了证实。Costa 等将 $Nf1^{+/-}$ 小鼠与杂合子 Ras 敲除小鼠（$K-ras^{+/-}$ 或 $N-Ras^{+/-}$）杂交，从遗传学角度降低 Ras 活性（Costa et al. 2002）。$Nf1^{+/-}$ 和 $K-ras^{+/-}$ 突变均会损害在水迷宫中测试的空间学习能力。然而，同时有这两种突变的小鼠具有正常的空间学习能力！此外，$Nf1^{+/-}$ 小鼠的空间学习障碍也可以通过法尼基转移酶抑制剂（farnesyl transferase inhibitor，FTI）的治疗得到好转（Costa et al. 2002）。FTI 通过阻断法尼基化（一种 Ras 激活所需的翻译后修饰）来减弱 Ras 信号转导。这些数据表明成年期 Ras 信号的增加是 $Nf1$ 突变小鼠海马依赖性认知障碍的原因。

重要的是，药物干预能够改善成人 NF1 患者的认知表型（see also Brown et al. 2010; Li et al. 2005），这表明这些行为缺陷并非完全由不可逆的发育变化引起，而是可以在成年期进行治疗。神经纤维瘤蛋白可以调节 trophic factor 信号通路，该通路和发育过程中 Nf1 突变产生的其他效应被认为是 $Nf1$ 突变小鼠产生认知缺陷的核心原因。基于这些 Nf1 研究，其他既往被认为完全由神经发育来源的表型也得以治疗，如脆性 X 综合征、唐氏综合征、Rett 综合征和结节性硬化症等（Dolen et al. 2007; Ehninger et al. 2008a, b; Fernandez et al. 2007; Guy et al. 2007）。因此，这些自 NF1 动物模型起始的研究极大促进了神经病理学和神经发育障碍治疗的进展。这些研究表明，尽管神经发育障碍有明确的发育原因（如源于产前发育的缺陷），但通过成年期分子水平和细胞水平的干预（如成年 $Nf1$ 小鼠的 Ras 信号增强），可以对与这些疾病相关的认知表型产生意想不到的积极作用。

为了寻找临床可持续且被 FDA 批准的治疗方法，Li 等检测了他汀类药物（如洛伐他汀）对 $Nf1^{+/-}$ 小鼠的影响。洛伐他汀不仅能降低胆固醇水平，还通过阻止 Ras 通路上的异戊二烯化来减少 Ras 的激活（Li et al. 2005）。与 FTI 类似，洛伐他汀治疗也改善了 $Nf1^{+/-}$ 小鼠的水迷宫缺陷。此外，洛伐他汀还能改善 $Nf1^{+/-}$ 小鼠的注意力缺陷，这表明这种治疗方法可能作用于与 NF1 相关的多个行为缺陷领域，包括注意力和空间认知（Li et al. 2005）。

$Nf1^{+/-}$ 小鼠学习和记忆缺陷的生理机制是什么？大量的证据表明，长期突触可塑性，尤其是海马的长时程增强效应（long-term potentiation，LTP），是空间学习和记忆的关键生理机制（Lee and Silva 2009; Matynia et al. 2002）。使 LTP 减弱的操作通常会导致空间学习障碍，而绝大多数（>90%）空间学习能力增强的突变小鼠也在海马 CA1 区显示出 LTP 的增强（Lee and Silva 2009）。重要的是，发生学习这一行为后，在海马中观察到类似 LTP 的变化（Whitlock et al. 2006）。而且，Ras-ERK 信号通路在海马 LTP 发挥着重要作用（Sweatt 2001）。$Nf1^{+/-}$ 小鼠的确在 θ 短阵快速脉冲刺激（TBS）诱导的海马 LTP 中显示出缺陷（Costa et al. 2002; Cui et al. 2008; Li et al. 2005）。引人注目的是，能够逆转 $Nf1^{+/-}$ 小鼠行为缺陷的操作也能够逆转这些小鼠的 LTP 缺陷。例如，K-Ras 敲除突变、FTI

和洛伐他汀治疗均能改善 $Nf1^{+/-}$ 小鼠的 LTP 缺陷（Costa et al. 2002；Cui et al. 2008；Li et al. 2005）。这些数据表明，Ras 激活的增加导致了 LTP 受损，从而导致了 $Nf1^{+/-}$ 小鼠的学习和记忆缺陷。

37.4.2.2 抑制增加：Ras 活性增加与 LTP 受损的联系

Ras 活性增强如何导致 $Nf1^{+/-}$ 小鼠的 LTP 缺陷？Ras 信号转导增加的细胞水平后果是什么？多方证据表明，Ras 信号增加导致 $Nf1^{+/-}$ 小鼠中 GABA 介导的抑制作用增加（Costa et al. 2002；Cui et al. 2008）。第一，海马 LTP 缺陷仅在 TBS 中出现（对 GABA 介导的抑制变化更为敏感）。第二，在使用 60 μA 突触刺激强度导致 GABA 介导的抑制作用增加时，$Nf1^{+/-}$ 小鼠显示出 LTP 缺陷；而在使用 35 μA 突触刺激强度无法导致抑制作用增加时，LTP 缺陷则不明显。第三，在使用 AMPA 和 NMDA 受体阻断剂时诱发的 IPSC 在 $Nf1^{+/-}$ 小鼠中更大。第四，木防己苦毒素（一种 $GABA_A$ 受体拮抗剂）逆转了 $Nf1^{+/-}$ 小鼠的海马 LTP 缺陷。

为了直接验证 GABA 假说，Cui 等使用了遗传学方法来研究敲除 Nf1 基因在特定类型神经元中的作用。他们使用 Cre-loxP 系统，在兴奋性神经元、抑制性神经元或神经胶质细胞中敲除了 Nf1 基因（Cui et al. 2008）。仅在抑制性神经元中杂合缺失 Nf1 会导致 Morris 水迷宫中的学习障碍，而在兴奋性神经元（杂合或纯合）或胶质细胞（杂合）中敲除 Nf1 则没有对学习产生同样的影响（没有空间学习缺陷）。相应地，只有在抑制性神经元中删除 Nf1 时，才会发现 LTP 缺陷，而在兴奋性神经元中敲除 Nf1 时并没有发现 LTP 缺陷。在 $Nf1^{+/-}$ 小鼠的海马中发现了活性依赖性的 GABA 释放增加，但没有发现谷氨酸释放增加，这证实了在 $Nf1^{+/-}$ 小鼠中抑制和兴奋之间失衡。重要的是，Ras/MEK/ERK 信号转导抑制剂阻断了 GABA 释放增加（Cui et al. 2008）。研究还发现在 $Nf1^{+/-}$ 小鼠的 ERK 位点的突触素 I 的磷酸化增加。目前已知这种磷酸化会导致更高水平的神经递质释放，这一发现提供了理解 $Nf1^{+/-}$ 小鼠学习缺陷机制的另外一个重要分子步骤。因此，这些小鼠具有更多的 Ras/ERK 信号转导、更高水平的突触素 I ERK 磷酸化，进而导致更高水平的 GABA 释放，从而导致 LTP 缺陷及其学习缺陷。重要的是，亚阈值剂量的木防己苦毒素可以逆转 $Nf1^{+/-}$ 小鼠的海马行为缺陷（如空间学习能力）（Cui et al. 2008）。

37.4.2.3 抑制增加与皮质-纹状体功能

在其他脑区（如皮质和纹状体）中，抑制功能也发挥着重要作用。这些脑区涉及注意力和工作记忆，而 NF1 患者的这些功能也会受到影响。Shilyansky 等研究了 $Nf1^{+/-}$ 小鼠的工作记忆缺陷是否由相同的机制（抑制增加）导致（Shilyansky et al. 2010a）。电生理分析显示，与同窝野生型小鼠相比，$Nf1^{+/-}$ 小鼠的内侧前额叶皮质（medial prefrontal cortex，mPFC）和纹状体中的活动依赖性 GABA 释放增加。同海马中一样，谷氨酸释放没有差异。在由 Cre 介导的抑制性神经元特异性缺失的 Nf1 突变体的内侧前额叶皮质（mPFC）中也发现了这种抑制作用的增强，这表明 Nf1 可调节 mPFC 中间神经元的 GABA 释放（Shilyansky et al. 2010a）。与海马类似，在 mPFC 中 MEK 抑制剂 U0126 逆转了 $Nf1^{+/-}$ 小鼠的抑制增加，这表明增强的 Ras/MEK/ERK 信号转导介导了这些小鼠中更强的 GABA 抑制作用。

为了研究抑制增加是否为 NF1 工作记忆缺陷的基础，Shilyansky 等使用木防己苦毒素处理 $Nf1^{+/-}$ 小鼠，并在延迟胜利-转移放射状臂迷宫任务和延迟非匹配样本任务中对其进行了测试（Shilyansky et al. 2010a）。值得注意的是，在这些任务中，一定剂量的木防己苦毒素引发了野生型小鼠的工作记忆缺陷，但却使 $Nf1^{+/-}$ 小鼠在这两项任务中的工作记忆缺陷有所好转。

唐氏综合征、脆性 X 综合征和 Rett 综合征的小鼠模型也显示出抑制调节的改变（Dani et al. 2005；Fernandez et al. 2007；Gibson et al. 2008）。与 $Nf1^{+/-}$ 小鼠的研究结果一致，唐氏综合征小鼠模型中的行为缺陷（如 Morris 水迷宫中的空间学习缺陷）可以被 $GABA_A$ 拮抗剂木防己苦毒素所治疗（Fernandez et al. 2007；Rueda et al. 2008）。

37.4.2.4 其他机制

除了作为 Ras 信号转导的负调控因子外，神经纤维瘤蛋白还可作为小鼠和果蝇中腺苷酸环化酶

(adenylate cyclase，AC)的正调控因子(Guo et al. 2000；Tong et al. 2002)。Nf1 缺失的果蝇突变体表现出 AC 活性降低以及嗅觉学习缺陷。通过 rutabaga(一种组成型活化的 AC)的表达，这些果蝇的学习缺陷有所恢复，这表明 AC 活性降低导致了这种 Nf1 突变果蝇的学习缺陷(Guo et al. 2000)。神经纤维瘤蛋白还通过 AC-PKA 通路调节神经元结构。$Nf1^{+/-}$ 小鼠的海马和视网膜神经节细胞神经元表现出生长锥面积和神经突长度减少以及凋亡增加，这些现象均可被 cAMP 水平的提高逆转(Brown et al. 2012)。然而，AC-PKA 信号转导的减弱是否与 NF1 患者的认知障碍有关，目前尚不清楚。

37.5 其他 RAS 信号通路病相关动物模型的认知研究

37.5.1 类 NF1(Legius)综合征

SPRED1 基因敲除小鼠($Spred1^{-/-}$)表现出多种与 SPRED1 基因突变个体相似的表型，如体重较轻、面部缩短以及脾脏中黑色素沉积(Brems et al. 2007)。重要的是，$Spred1^{-/-}$ 小鼠在 Morris 水迷宫和视觉辨别 T 迷宫中表现出缺陷，这些任务都是依赖于海马的(Denayer et al. 2008)。这种突变体还表现出异常激活的 Ras-MAPK 信号转导和海马 LTP 损伤，说明 Ras 信号转导改变导致的 LTP 损伤是产生 Legius 综合征学习缺陷的基础。

37.5.2 努南综合征

通过敲除 NS 相关 Ptpn11、Sos1 或 Raf1 基因突变构建了几种 NS 小鼠模型(Araki et al. 2004, 2009；Chen et al. 2010；Wu et al. 2011)。在 $SHP-2^{D61G/+}$ 突变小鼠的新生海马和皮质中观察到了神经细胞命运的改变，这表明这种发育异常可能是 NS 中认知问题的原因(Gauthier et al. 2007)。然而，其对行为的影响有待进一步研究。

Pagani 等在果蝇中研究了一种 NS 相关突变对学习和记忆的影响(Pagani et al. 2009)。功能获得性 corkscrew(csw)基因[果蝇 Ptpn11(SHP-2)基因的同源基因]的过表达导致了间隔训练后的长时记忆缺陷。这种缺陷可以通过使用阈值下剂量的磷酸酶抑制剂 NSC-87877 或延长训练间隔来改善。该研究表明，csw 通过调节 ERK 激活改变来调控休息间隔的持续时间对学习的影响(Pagani et al. 2009)。

37.5.3 Costello 综合征

$H-Ras^{G12V}$ 基因敲入突变体被用作 Costello 综合征的小鼠模型(Schuhmacher et al. 2008)。这种突变体表现出 Costello 综合征患者的一些症状，如面部畸形和心肌病(Schuhmacher et al. 2008)。纯合基因敲入小鼠($H-Ras^{G12V/G12V}$)在依赖海马的 Morris 水迷宫和情境恐惧条件反射任务中表现出缺陷，但在依赖皮质的新物体识别任务中表现正常。杂合小鼠则没有表现出任何学习缺陷。因此，与患者一样，这些小鼠的认知缺陷也是轻度至中度(Viosca et al. 2009)。

37.6 小鼠模型之后：在人体中的机制与治疗

基于动物模型的研究发现为转化研究提供了机会，以探究人类认知缺陷是否具有相同的机制，以及类似的治疗策略是否可用于 NF1 患者。

37.6.1 NF1 患者中的皮质-纹状体功能障碍

对 $Nf1^{+/-}$ 小鼠的研究表明，皮质和纹状体中的抑制作用增加是导致工作记忆缺陷的原因。Shilyansky 等利用行为任务和 fMRI，检查了 NF1 患者的工作记忆和皮质-纹状体功能(Shilyansky et al. 2010a)。NF1 患者在两项工作记忆任务[空间工作记忆维持和操作(spatial working memory maintenance and manipulation，stMNM)、空间工作记忆容量的参数化探测(parametric probe of spatial working memory capacity，SCAP)]中表现出明显缺陷，这两项任务是视觉空间工作记忆任务，与对 $Nf1^{+/-}$ 小鼠所使用的操作性延迟非匹配样本任务对应。fMRI 分析重点关注背外侧前额叶皮质(DLPFC)，该区域与啮齿动物的内侧前额叶皮质

(mPFC)同源，也集中在纹状体区域。与对照组相比，NF1 患者在 stMNM 任务中表现出皮质和纹状体区域的神经活动显著减少。相应地，NF1 患者在 SCAP 任务中也表现出与维持工作记忆中空间信息密切相关的皮质区域中的神经活动减少。此外，DLPFC 低激活程度与工作记忆表现显著相关，这表明皮质-纹状体功能障碍与人类 NF1 中的工作记忆缺陷直接相关（Shilyansky et al. 2010a）。小鼠和人类 NF1 的工作记忆缺陷极有可能具有相似的机制：抑制增加导致神经激活减少。

37.6.2 他汀对 NF1 患者认知功能的影响

尽管长期以来人们一直认为神经发育障碍在成人中不可逆转，但前述研究表明，通过逆转潜在的信号转导缺陷，可以治疗成年 $Nf1^{+/-}$ 小鼠的行为和生理表型。尽管 NF1 可能影响发育，但它也会影响成年后的功能，逆转小鼠成年后的缺陷足以逆转其学习和记忆表型。值得注意的是，一项果蝇的脆性 X 综合征研究表明，药物治疗可以逆转这种突变果蝇的关键表型（McBride et al. 2005）。那么，类似的成年期治疗是否对脆性 X 综合征或 NF1 患者有效？虽然目前下结论还为时尚早，但针对脆性 X 综合征和 NF1 的初步临床研究结果令人鼓舞。

Krab 等进行了一项随机、双盲、安慰剂对照临床试验，该试验涉及 62 名 NF1 患儿（Krab et al. 2008）。为了检验小鼠中关于他汀类药物的发现是否可以应用在 NF1 患者身上，NF1 患儿分别接受了为期 12 周的辛伐他汀或安慰剂治疗，并在治疗前后进行评估。重要的是，结果显示这种治疗方案在这一人群未出现不良反应。认知功能测试重点关注非语言长期记忆，注意力和小脑功能被设为主要结局指标。此外，对于在注意力和视觉-空间能力测试中基线评分小于等于平均值 1 个标准差的个体，还需评估次要结局指标。与安慰剂相比，辛伐他汀治疗似乎对主要结局指标没有额外作用。不过，辛伐他汀组在物体组装测试中的得分（次要结局指标之一）显著提高。该测试可以反映包括视觉综合和工作记忆在内的多个认知领域。辛伐他汀相对于安慰剂的治疗效果仅在 NF1 认知缺陷儿童中观察到，而对于初始得分在正常范围内患儿未观察到组间差异。

此外，一项以评估洛伐他汀在 24 名 NF1 患儿中安全性和耐受性为目的的 I 期研究还评估了其治疗前后的认知差异（Acosta et al. 2011）。研究结果除了确认洛伐他汀在这一儿童群体中的安全性外，还表明该治疗方法能够改善 NF1 患儿的言语和非言语记忆以及视觉注意力和视觉效率（Acosta et al. 2011）。然而，需要注意的是，上述两项研究并未按照有效性试验来设计。不过，美国和其他国家正在进行其他几项他汀类药物的临床试验，专门用于测试他汀对 NF1 认知表型的疗效。这些研究的结果可能会提供关于他汀类药物对 NF1 患儿甚至是在成人疗效的令人期待的信息。如果取得成功，这些研究自然会继续下去，进一步测试他汀类药物是否也能帮助受其他 RAS 信号通路相关疾病影响的儿童。

37.7 结论

动物模型是研究 NF1 和其他 RAS 信号通路相关疾病认知障碍的分子学和细胞学机制的重要工具。在过去的 20 年中，NF1 研究从明确致病基因，到揭示相关认知缺陷的分子学和细胞学机制，再到临床试验，已经取得了长足发展。这些研究的发现之路不仅作用于 NF1，也影响着其他具有认知表型的遗传性疾病。例如，通过对 NF1 的研究，我们认识到神经发育障碍患者开发成年期治疗方法是有可能的。这一发现改变了我们对神经发育障碍治疗的看法，目前有许多来自其他神经发育障碍动物模型的证据表明，成年期的治疗可以对与这类疾病相关的认知表型产生意想不到的重大影响。此外，在某些情况下，这些动物模型研究已经被转化为临床干预措施，尽管尚未得到明确结论，但到目前为止取得的结果非常令人鼓舞。在理解认知障碍和开发治疗方法方面，非常需要基础神经科学家、临床医师和患者组织之间的密切合作和互动。RAS 信号通路相关疾病的研究也适合这种协作方法，因为许多相关致病基因已被发现，有合适的动物模型，还有尽职且高效的患者组织，这些组织促进了招募工作，还非常高效地对家长及患者进行了告知与教育。最重要的是，这种相互关系带来了前所未有的科学和临床的协同,这对于解决认知障碍治疗所面临的诸多困难和挑战至关重要。新兴的技术,如从人体组织取得的iPS(诱导多能干细胞)为补充和加强当前的动物模型方法提供了新的视野(Carvajal-Vergara et al. 2010)。此外,基因组学革命为我们理解这些复杂的情况提供了有力的工具和必需的遗传学信息。尽管挑战重重,前路仍充满希望:我们比以往任何时候都更接近于找到治疗医学重大挑战之一——理解和治疗那些影响我们人类内核、自我认知的疾病的方法。

(朱以诚,付瀚辉,张明路 译)

参考文献

[1] Acosta MT, Kardel PG, Walsh KS, Rosenbaum KN, Gioia GA, Packer RJ (2011) Lovastatin as treatment for neurocognitive deficits in neurofibromatosis type 1: phase I study. Pediatr Neurol 45: 241-245

[2] Alfieri P, Cesarini L, Mallardi M, Piccini G, Caciolo C et al (2011) Long term memory profile of disorders associated with dysregulation of the RAS-MAPK signaling cascade. Behav Genet 41: 423-429

[3] Araki T, Mohi MG, Ismat FA, Bronson RT, Williams IR et al (2004) Mouse model of Noonan syndrome reveals cell type- and gene dosage-dependent effects of Ptpn11 mutation. Nat Med 10: 849-857

[4] Araki T, Chan G, Newbigging S, Morikawa L, Bronson RT, Neel BG (2009) Noonan syndrome cardiac defects are caused by PTPN11 acting in endocardium to enhance endocardial-mesenchymal transformation. Proc Natl Acad Sci USA 106: 4736-4741

[5] Aron AM, Rubenstein AE, Wallace SA, Halperin JC (1990) Learning disabilities in neurofibro-matosis. In: Rubenstein AE, Korf BR (eds) Neurofibromatosis: a handbook for patients, families and healthcare professionals. Thieme, New York, pp 55-58

[6] Axelrad ME, Schwartz DD, Katzenstein JM, Hopkins E, Gripp KW (2011) Neurocognitive, adaptive, and behavioral functioning of individuals with Costello syndrome: a review. Am J Med Genet C Semin Med Genet 157: 115-122

[7] Bernards A, Snijders AJ, Hannigan GE, Murthy AE, Gusella JF (1993) Mouse neurofibromatosis type 1 cDNA sequence reveals high degree of conservation of both coding and non-coding mRNA segments. Hum Mol Genet 2: 645-650

[8] Brems H, Chmara M, Sahbatou M, Denayer E, Taniguchi K et al (2007) Germline loss-of-function mutations in *SPRED1* cause a neurofibromatosis 1-like phenotype. Nat Genet 39: 1120-1126

[9] Brown JA, Emnett RJ, White CR, Yuede CM, Conyers SB et al (2010) Reduced striatal dopamine underlies the attention system dysfunction in neurofibromatosis-1 mutant mice. Hum Mol Genet 19: 4515-4528

[10] Brown JA, Diggs-Andrews KA, Gianino SM, Gutmann DH (2012) Neurofibromatosis-1 hetero-zygosity impairs CNS neuronal morphology in a cAMP/PKA/ROCK-dependent manner. Mol Cell Neurosci 49: 13-22

[11] Carvajal-Vergara X, Sevilla A, D'Souza SL, Ang YS, Schaniel C et al (2010) Patient-specific induced pluripotent stem-cell-derived models of LEOPARD syndrome. Nature 465: 808-812

[12] Cesarini L, Alfieri P, Pantaleoni F, Vasta I, Cerutti M et al (2009) Cognitive profile of disorders associated with dysregulation of the RAS/MAPK signaling cascade. Am J Med Genet 149A: 140-146

[13] Chen PC, Wakimoto H, Conner D, Araki T, Yuan T et al (2010) Activation of multiple signaling pathways causes developmental defects in mice with a Noonan syndrome-associated Sos1 mutation. J Clin Invest 120: 4353-4365

[14] Costa RM, Yang T, Huynh DP, Pulst SM, Viskochil DH et al (2001) Learning deficits, but normal development and tumor predisposition, in mice lacking exon 23a of Nf1. Nat Genet 27: 399-405

[15] Costa RM, Federov NB, Kogan JH, Murphy GG, Stern J et al (2002) Mechanism for the learning deficits in a mouse model of neurofibromatosis type 1. Nature 415: 526-530

[16] Cui Y, Costa RM, Murphy GG, Elgersma Y, Zhu Y et al (2008) Neurofibromin regulation of ERK signaling modulates GABA release and learning. Cell 135: 549-560

[17] Dani VS, Chang Q, Maffei A, Turrigiano GG, Jaenisch R, Nelson SB (2005) Reduced cortical activity due to a shift in the balance between excitation and inhibition in a mouse model of Rett syndrome. Proc Natl Acad Sci USA 102: 12560-12565

[18] Denayer E, Ahmed T, Brems H, Van Woerden G, Borgesius NZ et al (2008) Spred1 is required for synaptic plasticity and hippocampus-dependent learning. J Neurosci 28: 14443-14449

[19] Dileone M, Profice P, Pilato F, Alfieri P, Cesarini L et al (2010) Enhanced human brain associative plasticity in Costello syndrome. J Physiol 588: 3445-3456

[20] Dolen G, Osterweil E, Rao BS, Smith GB, Auerbach BD et al (2007) Correction of fragile X syndrome in mice. Neuron 56: 955-962

[21] Ehninger D, Han S, Shilyansky C, Zhou Y, Li W et al (2008a) Reversal of learning deficits in a $Tsc2^{+/-}$ mouse model of tuberous sclerosis. Nat Med 14: 843-848

[22] Ehninger D, Li W, Fox K, Stryker MP, Silva AJ (2008b) Reversing neurodevelopmental disorders in adults. Neuron 60: 950-960

[23] Eliason MJ (1986) Neurofibromatosis: implications for learning and behavior. J Dev Behav Pediatr 7: 175-179

[24] Eliason MJ (1988) Neuropsychological patterns: neurofibromatosis compared to developmental learning disorders. Neurofibromatosis 1: 17-25

[25] Fernandez F, Morishita W, Zuniga E, Nguyen J, Blank M et al (2007) Pharmacotherapy for cognitive impairment in a mouse model of Down syndrome. Nat Neurosci 10: 411-413

[26] Ferner RE, Hughes RA, Weinman J (1996) Intellectual impairment in neurofibromatosis 1. J Neurol Sci 138: 125-133

[27] Frankland PW, Cestari V, Filipkowski RK, McDonald RJ, Silva AJ (1998) The dorsal hippocampus is essential for context discrimination but not for contextual conditioning. Behav Neurosci 112: 863-874

[28] Gauthier AS, Furstoss O, Araki T, Chan R, Neel BG et al (2007) Control of CNS cell-fate decisions by SHP-2 and its dysregulation in Noonan syndrome. Neuron 54: 245-262

[29] Gibson JR, Bartley AF, Hays SA, Huber KM (2008) Imbalance of neocortical excitation and inhibition and altered UP states reflect network hyperexcitability in the mouse model of fragile X syndrome. J Neurophysiol 100: 2615-2626

[30] Guo HF, Tong J, Hannan F, Luo L, Zhong Y (2000) A neurofibromatosis-1-regulated pathway is required for learning in Drosophila. Nature 403: 895-898

[31] Guy J, Gan J, Selfridge J, Cobb S, Bird A (2007) Reversal of neurological defects in a mouse model of Rett syndrome. Science 315: 1143-1147

[32] Hajra A, Martin-Gallardo A, Tarle SA, Freedman M, Wilson-Gunn S et al (1994) DNA sequences in the promoter region of the NF1 gene are highly conserved between human and mouse. Genomics 21: 649-652

[33] Hofman KJ, Harris EL, Bryan RN, Denckla MB (1994) Neurofibromatosis type 1: the cognitive phenotype. J Pediatr 124: S1-S8

[34] Hyman SL, Shores A, North KN (2005) The nature and frequency of cognitive deficits in children with neurofibromatosis type 1. Neurology 65: 1037-1044

[35] Jacks T, Shih TS, Schmitt EM, Bronson RT, Bernards A, Weinberg RA (1994) Tumour predisposition in mice heterozygous for a targeted mutation in Nf1. Nat Genet 7: 353-361

[36] Jentsch JD, Aarde SM, Seu E (2009a) Effects of atomoxetine and methylphenidate on performance of a lateralized reaction time task in rats. Psychopharmacology 202: 497-504

[37] Jentsch JD, Trantham-Davidson H, Jairl C, Tinsley M, Cannon TD, Lavin A (2009b) Dysbindin modulates prefrontal cortical glutamatergic circuits and working memory function in mice. Neuropsychopharmacology 34: 2601-2608

[38] Kelly DP (2004) Neurodevelopmental dysfunction in the school-aged child, chap 29. Saunders, Amsterdam

[39] Krab LC, de Goede-Bolder A, Aarsen FK, Pluijm SM, Bouman MJ et al (2008) Effect of simvastatin on cognitive functioning in children with neurofibromatosis type 1: a randomized controlled trial. JAMA 300: 287-294

[40] Lee YS, Silva AJ (2009) The molecular and cellular biology of enhanced cognition. Nat Rev Neurosci 10: 126-140

[41] Lee DA, Portnoy S, Hill P, Gillberg C, Patton MA (2005) Psychological profile of children with Noonan syndrome. Dev Med Child Neurol 47: 35-38

[42] Li W, Cui Y, Kushner SA, Brown RA, Jentsch JD et al (2005) The HMG-CoA reductase inhibitor lovastatin reverses the learning and attention deficits in a mouse model of neurofibromatosis type 1. Curr Biol 15: 1961-1967

[43] Matynia A, Kushner SA, Silva AJ (2002) Genetic approaches to molecular and cellular cognition: a focus on LTP and learning and memory. Annu Rev Genet 36: 687-720

[44] Mautner VF, Kluwe L, Thakker SD, Leark RA (2002) Treatment of ADHD in neurofibromatosis type 1. Dev Med Child Neurol 44: 164-170

[45] McBride SM, Choi CH, Wang Y, Liebelt D, Braunstein E et al (2005) Pharmacological rescue of synaptic plasticity, courtship behavior, and mushroom body defects in a Drosophila model of fragile X syndrome. Neuron 45: 753-764

[46] Morris RG, Garrud P, Rawlins JN, O'Keefe J (1982) Place navigation impaired in rats with hippocampal lesions. Nature 297: 681-683

[47] Noonan JA (1994) Noonan syndrome. An update and review for the primary pediatrician. Clin Pediatr 33: 548-555

[48] North K, Joy P, Yuille D, Cocks N, Mobbs E et al (1994) Specific learning disability in children with neurofibromatosis type 1: significance of MRI abnormalities. Neurology 44: 878-883

[49] Pagani MR, Oishi K, Gelb BD, Zhong Y (2009) The phosphatase SHP2 regulates the spacing effect for long-term memory induction. Cell 139: 186-198

[50] Papadopoulou E, Sifakis S, Sol-Church K, Klein-Zighelboim E, Stabley DL et al (2011) CNS imaging is a key diagnostic tool in the evaluation of patients with CFC syndrome: two cases and literature review. Am J Med Genet 155A: 605-611

[51] Park CS, Zhong L, Tang SJ (2009) Aberrant expression of synaptic plasticity-related genes in the $NF1^{+/-}$ mouse hippocampus. J Neurosci Res 87: 3107-3119

[52] Pasmant E, Sabbagh A, Hanna N, Masliah-Planchon J, Jolly E et al (2009) SPRED1 germline mutations caused a neurofibromatosis type 1 overlapping phenotype. J Med Genet 46: 425-430

[53] Phillips RG, LeDoux JE (1992) Differential contribution of amygdala and hippocampus to cued and contextual fear conditioning. Behav Neurosci 106: 274-285

[54] Pierpont EI, Pierpont ME, Mendelsohn NJ, Roberts AE, Tworog-Dube E, Seidenberg MS (2009) Genotype differences in cognitive functioning in Noonan syndrome. Genes Brain Behav 8: 275-282

[55] Pierpont EI, Weismer SE, Roberts AE, Tworog-Dube E, Pierpont ME et al (2010) The language phenotype of children and adolescents with Noonan syndrome. J Speech Lang Hear Res 53: 917-932

[56] Ratner N, North K (2003) The central nervous system in neurofibromatosis type 1. In: Fisch GS (ed) Contemporary clinical neuroscience: genetics and genomics of neurobehavioral disorders. Humana, Totowa, NJ, pp 97-131

[57] Romano AA, Allanson JE, Dahlgren J, Gelb BD, Hall B et al (2010) Noonan syndrome: clinical features, diagnosis, and management guidelines. Pediatrics 126: 746-759

[58] Rueda N, Florez J, Martinez-Cue C (2008) Chronic pentylenetetrazole but not donepezil treatment rescues spatial cognition in Ts65Dn mice, a model for Down syndrome. Neurosci Lett 433: 22-27

[59] Schuhmacher AJ, Guerra C, Sauzeau V, Canamero M, Bustelo XR, Barbacid M (2008) A mouse model for Costello syndrome reveals an Ang II-mediated hypertensive condition. J Clin Invest 118: 2169-2179

[60] Shen MH, Harper PS, Upadhyaya M (1996) Molecular genetics of neurofibromatosis type 1 (NF1). J Med Genet 33: 2-17

[61] Shilyansky C, Karlsgodt KH, Cummings DM, Sidiropoulou K, Hardt M et al (2010a) Neurofibromin regulates corticostriatal inhibitory networks during working memory performance. Proc Natl Acad Sci USA 107: 13141-13146

[62] Shilyansky C, Lee YS, Silva AJ (2010b) Molecular and cellular mechanisms of learning disabilities: a focus on NF1. Annu Rev Neurosci 33: 221-243

[63] Silva AJ, Frankland PW, Marowitz Z, Friedman E, Laszlo GS et al (1997) A mouse model for the learning and memory deficits associated with neurofibromatosis type I. Nat Genet 15: 281-284

[64] Squire LR (1992) Memory and the hippocampus: a synthesis from findings with rats, monkeys, and humans. Psychol Rev 99: 195-231

[65] Sweatt JD (2001) The neuronal MAP kinase cascade: a biochemical signal integration system subserving synaptic plasticity and memory. J Neurochem 76: 1-10

[66] Tartaglia M, Gelb BD (2005) Noonan syndrome and related

disorders: genetics and pathogenesis. Annu Rev Genomics Hum Genet 6: 45-68

[67] Thomson SA, Fishbein L, Wallace MR (2002) NF1 mutations and molecular testing. J Child Neurol 17: 555-561 (discussion 71-72, 646-651)

[68] Tong J, Hannan F, Zhu Y, Bernards A, Zhong Y (2002) Neurofibromin regulates G proteinstimulated adenylyl cyclase activity. Nat Neurosci 5: 95-96

[69] van der Burgt I, Thoonen G, Roosenboom N, Assman-Hulsmans C, Gabreels F et al (1999) Patterns of cognitive functioning in school-aged children with Noonan syndrome associated with variability in phenotypic expression. J Pediatr 135: 707-713

[70] Verhoeven W, Wingbermuhle E, Egger J, Van der Burgt I, Tuinier S (2008) Noonan syndrome: psychological and psychiatric aspects. Am J Med Genet 146A: 191-196

[71] Viosca J, Schuhmacher AJ, Guerra C, Barco A (2009) Germline expression of H-Ras (G12V) causes neurological deficits associated to Costello syndrome. Genes Brain Behav 8: 60-71

[72] Weiss B, Bollag G, Shannon K (1999) Hyperactive Ras as a therapeutic target in neurofibromatosis type 1. Am J Med Genet 89: 14-22

[73] Whitlock JR, Heynen AJ, Shuler MG, Bear MF (2006) Learning induces long-term potentiation in the hippocampus. Science 313: 1093-1097

[74] Wieczorek D, Majewski F, Gillessen-Kaesbach G (1997) Cardio-facio-cutaneous (CFC) syndrome—a distinct entity? Report of three patients demonstrating the diagnostic difficulties in delineation of CFC syndrome. Clin Genet 52: 37-46

[75] Wingbermuehle E, Egger J, van der Burgt I, Verhoeven W (2009) Neuropsychological and behavioral aspects of Noonan syndrome. Horm Res 72(Suppl 2): 15-23

[76] Wingbermuhle E, Egger JI, Verhoeven WM, van der Burgt I, Kessels RP (2011) Affective functioning and social cognition in Noonan syndrome. Psychol Med 11: 1-8

[77] Wu X, Simpson J, Hong JH, Kim KH, Thavarajah NK et al (2011) MEK-ERK pathway modulation ameliorates disease phenotypes in a mouse model of Noonan syndrome associated with the Raf1(L613V) mutation. J Clin Invest 121: 1009-1025

[78] Zenker M (2011) Clinical manifestations of mutations in RAS and related intracellular signal transduction factors. Curr Opin Pediatr 23: 443-451

[79] Zenker M, Buheitel G, Rauch R, Koenig R, Bosse K et al (2004) Genotype-phenotype correlations in Noonan syndrome. J Pediatr 144: 368-374

[80] Zhu Y, Romero MI, Ghosh P, Ye Z, Charnay P et al (2001) Ablation of NF1 function in neurons induces abnormal development of cerebral cortex and reactive gliosis in the brain. Genes Dev 15: 859-876

第38章 恶性周围神经鞘膜瘤中 Ras 信号通路的生物学特点及相关疗法

Ras Signaling Pathway in Biology and Therapy of Malignant Peripheral Nerve Sheath Tumors

Faris Farassati

38.1 Ras 原癌基因及其信号通路的介绍

鸟嘌呤核苷酸结合蛋白（G 蛋白）的 Ras 家族在过去的 30 年里被认为是最重要的原癌基因家族，参与了超过 35% 的人类恶性肿瘤（Bollag et al. 2003；Campbell and Der 2004；Cox and Der 2002；Downward 2003；Jones et al. 2001）。虽然在一些人类癌症中已经发现了涉及 Ras 通路的基因突变（Bodemann and White 2008；Fernandez-Medarde and Santos 2011；Hamad et al. 2002；Lundquist 2006；van Dam and Robinson 2006；Yamamoto et al. 1999），但在没有基因改变的情况下，该通路中信号蛋白的过度激活可导致肿瘤进展（Bodempudi et al. 2009；De Luca et al. 2012）。Ras 蛋白的下游，一个扩展的激酶家族称为丝裂原活化蛋白激酶（mitogen-activated protein kinase，MAPK）（Buday and Downward 2008；Lawrence et al. 2008；Molina and Adjei 2006；Sundaram 2006）通过细胞质传递信号，导致细胞核中一系列转录因子的激活。在这种情况下，广泛的基因表达事件导致细胞生物学特性的剧烈变化（图 38.1）。Ras 激活导致不同的

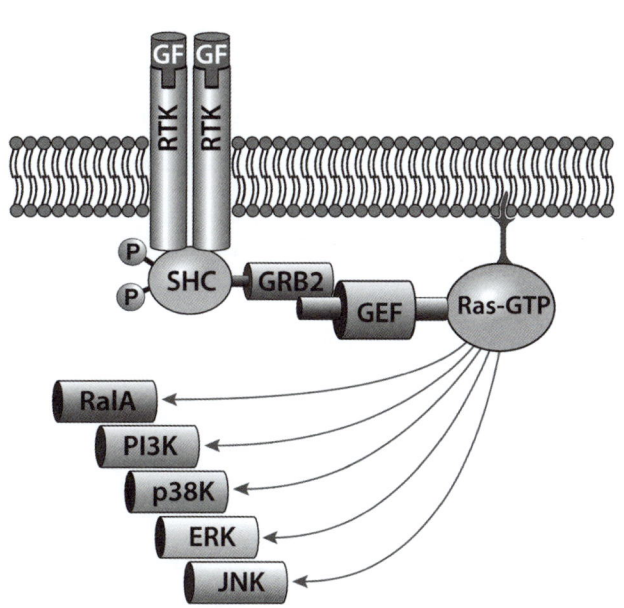

图 38.1 RTK 下游 Ras 的激活：受体酪氨酸激酶（RTK）的激活导致 GRB2 等接头蛋白的激活，从而激活 Ras-GEF，进一步导致 Ras 的激活。Ras 的激活反过来会导致许多效应通路的激活，如 ERK、JNK、p38 激酶、PI3K 和 RAL

MAPK 的激活，这些 MAPK 参与一系列细胞功能，如增殖、细胞周期进程、血管生成、细胞迁移和存活（Alvarado and Giles 2007；Chambard et al. 2007；McCubrey et al. 2007；Meloche and Pouyssegur

F. Farassati
Molecular Medicine Laboratory, Department of Medicine, The University of Kansas Medical School, Kansas City, KS, USA
e-mail: ffarassati@kumc.edu

2007；Murphy and Blenis 2006；Roberts and Der 2007；Shelton et al. 2003；Sundaram 2006；Zebisch et al. 2007）。Ras/MAPK 机制通过激活一系列不同的质膜受体，如酪氨酸激酶受体（RTK）（Daub et al. 1997）或 G 蛋白偶联受体（GPCRs）（Chiariello et al. 2010；Daub et al. 1996）对外部刺激做出反应。此外，物理信号，如紫外线（UV）也可以诱导 Ras 下游效应因子，如 p38 激酶途径（Muthusamy and Piva 2010）（图 38.2）。Ras 下游的主要效应信号通路包括细胞外信号相关激酶（extracellular signal-related kinase，ERK）（Brannan et al. 1994）、Jun 氨基末端激酶（Jun amino-terminal kinase，JNK）、p38 激酶和磷脂酰肌醇 3-激酶（p38 kinase，and phosphatidylinositol 3-kinase，PI3K）、Ral 蛋白（Ras like，Ral）（Downward 2003；Giehl 2005；Goldfinger 2008；Harrisingh and Lloyd 2004；Harrisingh et al. 2004；Rajalingam et al. 2007）和磷酸酯酶 Ce（phospholipase-C epsilon，PLCe）（Gresset et al. 2012；Song et al. 2001）（图 38.3）。这些效应因子通路的激活导致一系列转录因子的诱导，如 FOS、ELK、JUN、STAT、ATF2、CREB、SP1 和 MYC（Esfandyari et al. 2009；Hazzalin and Mahadevan 2002；Keren et al. 2006；O'Donnell et al. 2012；Plotnikov et al. 2011；Terada et al. 1999），启动了广泛的基因表达活性（图 38.2）。例如，Ras/Raf/ERK1/2 通路导致丝氨酸/苏氨酸激酶 ERK1/2 磷酸化（在其他底物中）核转录因子 ELK（Davis 1995；Kyosseva 2004）。磷酸化的 ELK 与血清反应因子（SRF）协同，与 c-fos 启动子中被称为血清反应元件（SRE）的特定结合元件结合，从而诱导许多参与增殖和分化等重要细胞功能的基因的转录（Cruzalegui et al. 1999；Whitmarsh et al. 1995）（图 38.4）。

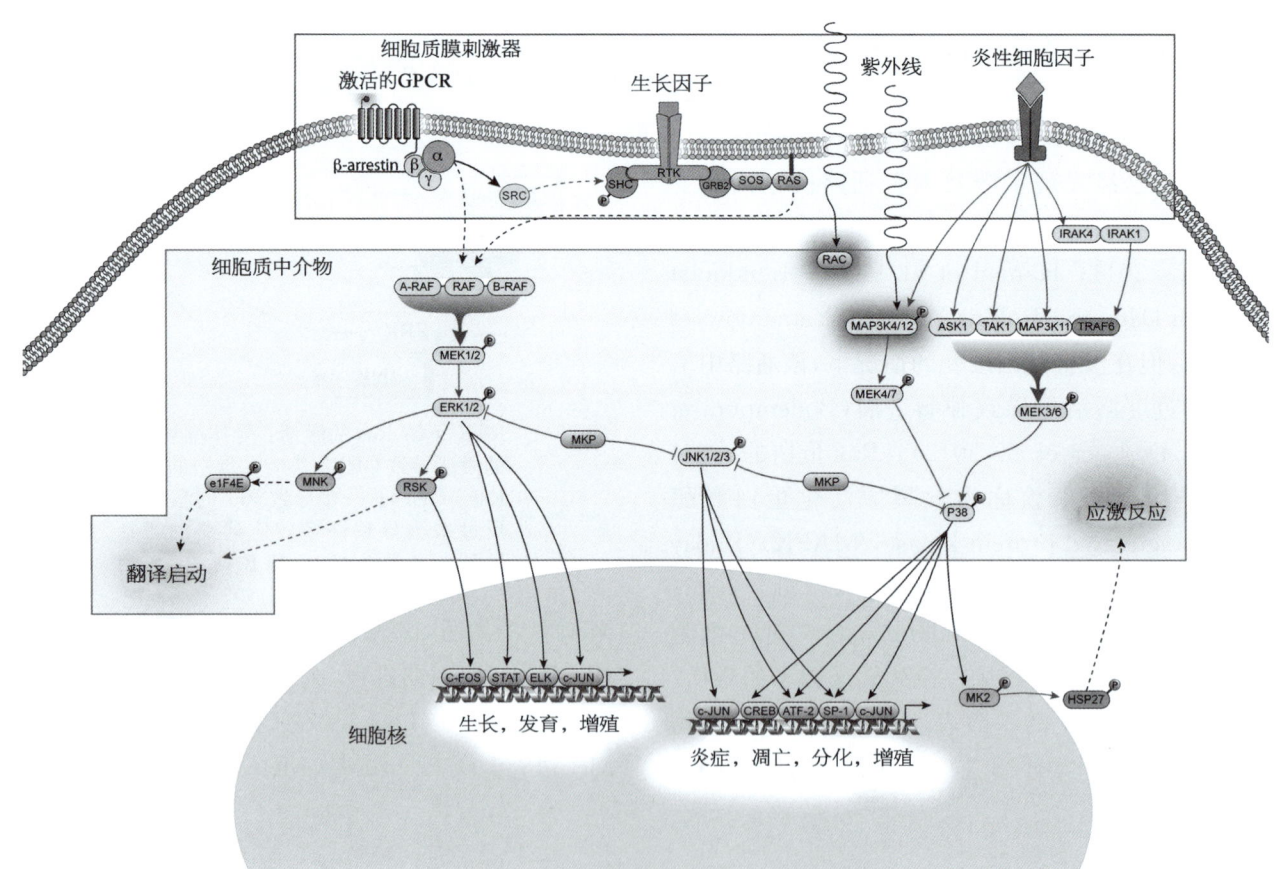

图 38.2 Ras 信号通路：从细胞膜到细胞核的信息流：在细胞膜水平上，不同的受体，如 G 蛋白偶联受体（GPCR）、受体酪氨酸激酶（RTK）和炎症因子受体可以刺激 Ras 信号通路的激活。在细胞质水平上，一系列的细胞质介质将信号转移到细胞核。许多转录因子的激活会影响细胞的生理环境。虽然 Ras 下游有许多通路被激活，但该图主要描述了参与 Ras 信号通路三个模块（质膜起诱导作用的受体、细胞质的中间介导者和核转录因子）的一些信号分子

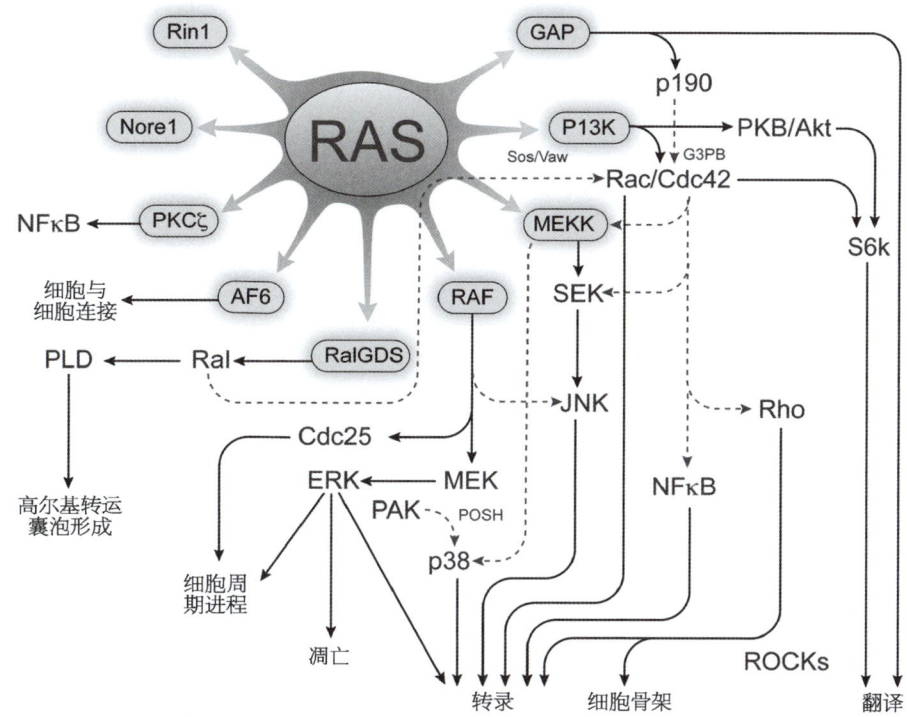

图 38.3 Ras 效应伙伴：Ras 下游被诱导，影响细胞生物学的不同方面。由于对细胞调控的广泛参与，癌症中 Ras 信号通路的下调是肿瘤产生恶性表型的重要一环

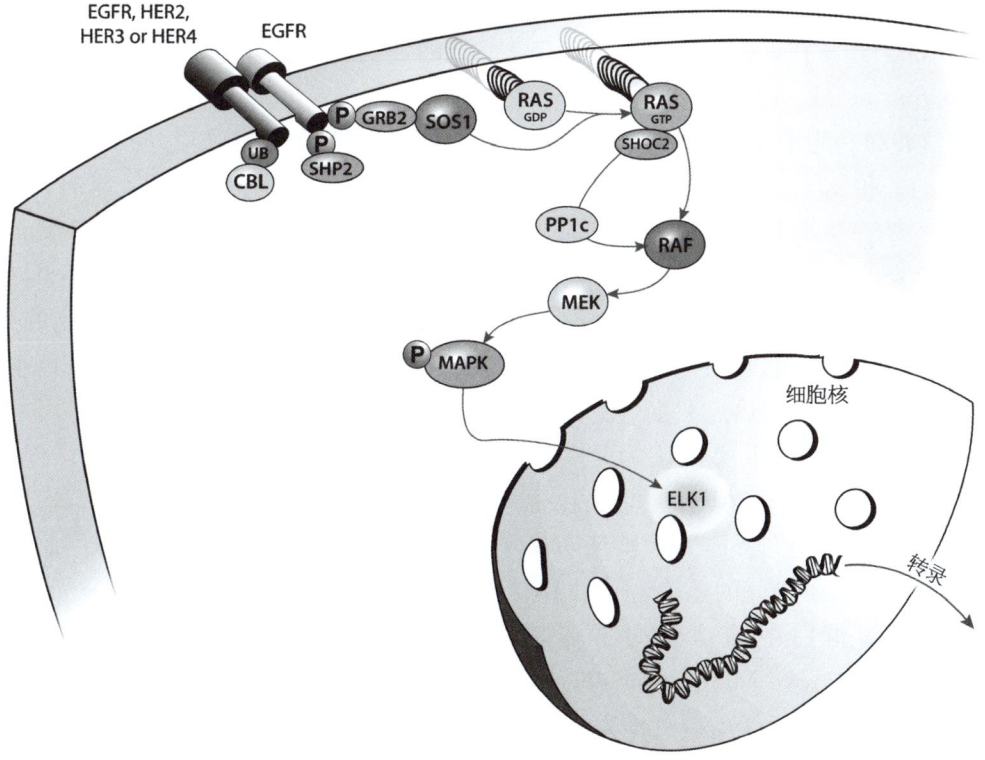

图 38.4 Ras/ERK 信号通路诱导转录事件：一个经典的 Ras 下游效应分子，Ras/Raf/ERK 通路的过度激活，已被证明参与了许多癌症，并导致转录因子 ELK 的激活

38.2 神经纤维瘤病、MPNST 和 Ras 信号通路

在家族性癌症易感综合征中,1型神经纤维瘤病(NF1)以 1∶3 000～1∶2 500 的出生发病率排名第一(Cawthon et al. 1991)。NF1 是一种常染色体显性遗传性疾病,恶性肿瘤发生率较高(Sorensen et al. 1986;Zoller et al. 1995)。NF1 患者的一个特征是不同恶性肿瘤的发病率增加,如恶性周围神经鞘膜瘤(malignant peripheral nerve sheath tumor, MPNST)、星形细胞瘤、嗜铬细胞瘤和儿童慢性髓系白血病(Shannon et al. 1994)。

良性神经纤维瘤恶性转化为 MPNST 的分子事件尚不完全清楚。这些肿瘤由紧密排列的深色梭形细胞组成,有丝分裂比例升高,经常发生在 30～60 岁之间(Laycock-van Spyk et al. 2011;Parrinello and Lloyd 2009)。1 型神经纤维瘤病基因(NF1)的两个等位基因的失活已在人类良性神经纤维瘤中被证实,并在小鼠模型中被证明会导致肿瘤(Serra et al. 1997)。NF1 和 P53 的杂合性缺失(loss of heterozygosity, LOH)经常在人类 MPNST 的病例中被观察到(Legius et al. 1994;Menon et al. 1990;Rey et al. 1992)。为了证实这一点,研究者利用携带失活的 nf1 和 p53 等位基因的转基因小鼠($cis-nf1^{+/-};p53^{+/-}$),证明了 nf1 和 p53 基因同时缺失在 MPNST 病因学中的累积效应(Cichowski et al. 1999;Vogel et al. 1999)。

NF1 是一个非常大的基因,具有一系列已确定的突变类型,但没有发现特定的热点突变(Li et al. 1995)。虽然神经纤维瘤蛋白主要被认为是一种 Ras-GTPase 激活蛋白(Ras-GAP),但它也包含一个 SEC14 结合域。虽然酵母 SEC14p 被证明参与调节细胞内蛋白质和脂质成分的运输,但其同源结构域在神经纤维瘤蛋白中的功能尚不清楚(Mousley et al. 2006;Trovo-Marqui and Tajara 2006)。我们最近提供了神经纤维瘤蛋白作为 RalA 的失活剂的新作用的证据(Bodempudi et al. 2009)。Ras 的激活状态是 Ras 鸟嘌呤核苷酸交换因子(Ras guanine nucleotide exchange factor, Ras-GEF)之间的平衡功能,Ras 通过将 Ras 转化为其 GTP 结合体(活性形式)和 Ras-GAP(如神经纤维瘤蛋白)来激活 Ras。这个过程会诱导 Ras-GTP 水解回 Ras-GDP(非活性形式)(Bos 1997;Cichowski and Jacks 2001;Vigil et al. 2010)。因此,我们假设 NF1 的主要分子信号异常导致神经纤维瘤蛋白的功能丧失(Harrisingh and Lloyd 2004;Katz et al. 2009)。在 MPNST 的病例中,通过研究来自 MPNST 患者的细胞证明了这一点,这些细胞显示缺乏神经纤维瘤蛋白表达和 Ras-GTP 水平升高(Basu et al. 1992;DeClue et al. 1992)。在此基础上,人们继续努力使用一系列 Ras 途径阻断剂,包括法炔基转移酶抑制剂(farnesyl transferase inhibitor, FTI),将抑制 Ras 途径作为 MPNST 的治疗策略(Wojtkowiak et al. 2008;Yan et al. 1995)。

38.3 MPNST 中 MAPK 信号通路的生物学特点及相关疗法

一系列的研究都集中在研究 MAPK 通路的激活及其靶向 MPNST 细胞的转化潜力上。例如,最近的一项研究表明,神经纤维瘤蛋白缺陷的 MPNST 细胞当暴露于 FTS(s-反式-法氨基硫代水杨酸)与 TGF-b 和骨形态发生蛋白(bone morphogenetic protein, BMP)的特定抑制剂时,发生表型逆转(Barkan et al. 2011)。另外,Ras/Raf/ERK 通路阻断剂索拉非尼特异性作用于 B-Raf,抑制磷酸化的 MEK 和 ERK,导致 MPNST 细胞的细胞周期受阻(Ambrosini et al. 2008)。在 MEK 水平的 ERK 通路抑制剂也被发现可以诱导三种不同的恶性神经鞘瘤和 MPNST 细胞的选择性凋亡(Mattingly et al. 2006)。此外,转录因子 AP1 是 ERK 和 JNK 通路的下游效应因子,它与人类 MPNST 细胞中的神经纤维瘤蛋白缺陷直接相关(Kraniak et al. 2010)。我们的团队广泛研究了小鼠和人类来源的 MPNST 细胞中 Ras 的激活模式及其下游通路(Farassati et al. 2008;Mashour et al. 2005;Yamoutpour et al. 2008)。从小鼠品系中获得了不同的 MPNST 细胞,这些品系含有失活的 nf1 和 p53 等位基因(Cichowski et al. 1999;Vogel et al. 1999)。从 Ras 通路信号转导的

角度来看,这些细胞可以分为两类(Farassati et al. 2008):一类是 Ras 激活增强,导致 MAPK 信号通路激活升高如 ERK、JNK、p38 激酶和 PI3K 通路,第二类是通路包含与非恶性施万细胞相同水平的 Ras 信号活性(Farassati et al. 2008)。有趣的是,这些细胞中 Ras 信号通路的激活增加导致对溶瘤单纯疱疹病毒突变体 G207 的接受增强(Farassati et al. 2008)。这与我们之前关于 Ras 转化对病毒耐受性影响的研究一致(Farassati and Lee 2003;Farassati et al. 2001;Norman et al. 2001)。然而,一项独立的研究声称,在人类 MPNST 细胞中没有观察到这种关系(Mahller et al. 2006)。但是,从 Ras 信号的角度和影响 Ras 激活的遗传背景来看,这项研究中的细胞并没有充分地被表征出来。

38.4 RalA 信号通路和 MPNST:一个治疗开发的新平台

Ral 鸟嘌呤核苷酸交换因子(Ral guanine nucleotide exchange factor,Ral‐GEF)将激活信号从 Ras 传递到 Ral,使 Ral 通路成为 Ras 的下游效应物(图 38.5)(Bodemann and White 2008;Neel et al. 2011)。Ral‐GEF 由两组不同的蛋白质组成:由于其羧基末端 Ras 结合域(RalGDS,RGL1,RGL2)而被 Ras 激活的蛋白质,以及另一种,主要通过 C 端 plecstrin 同源(PH)结构域(RALGPS1,PALGPS2)被 PI3K 底物激活的蛋白质(Feig 2003)。Ral 蛋白(RalA 和 RalB)通过明显不同的效应因子发出信号,通过与 ZO1 相关的核酸结合蛋白(ZO‐1 associated nucleic acid binding protein,ZONAB)和 RalA 结合蛋白 1(RalA binding protein 1,RalBP1)的相互作用来影响基因的表达和翻译(Cantor et al. 1995;Frankel et al. 2005;Jullien-Flores et al. 1995)。RalA 被 Aurora 激酶 A(Aurora kinase A,AKA)磷酸化/激活(Bodemann and White 2008)。RalB 直接与外囊体的 SEC5 亚基相互作用,以促进宿主的防御反应(Moskalenko et al. 2002;Sugihara et al. 2002)。RalBP1 虽然是促癌信号通路的汇聚点,但它作为 CDC42/Rac‐ GTPase 激活蛋白发挥作用连接 Ral 和 Rho(Jullien-Flores et al. 1995)。由于神经纤维瘤蛋白的 Ras‐GAP 功能在这些 MPNST 细胞系中丢失,所以值得注意的是,只有一小部分 MPNST 细胞显示 Ras 水平升高,而 RalA 在所有 MPNST 细胞系中仍然过度活跃(图 38.6)。在我们的研究中发现,RalA 通路在其他神经系统恶性肿瘤中,如胶质瘤和髓母细胞瘤中也被过度激活(数据未显示)。

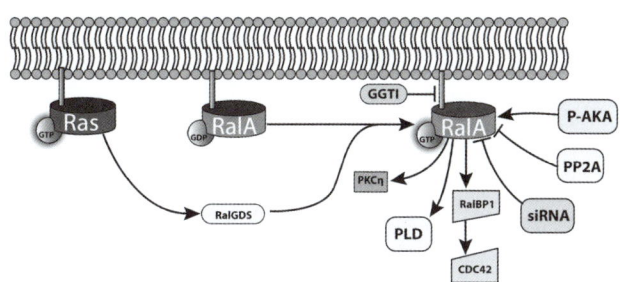

图 38.5 　 RalA 信号通路:Ras 的激活通过 RalGDS 蛋白的介导导致 RalA 的激活。下一步,RalA 的激活会触发一些促肿瘤的下游效应因子,如 PLD、RalBP1 和 PKC。虽然 P‐AKA 激活 RalA,但这个小 GTP 蛋白可以被 PP2A、GGTI 或抑制 siRNA 抑制

38.5 在 MPNST 细胞中沉默 RalA 的生物学结局

38.5.1 存活和侵袭性降低

考虑到缺乏针对 Ral 的特异性抑制剂,我们利用基因特异性沉默来评估抑制 RalA 对 MPNST 细胞恶性表型的影响(Bodempudi et al. 2009)。用沉默 Ral 的 siRNA 处理 MPNST 小鼠细胞可显著降低这些细胞的增殖和侵袭性。在这种情况下,一系列 EMT 标志物的表达发生了改变。

38.5.2 "钙黏蛋白开关"的反转

在获得侵袭性表型的过程中,一个重要的步骤是"Eton‐钙黏蛋白开关",其中抗侵袭性钙黏蛋白(e‐钙黏蛋白)减少,而促侵袭性钙黏蛋白(n‐钙黏蛋白)增加。这一过程也会受到 RalA 沉默的影响,导致 n‐钙黏蛋白水平显著降低,而 e‐钙黏蛋白水平没有明显改变,有效地逆转 Eton‐钙黏蛋白开关。

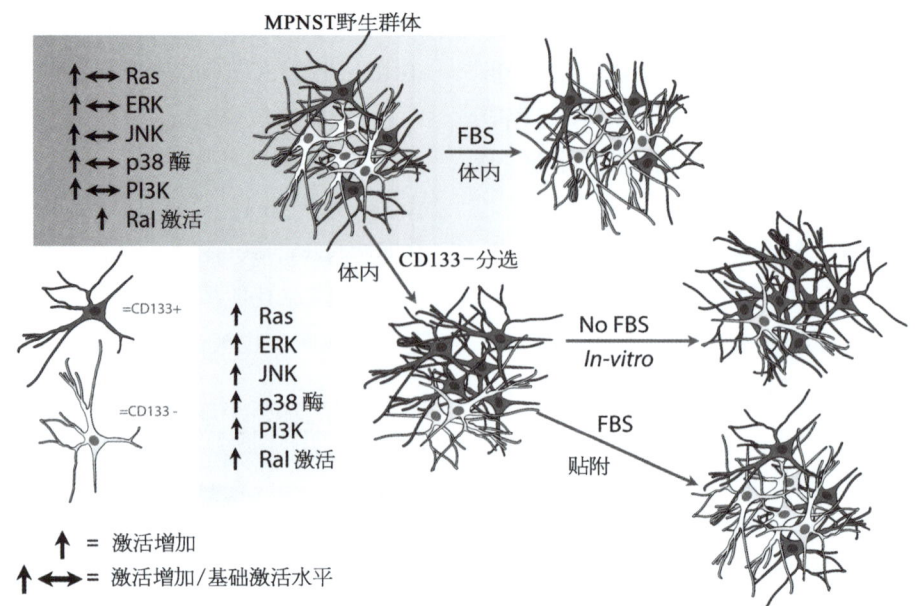

图 38.6 分化的和来自 MPNST 来源的 CSC 中的 Ras 信号通路：当研究野生型（未分类的）人类 MPNST 细胞群体时，与非恶性的施万细胞相比，Ras 信号通路及其下游效应物的水平可能会增加或处于基础水平。然而，RalA 似乎是一种豁免，因为它被发现持续激活。一旦这些群体富集了 CD133（作为 CSC 的标志物），Ras 及其下游的效应物与其他未分类的群体相比是显著的过度激活的

38.5.3 体内致瘤性的丧失

RalA-siRNA 通过电穿孔转染到 MPNST 细胞并注射到严重联合免疫缺陷（severe combined immunodeficient，SCID）小鼠皮下，观察到肿瘤的生长明显迟缓，其体积减小。与对照组 siRNA 治疗的肿瘤相比，经过治疗的肿瘤提取到的 RalA-GTP 显示水平降低（Bodempudi et al. 2009）。

38.6 用其他方法抑制 RalA 的激活

在我们的研究中，我们采用了另外两种方法来抑制 RalA 的激活。首先，我们使用 RalA 的显性阴性版本（S28N）来抑制 RalA 的激活。S28N 的瞬时表达显著降低了人 MPNST 细胞中 RalA-GTP 水平、活力和侵袭性。我们还很感兴趣的是，抑制香叶基-香叶基化（一种 RalA 激活所必需的翻译后修饰）是否会影响 MPNST 细胞的增殖。这是通过使用香叶基-香叶基转移酶抑制剂 2147（GGTI-2147）完成的，这是一种细胞渗透的非硫醇拟肽，作为香叶基-香叶基转移酶 I（geranyl-geranyl transferase I, GGTase I）的有效选择性抑制剂（Bernot et al. 2003；Vasudevan et al. 1999）。鉴于香叶基化也会影响包括 Ras 在内的其他蛋白质，我们使用 250 nM 浓度的 GGTI-2147 来减少对 Ras 的抑制作用。在此浓度下，观察到 RalA 活性和活力的丧失。

38.7 神经纤维瘤蛋白 gap 相关结构域（NF1-GRD）的表达降低了 RalA 的激活

为了研究 RalA 激活的潜在机制，我们在人 MPNST 细胞系中表达了 NF1-GRD，并评估了这种对 RalA-GTP 的调控结果，以及这些细胞的活力和侵袭性。虽然 RalA-GTP 水平降低，但这种处理导致了 MPNST 细胞的活力和侵袭性的丧失。这被认为是神经纤维瘤蛋白作为 RalA-GAP 蛋白的潜在作用的证据（Bodempudi et al. 2009）。然而，神经纤维瘤蛋白的这种作用有待进一步的研究证实。在人 MPNST 细胞中招募 NF1-GRD 表达的其他影响包括细胞周期 G1 期细胞比例的减少，G2/S 细胞比例的增加，以及这些细胞的凋亡亚群比

例的升高。这些变化显示通过 NF1-GRD 的表达所实现的 RalA 激活的减少带来的整体生长抑制结果。

38.8 MPNST 癌症干细胞中的 Ras 信号通路

根据新的理论，每个肿瘤中的一小部分细胞通过作为癌症干细胞（CSC）来再生肿瘤组织。CSC 的理论最初是在 19 世纪发展起来的（Reya et al. 2001）。然而，研究这些细胞的工具在大约 10 年前才出现（Bignold et al. 2006）。本质上，这一理论提出了肿瘤中存在一个具有多能能力的细胞亚群，即在肿瘤中产生所有类型的细胞（Akhtar et al. 2009；Costa et al. 2007；D'Amour and Gage 2002；Meeker and Coffey 1997；Mimeault and Batra 2006；Pan and Huang 2008；Rudland et al. 1980；Sagar et al. 2007；Singh et al. 2004；Spillane and Henderson 2007；Trosko 2009）。CSC 被认为对目前的抗肿瘤方式具有耐药性（Polyak and Hahn 2006；Singh et al. 2004），因此，迫切需要从生物学和细胞信号转导的角度来描述 CSC，以找到有效的靶点。

38.9 CSC 标志物

一系列的细胞表面标志物被认为反映了 CSC 的不成熟性和干细胞性。这些标志物也可能在正常组织中发现，通常表达水平较低，组织学模式更有限。

某些标志物，如 CD133（也称为突起蛋白 1）（Corbeil et al. 2001a，b；Mehra et al. 2006；Miraglia et al. 1997），被广泛认为是 CSC 的指示性指标；然而，这些细胞的详细生物学特征，包括它们的细胞信号谱仍未被大量研究。在此基础上，我们试图研究 CSC 在原代 MPNST 细胞中的存在，并评估其促癌细胞信号转导的特征。我们使用非恶性的人类施万细胞（human Schwann cell，HSC）作为这些细胞的健康对照进行分析。CD133 由于其在包括多种肿瘤类型的 CSC 中高表达，受到了相当程度的关注（Corbeil et al. 2001a、b；Mehra et al. 2006；Miraglia et al. 1997），包括髓母细胞瘤（Singh et al. 2004）、胶质母细胞瘤（Salmaggi et al. 2006）、黑色素瘤（Monzani et al. 2007）、结直肠癌（O'Brien et al. 2007）和前列腺癌（Collins et al. 2005）。虽然 CD133 的功能尚不清楚，但已有人提出，编码 Notch 和 Hedgehog/Gli 信号通路的基因在 CD133$^+$ 胶质瘤细胞中过表达（Clement et al. 2007；Hambardzumyan et al. 2006；Neuzil et al. 2007）。也有报道称，高水平的 CD133 表达与 CSC 对细胞凋亡的抵抗有关（Bao et al. 2006；Frank et al. 2005；Hambardzumyan et al. 2006）。

38.10 MPNST 细胞和肿瘤组织表达 CSC 标志物

我们报道了 5 种不同的人 MPNST 细胞系（S805、94.3 和 S462、T530 和 T532）中大量 CSC 标志物的表达，包括 CD24、CD34、CD44、CD90、CD133 和 EpCAM。在这些标志物中，CD24、CD44 和 CD90 似乎在 MPNST 和 HSC 中均有表达，而 CD133 和 CD34 似乎在 MPNST 细胞中优先表达。此外，人类 MPNST 组织，以及从 MPNST 小鼠模型中获得的细胞（Vogel et al. 1999）也发现 CD133 阳性。

38.11 CD133$^+$ MPNST 细胞

我们的团队（Borrego-Diaz et al. 2012）以及其他团队（Spyra et al. 2011）已经研究了 CD133$^+$ MPNST 细胞在赋予多潜能特性方面的功能。在我们的研究中，与野生型（未分选）的 MPNST 细胞相比，CD133$^+$ MPNST 细胞在低附着条件下形成了更多的细胞球。此外，以这种方式形成的细胞球 CD133 高表达，一旦在正常条件下培养，就能够产生 CD133 阴性细胞。Demestre 等的研究也证明了这些细胞在体内致瘤的能力增强是其干细胞性的一个标志（Spyra et al. 2011）。在本研究中，从人 MPNST 细胞系中建立的克隆细胞球的干细胞标志物 CD133、Oct4（八聚体结合转录因子 4）、巢蛋白和 NGFR（神经生长因子受体）的表达增加，成熟标志物 CD90 和 NCAM（神经细胞黏附分子）的表达降低。

38.12 CD133⁺ MPNST CSC 中的 Ras 信号通路

通过结合磁性细胞分选富集 CD133⁺ MPNST 细胞，我们评估了分选的和野生的 MPNST 细胞群体中 Ras 信号通路的激活情况。CD133⁺ 组分的三倍富集（45% CD133⁺）不仅显著增加了 Ras-gtp（活性 Ras）的水平，而且还显著提高了 Ras 下游效应物如 ERK、JNK、PI3K、p38 激酶和 RalA 的激活水平，这是通过体外激酶和亲和沉淀测定的（图 38.6）（Borrego-Diaz et al. 2012）。这一观察结果特别重要，因为它解释了靶向 MPNST CSC 策略的关键特征。假设这些细胞对 Ras 通路的药理抑制产生更高的耐药性。为了证明这一点，我们将 CD133 富集和野生型 MPNST 细胞暴露于 ERK 通路抑制剂中，并测量了暴露后 36 小时的细胞活力。CSC 富集的群体受到这种治疗的影响较小，这意味着他们的耐药性增加（Borrego-Diaz et al. 2012）。总之，我们建议也应该对 CSC 富集群体进行 MPNST 细胞对不同治疗药物的敏感性的研究，以找到一个能够有效靶向这一部分群体的最佳方案。

38.13 CD133⁺ MPNST CSC 的其他生物学和信号传导特征

38.13.1 侵袭性增加

通过体外实验，CD133⁺ MPNST CSC 表现出显著的侵袭性水平升高（$P<0.05$），同时 b-连环蛋白、snail 蛋白和桩蛋白的表达增加。注意 snail 蛋白对 e-钙黏蛋白的抑制作用（Cano et al. 2000），我们预计 CD133⁺ 细胞能表达较低水平的这种抗侵袭蛋白。此外，b-连环蛋白水平的增加，可能是 MPNST 中异常信号转导的直接结果，或者是 e-钙黏蛋白减少的产物（Kato et al. 2007），可导致 EMT 的进展和基质金属蛋白酶（如基质金属蛋白酶 7 或 MM7）的表达增强，作为增强转移能力的基础（McGuire et al. 2003；Zheng et al. 2009）。所观察到的 EMT 侵袭性表型和分子标志物的增强反映了 CD133⁺ 细胞可能成为 MPNST 转移灶建立的必要组成部分。通过研究来自转移灶获得的组织的 CD133⁺ 细胞，或像探索其他模型那样探索 CD133⁺ 循环 CSC 的存在性和生物学行为，可以进一步研究这些可能性（Maheswaran and Haber 2010；Monteiro and Fodde 2010）。

38.13.2 CD133⁺ MPNST CSC 细胞中的内质网应激标志物

未折叠蛋白的积累诱导了一种反应，称为 UPR（未折叠蛋白反应），这在所有哺乳动物物种以及酵母和线虫蠕虫之间都很常见（Hetz 2012）。UPR 是一种应激反应，随着内质网（endoplasmic reticulum, ER）腔内未折叠或错误折叠蛋白的积累而被激活（Parmar and Schroder 2012）。为了纠正这种情况，UPR 启动了减少蛋白质翻译以及增加可诱导蛋白质折叠的伴侣蛋白的机制。UPR 反应的第三种也是最后一种方法是在上述措施失败后诱导细胞凋亡（Treglia et al. 2012）。

参与内质网应激信号转导的蛋白包括内质网膜和钙伏结合蛋白，钙连接蛋白（Bergeron et al. 1994），它将新合成的糖蛋白保留在内质网内进行适当的折叠；分子伴侣蛋白（BIP），它通过与未展开的蛋白质结合来抑制聚集物的形成（Kohno et al. 1993）；蛋白质二硫异构酶（PDI），它催化二硫键的形成和异构化（Ellgaard and Ruddock 2005）；内质网膜相关的 n-糖蛋白，Ero1-La，它协助氧化蛋白折叠（Cabibbo et al. 2000）；蛋白激酶/核糖核酸内切酶，IRE 1a，它控制着未折叠蛋白的反应，以中和蛋白质的错误折叠（Cox et al. 1993）；以及跨膜蛋白 PERK，它将内质网应激信号与蛋白质翻译的抑制结合起来（Harding et al. 1999；Kigawa et al. 1998）。而这些标记在 CD133 富集群体和野生群体之间没有变化（Borrego-Diaz et al. 2012），CD133⁺ 群体中 IRE1a 降低。这可能导致 CD133⁺ 细胞对错误折叠蛋白的积累敏感，从而对针对内质网应激通路的药物产生潜在的治疗影响。

38.13.3 CD133$^+$ MPNST CSC 中的细胞凋亡调节因子

细胞的凋亡能力是由一系列促凋亡蛋白如 Bcl-2(B 细胞淋巴瘤 2)和抗凋亡蛋白如 Bad(bcl-2 相关死亡启动子)控制的(Munoz-Pinedo 2012)。对这两个重要的凋亡调节因子的表达水平的评估并没有发现任何 CD133 富集和野生型细胞群之间主要的差异(Borrego-Diaz et al. 2012),然而,需要进一步研究其他凋亡调节因子,以及测量其对促凋亡信号的生物学反应,以充分揭示 MPNST CSC 对促凋亡信号的程序性细胞死亡的特性。图 38.7 总结了 MPNST CD133$^+$ CSC 的生物学特征。

38.14 针对 MPNST 的溶瘤病毒

目前正在研究溶瘤病毒的使用(能够以特定方式靶向癌细胞的复制能力病毒)(Borrego-Diaz et al. 2011)作为不同群体靶向 MPNST 的可能性(Farassati et al. 2008;Liu et al. 2006a,b;Mahller et al. 2006,2007;Maldonado et al. 2010;Messerli et al. 2006;Prabhakar et al. 2010)。在 Ras 信号转导领域,我们已经证明了 Ras 的过度激活诱导了对溶瘤性疱疹病毒的接受性增强(Esfandyari et al. 2009;Farassati and Lee 2003;Farassati et al. 2001,2008)。此外,我们已经开发出了能够以特定方式靶向 Ras 信号通路和 CD133$^+$ 细胞的溶瘤病毒(Borrego-Diaz et al. 2011;Pan et al. 2009)。目前正在进行新的研究,以评估利用这些抗癌病毒靶向 MPNST 的可能性。

38.15 我们的结论和未来的发展方向

本章提供的信息回顾将 Ras 信号通路描述为研究 MPNST 的一个重要平台。简而言之:

• Ras 信号控制着 MPNST 来源的分化完成的细胞和干细胞的重要生物学特征。

• 与非恶性施万细胞相比,部分 MPNST 细胞中 Ras 的不同下游通路被过度激活。

• Ras 信号可作为 MPNST 细胞治疗的一个靶点。

• RalA 引导了一个重要的信号通路,包括在 MPNST 来源的分化细胞和肿瘤干细胞层面。

• 与分化的 MPNST 细胞相比,来自 MPNST 来源的 CD133$^+$ 细胞不仅表现出 CSC 特征,而且表现出更高水平的 Ras 信号激活。

未来的研究可以包括使用下游效应因子的特定抑制剂(包括 RalA 通路)来测试 Ras 信号通路抑制的结果,或使用可重复和不可重复的模型研究基因治疗策略。

致谢:这项工作是献给 Rivka Buchbinder 和她的父母的。我们要感谢 Sarah Ann Martin 提供的科学编辑服务,以及 Stanton Fernald 为本章提供的医学插图服务。

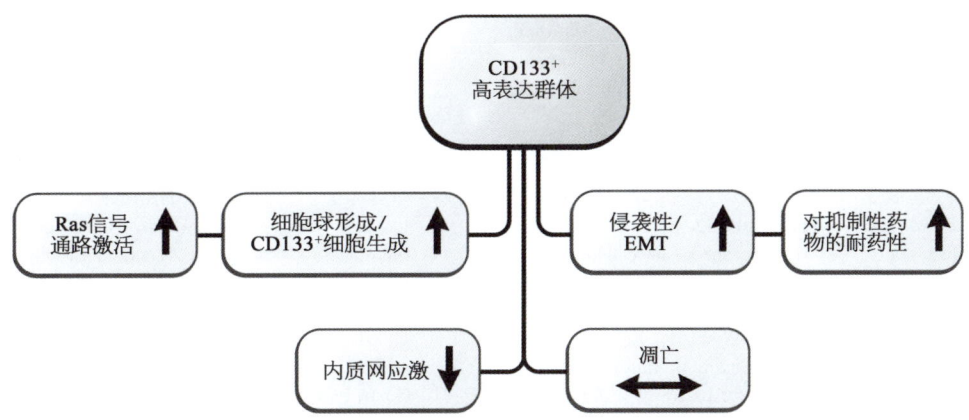

图 38.7 CD133$^+$ 人 MPNST 细胞的生物学特性:虽然 Ras 信号通路、细胞球形成、侵袭性和再生能力均得到增强,但应对内质网应激的能力可能会降低。重要的凋亡调节因子的表达保持不变

(吴浩,张雷 译)

参考文献

[1] Akhtar K, Bussen W, Scott SP (2009) Cancer stem cells—from initiation to elimination, how far have we reached? (Review). Int J Oncol 34(6): 1491-1503

[2] Alvarado Y, Giles FJ (2007) Ras as a therapeutic target in hematologic malignancies. Expert Opin Emerg Drugs 12(2): 271-284

[3] Ambrosini G, Cheema HS, Seelman S, Teed A, Sambol EB, Singer S, Schwartz GK (2008) Sorafenib inhibits growth and mitogen-activated protein kinase signaling in malignant peripheral nerve sheath cells. Mol Cancer Ther 7(4): 890-896

[4] Bao S, Wu Q, McLendon RE, Hao Y, Shi Q, Hjelmeland AB, Dewhirst MW, Bigner DD, Rich JN (2006) Glioma stem cells promote radioresistance by preferential activation of the DNA damage response. Nature 444(7120): 756-760

[5] Barkan B, Kloog Y, Ehrlich M (2011) Phenotypic reversion of invasive neurofibromin-deficient schwannoma by FTS: Ras inhibition reduces BMP4/Erk/Smad signaling. Mol Cancer Ther 10(8): 1317-1326

[6] Basu TN, Gutmann DH, Fletcher JA, Glover TW, Collins FS, Downward J (1992) Aberrant regulation of ras proteins in malignant tumour cells from type 1 neurofibromatosis patients. Nature 356(6371): 713-715

[7] Bergeron JJ, Brenner MB, Thomas DY, Williams DB (1994) Calnexin: a membrane-bound chaperone of the endoplasmic reticulum. Trends Biochem Sci 19(3): 124-128

[8] Bernot D, Benoliel AM, Peiretti F, Lopez S, Bonardo B, Bongrand P, Juhan-Vague I, Nalbone G (2003) Effect of atorvastatin on adhesive phenotype of human endothelial cells activated by tumor necrosis factor alpha. J Cardiovasc Pharmacol 41(2): 316-324

[9] Bignold LP, Coghlan BL, Jersmann HP (2006) Hansemann, Boveri, chromosomes and the gametogenesis-related theories of tumours. Cell Biol Int 30(7): 640-644

[10] Bodemann BO, White MA (2008) Ral GTPases and cancer: linchpin support of the tumorigenic platform. Nat Rev Cancer 8(2): 133-140

[11] Bodempudi V, Yamoutpoor F, Pan W, Dudek AZ, Esfandyari T, Piedra M, Babovick-Vuksanovic D, Woo RA, Mautner VF, Kluwe L et al (2009) Ral overactivation in malignant peripheral nerve sheath tumors. Mol Cell Biol 29(14): 3964-3974

[12] Bollag G, Freeman S, Lyons JF, Post LE (2003) Raf pathway inhibitors in oncology. Curr Opin Investig Drugs 4(12): 1436-1441

[13] Borrego-Diaz E, Mathew R, Hawkinson D, Esfandyari T, Liu Z, Lee PW, Farassati F (2011) Pro-oncogenic cell signaling machinery as a target for oncolytic viruses. Curr Pharm Biotechnol 13(9): 1742-1749

[14] Borrego-Diaz E, Terai K, Lialyte K, Wise AL, Esfandyari T, Behbod F, Mautner VF, Spyra M, Taylor S, Parada LF et al (2012) Overactivation of Ras signaling pathway in CD133+ MPNST cells. J Neurooncol 108(3): 423-434

[15] Bos JL (1997) Ras-like GTPases. Biochim Biophys Acta 1333(2): M19-M31

[16] Brannan CI, Perkins AS, Vogel KS, Ratner N, Nordlund ML, Reid SW, Buchberg AM, Jenkins NA, Parada LF, Copeland NG (1994) Targeted disruption of the neurofibromatosis type-1 gene leads to developmental abnormalities in heart and various neural crest-derived tissues. Genes Dev 8(9): 1019-1029

[17] Buday L, Downward J (2008) Many faces of Ras activation. Biochim Biophys Acta 1786(2): 178-187

[18] Cabibbo A, Pagani M, Fabbri M, Rocchi M, Farmery MR, Bulleid NJ, Sitia R (2000) ERO1-L, a human protein that favors disulfide bond formation in the endoplasmic reticulum. J Biol Chem 275(7): 4827-4833

[19] Campbell PM, Der CJ (2004) Oncogenic Ras and its role in tumor cell invasion and metastasis. Semin Cancer Biol 14(2): 105-114

[20] Cano A, Perez-Moreno MA, Rodrigo I, Locascio A, Blanco MJ, del Barrio MG, Portillo F, Nieto MA (2000) The transcription factor snail controls epithelial-mesenchymal transitions by repressing E-cadherin expression. Nat Cell Biol 2(2): 76-83

[21] Cantor SB, Urano T, Feig LA (1995) Identification and characterization of Ral-binding protein 1, a potential downstream target of Ral GTPases. Mol Cell Biol 15(8): 4578-4584

[22] Cawthon RM, Andersen LB, Buchberg AM, Xu GF, O'Connell P, Viskochil D, Weiss RB, Wallace MR, Marchuk DA, Culver M et al (1991) cDNA sequence and genomic structure of EV12B, a gene lying within an intron of the neurofibromatosis type 1 gene. Genomics 9(3): 446-460

[23] Chambard JC, Lefloch R, Pouyssegur J, Lenormand P (2007) ERK implication in cell cycle regulation. Biochim Biophys Acta 1773(8): 1299-1310

[24] Chiariello M, Vaque JP, Crespo P, Gutkind JS (2010) Activation of Ras and Rho GTPases and MAP Kinases by G-protein-coupled receptors. Methods Mol Biol 661: 137-150

[25] Cichowski K, Jacks T (2001) NF1 tumor suppressor gene function: narrowing the GAP. Cell 104(4): 593-604

[26] Cichowski K, Shih TS, Schmitt E, Santiago S, Reilly K, McLaughlin ME, Bronson RT, Jacks T (1999) Mouse models of tumor development in neurofibromatosis type 1. Science 286(5447): 2172-2176

[27] Clement V, Sanchez P, de Tribolet N, Radovanovic I, Ruiz i Altaba A (2007) HEDGEHOG-GLI1 signaling regulates human glioma growth, cancer stem cell self-renewal, and tumorigenicity. Curr Biol 17(2): 165-172

[28] Collins AT, Berry PA, Hyde C, Stower MJ, Maitland NJ (2005) Prospective identification of tumorigenic prostate cancer stem cells. Cancer Res 65(23): 10946-10951

[29] Corbeil D, Fargeas CA, Huttner WB (2001a) Rat prominin, like its mouse and human orthologues, is a pentaspan membrane glycoprotein. Biochem Biophys Res Commun 285(4): 939-944

[30] Corbeil D, Roper K, Fargeas CA, Joester A, Huttner WB (2001b) Prominin: a story of cholesterol, plasma membrane protrusions and human pathology. Traffic 2(2): 82-91

[31] Costa FF, Le Blanc K, Brodin B (2007) Concise review: cancer/testis antigens, stem cells, and cancer. Stem Cells 25(3): 707-711

[32] Cox AD, Der CJ (2002) Ras family signaling: therapeutic targeting. Cancer Biol Ther 1(6): 599-606

[33] Cox JS, Shamu CE, Walter P (1993) Transcriptional induction of genes encoding endoplasmic reticulum resident proteins requires a transmembrane protein kinase. Cell 73(6):

[34] Cruzalegui FH, Cano E, Treisman R (1999) ERK activation induces phosphorylation of Elk-1 at multiple S/T-P motifs to high stoichiometry. Oncogene 18(56): 7948-7957

[35] D'Amour KA, Gage FH (2002) Are somatic stem cells pluripotent or lineage-restricted? Nat Med 8(3): 213-214

[36] Daub H, Weiss FU, Wallasch C, Ullrich A (1996) Role of transactivation of the EGF receptor in signalling by G-protein-coupled receptors. Nature 379(6565): 557-560

[37] Daub H, Wallasch C, Lankenau A, Herrlich A, Ullrich A (1997) Signal characteristics of G protein-transactivated EGF receptor. EMBO J 16(23): 7032-7044

[38] Davis RJ (1995) Transcriptional regulation by MAP kinases. Mol Reprod Dev 42(4): 459-467

[39] De Luca A, Maiello MR, D'Alessio A, Pergameno M, Normanno N (2012) The RAS/RAF/MEK/ERK and the PI3K/AKT signalling pathways: role in cancer pathogenesis and implications for therapeutic approaches. Expert Opin Ther Targets 16(Suppl 2): S17-S27

[40] DeClue JE, Papageorge AG, Fletcher JA, Diehl SR, Ratner N, Vass WC, Lowy DR (1992) Abnormal regulation of mammalian p21ras contributes to malignant tumor growth in von Recklinghausen (type 1) neurofibromatosis. Cell 69(2): 265-273

[41] Downward J (2003) Targeting RAS signalling pathways in cancer therapy. Nat Rev Cancer 3(1): 11-22

[42] Ellgaard L, Ruddock LW (2005) The human protein disulphide isomerase family: substrate interactions and functional properties. EMBO Rep 6(1): 28-32

[43] Esfandyari T, Tefferi A, Szmidt A, Alain T, Zwolak P, Lasho T, Lee PW, Farassati F (2009) Transcription factors down-stream of Ras as molecular indicators for targeting malignancies with oncolytic herpes virus. Mol Oncol 3(5-6): 464-468

[44] Farassati F, Lee PW (2003) Ras signalling pathway: a gateway for HSV-1 infection. ScientificWorldJournal 3: 533-535

[45] Farassati F, Yang AD, Lee PW (2001) Oncogenes in Ras signalling pathway dictate host-cell permissiveness to herpes simplex virus 1. Nat Cell Biol 3(8): 745-750

[46] Farassati F, Pan W, Yamoutpour F, Henke S, Piedra M, Frahm S, Al-Tawil S, Mangrum WI, Parada LF, Rabkin SD et al (2008) Ras signaling influences permissiveness of malignant peripheral nerve sheath tumor cells to oncolytic herpes. Am J Pathol 173(6): 1861-1872

[47] Feig LA (2003) Ral-GTPases: approaching their 15 minutes of fame. Trends Cell Biol 13(8): 419-425

[48] Fernandez-Medarde A, Santos E (2011) Ras in cancer and developmental diseases. Genes Cancer 2(3): 344-358

[49] Frank NY, Margaryan A, Huang Y, Schatton T, Waaga-Gasser AM, Gasser M, Sayegh MH, Sadee W, Frank MH (2005) ABCB5-mediated doxorubicin transport and chemoresistance in human malignant melanoma. Cancer Res 65(10): 4320-4333

[50] Frankel P, Aronheim A, Kavanagh E, Balda MS, Matter K, Bunney TD, Marshall CJ (2005) RalA interacts with ZONAB in a cell density-dependent manner and regulates its transcriptional activity. EMBO J 24(1): 54-62

[51] Giehl K (2005) Oncogenic Ras in tumour progression and metastasis. Biol Chem 386(3): 193-205

[52] Goldfinger LE (2008) Choose your own path: specificity in Ras GTPase signaling. Mol Biosyst 4(4): 293-299

[53] Gresset A, Sondek J, Harden TK (2012) The phospholipase C isozymes and their regulation. Subcell Biochem 58: 61-94

[54] Hamad NM, Elconin JH, Karnoub AE, Bai W, Rich JN, Abraham RT, Der CJ, Counter CM (2002) Distinct requirements for Ras oncogenesis in human versus mouse cells. Genes Dev 16(16): 2045-2057

[55] Hambardzumyan D, Squatrito M, Holland EC (2006) Radiation resistance and stem-like cells in brain tumors. Cancer Cell 10(6): 454-456

[56] Harding HP, Zhang Y, Ron D (1999) Protein translation and folding are coupled by an endoplasmic-reticulum-resident kinase. Nature 397(6716): 271-274

[57] Harrisingh MC, Lloyd AC (2004) Ras/Raf/ERK signalling and NF1. Cell Cycle 3(10): 1255-1258

[58] Harrisingh MC, Perez-Nadales E, Parkinson DB, Malcolm DS, Mudge AW, Lloyd AC (2004) The Ras/Raf/ERK signalling pathway drives Schwann cell dedifferentiation. EMBO J 23(15): 3061-3071

[59] Hazzalin CA, Mahadevan LC (2002) MAPK-regulated transcription: a continuously variable gene switch? Nat Rev Mol Cell Biol 3(1): 30-40

[60] Hetz C (2012) The unfolded protein response: controlling cell fate decisions under ER stress and beyond. Nat Rev Mol Cell Biol 13(2): 89-102

[61] Jones HA, Hahn SM, Bernhard E, McKenna WG (2001) Ras inhibitors and radiation therapy. Semin Radiat Oncol 11(4): 328-337

[62] Jullien-Flores V, Dorseuil O, Romero F, Letourneur F, Saragosti S, Berger R, Tavitian A, Gacon G, Camonis JH (1995) Bridging Ral GTPase to Rho pathways. RLIP76, a Ral effector with CDC42/Rac GTPase-activating protein activity. J Biol Chem 270(38): 22473-22477

[63] Kato N, Shimmura S, Kawakita T, Miyashita H, Ogawa Y, Yoshida S, Higa K, Okano H, Tsubota K (2007) Beta-catenin activation and epithelial-mesenchymal transition in the pathogenesis of pterygium. Invest Ophthalmol Vis Sci 48(4): 1511-1517

[64] Katz D, Lazar A, Lev D (2009) Malignant peripheral nerve sheath tumour (MPNST): the clinical implications of cellular signalling pathways. Expert Rev Mol Med 11: e30

[65] Keren A, Tamir Y, Bengal E (2006) The p38 MAPK signaling pathway: a major regulator of skeletal muscle development. Mol Cell Endocrinol 252(1-2): 224-230

[66] Kigawa T, Endo M, Ito Y, Shirouzu M, Kikuchi A, Yokoyama S (1998) Solution structure of the Ras-binding domain of RGL. FEBS Lett 441(3): 413-418

[67] Kohno K, Normington K, Sambrook J, Gething MJ, Mori K (1993) The promoter region of the yeast KAR2 (BiP) gene contains a regulatory domain that responds to the presence of unfolded proteins in the endoplasmic reticulum. Mol Cell Biol 13(2): 877-890

[68] Kraniak JM, Sun D, Mattingly RR, Reiners JJ Jr, Tainsky MA (2010) The role of neurofibromin in N-Ras mediated AP-1 regulation in malignant peripheral nerve sheath tumors. Mol Cell Biochem 344(1-2): 267-276

[69] Kyosseva SV (2004) Mitogen-activated protein kinase signaling. Int Rev Neurobiol 59: 201-220

[70] Lawrence MC, Jivan A, Shao C, Duan L, Goad D, Zaganjor E, Osborne J, McGlynn K, Stippec S, Earnest S et al (2008) The roles of MAPKs in disease. Cell Res 18(4): 436-442

[71] Laycock-van Spyk S, Thomas N, Cooper DN, Upadhyaya M (2011) Neurofibromatosis type 1-associated tumours: their somatic mutational spectrum and pathogenesis. Hum Genomics 5(6): 623-690

[72] Legius E, Dierick H, Wu R, Hall BK, Marynen P, Cassiman

JJ, Glover TW (1994) TP53 mutations are frequent in malignant NF1 tumors. Genes Chromosomes Cancer 10(4): 250-255

[73] Li Y, O'Connell P, Breidenbach HH, Cawthon R, Stevens J, Xu G, Neil S, Robertson M, White R, Viskochil D (1995) Genomic organization of the neurofibromatosis 1 gene (NF1). Genomics 25(1): 9-18

[74] Liu TC, Zhang T, Fukuhara H, Kuroda T, Todo T, Canron X, Bikfalvi A, Martuza RL, Kurtz A, Rabkin SD (2006a) Dominant-negative fibroblast growth factor receptor expression enhances antitumoral potency of oncolytic herpes simplex virus in neural tumors. Clin Cancer Res 12(22): 6791-6799

[75] Liu TC, Zhang T, Fukuhara H, Kuroda T, Todo T, Martuza RL, Rabkin SD, Kurtz A (2006b) Oncolytic HSV armed with platelet factor 4, an antiangiogenic agent, shows enhanced efficacy. Mol Ther 14(6): 789-797

[76] Lundquist EA (2006) Small GTPases. WormBook Jan: 1-18

[77] Maheswaran S, Haber DA (2010) Circulating tumor cells: a window into cancer biology and metastasis. Curr Opin Genet Dev 20(1): 96-99

[78] Mahller YY, Rangwala F, Ratner N, Cripe TP (2006) Malignant peripheral nerve sheath tumors with high and low Ras-GTP are permissive for oncolytic herpes simplex virus mutants. Pediatr Blood Cancer 46(7): 745-754

[79] Mahller YY, Vaikunth SS, Currier MA, Miller SJ, Ripberger MC, Hsu YH, Mehrian-Shai R, Collins MH, Crombleholme TM, Ratner N et al (2007) Oncolytic HSV and erlotinib inhibit tumor growth and angiogenesis in a novel malignant peripheral nerve sheath tumor xenograft model. Mol Ther 15(2): 279-286

[80] Maldonado AR, Klanke C, Jegga AG, Aronow BJ, Mahller YY, Cripe TP, Crombleholme TM (2010) Molecular engineering and validation of an oncolytic herpes simplex virus type 1 transcriptionally targeted to midkine-positive tumors. J Gene Med 12(7): 613-623

[81] Mashour GA, Drissel SN, Frahm S, Farassati F, Martuza RL, Mautner VF, Kindler-Rohrborn A, Kurtz A (2005) Differential modulation of malignant peripheral nerve sheath tumor growth by omega-3 and omega-6 fatty acids. Oncogene 24(14): 2367-2374

[82] Mattingly RR, Kraniak JM, Dilworth JT, Mathieu P, Bealmear B, Nowak JE, Benjamins JA, Tainsky MA, Reiners JJ Jr (2006) The mitogen-activated protein kinase/extracellular signal-regulated kinase kinase inhibitor PD184352 (CI-1040) selectively induces apoptosis in malignant schwannoma cell lines. J Pharmacol Exp Ther 316(1): 456-465

[83] McCubrey JA, Steelman LS, Chappell WH, Abrams SL, Wong EW, Chang F, Lehmann B, Terrian DM, Milella M, Tafuri A et al (2007) Roles of the Raf/MEK/ERK pathway in cell growth, malignant transformation and drug resistance. Biochim Biophys Acta 1773(8): 1263-1284

[84] McGuire JK, Li Q, Parks WC (2003) Matrilysin (matrix metalloproteinase-7) mediates E-cadherin ectodomain shedding in injured lung epithelium. Am J Pathol 162(6): 1831-1843

[85] Meeker AK, Coffey DS (1997) Telomerase: a promising marker of biological immortality of germ, stem, and cancer cells: a review. Biochemistry (Mosc) 62(11): 1323-1331

[86] Mehra N, Penning M, Maas J, Beerepoot LV, van Daal N, van Gils CH, Giles RH, Voest EE (2006) Progenitor marker CD133 mRNA is elevated in peripheral blood of cancer patients with bone metastases. Clin Cancer Res 12(16): 4859-4866

[87] Meloche S, Pouyssegur J (2007) The ERK1/2 mitogen-activated protein kinase pathway as a master regulator of the G1- to S-phase transition. Oncogene 26(22): 3227-3239

[88] Menon AG, Anderson KM, Riccardi VM, Chung RY, Whaley JM, Yandell DW, Farmer GE, Freiman RN, Lee JK, Li FP (1990) Chromosome 17p deletions and p53 gene mutations associated with the formation of malignant neurofibrosarcomas in von Recklinghausen neuro-fibromatosis. Proc Natl Acad Sci USA 87(14): 5435-5439

[89] Messerli SM, Prabhakar S, Tang Y, Mahmood U, Giovannini M, Weissleder R, Bronson R, Martuza R, Rabkin S, Breakefield XO (2006) Treatment of schwannomas with an oncolytic recombinant herpes simplex virus in murine models of neurofibromatosis type 2. Hum Gene Ther 17(1): 20-30

[90] Mimeault M, Batra SK (2006) Concise review: Recent advances on the significance of stem cells in tissue regeneration and cancer therapies. Stem Cells 24(11): 2319-2345

[91] Miraglia S, Godfrey W, Yin AH, Atkins K, Warnke R, Holden JT, Bray RA, Waller EK, Buck DW (1997) A novel five-transmembrane hematopoietic stem cell antigen: isolation, characterization, and molecular cloning. Blood 90(12): 5013-5021

[92] Molina JR, Adjei AA (2006) The Ras/Raf/MAPK pathway. J Thorac Oncol 1(1): 7-9

[93] Monteiro J, Fodde R (2010) Cancer stemness and metastasis: therapeutic consequences and perspectives. Eur J Cancer 46(7): 1198-1203

[94] Monzani E, Facchetti F, Galmozzi E, Corsini E, Benetti A, Cavazzin C, Gritti A, Piccinini A, Porro D, Santinami M et al (2007) Melanoma contains CD133 and ABCG2 positive cells with enhanced tumourigenic potential. Eur J Cancer 43(5): 935-946

[95] Moskalenko S, Henry DO, Rosse C, Mirey G, Camonis JH, White MA (2002) The exocyst is a Ral effector complex. Nat Cell Biol 4(1): 66-72

[96] Mousley CJ, Tyeryar KR, Ryan MM, Bankaitis VA (2006) Sec14p-like proteins regulate phosphoinositide homoeostasis and intracellular protein and lipid trafficking in yeast. Biochem Soc Trans 34(Pt 3): 346-350

[97] Munoz-Pinedo C (2012) Signaling pathways that regulate life and cell death: evolution of apoptosis in the context of self-defense. Adv Exp Med Biol 738: 124-143

[98] Murphy LO, Blenis J (2006) MAPK signal specificity: the right place at the right time. Trends Biochem Sci 31(5): 268-275

[99] Muthusamy V, Piva TJ (2010) The UV response of the skin: a review of the MAPK, NFkappaB and TNFalpha signal transduction pathways. Arch Dermatol Res 302(1): 5-17

[100] Neel NF, Martin TD, Stratford JK, Zand TP, Reiner DJ, Der CJ (2011) The RalGEF-Ral effector signaling network: the road less traveled for anti-Ras drug discovery. Genes Cancer 2(3): 275-287

[101] Neuzil J, Stantic M, Zobalova R, Chladova J, Wang X, Prochazka L, Dong L, Andera L, Ralph SJ (2007) Tumour-initiating cells vs. cancer 'stem' cells and CD133: what's in the name? Biochem Biophys Res Commun 355(4): 855-859

[102] Norman KL, Farassati F, Lee PW (2001) Oncolytic viruses and cancer therapy. Cytokine Growth Factor Rev 12(2-3): 271-282

[103] O'Brien CA, Pollett A, Gallinger S, Dick JE (2007) A human colon cancer cell capable of initiating tumour growth in immunodeficient mice. Nature 445(7123): 106-110

[104] O'Donnell A, Odrowaz Z, Sharrocks AD (2012) Immediate-early gene activation by the MAPK pathways: what do and don't we know? Biochem Soc Trans 40(1): 58-66

[105] Pan Y, Huang X (2008) Epithelial ovarian cancer stem cells-a review. Int J Clin Exp Med 1(3): 260-266

[106] Pan W, Bodempudi V, Esfandyari T, Farassati F (2009) Utilizing ras signaling pathway to direct selective replication of herpes simplex virus-1. PLoS One 4(8): e6514

[107] Parmar VM, Schroder M (2012) Sensing endoplasmic reticulum stress. Adv Exp Med Biol 738: 153-168

[108] Parrinello S, Lloyd AC (2009) Neurofibroma development in NF1-insights into tumour initiation. Trends Cell Biol 19(8): 395-403

[109] Plotnikov A, Zehorai E, Procaccia S, Seger R (2011) The MAPK cascades: signaling components, nuclear roles and mechanisms of nuclear translocation. Biochim Biophys Acta 1813(9): 1619-1633

[110] Polyak K, Hahn WC (2006) Roots and stems: stem cells in cancer. Nat Med 12(3): 296-300

[111] Prabhakar S, Brenner GJ, Sung B, Messerli SM, Mao J, Sena-Esteves M, Stemmer-Rachamimov A, Tannous B, Breakefield XO (2010) Imaging and therapy of experimental schwannomas using HSV amplicon vector-encoding apoptotic protein under Schwann cell promoter. Cancer Gene Ther 17(4): 266-274

[112] Rajalingam K, Schreck R, Rapp UR, Albert S (2007) Ras oncogenes and their downstream targets. Biochim Biophys Acta 1773(8): 1177-1195

[113] Rey JA, Pestana A, Bello MJ (1992) Cytogenetics and molecular genetics of nervous system tumors. Oncol Res 4(8-9): 321-331

[114] Reya T, Morrison SJ, Clarke MF, Weissman IL (2001) Stem cells, cancer, and cancer stem cells. Nature 414(6859): 105-111

[115] Roberts PJ, Der CJ (2007) Targeting the Raf-MEK-ERK mitogen-activated protein kinase cascade for the treatment of cancer. Oncogene 26(22): 3291-3310

[116] Rudland PS, Ormerod EJ, Paterson FC (1980) Stem cells in rat mammary development and cancer: a review. J R Soc Med 73(6): 437-442

[117] Sagar J, Chaib B, Sales K, Winslet M, Seifalian A (2007) Role of stem cells in cancer therapy and cancer stem cells: a review. Cancer Cell Int 7: 9

[118] Salmaggi A, Boiardi A, Gelati M, Russo A, Calatozzolo C, Ciusani E, Sciacca FL, Ottolina A, Parati EA, La Porta C et al (2006) Glioblastoma-derived tumorospheres identify a population of tumor stem-like cells with angiogenic potential and enhanced multidrug resistance phenotype. Glia 54(8): 850-860

[119] Serra E, Puig S, Otero D, Gaona A, Kruyer H, Ars E, Estivill X, Lazaro C (1997) Confirmation of a double-hit model for the NF1 gene in benign neurofibromas. Am J Hum Genet 61(3): 512-519

[120] Shannon KM, O'Connell P, Martin GA, Paderanga D, Olson K, Dinndorf P, McCormick F (1994) Loss of the normal NF1 allele from the bone marrow of children with type 1 neurofibromatosis and malignant myeloid disorders. N Engl J Med 330(9): 597-601

[121] Shelton JG, Steelman LS, Lee JT, Knapp SL, Blalock WL, Moye PW, Franklin RA, Pohnert SC, Mirza AM, McMahon M et al (2003) Effects of the RAF/MEK/ERK and PI3K/AKT signal transduction pathways on the abrogation of cytokine-dependence and prevention of apoptosis in hematopoietic cells. Oncogene 22(16): 2478-2492

[122] Singh SK, Hawkins C, Clarke ID, Squire JA, Bayani J, Hide T, Henkelman RM, Cusimano MD, Dirks PB (2004) Identification of human brain tumour initiating cells. Nature 432(7015): 396-401

[123] Song C, Hu CD, Masago M, Kariyai K, Yamawaki-Kataoka Y, Shibatohge M, Wu D, Satoh T, Kataoka T (2001) Regulation of a novel human phospholipase C, PLCepsilon, through membrane targeting by Ras. J Biol Chem 276(4): 2752-2757

[124] Sorensen SA, Mulvihill JJ, Nielsen A (1986) Long-term follow-up of von Recklinghausen neurofibromatosis. Survival and malignant neoplasms. N Engl J Med 314(16): 1010-1015

[125] Spillane JB, Henderson MA (2007) Cancer stem cells: a review. ANZ J Surg 77(6): 464-468

[126] Spyra M, Kluwe L, Hagel C, Nguyen R, Panse J, Kurtz A, Mautner VF, Rabkin SD, Demestre M (2011) Cancer stem cell-like cells derived from malignant peripheral nerve sheath tumors. PLoS One 6(6): e21099

[127] Sugihara K, Asano S, Tanaka K, Iwamatsu A, Okawa K, Ohta Y (2002) The exocyst complex binds the small GTPase RalA to mediate filopodia formation. Nat Cell Biol 4(1): 73-78

[128] Sundaram MV (2006) RTK/Ras/MAPK signaling. WormBook Feb: 1-19

[129] Terada Y, Nakamura O, Inoshita S, Kuwahara M, Sasaki S, Marumo F (1999) Mitogen-activated protein kinase cascade and transcription factors: the opposite role of MKK3/6-p38K and MKK1-MAPK. Nephrol Dial Transplant 14(Suppl 1): 45-47

[130] Treglia AS, Turco S, Ulianich L, Ausiello P, Lofrumento DD, Nicolardi G, Miele C, Garbi C, Beguinot F, Di Jeso B (2012) Cell fate following ER stress: just a matter of "quo ante" recovery or death? Histol Histopathol 27(1): 1-12

[131] Trosko JE (2009) Review paper: cancer stem cells and cancer nonstem cells: from adult stem cells or from reprogramming of differentiated somatic cells. Vet Pathol 46(2): 176-193

[132] Trovo-Marqui AB, Tajara EH (2006) Neurofibromin: a general outlook. Clin Genet 70(1): 1-13

[133] van Dam EM, Robinson PJ (2006) Ral: mediator of membrane trafficking. Int J Biochem Cell Biol 38(11): 1841-1847

[134] Vasudevan A, Qian Y, Vogt A, Blaskovich MA, Ohkanda J, Sebti SM, Hamilton AD (1999) Potent, highly selective, and non-thiol inhibitors of protein geranylgeranyltransferase-I. J Med Chem 42(8): 1333-1340

[135] Vigil D, Cherfils J, Rossman KL, Der CJ (2010) Ras superfamily GEFs and GAPs: validated and tractable targets for cancer therapy? Nat Rev Cancer 10(12): 842-857

[136] Vogel KS, Klesse LJ, Velasco-Miguel S, Meyers K, Rushing EJ, Parada LF (1999) Mouse tumor model for neurofibromatosis type 1. Science 286(5447): 2176-2179

[137] Whitmarsh AJ, Shore P, Sharrocks AD, Davis RJ (1995) Integration of MAP kinase signal transduction pathways at the serum response element. Science 269(5222): 403-407

[138] Wojtkowiak JW, Fouad F, LaLonde DT, Kleinman MD, Gibbs RA, Reiners JJ Jr, Borch RF, Mattingly RR (2008) Induction of apoptosis in neurofibromatosis type 1 malignant peripheral nerve sheath tumor cell lines by a combination of novel farnesyl transferase inhibitors and lovastatin. J Pharmacol Exp Ther 326(1): 1-11

[139] Yamamoto T, Taya S, Kaibuchi K (1999) Ras-induced transformation and signaling pathway. J Biochem (Tokyo) 126(5): 799-803

[140] Yamoutpour F, Bodempudi V, Park SE, Pan W, Mauzy MJ, Kratzke RA, Dudek A, Potter DA, Woo RA, O'Rourke DM

et al (2008) Gene silencing for epidermal growth factor receptor variant III induces cell-specific cytotoxicity. Mol Cancer Ther 7(11): 3586-3597

[141] Yan N, Ricca C, Fletcher J, Glover T, Seizinger BR, Manne V (1995) Farnesyltransferase inhibitors block the neurofibromatosis type I (NF1) malignant phenotype. Cancer Res 55(16): 3569-3575

[142] Zebisch A, Czernilofsky AP, Keri G, Smigelskaite J, Sill H, Troppmair J (2007) Signaling through RAS-RAF-MEK-ERK: from basics to bedside. Curr Med Chem 14(5): 601-623

[143] Zheng G, Lyons JG, Tan TK, Wang Y, Hsu TT, Min D, Succar L, Rangan GK, Hu M, Henderson BR et al (2009) Disruption of E-cadherin by matrix metalloproteinase directly mediates epithelial-mesenchymal transition downstream of transforming growth factor-beta1 in renal tubular epithelial cells. Am J Pathol 175(2): 580-591

[144] Zoller M, Rembeck B, Akesson HO, Angervall L (1995) Life expectancy, mortality and prognostic factors in neurofibromatosis type 1. A twelve-year follow-up of an epidemiological study in Goteborg, Sweden. Acta Derm Venereol 75(2): 136-140

第39章 miRNA 与 1 型神经纤维瘤病肿瘤发生
MicroRNA and NF1 Tumorigenesis

Adrienne M. Flanagan and Nadège Presneau

39.1 历史和 miRNA 的生物发生

miRNA 是进化上保守的短（20～23 个核苷酸）内源性单链 RNA 分子，通过 mRNA 降解、翻译抑制和基于染色质的沉默机制调节基因功能（Bartel 2004）。最早发现的 miRNA 是秀丽隐杆线虫中的 miRNA lin-4 和 let-7，它们参与了幼虫的发育（Lee et al. 1993）。它们的功能机制来自发现 LIN4 编码两个小转录本（长度为 22 个和 61 个核苷酸），它们在 lin-14 mRNA 的 3′非翻译区（3′ untranslated region，3′ UTR）内包含多个保守位点的互补序列，并且正是这种互补性阻止了 lin-14 蛋白的翻译。从那时起，miRNA 被认为是一种保守的分子类别，在转录后水平上是基因表达的关键调节因子。

miRNA 基因存在于单个基因中，但约 30% 存在于基因簇中。在最新的 miRNA 库 miRbase version 18（2011 年 11 月发布）中，列出了 1 921 种独特的成年人类 miRNA（http://www.mirbase.org）。据估计，1/3 的蛋白质编码人类 mRNA 易受这种复杂的 miRNA 调控网络的影响。

近年的一些综述对 miRNA 的生物发生进行了详细的回顾，在这里不作详细的讨论（Calin and Croce 2006a, b; Krol et al. 2010; Van Kouwenhove et al. 2011）。miRNA 基因的特征是它们的中间 RNA 转录物折叠成发夹结构，由 miRNA 生物发生机制特异性识别和加工。这一过程如图 39.1 所示。

39.2 miRNA 在周围神经鞘膜瘤中的表达特征

只有少数关于 miRNA 在 1 型神经纤维瘤病中肿瘤发展中作用的报道。已发表的工作涉及神经鞘膜瘤的 miRNA 分析研究，包括比较 1 型神经纤维瘤患者的丛状神经纤维瘤与皮肤型神经纤维瘤以及非丛状神经纤维瘤与恶性周围神经鞘膜瘤的研究（Chai et al. 2010; Lee et al. 2011; Pasmant et al. 2011a; Presneau et al. 2012; Subramanian et al. 2010）。然而，并非所有这些研究都局限于这种综合征的患者的肿瘤。

39.2.1 p53 失活有助于 MPNST 的 miRNA 表达谱

miRNA 在神经鞘肿瘤中的首次研究涉及 23 个周围神经鞘膜瘤，包括 6 个 MPNST、11 个神经纤维瘤和 6 个神经鞘瘤。并非所有肿瘤都来自 1 型神经纤维瘤病患者。10 种 miRNA 在良恶性肿瘤中表达显著差异：5 种上调（miR-214、miR-377、miR-

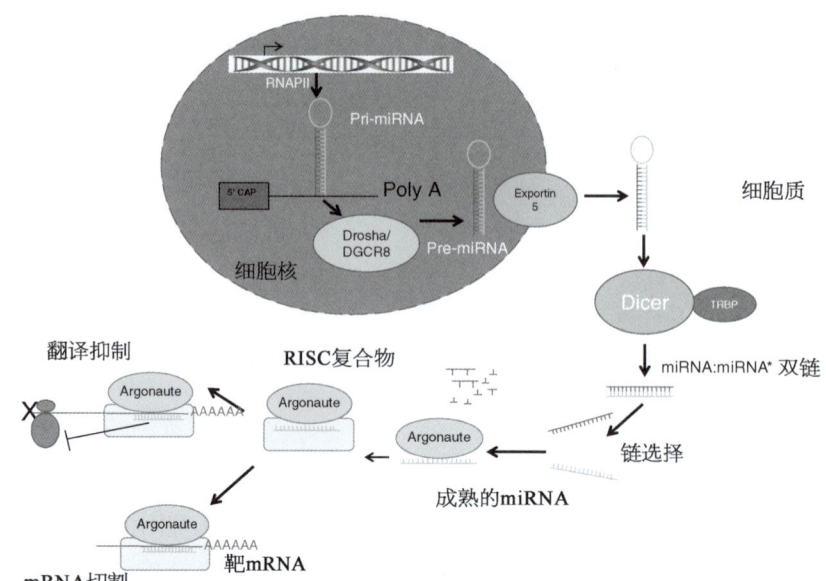

图 39.1 miRNA 的生物发生和功能示意图。miRNA 基因通过 RNAP Ⅱ 转录产生 primary-miRNA(pri-miRNA)，其结构为茎环，具有 5′端 CAP 结构，3′端 poly-a。这种茎环结构被核糖核酸内切酶 Drosha 及其 RNA 结合伙伴 DGCR8 识别。Drosha 将 pri-mRNA 转化为 miRNA 前体(pre-miRNA)(Denli et al. 2004；Gregory et al. 2004)。然后，这个发夹通过 export-5 以依赖于 Ran-GTP 的方式输出到细胞质中(Lund et al. 2004)。然后，它被另一种酶复合物 Dicer(一种 RNase Ⅲ 内切酶)与其 RNA 结合蛋白(RBP)伙伴 HIV-1 反激活反应(TAR)RNA 结合蛋白(TRBP)一起加工，切割发夹的环区，形成成熟的 20～23 个核苷酸的双链 RNA，称为 miRNA-miRNA* 双链(Hutvagner et al 2001)。两条链被分离：一条成为成熟的 miRNA，另一条被降解。成熟链被含 argonaute 复合物识别，产生 RNA 诱导的沉默复合物(RISC)，该复合物被认为通过识别靶 mRNA 导致 miRNA 介导的不稳定(mRNA 切割)或 miRNA 介导的翻译抑制(Chendrimada et al 2005；Filipowicz 2005；Gregory et al. 2005)

409-3p、miR-487b 和 miR-99b)，5 种下调(miR-517、miR-34a、miR-29a、miR-30e-5p 和 miR-27a)(Subramanian et al 2010)。本研究中选择的 6 个 MPNST 进行 miRNA 分析，表达 p53 失活基因表达特征，与良性肿瘤相比，miR-34a 是该肿瘤组中下调最显著的 miRNA，尽管尚不清楚这些肿瘤是否来自 1 型神经纤维瘤病患者。有充分证据表明，miR-34a 在多种肿瘤中是 p53 的直接靶点，包括结直肠癌和神经母细胞瘤，在这些肿瘤中，miR-34a 的低水平与抑制细胞凋亡有关。Subramanian 等(2010)研究了其在神经鞘肿瘤中的作用(Bommer et al. 2007；Dalgard et al. 2009；He et al. 2007a, b；Hermeking 2010)。

在缺乏 miR-34a 的 MPNST 细胞系中过度表达 miR-34a 导致细胞凋亡增加。此外，在同一细胞系中过度表达 p53 也会产生类似的效果，从而证明 p53 的表达通过 miR-34a 参与了其对细胞凋亡的影响。在细胞系中诱导 miR-34a 的高表达也导致一系列癌基因的表达降低，包括 *MYCN*、*E2F* 和 *CDK4*，这些都是已知的 miR-34a 的靶点。已知这些癌基因的激活可以减少细胞凋亡，这为 miR-34a 介导细胞凋亡的发现增加了分量(Hermeking 2010)。这些致癌基因在 MPNST 中的表达比在神经纤维瘤中的表达更高，这一发现为它们在该疾病中的病理生理作用提供了证据(Subramanian et al. 2010；Yu et al. 2011)。

Subramanian 等(2010)也表明，在 MPNST 细胞系中过度表达野生型 p53，除了 miR-34a 外，还导致 9 种 miRNA(miR-34b、miR-34c、miR-638、miR-373*、miR-492、miR-126、miR140、 miR-491和miR-293）的表达水平显著增加，所有这些miRNA都是由p53诱导的（Raver-Shapira et al. 2007）。除了miR-34家族外，这些p53诱导的6种mi-RNA（miR-638，miR-373，miR-492，miR-126，miR-140和miR-491）参与多种功能，包括肿瘤侵袭和增殖（miR-373，miR-126）（Huang et al. 2008；Sun et al. 2010），转移（miR-373，miR-492）（Huang et al 2008；von Frowein et al. 2011），通过PI3K途径抑制肿瘤生长（miR-126）（Guo et al. 2008），通过VEGF抑制血管完整性和血管生成（miR-126）（Wang et al. 2008），增殖、耐药（miR-140）（Song et al. 2009）和凋亡（miR-491）（Nakano et al. 2010）。这些发现与p53能够对几种介导一系列功能的miRNA发挥作用的认识一致，并解释了p53如何发挥其一系列抗癌作用（Feng et al. 2011）。

基于Subramanian等（2010）的功能研究结果，Lee及其团队采用计算生物学的方法，识别出一个涉及多个细胞周期相关基因模块的调控网络，包含E2F家族成员E2F7和E2F8（Lee et al. 2011）。由于E2F转录因子参与转录调控、DNA修复和细胞增殖，他们推测E2F7和E2F8的激活因子和抑制因子的表达变化，可能在恶性周围神经鞘膜瘤（MPNST）的形成中发挥作用，这与其他癌症中的相关报道类似（Endo-Munoz et al. 2009；Reimer et al. 2007）。研究结果表明，p53和miR-34a水平的下降会促进MPNST的发生。然而，并非所有MPNST都表现出p53功能丧失（Verdijk et al. 2010），因此可能还存在其他机制参与良性神经鞘瘤的恶性转化（Subramanian et al. 2010）。

一项更近的miRNA表达谱研究采用Agilent微阵列芯片，但未能证实Subramanian等（2010）的研究结果，即miR-34a在10个神经纤维瘤与9个MPNST之间存在显著差异表达（Presneau et al. 2012）。可能是患者群体的差异导致了两项研究结果的不一致。Subramanian等（2010）研究中的6个MPNST样本是基于p53基因失活的表达特征选择的，而Presneau等（2012）则基于患者患有1型神经纤维瘤病来选择病例。尚不清楚前一研究中的6名患者是否患有1型神经纤维瘤病，而后一研究中未进行基因表达谱分析。在此背景下，有趣的是，p53突变仅在约25%的MPNST中出现，其中仅少数（36%）出现在1型神经纤维瘤病患者的肿瘤中（Verdijk et al. 2010）。因此，推测miR-34a在良性和恶性神经鞘瘤中的差异表达至少部分依赖于p53的丧失，而p53的丧失可能受神经纤维瘤蛋白胚系突变的影响。另一个导致两项研究结果不一致的原因可能是他们使用了不同的miRNA微阵列平台，且样本量较小可能加剧差异。

39.2.2　MiR29c在周围神经鞘膜瘤进展中的失调

我们最近发现，来自1型神经纤维瘤病患者的10个神经纤维瘤和10个MPNST之间有16个miRNA表达显著差异（Presneau et al 2012）。其中，7个MPNST下调，包括miR-30e*、miR-29c*、miR-29c、miR-340*、miR-30c、miR-1395p和let-7g（q¼8.48E-03）。此外，芯片分析显示，大多数miR-29家族成员miR-29a、b、c*、b-1*的表达量在神经纤维瘤中转MPNST中明显下调。相比之下，与神经纤维瘤相比，miR-210（$q=4.1E-04$）在MPNST中上调。

计算机预测分析确定了miR-29家族的一系列靶基因，包括由多种胶原基因和肌腱蛋白组成的细胞外基质（extracellular matrix，ECM）基因，它们参与细胞迁移和侵袭（Daley et al. 2008；Newby. 2006）。细胞成分和分子功能的基因本体术语以及京都基因和基因组数据库（Kyoto Encyclopedia of Genes and Genomes，KEGG）分析也表明，预测的靶基因代表金属肽酶功能（$P=0.00461$）和ECM受体相互作用（$P=6.73\times10^{-10}$）。

这些miR-29c靶基因的选择，包括COL1A1、COL1A2、COL5A2、COL21A1、COL4A1、COL4A2、TGFB3和MMP2，被证明是由于在MPNST细胞系sNF96.2中使用合成寡核苷酸（模拟物）强制表达miR-29c而下调的，这表明内源性miR-29c的表达水平较低，从患者的MPNST样本中可以看出。功能分析显示，在transwell板和划痕/伤口愈合试验中评估的该细胞系的细胞运动性和侵袭性，在用miR-29c模拟物处理后显著降低。当使用各种检测方法(包括活细胞成像系统 IncuCyte、MTS 检测以及使用软琼脂在 3D 培养中培养细胞)进行评估时,转染 miR-29c 模拟物后,未发现对 sNF96.2 细胞的细胞生长/增殖有影响。

miR-29 家族的已知靶点 MMP2 的蛋白水解酶活性降低(Steele et al. 2010),导致 MPNST 细胞系中 miR-29c 的强制表达使迁移减少。这种 miRNA 的 mRNA 和蛋白质水平降低证明了这一点(Presneau et al 2012)。在同一实验中,虽然 MMP9 活性下降,但对蛋白质和 mRNA 的表达没有显著影响。这与 MMP9 不是 miR-29c 的直接靶点一致,表明 miR-29c 对 MMP9 酶的作用是间接的。

Presneau 等(2012)推测 MPNST 中 miR-29c 的低水平是通过激活 cMET/肝细胞生长因子受体介导的,cMET/肝细胞生长因子受体是一种通常在 MPNST 中被激活的蛋白质,约 20% 的病例是由于基因扩增所致(Mantripragada et al 2008)。cMET 的激活也可以由 p53 活性的丧失引起(Goldstein et al. 2011)。这一推测是基于 Torres 等(2011)的工作,他们表明 cMET 的高水平表达会导致体外 MPNST 中细胞运动性、侵袭性、血管生成增加,并诱导 MMP2 和 VEGF 的表达。cMET 的沉默在体外发挥相反的作用,并且在小鼠模型中也显著降低 MPNST 的局部和转移性生长(Torres et al. 2011)。此外,其他学者报道肝细胞生长因子通过诱导 miR-29a/b 抑制肝星状细胞中胶原 I 和 IV 的合成(Kwiecinski et al 2011);此外,通过迫使肝星状细胞中肿瘤生长因子 β 的表达,cMET 的表达增加,从而导致其配体肝细胞生长因子以及 miR-29a/b 的表达减少。与此一致的是,肝细胞生长因子的引入刺激了 miR-29 的表达,消除了肿瘤生长因子 β 的作用。

miR-29c 在 MPNST 中的低水平表达不太可能用染色体丢失来解释,因为用于研究 miR-29c 介导其作用机制的 MPNST 细胞系 sNF96.2[48,X,X 或 Y,+7,add(7)(p22)x2,+8,add(9)(p24),+mar]的核型并未显示 miR-29 家族成员所在的 1 号染色体和 7 号染色体上任何位点的丢失(Perrin et al 2007)。高甲基化也不太可能是 MPNST 中 miR-29c 失活的原因,因为神经纤维瘤和 MPNST 的甲基化分析[Presneau 等(2012)也对其 miRNA 进行了分析]显示,肿瘤组的甲基化状态几乎没有差异(Feber et al. 2011)。这些"合并"实验的结果在通过焦磷酸测序对相同样本进行基因体甲基化分析时得到了证实(Presneau et al 2012)。

总之,有证据表明,在 1 型神经纤维瘤病患者中出现的 MPNST 中 miR-29c 水平较低,至少部分是通过神经鞘膜瘤细胞迁移和侵袭增加介导的,这是通过胶原基因和金属蛋白酶介导的,miR-29c 靶向各自的转录本(Daley et al. 2008;Newby 2006;Presneau et al. 2012)。

39.2.3　MiR-214 与 TWIST1 在 MPNST 中的表达

在 Subramanian 等的 MPNST 队列中,miR-214 是表达最高的 miRNA。尽管在 Presneau 等的研究中并非如此,但他们也发现,与神经纤维瘤相比,这种 miRNA 在大多数 MPNST 中的表达水平更高。这种 miRNA 与许多不同癌症的肿瘤发生有关:在一些癌症中,它似乎是一种致癌基因,但在另一些癌症中,它是一种肿瘤抑制基因。具体来说,miR-214 在黑色素瘤细胞中的高表达导致黑色素瘤细胞转移行为增加(Penna et al. 2011);它通过靶向肿瘤抑制基因 PTEN 的 3' 末翻译区,从而抑制翻译,进而激活 Akt 通路,从而提高卵巢癌的细胞存活率和顺铂耐药性(Yang et al. 2008)。在胰腺癌标本中也发现了这种 miRNA 的上调,这与胰腺癌细胞对化学治疗的不良反应有关(Zhang et al. 2010)。相比之下,有报道称 miR-214 的下调通过上调 PTEN 诱导胃癌细胞周期阻滞(Xiong et al. 2011),其他人发现该 miRNA 在乳腺癌中的表达降低可能具有致瘤性(Derfoul et al. 2011)。最近,miR-214 被证明可以通过靶向 GALNT7 来抑制宫颈癌细胞的增殖、迁移和侵袭,这一发现得到了 GALNT7 沉默抑制宫颈癌细胞增殖、迁移和侵袭的支持(Peng et al. 2012)。

在许多癌症中,miR-214 的表达与 TWIST1 的表达呈正相关,TWIST1 是一种基本的螺旋-环-螺旋蛋白(Kwok et al. 2005;Lee et al. 2006,

2009),这一发现与该蛋白质在几乎所有 MPNST 中的高水平表达一致。TWIST1 的表达也与许多其他癌症的转移性疾病呈正相关,包括肝细胞癌(Lee et al. 2006)、前列腺癌(Kwok et al. 2005;Yuen et al. 2007)、乳腺癌(Kallergi et al. 2011)和头颈癌(Ou et al. 2008)。在 MPNST 细胞系 STS26T 中,当 siRNA 降低 TWIST1 的表达时,转移过程的关键组成部分趋化性被抑制,这一发现与上述发现一致(Miller et al. 2006)。因此,在周围神经鞘膜瘤中,mir-214 很可能作为一种致癌基因,尽管迄今为止尚未确定介导其作用的靶基因。

39.2.4 miRNA-10b 调控 1 型神经纤维瘤病的肿瘤发生

像神经纤维瘤蛋白(NF1)这样的真正的肿瘤抑制基因的定义是其双等位基因失活,通常是由肿瘤中一个等位基因突变和第二个野生型等位基因的染色体缺失引起的[关于肿瘤抑制基因失活的最新综述见 Berger 等(2011)]。Chai 及其同事提出假设,在 1 型神经纤维瘤病患者的肿瘤中,神经纤维瘤蛋白完全失活的两次打击之一,可能是由微 RNA(miRNA)的沉默作用导致的。有充分的证据表明,包括 p53 在内的其他肿瘤抑制基因也以这种方式沉默(Salmena et al. 2008;Swarbrick et al. 2010)。通过分析来自 1 型神经纤维瘤病患者的 MPNST 细胞系 ST88-14 中的 miRNA,并将其与来自散发性肿瘤的 MPNST 细胞系 STS26T 进行比较,发现前者的肿瘤细胞 miR-10b、miR155 和 miR-335 的表达明显高于后者。此外,与零星来源的 MPNST 细胞系相比,来自 1 型神经纤维瘤病患者的细胞中 let-7 家族,特别是 let-7a 和 let-7b 显著降低。

在 MPNST 细胞系 ST88-14 中,分别使用反义抑制对 miR-10b、miR-155、miR-335 和使用合成寡核苷酸模拟物对 let-7 进行功能表征,发现 miR-10b 显著降低细胞增殖、迁移和侵袭,而其他 miRNA 仅降低细胞的侵袭特性(Chai et al. 2010)。值得注意的是,在一组原发性良性和恶性周围神经鞘膜瘤中,只有 miR10b、let-7a 和 let-7b 存在差异表达。原发性肿瘤和细胞系中 miRNA 表达的差异可能反映了 MPNST 内部和之间存在组织学和遗传异质性(Burger and Scheithauer 2007)。只有研究更多的病例,并将 miRNA 谱与肿瘤的各种外观和行为联系起来,才能解决这个问题。

miR-10b 也被证明靶向神经纤维瘤蛋白,从而提供了在没有突变和染色体丢失的情况下沉默该基因表达的机制。与其他 miRNA 一样,mir-10b 也靶向许多其他基因(Thomas et al. 2010),包括 RAS 信号通路中的关键分子。这样,它也可能有助于外周非鞘性肿瘤的肿瘤发生(Chai et al. 2010)。

39.2.5 MPNST 中常见的 1.4 Mb 微缺失 1 型神经纤维瘤病区域的 miRNA

大约 5% 的 1 型神经纤维瘤病患者有 17q11.2 区域的微缺失,在大多数患者中涉及 1.4 Mb 的种系微缺失。这类患者发生 MPNST 的风险高于没有这种基因畸变的患者(Upadhyaya et al. 1998;Wu et al. 1995)。微缺失是由称为 NF1 低拷贝重复的两个高度同源片段之间的不等重组引起的。基因组分析显示,微缺失覆盖了完整的 350 kb 神经纤维瘤蛋白(NF1)基因,以及至少 16 个基因、4 个假基因和 2 个 miRNA(miR-193a 和 miR-365-2)。miR-193a 是特别有趣的,因为它在口腔鳞状细胞癌中作为肿瘤抑制基因(Kozaki et al. 2008)。它在口腔癌中下调是 DNA 超甲基化的结果(Kozaki et al. 2008),并且在含有 BRAF 突变的黑色素瘤中表达不良(Caramuta et al. 2010)。基因组学和机制研究表明,miR-193a-3p 通过富含丝氨酸/精氨酸的剪接因子 2 介导肝癌 5-FU 耐药中 caspase 2 促凋亡剪接形式的上调(Ma et al. 2012)。

miR-365 是微缺失中的第二个 miRNA,之所以引起人们的兴趣,是因为它在结肠癌中被下调,抑制细胞周期进程,促进结肠癌细胞凋亡,可能是通过靶向 cyclin D1 和 Bcl-2 来实现的(Nie et al. 2012)。

Pasmant 等(2011a)将皮肤型神经纤维瘤($n=23$)中 miR-193a 和 miR-365-2 的基因表达水平与丛状神经纤维瘤($n=13$)和 MPNST($n=13$)中的 miR-193a 和 miR-365-2 的基因表达水平进行了比较,该项目旨在测试 1.4 Mb 微缺失区间中的某些基因是否作为肿瘤抑制基因导致了恶性疾病的更大风险。结果采用实时 PCR 和 Human TaqMan® miRNA 检测试剂盒生成,未发现 miRNA 在不同组中表达差异的证据。非 1 型神经纤维瘤病患者的真皮神经纤维瘤作为对照,因为它们不会转化为 MPNST(Evans et al. 2002；King et al. 2000；Kleihues and Cavenee 2000；Pasmant et al. 2011a)。

39.3 非蛋白编码转录物在 1 型神经纤维瘤病中的作用

除了 miRNA 外,长链非编码 RNA(long non-coding RNA,lncRNA)是一类新的非编码 RNA。这些都与一系列生物功能的调节有关,而其中一些功能的破坏,如基因组印记和转录调节,在癌症的发展中起着关键作用(Gibb et al. 2011)。

Pasmant 及其同事使用高分辨率阵列比较基因组杂交技术发现,1 型神经纤维瘤患者中出现的丛状神经纤维瘤唯一复发性遗传改变是涉及染色体 9p21.3 的缺失(Pasmant et al. 2011b)。最小的常见缺失区域约为 0.5 Mb,包括 CDKN2A、CDKN2B 和 INK-4A/ARF,这些都是公认的肿瘤抑制基因,以及位于 INK-4A 位点的反义非编码 RNA ANRIL,该 RNA 已被证明可以调节 CDKN2A/B 位点的转录(Yap et al. 2010)。他们在 ANRIL 的 3rs2151280 内含子中发现了一个单核多态性,其中等位基因 T 与大量丛状神经纤维瘤显著相关。他们还发现这种多态性与 ANRIL mRNA 表达水平的降低显著相关,这表明 ANRIL 表达的改变可能介导了发生丛状神经纤维瘤的易感性。有趣的是,由于 $Cdkn2a/Arf$ 缺乏导致 $Nf1^{+/-}$ 背景小鼠中 MPNST 的形成,已经提出 9p21.3 区域参与 1 型神经纤维瘤病相关的肿瘤发生(Joseph et al. 2008)。这些数据表明 ANRIL 是 1 型神经纤维瘤病的修饰基因。然而,该研究存在局限性,ANRIL 与神经纤维瘤蛋白之间的相互作用尚未在生物学水平上得到证实。

39.4 结束语:未来的方向和前景,miRNA 作为 MPNST 的治疗靶点?

各种癌症的 miRNA 分析可以根据肿瘤的分化状态和起源细胞成功地对肿瘤进行分类(Lu et al. 2005；Volinia et al. 2006),在未来,它们可以作为诊断工具和预后指标。然而,到目前为止,这种工作仅限于实验室研究,并没有在临床实践中使用(Cummins and Velculescu 2006；Tricoli and Jacobson 2007；Visone and Croce 2009；Yanaihara et al. 2006)。

参与调节致癌基因和肿瘤抑制基因表达的 miRNA 是癌症治疗中靶向治疗的候选物(Nana-Sinkam and Croce 2011)。目前,miRNA/RNA-i 治疗领域尚处于起步阶段,但针对 miRNA 的几种方法正在开发中,包括抗 miRNA 寡核苷酸(Garzon et al. 2010),通过互补性阻断 miRNA(Garzon et al. 2010)。已通过各种给药途径测试了这些药物的输送,包括静脉注射和腹腔注射及吸入(Nana-Sinkam and Croce 2011)。初步研究表明,使用经肿瘤寻找抗体修饰的纳米颗粒分别递送相关的小干扰 RNA 和 miRNA,在体外和动物模型中显示出前景(Chen et al. 2010)。

(陈敏亮,徐潇 译)

参考文献

[1] Bartel DP (2004) MicroRNAs: genomics, biogenesis, mechanism, and function. Cell 116: 281-297
[2] Berger AH, Knudson AG, Pandolfi PP (2011) A continuum model for tumour suppression. Nature 476: 163-169
[3] Bommer GT, Gerin I, Feng Y et al (2007) p53-mediated activation of miRNA34 candidate tumor-suppressor genes. Curr Biol 17: 1298-1307
[4] Burger PC, Scheithauer BW (2007) AFIP atlas of tumor pathology, Series 4, Tumors of the central nervous system. American Registry of Pathology in collaboration with the Armed Forces Institute of Pathology. Armed Forces Institute of Pathology, Washington, DC
[5] Calin GA, Croce CM (2006a) MicroRNA signatures in human cancers. Nat Rev Cancer 6: 857-866
[6] Calin GA, Croce CM (2006b) MicroRNA-cancer connection: the beginning of a new tale. Cancer Res 66: 7390-7394
[7] Caramuta S, Egyhazi S, Rodolfo M et al (2010) MicroRNA expression profiles associated with mutational status and

survival in malignant melanoma. J Invest Dermatol 130: 2062-2070

[8] Chai G, Liu N, Ma J et al (2010) MicroRNA-10b regulates tumorigenesis in neurofibromatosis type 1. Cancer Sci 101: 1997-2004

[9] Chen Y, Zhu X, Zhang X et al (2010) Nanoparticles modified with tumor-targeting scFv deliver siRNA and miRNA for cancer therapy. Mol Ther 18: 1650-1656

[10] Chendrimada TP, Gregory RI, Kumaraswamy E et al (2005) TRBP recruits the Dicer complex to Ago2 for microRNA processing and gene silencing. Nature 436: 740-744

[11] Cummins JM, Velculescu VE (2006) Implications of microRNA profiling for cancer diagnosis. Oncogene 25: 6220-6227

[12] Daley WP, Peters SB, Larsen M (2008) Extracellular matrix dynamics in development and regenerative medicine. J Cell Sci 121: 255-264

[13] Dalgard CL, Gonzalez M, deNiro JE et al (2009) Differential microRNA-34a expression and tumor suppressor function in retinoblastoma cells. Invest Ophthalmol Vis Sci 50: 4542-4551

[14] Denli AM, Tops BB, Plasterk RH et al (2004) Processing of primary microRNAs by the microprocessor complex. Nature 432: 231-235

[15] Derfoul A, Juan AH, Difilippantonio MJ et al (2011) Decreased microRNA-214 levels in breast cancer cells coincides with increased cell proliferation, invasion and accumulation of the polycomb Ezh2 methyltransferase. Carcinogenesis 32: 1607-1614

[16] Endo-Munoz L, Dahler A, Teakle N et al (2009) E2F7 can regulate proliferation, differentiation, and apoptotic responses in human keratinocytes: implications for cutaneous squamous cell carcinoma formation. Cancer Res 69: 1800-1808

[17] Evans DG, Baser ME, McGaughran J et al (2002) Malignant peripheral nerve sheath tumours in neurofibromatosis 1. J Med Genet 39: 311-314

[18] Feber A, Wilson GA, Zhang L et al (2011) Comparative methylome analysis of benign and malignant peripheral nerve sheath tumors. Genome Res 21(4): 515-524

[19] Feng Z, Zhang C, Wu R et al (2011) Tumor suppressor p53 meets microRNAs. J Mol Cell Biol 3: 44-50

[20] Filipowicz W (2005) RNAi: the nuts and bolts of the RISC machine. Cell 122: 17-20

[21] Garzon R, Marcucci G, Croce CM (2010) Targeting microRNAs in cancer: rationale, strategies and challenges. Nat Rev Drug Discov 9: 775-789

[22] Gibb EA, Brown CJ, Lam WL (2011) The functional role of long non-coding RNA in human carcinomas. Mol Cancer 10: 38

[23] Goldstein I, Marcel V, Olivier M et al (2011) Understanding wild-type and mutant p53 activities in human cancer: new landmarks on the way to targeted therapies. Cancer Gene Ther 18: 2-11

[24] Gregory RI, Yan KP, Amuthan G et al (2004) The microprocessor complex mediates the genesis of microRNAs. Nature 432: 235-240

[25] Gregory RI, Chendrimada TP, Cooch N et al (2005) Human RISC couples microRNA biogenesis and posttranscriptional gene silencing. Cell 123: 631-640

[26] Guo C, Sah JF, Beard L et al (2008) The noncoding RNA, miR-126, suppresses the growth of neoplastic cells by targeting phosphatidylinositol 3-kinase signaling and is frequently lost in colon cancers. Genes Chromosomes Cancer 47: 939-946

[27] He L, He X, Lim LP et al (2007a) A microRNA component of the p53 tumour suppressor network. Nature 447: 1130-1134

[28] He X, He L, Hannon GJ (2007b) The guardian's little helper: microRNAs in the p53 tumor suppressor network. Cancer Res 67: 11099-11101

[29] Hermeking H (2010) The miR-34 family in cancer and apoptosis. Cell Death Differ 17: 193-199

[30] Huang Q, Gumireddy K, Schrier M et al (2008) The microRNAs miR-373 and miR-520c promote tumour invasion and metastasis. Nat Cell Biol 10: 202-210

[31] Hutvágner G, McLachlan J, Pasquinelli AE et al (2001) A cellular function for the RNA-interference enzyme Dicer in the maturation of the let-7 small temporal RNA. Science 293: 834-838

[32] Joseph NM, Mosher JT, Buchstaller J et al (2008) The loss of Nf1 transiently promotes self-renewal but not tumorigenesis by neural crest stem cells. Cancer Cell 13: 129-140

[33] Kallergi G, Papadaki MA, Politaki E et al (2011) Epithelial to mesenchymal transition markers expressed in circulating tumour cells of early and metastatic breast cancer patients. Breast Cancer Res 13: R59

[34] King AA, Debaun MR, Riccardi VM et al (2000) Malignant peripheral nerve sheath tumors in neurofibromatosis 1. Am J Med Genet 93: 388-392

[35] Kleihues P, Cavenee WK (2000) World Health Organization classification of tumours pathology and genetics of tumours of nervous system. International Agency for Research on Cancer (IARC), Lyon

[36] Kozaki K, Imoto I, Mogi S et al (2008) Exploration of tumor-suppressive microRNAs silenced by DNA hypermethylation in oral cancer. Cancer Res 68: 2094-2105

[37] Krol J, Loedige I, Filipowicz W (2010) The widespread regulation of microRNA biogenesis, function and decay. Nat Rev Genet 11: 597-610

[38] Kwiecinski M, Noetel A, Elfimova N et al (2011) Hepatocyte growth factor (HGF) inhibits collagen I and IV synthesis in hepatic stellate cells by miRNA-29 induction. PLoS One 6: e24568

[39] Kwok WK, Ling MT, Lee TW et al (2005) Up-regulation of TWIST in prostate cancer and its implication as a therapeutic target. Cancer Res 65: 5153-5162

[40] Lee RC, Feinbaum RL, Ambros V (1993) The C. elegans heterochronic gene lin-4 encodes small RNAs with antisense complementarity to lin-14. Cell 75: 843-854

[41] Lee TK, Poon RT, Yuen AP et al (2006) Twist overexpression correlates with hepatocellular carcinoma metastasis through induction of epithelial-mesenchymal transition. Clin Cancer Res 12: 5369-5376

[42] Lee YB, Bantounas I, Lee DY et al (2009) Twist-1 regulates the miR-199a/214 cluster during development. Nucleic Acids Res 37: 123-128

[43] Lee MJ, Cho JH, Galas DJ et al (2011) The systems biology of neurofibromatosis type 1—critical roles for microRNA. Exp Neurol 235(2): 464-468

[44] Lu J, Getz G, Miska EA et al (2005) MicroRNA expression profiles classify human cancers. Nature 435: 834-838

[45] Lund E, Güttinger S, Calado A et al (2004) Nuclear export of microRNA precursors. Science 303: 95-98

[46] Ma K, He Y, Zhang H et al (2012) DNA methylation-regulated miR-193a-3p dictates resistance of hepatocellular carcinoma to 5-fluorouracil via repression of SRSF2 expression. J Biol Chem 287: 5639-5649

[47] Mantripragada KK, Spurlock G, Kluwe L et al (2008) High-resolution DNA copy number profiling of malignant peripheral nerve sheath tumors using targeted microarray-based comparative genomic hybridization. Clin Cancer Res 14: 1015-1024

[48] Miller SJ, Rangwala F, Williams J et al (2006) Large-scale molecular comparison of human schwann cells to malignant peripheral nerve sheath tumor cell lines and tissues. Cancer Res 66: 2584-2591

[49] Nakano H, Miyazawa T, Kinoshita K et al (2010) Functional screening identifies a microRNA, miR-491 that induces apoptosis by targeting Bcl-X(L) in colorectal cancer cells. Int J Cancer 127: 1072-1080

[50] Nana-Sinkam SP, Croce CM (2011) MicroRNAs as therapeutic targets in cancer. Transl Res 157: 216-225

[51] Newby AC (2006) Matrix metalloproteinases regulate migration, proliferation, and death of vascular smooth muscle cells by degrading matrix and non-matrix substrates. Cardiovasc Res 69: 614-624

[52] Nie J, Liu L, Zheng W et al (2012) microRNA-365, down-regulated in colon cancer, inhibits cell cycle progression and promotes apoptosis of colon cancer cells by probably targeting Cyclin D1 and Bcl-2. Carcinogenesis 33: 220-225

[53] Ou DL, Chien HF, Chen CL et al (2008) Role of twist in head and neck carcinoma with lymph node metastasis. Anticancer Res 28: 1355-1359

[54] Pasmant E, Masliah-Planchon J, Levy P et al (2011a) Identification of genes potentially involved in the increased risk of malignancy in NF1-microdeleted patients. Mol Med 17: 79-87

[55] Pasmant E, Sabbagh A, Masliah-Planchon J et al (2011b) Role of noncoding RNA ANRIL in genesis of plexiform neurofibromas in neurofibromatosis type 1. J Natl Cancer Inst 103: 1713-1722

[56] Peng RQ, Wan HY, Li HF et al (2012) MicroRNA-214 suppresses the growth and invasiveness of cervical cancer cells by targeting UDP-N-acetyl-alpha-D-galactosamine: polypeptide N-acetylgalactosaminyltransferase 7. J Biol Chem 287: 14301-14309

[57] Penna E, Orso F, Cimino D et al (2011) microRNA-214 contributes to melanoma tumour progression through suppression of TFAP2C. EMBO J 30: 1990-2007

[58] Perrin GQ, Li H, Fishbein L et al (2007) An orthotopic xenograft model of intraneural NF1 MPNST suggests a potential association between steroid hormones and tumor cell proliferation. Lab Invest 87: 1092-1102

[59] Presneau N, Eskandarpour M, Shemais T et al (2012) MicroRNA profiling of peripheral nerve sheath tumours identifies miR-29c as a tumour suppressor gene involved in tumour progression. Br J Cancer (In Press)

[60] Raver-Shapira N, Marciano E, Meiri E et al (2007) Transcriptional activation of miR-34a contributes to p53-mediated apoptosis. Mol Cell 26: 731-743

[61] Reimer D, Sadr S, Wiedemair A et al (2007) Clinical relevance of E2F family members in ovarian cancer—an evaluation in a training set of 77 patients. Clin Cancer Res 13: 144-151

[62] Salmena L, Carracedo A, Pandolfi PP (2008) Tenets of PTEN tumor suppression. Cell 133: 403-414

[63] Song B, Wang Y, Xi Y et al (2009) Mechanism of chemoresistance mediated by miR-140 in human osteosarcoma and colon cancer cells. Oncogene 28: 4065-4074

[64] Steele R, Mott JL, Ray RB (2010) MBP-1 upregulates miR-29b that represses Mcl-1, collagens, and matrix-metalloproteinase-2 in prostate cancer cells. Genes Cancer 1: 381-387

[65] Subramanian S, Thayanithy V, West RB et al (2010) Genome-wide transcriptome analyses reveal p53 inactivation mediated loss of miR-34a expression in malignant peripheral nerve sheath tumours. J Pathol 220: 58-70

[66] Sun Y, Bai Y, Zhang F et al (2010) miR-126 inhibits non-small cell lung cancer cells proliferation by targeting EGFL7. Biochem Biophys Res Commun 391: 1483-1489

[67] Swarbrick A, Woods SL, Shaw A et al (2010) miR-380-5p represses p53 to control cellular survival and is associated with poor outcome in MYCN-amplified neuroblastoma. Nat Med 16: 1134-1140

[68] Thomas M, Lieberman J, Lal A (2010) Desperately seeking microRNA targets. Nat Struct Mol Biol 17: 1169-1174

[69] Torres KE, Zhu QS, Bill K et al (2011) Activated MET is a molecular prognosticator and potential therapeutic target for malignant peripheral nerve sheath tumors. Clin Cancer Res 17: 3943-3955

[70] Tricoli JV, Jacobson JW (2007) MicroRNA: potential for cancer detection, diagnosis, and prognosis. Cancer Res 67: 4553-4555

[71] Upadhyaya M, Ruggieri M, Maynard J et al (1998) Gross deletions of the neurofibromatosis type 1 (NF1) gene are predominantly of maternal origin and commonly associated with a learning disability, dysmorphic features and developmental delay. Hum Genet 102: 591-597

[72] Van Kouwenhove M, Kedde M, Agami R (2011) MicroRNA regulation by RNA-binding proteins and its implications for cancer. Nat Rev Cancer 11: 644-656

[73] Verdijk RM, den Bakker MA, Dubbink HJ et al (2010) TP53 mutation analysis of malignant peripheral nerve sheath tumors. J Neuropathol Exp Neurol 69: 16-26

[74] Visone R, Croce CM (2009) miRNAs and cancer. Am J Pathol 174: 1131-1138

[75] Volinia S, Calin GA, Liu CG et al (2006) A microRNA expression signature of human solid tumors defines cancer gene targets. Proc Natl Acad Sci USA 103: 2257-2261

[76] von Frowein J, Pagel P, Kappler R et al (2011) MicroRNA-492 is processed from the keratin 19 gene and up-regulated in metastatic hepatoblastoma. Hepatology 53: 833-842

[77] Wang S, Aurora AB, Johnson BA et al (2008) The endothelial-specific microRNA miR-126 governs vascular integrity and angiogenesis. Dev Cell 15: 261-271

[78] Wu BL, Austin MA, Schneider GH et al (1995) Deletion of the entire NF1 gene detected by the FISH: four deletion patients associated with severe manifestations. Am J Med Genet 59: 528-535

[79] Xiong X, Ren HZ, Li MH et al (2011) Down-regulated miRNA-214 induces a cell cycle G1 arrest in gastric cancer cells by up-regulating the PTEN protein. Pathol Oncol Res 17: 931-937

[80] Yanaihara N, Caplen N, Bowman E et al (2006) Unique microRNA molecular profiles in lung cancer diagnosis and prognosis. Cancer Cell 9: 189-198

[81] Yang H, Kong W, He L et al (2008) MicroRNA expression profiling in human ovarian cancer: miR-214 induces cell survival and cisplatin resistance by targeting PTEN. Cancer Res 68: 425-433

[82] Yap KL, Li S, Munoz-Cabello AM et al (2010) Molecular interplay of the noncoding RNA ANRIL and methylated histone H3 lysine 27 by polycomb CBX7 in transcriptional silencing of INK4a. Mol Cell 38: 662-674

[83] Yu J, Deshmukh H, Payton JE et al (2011) Array-based comparative genomic hybridization identifies *CDK4* and *FOXM1* alterations as independent predictors of survival in malignant peripheral nerve sheath tumor. Clin Cancer Res 17: 1924-1934

[84] Yuen HF, Chua CW, Chan YP et al (2007) Significance of TWIST and E-cadherin expression in the metastatic progression of prostatic cancer. Histopathology 50: 648-658

[85] Zhang XJ, Ye H, Zeng CW et al (2010) Dysregulation of miR-15a and miR-214 in human pancreatic cancer. J Hematol Oncol 3: 46

第40章 儿童和成人1型神经纤维瘤病的转化/临床研究

Translational/Clinical Studies in Children and Adults with Neurofibromatosis Type 1

Bruce Korf, Brigitte Widemann, Maria T. Acosta, and Roger J. Packer

40.1 引言

1型神经纤维瘤病（NF1）是一种由 *NF1* 基因突变引起的复杂疾病。已确定了数百种不同类型的 *NF1* 突变，这可能导致该疾病出现多变的临床表现，并在开发有效疗法时带来相当大的挑战。NF1 的儿童和成人都面临着疾病的急性和慢性临床表现的风险。治疗干预措施不仅要考虑治疗对急性症状的影响，还要考虑对疾病表现的慢性影响。大多数与 NF1 相关的并发症不会危及生命，但可能导致严重的长期不适和残疾。

当 NF1 首次被提出时，该疾病的一个特征是肿瘤围绕着神经组织周围生长。在过去的 20 年里，我们对 NF1 的理解有了很大提高，认识到 *NF1* 基因突变不仅会导致施万细胞异常，还会影响脑部发育以及其他器官（Zhu et al. 2002；Reilly et al. 2008）。疾病的临床表现范围广泛，从常见的慢性疾病（如皮肤型神经纤维瘤和学习障碍等）到急性、严重的并发症（如恶性周围神经鞘膜瘤和脑瘤），所有这些临床表现都是潜在的临床试验目标（Gutmann et al. 1997）。过去，针对儿童和成人 NF1 的治疗基本上是经验性的，使用具有类似临床表现的其他疾病的治疗方法。例如，由于瘙痒是皮肤型神经纤维瘤的常见特征，早期的研究使用抗组胺药来缓解症状并可能减少其他神经纤维瘤的相关症状（Riccardi and Mulvhill 1981；Riccardi 1993）。随着 NF1 的分子发病机制被逐步阐明，创新的靶向治疗方法成为可能。在对 NF1 患者进行治疗研究之前，评估这些新疗法所需的临床前和转化数据尚未明确。虽然对人体组织的分子分析已经产生深刻理解，但这些组织的获取通常有限，将人体组织转化为细胞系的能力也有限。各种 NF1 临床表现的小鼠模型增加了我们对这种疾病的理解，并确定了肿瘤中不同细胞类型、肿瘤微环境和肿瘤发展所需因素之间的重要相互作用；然而，小鼠建模有其自身的局限性，在很多情况下，并没有像最初希望的那样提供足够的信息。

将这些生物学进展转化为治疗方法还带来其他

挑战。尽管 NF1 是一种相对常见的遗传性疾病（特别是神经遗传），但对于某种类型的并发症，具有活动性疾病表现的患者数量可能很少，这使得大规模临床试验变得困难，尤其是那些需要对照组来证明疗效的试验。虽然这种疾病的临床表现非常严重，但通常是慢性的，要求成本效益比不仅要考虑治疗的短期效益，还要考虑长期的潜在影响。NF1 的某些并发症具有不规律的自然病程，使得疗效的评估变得困难。一些表现可能是终生的，然而与视神经胶质瘤患者情况一样，疾病的进展可能发生在离散的时间窗口内。此外，NF1 患者的治疗副作用也可能不同。

尽管存在这些限制和挑战，NF1 患者的管理已经进入了治疗时代。现在有大量的新药可以使用，可能会使患者受益。临床试验的基础设施已经建立起来，可以更有效和迅速地研究新的疗法，同时，结果测量也变得更加精细和有价值。例如，通过国防部的资助，美国自 2006 年起一直资助一个多中心、多学科的临床试验联盟。

本章将重点介绍一些与 NF1 相关的常见疾病的治疗方法，包括神经纤维瘤病（主要是丛状神经纤维瘤）、恶性周围神经鞘膜瘤、胶质瘤（主要是视神经胶质瘤）和学习障碍。还将简要讨论该疾病的其他并发症的治疗方法。将强调每种临床表现的机制，以及基于证据的临床治疗干预措施。

40.2 临床前建模的基本原则

临床前实验为 NF 患者的临床试验提供了识别潜在治疗靶点和方法的可能性。治疗方法可能包括重新利用现有药物以及发现新的化合物。尽管前者可以在不进行广泛临床前实验的情况下用于临床试验，但临床前实验提供了一种预筛选最有效化合物的方法，从而使资源集中在那些最有可能有效的化合物上。临床前实验系统包括体内和体外模型，每种模型都有其独特的优缺点。

体外模型包括细胞培养体系，细胞系可以从人或小鼠的恶性肿瘤，特别是恶性周围神经鞘膜瘤（MPNST）中获得（Fang et al. 2009；Hakozake et al. 2009；Wallace et al. 2000），可以无限传代。尽管肿瘤细胞系被用作研究模型，但细胞在体外经历持续的遗传进化，因此细胞系并不能完全反映原始肿瘤的特性。对非恶性组织（如成纤维细胞、黑色素细胞、施万细胞和发育不良的骨骼）的研究是在人或小鼠病变组织的原代细胞上进行的。某些情况下，可以培养具有生殖系 NF1 突变的施万细胞或具有获得性体细胞突变的双等位基因 NF1 突变的施万细胞。

各种实验指标可用于评估细胞模型。表型评估包括检测细胞增殖、存活和运动能力等。生化指标包括检测细胞信号蛋白如 RAS、MAPK 和 mTOR 等的激活情况。还可以在基因表达水平进行检测。细胞培养体系具有相对较低的成本和高效的优点，因此适合大规模筛选潜在的治疗化合物。还可以扩展到通过机器人系统大规模筛选化学库，用于发现一些新的治疗候选药物。然而，一个主要的缺点是体外系统可能无法准确反映 NF 表型的复杂性，尤其是那些涉及不同类型细胞之间相互作用的表型。此外，体外培养的细胞可能会继续进化，选择有利于培养生长而不是患者体内生长的特性。

动物模型则呈现相反的问题——成本更高、周期更慢，但更能准确反映疾病的生物学特性。除了一些关于牛丛状神经纤维瘤的报告，还没有其他天然的 NF 动物模型（Sartin et al. 1994）。科学家们已经通过基因工程技术在不同生物体中制备了 NF 动物模型，包括果蝇、斑马鱼和小鼠。果蝇具有低成本和能够在遗传水平上广泛研究的优势，有助于研究与 NF 基因产物相互作用的基因（Guo et al. 1997）。尽管果蝇中 NF 突变的表型与人类相差很大，但仍可用于药物筛选。斑马鱼模型因为较低的成本，以及其较短的繁殖时间也使其成为一个可用于研究 NF 的动物模型（Lee et al. 2010）。

小鼠一直是研究各种类型神经纤维瘤病最常用的模型（Brossier and Carroll 2011）。最初的杂合小鼠 Nf1 敲除模型（Brannan et al. 1994；Jacks et al. 1994）没有表现出类似 NF 的表型；小鼠发展成嗜铬细胞瘤，最终死于血液系统恶性肿瘤，但并未发展成神经纤维瘤。纯合子被发现是胚胎致死的，并伴有心血管系统的缺陷。在 $Nf1^{+/-}$ 背景下具有 $Nf1^{-/-}$ 细胞的嵌合动物确实发生了丛状神经纤维瘤（Cichowski et al. 1999），这是首次证明 NF1 具有抑癌基因的功能。后来的条件性敲除模型（一个等位基因受不同细胞类型中活化的 Cre 重组酶控制）已被证明可以复刻多种 NF1 的特征，包括丛状神经纤维瘤、皮肤型神经纤维瘤、视神经胶质瘤、骨骼发育不良和星形细胞瘤（Bajenaru et al. 2003；Kolanczyk et al. 2008；Lee et al. 2010；Parada et al. 2005；Reilly et al. 2000；Wang et al. 2011；Zhu et al. 2005）。Nf1 和 TP53 双敲除导致 MPNST 的发生（Cichowski et al. 1999）。除了这些基因工程模型，异种移植系统也被用于在小鼠中培养肿瘤移植体以进行相关的药物研究（Appenzeller et al. 1986；Babovic-Vuksanovic et al. 2004；Perrin et al. 2007）。

这些不同的模型为研究人员提供了多种药物测试及开发的工具。儿童肿瘤基金会资助了一个 NF 临床前联盟，可以在这些系统中对 NF1 和 NF2 中的良性和恶性肿瘤进行药物测试。

40.3 丛状神经纤维瘤

40.3.1 治疗挑战的概述

丛状神经纤维瘤（plexiform neurofibromas，PN）是一种组织学良性的神经鞘瘤，沿着神经生长并涉及神经的多个分支（Korf 1999）。高达 40% 的 NF 患者会患有这种肿瘤，因为相关的并发症如外观畸形、严重功能障碍以及手术切除的巨大挑战，使得其成为临床试验的主要候选对象（Canavese and Krajbich 2011；Korf 1999；Prada et al. 2012）。丛状神经纤维瘤最常见于儿童，通常在生命早期生长最快（Dombi et al. 2007；Friedrich et al. 2003）。它们可能在体外可见，导致软组织增生，或隐藏在体内深处，除非进行影像检查，否则可能无法诊断。眶面部丛状神经纤维瘤可导致面部畸形和视力或听力丧失，颈部肿瘤可导致气道受压，臂丛或腰丛肿瘤可导致周围神经功能障碍，纵隔肿瘤可导致肺阻塞，腹部肿瘤可导致肠梗阻，盆腔丛状神经纤维瘤可能阻塞输尿管或膀胱，脊柱任何部位的丛状神经纤维瘤都可能侵入神经孔并压迫脊髓。丛状神经纤维瘤常伴有骨发育不良，包括眼眶肿瘤导致蝶骨缺损、脊柱肿瘤导致脊柱侧凸以及四肢肿瘤导致骨畸形等。此外，8%～13% 的丛状神经纤维瘤进展为恶性周围神经鞘膜瘤，其特点是高侵袭性和高死亡率（Evans et al. 2002）。

目前治疗丛状神经纤维瘤的唯一方法是手术，但手术操作困难并且效果通常不佳。除非肿瘤能完全切除，否则很可能复发（Needle et al. 1997），但丛状神经纤维瘤形态大且不规则，通常无法完全切除。其血管丰富，手术期间有出血风险，并且很难确定肿瘤边界。在某些情况下，会栓塞供血血管以减少手术期间的失血量（Canavese and Krajbich 2011；Tanaka et al. 2005）。

迫切需要开发有效的药物疗法，以阻止丛状神经纤维瘤的生长、减小其大小并降低发病率。科学家们在丛状神经纤维瘤的发病机制、分子生物学和自然病史方面的研究取得了实质性的进展，再加上对丛状神经纤维瘤临床试验设计和这些复杂肿瘤图像分析的专业知识不断增加，使得开发靶向性药物成为可能。

40.3.2 临床转化

丛状神经纤维瘤由致瘤性施万细胞、成纤维细胞、神经束膜细胞和肥大细胞组成。致瘤性施万细胞缺乏 NF1 基因表达，神经纤维瘤蛋白的缺失与活化的 RAS 水平升高有关（Kluwe et al. 1999；Serra et al. 2000）。RAS 激活可引发一系列信号转导，如 RAF/MEK/MAPK 和 PI3K/AKT/mTOR 的激活（Dasgupta et al. 2005；Johannessen et al. 2005；Lau et al. 2000）。PN 的生长因子和生长因子受体表达增加，包括血管内皮生长因子（vascular endothelial growth factor，VEGF）、表皮生长因子受体（epidermal growth factor receptor，EGFR）和血小板衍生生长因子受体（platelet-derived growth factor receptor，PDGFR）等，这些可能会促进肿瘤的发生、发展（DeClue et al. 2000；Kawachi et al. 2003；Kim et al. 1997；Ling et al. 2005）。虽然施万细胞 NF1 的缺失足以产生肿瘤，但完全由 NF1 介导的肿瘤发生需要两方面：一是肿瘤细胞的 NF1 缺失，二是非肿瘤细胞中的杂合性缺失，这表明肿瘤微环境在神经纤维瘤发展中起着重要作用（Zhu et al. 2002）。有研究证明了这一点，$NF1^{+/-}$ 肥大细胞在神经纤维瘤发展中发挥着作用，这是由于 NF1 缺失的施万细胞分泌 kit 配体所致（Yang et al. 2003，2006，2008）。

丛状神经纤维瘤治疗的很多潜在靶点与正在开发的肿瘤新药是相同的，如 RAS、血管生成相关蛋白和 mTOR 等。随着丛状神经纤维瘤转基因小鼠模型的建立，新药的临床前评估已变得可行（Cichowski et al. 1999；Gutmann et al. 2002；Wu et al. 2008；Yang et al. 2008），进而合理地进行靶向药物的临床试验。例如，C-kit 和 PDGFR 抑制剂甲磺酸伊马替尼在丛状神经纤维瘤小鼠模型中的应用，促成伊马替尼用于治疗无法手术的丛状神经纤维瘤的临床试验（Yang et al. 2008），在一些患者中观察到症状改善和肿瘤缩小（Robertson et al. 2011）。

40.3.3 临床试验

最初的丛状神经纤维瘤临床试验采用与肿瘤学临床试验类似的设计，但 NF1 和 PN 的一些情况与难治性肿瘤不同，需要采用新的药物开发方法（Kim et al. 2009；Packer et al. 2002）。例如，用于测量肿瘤大小和评估实验反应的标准方法（一维 RECIST 和二维 WHO 标准）（Miller et al. 1981；Therasse et al. 2000）不足以量化 PN 有临床意义的变化（Widemann et al. 2006）。近年来，体积磁共振成像分析得到了发展（Cai et al. 2009；Poussaint et al. 2003；Solomon et al. 2004），并应用于临床试验（Babovic-Vuksanovic et al. 2006，2007；Jakacki et al. 2011a、b），能够更灵敏和可重复地记录肿瘤的生长。

临床试验的开展侧重于开发靶向性、基于生物学的治疗方法，目前只有一项针对化学治疗药物（甲氨蝶呤和长春新碱）的临床试验正在进行中。表 40.1 总结了已完成和正在进行的针对 PN 的靶向药物的临床试验。由于 NF1 患者和难治性肿瘤患者对药物的耐受性存在差异，因此对 NF1 丛状神经纤维瘤的几种药物进行了单独的 I 期临床试验。NF1 丛状神经纤维瘤的 I 期临床试验是安全的，并且与儿童或成人难治性肿瘤相比，其毒性在可耐受的剂量下是可接受的，除了索拉非尼（sorafenib）的儿童 I 期试验之外（Kim et al. 2009），该试验在 NF1 儿童中的耐受性低于难治性癌症儿童（Widemann et al. 2009a，b），是因为在使用索拉非尼治疗期间出现严重的丛状神经纤维瘤疼痛。与难治性癌症儿童相比，NF1 儿童在临床试验中接受实验性药物的时间更长，并且他们在参加临床试验时年龄更小（Kim et al. 2009）。因此，对于丛状神经纤维瘤的临床试验，必须仔细、纵向的评估潜在累积的毒性（Kim et al. 2009），这些毒性可能在药物暴露时间较短的年长儿童或成人中无法检测到。

利用体积 MRI 分析 PN 肿瘤缩小和疾病进展已成为多个 II 期临床试验的主要终点。一项随机、双盲、安慰剂对照、法尼基转移酶抑制剂替比法尼交叉 II 期临床试验的安慰剂组（Widemann et al. 2009a、b）已在后续多项实验中被用作对照组，以确定药物活性。与安慰剂相比，替比法尼并未使进展时间加倍。在替比法尼试验中，进行性丛状神经纤维瘤患者在试验开始时的中位进展时间为 10.6 个月，这突显与癌症肿瘤相比，记录丛状神经纤维瘤疾病进展所需的时间要更长。

虽然目前尚未确定标准的药物治疗方法，但在多项实验中观察到丛状神经纤维瘤缩小和症状改善（Babovic-Vuksanovic et al. 2006；Gupta et al. 2003；Jakacki et al. 2011a、b；Robertson et al. 2011）。因此，随着 NF 临床前和临床试验联盟的发展，有望大大加速丛状神经纤维瘤有效治疗方法的开发。

40.4 神经胶质瘤

40.4.1 治疗挑战的概述

神经胶质瘤在 NF1 的儿童和成人中并不罕见，超过 20% 的患者在其一生中会患有神经胶质瘤（Listernick et al. 1989，1997）。神经胶质瘤出现在大脑的不同区域，迄今为止最常见的是发生在 5 岁以下儿童的视觉通路。这种病变通常明显累及视交叉、视束和视放射。在筛查中可能会发现视觉通

表 40.1 已完成和正在进行的靶向治疗 NF1 相关丛状神经纤维瘤（PN）的临床试验

药物	作用靶点	阶段	数量	计划	入组条件	试验终止	反应评估	结果	参考文献
13-顺式维甲酸（CRA）或干扰素 α、干扰素 2α（IFN）	血管分化	II	57	CRA 口服，每天 1 次×21 天，28 天一周期 IFN 皮下注射，每天 1 次	进展型 PN；儿童和成人	缓解，TTP	2D	86% CRA 和 96% IFN 治疗者 18 个月内病情稳定；3 名 CRA 和 2 名 IFN 治疗者肿瘤缩小 10%~20%；3 名 CRA 和 5 名 IFN 治疗者症状改善	Packer 等（2002）
沙利度胺	血管生成	I	20	连续口服	进展型 PN；>5 岁	毒性	2D	最大剂量 200 mg/天；4 名患者肿瘤缩小幅度<25%；8 名症状改善	Gupta 等（2003）
替吡法尼	FTase	I	17	口服，每天 2 次，21 天，28 天一周期	无法手术的 PN；3~21 岁	毒性；PK, PD	WHO	最大耐受剂量 200 mg/(m²·d)，每天 2 次，21 d，28 天一周期，未观察到累积毒性	Widemann 等（2006）
		II	60	口服，每天 2 次，21 天，28 天一周期	进展型 PN；3~25 岁	TTPª（PN 体积增加 20%）	3D MRI	与安慰剂相比，TTP 没有增加 1 倍	Widemann 等（2009a, b）
吡非尼酮	成纤维细胞	I	24	连续口服	无法手术的 PN；成人	缓解	3D MRI	7 名患者肿瘤缩小幅度>15%；14 名患者症状改善	Babovic-Vuksanovic 等（2006）
		I	16	连续口服	无法手术的 PN；3~21 岁	毒性；PK	3D MRI	最佳剂量 500 mg/m²，3 次；无缓解	Babovic-Vuksanovic 等（2007）
		II	36	连续口服	进展型 PN；3~21 岁	TTPª	3D MRI	与安慰剂相比，TTP 没有增加 1 倍	Widemann 等（2009a, b）
聚乙二醇干扰素 α-2β	免疫，血管生成	I	30	皮下注射，每周 1 次	无法手术的 PN；1.3~21 岁	MTD	Who-3D MRI	最大耐受剂量 1 mg/kg 每周皮下注射；5/16 人疼痛改善；11/17 人 PN 体积缩小 15%~22%	Jakacki 等（2011a, b）
		II	—	皮下注射，每周 1 次	无法手术的，有症状的进展型 PN	TTPª；缓解ᵇ（PN 体积减小 20%）	临床 3D MRI	正在进行	—

续 表

药 物	作用靶点	阶段	数量	计 划	入组条件	试验终止	反应评估	结 果	参考文献
伊马替尼	C-Kit PDGFR VEGFR	II	36	儿童：440 mg/(m²·d) 成人：800 mg/天	儿童和成人	缓解；横截面积减小≥5%	2D	9/24 人缓解；7/24 人症状改善	Robertson 等(2011)
雷帕霉素	mTOR	II	—	连续口服	≥3岁；无法手术的 PN；放射学进展或稳定	进展型 PN：TTP[a] 稳定型 PN：缓解[b]	3D MRI	进展型 PN：正在进行中 稳定型 PN：无反应	Weiss 等(2010)
AZD2171	VEGFR2	II	—	连续口服	无法手术的 PN 或进展型 PN；成人	缓解	3D MRI	正在进行中	—
索拉非尼	C-Raf, B-Raf, VEGFR, C-Kit, PDGFR	I	6	连续口服	无法手术的 PN；3～21岁	毒性；PK,PD,DEMRI	3D MRI	与儿童实体瘤剂量相比，低剂量限制 PN 疼痛	Kim 等(2009)
尼洛替尼	C-Kit	II	—	—	成人	缓解	RECIST	正在进行中	—
AZD6244	MEK	I	—	连续口服	12～18岁	毒性，PK,PD	3D	正在进行中	—
舒尼替尼	VEGFR, PDGFR	II	—	—	儿童，成人	缓解	RECIST	即将开始	—

注：2D，二维；3D，三维；TTP，进展时间；PK，药代动力学；PD，药效学。[a] 定义为丛状神经纤维瘤体积增加≥20%的时间。[b] 定义为丛状神经纤维瘤体积减小≥20%。

路肿瘤，MRI 显示的肿瘤大小和范围可能与临床表现（包括视力和视野异常）不匹配。从 MRI 视觉通路和周围组织的异常信号强度区分活动性肿瘤是十分困难的。有时，MR 的异常会延伸到下丘脑、丘脑和大脑的其他周围区域，目前尚不清楚应针对病变的哪个部分进行治疗。视路胶质瘤的自然病程不稳定，增加了治疗的复杂性。尽管肿瘤晚期进展与视力减退有关，但大多数患者的肿瘤进展发生在疾病最初的几年。

发生在视觉通路以外部位的神经胶质瘤并不典型。局灶性和弥漫性神经胶质瘤似乎都倾向于起源于脑干，尽管在生命后期，皮质病变（包括涉及胼胝体的病变）发生的频率更高。同样，非视路神经胶质瘤的表现可能并不明显，这使得是否需要治疗变得难以决策。

大多数 NF1 相关神经纤维瘤是毛细胞星形细胞瘤，但也可能出现 2 级和恶性神经胶质瘤（Listernick et al. 1997，2007）。由于肿瘤位置以及此类肿瘤极有可能是毛细胞星形细胞瘤，手术干预，包括活检，通常被认为是不必要的或可能对视力或其他神经功能造成潜在伤害，因此患者通常在没有组织学确认的情况下接受治疗。对于视觉通路和脑干病变尤其如此（Pollack et al. 1996）。手术更常用于皮质肿物，以获得组织进行组织学诊断，并在特定情况下进行肿瘤的治疗。人体组织的缺乏限制了进行生物学研究的能力。治疗方法通常基于非 NF1 相关肿瘤的研究，因为大约 50% 的儿童视通路胶质瘤发生在非 NF1 患者中，并且比 NF1 相关病变更具侵袭性（Ater et al. 2011）。

40.4.2 临床转化

散发性毛细胞星形细胞瘤的分子发病机制最近得到了更好的阐明（Zhu et al. 2002；Gutmann et al. 2002；Hegedus et al. 2007）。60%～90% 的散发性肿瘤在组织学上和毛细胞星形细胞瘤一致，含有 RAS 信号通路中原癌基因 *BRAF* 的突变（Pfister et al. 2008）。大多数肿瘤是由于激活 *BRAF* 和 *KIAA* 的融合突变引起，少数肿瘤是由 *BRAF* 点突变引起。这些突变在 NF 相关的神经胶质瘤中尚未发现，NF1 患者的肿瘤发生需要双等位基因 *NF1* 基因失活（Gutmann et al. 2002）。*NF1* 基因表达的缺失并不发生在散发性肿瘤中。最近的全基因组关联研究表明，与散发性肿瘤相比，NF1 相关的毛细胞星形细胞瘤的基因表达谱存在差异。NF1 相关肿瘤的表达谱与培养的正常人类胎儿星形胶质细胞相似，而散发性毛细胞星形细胞瘤的表达谱通常与少突胶质细胞谱系有关（Lee et al. 2010）。

由于可供研究的人体组织相对缺乏，小鼠建模在开发用于治疗 NF1 患者神经胶质瘤（尤其是视路神经胶质瘤）的新分子靶向方法方面发挥了重要作用（Gutmann et al. 2002；Zhu et al. 2002）。目前只有少数基因敲除小鼠模型。这些模型显示视神经增生，其中一些发展为视通路神经胶质瘤（Hegedus et al. 2009；Zhu et al. 2005）。这些模型证实了 *NF1* 双等位基因缺失是肿瘤形成所必需的，但也揭示了单独的 *NF1* 缺失不足以形成星形细胞瘤，其他遗传因素或肿瘤微环境也会影响 NF1 相关神经胶质瘤的发生（Hegedus et al. 2009；Warrington et al. 2010；Lee et al. 2010）。*NF1* 杂合性会改变小胶质细胞的功能，导致其增殖和运动能力增强，并增加促生长分子的产生。此外，环磷酸腺苷的抑制会诱发 NF1 小鼠模型中神经胶质瘤的形成；这种抑制发生在视觉通路区域的发育时间窗中，可能部分解释了 NF1 儿童视觉通路肿瘤发生的时间（Zhu et al. 2005；Warrington et al. 2010；Sun et al. 2010）。神经纤维瘤蛋白的缺失与肿瘤微环境中其他促生长分子（如 CXCL12）的功能之间存在复杂的相互作用（Bajenaru et al. 2002，2003）。除其他变化外，这种相互作用还会影响 CXCR4 信号转导并诱导环磷酸腺苷水平的持续抑制（Dasgupta et al. 2003）。尽管已发现 CXCL12 单独表达不足以引起神经胶质瘤形成，但该通路的改变似乎对肿瘤生长极为重要（Sun et al. 2010）。已有研究证明，使用 PED4 抑制剂（罗利普仑）可以通过升高环磷酸腺苷抑制视神经胶质瘤的生长。

随着对视觉通路肿瘤发生发展的进一步研究，迄今为止，针对 NF 患儿神经胶质瘤的分子靶向治疗大多都是以 RAS 通路为靶点。这是基于前面讨论过的一个广为接受的观点，即神经纤维瘤蛋白作为 RAS 细胞内信号通路的负调节剂发挥作用，神经纤维瘤蛋白减少会导致 RAS 通路激活增加（Hegedus et al. 2007）。RAS 信号增加与哺乳动物星形胶质细胞中雷帕霉素（mammalian targeting of rapamycin，mTOR）的增加有关（Dasgupta et al. 2005）。小鼠模型显示，神经纤维瘤蛋白的缺失会导致胚胎形成过程中神经胶质祖细胞以 RAS 和 AKT 依赖的方式增殖（Hegedus et al. 2007）。mTOR/Rictor 介导的 AKT 激活是这种增殖的关键驱动因素。NF1 缺失的星形胶质细胞中 mTOR 的激活依赖 RAS 和 PI3K 信号的传导。

这些研究结果促进了临床试验的发展，然而，NF1 星形细胞瘤中信号通路的复杂性及可能存在的上下游生物反馈通路使得治疗更具挑战性。在肿瘤细胞中已经发现 mTOR 和 AKT 之间存在负反馈调控通路（Hidalgo 2012）。在对 mTOR 抑制敏感的细胞系中，已经注意到 AKT 的过度磷酸化和 AKT 激酶活性的增加。由于 AKT 信号与细胞存活途径相关，mTOR 对肿瘤生长的抑制可能会减弱。

克服由抑制负反馈通路造成的逃逸机制的一种可能方法（理论上可通过抑制 mTOR）是联合疗法，尝试阻断上游或其他信号靶标。研究表明，星形胶质细胞瘤过度表达表皮生长因子受体（epidermal growth factor receptor，EGFR）和磷酸化的 EGFR，使 EGFR 成为可能的上游靶标（Thorarinsdottir et al. 2008）。其他潜在靶标包括 PDGFR 和 VEGFR（McLaughlin et al. 2003）。在小鼠模型中，mTOR 和 PI3K 双抑制剂已显示出作为肿瘤抑制剂的潜在功效。还有一种方法是将生物制剂与化学治疗相结合以提高治疗效果。

40.4.3 临床试验

过去 20 年，研究者们已经针对毛细胞星形细胞瘤的儿童（包括 NF1 的儿童）进行了多项临床试验（Campagna et al. 2010；Gnekow et al. 2004；Gururangan et al. 2002, 2007；Hornstein et al. 2011；Jakacki et al. 2011a, b；Kadota et al. 1999；Lafay-Cousin et al. 2005；Lathier et al. 2003；Mahoney et al. 2000；Massimino et al. 2002a, b, 2010；McLaughlin et al. 2003；Mishra et al. 2010；Packer et al. 1993, 1997, 2009；Pons et al. 1992）（表 40.2）。开展此类试验的主要原因包括：NF1 相关星形细胞瘤和散发性星形细胞瘤患儿的诊断年龄较小；无法安全、广泛地切除中线肿瘤；以及担心放射治疗可能会对年幼患者造成严重的、不可逆的神经损伤，尤其是神经认知损伤。这些担忧在 NF1 相关视路胶质瘤的儿童中尤为突出，并且因为 NF1 相关辐射诱变和脑血管损伤的风险增加而加剧。这导致大多数（但并非所有）研究人员避免对进展期 NF1 相关低级别胶质瘤使用放射治疗。在为 NF1 患儿制订化学治疗方案时，一个值得关注的问题是人们不愿使用烷化剂或其他诱变性相对较高的药物，因为理论上担心会增加突变和继发性肿瘤（尤其是白血病）的发生。

表 40.2 部分儿童 NF1 和低级别胶质瘤的化学治疗试验

研 究	NF1 患者/所有研究患者	治疗时患者状态	肿瘤位置	客观缓解率：NF1/所有研究患者	PFS 或 EFS/所有 NF/所有研究患者
Packer 等（1993）卡铂/长春新碱	5/60	复发和 ND	所有	NG/58%	NG
Packer 等（1997）卡铂/长春新碱	15/63	ND	所有	50%/56%	2 年 PFS 79%±11%/75%±6%
Ater 等（2011）卡铂/长春新碱	127/401	ND	视觉通路	NG	5 年 EFS 69%/53%
Gnekow 等（2004）卡铂/长春新碱	36/123	ND	所有	NG	5 年 PFS 80%/53%

续 表

研 究	NF1患者/所有研究患者	治疗时患者状态	肿瘤位置	客观缓解率：NF1/所有研究患者	PFS或EFS/所有NF/所有研究患者
Laithier等(2003) 甲基苄肼、卡铂、依托泊苷、环磷酰胺、长春新碱	23/85	ND	视觉通路	NS/60%	2年PFS 82%/51%
Gururangan等(2002) 卡铂	22/81	复发和ND	所有	NS/28%	3年PFS 72%/62%
Mahoney等(2000) 卡铂	21/50	ND	视觉通路	2%/4%	3年PFS 67%/52%
Massimino等(2002a,b) 顺铂/依托泊苷	8/34	ND	所有	NG/70%	3年PFS 100%/78%
Massimino等(2010) 顺铂/依托泊苷	7/37	ND	所有	NG/64%	3年PFS NS/65%
Mishra等(2010) 硫代鸟嘌呤、洛莫司汀、长春新碱、甲基苄肼、二溴卫矛醇	6/33	ND	所有	NG	NG/30.3%

注：ND，新诊断；NG，未提供；NS，无显著差异；PFS，无进展生存期；EFS，无事件生存期。

到目前为止，在NF1相关神经胶质瘤患儿中，使用最多的疗法是卡铂和长春新碱的联合治疗(Packer et al. 1993, 1997)。这种联合用药是从放线菌素和长春新碱治疗儿童脑坏死症的经验中发展而来，最初经验性地应用于幼儿，主要是5岁以下的新诊断和复发的视路神经胶质瘤。对数百名NF1进展型低级别胶质瘤的青春期前儿童进行的研究显示，肿瘤的客观缓解率(不同研究定义不同，但至少要求肿瘤最大直径缩小25%)高达60%(Gnekow et al. 2004)。35%~40%的患者出现部分缓解和完全缓解，90%以上的患者在接受治疗期间病情趋于稳定。对于新诊断的进展期低级别胶质瘤患者，散发性毛细胞星形细胞瘤患者的疾病控制时间似乎与NF1相关肿瘤患者不同。虽然只有大约1/3的散发性肿瘤患者在接受卡铂和长春新碱方案治疗12~15个月后能维持治疗反应，但在开始治疗后3~5年内，近70%~80%的NF1相关肿瘤患儿能保持疾病缓解(Ater et al. 2011)。NF1合并脑干病变的患者也观察到了治疗反应。

在这些令人鼓舞的研究结果中，需要注意的是，尽管绝大多数患者在治疗期间病情会稳定或肿瘤缩小，而有些患者虽然放射学表现有所改善，但视力却会继续恶化(Campagna et al. 2010)。目前尚不清楚这是由于治疗效果不佳还是原有肿瘤对视觉功能的延迟影响。迄今为止，大多数研究都集中在放射学上的疾病反应和控制，而没有对视力进行评估。虽然卡铂和长春新碱治疗的耐受性相对较好，目前也未发现任何明显的突变增加，但这种疗法确实存在固有的副作用，包括与长春新碱相关的周围神经病变和与卡铂相关的骨髓抑制。在一些研究中，高达20%的患者会出现卡铂相关过敏的副作用，导致治疗提前终止。

如表40.2所示，NF1进展型视路和其他胶质瘤患者已经使用了替代化学治疗药物和药物治疗方案。如前所述，对于NF1儿童，人们不愿使用基于烷化剂的疗法，如TPDCV方案(6-硫代鸟嘌呤、甲基苄肼、二溴卫矛醇、洛莫司汀和长春新碱)或替莫唑胺(Ater et al. 2011; Gnekow et al. 2004)。同样，避免使用含依托泊苷的方案，即单独使用依托泊苷或联合使用依托泊苷。法国一个合作小组已使用甲基苄肼联合卡铂、依托泊苷联合顺铂和长春新碱联合环磷酰胺等积极化学治疗方案治疗NF1患者，效果和卡铂联合长春新碱治疗患者相似（Laithier et al. 2003）。除卡铂联合长春新碱方案外，使用最多的是长春新碱，特别是对卡铂过敏和单独使用卡铂的患者（Lafay-Cousin et al. 2005）。两种单药均显示出良好的效果，主要是延长疾病的稳定期。其他化学治疗方法包括使用长春瑞滨和低剂量顺铂及依托泊苷（Massimino et al. 2010）。后一种方案显示出较高的反应率，但人们担心它不适合用于视力已受损的儿童（因为顺铂会导致听力损失），也担心在NF1患者群体中使用依托泊苷。

对于NF1相关肿瘤的儿童，已经采用了分子靶向治疗，尽管大多数实验仍处于相对早期的发展阶段。贝伐单抗和伊立替康联合疗法在患和不患1型神经纤维瘤病的儿童中均显示出近70%的客观缓解率（Packer et al. 2009）。随后，儿童脑瘤联盟（Pediatric Brain Tumor Consortium）进行的一项前瞻性全国研究证实了3名NF1患儿初步获益。有趣的是，在这项有限的研究中，10名患儿中有7名不仅出现了客观缓解，并且视力得到恢复以及神经系统等症状得到明显改善。雷帕霉素和依维莫司等mTOR抑制剂目前正在临床试验中。雷帕霉素和塔西瓦联合使用用于克服因mTOR抑制导致的上游信号转导的反馈增加，对散发性低级别胶质瘤的疗效有限，但可延长NF1患者的病情稳定期，1名NF1患者有疾病缓解（Packer et al. 2010）。

40.5 神经认知功能障碍

40.5.1 治疗挑战的概述

虽然肿瘤易感性是NF1患者的主要问题，但一些更普遍的特征与肿瘤没有直接关系（Acosta et al. 2006）。40%～80%的NF1患者会出现认知功能障碍和学习困难（North et al. 1997；Hyman et al. 2006；Krab et al. 2008）。这些并发症影响患儿的日常生活，是NF1患者终生患病的最大原因（Acosta et al. 2006）。这些缺陷还会影响患者对社会的长期适应，导致生命质量低下（Acosta et al. 2006；Barton and North 2007；Krab et al. 2008）。

NF1的认知缺陷在过去20年才开始得到系统研究。早期对NF1人群智力功能的评估由于缺乏诊断标准，纳入了颅内肿瘤的患者，存在确认偏差以及使用非标准化心理测量评估，过高地评估了智力低下的发生率。最近的研究使用了更多的患者，仔细排除了颅内病变影响的病例，并仔细挑选对照人群（Hyman and North 2005；Acosta et al. 2006）。目前正在评估更可靠的表型（Acosta et al. 2006）。近年来，对NF1认知缺陷的临床和分子方面的研究取得了进展，以及神经影像学和分子遗传学技术的发展，都有可能对这些患者进行有效的干预（Costa et al. 2002；Li et al. 2005；Acosta et al. 2006）。

对该人群认知缺陷的经典描述包括以视觉空间学习缺陷作为主要特征，然而，如今很明显，NF1人群的认知缺陷表型比以前描述的更为复杂。随着从小鼠模型、基于生物学的观察和对大量患者的神经认知测试中获得的知识相结合，研究重点已转移到那些可能从生物学干预中获益的领域。识别患者的特定认知缺陷并应用生物和分子模型来研究影响小鼠模型中类似缺陷的潜在机制可能是一种有效的策略。降胆固醇药物洛伐他汀被证明可用于逆转NF1小鼠模型中的注意力缺陷（Li et al. 2005）。一项小规模试验的结果为正在进行的随机、双盲、安慰剂对照临床试验奠定了基础（Acosta et al. 2011）。随着该领域研究的不断深入，显然还有更多的研究机会。

对NF1儿童进行临床观察，结果显示注意缺陷多动障碍高发、与自闭症谱系障碍有关以及执行功能频繁受损，随后研究人员在小鼠模型上进行了生物实验，试图确定这些临床表现的分子基础。一旦确定了这些机制，下一步就是在患者身上验证这些机制。

40.5.2 临床前研究

$NF1^{+/-}$小鼠模型有助于测试与该疾病相关的几种表现的潜在治疗干预措施（Li et al. 2005；Cui et al. 2008，Hegedus et al. 2008），以及了解临床表现的生物学基础（Brown et al. 2010，2011）。尽管小鼠和人类之间存在明显差异，但分子和细胞研究表明，$NF1$基因突变导致的学习障碍在这两个物种中具有显著的相似性（Costa and Silva 2003）。*NF1* 基因突变对某些大脑功能的影响大于其他功能。例如，视觉空间学习（Silva et al. 1997）、注意力和运动协调能力都会受到影响，而各种学习形式（如经典条件反射）似乎并未受到影响。只有 40%～60% 的突变携带者受到影响，而补救训练可以缓解学习障碍（Silva et al. 1997）。NF1 认知表型的严重程度受遗传变异的影响，遗传变异会加剧 NF1 患者的问题，但对正常兄弟姐妹没有明显影响（Silva et al. 1997；Costa and Silva 2003）。与此相一致，研究表明，编码 N-甲基-D-天冬氨酸受体基因的杂合突变会增加同卵对照组学习障碍的严重程度。此外，遗传背景也会影响 $Nf1^{+/-}$ 小鼠学习障碍的发生率。这些相似性对研究 NF1 相关学习障碍的机制非常重要。表 40.3 展示了 NF1 小鼠模型的一些认知表型。

表 40.3 NF 小鼠模型的认知表型

动物模型	行为表型/其他生物学改变	与人类症状的比较	参考文献
$NF1^{+/-}$	Morris 水迷宫 恐惧条件反射 侧向反应时间任务 脉冲前抑制 延迟 win-shift 径向臂迷宫	视觉空间学习障碍 注意力障碍 工作记忆障碍	Silva 等（1997） Cui 等（2008） Li 等（2005） Shilyansky 等（2010）
$NF1\ 23a^{-/-}$	Morris 水迷宫 情境辨别 转棒实验	视觉空间学习障碍 运动障碍	Costa 等（2002）
NF1 flox/+;Synl-cre NF1 flox/+;Dlx 5/6-cre	Morris 水迷宫	视觉空间学习障碍	Cui 等（2008）
NF1 flox/flox	桶状皮质形成	自闭症谱系行为？	Lush 等（2008）
NF1 -/+ OPG	Morris 水迷宫中出现轻度空间学习/记忆障碍 注意力系统功能明显缺陷	注意力缺陷但不伴多动症	Brown 等（2010,2011）

40.5.3 临床转化和临床试验

治疗 NF1 患者认知缺陷的首个转化研究是使用降胆固醇药物洛伐他汀来逆转 NF1 儿童的认知缺陷。其理论依据是：*NF1* 基因突变导致 p21RAS 活性增加，这与在 NF1 小鼠和人类身上观察到的学习缺陷有关，从而提出了抑制 RAS 活性可逆转这些认知缺陷的假设（Silva et al. 1997；Costa and Silva 2003）。由于 p21RAS 发挥功能需要翻译后被法尼基化修饰，因此法尼基化被认为是 NF1 认知缺陷的药物治疗靶点。洛伐他汀是一种 3-羟基-3-甲基戊二酰辅酶 A 还原酶抑制剂，它能抑制 p21RAS 的异戊烯化和活性（Li et al. 2005）。Li 等研究了洛伐他汀对认知缺陷的影响，结果显示洛伐他汀可有效降低 p21RAS 活性并逆转 $Nf1^{+/-}$ 小鼠的注意力和学习能力缺陷（Li et al. 2005）。

虽然他汀类药物在小鼠模型中的治疗结果令人鼓舞，但辛伐他汀在人类身上并没有产生积极的结果（Krab et al. 2008）。值得注意的是，辛伐他汀试验并没有筛查特定的学习障碍，也没有排除智力迟钝的患者。最近完成的一项洛伐他汀 1 期开放安全临床试验显示（Acosta et al. 2011），在洛伐他汀治疗前后，患儿的认知能力明显改善，这表明洛伐他汀可能对治疗 NF1 儿童的认知障碍有效。由美国国防部资助的 NF 临床试验联盟正在进行一项多中心、Ⅱ 期、双盲、安慰剂对照临床试验，以在更大的儿童群体中对这些观察结果进行前瞻性研究。

目前正在小鼠模型中探索的其他神经认知障碍

包括多动症样症状、执行功能、工作记忆缺陷和自闭症谱系障碍,这些都有可能转化为人类干预措施。据报道,多达60%的NF1患者有类似多动症的症状(Brown et al. 2010),使用NF1视神经胶质瘤基因工程小鼠模型(GEM模型),报告了非选择性和选择性注意力缺陷,但没有伴随多动表型。与NF1的儿童相似,这些小鼠的注意力系统功能障碍在使用哌醋甲酯(methylphenidate,MPH)治疗后得到逆转,这表明大脑儿茶酚胺稳态存在失调,包括纹状体中多巴胺(dopamine,DA)水平降低。儿茶酚胺稳态在MPH或左旋多巴给药后恢复正常,被认为是NF1 GEM中注意力系统功能障碍的原因(Brown et al. 2010)。此外,利用神经影像学技术进行的PET研究显示纹状体多巴胺能稳态存在突触前缺陷。虽然哌甲酯和L-去甲肾上腺素能纠正PET成像显示的纹状体多巴胺水平和纠正NF1突变小鼠注意力系统功能的缺陷,但不能纠正这些小鼠中失调的环磷酸腺苷和RAS信号的转导。这些研究为评估治疗NF1相关多动症的药物建立了一个可靠的临床前模型。这些研究还支持临床观察,即兴奋剂药物可能有助于治疗与该人群多动症诊断相关的行为表现(Mautner et al. 2002),并进一步揭示了这些表现的病理生理学基础。

自闭症谱系障碍最近被认为是NF1患者认知谱系的一部分(Marui et al. 2004)。Lush等证实,神经纤维瘤蛋白是皮质桶状结构正常形成所必需的。复杂的遗传因素网络调节着皮质的发育。桶状皮质的改变与感觉融合失调和感觉调节过程有关,其中许多与自闭症谱系障碍有关。尽管在这一领域取得了初步成果,但进一步探索神经纤维瘤蛋白缺失与自闭症的生物学和临床相关性之间的生物学关联是研究干预措施的第一步。这是一个尚未得到系统探索的领域。最近在基于人群的系统评估中描述了对自闭症谱系障碍表现的识别和认识,行为问题、沟通和语言障碍是这一人群中经常出现的问题(Barton and North 2004)。自闭症谱系障碍在这一人群中的识别可能会为推进对这一人群的干预创造机会,并提高对可能产生自闭症表现的生物学基础改变的理解。

作为NF1患者认知表型的一部分,执行功能障碍已被广泛报道。在NF1小鼠模型中发现的工作记忆缺陷为更好地了解额叶发育过程中神经纤维瘤蛋白缺乏的影响打开了大门(Shilyansky et al. 2010)。神经纤维瘤蛋白调节前额叶和纹状体抑制网络,特别是活动依赖性GABA的释放,是工作记忆表现所必需的。这种机制被认为是$NF1^{+/-}$小鼠出现抑制依赖性工作记忆缺陷的原因。在对人类NF1受试者进行功能磁共振成像(fMRI)研究时,工作记忆评估显示皮质纹状体网络激活不足,工作记忆表现受损(Shilyansky et al. 2010)。这些小鼠和人的研究结果揭示了导致NF1工作记忆缺陷的相似分子和细胞机制,并可能带来针对工作记忆缺陷的干预措施。

在设计以认知缺陷为目标的生物临床试验时,大的挑战之一是使用可靠的测量方法。小鼠模型中使用的认知测量方法与人类认知领域中的等效测量方法需要仔细比对,这样才能验证分子靶点和干预措施。在某些情况下,基本认知机制可能具有可比性,如简单的注意力技能、定向或记忆。在其他情况下,执行功能任务、行为反应或社会互动可能难以在物种间进行比较。例如,在动物模型中,注意力、海马相关学习和视觉空间定向的测量结果与人类的某些相关功能是相关的。其他"人类特有的行为",如语言、社会交往和执行功能可能更为复杂,难以在物种间进行比较。为了将动物模型中的行为测试与人类行为关联起来,人们开发了大量的行为测试工具。正如对此类和其他遗传疾病引起的认知缺陷的潜在药物干预的评估一样,目前也需要对行为测量进行重新定义,并为物种间比较提供强有力的验证。

新技术可能提供一个观察功能变化的机会,这些功能变化可能比认知和行为异常更早被发现。神经成像技术可促进人们对动物模型和人类大脑功能的理解,并在使用明确的行为或认知测试之前就了解干预措施的影响。静息状态功能连接(resting state functional connectivity,RSFC)方法可以在没有外部刺激的情况下成功描绘功能性大脑网络(Chabernaud et al. 2012)。通过自发、低频大脑活动的同步模型,可以揭示无数的功能网络,这些网络与基于任务的fMRI方法中观察到的功能网络极为相似。此外,这项新技术还有可能用于多中心研究，利用现有的联盟促进临床试验的数据收集。最近由美国国立卫生研究院神经科学研究蓝图、神经成像信息工具和资源交换中心（NITRC）资助的一项试验（http：//www. NITRC. org），为功能和结构神经成像分析寻找和比较神经成像资源提供了便利。

40.6 恶性周围神经鞘膜瘤

40.6.1 治疗挑战的概述

恶性周围神经鞘膜瘤（malignant peripheral nerve sheath tumors，MPNST）也称为神经源性肉瘤、恶性神经鞘瘤或神经纤维肉瘤，是源自周围神经的软组织肉瘤，具有较高的局部复发和转移风险（Ferner and Gutmann 2002），占所有软组织肉瘤的10％。50％的MPNST发生在NF1患者身上，NF1患者一生中MPNST的发病率为8％～13％（Evans et al. 2002）。在NF1中，大多数但并非所有的MPNST都发生在原有的丛状神经纤维瘤中（King et al. 2000）。MPNST的早期诊断至关重要，因为只有完全手术切除才能治愈。NF1中MPNST的诊断可能难以确定或延迟，因为恶性肿瘤的临床指标（如疼痛、肿块增大和神经系统病变等）也可能是原有良性丛状神经纤维瘤的特征（Kim et al. 2009；Korf 1999）。MRI特征（Friedrich et al. 2005）和FDG-PET（Ferner et al. 2000，2008）可能有助于MPNST的诊断；然而，良性神经纤维瘤的FDG摄取率较高，需要进行活检才能确诊MPNST。必须仔细规划活检，以对MPNST最相关的肿瘤区域进行取样，并且可能需要进行多次活检。从组织学上看，大多数MPNST都是高级别的，其特点是高增殖指数、有丝分裂率和坏死（Costa et al. 1984；Trojani et al. 1984）。对于NF1患者，高肿瘤负荷（Mautner et al. 2008）、微缺失（De Raedt et al. 2003；Leppig et al. 1997）和之前接受过放射治疗可能会增加MPNST的发病风险。肿瘤体积大（>5 cm）、位置深、有远处转移是预后不良的特征（Scaife and Pisters 2003）。此外，大多数研究都显示NF1相关MPNST的总体生存率低于散发型MPNST，但原因尚不明确。例如，Carli等报道，29名NF1相关MPNST儿童的5年总生存率为32％，而138名散发性MPNST患者的5年总生存率为55％。同样，在最近的一项研究中，Ferrari等报告了27名NF1相关MPNST儿童的5年总生存率为11％，而44名散发性MPNST患者的5年总生存率为48％。与其他类型软组织肉瘤相比，MPNST的肉瘤特异性死亡风险最高（Ferrari et al. 2011；Kattan et al. 2002）。

MPNST的治疗方法与其他成人软组织肉瘤的治疗方法相同。只有完整的手术切除才能达到治愈的效果，这仍然是治疗的基石（Abbas et al. 1981；Scaife and Pisters 2003）。MPNST的局部复发率很高，从32％到65％不等（Gupta et al. 2008）。除手术外，放射治疗已被证实可改善成人软组织肉瘤的局部控制（Pisters et al. 1996；Yang et al. 1998），并且可用于改善>5 cm的高级别MPNST和边缘肿瘤切除术后的局部控制（Wong et al. 1998）。

化学治疗对MPNST的作用至今尚未明确。在成人软组织肉瘤中，只有多柔比星、达卡巴嗪和异环磷酰胺的缓解率始终保持在20％或以上，异环磷酰胺和多柔比星联合治疗的缓解率高达46％（Verma and Bramwell 2002）。以多柔比星为基础的辅助化学治疗并未在统计学上显示出总体生存率的显著提高（Verma and Bramwell 2002）。迄今为止，在组织学特异性实验中，尚未确定MPNST对用于治疗儿童和成人肉瘤的化学治疗药物的缓解率。两项研究表明，与散发性MPNST相比，NF1相关的MPNST对化学治疗的反应有所降低（Carli et al. 2005；Ferrari et al. 2011）。一项对167名MPNST儿童进行的大型回顾性分析中，47名散发性MPNST患者中有26名（55.3％）对化学治疗有反应，而17名NF1相关MPNST患者中有3名（17.6％）对化学治疗有反应（Carli et al. 2005）。第二项研究是来自几项临床试验前瞻性招募的患者，针对未转移未切除的儿童非横纹肌肉瘤软组织肉瘤，研究报告，与散发性MPNST[44例患者中有25例（34％）缓解]相比，NF1相关MPNST[27例患者中2例（7％）缓解]的化学治疗反应和总生存率下降（Ferrari et al.

2011)。确定散发性和 NF1 相关 MPNST 对标准肉瘤化学治疗的反应率是国防部正在进行的临床试验的主要目标。有不可切除或转移性 MPNST 且未接受过针对 MPNST 的化学治疗的患者,将根据散发性或 NF1 相关 MPNST 进行分层,并接受相同的化学治疗,包括异环磷酰胺、阿霉素和依托泊苷。根据结果,这项试验可能成为未来将化学治疗与靶向疗法相结合的试验平台。

由于 NF1 中 MPNST 的发病率高、治疗方案有限、死亡率高,迫切需要开发能够更早诊断 MPNST 的方法以及更有效的治疗方法。

40.6.2 临床转化

研究重点是开发能够更早发现 MPNST 的方法。例如,使用全身 MRI 进行纵向评估作为一种检测肿瘤负荷变化的工具,可以反映肿瘤的恶变(Tucker et al. 2009)。其他研究旨在识别生物标志物(Hummel et al. 2010),这可能有助于监测 NF1 患者是否发展为 MPNST。另外一个研究重点是更好地了解 MPNST 的发病机制。最近一项研究有力地支持了 MPNST 是通过 CDKN2A/B 缺失从非典型神经纤维瘤发展而来的,而 CDKN2A/B 缺失是发展为 MPNST 的第一步(Beert et al. 2011)。此外,多项研究旨在确定丛状神经纤维瘤和 MPNST 之间的差异,以确定 MPNST 的生物学治疗靶点。其中,p53、p16 和 p27(Beert et al. 2011; Perry et al. 2002)、EGFR(Li et al. 2002; Ling et al. 2005)、TWIST1(Miller et al. 2006)、SOX9(Miller et al. 2006)、mTOR(Johannessen et al. 2005, 2008; Johansson et al. 2008)、PDGFR(Holtkamp et al. 2006)、C-Kit(Holtkamp et al. 2006)、TOP2A(Skotheim et al. 2003)、IGF1R(Torres et al. 2011a, b; Yang et al. 2008)、MET(Torres et al. 2011a, b)和 HSP90(De Raedt et al. 2011)与 MPNST 的发病机制有关。MPNST 的异种移植(Johansson et al. 2008)和转基因小鼠模型(McClatchey and Cichowski 2001; Reilly et al. 2000)已经面世,在这些模型中进行的临床前试验可能对合理开展靶向药物临床试验具有重要意义。例如,mTOR 抑制剂在转基因动物(Johannessen et al. 2008)和异种移植(Johansson et al. 2008)中显示出活性。

基于这些发现,一项针对难治性 MPNST 患者的 mTOR 抑制剂联合血管生成抑制剂的临床试验已经启动,该试验可用于验证临床前的发现。

40.6.3 临床试验

表 40.4 总结了针对 MPNST 进行的几项组织特异性靶向药物的临床试验。EGFR 抑制剂厄洛替尼的 II 期临床试验是第一个针对 NF1 相关和散发型 MPNST 患者完成的靶向药物的临床试验(Albritton et al. 2006)。来自 13 家机构的 24 名患者在 22 个月内入组。大多数患者的病情进展迅速,厄洛替尼在 MPNST 中未显示活性。该试验表明,及时完成 MPNST 特异性试验是可行的。随后,一项针对包括成人 MPNST 在内的多种软组织肉瘤的 RAF 激酶和受体酪氨酸激酶抑制剂索拉非尼的 II 期临床试验启动(Maki et al. 2009)。索拉非尼对 MPNST 未表现出疗效,并且 MPNST 的中位无进展生存期(1.7 个月)和总生存期(4.9 个月)均短于所研究的其他软组织肉瘤,证实了与其他软组织肉瘤相比,MPNST 的预后较差。在随后的两项针对包括 MPNST 在内的软组织肉瘤亚型的试验中,伊马替尼(Chugh et al. 2009)或达沙替尼(Schuetze et al. 2010)均未见明显效果,大多数 MPNST 患者的病情进展迅速。鉴于 MPNST 的进展普遍较快,未来的试验除了放射学反应外,还可能将长期病情稳定性作为反应标准。在 MPNST 的临床试验中,靶向药物的组合以及在细胞毒性化学治疗中添加靶向药物可能会提高药物反应率和治疗效果。例如,最近在转基因 MPNST 小鼠模型中的研究表明,mTOR 抑制剂与 HSP90 抑制剂联合使用可使肿瘤体积大幅缩小,而单独使用其中一种药物则无法观察到这种效果(De Raedt et al. 2011)。MPNST 专项试验需要多个具有肉瘤研究经验的研究机构参与才能完成。临床前 NF 联盟与国防部赞助的 NF 临床试验联盟以及肉瘤专科联盟的合作将有助于及时将临床前研究结果转化为最有前景的药物临床试验的开发,并及时开展和完成针对 MPNST 患者的试验。

表 40.4　已完成和正在进行的针对恶性周围神经鞘膜瘤（MPNST）患者的靶向药物临床试验

药物	作用靶点	阶段	数量	计划	入组条件	试验终止	反应评估	结果	参考文献
厄洛替尼	EGFR	II	24	连续口服	难治性；成人	缓解	2D	19/20人2个月缓解，1人病情稳定	Albritton等（2006）
索拉非尼	CRAF, BRAF, VEGFR2, C-Kit, PDGFR	II	12	连续口服	难治性；成人	缓解	RECIST	无反应；中位无进展生存期1.7个月	Maki等（2009）
伊马替尼	C-Kit, PDGFR, VEGFR	II	7	连续口服 300 mg BID	难治性；>10岁	缓解	RECIST	无反应；1人病情稳定	Chugh等（2009）
达沙替尼	C-Kit, SRC	II	14	连续口服 70~100 mg/天	难治性	缓解	Choi	无反应或病情稳定	Schuetze等（2010）
贝伐单抗/RAD001	血管生成/mTOR	II	—	每14天1次，连续口服	难治性	缓解	WHO	即将开始	—

40.7 骨骼发育不良

40.7.1 治疗挑战的概述

NF1 相关骨骼发育不良包括蝶骨发育不良、长骨发育不良、非骨化性囊肿和脊柱侧弯。在儿童和成人中也有广泛性骨质减少的报道（Dulai et al. 2007；Kuorilehto et al. 2005；Petramala et al. 2011；Stevenson et al. 2011）。蝶骨发育不良通常与眼眶丛状神经纤维瘤同时发生，并导致面部畸形。脊柱侧弯很常见，但一小部分患者为营养不良型，需要手术矫正（Crawford and Herrera-Soto 2007）。最常见的长骨发育不良累及胫骨，有时也累及腓骨，可导致骨折和假关节形成。非骨化性囊肿可导致疼痛和骨折，但通常无症状。骨质减少可能会导致骨折和骨科术后愈合缓慢。这些不同病变的发病率使其成为治疗发展的合适目标（Elefteriou et al. 2009）。

40.7.2 转化和临床试验

胫骨发育不良通常通过佩戴支具治疗，以避免骨折。对于发生骨折的骨骼，人们尝试了多种不同的矫形手术，但大多数情况下效果都不理想。因此，人们对开发新的治疗方法产生了浓厚的兴趣。基于针对骨骼的条件性敲除技术，人们构建了长骨发育不良的小鼠模型。尽管小鼠不会自发发生胫骨弯曲或骨折（可能是由于负重较少），但可以通过对转基因骨骼进行创伤性损伤后的修复来模拟异常骨愈合。大剂量洛伐他汀全身治疗或局部治疗已被证明可改善这些模型的愈合（Kolanczyk et al. 2008）。Schindeler 等利用杂合 NF1 小鼠模型监测胫骨骨折的修复情况。他们发现，骨形态发生蛋白（bone morphogenetic protein，BMP）和双磷酸盐唑来膦酸联合使用可使约 63% 的骨折愈合，而仅使用 BMP 治疗的骨折愈合率为 25%。这促使研究人员对 7 名胫骨假关节患者进行了 BMP 加双磷酸盐治疗实验，其中 6 名患者患有 NF1。接受治疗的 8 名患者中有 6 名实现了一期愈合（其中 1 名患者为双侧疾病）。

成人和儿童 NF1 患者骨密度降低的临床意义一直难以解释，部分原因是接受测试的患者数量较少。Seitz 等用维生素 D 治疗了 4 名 NF1 患者，结果显示他们的骨密度有所增加。在另外一项研究中（Brunetti-Pierri et al. 2008），8 名患者接受了维生素 D 治疗，但 BMD 并未改善。因此，维生素 D 是否会改善 NF1 患者的临床结果仍未得到解决，有待进一步的临床试验。

40.8 皮肤型神经纤维瘤

40.8.1 治疗挑战的概述

皮肤型神经纤维瘤是 NF1 常见的并发症之一，有些患者全身长有巨大数量的肿瘤。虽然皮肤型神经纤维瘤不是导致重大医学疾病的原因，但其对外貌造成的损伤可能是巨大的，并对生命质量产生重大影响（Wolkenstein et al. 2001）。皮肤型神经纤维瘤可能突出于皮肤表面，也可能存在于真皮层内，或在真皮层下触及。其多发生在青春期（Huson et al. 1988）或孕期（Dugoff and Sulansky 1996），提示激素可能影响肿瘤生长。

40.8.2 转化和临床试验

皮肤型神经纤维瘤的临床治疗仅限于手术切除肿瘤，其他方法包括激光治疗（Elwakil et al. 2007）或电外科手术（Levine et al. 2008）。尚未进行正式的临床试验来评估这些方法的疗效。Riccardi 根据神经纤维瘤中发现的肥大细胞，对抗组胺药酮替芬进行了临床试验。研究显示疼痛和瘙痒感主观改善，但客观上肿瘤并未缩小。目前正在进行雷帕霉素或雷尼珠单抗局部应用的临床试验（基于 http://www.clinicaltrials.gov，12 月 2 日访问），但至今尚未公布结果。在丛状神经纤维瘤的临床试验过程中，真皮神经纤维瘤的反应没有被密切监测，尽管没有明显减少真皮肿瘤负担的报道。研究者们基于皮肤来源的前体细胞中 NF1 的敲除建立了皮肤型神经纤维瘤小鼠模型，这可能有助于未来皮肤型神经纤维瘤的临床前研究。

（吴南，谢婧怡 译）

参考文献

[1] Abbas JS, Holyoke ED, Moore R, Karakousis CP (1981) The surgical treatment and outcome of soft-tissue sarcoma. Arch Surg 116: 765-769

[2] Acosta MT, Gioia GA, Silva AJ et al (2006) Neurofibromatosis type 1: new insights into neurocognitive issues. Curr Neurol Neurosci Rep 6: 136-143

[3] Acosta MT, Kardel PG, Walsh KS et al (2011) Lovastatin as treatment for neurocognitive deficits in neurofibromatosis type 1: phase I study. Pediatr Neurol 45: 241-245

[4] Albritton K, Rankin C, Coffin C, Ratner N, Budd T, Schuetze S, Randall R, DeClue J, Borden E(2006) Phase II trial of erlotinib in metastatic or unresectable malignant peripheral nerve sheath tumor (MPNST). ASCO 24: 9518

[5] Appenzeller O, Kornfeld M, Atkinson R et al (1986) Neurofibromatosis xenografts: contribution to pathogenesis. J Neurol Sci 74(1): 69-77

[6] Ater J, Zhou T, Holmes E et al (2011) Treatment of progressive hypothalamic/optic pathway gliomas in children with neurofibromatosis type 1: a report from the Children's Oncology Group (COG). In: Proceedings of the Children's Tumor Foundation Conference, Jackson Wole, Wyoming, June 11-14, p 28

[7] Babovic-Vuksanovic D, Ballman K, Michels V et al (2006) Phase II trial of pirfenidone in adults with neurofibromatosis type 1. Neurology 67: 1860-1862

[8] Babovic-Vuksanovic D, Petrovic L, Knudsen BE et al (2004) Survival of human neurofibroma in immunodeficient mice and initial results of therapy with Pirfenidone. J Biomed Biotechnol 2004(2): 79-85

[9] Babovic-Vuksanovic D, Widemann BC, Dombi E et al (2007) Phase I trial of pirfenidone in children with neurofibromatosis 1 and plexiform neurofibromas. Pediatr Neurol 36: 293-300

[10] Bajenaru ML, Zhu Y, Hedrick NM et al (2002) Astrocyte-specific inactivation of the neurofibro-matosis 1 gene (NF1) is insufficient for astrocytoma formation. Mol Cell Biol 22: 5100-5113

[11] Bajenaru ML, Hernandez MR, Perry A et al (2003) Optic nerve glioma in mice requires astrocyte Nf1 gene inactivation and Nf1 brain heterozygosity. Cancer Res 63: 8573-8577

[12] Barton B, North K (2004) Social skills of children with neurofibromatosis type 1. Dev Med Child Neurol 46: 553-563

[13] Barton B, North K (2007) The self-concept of children and adolescents with neurofibromatosis type 1. Child Care Health Dev 33: 401-408

[14] Beert E, Brems H, Daniels B et al (2011) Atypical neurofibromas in neurofibromatosis type 1 are premalignant tumors. Genes Chrom Cancer 50: 1021-1032

[15] Brannan C, Perkins A, Vogel K et al (1994) Targeted disruption of the neurofibromatosis type-1 gene leads to developmental abnormalities in heart and various neural crest-derived tissues. Genes Dev 8: 1019-1029

[16] Brossier NM, Carroll SL (2011) Genetically engineered mouse models shed new light on the pathogenesis of neurofibromatosis type I-related neoplasms of the peripheral nervous system. Brain Res Bull 88: 58-71

[17] Brown JA, Emnett RJ et al (2010) Reduced striatal dopamine underlies the attention system dysfunction in neurofibromatosis-1 mutant mice. Hum Mol Genet 19: 4515-4528

[18] Brown JA, Xu J et al (2011) PET imaging for attention deficit preclinical drug testing in neurofibromatosis-1 mice. Exp Neurol 232: 333-338

[19] Brunetti-Pierri N, Berg JS, Scaglia F et al (2008) Recurrent reciprocal 1q21.1 deletions and duplications associated with microcephaly or macrocephaly and developmental and behavioral abnormalities. Nat Genet 40: 1466-1471

[20] Cai W, Kassarjian A, Bredella MA et al (2009) Tumor burden in patients with neurofibromatosis types 1 and 2 and schwannomatosis: determination on whole-body MR images. Radiology 250: 665-673

[21] Campagna M, Opocher E, Viscardi E et al (2010) Optic pathway glioma: Long-term visual outcome in children without neurofibromatosis type-1. Pediatr Blood Cancer 55: 1083-1088

[22] Canavese F, Krajbich J (2011) Resection of plexiform neurofibromas in children with neurofibromatosis type 1. J Pediatr Orthop 31: 303-311

[23] Carli M, Ferrari A, Mattke A et al (2005) Pediatric malignant peripheral nerve sheath tumor: the Italian and German soft tissue sarcoma cooperative group. J Clin Oncol 23: 8422-8430

[24] Chabernaud C, Mennes M, Kardel PG et al (2012) Lovastatin regulates brain spontaneous low-frequency brain activity in Neurofibromatosis type 1. Neurosci Lett 515(1): 28-33

[25] Chugh R, Wathen JK, Maki RG et al (2009) Phase II multicenter trial of imatinib in 10 histologic subtypes of sarcoma using a bayesian hierarchical statistical model. J Clin Oncol 21: 3148-3153

[26] Cichowski K, Shih TS, Schmitt E et al (1999) Mouse models of tumor development in neurofi-bromatosis type 1. Science 286: 2172-2176

[27] Costa RM, Silva AJ (2003) Mouse models of neurofibromatosis type I: bridging the GAP. Trends Mol Med 9: 19-23

[28] Costa J, Wesley RA, Glatstein E, Rosenberg SA (1984) The grading of soft tissue sarcomas. Results of a clinicohistopathologic correlation in a series of 163 cases. Cancer 53: 530-541

[29] Costa RM, Federov NB, Kogan JH et al (2002) Mechanism for the learning deficits in a mouse model of neurofibromatosis type 1. Nature 415: 526-530

[30] Crawford AH, Herrera-Soto J (2007) Scoliosis associated with neurofibromatosis. Orthop Clin North Am 38(4): 553-562

[31] Cui Y, Costa RM, Murphy GG et al (2008) Neurofibromin regulation of ERK signaling modulates GABA release and learning. Cell 135: 549-560

[32] Dasgupta B, Dugan LL, Gutmann DH (2003) The neurofibromatosis 1 gene product neurofibromin regulates pituitary adenylate cyclase-activating polypeptide-mediated signaling in astrocytes. J Neurosci 23: 8949-8954

[33] Dasgupta B, Yi Y, Chen DY et al (2005) Proteomic analysis reveals hyperactivation of the mammalian target of rapamycin pathway in neurofibromatosis 1-associated human and mouse brain tumors. Cancer Res 65: 2755-2760

[34] De Raedt T, Brems H, Wolkenstein P et al (2003) Elevated risk for MPNST in NF1 microdeletion patients. Am J Hum Genet 72: 1288-1292

[35] De Raedt T, Walton Z, Yecies JL et al (2011) Exploiting

cancer cell vulnerabilities to develop a combination therapy for ras-driven tumors. Cancer Cell 20：400-413
[36] DeClue JE, Heffelfinger S, Benvenuto G et al (2000) Epidermal growth factor receptor expression in neurofibromatosis type 1-related tumors and NF1 animal models. J Clin Invest 105：1233-1241
[37] Dombi E, Solomon J, Gillespie AJ et al (2007) NF1 plexiform neurofibroma growth rate by volumetric MRI：relationship to age and body weight. Neurology 68：643-647
[38] Dugoff L, Sulansky E (1996) Neurofibromatosis type 1 and pregnancy. Am J Med Genet 66(1)：7-10
[39] Dulai S, Briody J, Schindeler A et al (2007) Decreased bone mineral density in neurofibromatosis type 1：results from a pediatric cohort. J Pediatr Orthop 27(4)：472-475
[40] Elwakil TF, Samy NA, Elbasiouny MS (2008) Non-excision treatment of multiple cutaneous neurofibromas by laser photocoagulation. Lasers Med Sci 23(3)：301-306
[41] Evans DG, Baser ME, McGaughran J et al (2002) Malignant peripheral nerve sheath tumours in neurofibromatosis 1. J Med Genet 39：311-314
[42] Fang Y, Elah A, Denley RC et al (2009) Molecular characterization of permanent cell lines from primary, metastatic and recurrent malignant peripheral nerve sheath tumors (MPNST) with underlying neurofibromatosis-1. Anticancer Res 29(4)：1255-1262
[43] Ferner RE, Gutmann DH (2002) International consensus statement on malignant peripheral nerve sheath tumors in neurofibromatosis. Cancer Res 62：1573-1577
[44] Ferner RE, Lucas JD, O'Doherty MJ et al (2000) Evaluation of (18) fluorodeoxyglucose positron emission tomography ((18)FDG PET) in the detection of malignant peripheral nerve sheath tumours arising from within plexiform neurofibromas in neurofibromatosis 1. J Neurol Neurosurg Psychiatry 68：353-357
[45] Ferner RE, Golding JF, Smith M et al (2008) [18F]2-fluoro-2-deoxy-D-glucose positron emission tomography (FDG PET) as a diagnostic tool for neurofibromatosis 1 (NF1) associated malignant peripheral nerve sheath tumours (MPNSTs)：a long-term clinical study. Ann Oncol 19：390-394
[46] Ferrari A, Miceli R, Rey A et al (2011) Non-metastatic unresected paediatric nonrhabdomyosarcoma soft tissue sarcomas：results of a pooled analysis from United States and European groups. Eur J Cancer 47：724-731
[47] Friedrich RE, Korf B, Funsterer C, Mautner VF (2003) Growth type of plexiform neurofibromas in NF1 determined on magnetic resonance images. Anticancer Res 23：949-952
[48] Friedrich RE, Kluwe L, Funsterer C, Mautner VF (2005) Malignant peripheral nerve sheath tumors (MPNST) in neurofibromatosis type 1 (NF1)：diagnostic findings on magnetic resonance images and mutation analysis of the NF1 gene. Anticancer Res 25：1699-1702
[49] Friedrich RE, Stelljes C, Hagel C et al (2010) Dysplasia of the orbit and adjacent bone associated with plexiform neurofibroma and ocular disease in 42 NF-1 patients. Anticancer Res 30(5)：1751-1764
[50] Gnekow AK, Kortmann R-D, Pietsch T, Emser A (2004) Low grade chiasmatic-hypothalamic glioma—carboplatin and vincristin chemotherapy effectively defers radiotherapy within a comprehensive treatment strategy. A report from the Multicenter Treatment Study for Children and Adolescents with a Low Grade Glioma—HIT-LGG 1996—of the Society of Pediatric Oncology and Hematology (GPOH). Klin Padiatr 216：331-342
[51] Guo H-F et al (1997) Requirement of *Drosophila NF1* for activation of adenylyl cyclase by PACAP38-like neuropeptides. Science 276(5313)：795-798
[52] Gupta A, Cohen BH, Ruggieri P et al (2003) Phase I study of thalidomide for the treatment of plexiform neurofibroma in neurofibromatosis 1. Neurology 60：130-132
[53] Gupta G, Mammis A, Maniker A (2008) Malignant peripheral nerve sheath tumors. Neurosurg Clin N Am 19：533-543
[54] Gururangan S, Cavazos CM, Ashley D et al (2002) Phase II study of carboplatin in children with progressive low-grade gliomas. J Clin Oncol 20：2941-2958
[55] Gururangan S, Fisher MJ, Allen JC et al (2007) Temozolomide in children with progressive low-grade glioma. Neuro-oncol 9：161-168
[56] Gutmann DH, Aylsworth A, Carey JC et al (1997) The diagnostic evaluation and multidisciplinary management of neurofibromatosis 1 and neurofibromatosis 2. JAMA 278(1)：51-57
[57] Gutmann DH, Hedrick NM, Li J et al (2002) Comparative gene expression profile analysis of neurofibromatosis 1-associated and sporadic pilocytic astrocytomas. Cancer Res 62：2085-2091
[58] Hakozaki M, Hojo H, Sato M et al (2009) Establishment and characterization of a novel human malignant peripheral nerve sheath tumor cell line, FMS-1, that overexpresses epidermal growth factor receptor and cyclooxygenase-2. Virchows Arch 455(6)：517-526
[59] Hegedus B, Dasgupta B, Shin JE et al (2007) Neurofibromatosis-1 regulates neuronal and glial cell differentiation from neuroglial progenitors in vivo by both cAMP- and ras-dependent mechanisms. Cell Stem Cell 1：443-457
[60] Hegedus B et al (2008) Preclinical cancer therapy in a mouse model of neurofibromatosis-1 optic glioma. Cancer Res 68：1520-1528
[61] Hegedus B, Hughes WF, Garbow JR et al (2009) Optic nerve dysfunction in a mouse model of neurofibromatosis-1 optic glioma. J Neuropathol Exp Neurol 68：542-551
[62] Hidalgo M (2012) From node to pathway blockade：Lessons learned from targeting mammalian target of rapamycin. J Clin Oncol 30：85-87
[63] Holtkamp N, Okuducu AF, Mucha J et al (2006) Mutation and expression of PDGFRA and KIT in malignant peripheral nerve sheath tumors, and its implications for imatinib sensitivity. Carcinogenesis 27：664-671
[64] Hornstein SH, Kortmann R-D, Pietsch T et al (2011) Impact of chemotherapy on disseminated low-grade glioma in children and adolescents：report from the HIT-LGG 1996 trial. Pediatr Blood Cancer 56：1046-1054
[65] Hummel TR, Jessen WJ, Miller SJ et al (2010) Gene expression analysis identifies potential biomarkers of neurofibromatosis type 1 including adrenomedullin. Clin Cancer Res 16：5048-5057
[66] Huson SM, Harper PS, Compston DAS (1988) Von Recklinghausen neurofibromatosis. A clinical and population study in south-east Wales. Brain 111(6)：1355-1381
[67] Hyman SL, North KN (2005) The nature and frequency of cognitive deficits in children with neurofibromatosis type 1. Neurology 65：1037-1044
[68] Hyman SL, Shores EA, North KN et al (2006) Learning disabilities in children with neurofibromatosis type 1：subtypes, cognitive profile, and attention-deficit-hyperactivity

[69] Jacks T et al (1994) Tumorigenie and developmental consequences of a targeted Nf1 mutation in the mouse. Nat Genet 7: 353-361

[70] Jakacki RI, Bouffet E, Adamson PC et al (2011a) A phase 1 study of vinblastine in combination with carboplatin for children with low-grade gliomas: a Children's Oncology Group phase 1 consortium study. Neuro Oncol 13: 910-915

[71] Jakacki RI, Dombi E, Potter DM et al (2011b) Phase I trial of pegylated interferon-alpha-2b in young patients with plexiform neurofibromas. Neurology 76: 265-272

[72] Johannessen CM, Reczek EE, James MF et al (2005) The NF1 tumor suppressor critically regulates TSC2 and mTOR. Proc Natl Acad Sci USA 102: 8573-8578

[73] Johannessen CM, Johnson BW, Williams SM et al (2008) TORC1 is essential for NF1-associated malignancies. Curr Biol 18: 56-62

[74] Johansson G, Mahller YY, Collins MH et al (2008) Effective in vivo targeting of the mammalian target of rapamycin pathway in malignant peripheral nerve sheath tumors. Mol Cancer Ther 7: 1237-1245

[75] Kadota RP, Kun LE, Langston JW et al (1999) Cyclophosphamide for the treatment of progressive low-grade astrocytoma: a Pediatric Oncology Group phase II study. J Pediatr Hematol Oncol 21: 198-202

[76] Kattan MW, Leung DH, Brennan MF (2002) Postoperative nomogram for 12-year sarcomaspecific death. J Clin Oncol 20: 791-796

[77] Kawachi Y, Xu X, Ichikawa E et al (2003) Expression of angiogenic factors in neurofibromas. Exp Dermatol 12: 412-417

[78] Kim HA, Ling B, Ratner N et al (1997) NF1-deficient mouse Schwann cells are angiogenic and invasive and can be induced to hyperproliferate: reversion of some phenotypes by an inhibitor of farnesyl protein transferase. Mol Cell Biol 17: 862-872

[79] Kim A, Gillespie A, Dombi E et al (2009) Characteristics of children enrolled in treatment trials for NF1-related plexiform neurofibromas. Neurology 73: 1273-1279

[80] King AA, Debaun MR, Riccardi VM, Gutmann DH (2000) Malignant peripheral nerve sheath tumors in neurofibromatosis 1. Am J Med Genet 93: 388-392

[81] Kluwe L, Friedrich R, Mautner VF (1999) Loss of NF1 allele in Schwann cells but not in fibroblasts derived from an NF1-associated neurofibroma. Genes Chromosomes Cancer 24: 283-285

[82] Kolanczyk M, Kühnisch J, Kossler N et al (2008) Modeling neurofibromatosis type 1 tibial dysplasia and its treatment with lovastatin. BMC Med 6: 21

[83] Korf BR (1999) Plexiform neurofibromas. Am J Med Genet 89: 31-37

[84] Krab LC, Aarsen FK, deGoede-Bolder A et al (2008) Impact of neurofibromatosis type 1 on school performance. J Child Neurol 23: 1002-1010

[85] Kuorilehto T, Ekholm E, Nissinen M et al (2005) Nf1 gene expression in mouse fracture healing and in experimental rat pseudarthrosis. J Histochem Cytochem 54: 363

[86] Lafay-Cousin L, Holm S, Qaddoumi I et al (2005) Weekly vinblastine in pediatric low-grade glioma patients with carboplatin allergic reaction. Cancer 103: 2636-2642

[87] Laithier V, Grill J, Le Deley M-C et al (2003) Progression-free survival in children with optic pathway tumors: dependence on age and the quality of the response to chemotherapy—Results of the first French prospective study for the French Society of Pediatric Oncology. J Clin Oncol 21: 4572-4578

[88] Lau N, Feldkamp M, Roncari L et al (2000) Loss of neurofibromin is associated with activation of RAS/MAPK and PI3-K/AKT signaling in neurofibromatosis 1 astrocytoma. J Neuropathol Exp Neurol 59: 759-767

[89] Lee DY, Yeh T-H, Emnett RJ et al (2010) Neurofibromatosis-1 regulates neuroglial progenitor proliferation and glial differentiation in a brain region-specific manner. Genes Dev 24: 2317-2329

[90] Leppig KA, Kaplan P, Viskochil D et al (1997) Familial neurofibromatosis 1 microdeletions: cosegregation with distinct facial phenotype and early onset of cutaneous neurofibromata. Am J Med Genet 73: 197-204

[91] Levine SM, Levine E, Taubb PJ et al (2008) Electrosurgical excision technique for the treatment of multiple cutaneous lesions in neurofibromatosis type I. J Plast Reconstr Aesthet Surg 61(8): 958-962

[92] Li H, Velasco-Miguel S, Vass WC et al (2002) Epidermal growth factor receptor signaling pathways are associated with tumorigenesis in the Nf1: p53 mouse tumor model. Cancer Res 62: 4507-4513

[93] Li W, Cui Y et al (2005) The HMG-CoA reductase inhibitor lovastatin reverses the learning and attention deficits in a mouse model of neurofibromatosis type 1. Curr Biol 15: 1961-1967

[94] Ling BC, Wu J, Miller SJ et al (2005) Role for the epidermal growth factor receptor in neurofibromatosis-related peripheral nerve tumorigenesis. Cancer Cell 7: 65-75

[95] Listernick R, Charrow J, Greenwald MJ, Esterly NB (1989) Optic gliomas in children with neurofibromatosis type 1. J Pediatr 114: 788-792

[96] Listernick R, Louis DH, Packer RJ et al (1997) Optic pathway gliomas in children with neurofi-bromatosis 1: consensus statement from the NF1 Optic Pathway Glioma Task Force. Ann Neurol 441: 143-149

[97] Listernick R, Ferner RE, Liu GT, Gutmann DH (2007) Optic pathway gliomas in neurofibromatosis-1: controversies and recommendations. Ann Neurol 61: 189-198

[98] Lush ME, Li Y, Kwon C-H et al (2008) Neurofibromin is required for barrel formation in the mouse somatosensory cortex. J Neurosci 28: 1580-1587

[99] Mahoney DH Jr, Cohen ME, Friedman HS et al (2000) Carboplatin is effective therapy for young children with progressive optic pathway tumors: a Pediatric Oncology Group phase II study. Neuro Oncol 2: 213-220

[100] Maki RG, D'Adamo DR, Keohan ML et al (2009) Phase II study of sorafenib in patients with metastatic or recurrent sarcomas. J Clin Oncol 27: 3133-3140

[101] Marui T, Hashimoto O, Nanba E et al (2004) Association between the neurofibromatosis-1 (NF1) locus and autism in the Japanese population. Am J Med Genet 131B: 43-47

[102] Massimino M, Spreafico F, Cefalo G et al (2002a) High response rate to cisplatin/etoposide regimen in childhood low-grade glioma. J Clin Oncol 20: 4209-4216

[103] Massimino M, Spreafico F, Riva D et al (2002b) Treatment of ADHD in neurofibromatosis type 1. Dev Med Child Neurol 44: 164-170

[104] Massimino M, Spreafico F, Riva D et al (2010) A lower-dose, lower-toxicity cisplatinetoposide regimen for childhood progressive low-grade glioma. J Neurooncol 100: 65-71

[105] Mautner VF (2012) Impact of ADHD in adults with neurofibromatosis type 1: associated psychological and social problems. J Atten Disord doi: 10.1177/1087054712450749.

Published online before print July 10, 2012

[106] Mautner VF, Asuagbor FA, Dombi E et al (2008) Assessment of benign tumor burden by whole-body MRI in patients with neurofibromatosis 1. Neuro Oncol 10: 593-598

[107] Mautner V-F, Lan KL, Thakker SD, Leark SA (2002) Treatment of ADHD in neurofibromatosis type 1. Dev Med Child Neurol 44(3): 164-170

[108] McClatchey AI, Cichowski K (2001) Mouse models of neurofibromatosis. Biochim Biophys Acta 1471: M73-M80

[109] McLaughlin ME, Robson CD, Kieran MW et al (2003) Marked regression of metastatic pilocytic astrocytoma during treatment with imatinib mesylate (STI-571, Gleevec): a case report and laboratory investigation. J Pediatr Hematol Oncol 25: 644-648

[110] Miller AB, Hoogstraten B, Staquet M, Winkler A (1981) Reporting results of cancer treatment. Cancer 47: 207-214

[111] Miller SJ, Rangwala F, Williams J et al (2006) Large-scale molecular comparison of human Schwann cells to malignant peripheral nerve sheath tumor cell lines and tissues. Cancer Res 66: 2584-2591

[112] Mishra KK, Squire S, Lamborn K et al (2010) Phase II TPDCV protocol for pediatric low-grade hypothalamic/chiasmatic gliomas: 15-year update. J Neurooncol 100: 121-127

[113] Needle MN, Cnaan A, Dattilo J et al (1997) Prognostic signs in the surgical management of plexiform neurofibroma: the Children's Hospital of Philadelphia experience, 1974-1994. J Pediatr 131: 678-682

[114] North KN, Riccardi V, Samango-Sprouse C et al (1997) Cognitive function and academic performance in neurofibromatosis 1: consensus statement from the NF1 Cognitive Disorders Task Force. Neurology 48: 1121-1127

[115] Packer RJ, Lange B, Ater J et al (1993) Carboplatin and vincristine for recurrent and newly diagnosed low-grade gliomas of childhood. J Clin Oncol 11: 850-856

[116] Packer RJ, Ater J, Allen J et al (1997) Carboplatin and vincristine chemotherapy for children with newly diagnosed progressive low-grade gliomas. J Neurosurg 86: 747-754

[117] Packer R, Gutmann D, Rubenstein A et al (2002) Plexiform neurofibromas in NF1: toward biologic-based therapy. Neurology 58: 1461-1470

[118] Packer RJ, Jakacki R, Horn M et al (2009) Objective response of multiply recurrent low-grade gliomas to bevacizumab and irinotecan. Pediatr Blood Cancer 52: 791-795

[119] Packer RJ, Yalon M, Rood BR et al (2010) Phase I/II study of tarceva/rapamycin for recurrent pediatric low-grade gliomas (LGG). Neuro Oncol 12: ii20

[120] Parada LF, Kwon C-H, Zhu Y (2005) Modeling neurofibromatosis type 1 tumors in the mouse for therapeutic intervention. Cold Spring Harb Symp Quant Biol 70: 173-176

[121] Perrin GQ, Fishbein L, Thomson SA et al (2007) Plexiform-like neurofibromas develop in the mouse by intraneural xenograft of an NF1 tumor-derived Schwann cell line. J Neurosci Res 85(6): 1347-1357

[122] Perry A, Kunz SN, Fuller CE et al (2002) Differential NF1, p16, and EGFR patterns by interphase cytogenetics (FISH) in malignant peripheral nerve sheath tumor (MPNST) and morphologically similar spindle cell neoplasms. J Neuropathol Exp Neurol 61: 702-709

[123] Petramala L, Giustini S, Zinnamosca L et al (2012) Bone mineral metabolism in patients with neurofibromatosis type 1 (von Recklingausen disease). Arch Dermatol Res 304: 325-331

[124] Pfister S, Janzarik WG, Remke M et al (2008) BRAF gene duplication constitutes a mechanism of MAPK pathway activation in low-grade astrocytomas. J Clin Invest 1218: 1739-1749

[125] Pisters PW, Leung DH, Woodruff J et al (1996) Analysis of prognostic factors in 1,041 patients with localized soft tissue sarcomas of the extremities. J Clin Oncol 14: 1679-1689

[126] Pollack IF, Shultz B, Mulvihill JJ (1996) The management of brainstem gliomas in patients with neurofibromatosis 1. Neurology 46: 1652-1660

[127] Pons MA, Finlay JL, Walker RW et al (1992) Chemotherapy with vincristine (VCR) and etoposide (VP-16) in children with low-grade astrocytoma. J Neurooncol 14: 151-158

[128] Poussaint TY, Jaramillo D, Chang Y, Korf B (2003) Interobserver reproducibility of volumetric MR imaging measurements of plexiform neurofibromas. Am J Roentgenol 180: 419-423

[129] Prada CE, Rangwala FA, Martin LJ et al (2012) Pediatric plexiform neurofibromas: impact on morbidity and mortality in neurofibromatosis type 1. J Pediatr 160: 461-467

[130] Reilly K, Loisel D, Bronson R et al (2000) *Nf1*; *Trp53* mutant mice develop glioblastoma with evidence of strain specific effects. Nat Genet 26: 109-113

[131] Reilly KM, Rubin JB, Gilbertson RJ et al (2008) Re-thinking brain tumors: the fourth mouse models of Human Cancers Consortium Nervous System Tumors Workshop. Cancer Res 68: 5508-5511

[132] Riccardi VM (1993) A controlled multiphase trial of ketotifen to minimize neurofibroma-associated pain and itching. Arch Dermatol 129: 577-581

[133] Riccardi VM, Mulvihill JJ (eds) (1981) Neurofibromatosis (von Recklinghausen disease) genetics, cell biology and biochemistry. Adv neurol 29: 1-282

[134] Robertson K, Bowers D, Yang F et al (2011) Phase II pilot study of imatinib mesylate in neurofibromatosis (NF1) patients with plexiform neurofibromas. ASCO, Chicago, IL (J Clin Oncol 29: 2011 suppl: abstr 10030)

[135] Sartin EA, Doran SE, Riddell MG et al (1994) Characterization of naturally occurring cutaneous neurofibromatosis in Holstein cattle. A disorder resembling neurofibromatosis type 1 in humans. Am J Pathol 145(5): 1168-1174

[136] Scaife CL, Pisters PW (2003) Combined-modality treatment of localized soft tissue sarcomas of the extremities. Surg Oncol Clin N Am 12: 355-368

[137] Schindeler A, Birke O, Yu C et al (2011) Distal tibial fracture repair in a neurofibromatosis type 1-deficient mouse treated with recombinant bone morphogenetic protein and a bisphosphonate. J Bone Joint Surg Br 93-B(8): 1134-1139

[138] Schuetze S, Wathen S, Choy E et al (2010) Results of a sarcoma alliance for research through collaboration (SARC) phase II trial of dasatinib in previously treated, high-grade, advanced sarcoma. ASCO, Chicago, IL [J Clin Oncol 28: 15s (suppl: abstr 10009)]

[139] Serra E, Rosenbaum T, Winner U et al (2000) Schwann cells harbor the somatic NF1 mutation in neurofibromas: evidence of two different Schwann cell subpopulations. Hum Mol Genet 9: 3055-3064

[140] Shilyansky C, Karlsgodt KH, Cummings DM et al (2010)

Neurofibromin regulates corticostriatal inhibitory networks during working memory performance. Proc Natl Acad Sci USA 107: 13141-13146

[141] Silva AJ, Frankland PW, Marowitz Z et al (1997) A mouse model for the learning and memory deficits associated with neurofibromatosis type I. Nat Genet 15: 281-284

[142] Skotheim RI, Kallioniemi A, Bjerkhagen B et al (2003) Topoisomerase-II alpha is upregulated in malignant peripheral nerve sheath tumors and associated with clinical outcome. J Clin Oncol 21: 4586-4591

[143] Solomon J, Warren K, Dombi E et al (2004) Automated detection and volume measurement of plexiform neurofibromas in neurofibromatosis 1 using magnetic resonance imaging. Comput Med Imaging Graph 28: 257-265

[144] Stevenson DA, Yan J, He Y et al (2011) Multiple increased osteoclast functions in individuals with neurofibromatosis type 1. Am J Med Genet 155(5): 1050-1059

[145] Sun T, Gianinoo SM, Jackson E et al (2010) CXCL12 alone is insufficient for gliomagenesis in NF1 mutant mice. J Neuroimmunol 224: 108-113

[146] Tanaka J, Kuramochi A, Nishi N et al (2005) Preoperative transarterial embolization enhances the surgical management of diffuse plexiform neurofibroma: a case report. Cardiovasc Intervent Radiol 28: 686-688

[147] Therasse P, Arbuck S, Eisenhauer E et al (2000) New guidelines to evaluate the response to treatment in solid tumors. J Natl Cancer Inst 92: 205-216

[148] Thorarinsdottir HK, Santi M, McCarter R et al (2008) Protein expression of platelet-derived growth factor receptor correlates with malignant histology and PTEN with survival in childhood gliomas. Clin Cancer Res 14: 3386-3394

[149] Torres KE, Liu J, Young E et al (2011a) Expression of 'drugable' tyrosine kinase receptors in malignant peripheral nerve sheath tumour: potential molecular therapeutic targets for a chemoresistant cancer. Histopathology 59: 156-159

[150] Torres KE, Zhu QS, Bill K et al (2011b) Activated MET is a molecular prognosticator and potential therapeutic target for malignant peripheral nerve sheath tumors. Clin Cancer Res 17: 3943-3955

[151] Trojani M, Contesso G, Coindre JM et al (1984) Soft-tissue sarcomas of adults; study of pathological prognostic variables and definition of a histopathological grading system. Int J Cancer 33: 37-42

[152] Tucker T, Friedman JM, Friedrich RE et al (2009) Longitudinal study of neurofibromatosis 1 associated plexiform neurofibromas. J Med Genet 46: 81-85

[153] Verma S, Bramwell V (2002) Dose-intensive chemotherapy in advanced adult soft tissue sarcoma. Expert Rev Anticancer Ther 2: 201-215

[154] Wallace MR, Rasmussen SA, Lim IT et al (2000) Culture of cytogenetically abnormal Schwann cells from benign and malignant NF1 tumors. Genes Chromosomes Cancer 27: 117-1230

[155] Wang W et al (2011) Mice lacking Nf1 in osteochondroprogenitor cells displays skeletal dysplasia similar to patients with neurofibromatosis type 1. Hum Mol Genet 20(20): 3910-3924

[156] Warrington NM, Gianino SM, Jackson E et al (2010) Cyclic AMP suppression is sufficient to induce gliomagenesis in a mouse model of neurofibromatosis-1. Cancer Res 70: 5717-5727

[157] Weiss B, Fisher M, Dombi E et al (2010) Phase II study of the mTOR inhibitor sirolimus for nonprogressive NF1-associated plexiform neurofibromas: a Neurofibromatosis Consortium Study. ISPNO, Vienna, Austria, pp ii43

[158] Widemann BC, Salzer WL, Arceci RJ et al (2006) Phase I trial and pharmacokinetic study of the farnesyltransferase inhibitor tipifarnib in children with refractory solid tumors or neurofibromatosis type I and plexiform neurofibromas. J Clin Oncol 24: 507-516

[159] Widemann B, Dombi E, Gillespie A et al (2009) Phase II randomized, flexible cross-over, double-blinded, placebo-controlled trial of the farnesyltransferase inhibitor (FTI) tipifarnib (R115777) in pediatric patients (pts) with neurofibromatosis type 1 (NF1) and progressive plexiform neurofibromas (PN). Children's Tumor Foundation, Portland, OR

[160] Widemann B, Fox E, Adamson P et al (2009) Phase I study of sorafenib in children with refractory solid tumors: a Children's Oncology Group Phase I Consortium Trial. ASCO, Orlando, FL Wolkenstein P, Zeller J, Revuz J et al (2001) Quality-of-life impairment in neurofibromatosis type 1: a cross-sectional study of 128 cases. Arch Dermatol 137 (II): 1421-1425

[161] Wong WW, Hirose T, Scheithauer BW et al (1998) Malignant peripheral nerve sheath tumor: analysis of treatment outcome. Int J Radiat Oncol Biol Phys 42: 351-360

[162] Wu J, Williams JP, Rizvi TA et al (2008) Plexiform and dermal neurofibromas and pigmentation are caused by Nf1 loss in desert hedgehog-expressing cells. Cancer Cell 13: 105-116

[163] Yang JC, Chang AE, Baker AR et al (1998) Randomized prospective study of the benefit of adjuvant radiation therapy in the treatment of soft tissue sarcomas of the extremity. J Clin Oncol 16: 197-203

[164] Yang FC, Ingram DA, Chen S et al (2003) Neurofibromin-deficient Schwann cells secrete a potent migratory stimulus for $Nf1^{+/-}$ mast cells. J Clin Invest 112: 1851-1861

[165] Yang FC, Chen S, Clegg T et al (2006) $Nf1^{+/-}$ mast cells induce neurofibroma like phenotypes through secreted TGF-beta signaling. Hum Mol Genet 15: 2421-2437

[166] Yang FC, Ingram DA, Chen S et al (2008) Nf1-dependent tumors require a microenvironment containing $Nf1^{+/-}$ and c-kit-dependent bone marrow. Cell 135: 437-448

[167] Yang J, Ylipaa A, Sun Y et al (2011) Genomic and molecular characterization of malignant peripheral nerve sheath tumor identifies the IGF1R pathway as a primary target for treatment. Clin Cancer Res 17: 7563-7573

[168] Zhu Y, Ghosh P, Charnay P et al (2002) Neurofibromas in NF1: Schwann cell origin and role of tumor environment. Science 296: 920-922

[169] Zhu Y, Harada T, Liu L et al (2005) Inactivation of NF1 in CNS causes increased glial progenitor proliferation and optic glioma formation. Development 132: 5577-5588

第41章 1型神经纤维瘤病民间基金会的作用：未来愿景

The Role of NF1 Lay Foundations: Future Vision

Kim Hunter-Schaedle

41.1 引言

41.1.1 NF1：一种罕见的疾病

1型神经纤维瘤病（NF1）估计影响到全世界1/3 000的人，即全世界有超过200万人受到影响。NF1在全美的影响率低于20万人，因而被归类为一种罕见疾病。它实际上是一种更"常见"的罕见病，但尽管如此，NF1并没有一个明确的公众"角色"。与更容易被公众所熟知的囊性纤维化等罕见病不同，NF1通常是闻所未闻的。这种情况的一个原因可能是，像囊性纤维化等许多罕见的疾病都有一个相当标准的临床进展。相比之下，NF1则是以无数种方式影响个体。有些NF1患者会有神经肿瘤，这些肿瘤在皮肤上表现为多个"肿块"，或在面部或其他地方表现为更大的生长。另外一些人会有身体内部肿瘤，这些肿瘤虽然临床上常常是毁灭性的损害，但是却无法被看到。NF1可导致骨骼发育不良，通常在儿童早期需要截肢。2/3的NF1患者会有某种形式的学习障碍，可能是轻微的，也可能是严重的，可能与注意力缺陷障碍、自闭症或其他众所周知的疾病有共同的特征。换句话说，NF1没有单一的公共"面孔"。此外，由于大多数NF1病例是慢性的和终身的，所以NF1患者从婴儿期到老年期都有存在。因此，NF1作为一个具有挑战性的疾病被告知大众；而这一挑战成为民间基金会的重要工作。

41.1.2 为何及如何建立民间基金会

医疗基金会可以采取多种形式，但它们的基本目标几乎都是为那些受疾病或医疗条件影响的人充当了倡导者和资讯点的角色。有时，新的基金会是为关注某种疾病或病症而成立的，因为这种疾病或病症没有现有的基金会。有时，新的基金会是针对已经存在的疾病或病症而创建的，这些基金会是由希望采取与现有基金会不同的方法的个人建立的。有些基金会是由一个或多个人建立的，旨在吸引广泛的选民基础。另一些则是由一个家族设立的，可能仅仅是为了用于某一特定疾病领域医学研究的慈善事业，也可能是为了某一特定机构或研究者。

设立基金会对于NF1等罕见疾病有着重要作用，因为被诊断患有这种疾病的人可能不认识任何其他NF1的病友，也不知道从哪里找到信息。许多以罕见病为重点的基金会的建立仅仅是为患者提供一个连接点和支持源头。然而，许多注重疾病的基

Dr. Hunter-Schaedle was the Chief Scientific Officer of the Children's Tumor Foundation from 2005 to 2011.

K. Hunter-Schaedle (*)
Children's Tumor Foundation, 95 Pine Street, New York, NY 10005, USA
e-mail: khsphd@yahoo.com

金会已经从这样一个小的开始发展到一个复杂的形式,特别是一旦基金会开始资助医学研究。有些基金会开始时根基不牢固,后来发展成为推动特定疾病领域研究议程的强大国际力量。一个例子是青少年糖尿病研究基金会(The Juvenile Diabetes Research Foundation,JDRF),它专注于1型糖尿病。JDRF 的根源是成立于 20 世纪 70 年代的一个家族操控的实体。如今,JDRF 是 1 型糖尿病领域国际领先的研究资助机构。JDRF 已承诺为医学研究投入超过 10 亿美元,与包括制药和生物技术公司在内的其他实体建立了众多伙伴关系,同时建立了国际分支机构和合作关系,并大力倡导为 1 型糖尿病研究提供联邦资金。这说明了一个民间基金会的潜在影响,即使是一个由草根发起的基金会。

41.1.3　NF1 民间基金会的形势

在美国,两个最大的 NF1 民间基金会是儿童肿瘤基金会和神经纤维瘤病网络。儿童肿瘤基金会成立于 1978 年,前身为国家神经纤维瘤病基金会,2004 年更名为儿童肿瘤基金会。神经纤维瘤病网络成立于 1988 年,前身为神经纤维瘤病集团,并于 2011 年更名为神经纤维瘤病网络。儿童肿瘤基金会是一个总部设在纽约的全国性组织;神经纤维瘤病网络是一个联盟组织,包括一些独立运作的区域团体。两个基金会都为那些受 NF1 影响的人提供信息、支持和社会共同体,两个基金会都主张为 NF1 研究提供联邦资金。这两个基金会都资助研究和医疗项目,但都逐渐形成了不同的方法。儿童肿瘤基金会在全国范围内募集资金;资金集中在纽约,用于资助世界各地的科学研究项目,并通过竞争性申请和评审程序进行选择。NF 网络在其联盟下的每个区域内筹集资金,这些资金可在当地支付给选定的研究项目。除了这两个基金会之外,在美国和全球还有其他 NF1 相关的基金会(国际 NF 基金会列表),为那些受到 NF1 影响的群体提供支持和保护,并在某些情况下独立资助研究。

41.2　NF1 民间基金会的多面性

为了调查 NF1 民间基金会的多面性,本节将重点介绍儿童肿瘤基金会:它的使命和职责、资源和工具,以及它最近为帮助影响和推动 NF1 研究进展而采取的举措。

41.2.1　NF1 民间基金会的角色和职责

儿童肿瘤基金会的倡议涵盖了神经纤维瘤病的所有种类,包括 NF1、NF2 和神经鞘瘤病。在这里,我们将重点介绍基金会的 NF1 相关项目。

儿童肿瘤基金会有四个任务领域,每个领域都可以在 NF1 诊断和进展过程中的某个节点解决问题,这对所有受 NF1 影响的个体都很重要。这四个任务领域,它们所处理的问题,以及基金会如何尽力解决这些问题,将在下面加以阐述。

任务领域 1:为 NF 患者及其家人提供信息和支持
问题解答:"NF1 是什么?还有谁会受到影响?"
当一个人被新诊断为 NF1 时,对他们和他们的家人来说,最紧迫的问题通常是如何更好地理解这种诊断意味着什么。因此,访问当前且易于搜索的 NF1 资源至关重要。儿童肿瘤基金会制订了一系列患者手册(儿童肿瘤基金会患者手册),介绍 NF1 患者生活的不同方面。这些小册子由 NF1 临床护理专家撰写,针对受影响的个人及其家庭量身定制,解决了许多即将面临的最紧迫的问题。有一份针对 NF1 儿童教师的"教育工作者指南",这种小册子,以及配套的"NF1 学习障碍"小册子,是非常重要的资源,可以带到儿童学校,用来解释 NF1 是什么以及它可能如何影响孩子的课堂需求。

儿童肿瘤基金会还为 NF1 患者提供了一个社团,让他们与其他受 NF1 影响的个人和家庭建立联系。这包括各种在线资源(NF 资源共存),如社交媒体交流;面对面的活动,如区域互助小组,全国 NF 家庭论坛;为 NF1 的儿童和年轻人举办的年度夏令营;以及纸本和电子刊物,包括每季度一份的 NF 通讯。这些资源将受 NF1 影响的人与信息和新的支持网络联系起来——在 NF1 诊断后的早期,这两者都是非常需要的。

任务领域 2:为 NF 患者创造获得优质健康保健的更好途径
问题解答:"我的孩子在哪里可以得到临床关怀?"
许多儿童将在儿科医师办公室得到 NF1 的诊

断，又或通过转诊给遗传学专家而诊治。当碰到医疗机构有 1 位了解 NF1 或能够转诊到专科诊所的医师时，这个家庭可能是很幸运的。然而，由于 NF1 很少见，所以这种专业知识并不总是可用的。许多"新诊断"的家庭联系儿童肿瘤基金会，为了寻求他们所在地区的 NF1 专家或诊所。2007 年，基金会建立了第一个国家级 NF 诊所网络。基金会的临床护理咨询委员会制订了一套"临床准则"——NF 诊所对寻求治疗的患者应该期望的指导方针，例如为儿童和成人 NF 患者提供（或转诊当地）对所有临床表现的护理的能力。这是一项相当艰巨的任务，因为 NF1 可以导致无数的颅脑和周围神经肿瘤类型以及其他表现，但这也意味着 NF1 患者由一位在 NF1 方面有经验的医师来治疗是非常重要的，并且可以有一个全面的护理团队来解决专业需求。基金会邀请美国所有治疗 NF 患者的诊所在 NF 诊所网络中申请附属诊所地位。接受的条件是基于诊所是否符合"诊所准则"。NF 诊所现在有 44 家附属诊所，基金会正在与一些诊所合作，帮助它们达到附属诊所的标准。在基金会的网站上，NF1 患者个人和他们的家人可以访问"找医师"（http://www.ctf.org/Living-with-NF/find-a-doctor.html）的信息，这些信息是关于美国所有治疗 NF 患者的诊所的，这个列表也突出了那些 NF 网络附属诊所。

事实证明，NF 诊所网络在整合 NF 临床护理信息方面是成功的，也是追踪每年有多少 NF 患者就诊的一个极好的方法。每年，基金会要求附属诊所提交一份详细的年度报告，其中包括患者数量。2010 年，NF 诊所网络报告了超过 10 000 例 NF 患者。尽管 NF 诊所网络在完全发展之前还有很长的路要走，但许多患者和家属赞扬了这种为整合 NF 临床护理信息所做的努力，这种方式之前都是不可用的。

任务领域 3：鼓励和支持 NF 研究寻找治疗和治愈的方法

问题解答："什么时候能治愈 NF1？"

一旦 NF1 患者及其家人了解了诊断并建立了 NF1 临床护理的"规范"，他们通常会参与监测 NF1 医学研究进展，并希望通过筹款支持研究来帮助实现这一目标。儿童肿瘤基金会是世界上主要的非政府性 NF 研究资助机构。基金会自成立之初即作为国家神经纤维瘤病基金会资助了 NF 研究，自 2006 年以来，通过制订和实施一项经过深思熟虑和详细的战略计划，确定了最需要资金的研究领域，以加速寻找有效的 NF 治疗方法，从而增加了其研究项目组合。因此，那些有兴趣通过基金会支持 NF1 研究的人是在与其他筹款人或"投资者"的资金一起"投资"战略计划。通过支持一个集中的战略计划和利用其他捐赠，投资的美元可能会产生最大的影响。儿童肿瘤基金会的研究计划和资助过程将在本章后面更详细地描述。

除了直接资助研究外，儿童肿瘤基金会还鼓励联邦政府支持 NF 研究。美国国立卫生研究院（National Institutes of Health，NIH）是美国最大的医学研究资助者。由于 NF 临床表现的广泛影响了各种器官系统，美国国立卫生研究院通过其至少 10 个研究所资助 NF 研究，包括国家癌症研究所、国家神经疾病和卒中研究所和国家精神卫生研究所。

虽然美国国立卫生研究院是美国最大的医学研究资助者，但自 1996 年以来，大多数 NF 研究都是由国会指导的医学研究计划神经纤维瘤病研究计划（Congressionally Directed Medical Research Program Neurofibromatosis Research Program，CDMRP NFRP）资助的。CDMRP NFRP 资助对 NF 研究的进步至关重要，因为其目标每年都由包括临床医师、研究人员和 NF 患者倡导者在内的整合小组更新。整合小组每年都可以评估当时最需要资金的地方，以最迅速的方式加速 NF 研究，然后在这些领域申请资金。在过去，这种明确的方法促使了由 9 个学术医学中心组成的国家 NF 临床试验联盟的建立，并导致了 NF 基因工程小鼠模型的发展。

CDMRP NFRP 资金每年由国会推荐，为期 1 年，该资金每年都有被削减的风险。在鼓励当选官员支持 CDMRP NFRP，并表明该计划对他们自己、他们的孩子或爱人有多重要方面，NF 民间基金会和选民基础发挥着非常重要的作用。确保 CDMRP NFRP 的持续性是基金会的优先事务，也是每个人都可以提供帮助的领域。

任务领域 4：提高公众对 NF 的认识度和接受度

问题解答："为什么这么多人从未听说过 NF1？"

在 NF1 患者的一生当中会遇到对这种疾病感到好奇的人，而且他们可能从未听说过这种疾病。许多 NF1 的人都经历过这样的询问，不幸的是，这可能会发展为社交困难，甚至导致真实的或感观的歧视。这可能是由于 1 个人的外表，比如身体上存在毁容的外部肿瘤或者是沟通障碍，因为 2/3 的 NF1 患者有学习障碍，这可能会导致社交困难。令人担忧的是，许多人从未听说过 NF1。许多关注 NF1 的基金会努力宣传 NF1 的真相，特别是消除 NF1 是"象人病"的误解（尽管事实证明这是 Proteus 综合征，但仍然会与 NF1 混淆）(Legendre et al. 2011)。Reggie Bibbs 先生是一个特别成功的独立的变革推动者，他是一名患 NF1 的年轻人，他通过他的基金会(Just Ask 基金)和"Just Ask"的信息，邀请了关于 NF1 的公开讨论。儿童肿瘤基金会通过各种渠道努力提高公众对 NF 的认识。然而，向公众解释 NF1 仍然是一个巨大的挑战。

41.2.2 NF1 民间基金成为进步的催化剂

即使是最成功的民间基金会也只能获得有限的资金。然而，经过精心规划，民间基金会可以对医学研究的进展产生巨大的影响，NF1 也不例外。儿童肿瘤基金会提供了一个如何实现这一目标的例子。直到 2006 年，儿童肿瘤基金会的研究资金主要集中在支持青年研究者奖(Young Investigator Awards，YIA)上。这些奖项致力于 NF 研究事业，并为有可能从事 NF 研究的博士和博士后科学家提供 2 年的薪水。这个项目仍然是一项有价值的投资，它帮助发展了一些当今领先的 NF 研究人员和临床医师的职业生涯(儿童肿瘤基金会青年研究者奖)。2006 年，基金会寻求将其研究支持从 YIA 扩展到更广泛的项目，其目标是开发 NF 的有效治疗方法并改善这种疾病患者的生命质量。

基金会首先分析了 NF 研究的整体"形势"，以评估哪些类型的 NF 研究得到了资助。这项分析的目的是确定那些可能对研究进展有重大影响但却被忽视和没有得到资助的研究领域。基金会分析了由 CDMRP NFRP、美国国立卫生研究院和儿童肿瘤基金会资助的 NF 研究，这 3 个基金会是 NF 研究的最大资助者。分析了 1996—2005 年的基金资助情况。所有资助的拨款都被分配到"箱子"中，这是由研究的重点从基础到临床的途径所决定的。超过 2.2 亿美元的 NF 研究资金被计划投入进 NF 研究形势中。随之而来的是基金会主办了一个由来自 NF 研究、生产制造、其他基金会和 NF 民间团体的专家组成的智囊团，以检查 NF 研究前景，确定被忽视的领域，并为基金会提出新的研究建议。

由此产生的 2006 年战略计划（2006 年儿童肿瘤基金会）建议实施一系列新举措，包括临床前药物测试、临床试验试点和国家 NF 临床网络(在本章前面描述)。因此，儿童肿瘤基金会在 2006—2011 年的 5 年期间实施了 1 000 万美元的新研究投资。考虑到在同一时期 CDMRP 和 NIH 在 NF 研究上总共投资了 1 亿多美元，因此这并不是一笔很大的投资。但是，新的基金会项目是具有催化作用的新型种子资金，包括具有一定风险的新想法，存在很高的潜力，但缺乏需要联邦资助的初步数据。

儿童肿瘤基金会催化种子基金项目的一个成功例子是药物发现倡议（Drug Discovery Initiative，DDI）奖。DDI 奖于 2006 年启动，为支持候选 NF 药物的临床前试验阶段提供种子资金。大多数 DDI 奖项的金额为 3 万美元或更少。资助的 DDI 奖评估了 NF 肿瘤外植体、原代细胞和细胞系的药物；异种移植和转基因小鼠模型；以及果蝇基因工程和斑马鱼的 NF 模型。NF1 的表现包括肿瘤、学习障碍、骨发育不良和心血管缺陷。对于所有的基金会项目，DDI 奖申请由基金会研究顾问理事会的一个委员会进行审查。DDI 奖申请不需要初步数据，委员会负责平衡彻底审查的风险和潜力。此外，DDI 奖的申请很简短，只有 3 页，基金会致力于快速审查这些申请。在大多数情况下，审查需要几周的时间，这与联邦拨款申请审查需要几个月的时间形成鲜明对比。

由于 DDI 奖励计划是独一无二的，基金会对一系列结果指标进行监测，以评估其成功与否。为了监测这笔资金的长期影响，基金会在 DDI 奖结束后很长一段时间内对资助的研究人员进行了跟踪。目的是跟踪研究在DDI奖结束后是否继续进行；DDI奖资助的数据是否发表；是否建立了任何行业合作；以及在DDI奖结束后，是否从其他来源获得后续资金以继续研究。目前对DDI奖项5年（2006—2011）的评估显示，大约有50笔津贴得到了资助，总投资约为100万美元。大约一半的DDI资助项目显示出"积极"的结果，即药物测试对NF表现有影响（例如肿瘤缩小）。获奖者发表了大约20篇关于DDI研究的论文；大约有20家还形成了产业（生物技术或制药）合作。也许最值得注意的是，根据DDI奖从不同来源（包括NIH、CDMRP、机构基金、行业赠款和基金会赠款）获得的数据，先前的获奖者总共获得了超过500万美元的后续资金。许多获得DDI奖的人表示，如果没有最初的DDI奖资助，他们的项目可能永远无法启动。

总而言之，DDI奖励计划通过为新的和未经测试的想法提供初始资金，达到了成功催化种子资金计划的标准。总的来说，DDI奖励计划帮助了NF临床前药物测试研发，并证明了少量的种子资金实际上可以对研究领域产生巨大的影响。

41.2.3　NF1民间基金会的媒介作用

医疗民间基金会有一个重要、独特的作用，即促成并建立与各种可能有助于基金会工作的组织机构之间的关系。由于民间基金会代表着大众的声音，因此往往能在这些关系网的建立中发挥独特的优势，并确保大家的目标清晰一致。以下内容简介了NF1基金会可能作为媒介的一些情形。

41.2.3.1　建立NF1研究者与临床医师之间的共识与协作

NF1专业群体包括在世界各地工作的研究人员和临床医师，但这实际上包含了相当少的个人。为了确保NF1研究取得进展，研究人员和临床医师在这一领域的持续沟通和及时分享研究进展是很重要的。NF1基金会可以在促进这方面发挥重要作用，儿童肿瘤基金会在这方面取得了重大成功。25年来，基金会每年为来自世界各地的NF科学家和临床医师组织一次会议，作为分享研究和医学进步以及讨论需要关注的问题的论坛。这一活动在过去几年中不断发展，除了长期关注研究发现之外，还越来越关注临床问题，自2005年以来，会议规模几乎增加了两倍，在2011年NF会议吸引了300多名参会者。在过去的几年里，基金会还出版了NF会议的专业报告，从而进一步增加了专业听众，他们可以从这个重要会议的演讲和讨论中受益（Kalamarides et al. 2012）。

有时候，NF研究的一个领域需要特别关注，以便充分了解该领域的现状并确定未来的优先事务。儿童肿瘤基金会举办了一系列的"研讨会"——智囊团专注于特定的肿瘤领域。这些研讨会通常包括来自该领域的25~30名专家，并总结该领域的现状、关键挑战以及如何解决这些挑战以推进该领域的研究进展。与NF会议一样，过去几年这些研讨会的成果报告已经出版，以供NF专业群体的其他人使用（Elefteriou et al. 2009）。

41.2.3.2　让产业界参与NF1事务

在过去，与许多其他罕见疾病一样，让生物技术和制药公司参与NF1事务一直具有挑战性。现在这种情况正在改变，因为公司认识到NF1的潜在商业机会，因为NF1需要终身治疗且没有批准的药物。然而，吸引行业参与的第一步仍然具有挑战性。为了解决这个问题，儿童肿瘤基金会创建了研究项目，为产业界提供了一个进入NF1研究的机会，而无须承担重大成本或风险。

如前所述，DDI奖励计划用来资助试点阶段的临床前药物测试。一些DDI获奖者已经能够从产业界获得测试药物。为DDI研究提供药物对公司来说几乎没有责任或风险。为了促进这些合作，儿童肿瘤基金会建立了DDI工具箱（药物发现倡议工具箱），一个公司可以列出他们愿意为NF研究提供的药物的网页。如果研究者对某一特定药品感兴趣，则公司与研究者所在机构签署必要的材料法律文件。

为了将DDI理念提升到一个新的水平，2008年，儿童肿瘤基金会建立了NF临床前联盟（NF Preclinical Consortium，NFPC），该联盟由6个学术研究中心组成，每个中心都专注于不同的NF肿瘤类型，并使用代表这些肿瘤的经过验证的小鼠模型。NFPC的目标是从业界获得药物，并在多个NF肿瘤小鼠模型中测试它们，以比较不同肿瘤类型对同一药物的反应。NFPC 由一个具有产业经验的科学家组成的外部顾问理事会监督。NFPC 是一项宏伟的事业，2008—2011 年它的初始成本为 400 万美元（NF 临床前联盟）。然而，事实证明它对产业界很有吸引力，因为它提供了在 NF 模型中对药物进行全面测试的方法。NFPC 也面临着挑战，尤其是为了每项研究而与多家机构签署法律协议的复杂之处。2011 年，基金会又重新将 NFPC 延长了 2 年，在结束的时候看看总体上完成了什么将会很有趣。

41.2.3.3 与其他 NF1 资金实体合作，实现互利共赢

正如本章前面所强调的，有许多 NF1 的民间基金会。这些实体是否有机会为了 NF1 患者群体的利益而进行合作？儿童肿瘤基金会和得克萨斯州 NF 基金会近期证明了这是可以做到的。在 2010 年和 2011 年，得克萨斯州 NF 基金会分别通过儿童肿瘤基金会资助了 1 个 NF1 青年研究者奖和 1 个 NF1 药物发现倡议奖。这两个项目都是通过儿童肿瘤基金会的审查程序推荐资助的。这是一个很好的例子，说明两个 NF1 民间基金会可以以一种切实可行的方式一起工作，希望它为今后这类合作奠定基础。

41.3 未来视野：NF1 民间基金会的演变

现今，新诊断为 NF1 的儿童比 10 年前诊断为 NF1 的儿童有非常大的希望前景。对于 NF1 患者来说，这是一个"希望的年代"。NF1 的临床诊断和治疗方法已经得到改善，并且 NF1 的候选药物治疗正在进行临床测试。但民间基金会在多大程度上能够或者应该为 NF1 患者带来希望呢？在哪些方面应该保持乐观，在进展消息传递中对于哪些方面应保持谨慎？NF1 民间基金会在展望未来时，还需要注意其他问题吗？最重要的是，NF1 民间基金会如何确保它们能够继续满足受 NF1 影响的个人及其家庭的需要？

41.3.1 NF1 的进展：在希望年代中平衡乐观和谨慎

NF1 的临床诊断和治疗选择在过去几年中取得了重大进展。目前已经对 NF1 的临床进展有了更好的了解，早期发现 NF1 临床表现的方法（如肿瘤成像技术）使 NF1 患者能够接受更警醒的临床监测，以便及早发现需要注意的医疗问题。基因检测现在广泛用于诊断和计划生育。除了手术干预外，现在有一系列 NF1 临床试验药物用于治疗 NF1 相关肿瘤、学习障碍和骨发育不良。NF1 临床前药物研发系统也在发展，很可能在不久的将来会有更多的药物进入临床试验。所有这些都意味着，与 5 年前相比，NF1 患者可以选择更大范围的治疗或试验。用不了多久，NF1 患者可能会被可用的选择所淹没。然而，重要的是要记住，大多数进入临床试验的药物最终都不会获得批准，参与临床试验并不能保证药物的成功。如果试验是盲法及安慰剂对照法，患者必须接受这样一个事实，即他们在试验期间甚至可能没有接受有效药物。虽然这肯定不仅仅是 NF1 基金会的责任，但对于基金会来说，尽可能多地告知个人和家庭这些潜在的问题，并提供尽可能多的关于所有可用治疗方式的最新信息是很重要的。

41.3.2 "患者力量"的兴起及其对未来 NF1 民间基金会的影响

NF1 民间基金会的核心是患者和家属，为这些人服务是民间基金会的主要责任。传统上，民间基金会一直是这些个人信息的来源和守护者，但是近几年已经看到了这种变化。有关研究和临床试验的信息现在可以在互联网上免费获得；许多患者对自己的病情进行了深度的研究，然后许多人利用这些信息来决定选择护理和治疗方案。因此，许多新诊断为 NF1 的人或他们的家人在第一次接触民间基金会时往往得到了广泛的信息。这使得基金会受到了比过去更多的审查，基金会需要为此做好准备。

许多患者和家庭开始参与管理自己的医疗保健，特别是对于像 NF1 这样临床进展可能相当复杂的罕见疾病。

在美国，健康保险流通与责任法案（像我这样的患者）对医师利用患者信息进行研究的能力产生了影响，尽管这种研究可能会更好地了解疾病或潜在

的治疗方法。相比之下，患者自己可以自由地分享他们的数据。在 PatientsLikeMe 网站上，个人可以分享他们的病史和治疗方案，并与其他有相同病情的人组成小组。PatientsLikeMe 包括患者的临床资源，并作为制药和生物技术公司的连接器来寻求和了解特定的患者群体。

随着个人在决定自己的临床护理路径方面发挥更积极的作用，这种演变被称为"患者力量"。随着基因组学在临床管理中的作用日益显现，直接接触患者本身将是非常有价值的，并可能对研究进展的速度产生重大影响。民间基金会非常清楚这一点，一些基金会正在将这些变化融入他们自己的项目中。例如，传统上民间基金会资助临床数据库的开发，这些数据库由临床中心维护和持有。最近，反而出现了一种由患者登记注册的趋势。儿童肿瘤基金会将在 2012 年推出这样的登记系统。患者驱动性的注册消除了通过诊所收集数据的限制，并有望更快地招募注册参与者。这是民间基金会拥有"患者力量"的一个例子，它也可以作为一种激励工具，使患者与基金会更紧密地联系在一起。

"患者力量"的兴起也会影响 NF1 民间基金会与那些为基金会的研究项目捐赠资金者之间的关系，因为许多新的捐助者希望密切参与他们所支持的研究。由于大多数民间基金会代表了一个非常广泛的组成基础，基金会为这些不断发展的关系建立界限和指导方针，以满足捐赠者和基金会的需求，这将是非常重要的。

41.4 结论

NF1 民间基金会对有这种罕见疾病的患者起着重要作用。这些作用包括筹集和分配研究资金以支持 NF1 研究和临床进展，这将对寻找 NF1 的治疗方法产生最大影响；向受 NF1 影响的人士提供尽可能多的资料，以便他们就临床护理等事宜做出明智的决定；在与资助 NF1 研究的其他实体联络时，作为 NF1 的倡导者和经纪人，可以推进民间基金会的任务，并最终改善 NF1 患者的生活。其核心是，通过支持有可能对 NF1 形势产生重大影响的新想法和概念，NF1 民间基金会应发挥催化剂的作用。

NF1 民间基金会确实需要意识到民众获取 NF1 信息和做出有关筹款决策的方式的演变，并准备好随着这些变化而发展。

（王广宇　译）

参考文献

[1] Children's Tumor Foundation Patient Brochures. http://www.ctf.org/Living-with-NF/patient-information-brochures.html

[2] Children's Tumor Foundation Young Investigator Awards. http://www.ctf.org/For-Scientists/young-investigator-awards.html

[3] Congressionally Directed Medical Research Program Neurofibromatosis Research Program. http://cdmrp.army.mil/nfrp/default.shtml

[4] Elefteriou F, Kolanczyk M, Schindeler A, Viskochil DH, Hock JM, Schorry EK, Crawford AH, Friedman JM, Little D, Peltonen J, Carey JC, Feldman D, Yu X, Armstrong L, Birch P, Kendler DL, Mundlos S, Yang FC, Agiostratidou G, Hunter-Schaedle K, Stevenson DA (2009) Skeletal abnormalities in neurofibromatosis type 1: approaches to therapeutic options. Am J Med Genet A 149A(10): 2327–2338

[5] Find an NF doctor. http://www.ctf.org/Living-with-NF/find-a-doctor.html

[6] Kalamarides M, Acosta MT, Babovic-Vuksanovic D, Carpen O, Cichowski K, Gareth Evans D, Giancotti F, Oliver Hanemann C, Ingram D, Lloyd AC, Mayes DA, Messiaen L, Morrison H, North K, Packer R, Pan D, Stemmer-Rachamimov A, Upadhyaya M, Viskochil D, Wallace MR, Hunter-Schaedle K, Ratner N (2012) Neurofibromatosis 2011: a report of the Children's Tumor Foundation Annual Meeting. Acta Neuropathol 123(3): 369–380

[7] Legendre CM, Charpentier-Côté C, Drouin R, Bouffard C (2011) Neurofibromatosis type 1 and the "elephant man's" disease: the confusion persists: an ethnographic study. PLoS One 6(2): e16409

[8] List of international NF foundations. http://www.neurofibromatosis-network.org

[9] "Living with NF" resources. http://www.ctf.org/About-the-Foundation/living-with-nf-info.html

[10] National Institutes of Health. http://www.nih.gov

[11] Patients Like Me. http://www.patientslikeme.com/

[12] The Children's Tumor Foundation. http://www.ctf.org

[13] The Children's Tumor Foundation 2006 Strategic Plan. http://www.ctf.org/pdf/professionals/STRAT_PLAN_WEBPAGE.pdf

[14] The Drug Discovery Initiative Award Program. http://www.ctf.org/For-Scientists/ddi-awards.html

[15] The Drug Discovery Initiative Toolbox. http://www.ctf.org/

For-Scientists/ddi-toolbox. html
[16] The Just Ask Foundation. http://www. justaskfoundation. org
[17] The Juvenile Diabetes Research Foundation. http://www. jdrf. org
[18] The Neurofibromatosis Network. http://www. nfnetwork. org
[19] The NF Preclinical Consortium. http://www. ctf. org/For-Scientists/ddi-nf-preclinical-consortium. html
[20] The Texas NF Foundation. http://texasnf. org/

第42章 1型神经纤维瘤病中的社会污名化
Social Stigma in Neurofibromatosis 1
Joan Ablon

42.1 引言

几乎没有临床医师有时间或机会去了解 NF1 患者的日常生活的系统经验和这些经验对其情感健康的影响。那些致力于解开遗传学、分子生物学和 NF1 周围其他错综复杂的技术领域的科学家们与受此疾病折磨的人的生活经历十分遥远。在本章中，我努力提供一个窗口，让大家可以了解影响患者个体在其生命过程中面临的围绕 NF1 的一些个人和家庭问题。

我将重点关注 Riccardi 所描述的 NF1 的"社会心理社会负担"的一个方面："NF1 对患者的情感和社会生活有明显不利的影响"（Riccardi 1992, p.198）。在过去 10 年间，关于 NF1 患者的"生命质量"问题的新兴文献开始出现（see the review of this literature by Birch and Friedman, Chap.8）。在此之前，很少有研究探讨 NF1 患者生活中的心理社会问题。Messner 和 Neff Smith (1986) 在报告中提到，从对国际文献的广泛回顾来看，个人和家庭的适应只是被"浅尝辄止"。事实上，Messner 和她的同事们发表了这个不被关注的领域内的大部分研究，他们发现了 NF1 患者的个人情绪适应和负面自我形象的表现，这通常是由于社会对他们的侮辱造成的（Messner and Neff Smith 1986；Messner et al. 1985a, b）。*Neurofibromatosis: A Handbook for Patients, Families and Health Care Professionals* (Rubenstein and Korf 1990) 一书中的一些章节对 NF1 的心理社会问题进行了概述，而 Ablon (1999) 做了迄今为止对这些问题最全面的探索。

虽然临床医师可能认为大多数 NF1 患者没有也不会受到严重的社会因素影响，Bejemain 等（1993）发现，在他们的研究中，大多数 NF1 患者认为他们的病情比临床医师判断的更严重。临床评估通常不考虑症状的心理社会影响，例如可能是非常小的外部神经纤维瘤和学习障碍，这些症状可能具有或不具有临床威胁性，但却可能对患者有着广泛的影响，不仅影响日常生活体验，还影响整个生命过程中的主要期望、机会和决策。社会污名化和社会排斥似乎比患者身体症状更频繁地给受试者带来心理和社会负担。各种形式的社会污名可能常伴在受影响者的日常生活左右。此外，长期以来被误诊为 NF1 的"象人"的幽灵在许多成年人的童年和青少年时期萦绕不去。

42.2 污名化的概念

在经典著作《污名化》（*Stigma*）中，Goffman

J. Ablon
Medical Anthropology Program, Department of Anthropology, History, and Social Medicine, School of Medicine, University of California, San Francisco, CA, USA
e-mail: ablonj@aol.com

M. Upadhyaya and D. N. Cooper (eds.), *Neurofibromatosis Type 1*,
DOI 10.1007/978-3-642-32864-0_42, # Springer-Verlag Berlin Heidelberg 2012

(1963)提供了将污名化作为一种社会和文化现象来解决的第一个指导:

社会建立了分类人的方法,并规定了每个类别成员应具备的普通和自然的属性。……当陌生人在我们面前时,可能会出现证据表明他拥有一种属性,使他与其他人不同……并且是较不受欢迎的那种——极端情况下,一个人可能非常坏、危险或软弱。……因此,在我们的脑海中,他从一个普通的人变成了一个有污点、被轻视的人。这种属性是一种耻辱,尤其是当它的诋毁效果非常广泛时:有时它也被称为失败、缺点、障碍。(第2~3页)

污名是社会的创造和产物。关于什么构成身体正常或审美上可接受的人的定义是任意的,并受到文化和社会背景的影响。美国的价值观包括对"美""丑"和"健康"的重要且往往正式的外貌和社会规范。这些处方通过媒体的描绘以及生活的社会、经济和政治层面的选择得到了系统的强化。社会成功有利于个人成就、良好的身体健康、外在美以及职业和运动成就。对可能无法满足此类处方的身体或精神上不同的人的负面态度已有很好的记录(among many such writings are those of Goffman 1963; Eisenberg et al. 1982; Graham and Kligman 1985; Murphy 1990; Ablon 1998; Hatfield and Sprecher 1986; Grealy 1994)。导致明显特征被视为缺陷的情况,如NF1的情况,可能会给受影响的人带来严重的负担。Murphy(1990)指出:"一个人充分参与这个社会的最大障碍不是他的身体缺陷,而是社会对他们的神话、恐惧和误解。"(Murphy 1990, pp. 112-113)

Goffman(1963)提出,可见和不可见的污名会导致其持有者名誉扫地或不可信任。例如,那些身体上可见污名的人可能会立即名誉扫地,但如果污名特征被揭示,那些在日常互动中不可见的污名的人则可能被认为是不可信的。当一个人的耻辱感不易察觉时,对信息的控制可能成为个人的主要问题。对于NF1不易看到的人来说,仍然可能存在是否披露其状况的负担。一些最引人注目的披露时间可能是在一段新关系的发展阶段,或者是在第一次亲密接触的时候。管理一个潜在的不光彩的属性可能会非常令人焦虑,并严重影响一个人对自我的定义。

Quaid(1994)指出:

遗传信息被广泛认为是在某种基本的(如果没有表达的话)层面上说一个人是谁。特别是在这个意义上,人们似乎因暴露其遗传信息而感到污名化,而其他人可能更容易因此而受到污名化。在某些情况下,即使是医疗专业人员也倾向于以不同于治疗其他疾病的方式治疗已证实的遗传性疾病,对处于危险中的个体产生可预测的影响。(第6页)

尽管今天在互联网和各种媒体上获得的关于NF1的信息比以往任何时候都多,但很明显,多年来NF1的儿童和成年人面临的主要生活问题一直没有改变。社会对被视为负面的差异的反应在生活的大多数领域都很常见。例如,请注意新命名的"欺凌"现象的出现,以及近年来涉及这一主题的书籍、电影和研讨会。事实上,一个戏剧性的名字现在被赋予到古老的行为上,这种行为负面地挑战了许多类型的差异。

42.3 方法

这里提供的受影响个人的数据和陈述是基于我在20世纪90年代在加利福尼亚州参加的定性开放式访谈和支持小组会议以及近年来的后续访谈。我最初采访了54名NF1成年人,他们从3个来源招募:① 参加加利福尼亚州北部三个地区和国家支持团体的人群,② 对这些组织在当地邮寄公告中发布的通知做出回应的人群,以及③ 两个主要大都市医院遗传学部门的病例量。我不能说这里报告的对象代表了所有受NF1影响的人,因为NF1患者群像的确切构成尚不清楚。然而,我相信这些受试者公平地代表了成千上万参加支持小组、收到通知但未参加以及参加医院项目的人中的许多人。然而,应该指出的是,这些来源可能会吸引受影响人群和受影响人群中较为严重的家庭。

在大多数情况下,我的采访是在受试者的家中进行的,在少数情况下是在餐馆进行的。34名受试者接受了一次访谈;11名受试者接受了两次访谈;另外9人接受了3次或3次以上的采访,其中一些人在多年内接受了5~6次采访。在NF支持小组会议和电话交谈中也收集了材料。受试者慷慨地与我分享了他们的生活经历和对 NF1 的态度。面试往往持续至少 3 个小时,许多面试持续 4 个或 5 个小时或更长时间。许多人表示,他们以前从未坦率地与他人谈论过自己的病情以及他们认为病情对他们生活的影响。关于访谈的更多细节,见脚注 1[①](Ablon 1999)。

42.4 NF1 的污名化

一个接一个的患者谈论着他们对身上肿瘤的担忧,即使他们的肿瘤在穿着衣服时看不见。NF1 在受影响者生活中的残酷在一个年轻人的痛苦陈述中得到了很好的体现,他英俊的脸上有许多小肿瘤。

我可以应对手术和震耳欲聋、失明和瘫痪的威胁——这是一回事。但是,这似乎是徒劳的,困扰我的是毁容。从社会角度来看,这是最令人压抑的事情。如果我每隔几年做一两次手术,人们不会因此而避开我。但如果你看起来皮肤状况很糟糕,人们真的会很残忍。我曾有过这样的幻想——如果我能在没有 NF 的情况下度过 24 小时。只是为了感受它是什么样子!即使没有人能看到我,我只看到了自己!这是一个奇怪的幻想。只是想知道没有它我会是什么样子!我试着不去想,如果我没有这个,我的生活会有多么不同。我尽量不去说"如果",因为如果我这样做,我现在就失去了宝贵的时间。

尽管这名男子之前曾因颈部和背部的大型内部肿瘤接受过非常危险的手术,但他在我们采访中的重点仍旧是他因外表而遭受的社会排斥。他对外表的强调最终变成了一个悲剧性的讽刺,因为他在我们采访的 2 个月后因为一个未被发现的巨大脑瘤而去世了。

42.5 污名化的主要来源

电视、电影和其他公共媒体为我们生动描绘了具有局限性的文化和社会价值观,他们往往为美丽和健康创造了无法达到的标准。对于有明显 NF1 的人来说,负面行为、态度和好奇心可能会出现在商场等公共场所以及日常生活的一般互动中。被误诊为"象人病"的 Joseph Merrick 令人难忘的形象在印刷品、戏剧和电影中广泛流行(Montagu 1971;Graham and Oehlschlaeger 1992),对许多 NF1 患者的羞耻和压抑的发展产生了非常大的影响。同样,医师告诉患者和家属这种"罕见"和"可怕"的疾病可能导致严重残疾的浮夸辞藻,是许多受试者对其病情产生负面心态的重要因素。

1 位看过许多 NF1 患者的神经科医师说:"这吓坏了患者,尤其是那些疯狂地认为自己的孩子会长成这个怪物的父母。"1 位遗传顾问说:"我认为《象人》是对 NF1 患者最大的伤害。""每个人都想知道他们是否会这样。"在病情不可预测的背景下,医师早期的可怕陈述,再加上媒体对象人的描述,极大地加剧了受试者的恐惧(Ablon 1995)。一位描述自己无法规划教育或职业未来的女性告诉我:"我现在明白了,这一切都是一个大错误。我瘫痪了好几年。我以为我会成为'大象夫人'。"

父母最大的创伤发生在与第一次诊断相关时的记忆中。一位母亲说:

当医师告诉我 Karen 患有象人病时,我晕倒在他的地板上。那天晚些时候,当我告诉丈夫时,我又晕倒了。

另一位母亲:

我直接去了大学和 Harper 医院的医学图书馆。

(你的反应是什么?)

恐怖,恐怖。

令人遗憾的是,许多医师甚至在今天仍然继续告诉患者及其家属 NF1 是象人病,尽管大约 26 年前,医学期刊甚至流行文献都明确公开宣布了这一误诊(Tibbles and Cohen 1986)。Legendre 等

---

① 研究参与者是从国家神经纤维瘤病基金会股份有限公司赞助的支持团体招募的,该基金会现已更名为儿童肿瘤基金会和现在的组织加利福尼亚神经纤维瘤症网络。目前,还有一些团体得到了加利福尼亚股份有限公司神经纤维瘤病的支持。采访了 54 名受影响的成年人,其中 32 名是女性,22 名是男性。15 人的父母患有 NF1。20 名儿童受到影响。10 人是少数民族成员:5 名西班牙裔、3 名非裔美国人、1 名中国人和 1 名菲律宾人。第一次面试时,受试者的年龄从 19 岁到 70 岁不等。教育水平从高中毕业到博士级研究生课程入学不等。受试者的职业如此多样化,以至于他们的人数几乎与受试者人数相等。职业包括专业人员、劳动者、退休人员以及依靠临时和永久残疾福利生活的人。

(2011)在最近的一项研究中报告称,一些加拿大医师继续将象人病与NF1混淆。此外,这种混淆仍然发生在媒体上,即使是在引用的词典条目中。这些作者表示:

> 将NF1与象人的病情混淆会损害NF1患者的利益,尤其是因为众所周知,NF1患者在建立社会关系和培养良好自尊方面遇到了困难……他们的病情被误认为是象人病,因此背负着其他人认为他们会随着时间的推移而严重毁容的观念,只会增加这些困难,损害他们实现正常社会生活、找到感兴趣的工作、享受持久的浪漫关系和生孩子的希望。(第113页)

家庭、学校、同事和医务人员可能会对NF1患者进行污名化和表达。消极的家庭态度尤其具有破坏性,会造成早期糟糕的自我形象,抑制自信心和积极应对技能的发展。早期的学校经历可能具有破坏性。入学通常是儿童与社会规范和公众监督的第一次重大对抗。其他孩子的教导、歧视甚至身体虐待,现在通常被称为"欺凌"行为,可能会让孩子对他或她余生中预期的社会行为有一个预览。同样,主管和同事在工作场所的负面态度和系统性歧视给成年人带来了士气低落的工作环境,他们可能已经因为学习障碍而受到不良学业的阻碍。

我在这里要强调,与医务人员的负面互动可能是污名的主要来源。许多NF1患者向我讲述了他们认为污名化的医师和其他医务人员的陈述和态度,一些医务人员公开对患者的外表表示厌恶。1名男子说,他一直觉得自己是个"基因怪胎",总是对学生和医学同事开放,但很快就被解雇了,因为他无法治愈。

许多人对他们的医师表示非常不满,他们认为医师通常对自己或孩子的医疗护理不感兴趣或关心。虽然从业者将患者描述为"顺从""温和""渴望接受"和"不为自己的病情感到痛苦"(e. g., Trevisani et al. 1982),但这种外表可能是由于患者的被动性造成的,这种被动性是基于他们对一生糟糕的医疗护理和对未来医疗互动的低期望。此外,学习障碍和其他与NF1相关的压力产生因素的影响对他们的自我形象和应对技能产生了不利影响,医师有时会错误地解释这种被动性。事实上,在他们与我的谈话和支持小组会议中,受影响的人在许多情况下对他们的护理有非常负面的看法,但不会在医疗互动中公开表达这些看法。

由于NF1的不可预测性,受影响者可能一生都生活在可能出现的多种症状的恐惧中,医师对患者病情的初步或唯一可能的预测的任何评论,多年以后都有可能不可摆脱地困扰着患者。这种超敏反应提醒我们,医师应该意识到他们的陈述的效力,以及对清晰和支持性沟通的特殊需求。例如,几位母亲报告说,儿科医师告诉她们,根据婴儿身上咖啡牛奶斑的数量,孩子可能患有NF1,即象人病,但由于诊断可能几年后才知道,她们不应该担心。但这样的叙述反而让这些母亲心中充满了恐惧,并且这种恐惧将一直伴随着她们。

42.6 对生活的主要领域的影响

社会污名可能会严重影响受影响的人的教育和经济经历,并剥夺他们对亲密关系(性、约会、婚姻和生育)的正常期望。

42.6.1 教育和就业

学习障碍在NF1患者中相对常见,对受影响的人来说往往是毁灭性的,因为这为糟糕的学校职业生涯以及学校的歧视和鄙视奠定了基础。在目前普遍存在的学习和注意力缺陷障碍以及针对这些障碍的特殊教育计划的发展之前,有此类学校经历的成年人可能经受了特别严重的损害。许多人被告知他们只是"愚蠢"。糟糕的学习成绩和围绕学校经历的沮丧往往导致他们获得满意或高薪工作的机会受到严重限制。在求职时,像NF1这样有特殊健康状况的人会发现自己因外表、医疗问题以及医师就诊或治疗需求的缺失而处于双重或三重劣势之中。我采访的许多人都很少得到基于残疾人辅助的各种项目的支持。即使是在中产阶级或舒适的家庭环境中长大的人,也发现自己作为成年人已经处在了边缘人生活环境中的"边缘"了。

42.6.2 亲密关系与婚姻关系

NF1患者所描述的亲密关系是最令人心酸和

敏感的。僵化的社会对外表和成就的规定可能会阻碍NF1患者寻找潜在的伴侣，并在受影响的人中产生低自我价值的态度，从而在这个最个人化的生活领域中经历强烈的负面打击。社会对美丽和健康的处方往往与浪漫的成功有关，尽管主流社会中能够达到这些处方的人相对较少。那些明显不同的人可能会被个人失败和不足的感觉所压倒。

我的研究发现，女性在寻求性接触和约会的机会时表现得更具攻击性。男性往往对自己的失败更加气馁，更有可能退出对伴侣的寻找。对于那些穿衣服时NF1不明显的人来说，在亲密的情况下暴露身体上的肿瘤是一个巨大的挑战。许多找到了与他们结婚的特殊人士的人同样面临着其他挑战，比如，是否生孩子和是否有可能因病情而去世等。女性则需要面对孩子的遗传病风险以及妊娠带来新肿瘤的可能。

年长女性虽然也会受到NF1带来的生活影响，但并不像许多年轻女性那样明显地受到病情的困扰。她们与丈夫有着长期稳定的婚姻，丈夫接受她们的NF1是她们身体中不起眼的一部分。今天的年轻人，无论是男性还是女性，都更容易受到媒体和其中描绘的耀眼的美丽，他们更清楚自己的差异。即使他们有一个充满爱、乐于接受的伴侣在场，也可能无法减轻他们的痛苦。事实上，他们可能更加担心配偶会离开他们，他们将无法找到另一个能够忍受他们的外表或医疗问题的人。

42.7 成功应对污名化的因素

我对具有导致身体差异的不同遗传状况的人（侏儒症，Ablon 1984，1988；NF1，Ablon 1999；成骨不全，Ablon 2010）进行的访谈表明，在大多数情况下，那些成功应对污名化健康状况的人表现出生物特征和意识形态的共性。

（1）最重要的特征是无条件的家庭支持和明确的家庭内部沟通。拥有强大的家庭支持，能够在生命的早期向个人灌输信心和安全感。拥有一个坚定支持并善于鼓励的家庭能够在个人被诊断后表现出更好的应对，为应对生活带来的任何挑战奠定了基础。这些家庭积极而批判性地为他们的孩子寻求最好的医疗服务，并始终提供实际和情感支持。在健康状况不佳的时期，家庭成员能够陪同儿童或成人去看医师，就治疗方案做出决定，住院时总是陪在床边。积极的父母沟通也至关重要，对于父母有同样情况的人来说，这种沟通似乎至关重要。如果这些父母尽一切努力教育孩子了解他们的病情，并愿意谈论他们表达或未表达的恐惧和担忧，这种氛围将预示着更明智和有效的应对方式。

（2）事实证明，参加NF支持小组对许多人特别有帮助，这让他们有难得的机会与他人见面，了解最新的临床和科学发现。在分享和讨论小组中，受影响的人有机会表达他们的担忧、恐惧和问题，并且往往能够从他人的经验和策略中学习。在区域和国家信息活动中，演讲者通常是临床医师、遗传学家和遗传顾问，他们可以报告最新的治疗方法和科学发现；因此，参会者可以特别地接触到NF1专家，专家可以回答他们的具体问题。对现有治疗方案的深入了解往往可以缓解他们的担忧，而与克服了自己挑战的其他人会面，可以建立对成功应对未来可能带来的能力的自信。

（3）促进成功应对污名化条件的第三个特征是一种哲学，它否认身体差异是污名化或较低身份的基础。这使人们认识到，像NF1这样的特殊健康状况不会削弱他们的天生能力，不会使他们成为低人一等的人，也不应该以任何方式自动剥夺他们享有主流社会期望和利益的权利。这一理念是残疾人权利运动的基础，该运动强调"残疾"和特殊健康状况（如NF1）的主要问题在于剥夺受影响者平等权利和机会的社会、文化、经济和政治制度，而不是个人差异或不足。此外，这些问题可以更好地理解为对社会难以接受的少数群体的偏见的民权问题。内化这一哲学的人可能会更加积极，更有信心和控制感，因为通过共同努力，社会和文化环境可以而且将会改变。父母、教师、工作主管和医务人员帮助那些可能被社会标记为污名的人发展、维护和体现这一理念，将确保他们有可能过上更满意、更成功的生活。

致谢：我非常感谢美国国家科学基金会（批准号：BN58819633）和旧金山加利福尼亚大学学术参议院研究资助，这使我能够进行本章所基于的实地研究。

（王达辉，钱闯　译）

参考文献

[1] Ablon J (1984) Little people in America: the social dimensions of dwarfism. Praeger, New York

[2] Ablon J (1988) Living with difference: families with dwarf children. Praeger, New York

[3] Ablon J (1995) "The Elephant Man" as "self" and "other": The psycho-social costs of a misdiagnosis. Soc Sci Med 40 (11): 1481-1489

[4] Ablon J (1998) Coping with visible and invisible stigma: Neurofibromatosis 1. In: Makas E, Haller B, Doe T (eds) Accessing the issues: current research in disability studies. The Society for Disability Studies, Edmund S. Muskie Institute of Public Affairs, Lewiston, ME, pp 45-49

[5] Ablon J (1999) Living with genetic disorder. Auburn House, Westport, CT

[6] Ablon J (2010) Brittle bones, stout hearts and minds: adults with Osteogenesis Imperfecta. Jones & Bartlett, Sudbury, MA

[7] Benjamin CM, Colley A, Donnai D, Kingston H, Harris R, Kerzin-Storrar L (1993) Neurofibro-matosis type 1 (NF1): knowledge, experience, and reproductive decisions of affected patients and families. J Med Genet 30: 567-574

[8] Eisenberg M, Griggins C, Duval R (eds) (1982) Disabled people as second class citizens. Springer, New York

[9] Goffman I (1963) Stigma: notes on the management of spoiled identity. Prentice-Hall, Englewood, NJ

[10] Graham J, Kligman A (1985) The psychology of cosmetic treatment. Praeger, New York

[11] Graham PW, Oehlschlaeger FH (1992) Articulating the Elephant Man: Joseph Merrick and his interpreters. The Johns Hopkins University Press, Baltimore, MD

[12] Grealy L (1994) Autobiography of a face. Houghton Mifflin, Boston, MA

[13] Hatfield E, Sprecher S (1986) Mirror, mirror ... The importance of looks in everyday life. State University of New York Press, Albany, NY

[14] Legendre C-M, Charpentier-Côté C, Drouin R (2011) Neurofibromatosis type 1: persisting misidentification of the "Elephant Man" disease. J Am Board Fam Med 24(1): 112-114

[15] Messner RL, Neff Smith M (1986) Neurofibromatosis: relinquishing the masks: a quest for quality of life. J Adv Nurs 11: 459-464

[16] Messner RL, Gardner S, Messner MR (1985a) Neurofibromatosis—an international enigma: a framework for nursing. Cancer Nurs 8(6): 314-322

[17] Messner RL, Messner MR, Lewis SJ (1985b) Neurofibromatosis: a familial and family disorder. J Neurosurg Nurs 17(4): 221-228

[18] Montagu A (1971) The Elephant Man: a study in human dignity. Outerbridge and Dienstfrey, New York (Distributed by E. P. Dutton)

[19] Murphy R (1990) The body silent. W. W. Norton, New York

[20] Quaid KA (1994) A few words from a "wise" woman. In: Weir RF, Lawrence SC, Fales E (eds) Genes and human self-knowledge. University of Iowa Press, Iowa City, IA, pp 3-17

[21] Riccardi VM (1992) Neurofibromatosis, phenotype, natural history, and pathogenesis. The Johns Hopkins University Press, Baltimore

[22] Rubenstein A, Korf B (eds) (1990) Neurofibromatosis: a handbook for patients, families and health-care professionals. Thieme Medical Publishers, New York

[23] Tibbles J, Cohen M (1986) The Proteus syndrome: the Elephant Man diagnosed. Br Med J (Clin Res Ed) 293(6548): 683-685

[24] Trevisani TP, Pohl AL, Matloub HS (1982) Neurofibroma of the ear: function and aesthetics. Plast Reconstr Surg 70(2): 217-219

第43章 1型神经纤维瘤病的个性化诊疗
Personalized Medicine in NF1

David Viskochil

43.1 引言

个性化诊疗是指利用临床上潜在的或尚未被认识的特征，对患者进行个体化的医疗服务。通常这一概念适用于大多数人群，建立的诊断能以个性化的形式指导医疗服务。研究者们启动了一项针对NF1的终身监测计划，以发现在普通人群中无法预测的医疗事件。NF1的诊断是个性化诊疗的最佳案例，它改变了那些被诊断为NF1患者的管理方式和治疗方案。一旦确诊NF1，个性化诊疗原则便可以应用于这些患者。

43.2 NF1的预期性指导

NF1患儿的家人和医护人员对潜在的并发症常常感到焦虑，不知何时需要警惕，何时可以放松。充分应用个性化诊疗原则可以减少医务人员对NF1常规预期性指导的依赖，专注于更可能影响特定临床、遗传和环境特征个体的医疗问题，从而制订个性化的健康管理计划。例如，表43.1列出了不同年龄段可能出现的NF1临床表现的预期性指导原则。通过识别特定年龄的临床症状，就可以基于年龄因素优化影像学或诊断学检查的时间安排，作为

表43.1 年龄相关的NF1多种临床表现的预期性指导原则（Adopted from Viskochil, D. 2010. Neurofibromatosis type 1. In: Management of Genetic Syndromes）

针对年龄相关的特定临床表现的干预指南
胫骨弓：长骨发育不良/童年早期假关节
营养不良性脊柱侧凸：童年早期
视神经通路肿瘤：童年早期至中期；具有种族因素
言语和语言障碍：童年早期至中期
认知损害：童年早期至中期
社交能力障碍：童年/青春期
恶性周围神经鞘膜瘤：青少年晚期/成年期
真皮神经纤维瘤：童年晚期/青春期

注：我们需要时刻关注的临床表现：丛状神经纤维瘤、肉瘤、血管异常、不明确的精神异常。

个性化诊疗保健的一部分。由于NF1临床表现多样，所以很难提供更详细的干预指导。因此开发和应用标志物十分重要，这些标志物能够帮助医务人员在症状出现前就识别出某种症状的高危和低危个体，也能够更可靠地记录疾病的进展，对标志物的应用可以优化治疗措施并节省医疗费用。在NF1个

性化诊疗背景下，疾病标志物不仅包括传统意义上的基因标记，如 *NF1* 基因型、功能多态性和实验室检测的生物标志物，还包括影像学研究、血压监测、临床检查和谱系分析。

在确诊 NF1 的面诊及此后的每次随访中，患者的家人常常会问一个关键问题："我的孩子会经历一段艰难的时期吗？还是我们可以放松一点，把担忧转移到其他事情上？"无论答案如何，帮助父母做好心理准备并建立合理的预期，可以大大减轻患者和家属所感受到的"定时炸弹"般的压力。应用疾病标志物可以改进对个体风险的定义，以减轻家长和医护人员在面对孩子可能出现的临床症状的焦虑：视神经通路肿瘤的发生率为 15%，胫骨假关节的发生率为 2%，丛状神经纤维瘤的发生率为 25%，恶性周围神经鞘膜瘤的发生率为 10%。治疗方案不确定性带来的焦虑也可以得到缓解，例如，何时以及多久进行一次影像学检查、治疗干预的时机和对治疗的预期反应等。

43.3　个性化诊疗的应用

循证医学被广泛应用于个性化诊疗，其定义是在临床干预之前对系统性收集的证据进行批判性分析，并进一步评估临床结果的过程（Willard and Ginsburg 2009）。这一过程通常耗时较长，平均需要 17 年才能将成果完全应用于临床（Balas and Boren 2000）。因此，当前对 NF1 某项特定症状的成功干预进行集中分析，其结果预计需要十几年才能纳入最佳实践指南。这主要适用于显性的临床症状。更难研究的是预防临床症状的干预措施，因为 NF1 临床表现的高度异质性，很难确定哪些人有可能出现众多临床表现中的任何一种。个性化诊疗的实践包含了健康风险评估，以确定患病的可能性或者患者的临床表现（Ginsburg and Willard 2009）。这种风险分层可以基于对相关发现的临床识别、谱系分析、分子研究（生物标志物）和影像学检查等信息建立起来。当使用临床决策支持系统处理这些信息时（Osheroff et al. 2007），医务人员可以为患者制订更好的个性化医疗服务，以实现患者的目标。

43.4　个性化诊疗在 NF1 诊疗中的应用

在 NF1 个性化诊疗中的一个简单例子是血压监测。一个临床上看不见的发现，即通过血压监测发现的儿童高血压，可以指向不同的医疗选择。如果在三次重复测量中血压均高于同年龄、身高和性别的标准，就应当进行影像学检查以确定是否存在肾动脉狭窄。像血压这种基本的临床信息就可以带来有效的个体化诊疗。然而，医务人员必须确定最有效的干预措施，这就需要结合全面的循证医学证据、健康风险评估和临床决策支持系统，来提供一系列干预建议和时机的选择。这种选择综合考虑了多种因素，并体现了个性化诊疗的艺术。

基因型-表型的相关性始终是应用个性化诊疗时需要考虑的重要因素，大多数医务人员也常将这一因素与"个性化诊疗"这一泛用的术语联系起来。*NF1* 基因座有一些致病突变，可用来预测可能的临床症状和严重程度。全基因 *NF1* 缺失（Kayes et al. 1994；Pasmant et al. 2010）提示恶性周围神经鞘膜瘤风险增加（De Raedt et al. 2003；Mautner et al. 2010），因此需要加强肿瘤监测。22 号外显子中的第 3 碱基对缺失（Stevenson et al. 2006）与恶性程度较低的肿瘤表型相关（Upadhyaya et al. 2007），因此可以减少监测。此外，可以为携带者提供优化的生殖风险咨询，以预防下一代出现更严重的临床症状。*NF1* 基因座的胚系突变遍布在这个包含有 60 个外显子的基因中，通常会导致单倍体不足，从而解释了这种情况下缺乏基因型与临床症状之间的相关性。某些错义突变是例外，例如识别参与调节 Ras 通路活性的神经纤维瘤蛋白的特定结构域。然而，即使在同一家族中的错义突变，也可以导致多种 NF1 临床表型。总的来说，NF1 突变筛查并没有为健康风险评估提供很大的帮助。

个性化诊疗在 NF1 中的另一个创新应用，是通过全身 MRI 评估肿瘤负荷来进行风险分层（Mautner et al. 2008；Plotkin et al. 2012）。该 MRI 成像方案运用了一种生物标志物，利用影像学检查评估全身肿瘤负荷，从而为可能发展为 MPNST 的 NF1 患者提供更加合理的监测方案（Mautner et al. 2008）。

肿瘤体积增大的风险因素包括皮下神经纤维瘤数量和女性性别（Plotkin et al. 2012）。这些数据代表了NF1循证医学的早期阶段，方案实施尚未正式纳入普遍的临床指南。随着更多的临床中心将全身影像学检查纳入肿瘤监测方案，该检查对NF1患者筛查的效果将会得到进一步评估。这也展示了个性化诊疗应用的另一个组成部分，即对医疗服务成本的评估，以确保采取的诊疗方案在不同患者之间取得平衡，在不过多占用医疗资源的情况下，最大限度地提高个人的医疗获益。

NF1与视神经通路肿瘤相关，肿瘤学家发现NF1患者的视神经肿瘤侵袭性低于非NF1患者。这就为患者制订下丘脑-视神经低级别胶质瘤的标准治疗方案提供了预后信息。一个尚未充分解释的有趣现象是，日本血统的NF1患者视神经通路肿瘤发病率较低［Niimura Personal communication（日本患者约为1.5%，而欧洲和北美患者约为15% Rosenfeld et al. 2010）］。人们推测，日本人群中可能存在修饰基因或功能多态性，一旦其中的规律被揭开，医务人员可以将健康风险评估算法应用到视神经胶质瘤相关的个性化风险分层中，从而改变常规眼科和脑MRI检查的策略，以便早期对低级别视神经通路胶质瘤检测和治疗。然而，日本较低患病率的这一观察结果尚未通过循证医学的审查，因此尚未纳入NF1的预期性指导中。

NF1患者认知障碍非常常见，超过60%的患者存在某种形式的障碍，包括但不限于言语困难、执行功能问题、注意力缺陷、短期记忆困难和社交障碍等问题。这一认识促使大家更加重视神经心理学测试和干预措施，希望以此改善患者的学业状况（Krab et al. 2008）。由于认知障碍的临床表现差异较大，早期诊断策略将有助于制订合适的学业状况的干预措施。使用最先进的影像学技术，如功能性MRI成像的静息状态连接（Chabernaud et al. 2012），有助于识别特定的认知障碍，评估行为和药物干预等的治疗反应。

流行病学研究表明，NF1与早期死亡率（Rasmussen et al. 2001）、脑癌（Walker et al. 2006）和乳腺癌（Sharif et al. 2007）的风险增加有关。这些报告已通过循证医学审查，并成为鉴定NF1患者携带更高恶性的MPNST（即全基因NF1缺失）、胶质母细胞瘤（即PTEN-AKT通路中的功能多态性）、乳腺癌（即表观遗传学变化）或血管疾病（即炎症循环标志物）发展风险的生物标志物。找出这些生物标志物对健康风险评估的准确度来说至关重要，以便在症状出现前就识别出潜在的严重症状的个体。这些研究才刚刚起步，临床决策支持系统的建立还有很长的路要走。然而，DNA、血清和尿液样本的收集，以及来自患者病史的纵向临床信息，将为NF1患者的个性化诊疗应用开辟道路。

需要注意的是，个性化诊疗并不总是意味着识别血液、尿液生物标志物或基因组变化，还可以通过对临床症状和体征进行详细分析来实现。除了专注于肿瘤筛查的开发，我们还应该重视家族谱系信息、病史文书（包括系统回顾、体格检查）、预后转归（特别是有治疗措施）。Sbidian等（2010）确定了四个变量来筛查有椎旁肿瘤倾向的NF1患者：两个或多个皮下神经纤维瘤、无皮肤型神经纤维瘤、少于6个咖啡牛奶斑，年龄在30岁或以下。临床上，这一评分可能只对一小部分NF1患者适用，以确定谁应该接受更密切的恶性肿瘤监测。只有通过持续收集旨在提升医疗决策系统的数据，才能最终改变临床诊疗方案。

43.5 结论

个性化诊疗的发展是一条漫长的道路，但在特定疾病中已经取得了进展，例如Poon和Hamid（2012）所述的哮喘治疗中，通过对哮喘患者人群进行内在分型，已促成了针对特定分型的更为有效的治疗方案的发展。与其他疾病一样，NF1的最佳临床指南已经制订出来，并随着新知识的不断积累而不断更新，以指导家人和医务人员根据患者的临床表现和需求量身定制诊疗方案。结合现有的临床指南与分子生物标志物，将为基于生物学的干预措施提供机遇，从而加快循证医学在个性化诊疗中的应用进程。

（顾建英，卫传元 译）

参考文献

[1] Balas E, Boren S (2000) Managing clinical knowledge for health care improvement. In: Bemmel J, McCray AT (eds) Yearbook of medical informatics 2000: patient-centered systems. Schattauer, Stuttgart, pp 65–70

[2] Chabernauda C, Mennes M, Kardelb P, Gaillardc W, Kalbfleischd M, VanMeter J, Packer R, Milham M, Castellanos F, Acosta M (2012) Lovastatin regulates brain spontaneous low-frequency brain activity in neurofibromatosis type 1. Neurosci Lett 515: 28–33

[3] De Raedt T, Brems H, Wolkenstein P, Vidaud D, Pilotti S, Perrone F, Mautner V, Frahm S, Sciot R, Legius E (2003) Elevated risk for MPNST in NF1 microdeletion patients. Am J Hum Genet 72: 1288–1292

[4] Ginsburg G, Willard H (2009) Genomic and personalized medicine: foundations and applications. Transl Res 154: 277–287

[5] KayesLM BW, Riccardi VM, Bennett R, Ehrlich P, Rubenstein A, Stephens K (1994) Deletions spanning the neurofibromatosis 1 gene: identification and phenotype of five patients. Am J Hum Genet 54: 424–436

[6] Krab L, Aarsen F, de Goede-Bolder A, Catsman-Berrevoets C, Arts W, Moll H, Elgersma Y (2008) Impact of neurofibromatosis type 1 on school performance. J Child Neurol 23: 1002–1010

[7] Mautner V-F, Asuagbor F, Dombi E, Funsterer C, Kluwe L, Wenzel R, Widemann B, Friedman J (2008) Assessment of benign tumor burden by whole-body MRI in patients with neurofibro-matosis 1. Neuro Oncol 10: 593–598

[8] Mautner VF, Kluwe L, Friedrich RE, Roehl AC, Bammert S, Högel J, Spöri H, Cooper DN, Kehrer-Sawatzki H (2010) Clinical characterisation of 29 neurofibromatosis type-1 patients with molecularly ascertained 1.4 Mb type-1 NF1 deletions. J Med Genet 47: 623–630

[9] Osheroff J, Teich J, Middleton B, Steen E, Wright A, Detmer D (2007) A roadmap for national action on clinical decision support. J Am Med Inform Assoc 14: 141–145

[10] Pasmant E, Sabbagh A, Spurlock G, Laurendeau I, Grillo E, Hamel MJ, Martin L, Barbarot S, Leheup B, Rodriguez D, Lacombe D, Dollfus H, Pasquier L, Isidor B, Ferkal S, Soulier J, Sanson M, Dieux-Coeslier A, Bièche I, Parfait B, Vidaud M, Wolkenstein P, Upadhyaya M, Vidaud D, Members of the NF France Network (2010) NF1 microdeletions in neurofibromatosis type 1: from genotype to phenotype. Hum Mutat 31: E1506–E1518

[11] Plotkin S, Bredella M, Cai W, Kassarjian A, Harris G, Esparza S, Merker V, Munn L, Muzikansky A, Askenazi M, Nguyen R, Wenzel R, Mautner V (2012) Quantitative assessment of whole-body tumor burden in adult patients with neurofibromatosis. PLoS One 7: e35711

[12] Poon A, Hamid Q (2012) Personalized medicine for asthma: are we there yet? Ann Thorac Med 7: 55–56

[13] Rasmussen S, Yang Q, Friedman J (2001) Mortality in neurofibromatosis 1: an analysis using U.S. death certificates. Am J Hum Genet 68: 1110–1118

[14] Rosenfeld A, Listernick R, Charrow J, Goldman S (2010) Neurofibromatosis type 1 and high-grade tumors of the central nervous system. Childs Nerv Syst 25: 663–667

[15] Sbidian E, Wolkenstein P, Valeyrie-Allanore L, Rodriguez D, Hadj-Rabia S, Ferkal S, Lacour J-P, Leonard J-C, Taillandier L, Sportich S, Berbis P, Bastuji-Garin S, Members of the NF France Network (2010) NF-1Score: a prediction score for internal neurofibromas in neurofibromatosis-1. J Invest Derm 130: 2173–2178

[16] Sharif S, Moran A, Huson S, Iddenden R, Shenton A, Howard E, Evans D (2007) Women with neurofibromatosis 1 are at a moderately increased risk of developing breast cancer and should be considered for early screening. J Med Genet 44: 481–484

[17] Stevenson D, Viskochil D, Rope A, Carey J (2006) Clinical and molecular aspects of an informative family with neurofibromatosis type 1 and Noonan phenotype. Clin Genet 69: 246–253

[18] Upadhyaya M, Huson SM, Davies M, Thomas N, Chuzhanova N, Giovannini S, Evans DG, Howard E, Kerr B, Griffiths S, Consoli C, Side L, Adams D, Pierpont M, Hachen R, Barnicoat A, Li H, Wallace P, Van Biervliet JP, Stevenson D, Viskochil D, Baralle D, Haan E, Riccardi V, Turnpenny P, Lazaro C, Messiaen L (2007) An absence of cutaneous neurofibromas associated with a 3-bp inframe deletion in exon 17 of the NF1 gene (c.2970–2972 delAAT): evidence of a clinically significant NF1 genotype-phenotype correlation. Am J Hum Genet 80: 140–151

[19] Viskochil D (2010) Neurofibromatosis Type 1. In: Allanson J, Cassidy S (eds) Management of genetic syndromes. Wiley, New York

[20] Walker L, Thompson D, Easton D, Ponder B, Ponder M, Frayling I, Baralle D (2006) A prospective study of neurofibromatosis type 1 cancer incidence in the UK. Br J Cancer 95: 233–238

[21] Willard HF, Ginsburg GS (eds) (2009) Genomic and personalized medicine. vols. 1 and 2. Academic, Amsterdam

第44章 1型神经纤维瘤病：未来的方向（我们该何去何从？）

Neurofibromatosis Type 1: Future Directions (Where Do We Go from Here?)

Luis F. Parada

44.1 引言

Francis Collins 和 Ray White 的实验室在 1990 年成功克隆了 NF1 基因，从此开启了 1 型神经纤维瘤病波澜壮阔的研究时代（Ballester et al. 1990；Cawthon et al. 1990；Wallace et al. 1990）。通过分子分析，研究者很快发现了一种序列，可用于预测假定编码酶的活性，该序列也可解释 NF1 作为肿瘤抑制因子的作用（Buchberg et al. 1990）。事实上，研究者发现神经纤维瘤蛋白作为高分子量编码蛋白，含有功能性 Ras GTPase 激活域（GTPase activating domain，GAP）。因此，NF1 功能丧失将导致 Ras 蛋白负调控能力丧失（Bollag et al. 1996；Martin et al. 1990；Xu et al. 1990）。时至今日，这仍然是研究者对于 NF1 了解最彻底的功能，并且可以很好地解释它的全部活性。

本书众多章节总结了对于该疾病广泛深入的研究与进展，以便人们更好地理解这一多效性疾病。在这个坚实的基础上，我们期待进一步的研究进展，不仅可以更为清晰地了解疾病，还有望对 NF1 相关临床表现进行干预。

44.2 神经纤维瘤蛋白

神经纤维瘤蛋白是一种高分子量蛋白质，其序列保守度超过了 Ras‐GAP 结构域，在许多物种中都存在，包括哺乳动物、斑马鱼和果蝇（Bernards et al. 1993；Padmanabhan et al. 2009；1997）。这种强烈的序列保守性使得 Ras‐GAP 结构域外的区域依然可以发挥重要功能，保留蛋白质的整体活性。然而，对于神经纤维瘤蛋白潜在的其他调控功能的研究成果有限，有时还存在争议性结论（Johnson et al. 1994；The et al. 1997；Tong et al. 2002）。显然，我们对其理解仍然存在不足，还有很多路要走。基于果蝇和斑马鱼的模式动物基因研究可能会对这个领域做出很大贡献。同样重要的是，全长 cDNA 最近被成功克隆（Frank McCormick, personal communication）。尽管该基因在 22 年前就被克隆出来，但全长 cDNA 的分离一直存在技术障碍。因此，对 NF1 基因的整个编码区进行直接的结构/功能分析仍然是不可能实现的。现在，随着全长 cDNA 的成功克隆，上述分析

L. F. Parada (*)
Department of Developmental Biology, University of Texas Southwestern Medical Center, Dallas, TX, USA
e-mail: luis.parada@utsouthwestern.edu

已经有可能实现,并有助于揭示神经纤维瘤蛋白除 Ras 调节活性之外其他结构域的功能活性。通过实验直接分析可以揭示独立结构域是否具有信号转导能力。当然,神经纤维瘤蛋白其他区域的重要特性也将被揭开面纱。例如,很可能存在关键的蛋白质或脂质相互作用的结构域,这些结构域可能决定蛋白质的特异性,例如在何处、何时以及如何在细胞内执行其功能。目前,研究已经报道了几种神经纤维瘤蛋白下游的效应蛋白,包括 Erk、PI3-Kinase、mTOR、ral 和 PKA 通路(Bodempudi et al. 2009;Bollag et al. 1996;Brown et al. 2012;Dasgupta et al. 2005;Johannessen et al. 2005;Klesse & Parada 1998)。在不同的细胞环境中,这些通路的相对活性是如何调控的?对于不同的病理环境,同样的问题也必须得到解决。因此,上述最新的研究进展大大增加了实验研究细胞内神经纤维瘤蛋白作用机制的可行性,并产生深远影响。

44.3 动物模型

1 型神经纤维瘤病是一种单基因疾病,这极大地方便了在动物模型中多方面再现该疾病。相较于许多由更复杂的突变组合发展而来的其他疾病和癌症,NF1 动物模型具有显著优势。20 世纪 90 年代中期,在班伯里会议中心举行的神经纤维瘤病会议上,首次报道了 NF1 肿瘤小鼠模型的成功建立以及基因敲除条件(Brannan et al. 1994;Jacks et al. 1994;Zhu et al. 2001)。在那次会议上,冷泉港实验室主席 Bruce Stillman 宣布,NF1 动物模型预示着基因工程小鼠有望成功构建,用于研究总结、理解和治愈人类疾病。他的乐观态度无疑被证明是正确的,因为没有哪个研究领域比他更积极地应用小鼠和其他物种的动物模型来了解疾病的广度和深度。果蝇的学习与记忆障碍模型已经被成功构建(Guo et al. 2000;Ho et al. 2007),该系统的遗传性可以对信号通路产生持续渗透。上述研究的后续进展将会对该领域做出重大贡献。同样,斑马鱼现在也能够复现 NF1 相关的肿瘤,并且可以进行遗传研究以及更为重要的中低通量治疗手段的开发(Lee et al. 2010)。这个强大的新工具将为 NF1 研究的临床转化做出重要贡献。

虽然模式动物众多,但是实验小鼠已经一再被证明是 NF1 实验研究的主力,在过去、现在和未来的 NF1 研究和发现中都是最重要的贡献者。许多实验室正在使用小鼠模型来研究神经纤维瘤病的各种不同病理表现。其包括:丛状和真皮神经纤维瘤、恶性周围神经鞘膜瘤、视神经胶质瘤、髓系白血病、学习和记忆缺陷、骨骼异常,以及最近与自闭症谱系障碍相关的认知障碍(Acosta et al. 2006;Bajenaru et al. 2003;Bollag et al. 1996;Cichowski et al. 1999;Keng et al. 2012;Kolanczyk et al. 2008;Le et al. 2004;Silva et al. 1997;Vogel et al. 1999;Zhu et al. 2002,2005)。此外,小鼠遗传模型已被应用于研究 NF1 基因的修饰因子(Amlin-VanSchaick et al. 2012a、b)。在最近几年,通过此类模型的成功开发,小鼠模型已进入临床前研究,以开发潜在的新疗法(De Raedt et al. 2011;Kalamarides et al. 2012;Kolanczyk et al. 2008;Yang et al. 2008)。目前各个研究小组通力合作,共同推进 NF1 研究的转化,使其具有良好的应用前景。坦率地说,目前 NF1 研究人员存在一种共识,即在未来几年,他们将见证近期临床前"证实疾病原理"相关研究的深入与拓展。对于迅速产生的新有效疗法而言,目前的研究仅仅只是触及其表面。这些未来的进步将大大提高 NF1 患者的生命质量。

通过小鼠模型,研究者可以详尽地探索病理状态自然发展的病史。就肿瘤而言,这是非常有用的,因为只有了解肿瘤细胞来源,我们才可以对肿瘤在发生前与发展期间的基因与表观遗传变化进行详细直接的比较。正是通过这些直接比较,我们有可能发现在瘤前状态和完全成瘤状态的细胞中出现的基因表达变化。这些研究自然不可能在患者或已建立的细胞系中进行。这种实验策略将揭示 NF1 相关肿瘤特有的基因、细胞代谢和信号转导途径的重要新信息。识别这些独特的通路将有助于设计靶向治疗方案,以阻止或逆转肿瘤的发展,同时对正常细胞的影响很小。此类研究将对神经纤维瘤、视神经胶质瘤和恶性周围神经鞘膜瘤的诊疗产生重要影响,上述肿瘤均可以在小鼠模型中复现,且与在患者身上观察到的肿瘤具有显著的一致性。

关于假性关节、发育性骨异常以及NF1综合征的许多低外显率方面的研究进展如何呢？这些领域的研究滞后于肿瘤研究。尽管如此，最近还是有相关研究报道了NF1相关的骨异常小鼠模型的成功构建（Elefteriou et al. 2006；Kolanczyk et al, 2008；Kuorilehto et al. 2004；Wang et al. 2011）。目前的研究也将同样面临肿瘤建模研究中的复杂情况。引起异常的致病突变位于何处？理解"细胞起源"将有助于我们在正常和病理状态之间进行基因组、细胞和分子比较。与更高级的肿瘤研究类似，此类持续研究将有助于揭示异常发育的关键阶段，并提供治疗靶点的参考，届时小鼠将再次成为强大的临床前研究工具。

围绕NF1和大脑发育的讨论也持续获得研究者关注。NF1个体易患智力缺陷和情绪障碍（Acosta et al. 2006；Huson et al. 1988；Hyman et al. 2006；North et al. 1994）。然而，人们对其潜在的神经病理学仍然知之甚少。除了NF1脑中的一些异常成像外，特定脑区域的异常与特定神经认知表型的因果关系仍不明确。在这方面，小鼠模型具有很大的应用前景。定向突变大脑特定解剖区域构建NF1的方法已经获得新进展，甚至有望提供可能的治疗策略（Acosta et al. 2006）。更精准的方法可以在时间和空间上靶向实现NF1功能丧失，加上目前小鼠行为和分析领域研究的不断成熟，这些成果为有效识别大脑的易感细胞类型、系统和区域带来了巨大的希望。上述研究进展将促使我们开展恰当的临床前研究。这一研究领域还有很多值得期待的地方。

总之，与NF1病理各方面相关的小鼠模型正变得日益复杂，在生理学方面也更为先进。随着临床和基础研究的融合，该模型可以为当前和未来的临床试验带来巨大的希望，这些临床试验基于严格的假设，将更为可靠。

44.4 临床实践

在过去，NF1患者的诊疗完全依赖于他们的主要护理人员、医师、遗传和心理咨询师的医疗专业知识、经验、奉献精神和同情心。除了基因分型和遗传咨询外，基础科学对这一问题的实际贡献现在才开始慢慢显现。然而，在NF社区中，将基础科学家、临床研究人员和临床医师正式聚集在一起进行讨论，必然会对神经纤维瘤患者的诊疗产生实质性的益处，即使是非专业人士也一样。这些讨论使临床观察到的现象更有意义，并为基础科学家提供更多的医学研究关联与研究方向。

作为一个范例，最近NF1研究人员和临床医师开展合作，收集、重新检查和分析NF1中自闭症谱系障碍的发病率。该研究由Maria Acosta和Susan Huson以及该领域的许多同事牵头，商定使用了标化的分析方法，揭示了这一合并症的严峻发病率。这一合并症概念的明确将促进临床研究新方向的产生，而对于其治疗方法的研发必将激励小鼠建模领域学者的积极加入。从基因型/表现型研究到发生率较低但仍然重要的嵌合体病例，以及渗透性较低的病理表现和治疗，临床研究人员也一直在不停地获得研究进展。从基础到临床，NF1相关研究不断进行交叉与统一，这有利于患者的治疗，提高生命质量。正在进行的丛状神经纤维瘤临床试验进展顺利，其他类型的肿瘤也将会很快跟进。基于前文讨论的分子和动物模型研究的预期进展，这一代患者将会见证NF1治疗方法与质量的大幅提升。

44.5 除1型神经纤维瘤病外的其他疾病

NF1基因的胚系突变可导致多种缺陷，其中最重要的是癌症易感性，它是由1型神经纤维瘤病中公认的肿瘤抑制基因突变导致的。受到癌症基因组图谱计划（Cancer Genome Atlas Project，TCGA）的推动以及动物模型的支持，近期癌症基因组学研究获得了爆发式的成果（Chen et al. 2012；Llaguno et al. 2008；TCGAR Network 2008；Parada et al. 2005），由此将NF1归类为真正的通用肿瘤抑制基因。特发性恶性胶质母细胞瘤中，NF1很大概率发生突变，是这种绝症中高发的癌症相关突变基因之一（Chen et al. 2012；TCGAR Net-work 2008）。此外，在结肠癌、肺癌和嗜铬细胞瘤中也检测到

NF1基因突变（Bausch et al. 2006；Cacev et al. 2005；Ding et al. 2008）。随着这些研究的进一步完善，更多联系可能会出现。因此，NF1基因可以与p53、PTEN和Ras等更著名的对应基因一起被认作常见的癌症可疑基因。

小鼠研究也揭示了微环境与神经纤维瘤瘤细胞之间复杂的相互作用（Zhu et al. 2002；Yang et al. 2008）。借助动物模型和细胞系统，我们可以明确肥大细胞、神经元、成纤维细胞、内皮细胞和施万细胞祖细胞如何通过相互作用，构建促肿瘤环境。这些成果将在未来为神经纤维瘤提供新的潜在治疗策略。癌症与微环境是当前研究的热点。NF1肿瘤相关研究的诸多成果也可能揭示肿瘤细胞-基质间相互作用的重要共性特征，有望应用于散发性实体瘤。因此，过去NF1研究领域的所有成果都将对未来的进步做出贡献，不仅有助于改进神经纤维瘤病的治疗方法，而且还将对许多散发性体细胞癌症的分子分类、预后和治疗方法的改进产生更广泛的影响。NF1领域的研究已经走过了漫长的道路，但还有很长的路要走。

致谢：LFP是发育生物学系的教授和主席，并担任Diana与Richard C. Strauss发育生物学杰出主席。他是美国癌症协会的教授，并得到了NCI、NINDS、CPRIT、Simons基金会和Goldhirsh基金会的资助。LFP感谢Renée M. McKay协助本文书写，并对无意中遗漏的相关主题或参考文献表示歉意。

（王旭东，吴昊 译）

参考文献

[1] Acosta MT, Gioia GA, Silva AJ (2006) Neurofibromatosis type 1: new insights into neurocognitive issues. Curr Neurol Neurosci Rep 6: 136-143

[2] Amlin-Van Schaick J, Kim S, Broman KW, Reilly KM (2012a) Scram1 is a modifier of spinal cord resistance for astrocytoma on mouse Chr 5. Mamm Genome 23: 277-285

[3] Amlin-Van Schaick JC, Kim S, DiFabio C, Lee MH, Broman KW, Reilly KM (2012b) Arlm1 is a male-specific modifier of astrocytoma resistance on mouse Chr 12. Neuro Oncol 14: 160-174

[4] Bajenaru ML, Hernandez MR, Perry A, Zhu Y, Parada LF, Garbow JR, Gutmann DH (2003) Optic nerve glioma in mice requires astrocyte Nf1 gene inactivation and Nf1 brain heterozygosity. Cancer Res 63: 8573-8577

[5] Ballester R, Marchuk D, Boguski M, Saulino A, Letcher R, Wigler M, Collins F (1990) The NF1 locus encodes a protein functionally related to mammalian GAP and yeast IRA proteins. Cell 63: 851-859

[6] Bausch B, Koschker AC, Fassnacht M, Stoevesandt J, Hoffmann MM, Eng C, Allolio B, Neumann HP (2006) Comprehensive mutation scanning of NF1 in apparently sporadic cases of pheo-chromocytoma. J Clin Endocrinol Metab 91: 3478-3481

[7] Bernards A, Snijders AJ, Hannigan GE, Murthy AE, Gusella JF (1993) Mouse neurofibromatosis type 1 cDNA sequence reveals high degree of conservation of both coding and non-coding mRNA segments. Hum Mol Genet 2: 645-650

[8] Bodempudi V, Yamoutpoor F, Pan W, Dudek AZ, Esfandyari T, Piedra M, Babovick-Vuksanovic D, Woo RA, Mautner VF, Kluwe L et al (2009) Ral overactivation in malignant peripheral nerve sheath tumors. Mol Cell Biol 29: 3964-3974

[9] Bollag G, Clapp DW, Shih S, Adler F, Zhang YY, Thompson P, Lange BJ, Freedman MH, McCormick F, Jacks T et al (1996) Loss of NF1 results in activation of the Ras signaling pathway and leads to aberrant growth in haematopoietic cells. Nat Genet 12: 144-148

[10] Brannan CI, Perkins AS, Vogel KS, Ratner N, Nordlund ML, Reid SW, Buchberg AM, Jenkins NA, Parada LF, Copeland NG (1994) Targeted disruption of the neurofibromatosis type-1 gene leads to developmental abnormalities in heart and various neural crest-derived tissues. Genes Dev 8: 1019-1029

[11] Brown JA, Diggs-Andrews KA, Gianino SM, Gutmann DH (2012) Neurofibromatosis-1 hetero-zygosity impairs CNS neuronal morphology in a cAMP/PKA/ROCK-dependent manner. Mol Cell Neurosci 49: 13-22

[12] Buchberg AM, Cleveland LS, Jenkins NA, Copeland NG (1990) Sequence homology shared by neurofibromatosis type-1 gene and IRA-1 and IRA-2 negative regulators of the RAS cyclic AMP pathway. Nature 347: 291-294

[13] Cacev T, Radosevic S, Spaventi R, Pavelic K, Kapitanovic S (2005) NF1 gene loss of heterozy-gosity and expression analysis in sporadic colon cancer. Gut 54: 1129-1135

[14] Cawthon RM, Weiss R, Xu GF, Viskochil D, Culver M, Stevens J, Robertson M, Dunn D, Gesteland R, O'Connell P et al (1990) A major segment of the neurofibromatosis type 1 gene: cDNA sequence, genomic structure, and point mutations. Cell 62: 193-201

[15] Chen J, McKay RM, Parada LF (2012) Malignant glioma: lessons from genomics, mouse models, and stem cells. Cell 149: 36-47

[16] Cichowski K, Shih TS, Schmitt E, Santiago S, Reilly K, McLaughlin ME, Bronson RT, Jacks T (1999) Mouse models of tumor development in neurofibromatosis type 1. Science 286: 2172-2176

[17] Dasgupta B, Yi Y, Chen DY, Weber JD, Gutmann DH (2005) Proteomic analysis reveals hyperactivation of the mammalian target of rapamycin pathway in neurofibromatosis 1-associated human and mouse brain tumors. Cancer Res 65: 2755-2760

[18] De Raedt T, Walton Z, Yecies JL, Li D, Chen Y, Malone CF, Maertens O, Jeong SM, Bronson RT, Lebleu V et al

(2011) Exploiting cancer cell vulnerabilities to develop a combination therapy for ras-driven tumors. Cancer Cell 20: 400-413

[19] Ding L, Getz G, Wheeler DA, Mardis ER, McLellan MD, Cibulskis K, Sougnez C, Greulich H, Muzny DM, Morgan MB et al (2008) Somatic mutations affect key pathways in lung adenocarcinoma. Nature 455: 1069-1075

[20] Elefteriou F, Benson MD, Sowa H, Starbuck M, Liu X, Ron D, Parada LF, Karsenty G (2006) ATF4 mediation of NF1 functions in osteoblast reveals a nutritional basis for congenital skeletal dysplasiae. Cell Metab 4: 441-451

[21] Guo HF, Tong J, Hannan F, Luo L, Zhong Y (2000) A neurofibromatosis-1-regulated pathway is required for learning in Drosophila. Nature 403: 895-898

[22] Ho IS, Hannan F, Guo HF, Hakker I, Zhong Y (2007) Distinct functional domains of neurofibromatosis type 1 regulate immediate versus long-term memory formation. J Neurosci 27: 6852-6857

[23] Huson SM, Harper PS, Compston DA (1988) von Recklinghausen neurofibromatosis. A clinical and population study in south-east Wales. Brain 111(Pt 6): 1355-1381

[24] Hyman SL, Arthur Shores E, North KN (2006) Learning disabilities in children with neurofibro-matosis type 1: subtypes, cognitive profile, and attention-deficit-hyperactivity disorder. Dev Med Child Neurol 48: 973-977

[25] Jacks T, Shih TS, Schmitt EM, Bronson RT, Bernards A, Weinberg RA (1994) Tumour predisposition in mice heterozygous for a targeted mutation in Nf1. Nat Genet 7: 353-361

[26] Johannessen CM, Reczek EE, James MF, Brems H, Legius E, Cichowski K (2005) The NF1 tumor suppressor critically regulates TSC2 and mTOR. Proc Natl Acad Sci USA 102: 8573-8578

[27] Johnson MR, DeClue JE, Felzmann S, Vass WC, Xu G, White R, Lowy DR (1994) Neurofibromin can inhibit Ras-dependent growth by a mechanism independent of its GTPase-accelerating function. Mol Cell Biol 14: 641-645

[28] Kalamarides M, Acosta MT, Babovic-Vuksanovic D, Carpen O, Cichowski K, Evans DG, Giancotti F, Hanemann CO, Ingram D, Lloyd AC et al (2012) Neurofibromatosis 2011: a report of the Children's Tumor Foundation annual meeting. Acta Neuropathol 123: 369-380

[29] Keng VW, Rahrmann EP, Watson AL, Tschida BR, Moertel CL, Jessen WJ, Rizvi TA, Collins MH, Ratner N, Largaespada DA (2012) PTEN and NF1 inactivation in Schwann cells produces a severe phenotype in the peripheral nervous system that promotes the development and malignant progression of peripheral nerve sheath tumors. Cancer Res 72(13): 3405-3413

[30] Klesse LJ, Parada LF (1998) p21 ras and phosphatidylinositol-3 kinase are required for survival of wild-type and NF1 mutant sensory neurons. J Neurosci 18: 10420-10428

[31] Kolanczyk M, Kuhnisch J, Kossler N, Osswald M, Stumpp S, Thurisch B, Kornak U, Mundlos S (2008) Modelling neurofibromatosis type 1 tibial dysplasia and its treatment with lovastatin. BMC Med 6: 21

[32] Kuorilehto T, Nissinen M, Koivunen J, Benson MD, Peltonen J (2004) NF1 tumor suppressor protein and mRNA in skeletal tissues of developing and adult normal mouse and NF1-deficient embryos. J Bone Miner Res 19: 983-989

[33] Le DT, Kong N, Zhu Y, Lauchle JO, Aiyigari A, Braun BS, Wang E, Kogan SC, Le Beau MM, Parada L et al (2004) Somatic inactivation of Nf1 in hematopoietic cells results in a progressive myeloproliferative disorder. Blood 103: 4243-4250

[34] Lee JS, Padmanabhan A, Shin J, Zhu S, Guo F, Kanki JP, Epstein JA, Look AT (2010) Oligoden-drocyte progenitor cell numbers and migration are regulated by the zebrafish orthologs of the NF1 tumor suppressor gene. Hum Mol Genet 19: 4643-4653

[35] Llaguno SA, Chen J, Kwon CH, Parada LF (2008) Neural and cancer stem cells in tumor suppressor mouse models of malignant astrocytoma. Cold Spring Harb Symp Quant Biol 73: 421-426

[36] Martin GA, Viskochil D, Bollag G, McCabe PC, Crosier WJ, Haubruck H, Conroy L, Clark R, O'Connell P, Cawthon RM et al (1990) The GAP-related domain of the neurofibromatosis type 1 gene product interacts with ras p21. Cell 63: 843-849

[37] North K, Joy P, Yuille D, Cocks N, Mobbs E, Hutchins P, McHugh K, de Silva M (1994) Specific learning disability in children with neurofibromatosis type 1: significance of MRI abnormalities. Neurology 44: 878-883

[38] Padmanabhan A, Lee JS, Ismat FA, Lu MM, Lawson ND, Kanki JP, Look AT, Epstein JA (2009) Cardiac and vascular functions of the zebrafish orthologues of the type I neurofibromatosis gene NF1. Proc Natl Acad Sci USA 106: 22305-22310

[39] Parada LF, Kwon CH, Zhu Y (2005) Modeling neurofibromatosis type 1 tumors in the mouse for therapeutic intervention. Cold Spring Harb Symp Quant Biol 70: 173-176

[40] Silva AJ, Frankland PW, Marowitz Z, Friedman E, Lazlo G, Cioffi D, Jacks T, Bourtchuladze R (1997) A mouse model for the learning and memory deficits associated with neurofibromatosis type I. Nat Genet 15: 281-284

[41] TCGAR Network (2008) Comprehensive genomic characterization defines human glioblastoma genes and core pathways. Nature 455: 1061-1068

[42] The I, Hannigan GE, Cowley GS, Reginald S, Zhong Y, Gusella JF, Hariharan IK, Bernards A (1997) Rescue of a Drosophila NF1 mutant phenotype by protein kinase A. Science 276: 791-794

[43] Tong J, Hannan F, Zhu Y, Bernards A, Zhong Y (2002) Neurofibromin regulates G protein-stimulated adenylyl cyclase activity. Nat Neurosci 5: 95-96

[44] Vogel KS, Klesse LJ, Velasco-Miguel S, Meyers K, Rushing EJ, Parada LF (1999) Mouse tumor model for neurofibromatosis type 1. Science 286: 2176-2179

[45] Wallace MR, Marchuk DA, Andersen LB, Letcher R, Odeh HM, Saulino AM, Fountain JW, Brereton A, Nicholson J, Mitchell AL et al (1990) Type 1 neurofibromatosis gene: identification of a large transcript disrupted in three NF1 patients. Science 249(4965): 181-186

[46] Wang W, Nyman JS, Ono K, Stevenson DA, Yang X, Elefteriou F (2011) Mice lacking Nf1 in osteochondroprogenitor cells display skeletal dysplasia similar to patients with neurofibromatosis type I. Hum Mol Genet 20: 3910-3924

[47] Xu GF, O'Connell P, Viskochil D, Cawthon R, Robertson M, Culver M, Dunn D, Stevens J, Gesteland R, White R et al (1990) The neurofibromatosis type 1 gene encodes a protein related to GAP. Cell 62: 599-608

[48] Yang FC, Ingram DA, Chen S, Zhu Y, Yuan J, Li X, Yang X, Knowles S, Horn W, Li Y et al (2008) Nf1-dependent tumors require a microenvironment containing $Nf1^{+/-}$ and c-kit-dependent bone marrow. Cell 135: 437-448

[49] Zhu Y, Romero MI, Ghosh P, Ye Z, Charnay P, Rushing EJ, Marth JD, Parada LF (2001) Ablation of NF1 function in

neurons induces abnormal development of cerebral cortex and reactive gliosis in the brain. Genes Dev 15: 859-876

[50] Zhu Y, Ghosh P, Charnay P, Burns DK, Parada LF (2002) Neurofibromas in NF1: Schwann cell origin and role of tumor environment. Science 296: 920-922

[51] Zhu Y, Harada T, Liu L, Lush ME, Guignard F, Harada C, Burns DK, Bajenaru ML, Gutmann DH, Parada LF (2005) Inactivation of NF1 in CNS causes increased glial progenitor proliferation and optic glioma formation. Development 132: 5577-5588